2

Basics of
ANESTHESIA

Basics of ANESTHESIA

SIXTH EDITION

Ronald D. Miller, MD

Professor of Anesthesia and Perioperative Care
University of California, San Francisco, School of Medicine
San Francisco, California, USA

Manuel C. Pardo, Jr. MD

Professor of Anesthesia and Perioperative Care
Director of Residency Programs
University of California, San Francisco, School of Medicine
San Francisco, California, USA

ELSEVIER
SAUNDERS

ELSEVIER
SAUNDERS

1600 John F. Kennedy Blvd.
Ste 1800
Philadelphia, PA 19103–2899

BASICS OF ANESTHESIA   ISBN: 978-1-4377-1614-6

Library of Congress Cataloging-in-Publication Data

Miller, Ronald D., 1939-
  Basics of anesthesia/Ronald D. Miller, Manuel C. Pardo Jr. – 6th ed.
      p. ; cm.
  Rev. ed. of: Basics of anesthesia/Robert K. Stoelting and Ronald D. Miller. 5th ed. c2007.
  Includes bibliographical references and index.
  ISBN 978-1-4377-1614-6 (hardcover: alk. paper)   1. Anesthesia.   I. Pardo, Manuel, 1965-   II. Stoelting, Robert K. Basics of anesthesia.   III.   Title.
  [DNLM: 1. Anesthesia. WO 200]
  RD81.S86 2011
  617.9'6–dc22

                                                        2011004283

Executive Publisher: Natasha Andjelkovic
Acquisitions Editor: Julie Goolsby
Publishing Services Manager: Patricia Tannian
Team Manager: Radhika Pallamparthy
Senior Project Manager: Sharon Corell
Project Manager: Joanna Dhanabalan
Design Direction: Louis Forgione

Printed in China
Last digit is the print number: 9   8   7   6   5   4   3

CONTRIBUTORS

Amr E. Abouleish, MD, MBA
Professor, Anesthesiology, University of Texas Medical Branch, Galveston, Texas, USA

Meredith C. B. Adams, MD
Pain Medicine Fellow, Anesthesiology and Critical Care Medicine, Johns Hopkins University, Baltimore, Maryland, USA

Dean B. Andropoulos, MD, MHCM
Professor, Anesthesiology and Pediatrics, Baylor College of Medicine, Chief, Pediatric Anesthesiology, Texas Children's Hospital, Houston, Texas, USA

James E. Baker, MD
Assistant Professor, Anesthesia, University of Toronto, Canada

Sheila Ryan Barnett, MD
Associate Professor, Anesthesiology, Harvard Medical School, Department of Anesthesia, Critical Care, and Pain Management, Beth Israel Deaconess Medical Center, Boston, Massachusetts, USA

Luca M. Bigatello, MD
Associate Professor, Anaesthesia, Massachusetts, General Hospital, and Chief, Anaesthesia and Critical Care Service, Veterans Administration Boston Healthcare System, Boston, Massachusetts, USA

Thomas J.J. Blanck, MD, PhD
Professor and Chairman, Anesthesiology, and Professor, Physiology and Neuroscience, New York University School of Medicine, New York, New York, USA

James Caldwell, MBChB
Professor, Anesthesia and Perioperative Care, University of California, San Francisco, San Francisco, California, USA

Lundy Campbell, MD
Associate Professor, Anesthesiology, Perioperative and Critical Care, University of California, San Francisco, San Francisco, California, USA

Lydia Cassorla, MD, MBA
Professor, Anesthesia and Perioperative Care, University of California, San Francisco, School of Medicine, San Francisco, California, USA

Daniel J. Cole, MD
Professor and Chair, Anesthesiology, Mayo Clinic Arizona, Phoenix, Arizona, USA

Adam B. Collins, MD
Associate Professor, Anesthesia and Perioperative Care, University of California, San Francisco, School of Medicine, San Francisco General Hospital, San Francisco, California, USA

Anil de Silva, MD
Professor, Anesthesia and Perioperative Care, University of California, San Francisco, School of Medicine, San Francisco, California, USA

Karen B. Domino, MD, MPH
Professor, and Vice Chair, Clinical Research Anesthesiology and Pain Medicine, University of Washington, Seattle, Washington, USA

Kenneth Drasner, MD
Professor, Anesthesia, and Perioperative Care, University of California, San Francisco, San Francisco General Hospital, San Francisco, California, USA

Talmage D. Egan, MD
Professor, Anesthesiology, and Director, Neuroanesthesia, University of Utah, Salt Lake City, Utah, USA

Helge Eilers, MD
Associate Professor, Anesthesia and Perioperative Care, University of California, San Francisco, School of Medicine, San Francisco, California, USA

John Feiner, MD
Professor, Anesthesia and Perioperative Care, University of California, San Francisco, School of Medicine, San Francisco, California, USA

Alana Flexman, BSc, MD
*Assistant Professor, Anesthesia and Perioperative Care,
University of California, San Francisco, School of Medicine,
San Francisco, California, USA*

Patricia Fogarty Mack, MD
*Associate Professor, Clinical Anesthesiology, Weill
Cornell Medical College, Associate Attending Anesthesiologist,
New York-Presbyterian Hospital, New York, New York, USA*

William R. Furman, MD
*Professor, Anesthesiology, and Vice Chair for Clinical Affairs,
Anesthesiology, Vanderbilt University School of Medicine,
Nashville, Tennessee, USA*

Steven Gayer, MD, MBA
*Associate Professor, Anesthesiology and Ophthalmology,
Miller School of Medicine, University of Miami, Associate
Medical Director, Surgery and Anesthesia, Bascom Palmer
Eye Institute, Miami, Florida, USA*

David Glick, MD, MBA
*Associate Professor, Anesthesia and Critical Care, University
of Chicago, Medical Director, PACU, University of Chicago
Hospital, Chicago, Illinois, USA*

Erin A. Gottlieb, MD
*Assistant Professor, Pediatrics and Anesthesiology,
Baylor College of Medicine, Attending Anesthesiologist,
Pediatric Anesthesiology, Texas Children's Hospital,
Houston, Texas, USA*

Tula Gourdin, MBA
*Analyst, Anesthesia and Perioperative Care, University of
California, San Francisco, San Francisco, California, USA*

Andrew T. Gray, MD, PhD
*Professor, Anesthesia and Perioperative Care, University of
California, San Francisco, School of Medicine, San Francisco
General Hospital, San Francisco, California, USA*

Michael Gropper, MD, PhD
*Professor, Anesthesia and Perioperative Care, and Professor,
Physiology, University of California, San Francisco, School of
Medicine, Director, Critical Care Medicine, University of
California, San Francisco, Medical Center, San Francisco,
California, USA*

Jin J. Huang, MD
*Assistant Professor, Anesthesia and Perioperative Care,
University of California, San Francisco, San Francisco,
California, USA*

Robert W. Hurley, MD, PhD
*Associate Professor, Anesthesiology, University of Florida,
Chief, Pain Medicine, Shands Hospital, Gainesville,
Florida, USA*

Steven Hyman, MD, MM
*Associate Professor, Anesthesiology, Vanderbilt University,
Nashville, Tennessee, USA*

Andrew Infosino, MD
*Professor, Anesthesia and Perioperative Care, University of
California, San Francisco, School of Medicine, San Francisco,
California, USA*

Alan David Kaye, MD, PhD
*Professor and Chairman, Department of Anesthesia,
Louisiana State University School of Medicine, Director,
Anesthesia Services, Anesthesia, University Hospital (LSU
Interim Hospital), New Orleans, Louisiana, USA*

Merlin D. Larson, MD
*Professor Emeritus, Anesthesia and Perioperative Care,
University of California, San Francisco, School of Medicine,
San Francisco, California, USA*

Jae-Woo Lee, MD
*Assistant Professor, Anesthesia and Perioperative Care,
University of California, San Francisco, School of Medicine,
San Francisco, California, USA*

Eric Y. Lin, MD
*Assistant Professor, Anesthesia and Perioperative Care,
University of California, San Francisco, School of Medicine,
San Francisco, California, USA*

Lawrence Litt, PhD, MD
*Professor, Anesthesia and Perioperative Care, University of
California, San Francisco, School of Medicine, San Francisco,
California, USA*

Linda L. Liu, MD
*Professor, Anesthesia and Perioperative Care, University of
California, San Francisco, School of Medicine, San Francisco,
California, USA*

Jennifer M. Lucero, MD
Instructor, Anesthesia and Perioperative Care, University of California, San Francisco, School of Medicine, San Francisco, California, USA

Vinod Malhotra, MD
Professor, Anesthesiology, and Clinical Director, Operating, Rooms, Weill Cornell Medical College and Medical Center, New York, New York, USA

Rachel Eshima McKay, MD
Associate Professor, Anesthesia and Perioperative Care, University of California, San Francisco, School of Medicine, San Francisco, California, USA

Pankaj Mehta, MD
Resident and Fellow, Anesthesia, Harvard Medical School, Department of Anesthesia, Critical Care, and Pain Medicine, Massachusetts General Hospital, Boston, Massachusetts, USA

Douglas G. Merrill, MD, MBA
Medical Director, Outpatient Surgery, Anesthesiology, Dartmouth-Hitchcock Medical Center, Lebanon, New Hampshire, USA

Ronald D. Miller, MD
Professor of Anesthesia and Perioperative Care, University of California, San Francisco, School of Medicine, San Francisco, California, USA

Dorre Nicholau, MD, PhD
Professor, Anesthesia, Perioperative Critical Care, University of California, San Francisco, School of Medicine, San Francisco, California, USA

Howard Palte, MD
Assistant Professor, Anesthesiology, Perioperative Medicine, and Pain Management, Miller School of Medicine, University of Miami, Miami, Florida, USA

Anup Pamnani, MD
Assistant Professor, Anesthesiology, Weill Cornell Medical College, New York, New York, USA

Manuel C. Pardo, Jr., MD
Professor of Anesthesia and Perioperative Care, Director of Residency Programs, University of California, San Francisco, School of Medicine, San Francisco, California, USA

James P. Rathmell, MD
Associate Professor, Anesthesia, Harvard Medical School, Chief, Division of Pain Medicine, Department of Anesthesia, Critical Care, and Pain Medicine, Massachusetts General Hospital, Boston, Massachusetts, USA

Mark D. Rollins, MD, PhD
Assistant Professor, Anesthesia and Perioperative Care, University of California, San Francisco, School of Medicine, San Francisco, California, USA

Andrew D. Rosenberg, MD
Professor and Executive Vice Chair, Department of Anesthesiology, New York University School of Medicine, Chief, Department of Anesthesiology, New York University Hospital for Joint Diseases, New York, New York, USA

Patricia Roth, MD
Professor, Anesthesia and Perioperative Care, University of California, San Francisco, School of Medicine, San Francisco, California, USA

Isobel A. Russell, MD, PhD, FACC
Professor, Anesthesia and Perioperative Care, University of California, San Francisco, School of Medicine, Chief, Cardiac Anesthesia Services, University of California, San Francisco, Medical Center, San Francisco, California, USA

Steven L. Shafer, MD
Professor, Anesthesiology, Columbia University, New York, New York, USA; Adjunct Professor, Anesthesia, Stanford University, Stanford, California, USA; Adjunct Professor, Biopharmaceutical Science, University of California, San Francisco, San Francisco, California, USA

David Shimabukuro, MDCM
Assistant Professor, Anesthesia and Perioperative Care, University of California, San Francisco, School of Medicine, San Francisco, California, USA

Venkatesh Srinivasa, MBBS, MD
Instructor, Anesthesiology, Harvard Medical School, Boston, Massachusetts, USA

Robin A. Stackhouse, MD
Professor, Anesthesia and Perioperative Care, University of California, San Francisco, School of Medicine, San Francisco, California, USA

Randoloh H. Steadman, MD
Vice Chair, Anesthesiology, David Geffen School of Medicine, University of California Los Angeles, Santa Monica-University of California, Los Angeles, Medical Center, Santa Monica, California, USA

Greg Stratmann, MD, PhD
Associate Professor, Anesthesia and Perioperative Care, University of California, San Francisco, School of Medicine, San Francisco, California, USA

Bobbie Jean Sweitzer, MD
Professor, Anesthesia and Critical Care, and Director, Anesthesia Perioperative Medicine Clinic, Anesthesia and Critical Care, University of Chicago Medical Center, Chicago, Illinois, USA

Pekka Talke, MD
Professor, Anesthesia and Perioperative Care, University of California, San Francisco, School of Medicine, San Francisco, California, USA

Art Wallace, MD, PhD
Professor, Anesthesiology and Perioperative Care, University of California, San Francisco, School of Medicine, Veterans Affairs Medical Center, San Francisco, California, USA

Victor W. Xia, MD
Associate Professor, Anesthesiology, David Geffen School of Medicine, University of California Los Angeles, Santa Monica-University of California, Los Angeles, Medical Center, Santa Monica, California, USA

William L. Young, MD
Professor, Anesthesiology and Perioperative Care, University of California, San Francisco, School of Medicine, San Francisco, California, USA

PREFACE

Basics of Anesthesia was first published in 1984 under the leadership of Robert K. Stoelting and Ronald D. Miller. Their consistent goal was to provide a concise source of information for the entire community of anesthesia learners, including medical students, residents, fellows, and other trainees. This sixth edition of *Basics of Anesthesia* continues the pursuit of that goal while evolving to meet the newest challenges of our specialty. This edition continues the development of a companion Expert Consult website, which contains the complete text and illustrations.

In this edition we also welcome Manuel C. Pardo, Jr., as one of the editors of the text, succeeding Dr. Stoelting. Dr. Stoelting's well-recognized, concise, and clear writing style was the major reason behind the success and popularity of *Basics of Anesthesia*. We are immensely grateful for the expert writing and editing skills he has contributed to the past editions. Dr. Pardo is the director of the anesthesia residency program at the University of California, San Francisco (UCSF), a member of the prestigious UCSF Academy of Medical Educators, and a campus leader in the use of simulators in medical education. His qualifications ensure that the *Basics of Anesthesia* will continue to provide contemporary information and approaches to the practice of anesthesiology.

Although multiple chapters have been restructured, we have maintained the style and format of the previous editions, including extensive use of color illustrations and tables, to ensure that *Basics of Anesthesia* continues to succinctly present pertinent and timely information relevant to anesthesiology. We have also expanded the geographic diversity of our chapter contributors by including 18 chapters in this edition that were contributed by authors from institutions other than UCSF. We are very grateful to all of the authors of the previous edition for providing a high standard that the current edition is proud to continue. In addition, all of the chapters have undergone extensive revisions to ensure content is completely current. Three new chapters also have been added: Chapter 32, "Anesthesia for Orthopedic Surgery"; Chapter 46, "Awareness Under Anesthesia"; and, consistent with the direction of medicine in general, a completely new chapter (Chapter 47) on "Quality of Care and Patient Safety," by Drs. Vinod Malhotra and Patricia Fogarty-Mack.

The editors gratefully acknowledge the editorial and administrative support of Tula Gourdin, as well as the professional guidance of Julie Goolsby and Natasha Andjelkovic at Elsevier Inc.

Ronald D. Miller
Manuel C. Pardo, Jr.

CONTENTS

Contents

INTRODUCTION

1 HISTORY OF ANESTHESIA

Merlin D. Larson

Although the ancient Greeks used ineffectual potions and poppy extracts to ablate surgical pain, the origin of anesthesia as we know it today dates to the late 18th century. Chemists at that time were beginning to query the nature of various gases that emerged during fermentation and from heating and acidifying metallic compounds. One of these curious individuals, Joseph Priestley, a schoolmaster and congregational minister, began to ponder the nature of the gas that emerged during fermentation, and he compared the differences in the properties of this "fixed air" with a gas obtained by heating mercuric oxide. Priestley did not recognize that one gas (carbon dioxide) was produced from the other gas (oxygen) during metabolism and combustion, but his curiosity concerning the nature of gases led him to discover an anesthetic (nitrous oxide) that is still in use today.

INHALED ANESTHETICS

By exposing a solution of brass to nitric acid, Priestley obtained a gas, which he called nitrous air (nitric oxide). He then exposed this gas to a mixture of iron filings and mercury, and named this gas "dephlogisticated nitrous air," a gas known today as nitrous oxide. Dephlogisticated meant that it would support combustion, a fact that has meaning even today because airway fires can be supported by nitrous oxide. Priestley learned that this gas would not support life and was unable to find any practical use for it, but he speculated that it might be insufflated rectally to cure intestinal diseases.

Nitrous Oxide

The study of nitrous oxide began with the young prodigy Humphry Davy, who was destined to become one of the great scientists of the 19th century. Davy began his education in the seaport of Penzance, England, but abandoned his formal education at an early age to study the works of Priestley and Antoine Lavoisier and to perform his own experiments on the nature of gases. He accepted the position as Superintendent of Research at the Beddoes Institute in Clifton, England, where he constructed an airtight room into which he would enter to breathe nitrous oxide. This was a bold undertaking by the young scientist because nitrous oxide at the time was thought to be a dangerous gas that could result in death if inhaled.

Davy's book on the subject[1] stated that nitrous oxide produced feelings of exhilaration and euphoria and also resulted in analgesia, leading him to observe, "As nitrous oxide . . . appears capable of destroying physical pain, it may probably be used with advantage during surgical operations in which no great effusion of blood takes place." Davy's work sparked an interest in nitrous oxide inhalation that spread throughout Europe and America, but the analgesic properties of the gas were ignored. Scientific exhibitions that traveled to various communities demonstrated the effects of electricity, magnetism, chemical reactions, and inhalation of nitrous oxide (Fig. 1-1). For almost 50 years after the discovery of the analgesic properties of gas inhalation, physicians were inattentive to the agonizing pain and terror of surgery (Fig. 1-2).

The early 19th century witnessed a change in cultural and social beliefs that allowed the idea of painless surgery to surface. One of the first physicians to focus attention on the ablation of surgical pain was Henry Hill Hickman, who demonstrated in 1824 that inhalation of carbon dioxide could produce analgesia in animals. At the same time, Anton Mesmer and his followers claimed that they were able to induce a trancelike state that would allow surgery without the use of drugs. Although these methods were eventually proved to be unsuccessful,

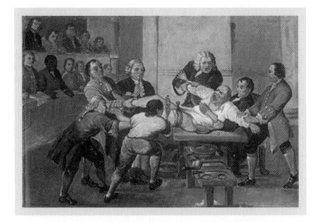

Figure 1-2 Leg amputation prior to introduction of general anesthesia. Artist unknown. (Reproduced with permission, Council of the Royal College of Surgeons of England.)

they initiated public awareness in the possibility of pain control and questioned the belief that only religious authorities could interpret and assuage pain.

One itinerant chemist and entrepreneur, Gardner Q. Colton, is thought by some to be the dominant figure in the eventual introduction of inhalation anesthesia. Colton, who had briefly attended medical school, designed an exhibit that included a demonstration of the effects of nitrous oxide inhalation. On the night of December 10, 1844, he exhibited in the community of Hartford, Connecticut, where a young man, Samuel A. Cooley, accidentally sustained an injury to his leg while under the influence of nitrous oxide. Horace Wells, a local dentist who had an interest in painless dentistry, observed this event and asked Cooley whether he felt any pain during the injury. When he answered that he had felt no pain while under the influence of nitrous oxide, Wells arranged for Colton to administer the gas on the next morning for the extraction of one of Well's own teeth, performed painlessly by a colleague, John M. Riggs.

Diethyl Ether

Wells was a tragic figure whose success was thwarted by an unsuccessful attempt to demonstrate the use of nitrous oxide for surgical anesthesia before an audience at the Massachusetts General Hospital. Wells became addicted to chloroform and committed suicide in 1848. The honor of a successful public demonstration of inhalation anesthesia instead went to his former colleague William Thomas Green Morton (Fig. 1-3), who used diethyl ether vapor instead of nitrous oxide in experiments on his pets and selected dental patients. Because of the inconsistency of nitrous oxide anesthesia, Morton had shifted his attention from nitrous oxide to ether at the advice of his

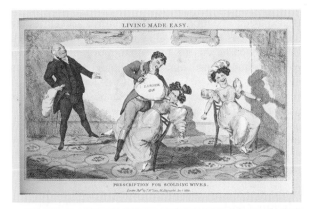

Figure 1-1 In the early 19th century, nitrous oxide provided novel entertainment for the middle class in Europe and America. Unfortunately, the analgesic properties of the gas were ignored for almost 50 years after Humphry Davy reported them. (Courtesy of the National Library of Medicine; originally published by T. McLean, 26 Haymaker, London, 1830.)

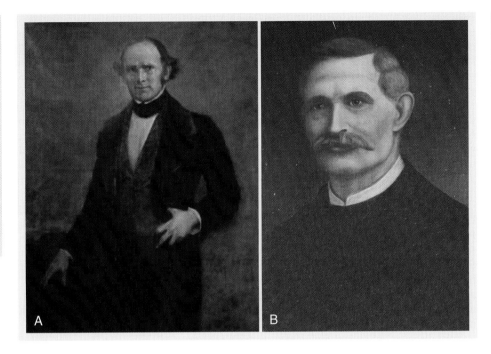

Figure 1-3 A, Horace Wells demonstrated the anesthetic properties of nitrous oxide in 1844. Portrait by Charles Noel Flagg. **B,** William T. G. Morton publicly demonstrated the use of ether anesthesia for operative surgery in 1846. Portrait by an unknown artist. (A courtesy of the Menczer Museum of Medicine and Dentistry, Hartford, Connecticut; B courtesy of Mr. Thomas E. Keys and Alan D. Sessler, M.D.)

chemistry professor, Charles A. Jackson. On October 16, 1846, Morton used ether to produce anesthesia for an excision of a neck mass by the dean of American surgery, John C. Warren (Fig. 1-4). The patient, Edward Gilbert Abbott, was insensitive to the surgical manipulation until near the end of the operation and he stated that he felt no pain.

Although some surgeons opposed the use of ether anesthesia, its use spread rapidly around the world after the October 16, 1846, demonstration. The Boston surgeons, who included Jacob Bigelow, George Hayworth, and John C. Warren, vigorously promoted the use of ether.[2] Several claims were made by others to have previously used ether vapor for the same purpose. Credit for the discovery of anesthesia has therefore been given to various individuals, including Charles A. Jackson, Horace Wells, Gardner Q. Colton, William T. G. Morton, and Crawford Long, a surgeon from Athens, Georgia, who administered ether to induce surgical anesthesia in 1842 but did not publish his report until 1849.[3]

Alternatives to Ether

Ether was a relatively safe inhaled anesthetic, but it had several disadvantages, which included flammability, prolonged induction of anesthesia, delayed emergence from anesthesia, and a high incidence of nausea and vomiting. In 1847, James Y. Simpson, an obstetrician from Edinburgh, Scotland, proposed chloroform as a suitable alternative to ether. John Snow, considered by many to be the first anesthesiologist, popularized chloroform, and the

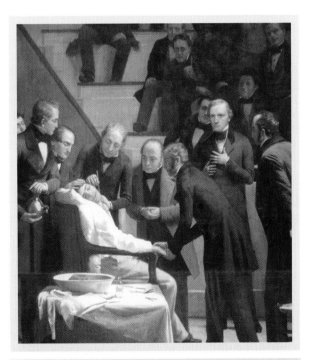

Figure 1-4 Robert Hinkley's painting from 1882 depicts the first ether anesthetic, provided on October 16, 1846, in Boston, Massachusetts. William T. G. Morton (*left*) is holding the globe inhaler, while the surgeon, John C. Warren, operates on the patient, Edward Gilbert Abbott. (Courtesy of the Francis A. Countway Library of Medicine, Boston Medical Library, Cambridge, MA.)

drug received further endorsement from Queen Victoria of England, who inhaled the chloroform during the delivery of two of her children.

A second alternative to ether, nitrous oxide was reintroduced by Colton, who returned to Connecticut in 1863 after a brief move to California and successfully administered thousands of nitrous oxide anesthetics for dental procedures. The addition of oxygen to nitrous oxide was popularized in the late 19th century, but even with this improvement, its relative impotency limited its use for prolonged surgical interventions.

LOCAL ANESTHETICS

Paralleling the recognition of the value of inhaled gases for anesthesia, there were significant advances to establish regional anesthesia as an alternative to general anesthesia. Although the first local anesthetic, cocaine, was applied topically, the field of regional anesthesia could not have progressed without the invention of the hollow needle and syringe. The momentum for this development was the discovery of several biologically active alkaloids, such as morphine, strychnine, atropine, and brucine, which were relatively inactive when administered orally but produced dramatic effects when deposited into an open wound. In 1844, Francis Rynd developed the precursor of the syringe with a device that deposited fluids by gravity flow into tissues through a lancet wound. Alexander Wood was the first to use the hollow needle and syringe combination for treatments of patients. In 1858, he reported the use of hypodermic injections of morphine for treatment of painful neuralgias. With parallel discoveries about bacterial sepsis and sterile techniques, the use of injections became relatively safe. Other physicians adopted the method and used hypodermic injections of diverse drugs for various ailments.[4]

Cocaine was isolated from the indigenous Andean medicinal plant *Erythroxylum coca* in 1856, and its ability to produce reliable local anesthesia of the corneal surface of the eye was demonstrated by Carl Koller in 1884.[5] Injections of cocaine directly into nerve trunks followed within a year.[6] The less toxic local anesthetic procaine was introduced in 1905 by Alfred Einhorn. Percutaneous blocks of the brachial plexus were first described in 1911, and the study and perfection of peripheral nerve blocks have continued to this day. Recent developments involve nerve localization via direct electrical stimulation or ultrasound visualization of selected mixed nerves.

NEURAXIAL BLOCK

Leonard Corning performed neuraxial block in 1885, but his technique was unsafe and poorly thought out. The first true spinal anesthetic based on an understanding of injections into the cerebrospinal fluid awaited the classic experimental studies of August Bier in 1899.[7] Neuraxial blocks were refined in the first few decades of the 20th century. Caudal anesthesia was introduced in 1901, and it was used by Fernand Cathelin for surgical anesthesia, but the technique was found to be unreliable for operations performed on the abdomen. Identification and injection of local anesthetics into the lumbar and thoracic epidural space was first described in 1921 by Fidel Pagés,[8] but it was not popularized until a decade later, when Achillo F. Dogliotti perfected the loss-of-resistance method to identify the epidural space. The epidural method was introduced in the mid-20th century as an improved analgesic regimen to ablate obstetric pain. Neuraxial blocks, including spinal anesthesia, and caudal, lumbar, and thoracic epidural anesthesia, remain popular methods to provide surgical anesthesia.

METHODS FOR DELIVERY OF GENERAL ANESTHESIA

During the time of discovery of neuraxial anesthesia, the techniques for delivery of general anesthesia and the drugs used for that purpose were little changed from what was available before the 20th century. Delivery of ether or chloroform vapors or of nitrous oxide and oxygen by facemask was the standard approach, although several attempts had been made to find more suitable anesthetics. Untrained personnel were assigned the task of delivering the anesthetics, and there was only a limited interest in promoting the study of anesthesia as a scientific discipline (Fig. 1-5). However, beginning in 1930 and for the next several decades, there were significant and rapid advances in general anesthetic methods, and these improvements threatened to diminish the importance of regional anesthesia.

Tracheal Intubation

Airway devices inserted into the trachea were available before the 19th century and were used during resuscitation from drowning. The skills to perform this procedure were perfected approximately 100 years ago by otorhinolaryngology specialists, who like Chevalier Jackson, were often called to remove foreign bodies from the airway. The Jackson laryngoscope[9] was designed for such a purpose but was quickly modified by anesthesiologists for inserting tracheal tubes. Arthur E. Guedel, Ralph M. Waters,[10] and Ivan Macintosh were quick to point out the advantages of the tracheal tube, which included protection of the patient's airway, controlled positive-pressure ventilation of the lungs, and convenient access to the surgical field for the head and neck surgeon.

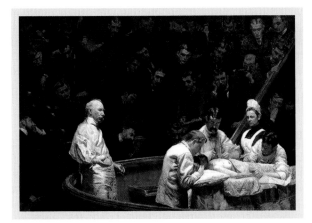

Figure 1-5 The Agnew Clinic (1889) was painted by Thomas Eakins. Young students or nurses, who had little or no prior training, usually administered anesthetics before 1900. This young anesthetist carefully observes the patient and palpates the superficial temporal artery. (Courtesy of the University of Pennsylvania, School of Medicine, Philadelphia, PA.)

DIFFICULT AIRWAY

Although the sequence of intravenous or facemask induction of anesthesia followed by tracheal intubation had numerous advantages, it was hazardous if the trachea could not be intubated. Various inventions were designed to deal with this problem, including airway devices that position above the glottis, lighted stylets (i.e., flexible light wands), and fiberoptic bronchoscopes (i.e., laryngoscopes). A new concept in airway management, the laryngeal mask airway (LMA) was introduced in 1983.[11] The device surrounds the glottic opening and is often used for maintaining ventilation in selected elective surgical procedures and as an alternative to tracheal intubation in cases of difficult airway management.

NEUROMUSCULAR BLOCKING DRUGS

Arrow poisons and blowguns were an integral part of many primitive cultures. Curiosity surrounding the ingredients of the South American arrow poisons attracted the attention of the Spanish conquistadors in the early 16th century as they entered the Amazonian basin. Their accounts gained the attention of members of the medical community in Europe, who performed limited studies on animals with the small quantities that they could obtain. Sir Walter Raleigh's party reported that the native hunters were surprisingly skilled with the blowgun and preferred to use their arrow poisons instead of Western firearms, which frightened the game. The eccentric English Squire Charles Waterton took specimens of the arrow poison to England from British Guinea in 1812. In collaboration with Sir Benjamin Brodie and Francis Sibson, Waterton determined that a donkey could survive the poison if artificial respiration was provided. The active principle of the arrow poison was eventually found to derive from the bark of certain lianas (vines) that grow in the primary forests of South America. Claude Bernard accomplished localization of the effect of the drug to the neuromuscular junction in 1857.[12]

For almost 200 years, the curare poison lacked a medical indication. During the 19th century, several physicians attempted to use unpurified extracts of the arrow poison to treat tetanus and rabies. However, the increased interest in tracheal intubation in the early 20th century and the use of controlled ventilation of the lungs stimulated interest in the use of curare during anesthesia. The development of tracheal intubation and the use of curare in anesthesia were complementary innovations that combined to radically change the practice of anesthesia.

The procurement of sufficient curare for clinical use resulted from the efforts of Richard Gill and his wife Ruth Gill, who had lived in Ecuador as owners of a hacienda near Banos, Ecuador, now a popular tourist attraction because of its natural hot springs. The Gills knew the native customs and were familiar with the arrow poisons of the Jivaro Indians, who live along the Pastaza and Napo rivers.

Richard Gill's interest in the drug arose after conversations with his neurologist, Walter Freeman, who suggested that Gill's obscure neurologic syndrome, characterized by intermittent spasticity, might be relieved if sufficient arrow poison could be procured for clinical testing. In 1938, Richard and Ruth Gill led an ambitious expedition into the interior jungle and returned 7 months later with 25 pounds of the curare paste. The crude preparation was delivered to the pharmaceutical company Squibb and Sons, who initially were unable to find clinicians to study the compound. Perplexed about what use it might have, they eventually delivered samples to Abram E. Bennett, a psychiatrist working in Omaha, Nebraska, and friend of Walter Freeman. Bennett first used the drug for spastic states with limited success, but his use of this compound to prevent the violent muscular contractions during Metrazol convulsive therapy gained acceptance as a means to prevent joint dislocations and fractures associated with these treatments.

Lewis H. Wright, an anesthesiologist and consultant to Squibb and Sons, sought out several anesthesiologists to try the drug form of curare known as Intocostrin for skeletal muscle relaxation during surgery. Initial clinical trials were unsuccessful, but in 1942, Harold R. Griffith and Enid Johnson reported their successful use of Intocostrin to relax abdominal skeletal muscles during cyclopropane anesthesia.[13] In their landmark paper, it is of interest that respiration was not assisted and the anesthetic was delivered by mask. Others quickly recognized the value of Intocostrin, and with the concomitant rise in popularity of tracheal intubation, the safe use of skeletal muscle paralysis during anesthesia was established. Subsequent years witnessed a refinement in the drugs that produce neuromuscular blockade by minimizing the autonomic side effects of the drugs and optimizing their pharmacodynamic properties (e.g., onset and duration of action, mechanism of clearance) to fit the anesthesiologist's needs.

IMPROVED INHALED AND INTRAVENOUS ANESTHETICS

A significant advance in the mid-20th century was the introduction of safe and nonflammable anesthetic vapors that gradually replaced chloroform (hepatotoxic) and ether and cyclopropane (flammable and explosive). This change occurred primarily because of advances in chemistry that allowed the halogenation of the hydrocarbon molecule. Potent nonflammable volatile liquids such as halothane,[14] enflurane, and isoflurane were all highly successful, but the newer anesthetics represented by desflurane and sevoflurane have similar safety records with more favorable pharmacodynamic properties.

Parallel advances in pharmacology and chemical research led to a progressive refinement of intravenous anesthetics ranging from chloral hydrate to short-acting barbiturates (thiopental) and, more recently, to etomidate and propofol. With propofol, it is possible to administer anesthesia without inhaled anesthetics.

ABLATION OF THE STRESS RESPONSE

The term *anesthesia* was suggested to William Morton by Oliver Wendell Holmes in 1846 based on its Greek origin meaning "without sensation." However, some rudimentary sensations persist even during deep anesthesia, and it is therefore more appropriate to think of anesthesia as an immobile state "without perception."

The Riva Rocci method of blood pressure measurement was described in 1896, and brief anesthetic records followed soon after. These early records revealed alarming hemodynamic responses to surgical stimuli in apparently adequately anesthetized patients.

Surgeons soon became aware of the stresses placed on the surgical patient and devised methods to ablate the autonomic and hormonal responses to surgery. George Crile championed the concept of stress-free anesthesia in his book *Anoci-association*, published in 1911. His anesthetic method was to combine procaine infiltration of the tissues with administration of nitrous oxide and oxygen by mask. The combination of central nervous system depression and peripheral nerve block was thought to result in significant benefits in the postoperative period. These ideas were widely disseminated at the time, but with the introduction of improved analgesics and neuromuscular blocking drugs, attention to perioperative stress reduction by combined local and general anesthesia diminished. Over the next decades, new definitions of the anesthetic state were proposed that included lack of movement, unconsciousness, and a poorly defined component of analgesia.

Balanced Anesthesia

In 1926, John S. Lundy, working at the Mayo Clinic, introduced the concept of balanced anesthesia. The concept emphasized the use of multiple drugs to produce unconsciousness and antinociception, provide skeletal muscle relaxation, and obliterate reflex responses. No single anesthetic drug could provide all the characteristics of an ideal general anesthesia, but a combination of intravenous analgesics, neuromuscular blocking drugs, and hypnotics given together produced the desired balanced anesthetic. Lower doses of each drug could be used because the different drugs tended to act synergistically.

Short-Acting Opioids

The introduction of short-acting opioids beginning in the 1960s had a profound influence on the practice of anesthesia. Before 1960, meperidine was commonly used during nitrous oxide–oxygen anesthesia to provide additional analgesia. Meperidine and morphine were relatively long-acting drugs and were associated with side effects that the newly developed short-acting opioids (e.g., fentanyl, sufentanil, alfentanil, remifentanil) did not produce. Today, opioids and β-adrenergic blocking drugs are widely used to control hemodynamic responses during and after surgery.

Subarachnoid Opioids

In 1979, it was reported that subarachnoid (intrathecal) and epidural opioids produced long-lasting and profound analgesia by acting on opioid receptors in the spinal cord. Combinations of local anesthetics and opioids in dilute concentrations are used commonly to provide prolonged (18 to 36 hours) postoperative pain relief with little effect on motor function or systemic blood pressure. Acute pain services, often directed by anesthesiologists, were created to provide a smooth transition from intraoperative to postoperative pain control.

RECENT DEVELOPMENTS

Increased sophistication in monitoring the vital signs during anesthesia accelerated during the second half of the 20th century, a trend that coincided with an increasing complexity of surgical procedures. Anesthesia machines evolved from simple bottles and tubes to portable gas tanks and then to the large stand-alone units (i.e., workstations) prevalent today. Flowmeters, respirometers, and ventilators were eventually attached to the anesthesia machine, allowing accurate delivery of known concentrations and volumes of inspired gases.

Evaluation of gas exchange and oxygen delivery was significantly enhanced through the introduction of blood gas analysis in 1959 and the pulse oximeter in 1974.[15] End-tidal gas analysis based on infrared spectroscopy allows instantaneous evaluation of alveolar gases such as oxygen, nitrous oxide, carbon dioxide, and volatile anesthetics. Together with the studies performed in the 1960s on the end-tidal concentrations (minimum alveolar concentration [MAC]) required to prevent movement in 50% of surgical subjects,[16] these measurements provide a useful estimate of anesthetic depth when using volatile anesthetics.

Transesophageal echocardiography, introduced in 1979 and applied during anesthesia in 1982, allows the motions and valvular functions of the heart to be continuously monitored and is mandatory for certain surgical procedures. Brain function monitors to evaluate the effects of anesthetic drugs on the target organ are among the most recent monitors to become available.

As the machines and equipment became more complex, it became apparent that universal standards and safety measures were necessary to prevent accidents from defective apparatus. Professional societies arose that accredited practitioners in the art of anesthesia and provided standards of care for anesthesia services. The first professional society of anesthesiologists was organized in England in 1893, but associations of physician-anesthesiologists did not have significant influence until the American Society of Anesthesiologists (ASA) and the Faculty of Anesthetists of the Royal College of Surgeons were founded in the 1940s. The ASA has been a leader in organized medicine in developing standards of practice and practice guidelines for delivery of anesthesia and perioperative care of patients. Since the Anesthesia Patient Safety Foundation was founded in 1985, it has been a progressive force in prevention of anesthetic accidents and use of anesthesia simulators (i.e., mannequins) to provide education and training.[17]

Even though anesthesia is remarkably safe today, unexpected complications still occur. Anesthesia remains a process of controlled poisoning, because all of the drugs are lethal if given improperly. Although the human brain appears to have intrinsic analgesic mechanisms, current techniques have not been able to consistently mobilize these mechanisms to combat surgical pain (Fig. 1-6).

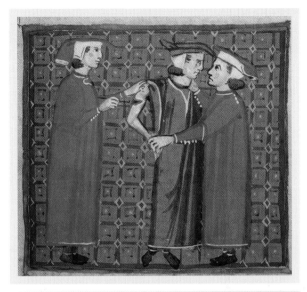

Figure 1-6 Attempts have been made over the past 500 years to control pain without drugs. In this 13th century painting, a surgeon operates while an assistant diverts the patient's attention with a fixed gaze. Mesmerism, hypnotism, and acupuncture are more recent examples of this approach to the control of surgical pain.

MODERN ANESTHESIOLOGY PRACTICE

Today's anesthesiologist is expected to suppress intraoperative pain, provide preoperative counseling, maintain the *milieu interne* during surgery, and facilitate the recovery process. For some procedures, massive transfusions and special techniques are required to sustain life. In these situations, the traditional roles of the anesthesiologist become complementary to those of maintaining fluid and electrolyte balance, preventing coagulopathy, and delivering sufficient oxygen to the vital organs. In the operating room, anesthesiologists often practice in a care team model, working with nurse anesthetists to provide intraoperative anesthesia care. Anesthesiologists also are experts in critical care, airway management, acute pain control, operating room management, and the direction of ambulatory surgery centers.

QUESTIONS OF THE DAY

1. What are the major disadvantages of ether as an anesthetic?
2. What were the earliest medical indications for the neuromuscular blocking drug curare? What were its initial uses in anesthesia care?
3. When was the concept of "balanced anesthesia" introduced? What was unique about this approach?

REFERENCES

1. Davy H: *Researches chemical and philosophical chiefly concerning nitrous oxide or dephlogisticated nitrous air, and its respiration*, London, Bristol, 1800, Biggs and Cottle.
2. Bigelow H: Insensibility during surgical operations produced by inhalation, *Boston Med Surg J* 35:309–317, 1846.
3. Raper H: *Man Against Pain: The Epic of Anesthesia*, New York, 1945, Prentice-Hall.
4. Fink BR: Leaves and needles: The introduction of surgical local anesthesia, *Anesthesiology* 63:77–83, 1985.
5. Koller C: On the use of cocaine for producing anaesthesia on the eye, *Lancet* 2:990–994, 1884.
6. Halsted W: Practical comments on the use and abuse of cocaine; suggested by its invariably successful employment in more than a thousand minor surgical operations, *N Y Med J* 42:294, 1885.
7. Bier A: Versuche uber Cocainisirung des Rückenmarkses, *Dtsch Z Chir* 51:361–369, 1899.
8. Pagés F: Anestesia metamérica, *Rev Sanid Milit* 11:351–365, 389–396, 1921.
9. Jackson C: *Tracheobronchoscopy, Esophagoscopy and Gastroscopy*, St Louis, 1907, CV Mosby.
10. Guedel A, Waters R: A new intratracheal catheter, *Anesth Analg* 7:238–239, 1928.
11. Brain A: The laryngeal mask: A new concept in airway management, *Br J Anaesth* 55:801–805, 1983.
12. Bernard C: *Lecons sur les Effects Des Substances Toxiques et Medicamenteues*, Paris, 1857, J.B. Bailliére.
13. Griffith H, Johnson G: The use of curare in general anesthesia, *Anesthesiology* 3:418–420, 1942.
14. Raventós J: The action of Fluothane—A new volatile anaesthetic, *Br J Pharmacol* 11:394–410, 1956.
15. Severinghaus J, Honda Y: Pulse oximetry, *Int Anesthesiol Clin* 25:205–214, 1987.
16. Merkle G, Eger E: A comparative study of halothane and halopropane anesthesia: Including method for determining equipotency, *Anesthesiology* 24:346–357, 1963.
17. Cooper JB, Gaba D: No myth: Anesthesia is a model for addressing patient safety, *Anesthesiology* 97:1335–1337, 2002.

2 SCOPE OF ANESTHESIA PRACTICE

Ronald D. Miller

In the early 19th century, the concept of providing analgesia and eventually anesthesia became increasingly possible (Chapter 1). This evolution was facilitated by the creativity of some curious individuals who developed several drugs that could produce analgesia and anesthesia. Accordingly, the specialty of anesthesiology began to evolve in a spontaneous manner. Originally, the major or even entire emphasis was on surgical anesthesia. As surgical procedures became more diverse and complex, other associated skills were developed. For example, airway management, including endotracheal intubation, was required to provide controlled ventilation to patients who had respiratory depression and paralysis from neuromuscular blocking drugs. These skills evolved into the development of critical care medicine (Chapter 41). The development of regional anesthesia created opportunities for treatment of some chronic pain syndromes (Chapters 40 and 43). Anesthesiology also evolved into a recognized medical specialty (as affirmed by the American Medical Association and the American Board of Medical Specialties), providing continuous improvement in patient care based on the introduction of new drugs and techniques made possible in large part by research in the basic and clinical sciences.

DEFINITION OF ANESTHESIOLOGY AS A SPECIALITY

A more formal definition of the specialty of anesthesiology is provided by The American Board of Anesthesiology's website, http://www.theaba.org. The ABA defines anesthesiology as a discipline within the practice of medicine "…dealing with but not limited to:

1. Assessment of, consultation for, and preparation of, patients for anesthesia.
2. Relief and prevention of pain during and following surgical, obstetric, therapeutic and diagnostic procedures.

3. Monitoring and maintenance of normal physiology during the perioperioperative period.
4. Management of critically ill patients.
5. Diagnosis and treatment of acute, chronic and cancer related pain.
6. Clinical management and teaching of cardiac and pulmonary resuscitation.
7. Evaluation of respiratory function and application of respiratory therapy.
8. Conduct of clinical, translational and basic science research.
9. Supervision, teaching and evaluation of performance of both medical and paramedical personnel involved in perioperative care.
10. Administrative involvement in health care facilities and organizations, and medical schools necessary to implement these responsibilities."

As with other medical specialties, anesthesiology is represented by professional societies (American Society of Anesthesiologists, International Anesthesia Research Society), scientific journals (Anesthesiology, Anesthesia and Analgesia), a residency review committee with delegated authority from the Accreditation Council for Graduate Medical Education to establish and ensure compliance of anesthesia residency training programs with published standards, and a medical specialty board, the American Board of Anesthesiology, that establishes criteria for becoming a certified specialist in anesthesiology. This describes the American system. Other countries and/or societies have their systems to certify specialists in anesthesiology.

EVOLUTION OF ANESTHESIA AS A MULTIDISCIPLINARY MEDICAL SPECIALTY

In the last 50 years, anesthesiology gradually began to extend its influence outside the operating rooms. Of prime emphasis was pain management (Chapter 43) and adult critical care medicine (Chapter 41). A common thread among these two rather disparate disciplines is that they are practiced by several specialties other than anesthesiology. In addition to Board Certification in Anesthesiology, the American Board of Anesthesiology has an additional certification process for pain management and critical care medicine. All of the other specialties are connected to critical care patients in some way.

Pain Management (Chapter 43)

A pain management center or pain clinic usually takes care of patients on an outpatient basis with occasional consultations in the hospital itself. Many specialties are involved, including neurology, neurosurgery, medicine, and psychiatry. Many other supportive services are required including physical therapy. Because pain management has rapidly become a specialty in its own right, it has its own formally recognized certification process. As an anesthesiologist, formal certification in both anesthesiology and pain management is increasingly required.

Acute pain management (Chapter 40) is primarily directed to postoperative pain. Many tertiary care centers have special teams that provide this type of pain management. In the last 20 years, postoperative pain management has become both more effective and more complex necessitating separate attention and even separate teams.

Critical Care Medicine (Chapter 41)

Critical care medicine can be even more complex than pain management with regard to medical personnel. First is the issue of "open versus closed" units. Usually a "closed" system means that full-time critical care physicians take care of the patients. An "open" system means that the patient's attending physician continues to provide the care in the intensive care unit (ICU). Also, ICUs can be specialty dictated (e.g., medical, surgical, pediatric, neurosurgical, cardiac). Because so many specialties are involved, multiple staffing approaches are used. Anesthesiologists are usually part of a multidisciplinary team all of whom are usually specifically certified and boarded. In many institutions, anesthesiologists are in leadership roles in critical care medicine in their local ICUs.

Pediatric Anesthesia (Chapter 34)

Pediatric anesthesia does not require separate certification to practice pediatric anesthesia in addition to being board certified in Anesthesiology. However, that additional certification has not become a reality yet. The American Board of Pediatrics and the American Board of Anesthesiology have announced commencement of a combined integrated training program in both pediatrics and anesthesiology that would take 5 years instead of the traditional 6 years. In pediatric hospitals, the role of pediatric anesthesiologists is very clear. However, the practice is more complex when pediatric and adult surgery is done in the same hospitals. Typical questions include how young must a patient be when only pediatric anesthesiologists (i.e., instead of anesthesiologists whose practice is mostly adult patients) deliver anesthesia? How should anesthesia be covered when there are no pediatric anesthesiologists? In a few hospitals, pediatric anesthesiologists also manage the pediatric ICUs.

Cardiac Anesthesia (Chapters 25 and 26)

Frequently, anesthesiologists with special cardiac anesthesia training serve both pediatric and adult cardiac patients. It is possible that separate certification processes will evolve.

Other Surgical Areas of Anesthesia (Chapters 27-33, 35, 36, and 42)

Anesthesia for the remaining surgical specialties is not associated with another certification process. With the possible exception of liver transplantation, anesthesia for the remaining surgical subspecialties is frequently delivered by anesthesiologists without additional special training other than that provided by a routine anesthesiology residency. Often, institutional patient volume dictates whether specialized anesthesia teams can deliver anesthesia. For example, institutions with large outpatient or neurosurgical surgery may have separate teams. Likewise institutions with large obstetric volumes will have a special obstetric anesthesia team giving anesthesia 24/7. Many of these specialties have their own anesthetic society (e.g., obstetric, neurosurgical, transplantation, and trauma).

PERIOPERATIVE PATIENT CARE

Preoperative Evaluation (Chapter 13)

Perioperative care includes preoperative evaluation, preparation in the immediate preoperative period, intraoperative care, postanesthesia care unit (PACU), acute postoperative pain management (Chapter 40), and possibly the ICU. About 15 years ago, most surgical patients were required to arrive the morning of surgery rather than the night before. This change dictated that the anesthesia preoperative evaluation be performed during the morning of surgery. However, with complex patient medical risks and surgical procedures, many institutions created a preoperative clinic that allowed patients to be evaluated before the day of surgery. These clinics have become quite sophisticated (see Chapter 13). Preoperative clinics are usually managed by anesthesiologists with involvement of nursing and, increasingly, hospitalists and even internists.

Operating Room Theaters (Chapter 45)

Operating room theaters are increasingly becoming management challenges. Matching operating room available time with predicted surgical complexity and length is an intellectual challenge in its own right.[1,2] "Throughput" is the term used to describe the efficiency of each patient's experience. Sometimes, the throughput is delayed not because of the operating room availability but because of insufficient beds in the PACU. There are numerous steps in the perioperative pathway (e.g., preoperative evaluation, the accuracy of predicting length and complexity of surgical care, and patient flow in and out of PACUs) that can delay a patient's progress as scheduled. Institutions are increasingly appointing perioperative or operating room directors who either manage the operating rooms or coordinate the entire perioperative process starting from the preoperative clinic until exit from the PACU. These positions can be administratively challenging and require considerable skill and clinical savvy. Such jobs are frequently held by an anesthesiologist, although sometimes the director might be a surgeon, nurse, or hospital administrator.

Postanesthesia Care Unit (Chapter 39)

In a tertiary care hospital, the role of the PACU is pivotal. Not only are patients recovering from anesthesia and surgery, they also are receiving direction for appropriate care after their PACU time that spans from ICU to discharge. Even now, insufficient PACU beds are often a cause of delayed throughput in operating room theaters.[1,2] In the future, as anesthesiologists take care of patients with more complex medical risks, more PACU beds will be required in hospitals. In addition to the quality of care, patient logistical management is key to the quality and efficiency of care in the perioperative period.

TRAINING AND CERTIFICATION IN ANESTHESIOLOGY

Postgraduate (Residency) Training in Anesthesiology

Postgraduate training in anesthesiology consists of 4 years of supervised experience in an approved program after the degree of doctor of medicine or doctor of osteopathy has been obtained. The first year of postgraduate training in anesthesiology consists of non-anesthesia experience (Clinical Base Year) in patient care–related specialties. The second, third, and fourth postgraduate years (Clinical Anesthesia years 1 to 3) are spent learning all aspects of clinical anesthesia, including subspecialty experience in obstetric anesthesia, pediatric anesthesia, cardiothoracic anesthesia, neuroanesthesia, anesthesia for outpatient surgery, recovery room care, regional anesthesia, and pain management. In addition to these subspecialty experiences, 4 months of training in critical care medicine is required.

The content of the educational experience during the clinical anesthesia years reflects the wide-ranging scope of anesthesiology as a medical specialty. Indeed, the anesthesiologist should function as the clinical pharmacologist and internist or pediatrician in the operating room. Furthermore, the scope of anesthesiology extends beyond the operating room to include acute and chronic pain management (see Chapters 40 and 43), critical care medicine (see Chapter 41), cardiopulmonary resuscitation (see Chapter 44), and research. More recently, anesthesia training programs have been given increasingly more flexibility. For example, options for a 5-year residency including the Clinical Base Year have been made available. These programs would be allowed to have 2 of those 5 years be devoted to critical care or research. These more specialized training programs have the opportunity to produce leaders in critical care medicine and research. Clearly anesthesia training programs are being encouraged to train anesthesiologists who can meet the challenges of the future.

Approximately 120 postgraduate training programs in anesthesiology are approved by the Accreditation Council for Graduate Medical Education. Approved postgraduate training programs are visited periodically (at least every 5 years) by a representative of the Anesthesia Residency Review Committee to ensure continued compliance with the published standards of quality medical education. The Anesthesia Residency Review Committee consists of members appointed by the American Medical Association, the American Society of Anesthesiologists, and the American Board of Anesthesiology.

American Board of Anesthesiology

The ABA was incorporated as an affiliate of the American Board of Surgery in 1938. After the first voluntary examination, 87 physicians were certified as diplomates of the ABA. The ABA was recognized as an independent board by the American Board of Medical Specialties in 1941. To date, more than 30,000 anesthesiologists have been certified as diplomates of the ABA based on completing an accredited postgraduate training program, passing a written and oral examination, and meeting licensure and credentialing requirements. These diplomates are referred to as "board-certified anesthesiologists," and the certificate granted by the ABA is characterized as the primary certificate. Starting on January 1, 2000, the ABA, like most other specialty boards, began to issue time-limited certificates (10-year limit). To recertify, all diplomates must participate in a program designated Maintenance of Certification in Anesthesiology (MOCA). Diplomates whose certificates are not time limited (any certificate issued before January 1, 2000) may participate voluntarily in MOCA. The MOCA program emphasizes continuous self-improvement (cornerstone of professional excellence) and evaluation of clinical skills and practice performance to ensure quality, as well as public accountability. The components include (1) a measure of professional standing (unrestricted state license), (2) a commitment to lifelong learning (formal and informal continuing medical education), (3) cognitive expertise (passing a secure written examination), and (4) evaluation of current practice. This final component, practice performance assessment and improvement, includes case evaluations and simulation education.

Along with several other specialties, ABA also issues certificates in Pain Management, Critical Care Medicine, and Hospice and Palliative Medicine to diplomates who complete 1 year of additional postgraduate training in the respective subspecialty, meet licensure and credentialing requirements, and pass a written examination. These certificates are time limited (10 years), and recertification is achieved by meeting licensure and credentialing requirements and passing a written examination.

Credentialing and Privileging

The credentialing and privileging process allows appropriate institutions (e.g., medical centers) to collect, verify, and evaluate all data regarding a clinician's professional performance. Recently, three new concepts were developed on a joint basis by the Accreditation Council for Graduate Medical Education and the American Board of Medical Specialties. First, General Competencies (i.e., Patient Care, Medical/Clinical Knowledge, Practiced-Based Learning and Improvement, Interpersonal and Communication Skills, Professionalism, and Systems-Based Practice) are used by the medical staff to evaluate clinicians. Also, Focused Professional Practice Evaluation can be used to provide more thorough information about an individual clinician. The last new concept is Ongoing Professional Practice Evaluation. In essence, processes need to be developed to identify a problem as soon as possible.

OTHER ANESTHETIC PROVIDERS

Certified Registered Nurse Anesthetists

Certified registered nurse anesthetists (CRNAs) probably participate in more than 50% of the anesthetics administered in the United States, most often under the supervision of a physician. To become a CRNA, the candidate must earn a registered nurse degree, spend 1 year as a critical care nurse, and then complete 2 to 3 years of didactic and clinical training in the techniques of administration of anesthetics in an approved nurse anesthesia training program. The American Association of Nurse Anesthetists is responsible for the curriculum of nurse anesthesia training programs, as well as the establishment of criteria for certification as a CRNA. The activities of CRNAs frequently concern the intraoperative care of patients during anesthesia while working under the supervision (medical direction) of an anesthesiologist. This physician-nurse anesthetist team approach ("anesthesia care team") is consistent with the concept that administration of anesthesia is the practice of medicine. In some situations CRNAs administer anesthesia without the supervision or medical direction of an anesthesiologist.

Anesthesiologist Assistants

Anesthesiologist assistants complete a graduate-level program (about 27 months) and receive a master of medical science in anesthesia from an accredited training program (currently Case Western Reserve University, Emory University School of Medicine, Nova Southeastern University, South University, and University of Missouri).[3] Anesthesiologist assistants work cooperatively under the direction of the anesthesiologist as members of the anesthesia care team to implement the anesthesia care plan.

QUALITY OF CARE AND SAFETY IN ANESTHESIA (See Also Chapter 47)

Continuous Quality Improvement

Quality is a difficult concept to define in the practice of medicine. It is generally agreed, however, that attention to quality will improve patient safety and satisfaction with anesthetic care. Although the specialty of anesthesiology has had such emphasis for a long time, the Institute of Medicine drew attention to these issues in medicine overall in 2000 with their report "To Err Is Human."[4] New frequently used words became a routine part of our vocabulary (e.g., metrics of competency, ongoing measurement, standardization, checklists, time-outs, system approaches, practice parameters).[5,6] Quality improvement programs in anesthesia are often guided by requirements of the Joint Commission on Accreditation of Healthcare Organizations (JCAHO). Quality of care is evaluated by attention to (1) structure (personnel and facilities used to provide care), (2) process (sequence and coordination of patient care activities such as performance and documentation of a preanesthetic evaluation, continuous attendance to and monitoring of the patient during anesthesia), and (3) outcome. A quality improvement program focuses on measuring and improving these three basic components of care. In contrast to quality assurance programs designed to identify "outliers," continuous quality improvement (CQI) programs take a "systems" approach in recognition of the fact that random errors are inherently difficult to prevent. System errors, however, should be controllable and strategies to minimize them should be attainable. A CQI program may focus on undesirable outcomes as a way to identify opportunities for improvement in the structure and process of care.

Improvement in quality of care is often measured by a decrease in the rate of adverse outcomes (see Chapter 47). However, the relative rarity of adverse outcomes in anesthesia makes measurement of improvement difficult. To complement outcome measurement, CQI programs may focus on critical incidents and sentinel events. Critical incidents (e.g., ventilator disconnection) are events that cause or have the potential to cause injury if not noticed and corrected in a timely manner. Measurement of the occurrence rate of important critical incidents may serve as a substitute for rare outcomes in anesthesia and lead to improvement in patient safety. Sentinel events are isolated events that may indicate a systematic problem (syringe swap because of poor labeling, drug administration error related to keeping unneeded medications on the anesthetic cart).

The key factors in the prevention of patient injury related to anesthesia are vigilance, up-to-date knowledge, and adequate monitoring. Clearly, it is important to follow the standards endorsed by the American Society of Anesthesiologists. In this regard, American anesthesiology has been a leader within organized medicine in the development and implementation of formal, published standards of practice. These standards have significantly influenced how anesthesia is practiced in the United States (e.g., practice parameters).[6]

The publicity and emphasis on quality and safety have been intense for several years, but sometimes the standards are not implemented as rapidly and completely as desired. Recently suggestions have been made to attach credentialing requirements and penalties for failure to adhere to the required practices.[7] Table 2-1 lists some examples of practices and penalties as published in the New England Journal of Medicine.

ORGANIZATIONS WITH EMPHASIS ON ANESTHESIA QUALITY AND SAFETY

Anesthesia Patient Safety Foundation

The Anesthesia Patient Safety Foundation (APSF) was established under the direction of Ellison C. Pierce, Jr., M.D., during his year as president of the American Society of Anesthesiologists.[8] Initial financial support for formation of the APSF was provided by the American Society of Anesthesiologists, and this financial support continues to the present. In addition, APSF receives financial support from corporations, specialty societies, and individual donors. The purpose of APSF is to "assure that no patient shall be harmed by anesthesia." To fulfill this mission, the APSF provides research grants to support investigations designed to provide a better understanding of preventable anesthetic injuries and promotes national and international communication of information and ideas about the causes and prevention of harm from anesthesia. A quarterly APSF newsletter is the most widely distributed anesthesia publication in the world and is dedicated to discussion of anesthesia patient safety issues. Anesthesiology is the only specialty in medicine with a foundation dedicated solely to issues of patient safety. The National Patient Safety Foundation, formed in 1997 by the American Medical Association, is modeled after the APSF.

Table 2-1 Examples of Patient Safety Practices, with Suggested Penalties for Failure to Adhere to Practice

Patient Safety Practice	Suggested Initial Penalty to Adhere to Practice*
Practicing hand hygiene	Education and loss of patient care privileges for 1 week
Following an institution's guidelines regarding provider-to-provider sign-out at the end of a shift	Education and loss of patient care privileges for 1 week
Performing a "time-out" before surgery	Education and loss of operating room privileges for 2 weeks
Marking the surgical site to prevent wrong-site surgery	Education and loss of operating room privileges for 2 weeks
Using the checklist when inserting central venous catheters	Counseling and review of evidence; loss of catheter insertion privileges for 2 weeks[†]

*These penalties would be applied only in cases in which a clinician did not respond to initial warnings and counseling. Continued failure to adhere to the practice after the initial penalty would lead to permanent loss of clinical privileges (for physicians) or firing, in keeping with the relevant medical staff or human resource policy. Stress management and other behavioral interventions should be considered as possible adjunct approaches when a caregiver chronically fails to adhere to agreed-upon safety standards.
[†]Provonost P, Needham D, Berenholtz S, et al. An intervention to decrease catheter-related bloodstream infections in the ICU. N Engl J Med 2006;355:2725-2732 (erratum, N Engl J Med 2007;356:2660). From Wachter RM, Pronovost PJ. Sounding board: Balancing "no blame" with accountability in patient safety. N Engl J Med 2009;361:1401-1406.

Anesthesia Quality Institute

The Anesthesia Quality Institute (AQI) was formed in 2008 for the purpose of being a primary source of information for quality improvement in the practice of anesthesiology. It maintains data that can be used to "assess and improve patient care." Eventually, the AQI will be able to provide quality and safety data that could be used to meet regulatory requirements. The AQI could also be a source of data for clinical care, research, and societies who have improving quality of care as a goal. The AQI website describes the structure of the National Anesthesia Clinical Outcomes Registry (NACOR) and how data flow into and out of the AQI (http://www.aqihq.org/Introduction.aspx).

American Society of Anesthesiology Closed Claims Project

The ASA established closed claims project is a retrospective analysis of legal cases with adverse outcomes. This ongoing investigation has helped identify patient and practice risk areas that tend to have difficulties and require added attention from the specialty with regard to quality and safety.[5]

Foundation for Anesthesia Education and Research

Although not directly involved with quality and safety, the Foundation for Anesthesia Education and Research (FAER) is an exceptionally important vehicle for support of research in the specialty of anesthesiology. FAER was established in 1986 with financial support from the American Society of Anesthesiologists. In addition, FAER receives financial support from corporations, specialty societies, and individual donors. The purpose of FAER is to encourage research, education, and scientific innovation in anesthesiology, perioperative medicine, and pain management. Over the years, FAER has funded numerous research grants and provided support for the development of academic anesthesiologists.

PROFESSIONAL LIABILITY

Because of intense dedication to quality and safety, malpractice claims have been reduced both in frequency and magnitude. As a result, malpractice premiums have dramatically decreased over the last 20 years. Nevertheless the fundamental principles need to be understood. First, litigation still occurs. For example, 93 claims were filed in the United Kingdom over the years 1995 to 2007.[9] Sixty-two claims involved alleged drug administration errors in which muscle relaxants were the most common issue. Also, 19 claims involved patients being awake and paralyzed (see Chapter 46). With proper labeling and double checking, such errors can be decreased. The anesthesiologist is clearly responsible for management and recovery from anesthesia. Physicians administering anesthetics are not expected to guarantee a favorable outcome to the patient, but are required to exercise ordinary and reasonable care or skill in comparison to other anesthesiologists. That the anticipated result does not follow or that complications occur does not imply negligence (practice below the standard of care). Furthermore, an anesthesiologist is not responsible for an error in judgment unless it is viewed as inconsistent with the skill expected of every physician. As a specialist, however, an anesthesiologist is responsible for making medical judgments that are consistent with national, not local, standards. Anesthesiologists maintain professional liability (malpractice) insurance that provides financial protection in the event of a court judgment against them. Also, CRNAs can be held legally responsible for the technical aspects of the administration of anesthesia. It is likely, however, that legal responsibility for the actions of the CRNA will be shared by the physician responsible for supervising the administration of anesthesia.

The best protection for the anesthesiologist against medicolegal action lies in the thorough and up-to-date practice of anesthesia, coupled with interest in the patient by virtue of preoperative and postoperative visits plus detailed records of the course of anesthesia (automated information systems provide the resource to collect and record real-time, actual data). Also, all anesthesia providers should be prepared to transition to anesthesia record keeping via automated information systems. However, this necessary transition is often not easy. In the United States, pressure is rapidly increasing to use electronic health records (EHR).[10] Specifically, use of automated anesthetic records should be fully integrated into one's medical center information technology system. Unfortunately, implementation of EHR is difficult, costly, time-consuming, and fraught with many unintended consequences, including not meeting safety standards. Fortunately, the current status of EHRs is recognized, which will lead to certification of appropriate EHR by an appropriate national agency such as from the office of the National Coordination for Health Information Technology.[10]

Adverse Events

In the event of an accident or complication related to the administration of anesthesia, the anesthesiologist should promptly document the facts on the patient's medical record (see the APSF website www.apsf.org) and immediately notify the appropriate agencies, especially one's own medical center administration and legal office. Patient treatment should be noted and consultation with other physicians sought when appropriate. The anesthesiologist should provide the hospital and the company that writes the physician's professional liability insurance with a complete account of the incident.

RISKS OF ANESTHESIA

Although patients may express a fear of dying during anesthesia, the fact is that anesthesia-related deaths have decreased dramatically in the last 2 decades.[11] Because fewer adverse events are being attributed to anesthesia, the professional liability insurance premiums paid by anesthesiologists have decreased.[12] The increased safety of anesthesia (especially for patients without significant coexisting diseases and undergoing elective surgery) is presumed to reflect the introduction of improved anesthesia drugs and monitoring (pulse oximetry, capnography), as well as the training of increased numbers of anesthesiologists. Despite the perceived safety of anesthesia, adverse events still occur, and not all agree that the mortality rate from anesthesia has improved as greatly as suggested. Improvement is based on a series of 244,000 surviving patients who underwent anesthesia and surgery. This series is the basis for estimating a mortality rate from anesthesia of 1 in 250,000.[13] It is likely

that the safety of anesthesia and surgery can be improved by persuading patients to stop smoking, lose weight, avoid excess intake of alcohol, and achieve optimal medical control of essential hypertension, diabetes mellitus, and asthma before undergoing elective operations.

When perioperative adverse events occur, it is often difficult to establish a cause-and-effect mechanism. In many instances it is impossible to separate an adverse event caused by an inappropriate action of the anesthesiologist ("lapse of vigilance," breach in the standard of care) from an unavoidable mishap (maloccurrence, coincidental event) that occurred despite optimal care.[14] Examples of adverse outcomes other than death include peripheral nerve damage, brain damage, airway trauma (most often caused by difficult tracheal intubation), intraoperative awareness, eye injury, fetal/newborn injury, and aspiration. Difficult airway management is perceived by anesthesiologists as the greatest anesthesia patient safety issue (Table 2-2).[15]

Improved monitoring of anesthetized patients hopefully will serve to further enhance the vigilance of the anesthesiologist and decrease the role of human error in anesthetic morbidity and mortality. Indeed, human error, in part resulting from lapses in attention (vigilance), accounts for a large proportion of adverse anesthesia events. A number of factors at work in the operating room environment serve to diminish the ability of the anesthesiologist to perform the task of vigilance. Prominent among these factors are sleep loss and fatigue with known detrimental effects on work efficiency and cognitive tasks (monitoring, clinical decision making). The Anesthesia Residency Review Committee mandates that anesthesia residents not be assigned clinical responsibilities the day after 24-hour in-hospital call. Recently, the Institute of Medicine has made very specific recommendations regarding resident work hours and will no doubt

Table 2-2 Ten Most Important Anesthesia Patient Safety Issues as Perceived by Anesthesiologists

1. Difficult airway management
2. Production pressures (decreased time between cases in the operating room ["turnover time"], desire to avoid cancellations)
3. Anesthesia delivery outside the operating rooms at remote sites in the hospital
4. Anesthesia delivery in physicians' offices
5. Neurologic deficit attributed to the anesthetic technique
6. Presence of coronary artery disease in patients
7. Occupational stress for the anesthesiologist
8. Anesthesiologist fatigue
9. Medication errors
10. Time available for preoperative evaluation

From Stoelting RK. APSF survey results identify safety issues priorities. APSF Newsletter 1999;spring vol:6-7; available at http://www.apsf.org.

make recommendations for physicians overall that could eventually be mandated. The emphasis on efficiency in the operating room ("production pressures") designed to improve productivity may supersede safety and provoke the commission of errors that jeopardize patient safety. At the same time, not all adverse events during anesthesia are a result of human error and therefore preventable.

HAZARDS OF WORKING IN THE OPERATING ROOM

Anesthesiologists spend long hours in an environment (operating room) associated with exposure to vapors from chemicals (volatile anesthetics), ionizing radiation, and infectious agents (hepatitis viruses, human immunodeficiency virus). There is psychological stress from demands of the constant vigilance required for the care of patients during anesthesia. Furthermore, interactions with members of the operating team (surgeons, nurses) may introduce varying levels of interpersonal stress. Removal of waste anesthetic gases (scavenging) has decreased exposure to trace concentrations of these gases, although evidence that this practice has improved the health of anesthesia personnel is lacking. Universal precautions are recommended in the care of every patient in an attempt to prevent the transmission of blood-borne infections, particularly by accidental needlestick injuries.

Increased exposure to latex gloves by virtue of adherence to universal precautions has been associated with a dramatic increase in the incidence of latex sensitivity among operating room personnel, especially anesthesiologists with a preexisting history of atopy. Sensitization to latex may be manifested as cutaneous sensitivity from direct contact with latex gloves or as airway changes from the inhalation of latex antigens, or both. Latex sensitivity is appropriately considered an occupational hazard of working in the operating room. Substance abuse, mental illness (depression), and suicide seem to occur with increased frequency among anesthesiologists, perhaps reflecting the impact of occupational stress.

Lastly, infection control for both patients and clinical personnel in the operating rooms require increasingly strict rules regarding specific procedures in the operating room such as washing hands (see Table 2-1).

SUMMARY AND FUTURE OUTLOOK

This chapter reflects the constantly evolving and changing practice of anesthesia. Our responsibilities have grown in magnitude, scope, and depth. Although anesthesia practice is partly based on outpatient activities (see Chapters 37 and 43), it has also become a leading specialty with regard to inpatient medicine, especially the perioperative period including critical care medicine (see Chapter 41). What does the future hold? How much will technology and computers be integrated into our practice? The answer to this question is "a lot." Are robots in the future?[16] The specialty will become even more valuable to medicine overall by attempting to anticipate future societal needs[14] and continuing to dedicate ourselves to the pursuit of excellence.[6]

QUESTIONS OF THE DAY

1. Which organizations are involved with the certification of individual anesthesia practitioners? Which organizations are involved with accreditation of training programs? What are the relationships between these accrediting and certifying organizations?

2. What organizations focus almost exclusively on quality and safety in anesthesia practice? How can their impact be measured?

3. What vehicle will increasingly be used to evaluate quality and safety?

4. Which specialties in anesthesiology require separate certification from the American Board of Anesthesiology?

ACKNOWLEDGMENT

The editors and publisher would like to thank Dr. Robert K. Stoelting for contributing a chapter on this topic to the prior edition of this work. It has served as the foundation for the current chapter.

REFERENCES

1. Sandberg WS: Engineering parallel processing perioperative systems for improved throughput, *ASA Newsl* 74:26–27, 2010.
2. Parker BM: Managing hospital and O.R. throughput, *ASA Newsl* 74:18–21, 2010.
3. American Academy of Anesthesiologist Assistants: Available at http://www.anesthetist.org.
4. Committee on Quality of Health Care in America, Institute of Medicine: *To Err Is Human*, Washington, DC, 2000, National Academy Press.
5. Spiess BD, Wahr JA, Nussmeier NA: Bring your life into FOCUS, *Anesth Analg* 110:283–287, 2010.
6. Miller RD: The pursuit of excellence. The 47th Annual Rovenstine Lecture, *Anesthesiology* 110:714–720, 2008.
7. Apfelbaum JL, Aveyard C, Cooper L, et al: Outsourcing anesthesia preparation, *Anesthesiol News* 1–6, 2009.
8. Pierce EC: The 34th Rovenstine Lecture: 40 years behind the mask: safety revisited, *Anesthesiology* 84:965–997, 1996.
9. Cranshaw J, Gupta KJ, Cook TM: Litigation related to drug errors in anaesthesia: an analysis of claims against the NHS in England 1995–2007, *Anaesthesia* 64:1317–1323, 2009.
10. Sittig DF, Classen DC: Safe electronic health record use requires a comprehensive monitoring and

evaluation framework, *JAMA* 303(5):450–451, 2010.

11. Cooper JB, Gaba DG: No myth: Anesthesia is a model for addressing patient safety, *Anesthesiology* 97:1335–1337, 2002.

12. Hallinan JT: Once seen as risky, one group of doctors changes its ways, *The Wall Street Journal* June 21, 2005.

13. Lagasse RS: Anesthesia safety: model or myth? A review of the published literature and analysis of current original data, *Anesthesiology* 97:1609–1617, 2002.

14. Miller RD: Report from the Task Force on Future Paradigms of Anesthesia Practice, *ASA Newsl* 69:2–6, 2005.

15. Stoelting RK: APSF survey results identify safety issues priorities, *APSF Newsletter* spring 6–7:1999. Available at http://www.apsf.org.

16. Berlinger NT: Robotic surgery: Squeezing into tight places, *N Engl J Med* 354:2099–2101, 2006.

3 APPROACH TO LEARNING ANESTHESIA

Manuel C. Pardo, Jr.

For the beginning trainee, learning perioperative anesthesia care can be anxiety provoking for a number of reasons (Table 3-1). There are no proven ways to decrease the stress of starting anesthesia training. Most training programs begin with close clinical supervision by an attending anesthesiologist. More experienced trainees may offer their perspectives and practical advice. Some programs use a mannequin-based patient simulator to recreate the operating room environment.[1] Learning to practice anesthesia involves the development of flexible patient care routines, factual and theoretical knowledge, manual and procedural skills, and the mental abilities to adapt to changing situations.[2]

COMPETENCIES

The anesthesia provider must be skilled in many areas. Over the last decade, the Accreditation Council for Graduate Medical Education (ACGME) developed its Outcome Project, which includes a focus on six core competencies: patient care, medical knowledge, professionalism, interpersonal and communication skills, systems-based practice, and practice-based learning and improvement (Table 3-2).[3] The American Board of Anesthesiology has adopted the competency framework in its Maintenance of Certification in Anesthesiology (MOCA) program.

STRUCTURED APPROACH TO ANESTHESIA CARE

Anesthesia providers care for the surgical patient in the preoperative, intraoperative, and postoperative periods (Table 3-3). Important patient care decisions reflect the preoperative evaluation, creating the anesthesia plan, preparing the operating room, managing the intraoperative anesthetic, and postoperative care and outcome.

Table 3-1 Anxiety-Provoking Aspects of Learning Perioperative Anesthesia

Unfamiliar work environment
    Anesthesia machine
    Electronic monitors
    Anesthetic drugs
    Equipment cart

Unfamiliar systems of care
    Patient safety procedures (e.g., "time-out")
    Documentation required by regulatory agencies such as The Joint Commission

Direct responsibility for patient management

Time pressure
    Routine procedural aspects of anesthesia care (e.g., intravenous line placement may require more time for beginning trainees)

Fear of an unknown or unpredictable critical event (e.g., dynamic nature of the operating room environment)
    Physiologic effects of surgery
    Sudden problem (e.g., hypotension)

Table 3-2 Competencies in Anesthesia Care

Procedure Event/Problem	Competency
Perform preoperative history and physical	Patient care, communication
Determine dose of induction drug	Medical knowledge
Perform laryngoscopy and tracheal intubation	Patient care
Interact with surgeons and nurses in operating room	Professionalism, communication
Manage maintenance and emergence from anesthesia	Patient care
Patient with dental injury: refer to quality assurance committee	Systems-based practice
Patient with postoperative nausea: compare prophylaxis strategy with published literature	Practice-based learning and improvement

Table 3-3 Phases of Anesthesia Care

Preoperative Phase
Preoperative evaluation
Choice of anesthesia
Premedication

Intraoperative Phase
Physiologic monitoring and vascular access
General anesthesia (i.e., plan for induction, maintenance, and emergence)
Regional anesthesia (i.e., plan for type of block, needle, local anesthetic)

Postoperative Phase
Postoperative pain control method
Special monitoring or treatment based on surgery or anesthetic course
Disposition (e.g., home, postanesthesia care unit, ward, monitored ward, step-down unit, intensive care unit)
Follow-up (anesthesia complications, patient outcome)

Preoperative Evaluation

The goals of preoperative evaluation include assessing the risk of coexisting diseases, modifying risks, addressing patients' concerns, and discussing options for anesthesia care (see Chapters 13 and 14). The beginning trainee should learn the types of questions that are the most important to understanding the patient and the proposed surgery. Some specific questions and their potential importance follow.

What is the indication for the proposed surgery? Is it elective or an emergency? The indication for surgery may have particular anesthetic implications. For example, a patient requiring esophageal fundoplication will likely have severe gastroesophageal reflux disease, which may require modification of the anesthesia plan (e.g., preoperative nonparticulate antacid, intraoperative rapid-sequence induction of anesthesia). A given procedure may also have implications for anesthetic choice. Hand surgery, for example, can be accomplished with local anesthesia, peripheral nerve blockade, general anesthesia, or sometimes a combination of techniques. The urgency of a given procedure (e.g., acute appendicitis) may preclude lengthy delay of the surgery for additional testing, without increasing the risk of complications (e.g., appendiceal rupture, peritonitis).

What are the inherent risks of this surgery? Surgical procedures have different inherent risks. For example, a patient undergoing coronary artery bypass graft has a significant risk of problems such as death, stroke, or myocardial infarction. A patient undergoing cataract extraction has a low risk of major organ damage.

Does the patient have coexisting medical problems? Does the surgery or anesthesia care plan need to be modified because of them? To anticipate the effects of a given medical problem, the anesthesia provider must understand the physiologic effects of the surgery and anesthetic and the potential interaction with the medical problem. For example, a patient with poorly controlled systemic hypertension is more likely to have an exaggerated hypertensive response to direct laryngoscopy to facilitate tracheal intubation. The anesthesia provider may change the anesthetic plan to increase the induction dose of intravenous anesthetic (e.g., propofol) and administer a short-acting β-adrenergic blocker (e.g., esmolol) before airway instrumentation. Depending on the medical problem, the anesthesia plan may require modification during any phase of the procedure.

Has the patient had anesthesia before? Were there complications such as difficult airway management? Does the patient have risk factors for difficult airway management? Anesthesia records from previous surgery can yield much useful information. The most important fact is the ease of airway management techniques such as direct laryngoscopy. If physical examination suggests some risk factors for difficult tracheal intubation, but the patient had a clearly documented uncomplicated direct laryngoscopy for recent surgery, the anesthesia provider may choose to proceed with routine laryngoscopy. Other useful historical information includes intraoperative hemodynamic and respiratory instability and occurrence of postoperative nausea.

Creating the Anesthesia Plan

After the preoperative evaluation, the anesthesia plan can be completed. The plan should list drug choices and doses in detail, as well as anticipated problems (Tables 3-4 and 3-5). Many variations on a given plan may be acceptable, but the trainee and the supervising anesthesia provider should agree in advance on the details.

Preparing the Operating Room

After determining the anesthesia plan, the trainee must prepare the operating room (Table 3-6). Routine operating room preparation includes tasks such as checking the anesthesia machine (see Chapter 15). The specific anesthesia plan may have implications for preparing additional equipment. For example, fiberoptic tracheal intubation requires special equipment that may be kept in a cart dedicated to difficult airway management.

Managing the Intraoperative Anesthetic

Intraoperative anesthesia management generally follows the anesthesia plan, but should be adjusted based on the patient's responses to anesthesia and surgery. The anesthesia provider must evaluate a number of different information pathways from which a decision on whether to change the patient's management can be made. The trainee must learn to process these different information sources and attend to multiple tasks simultaneously. The general cycle of mental activity involves observation, decision making, action, and repeat evaluation. Vigilance—being watchful and alert—is necessary for safe patient care, but vigilance alone is not enough.[4] The anesthesia provider must weigh the significance of each observation and can become overwhelmed by the amount of information or by rapidly changing information. Interpreting findings, processing information, diagnosing problems, and making management changes are often topics of discussion for the new trainee in the operating room.

Table 3-4 Sample General Anesthesia Plan

Case
A 47-year-old woman with biliary colic and well-controlled asthma requires anesthesia for laparoscopic cholecystectomy.

Preoperative Phase
Premedication
    Midazolam, 1-2 mg IV, to reduce anxiety
    Albuterol, two puffs, to prevent bronchospasm

Intraoperative Phase
Vascular access and monitoring
Vascular access: one peripheral IV catheter
Monitors: pulse oximetry, capnography, electrocardiogram, noninvasive blood pressure with standard adult cuff size, temperature
Induction
    Propofol, 2 mg/kg IV (may precede with lidocaine, 1.5 mg/kg IV)
    Neuromuscular blocking drug to facilitate tracheal intubation (succinylcholine, 1-2 mg/kg IV) or nondepolarizing neuromuscular-blocking drugs (rocuronium, 0.6 mg/kg)
Airway management
    Facemask: adult medium size
    Direct laryngoscopy: Macintosh 3 blade, 7.0-ID endotracheal tube
Maintenance
    Inhaled anesthetic: sevoflurane or desflurane
    Opioid-fentanyl: anticipate 2-4 µg/kg IV total during case
    Neuromuscular blocking drug titrated to train-of-four monitor (peripheral nerve stimulator) at the ulnar nerve*
Emergence
    Antagonize effects of nondepolarizing neuromuscular-blocking drug: neostigmine, 70 µg/kg, and glycopyrrolate, 14 µg/kg IV, titrated to train-of-four monitor
    Antiemetic: dexamethasone, 4 mg IV, at start of case; ondansetron, 4 mg IV, at end of case
    Tracheal extubation: when patient is awake, breathing, and following commands
Possible intraoperative problem and approach
    Bronchospasm: increase inspired oxygen and inhaled anesthetic concentrations, decrease surgical stimulation if possible, administer albuterol through endotracheal tube (5-10 puffs), adjust ventilator to maximize expiratory flow

Postoperative Phase
Postoperative pain control: patient-controlled analgesia—hydromorphone, 0.2 mg IV; 6-minute lock-out, no basal rate
Disposition: postanesthesia care unit, then hospital ward

---

*Nondepolarizing neuromuscular blocking drug choices include rocuronium, vecuronium, pancuronium, atracurium, and cisatracurium.

Table 3-5 Sample Regional Anesthesia Plan

Case

A 27-year-old man requires diagnostic right shoulder arthroscopy for chronic pain. He has no known medical problems.

Preoperative Phase

Premedication: midazolam, 1-2 mg IV, to reduce anxiety

Intraoperative Phase

Type of block: interscalene

Needle: 22-gauge, nerve-stimulator needle

Local anesthetic: 1.5% mepivacaine, 25 mL

Ancillary equipment: nerve stimulator with attached cable, electrocardiographic pad for grounding

Technique: povidone-iodine (Betadine) preparation, standard surface landmarks, proximity to brachial plexus identified by nerve stimulation at <0.5 mA current

Intraoperative sedation and analgesia

  Midazolam, 0.5-1 mg IV, given every 5-10 minutes as indicated

  Fentanyl, 25-50 μg IV, given every 5-10 minutes as indicated

Postoperative Phase

Postoperative pain control: when block resolves, may treat with fentanyl, 25-50 μg IV, as needed

Disposition: postanesthesia care unit, then home

Table 3-6 Operating Room Preparation

Components	Preparation Tasks/Supplies and Equipment
Basic Room Setup	
Suction (S)	Check that suction is connected, working, and near the head of the bed.
Oxygen (O)	Check oxygen supply pressures (pipeline of approximately 50 psi and E-cylinder of at least 2000 psi). Check anesthesia machine (do positive-pressure circuit test).
Airway (A)	Two laryngoscope blades and handles Two endotracheal tubes of different sizes (one with and one without a stylet) Two laryngeal mask airways (LMA 3 and LMA 4) Two oral airways Two nasal airways Lidocaine or K-Y Jelly Bite block and tongue depressor Tape
Intravenous access (I)	Two catheter sizes 1-mL syringe with 1% lidocaine Tourniquet, alcohol pads, gauze, plastic dressing, tape
Monitors (M)	Electrocardiographic pads Blood pressure cuff (correct size for patient) Pulse oximeter probe Capnography (breathe into circuit to confirm function) Temperature probe
Daily Drugs to Prepare	
Premedicants	Midazolam, 2 mL at 1 mg/mL
Opioids	Fentanyl, 5 mL at 50 μg/mL

Continued

Table 3-6 Operating Room Preparation—cont'd

Components	Preparation Tasks/Supplies and Equipment
Induction drugs	Propofol, 20 mL at 10 mg/mL *or* Thiopental, 20 mL at 25 mg/mL Etomidate, 20 mL at 2 mg/mL
Neuromuscular blocking drugs	Succinylcholine, 10 mL at 20 mg/mL Rocuronium, 5 mL at 10 mg/mL
Vasopressors	Ephedrine, 10 mL at 5 mg/mL (dilute 50 mg/mL in 9 mL of saline) Phenylephrine, 10 mL at 100 µg/mL (dilute 10 mg in 100 mL of saline)
Avoiding Drug Errors Tips for prevention	Look twice at the source vial being used to prepare your drug. Some vials look alike, and some drug names sound the same. Always label your drugs as soon as they are prepared. Write the following on the label: drug name and concentration, date, time, your initials. Discard unlabeled syringes.
Conversion of % to mg/mL	Move decimal point one place to the right (1.0% = 10 mg/mL). By definition, 1% = 1 g/100 mL. 1% lidocaine is 1000 mg/100 mL, or 10 mg/mL
Conversion of 1:200,000	Memorize: 1:200,000 is 5 µg/mL (1:1000 is 1000 µg/mL or 1 mg/mL)

Patient Follow-Up

The patient should be reassessed after recovery from anesthesia. This follow-up includes assessing general satisfaction with the anesthetic, as well as a review for complications such as dental injury, nausea, nerve injury, and intraoperative recall. There is increasing attention on the long-term impact of anesthesia, including the role of "deep" levels of anesthesia.[5]

Learning Strategies

Learning during supervised direct patient care is the foundation of clinical training. Because the scope of anesthesia practice is so broad (Chapter 2) and the competencies trainees are required to master are diverse, direct patient care cannot be the only component of the teaching program. Other modalities include lectures, group discussions, simulations, and independent reading. Lectures can be efficient methods for transmitting large amounts of information. A series of lectures on a given topic can offer increasing depth and complexity. However, the lecture format is not conducive to large amounts of audience interaction. Group discussions are most effective when they are small (less than 12 participants) and interactive. Journal clubs, quality assurance conferences, and problem-based case discussions lend themselves to this format. Simulations can take several forms: task-based simulators to practice discrete procedures such as laryngoscopy or intravenous catheter placement, mannequin-based simulators to recreate an intraoperative crisis such as malignant hyperthermia or cardiac arrest, and computer-based simulators designed to repetitively manage advanced cardiac life support algorithms. Independent reading should include basic textbooks and selected portions of comprehensive textbooks as well as anesthesia specialty journals and general medical journals.

The beginning trainee is typically focused on learning to care for one patient at a time, i.e., case-based learning. When constructing an individual anesthesia plan, the trainee should also set learning goals for a case. For example, the patient in Table 3-4 has a history of asthma and requires laparoscopic surgery. Several questions could become topics for directed reading before the case or discussion during the case. *What are the complications of laparoscopic surgery? What are the manifestations? How should they be treated? How will I assess the severity of the patient's asthma? What if she had wheezing and dyspnea in the preoperative area?* Trainees should regularly reflect on their practice and on how they can improve their individual patient care and their institution's systems of patient care.

QUESTIONS OF THE DAY

1. What are the Accreditation Council for Graduate Medical Education (ACGME) core competencies?
2. What are the components of a plan for general anesthesia? Regional anesthesia?
3. What are the basic steps in preparing the operating room for delivery of anesthesia care?

REFERENCES

1. Murray DJ, Boulet JR, Avidan M, et al: Performance of residents and anesthesiologists in a simulation-based skill assessment, *Anesthesiology* 107:705–713, 2007.
2. Smith A, Goodwin D, Mort M, et al: Expertise in practice: an ethnographic study exploring acquisition and use of knowledge in anaesthesia, *Br J Anaesth* 91:319–328, 2003.
3. Tetzlaff JE: Assessment of competency in anesthesiology, *Anesthesiology* 106:812–825, 2007.
4. Gaba DM: Anaesthesiology as a model for patient safety in health care, *BMJ* 320:785–788, 2000.
5. Lindholm ML, Träff S, Granath F, et al: Mortality within 2 years after surgery in relation to low intraoperative bispectral index values and preexisting malignant disease, *Anesth Analg* 108:508–512, 2009.

4 MEDICAL INFORMATICS

James Caldwell

*I*nformatics is a contraction of information science and is defined as "the collection, classification, storage, retrieval, and dissemination of recorded knowledge treated both as a pure and as an applied science."[1] Medical informatics is the science of informatics as it relates to the fields within health care and biomedicine. Medical informatics is a relatively new science (term was coined in the late 1970s) that serves as an umbrella term, encompassing more specific fields, such as bioinformatics (Table 4-1). Medical informatics has two components; one is purely scientific and the other applied. The pure science of medical informatics relates to theoretical aspects of information and knowledge management. The applied component deals with how information is used in the service of patients and clinicians.

Some confusion may be caused by other terms encountered, such as health informatics, medical information science, medical computer science, and computers in medicine. These designations are being superseded by the term *medical informatics*, or they are recognized as representing only a limited area within medical informatics.

PURPOSE OF MEDICAL INFORMATICS

The purpose of medical informatics may be described as the creation and implementation of structures and processes that facilitate the objective of gathering data and development of knowledge and the tools to permit the application of those data and that knowledge to the clinical decision-making process at any time and place when a decision needs to be made. Clinicians use information and knowledge to make diagnoses and decide on interventions, and medical informatics is a vital tool in optimizing this process. There are many examples of information that have not been used optimally, including analysis of medical errors and the over- and underuse of services. The judicious use of medical informatics will probably decrease medical errors.[2,3]

Table 4-1 Specialized Areas within Medical Informatics

Clinical informatics
Nursing informatics
Dental informatics
Bioinformatics
Imaging informatics
Public health informatics

Health care professionals with knowledge of informatics improve the quality of information processing, which in turn influences the quality of health care itself. For systematic processing of information in health care, health care professionals require some level of expertise in medical informatics.

COMPUTERS IN MEDICINE

Computers are the vehicles used to realize the goals of medical informatics. Medical informatics deals with the entire domain of medicine and health care, from computer-based patient records to image processing in practice areas ranging from primary care to individual hospitals to regional health care organizations. Some areas of the field are relatively fundamental; others have an applied character. After methods and systems have been developed and made operational for one medical specialty, they can also be transferred to other specialties.

The first example of the use of computational methods relevant to medical information occurred in the U.S. census in 1890, when a punch-card system was used to process the data. In the 1960s, an early decision-support system was developed at the University of Leeds to aid in the diagnosis of acute abdominal pain. In the 1970s, the arrival of the minicomputer put the power of computing at the level of individual departments. Software tools such as UNIX allowed individuals to develop their own applications. The microcomputer or personal computer era began in the 1980s. Since then, individual physicians have had access to personal computers of increasing power at decreasing cost, and the latest manifestation of this trend is the growing use of mobile handheld devices.[4]

Although many individuals and departments have been enthusiastic in developing and using computer-based systems in their practice, the health care industry as a whole has been relatively slow to adopt enterprise-wide systems of managing health information. For example, less than 15% of health care institutions in the United States use electronic medical records (EMRs). This situation is beginning to change, and the pace of change will accelerate. Strong external forces are driving the use of computers in health care. The Leapfrog Group is an alliance of large corporations that are major purchasers of health care, and they have strongly advocated the use of computerized physician order entry (CPOE) systems. The adoption of EMRs is being driven at both the state (specifically California) and federal government levels.

The most compelling reason to incorporate computer-based information systems in medicine is to effectively manage and use the already vast and increasing amount of information that is available. An example is the proliferation of medications and information regarding their interactions. An individual physician cannot keep details of drugs and their interactions in his or her head the way an earlier generation did. More tests and services are available and performed on patients than ever before. The result has been both overuse and underuse of tests and services. Turnover of patients in hospitals has increased, and resident work hours require multiple transfers of care in a single day. The only way to manage the array of data and to pass it on safely between the members of the care team is by electronic means. Reliance on memory and paper records will become a relic of the past.

Standards

The use of computers to manage and share information has many consequences. The first of these is that there needs to be common standards of information transfer. A simple definition of what constitutes a standard is that it is "what most people do." Standards familiar to most clinicians are the International Classification of Diseases (ICD), version 10 and the Current Procedural Terminology (CPT) standards for describing diseases and medical procedures, respectively. Standards may be developed in several ways. The simplest method requires the dominant vendor in an area to set the standard. An example of this is the Microsoft Windows operating system. Another approach is for a government agency such as the Center for Medicare and Medicaid Services (CMS) or National Institute for Standards and Technology (NIST) to mandate the use of an existing system. Groups of interested parties can meet and develop standards independently. If the process has been sufficiently open and rigorous, these recommendations are adopted as standards, such as the Health Level 7 (HL7) standard for clinical data interchange.

Standards have been developed and adopted in many areas of medicine, but in several crucial areas, they have not. The most complex problem is in the area of medical terminology. For example, the terms *heart attack*, *cardiac infarction*, and *myocardial infarction* mean the same thing to a clinician, but to a computer, they are three different entities. Structured systems such as the Unified Medical Language System (UMLS) and Systematized Nomenclature of Human and Veterinary Medicine (SNOMED) exist, but none has gained universal acceptance. The problem of developing standardized terminology is compounded because there need to be systems of nomenclature for all areas of health care, such as nursing. Terminology needs to be standardized within a system and across systems in different areas of health care. The Data Dictionary Task Force, sponsored by the Anesthesia Patient Safety Foundation, has developed a set of common anesthesia terms that have been adopted by SNOMED and licensed by the National Library of Medicine. Common anesthesia terms are essential for optimal use of automated information systems, including anesthesia records that will reflect real-time and accurate physiologic data.[5]

Heath Insurance Portability and Accountability Act

The Health Insurance Portability and Accountability Act (HIPAA) became law on August 21, 1996. Among its many provisions are several relating to the use of electronic health care information. The requirements of HIPAA apply to all covered entities. A covered entity is one in which any patient information is transmitted electronically, no matter how small a proportion it represents of the overall data management by the entity. Hospitals, physicians, other health care providers, health plan organizations, and their employees are covered entities. That means any clinician using any electronic means to apply or access patient information is covered by HIPAA, and the clinician must have some basic knowledge of its provisions. The two areas of most relevance are privacy and security.

Privacy

The use of computers for collecting, storing, and exchanging patient information opens up the possibility of those data falling into the wrong hands. All clinicians have an obligation to ensure that patient information is accessed only by those for whom it is appropriate in the conduct of that patient's care. An example of a breach of privacy is examination of medical information of a celebrity patient by curious health care workers.

PROTECTED HEALTH INFORMATION

If a covered entity transmits any data electronically, all protected health information (PHI), whether electronic or not, must be handled in accordance with the privacy rule. PHI is any information that can be matched to a patient, is created in the process of caring for the patient, and is kept or used in any manner—written, oral, or electronic (Table 4-2). Research records of patient care are also PHI. If all the patient identifiers are removed, the material is no longer PHI.

All patients must be provided with an official notice of privacy rights and practices, and a good faith attempt must be made to obtain a written acknowledgment of receipt of these materials. It is usually not the responsibility of an anesthesia provider to give this notice and obtain consent.

Table 4-2 Examples of Protected Health Information

Names

Geographic subdivisions smaller than a state

All elements of dates and the age of patients older than 89 years

Telephone and facsimile numbers, email or IP addresses, and URLs

Social Security numbers, medical record numbers, health plan numbers, account numbers

Device identifiers and serial numbers

Biometric identifiers (fingerprints, voiceprints)

Photographs of the face or other identifying objects (tattoos)

Any other unique identifying number, characteristic, or code

Thereafter, routine use of PHI for treatment, payment, or health care operations is permitted without further consents being necessary.

Authorization

Authorization is required for release of specific elements of PHI for specific purposes outside routine use or disclosure (e.g., application for insurance coverage, employment physical, marketing or fundraising, clinical research). The authorization document must be signed by the patient, and it must specify an expiration date or event.

Use and Disclosure

The clinician may use (i.e., share data within the institution) and disclose (i.e., share data outside the institution) PHI. An example of use of PHI is looking up results of tests in the clinical laboratory database. An example of disclosure of PHI is communicating with a patient's primary physician outside the clinician's institution. Although many exchanges of data are covered by the minimum necessary standard (i.e., do not transmit more information than is absolutely necessary), this standard does not apply to treatment-related exchanges between health care providers.

PATIENTS' RIGHTS UNDER THE HEALTH INSURANCE PORTABILITY AND ACCOUNTABILITY ACT

Patients have an unlimited right to restrict or amend the use or disclosure of PHI. However, the clinician is under no obligation to treat that patient if the restrictions are considered to compromise the quality of care delivery. Patients have a right to access their records if they are part of a designated record set, which is defined as any data that were used to make a decision about an individual.

Security

Security is required to ensure that PHI cannot be obtained by those not authorized to have access to it. A good security system emphasizes confidentiality, integrity, and

Table 4-3 Essential Practices for Maintaining Security of Electronic Protected Health Information

- Do not share passwords under any circumstances.
- Use a "strong" password (minimum of six characters, with at least three being a capital letter, number, or symbol).
- Log off computer stations when finished with use.
- Destroy all papers containing PHI in shredder or locked disposal bins (never in a trash can).
- Do not leave PHI, in any form, lying around.
- Do not send PHI over an unsecured email system (e.g., to your personal email account).
- Do not leave PHI messages on voicemail.
- Password-protect all personal electronic devices with PHI.

PHI, protected health information.

Table 4-4 Comparison of Paper and Electronic Medical Records

Feature	Paper Records	Electronic Records
Clinician comfort	High, because of familiarity	Wariness regarding new system
Accessibility	Only in one location	Multiple access points
Legibility	Variable, often poor	Excellent
Training required	Minimal	Extensive
Reliability	May be lost or misplaced	Must have stable infrastructure
Data entry	Almost infinite flexibility	Highly structured
Structured searching	Labor intensive	Easy
Viewing options	Limited	Almost infinite

availability. Confidentiality means that only the appropriately authorized individuals have access to PHI. Integrity means that data can be altered only by those authorized to do so. Availability means that data are readily accessible by those who need it.

The basis of security lies in creating a culture and an infrastructure that make security possible (Table 4-3). Security starts with an appropriate culture of human behavior; this leads to an appropriate computer policy, which determines the technical mechanisms (infrastructure) to be used. Inappropriate individual behavior can defeat even the best electronic security systems. An example of human behavior that can defeat the system is a physician who carries unprotected PHI in a personal digital assistant that is left in a public place. Another example is careless discussion about patients by providers in public areas. Unless the human or organizational culture changes first, technical solutions will fail to provide security.

Table 4-5 Reasons for Using Electronic Medical Records

Quality Control
Uniform data entry facilitated
Protocols and guidelines established and made accessible
Reporting of outcomes improved
Enhanced ability to benchmark performance

Patient Care
Improved accessibility of information
Computerized physician order entry
Evidence-based medicine and decision support facilitated
Errors decreased

Management and Planning
Medical records linked to other hospital systems to examine performance metrics
Revenue optimized
Forecasting improved

Research
Terminology standardized
Search capability much enhanced (identifying populations for study)
Large-scale epidemiologic studies facilitated

ELECTRONIC MEDICAL RECORD

A core function of computers in medicine is the electronic medical record, or computerized medical record. Computer databases eventually will replace paper records throughout health care. There is strong pressure from all areas of government and the private sector to implement electronic records (Tables 4-4 and 4-5). In the Veterans Administration, the medical records are almost entirely electronic; and electronic anesthesia records are now being implemented. This has resulted in decreased costs and improved outcomes. However, clinicians are wary of change, and paper records are familiar and difficult for some to relinquish.[4] An important benefit of computerization is facilitation of the adoption of evidence-based medicine (EBM).

EVIDENCE-BASED MEDICINE

EBM has been defined as "the conscientious, explicit, and judicious use of current best evidence in making decisions about the care of individual patients."[5] The practice of EBM means integrating individual clinical expertise with the best available external clinical evidence from systematic research. The optimal application of EBM requires clinical expertise in acquiring information from the patient by history, physical examination, and performance of appropriate tests, and it requires combining those results with the best available external knowledge (i.e., medical literature) and applying this knowledge to diagnosis and treatment. EBM gives less importance to intuition and more emphasis to a systematized approach to health care. This approach does not devalue individual clinical expertise, rather it supplements.

Information Retrieval

The first step in practicing EBM is retrieving relevant information from the vast available repository via the Internet. The days of poring over reference tomes such as the Index Medicus and then laboriously locating and photocopying the articles or chapters of interest are gone. Internet-based sources are usually updated frequently, in contrast to CD-based systems, which go out of date rapidly. A current scenario may be described as follows: (1) open your Web browser, (2) select a search engine, (3) type in some search terms, (4) identify the works of interest, and (5) save them directly into a citation manager or as full-text pdf files. When planning a search, the goal should be to optimize the sensitivity of the search (i.e., chance of finding what you want) and the specificity (i.e., avoid being inundated with irrelevant information).

TARGETED SEARCH STRATEGIES

A strategy for efficient searching is to start at a site that focuses on the type of information needed (Table 4-6). Alternatively, the search may be initiated at a site that deals with the specific disease entity or organ system (see Table 4-6). Another approach is to initiate the search at specific subspecialty websites (see Table 4-6).

GENERAL DATABASES
MEDLINE: The National Library of Medicine Website

Any person with a U.S. online account can have free access to PubMed (www.ncbi.nlm.nih.gov/PubMed). It is a comprehensive database of peer-reviewed biomedical information (see Table 4-6). To facilitate efficient searching, it has built-in search categories of therapy, diagnosis, etiology, and prognosis. Searching in PubMed is significantly enhanced by a working knowledge of its specific medical subject heading (MeSH) terms (http://www.nlm.nih.gov/mesh/MBrowser.html).

Commercial Sites

Merck Medicus (www.merckmedicus.com) is an example of a site that requires registration. It is free and provides access to a vast array of information, including online textbooks, MEDLINE, medical journals, and non-MEDLINE databases (see Table 4-6).

Table 4-6 Targeted Search Strategies
Evidence-Based Practices
Cochrane Library (www.cochrane.org) (database for systematic reviews and meta-analyses)
Agency for Health Care Research and Quality (www.ahrq.org)
National Guidelines Clearing House (www.guidelines.org)
Specific Disease Entity or Organ System
National Cancer Institute (www.cancer.gov)
Subspecialties
American Society of Anesthesiologists (www.asahq.org) (standards, guidelines, consensus statements)
American College of Cardiology (www.acc.org) (standards, guidelines, consensus statements)
General Databases
MEDLINE: The National Library of Medicine (PubMed) (www.ncbi.nlm.nih.gov)
Commercial Sites
Merck Medicus (www.merckmedicus.com)
Web Search Engines
Google Scholar (scholar.google.com)
MD Consult (www.mdconsult.com)
Scirus (www.scirus.com) (restricts searches to science-specific web pages)

WEB SEARCH ENGINES

There is so much information available through search engines that it is possible to be inundated (see Table 4-6). For example, in generic Google, typing the query "awareness under anesthesia" generates over 500,000 hits. Putting quotation marks around the phrase to limit the search to the exact phrase and using other modifiers, such as preceding the search phrase with "allintitle:" still produces almost 1000 hits. The hierarchy of the order in which the hits are presented may not match the quality of the content. Thankfully, by switching to the more specific search engine Google Scholar the same query results in only 18 hits. Judging the quality of the information recovered in searches is a necessary skill in this era of easy accessibility to vast quantities of information.

Critically Evaluating the Information

There are two general source types of medical literature. The first is a primary source, and it is characterized by some amount of experimentation and generation of data. An example of this type of source is an original research article. The second type is a secondary source, which is a compilation of information from a primary source. Examples of a secondary source are systematic reviews and meta-analyses.

PRIMARY SOURCES

Title and Introduction

The title should clearly convey the hypothesis, the study population, and the basic study design. The introduction must "sell" the study to the reader. There should be a clear description of the purpose of the study or the principal hypothesis to be tested. The primary and major secondary outcomes should be objective measures and appropriate to the study question. The authors should offer persuasive justification for performing the study. The reader should be made to feel that the study is important and that it can contribute to better patient care.

Methods

The methods must be focused on and capable of addressing the primary hypothesis. In particular, the study population must be appropriate, and the numbers of subjects justified by a priori power analysis. The conduct of the study must be ethical, with proper informed consent obtained.

Results

In presenting the results, the focus must continue to be on the primary and major secondary outcome variables. Statistics are useful, but the results should pass the "eyeball test." Significant and important differences are usually obvious to visual inspection. Beware of small "statistically significant" differences that are not obvious and of differences presented for minor variables that were not specified previously. Data should be clearly displayed, and individual data and summary statistics should be presented. All subjects should be accounted for. Significant numbers of "dropouts" that are not explained cast doubt on the validity of the results.

Discussion

The discussion should focus on the primary hypothesis or outcome. There should also be a critique of the methodology. No study is perfect, and a genuine discussion of weaknesses attests to the objectivity of the investigators. Authors are often tempted to extrapolate the results and make conclusions that are unjustified. Conclusions should relate only to the hypothesis or outcomes that were tested.

Source

Original research articles should be peer reviewed, and they are listed in databases such as MEDLINE or EMBASE. A consequence of the growth of the World Wide Web is the proliferation of non–peer-reviewed publications. Lack of peer review does not invalidate a study, nor does peer review necessarily guarantee quality. The source of funding for the work should be stated. Studies funded by independent bodies such as the National Institutes of Health or by university or clinical departments are likely to be unbiased. Industry-sponsored studies have a predisposition to bias.

SECONDARY SOURCES

For assessing secondary material, the source is the most important predictor of quality. Reliable databases include the Cochrane Collaboration, the American College of Physicians Journal Club/Evidence-Based Medicine site, and the Database of Abstracts of Reviews of Effectiveness (DARE). These sites use experts to evaluate the primary source material and provide generally unbiased conclusions. Professional societies may sponsor reviews or publish practice guidelines. The authors are independent experts appointed by the society. Less reliable are publications by self-appointed groups of experts, who could have a specific agenda to promote.

DECISION SUPPORT

Categories of Information

There are two general categories of information. Patient-specific information is generated from the care of an individual patient, and it includes results of a careful, thorough history and physical examination plus the results of all tests and interventions. In the computerized world, this information resides in the electronic medical record.

The other category is knowledge-based information, which consists of the scientific literature of health care. Computers provide the means for information retrieval and EBM. When those two information systems are combined, the result is a decision-support system. Decision support can also be defined as the application of information from knowledge-based systems to an individual patient. Although clinicians are initially wary of such systems, some design characteristics encourage acceptance.[6] The system should guide practice, not coerce it. The system should not block nor lock out the physician. Systems are perceived as helpful in compensating for human failure. Computer-based clinical decision–support systems can enhance drug dosing, reduce errors, enhance patient safety, and improve compliance with clinical guidelines.[2,3,7,8]

Examples of Decision Support in Anesthesia

PERIOPERATIVE CARDIOVASCULAR EVALUATION AND TESTING (Also See Chapter 13)

A clinician is performing a preoperative evaluation of a 59-year-old male patient, who is scheduled for unilateral total-hip arthroplasty. He has a history of essential hypertension, which is treated with a diuretic. His hip pain is managed with a nonsteroidal anti-inflammatory drug. He smoked cigarettes until 10 years ago, and he does not drink alcohol. His maternal grandfather died of a myocardial infarction when he was 63 years old; otherwise, there is no significant family medical history. He used to walk regularly and play golf twice each week. He no longer does so because of hip pain. He can climb two flights of stairs, with some slight shortness of breath.

His only previous anesthetic was 20 years earlier for an appendectomy. He is obese (132 kg), and his arterial blood pressure is 146/85 mm Hg. Laboratory results show fasting glucose level of 83 mg/dL and cholesterol level of 212 mg/dL. The physician is unsure about which preoperative tests should be ordered.

The physician goes to a computer and opens PubMed. Under the search terms "preoperative," "cardiac risk assessment," and "guidelines," several citations are found. On scanning the abstracts, guidelines for preoperative cardiovascular evaluation published by the American College of Cardiology and the American Heart Association were found. Upon opening Google, the home page for the American College of Cardiology is located. The pathway Quality and Science/Clinical Statements/Guidelines/Search Topics is followed, and a pdf file entitled "Perioperative Cardiovascular Evaluation and Care for Noncardiac Surgery: 2009 ACCF/AHA Focused Update on Perioperative Beta Blockade Incorporated into the ACC/AHA 2007 Guidelines"[9] is found.

This is a large and complex document, but gives the clinician the needed information. As a result, the clinician ordered a 12-lead electrocardiogram, which revealed a normal sinus rhythm at 82 beats per minute. No further tests of cardiac function are indicated. The option of preoperative β-blockade is discussed with the patient, and together they decide not to start therapy so close to his impending surgery. Although the clinician still had the final decision-making authority, the decision was guided by solid information and knowledge; this is the essence of decision support.

PROPHYLAXIS OF POSTOPERATIVE NAUSEA AND VOMITING (Also See Chapter 39)

An anesthesiologist is reading the preoperative clinic note for his patient for the next day. She is a 31-year-old woman scheduled for an outpatient gynecologic procedure. Written prominently on the chart is the fact that the patient's greatest concern is postoperative nausea and vomiting (PONV). According to the record, she had protracted PONV after a laparoscopic cholecystectomy 2 years earlier. She is a nonsmoker.

The physician's initial search in PubMed using the terms "postoperative nausea and vomiting" yields more than 1000 citations. Eventually, after using the additional terms "prophylaxis" and "risk factors," the number of results is narrowed to a manageable number. Two papers provide the needed information.[10,11] These articles suggest that this patient's risk of PONV is high and . that multimodal therapy is warranted. The clinician therefore decides to use ondansetron, droperidol, dexamethasone, and propofol and to avoid volatile anesthetics.

CONCLUSION

This brief chapter has focused on some practical areas of applied medical informatics. This area is still an immature field, and much of the research in support of electronic records, evidence-based medicine, and decision support is at an early stage. Regardless, the volume of information available to clinicians, and indeed the public, is increasing rapidly, and we need to avail ourselves of informatics tools to enable us to critically evaluate and use this information.

QUESTIONS OF THE DAY

1. What is the definition of "protected health information" (PHI) in the Health Insurance Portability and Accountability Act (HIPAA)?
2. What are the key components of a decision-support system?

REFERENCES

1. van Bemmel JH: The structure of medical informatics, *Med Inform (Lond)* 9:175–180, 1984.
2. Bates DW, Cohen M, Leape LL, et al: Reducing the frequency of errors in medicine using information technology, *J Am Med Inform Assoc* 8:299–308, 2001.
3. van Doormaal JE, van den Bemt PM, Zaal RJ, et al: The influence that electronic prescribing has on medication errors and preventable adverse drug events: an interrupted time-series study, *J Am Med Inform Assoc* 16:816–825, 2009.
4. Prgomet M, Georgiou A, Westbrook JI: The impact of mobile handheld technology on hospital physicians' work practices and patient care: a systematic review, *J Am Med Inform Assoc* 16:792–801, 2009.
5. Ahmadian L, Cornet R, van Klei WA, et al: Diversity in preoperative-assessment data collection, a literature review, *Stud Health Technol Inform* 136:127–132, 2008.
6. Phipps DL, Beatty PC, Parker D, et al: Motivational influences on anaesthetists' use of practice guidelines, *Br J Anaesth* 102:768–774, 2009.
7. Hunt DL, Haynes RB, Hanna SE, et al: Effects of computer-based clinical decision support systems on physician performance and patient outcomes: A systematic review. *JAMA* 280:1339–1346, 1998.
8. Shiffman RN, Liaw Y, Brandt CA, et al: Computer-based guideline implementation systems: A systematic review of functionality and effectiveness, *J Am Med Inform Assoc* 6:104–114, 1999.
9. Fleisher LA, Beckman JA, Brown KA, et al: 2009 ACCF/AHA focused update on perioperative beta blockade incorporated into the ACC/AHA 2007 guidelines on perioperative cardiovascular evaluation and care for noncardiac surgery: A report of the American College Of Cardiology Foundation/American Heart Association task force on practice guidelines, *Circulation* 120:e169–e276, 2009.
10. Apfel CC, Korttila K, Abdalla M, et al: A factorial trial of six interventions for the prevention of postoperative nausea and vomiting, *N Engl J Med* 350:2441–2451, 2004.
11. Gan TJ, Meyer TA, Apfel CC, et al: Society for Ambulatory Anesthesia guidelines for the management of postoperative nausea and vomiting, *Anesth Analg* 105:1615–1628, 2007.

PHARMACOLOGY AND PHYSIOLOGY

5 BASIC PHARMACOLOGIC PRINCIPLES

Steven L. Shafer

Medical students are typically asked during their interviews for residency why they want to become anesthesiologists. The answer is often a variant of "I like pharmacology and physiology." The answer may seem pedestrian to the practicing anesthesiologist, but it accurately reflects the profoundly close linkage between anesthesia and pharmacology.

This linkage consists of several components. We give drugs to patients, who proceed to "dispose" of the drugs through the processes of absorption, distribution, metabolism, and elimination. This process is called pharmacokinetics, and reflects what the body does to the drug. During its sojourn through the body the drug will interact with specific receptors in the body, producing the drug effect. This process is called pharmacodynamics, and reflects what the drug does to the body.

Our clinical practice teaches fundamental concepts in pharmacology: steady-state potency, which we call "MAC" (minimum alveolar concentration) for inhaled anesthetics (also see Chapter 8); the complex nature of drug accumulation, which we refer to as "context-sensitive half-times"; and plasma-effect site hysteresis. In many countries anesthesia care providers either do or will use computers to give anesthetic drugs, directly applying the principles of pharmacokinetics and pharmacodynamics. New clinical monitors solve the complex mathematics of drug uptake and distribution, and predict anesthetic drug concentration and anesthetic drug interactions using three-dimensional surfaces to help guide the clinician.

This chapter will present the basic pharmacokinetic and pharmacodynamic principles that govern anesthetic drug behavior.

PHARMACOKINETICS

Pharmacokinetics describes the processes of absorption, distribution, and elimination that link drug administration to drug concentration in the plasma and at the site of drug effect. Absorption is not relevant to intravenously administered drugs, but is relevant to all other routes of drug delivery. Distribution includes the instantaneous distribution (and dilution) into the blood volume and the subsequent partitioning of drug into peripheral compartments. Clearance describes elimination of the drug, typically through hepatic metabolism, renal elimination, or (in the case of inhaled anesthetics) removal via the lungs.

Physiologic Basis of Pharmacokinetics

ABSORPTION

Absorption of drugs is governed by the route of delivery, the bioavailability, and the possibility of first-pass metabolism. Outside of anesthesia most drugs are given orally. Orally administered tablets, pills, and liquids exhibit complex behavior, including transit delays, pH effects, food effects, and first-pass metabolism. These concepts are not particularly relevant to the practice of anesthesia. Several drugs, including fentanyl, are administered through the buccal mucosa. Transmucosal delivery is characterized by a rapid absorption phase through the buccal mucosa, which is not affected by food or first-pass metabolism, and a slower phase for drug swallowed into the stomach. Inhaled anesthetics are also "absorbed" through the lungs, typically with very rapid transit. Drug injected into tissues is also absorbed into the systemic circulation. Absorption from tissue is the process responsible for the offset of local anesthetic effect after nerve blocks. The skin may also be a site of drug absorption, for example with transdermal clonidine, scopolamine, nitroglycerin, and fentanyl. The skin (by design) presents a considerable barrier to absorption, and typically several hours are required for clinical effect to commence following transdermal delivery. The skin also provides a depot of drug, resulting in continued drug delivery even after the drug has been removed from the skin.

The fundamental concept of absorption is that the rate of transfer from the depot (stomach, lung, nerve bundle, transdermal patch) to the systemic circulation is directly proportional to the concentration gradient between the depot and the systemic circulation. When the rate of drug flow is proportional to the concentration gradient, it is called "first-order" transfer. A characteristic of first-order transfer is that the "shape" of the curve does not depend on the dose. If you double the dose, the curve will look the same, and peak at the same time, but the concentrations will be exactly twice as high at all times. However, the absorption rate has a considerable influence on the magnitude of the peak concentration. Basically, rapid absorption leads to high peaks, and slow absorption leads to smaller peaks. This is why nerve blocks at sites with rapid absorption (e.g., intercostal blocks) of local anesthetic drugs result in steeper and higher peaks, and a more frequent risk of toxicity, than nerve blocks at sites with slow absorption.

DISTRIBUTION

Distribution dilutes the drug from the highly concentrated solution injected into the body to the highly dilute concentration in the plasma. It is a process of mixing, initially with the blood, and then with the tissues of the body. If we measure the concentration of the drug, then we can readily calculate the mixing volume. Concentration is defined as amount/volume. If we measure concentration, and we know the amount injected, we can solve this equation for the volume of distribution:

$$\text{Volume} = \frac{\text{Amount(or dose)}}{\text{Concentration}} \qquad Eq.1$$

Central Volume of Distribution

The central volume of distribution is the apparent volume immediately after injecting a bolus of drug into the body. The concept is not exactly right, because there is a time lag of roughly half a minute between giving an intravenous bolus of drug and the appearance of drug in arterial blood. This time lag is typically and appropriately ignored. The central volume reflects the blood and tissue that the drug has had time to mix with during this rapid transit. Typically that might include the blood in the heart and great vessels, as well as drug uptake by the lungs. The central volume is often used to calculate the dose of drug that should be administered to obtain a given concentration by rearranging Equation 1:

$$\text{Dose} = \text{Desired Concentration} \times \text{Volume} \qquad Eq.2$$

Peripheral Volumes of Distribution

Anesthetic drugs are typically highly fat soluble, resulting in considerable distribution into peripheral tissues. These tissues comprise peripheral volumes of distribution, which are linked to the central volume of distribution. The size of the peripheral volumes of distribution relates to the solubility of the drug in the tissue, relative to the solubility in blood (or plasma). If the drug is highly soluble in a tissue, then it will have a large peripheral volume of distribution. For example, propofol is highly soluble in fat, resulting in a huge (>1000 L) peripheral volume of distribution. Rarely are the actual solubilities of drugs in peripheral tissues known, but that does not matter. By convention, pharmacokinetic models assume that the solubility of the drug in every tissue is the same as the solubility in blood or plasma, and that the tissue is correspondingly large when the drug is, in fact, highly soluble.

Peripheral volumes of distribution can be characterized several ways. There are highly detailed physiologic models for some drugs that account for each organ, the solubility of drug in each organ, and the flow of drug to organs.[1] These models are not particularly useful. A pseudophysiologic approach is to approximately divide the body into several tissue beds: "vessel-rich group" (e.g., brain, most organs), the muscle group, the fat group, and the "vessel-poor group" (skin, cartilage, ligaments). This scheme is often used for inhaled anesthetics. Another approach is to determine the number of compartments required to accurately predict drug concentration in pharmacokinetic models. Nearly all anesthetic drugs can be described by a model with one central compartment of distribution, and two peripheral volumes of distribution. In this latter approach, the compartments may be described using terms that sound physiologic (e.g., the rapidly equilibrating compartment), but the models are strictly empiric and do not describe underlying physiology.

CLEARANCE

Clearance is the process that removes drug from a tissue. Systemic clearance is the permanent removal of drug from the body, and "intercompartmental" clearance describes the movement of drug from one tissue to another. Clearance has units of flow: the volume "cleared" per unit of time (e.g., liters/minute). For example, consider propofol. The liver metabolizes virtually all of the propofol that enters the liver via the hepatic artery and portal vein. Thus, the clearance of propofol is liver blood flow. The liver clears only about half of the fentanyl that enters via the hepatic artery or portal vein, so fentanyl's clearance is half the liver blood flow. Similarly, if the kidneys remove every molecule that enters the kidney, then renal clearance would be the same as renal blood flow. However, if the kidneys only remove every molecule that is filtered at the glomerulus, then plasma clearance is the glomerular filtration rate.

Hepatic Metabolism

Most anesthetic drugs are removed from the body by hepatic biotransformation. The liver metabolizes drugs through oxidation and reduction via the cytochrome P-450 system. The most important cytochrome (CYP) for anesthetic drugs is CYP 3A4, which metabolizes acetaminophen, alfentanil, dexamethasone, fentanyl, lidocaine, methadone, midazolam, and sufentanil. Propofol is partly oxidized by CYP 3A4, but mostly by CYP 2B6. Cytochromes can be induced or inhibited by drugs and disease. For example, midazolam inhibits CYP 3A4, and thus might be expected to prolong the effect of drugs metabolized by CYP 3A4 (alfentanil, fentanyl). Propofol also inhibits CYP 3A4, although the clinical relevance is unclear.[2] CYP 3A4 is potently inhibited by grapefruit juice,[3] antifungal drugs, protease inhibitors, the "mycin" antibiotics, and several selective serotonin reuptake inhibitors (SSRIs). Conversely, rifampin, rifabutin, tamoxifen, glucocorticoids, carbamazepine, barbiturates, and the herb St. John's wort induce CYP 3A4, increasing the metabolism of 3A4 substrates.

CYP 2D6 is responsible for the conversion of codeine to morphine, which is the active metabolite of codeine. Many drugs inhibit CYP 2D6, including quinidine and the SSRIs. As a result, codeine, oxycodone, and hydrocodone are poor analgesic choices for patients receiving SSRIs.

The liver also metabolizes drugs through conjugation and hydrolysis. Conjugation transforms hydrophobic molecules into water-soluble molecules so the kidney can excrete the molecule. Hydrolysis splits molecules apart, typically at peptide or ester linkages. The metabolites of most anesthetic drugs are inactive, although morphine and midazolam have metabolites that are as potent as the parent drug.

Tissue Metabolism

Remifentanil, succinylcholine, and esmolol are cleared in the plasma and tissues via ester hydrolysis. These drugs vanish from the plasma incredibly quick, because esterases are ubiquitous in tissue and plasma. Additionally, drugs cleared by ester hydrolysis typically have highly predictable pharmacokinetics, because the esterase system is very robust. The exception is succinylcholine, whose metabolism by butycholinesterase (formerly called "pseudocholinesterase") is sometimes very slow when a genetic defect in butylcholinsterase metabolism occurs.

Metabolism and Clearance

Clearance is a fundamental biologic property. For example, propofol clearance is almost identical to hepatic blood flow. What does that say about the rate of drug removal from the liver? The rate at which propofol flows into the liver is obviously the propofol concentration times liver blood flow. If you double the propofol concentration, then you double the amount of propofol flowing into the liver. Because the liver removes all the propofol it detects, the rate of propofol metabolism must be proportional to propofol concentration as well. This is a general characteristic of all anesthetic drugs: the rate of metabolism is proportional to the drug concentration. When that is the case, the drug is described as having "linear" pharmacokinetics, meaning that if you exactly double the dose, you will double the blood concentrations as well.

The liver's metabolic rate to liver blood flow, Q, and the concentrations of drug flowing into and out of the liver (Fig. 5-1) can be calculated with a simple equation:

$$\text{Rate of drug metabolism} = R = Q(C_{\text{inflow}} - C_{\text{outflow}})$$

$$Eq.3$$

In the case of propofol, C_{outflow} is nearly 0, so metabolism is the rate of drug flowing into the liver: $Q = C_{\text{inflow}}$. Again, the liver metabolizes only about half of the fentanyl presented to it. In this case, C_{outflow} is about half of C_{inflow}.

If we divide both sides of Equation 3 by C_{inflow}, we get:

$$\frac{R}{C_{\text{inflow}}} = Q\left(\frac{C_{\text{inflow}} - C_{\text{outflow}}}{C_{\text{inflow}}}\right) = Q \times ER = \text{Clearance}$$

$$Eq.4$$

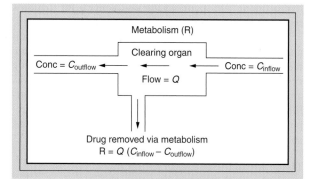

Figure 5-1 The rate of metabolism equals liver blood flow times the difference between the inflowing and outflowing drug concentrations. (Adapted from Shafer SL, Flood P, Schwinn DA: Basic Principles of Pharmacology. In Miller RD [ed]. Miller's Anesthesia, 7th ed. Philadelphia, Churchill Livingstone Elsevier, 2010, pp 479-513.)

Consider the expression

$$\left(\frac{C_{inflow} - C_{outflow}}{C_{inflow}} \right)$$

in Equation 4. This is the fraction of drug flowing into the liver that is removed during the passage. If $C_{outflow} = 0$ (propofol), this is 1. If $C_{outflow}$ is half of C_{inflow} (fentanyl), then this is 0.5. This term is often called the "extraction ratio," meaning the fraction (or ratio) of drug that is "extracted" from the drug flowing into the liver. In the third term, we have substituted ER for the explicit ratio. The resulting term, $Q \times ER$, is how clearance is typically defined.

Let's now consider the first term and last terms of Equation 4, but first rearrange by multiplying through by C_{inflow}:

$$R = Clearance \times C_{inflow} \qquad Eq.5$$

For most drugs used in anesthesia, the rate of metabolism is proportional to concentration. We now see that proportionality constant is clearance. This is the second common definition of clearance: the proportionality constant that links drug concentration to metabolic rate. If the extraction ratio is constant, it follows that the ratio

$$\frac{C_{outflow}}{C_{inflow}}$$

must also be constant. We can define another term, "intrinsic clearance," as the proportionality constant between the ratio of drug flowing in and flowing out of the liver:

$$\frac{C_{outflow}}{C_{inflow}}$$

and clearance is calculated as:

$$Clearance = Q \times ER = \frac{C_{outflow}}{C_{inflow}} \times Intrinsic\ clearance$$
$$Eq.6$$

With a little algebra, one can demonstrate that

$$Intrinsic\ clearance = \frac{Q \times ER}{1 - ER}.$$

Intrinsic clearance reflects the metabolic horsepower of the liver. We can use the concept of intrinsic clearance to relate extraction ratio, liver blood flow, and clearance, as shown in Figure 5-2. For drugs such as propofol, with an extraction ratio that is nearly 1 because the liver removes nearly all the drug that flows in, changes in liver blood flow produce proportional changes in clearance. These drugs are said to be "flow limited," in that clearance is limited only by the rate of blood flowing into the liver. An increase or decrease in liver blood flow produces a proportional increase or decrease in clearance. For drugs with low extraction ratios (e.g., alfentanil), clearance is limited by the capacity of the liver to metabolize the drug. Metabolism of such drugs is "capacity limited." For drugs with capacity limited metabolism, changes in liver blood flow do not affect clearance. The liver can only metabolize a fraction of the drug flowing in anyway, so it doesn't matter if more or less drug flows into the liver.

The liver does not have infinite capacity to metabolize drugs. There must be a point at which every cytochrome in every hepatocyte is working as hard as possible to metabolize the drug flowing in. At this point, metabolism is "saturated," and if additional drug flows into the liver, it will simply flow out again. If we define Vm as the maximum metabolic rate, and Km as the concentration of drug associated with half of the maximum metabolic rate, we can then modify Equation 4 to account for saturable metabolism:[4]

$$Rate\ of\ drug\ metabolism = R = Q(C_{inflow} - C_{outflow})$$
$$= Vm\frac{C_{outflow}}{Km + C_{outflow}}$$
$$Eq.7$$

Equation 7 permits calculation of the relationship among Vm, which measures the hepatic metabolic horsepower, clearance, and extraction ratio. Figure 5-3 shows how clearance will respond to changes in Vm, as might occur with enzyme inhibition, enzyme induction, or liver disease. Drugs with a high extraction ratio, such as propofol, are insensitive to changes in Vm. The liver has so much metabolic capacity for propofol that only massive liver destruction affects clearance. On the other hand, for drugs with low extraction ratios (e.g., alfentanil), changes in Vm produce proportional changes in clearance. That is why even minor induction or inhibition of CYP 3A4 might affect alfentanil clearance.

Figure 5-2 The relationship between liver blood flow (Q), clearance, and extraction ratio (ER), showing the response of flow limited drugs (ER > 0.6) versus capacity limited drugs (ER < 0.5) to changes in liver blood flow. (In Miller RD [ed]. Miller's Anesthesia, 7th ed. Philadelphia, Churchill Livingstone Elsevier, 2010, pp 479-513.)

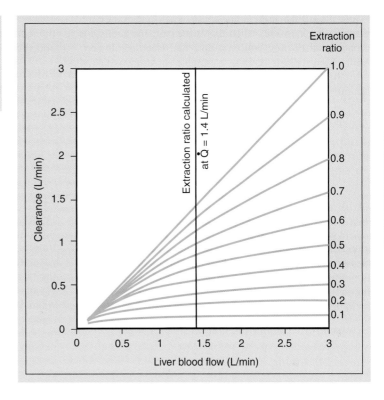

Figure 5-3 The relationship between liver blood flow (Q), clearance, and extraction ratio (ER), showing the response of flow limited drugs (ER > 0.6) versus capacity limited drugs (ER < 0.5) to changes in liver metabolic capacity. (From Miller RD [ed]. Miller's Anesthesia, 7th ed. Philadelphia, Churchill Livingstone Elsevier, 2010, pp 479-513.)

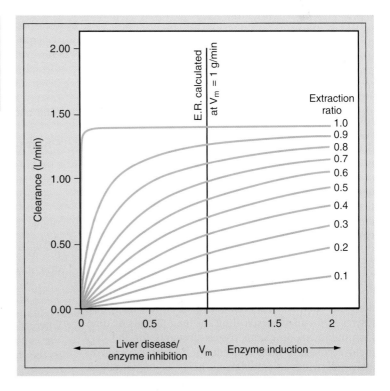

For most drugs used in anesthesia, $C_{outflow}$ in Equation 5 is much less than Km. When this is the case, metabolism is proportional to drug concentration, and clearance is constant. Some drugs exhibit saturable pharmacokinetics, meaning that the concentration of drug exceeds Km. The clearance of drugs with saturable metabolism (e.g., phenytoin) is a function of drug concentration, rather than a constant.

Renal Clearance

The steroidal muscle relaxants are among the few drugs used in anesthesia practice that are eliminated by the renal filtration. The kidneys eliminate about 85% of administered pancuronium, 20% to 30% of vecuronium, and 10% to 20% of rocuronium (see Chapter 12).

The kidneys remove drug from plasma by filtration at the glomerulus and direct transport into the tubules. Creatinine clearance is a useful approximation of the glomerular filtration rate, and can be predicted from age and weight according to the equation of Cockroft and Gault:[5]

Men:

$$\text{Creatinine clearance(ml/min)} = \frac{(140 - \text{age(yrs)}) \times \text{weight(kgs)}}{72 \times \text{serum creatinine(mg\%)}} \qquad Eq.8$$

Women: 85% of the above.

Equation 8 shows that age is an independent predictor of creatinine clearance, which stems in part from the reduction in renal blood flow with advancing age. The subtle clinical point is that elderly patients *with normal serum creatinine levels* still have decreased creatinine clearance. Decreased renal clearance will delay the offset of effect for renally excreted drugs, particularly pancuronium. In general, pancuronium should not be used in elderly patients because clearance will be decreased, even if the serum creatinine is normal.

Propofol's clearance is larger than hepatic blood flow, which is possible only if there are extrahepatic sites of propofol metabolism. The kidneys have been identified as one of the primary sites of extrahepatic propofol metabolism.[6] Renal propofol clearance is about 0.4 L/min, accounting for approximately a quarter of propofol clearance. Propofol is virtually entirely metabolized, with less than 1% appearing unchanged in the urine. The kidney is a metabolic organ for propofol, similar to the liver. Renal elimination of propofol is not a result of filtration.

Distribution Clearance

Distribution clearance is the transfer of drug between the blood and the peripheral tissues. Distribution clearance does not permanently remove drug from the body. However, it can sequester drug for long periods of time. Distribution of drug into tissues accounts for the very rapid decrease in drug concentration observed immediately following an intravenous bolus of an anesthetic drug. The rate of drug transfer is proportional to the concentration of drug in each tissue. At steady state, the concentration of drug in each tissue is the same, and there is no net transfer of drug between tissues.

PROTEIN BINDING

Many drugs are bound to plasma proteins, particularly to albumin and alpha 1-acid glycoprotein. The relationship between drugs and their binding proteins can be described as:

[Free drug]

$$+ \text{[Unbound protein binding sites]} \underset{k_{off}}{\overset{k_{on}}{\rightleftharpoons}} \text{[Bound drug]}$$

where [Free drug] is the free drug concentration, [Unbound protein binding sites] is the concentration of the available unbound protein binding sites, [Bound drug] is the concentration of drug bound to plasma proteins, k_{on} is the rate constant for binding of drug to plasma protein, and k_{off} is the rate constant for dissociation of bound drug from the plasma proteins. This binding occurs almost instantaneously when drug is administered. Plasma proteins have enormous capacity to bind anesthetic drugs, so that even for our least potent drugs (e.g., thiopental) the number of binding sites greatly exceeds the number of thiopental molecules. In this setting, the fraction of drug bound to plasma proteins is purely a function of the concentration of plasma protein.

Will changes in protein concentrations with age or disease affect the binding of anesthetic drugs? If the drug is highly bound, (e.g., free fraction is < 10%) then a 50% reduction in protein concentration will double the free fraction. This would increase the apparent potency of the drug, particularly after bolus administration prior to equilibration of the drug with peripheral tissues. However, changes in plasma protein concentration have virtually no effect on the potency at steady state, because it is the free concentration that equilibrates among tissues, and plasma proteins contribute very little to the total body binding capacity of the drug.

Pharmacokinetic Models

FIRST-ORDER PROCESSES

Your interest payment on your home mortgage is usually proportional to the outstanding balance (e.g., a 6% loan pays the bank 6% of the outstanding principal each year). When you drain your bathtub, the water leaves at a rate that is proportional to the amount (height) of water in the tub. These are first-order processes, and the rate is described by an equation of form:

$$\frac{dx}{dt} = k \cdot x,$$

where x has units of amount, and k has units of 1/time. We can calculate the amount of x at any point in time as the integral from time 0 to time t:

$$x(t) = x_0 \, e^{kt},$$

where x_0 is the value of x at time 0. If $k > 0$, $x(t)$ increases exponentially. If $k < 0$, $x(t)$ decreases exponentially.

This is the fundamental model for pharmacokinetics, because drug flows between tissues and is metabolized at a rate that is proportional to concentration. The rate constant, k, is negative because concentrations decrease over time. The minus sign is usually explicit, so k is expressed as a positive number, yielding the basic equation for drug elimination from a one-compartment model following bolus injection:

$$x(t) = x_0 \cdot e^{-kt}.$$

This relationship is shown in Figure 5-4 in the standard domain (upper graph) and in the log domain (lower graph).

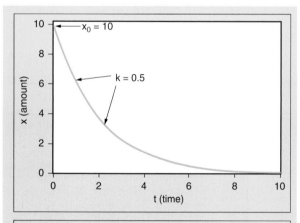

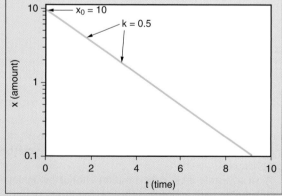

Figure 5-4 The top graph shows an exponential decay curve, as given by $x(t) = x_0 \, e^{-kt}$, plotted on standard axes, with $x_0 = 10$ and $k = 0.5$. The lower graph shows the same exponential decay curve plotted on a log y axis. (From Miller RD [ed]. Miller's Anesthesia, 7th ed. Philadelphia, Churchill Livingstone Elsevier, 2010, pp 479-513.)

How long will it take for x to go from some value, x_1, to half that value, $x_{1/2}$? One can substitute x_1, and $x_{1/2}$ into the exponential decay equation above and solve for time:

$$t_{1/2} = \frac{0.693}{k}.$$

This is the fundamental relationship between $t_{1/2}$, also called "half-life," and the rate constant k.

COMPARTMENT MODELS

Figure 5-5 shows conventional pharmacokinetic models of one, two, and three compartments. All of the models involve a central volume of distribution, termed V_1. The two- and three-compartment models have peripheral volume of distribution, termed V_2 and V_3, respectively. The rate constants relate the flow of drug to the amount in the driving compartment. Thus, the rate of flow from compartment 1 to compartment 2 is $A_1 \times k_{12}$, where A_1 is the amount of drug in compartment 1. The rate of flow from compartment 2 to compartment 1 is $A_2 \times k_{21}$. At steady state, there is no net rate of flow, and so $A_1 \times k_{12} = A_2 \times k_{21}$.

The rate constant for eliminating drug from the central compartment is k_{10}. Because this is a first-order process, the actual rate of drug elimination is $A_1 \times k_{10}$. What is the clearance of the drug? We know from Equation 5 that clearance = elimination rate / C. Substituting $A_1 \times k_{10}$ for the elimination rate, and A_1/V_1 for the concentration (by definition), we see that clearance = $k_{10} \times V_1$. This is a fundamental pharmacokinetic identity. It can also be shown that clearance = total systemic dose/area under the concentration versus time curve, often abbreviated as:

$$\frac{Dose}{AUC}.$$

For the one-compartment model, the bolus dose to achieve a given target concentration, C_T, can be calculated as $C_T \times V_1$, where C_T is the target concentration. Similarly, the infusion rate to maintain a given concentration is $C_T \times$ Clearance.

Unfortunately, no anesthetic drug is described by a one-compartment model. The plasma concentrations over time following an intravenous bolus resemble the curve in Figure 5-6. In contrast to Figure 5-4, Figure 5-6 is not a straight line even though it is plotted on a log Y-axis. For many drugs, three distinct phases can be distinguished, a "rapid distribution" phase (solid line), a "slow distribution" phase, and a "terminal phase" (dotted line) that is log linear. The presence of three distinct phases following bolus injection is a defining characteristic of a three-compartment pharmacokinetic model. The individual phases reflect the peripheral volumes initially filling with drug (distribution phases), and then discharging drug back to the plasma (terminal phase).

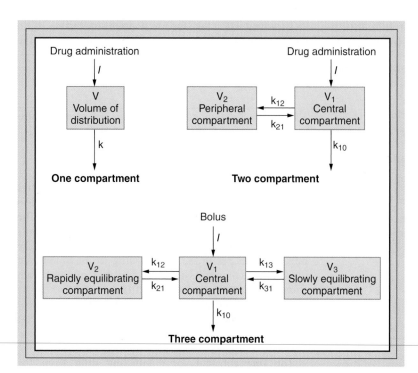

Figure 5-5 One-, two-, and three-compartment mammillary models. (From Miller RD [ed]. Miller's Anesthesia, 7th ed. Philadelphia, Churchill Livingstone Elsevier, 2010, pp 479-513.)

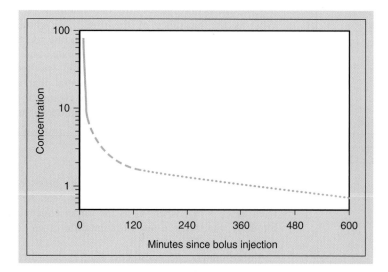

Figure 5-6 Concentration versus time relationship showing a very rapid initial decline after bolus injection. The terminal log-linear portion is seen only after most of the drug has left the plasma. This is characteristic of most anesthetic drugs. Different line types highlight the rapid, intermediate, and slow (log-linear) portions of the curve. (From Miller RD [ed]. Miller's Anesthesia, 7th ed. Philadelphia, Churchill Livingstone Elsevier, 2010, pp 479-513.)

The curve in Figure 5-6 can be described by a sum of negative exponentials:

$$C(t) = Ae^{-at} + Be^{-\beta t} + Ce^{-\gamma t} \qquad Eq.9$$

where t is the time since the bolus, $C(t)$ is the drug concentration following a bolus dose, and A, α, B, β, C, and γ are parameters of a pharmacokinetic model. A, B, and C are called coefficients, while α, β, and γ are called exponents. The main reason that polyexponential equations are used is that they describe the plasma concentrations observed after bolus injection. One can convert the parameters A, α, B, β, C, and γ, into V_1, k_{10}, k_{12}, k_{13}, k_{21}, and k_{31} seen in Figure 5-5, but the math is complicated.*

A steady-state drug concentration cannot be achieved with a bolus and a simple infusion for drugs described by multiple compartments. The infusion rate must initially be high enough to compensate for drug that flows into the peripheral compartments. Only after these compartments

---

*See http://www.nonmemcourse.com/convert.xls, last accessed April 22, 2010.

have come into equilibration can the infusion be set at $C_T \times$ Clearance. One can approximate such an infusion with various "cookbook" formulae, although the use of "target-controlled infusions" permits a computer to rapidly achieve, and sustain, a constant plasma drug concentration.[7]

THE TIME COURSE OF DRUG EFFECT

The plasma is not the site of drug effect for the anesthetic drugs except perhaps heparin and methylene blue. Anesthetic drugs must diffuse from the blood into the target tissue, which produces a delay in the onset of drug effect. For example, alfentanil has a more rapid onset than fentanyl. Figure 5-7 shows a study by Stanski and colleagues in

which patients received either fentanyl (top figure) or alfentanil (lower figure).[8] The circles show the rapid rise in arterial alfentanil or fentanyl concentrations. The time course of the electroencephalographic (EEG) response to fentanyl clearly lags several minutes behind the changes in arterial fentanyl concentration, but there is much less "hysteresis" between the rapidly changing arterial concentration and the EEG for alfentanil. The difference shows that alfentanil blood-brain equilibration is much faster than fentanyl blood-brain equilibration.

The relationship between plasma concentration and drug concentration at the site of drug effect can be described by adding an "effect site," as shown in

Figure 5-7 Fentanyl and alfentanil concentrations in arterial blood (*circles*) and the concurrent EEG (*spectral edge*) during and after an intravenous infusion. The time lag between rise and fall in plasma opioid concentration and EEG effect is much greater for fentanyl than for alfentanil, reflecting the slower plasma-effect site equilibration of alfentanil. EEG, electroencephalographic. (Modified from Scott JC, Ponganis KV, Stanski DR. EEG quantitation of narcotic effect: The comparative pharmacodynamics of fentanyl and alfentanil. Anesthesiology 1985;62:234-241.)

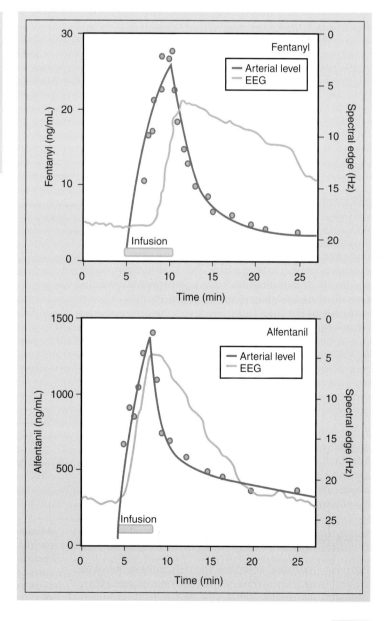

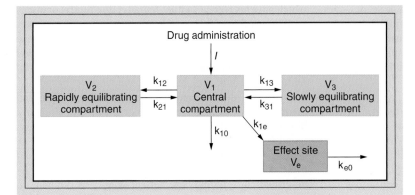

Figure 5-8 A three-compartment model with an effect site to account for the equilibration delay between arterial drug concentrations and drug effect. (From Miller RD [ed]. Miller's Anesthesia, 7th ed. Philadelphia, Churchill Livingstone Elsevier, 2010, pp 479-513.)

Figure 5-8. The site of drug effect is connected to the plasma by a first-order process, with the term k_{e0} representing the equilibration rate constant between the plasma and the site of drug effect; k_{e0} is most easily understood in terms of its reciprocal, $0.693/k_{e0}$, the half-time for equilibration between the plasma and the site of drug effect. Pharmacokinetic models must include k_{e0} to accurately predict the time course of drug effect.

THE OFFSET OF DRUG EFFECT

In medical literature the term "half-life" is often calculated based on the slowest elimination phase (i.e., 0.693/smallest exponent). Unfortunately, "half-life" is a useless concept for anesthetic drugs, and should be abandoned entirely. A better concept is the context-sensitive half-time that relates steady-state infusions of given durations to the time required for a 50% decrease in plasma drug concentration.[9] The context-sensitive half-time does not incorporate the equilibration delay,[10] so it is limited in the ability to characterize the offset of drug effect. The context-sensitive effect site decrement time specifically relates the time course of effect site concentration with the duration of drug delivery.[11] Figure 5-9 shows the context-sensitive half-time (top graph) and the 50% effect site decrement time (lower graph) for the intravenous opioids used in anesthesia practice. Morphine has rapid plasma pharmacokinetics, but very slow blood-brain equilibration. The upper graph suggests that morphine might be associated with recovery faster than alfentanil or sufentanil. The lower graph incorporates the very slow plasma-effect site equilibration of morphine, and suggests that it is not an appropriate drug for continuous infusion during anesthesia.

PHARMACODYNAMICS

Pharmacodynamics describes the relationship between plasma drug concentration and pharmacologic effect. Although the study of clinically important drug effects

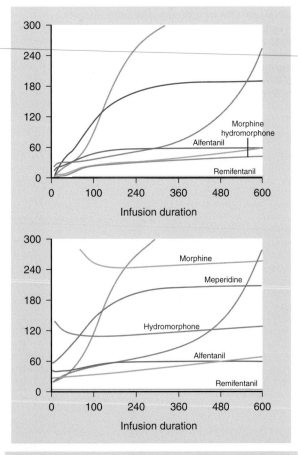

Figure 5-9 The top graph shows the context-sensitive half-life for fentanyl, meperidine, methadone, alfentanil, sufentanil, morphine, hydromorphone, and remifentanil. The lower graph shows the 50% effect site decrement curve for these same opioids. The effect site decrement curve incorporates the plasma-effect site equilibration delay.

is multifaceted, we will divide pharmacodynamics into two general areas: transduction of biologic signals (receptor theory and receptor types) and clinical evaluation of drug effects.

Transduction of Biologic Signals

RECEPTOR THEORY

The binding of a ligand, L, to its receptor, R, follows the laws of mass action:

$$[L] + [R] \underset{k_{off}}{\overset{k_{on}}{\rightleftarrows}} [LR],$$

where k_{on} is the rate constant for the ligand binding to the receptor, k_{off} is the rate constant for the ligand disassociating from the receptor, [L] is the concentration of the ligand, [R] is the concentration of the unbound receptor, and [LR] is the concentration of the bound receptor. The rate of formation of [LR] is

$$\frac{d[LR]}{dt} = [L][R]k_{on} - [LR]k_{off}.$$

At steady state, which is nearly instantaneous, the net rate of formation is 0, and thus

$$[L][R]k_{on} = [LR]k_{off},$$

K_d, the dissociation constant, is the ratio of k_{off} to k_{on}:

$$K_d = \frac{[L][R]}{[LR]} = \frac{k_{off}}{k_{on}}.$$

K_d has units of [L]. When 50% of the receptors are occupied (i.e., [R]=[LR]), K_d is equal to the drug concentration.

A low K_d indicates tight binding to the receptor, while a high K_d implies weak binding.

Full agonists are drugs that activate a receptor to the maximum capacity. Partial agonists are drugs that only partially activate a receptor, even at very high concentrations. Antagonists block other drugs, but on their own do not cause activation of the receptor. Inverse agonists have the opposite effect of agonists, which is usually thought to result from blockade of endogenous agonists. These relationships are shown in Figure 5-10. The difference between full agonists, partial agonists, antagonists, and inverse agonists results from differing intrinsic efficacy. Efficacy should not be confused with affinity. Two drugs can have identical affinity for a receptor (and therefore bind to the same extent at a given drug concentration), yet produce different levels of activation, no activation, or block an endogenous agonist. Antagonists can be either competitive, in which case they physically displace an agonist from the receptor site without blocking it, or noncompetitive, in which case they irreversibly bind to the receptor complex.

The binding of an agonist to a receptor has traditionally been thought to change the three-dimensional shape of the receptor, resulting in the drug effect. It is now known that receptors have many conformations, and that the conformation is in constant flux. It is likely that the binding of an agonist causes the receptor to favor one conformation more than when the agonist is not bound, increasing the amount of time the receptor spends in a particular conformation. By spending more time in a particular conformation, the protein facilitates a particularly biochemical cascade, resulting in the drug effect.

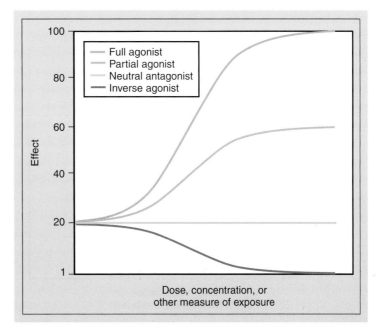

Figure 5-10 Dose or concentration versus response relationships for a full agonist, a partial agonist, a neutral antagonist, and an inverse agonist. (From Miller RD [ed]. Miller's Anesthesia, 7th ed. Philadelphia, Churchill Livingstone Elsevier, 2010, pp 479-513.)

RECEPTORS TYPES

Receptors are present in cell membranes, cytoplasm, organelles, and the nucleus. The receptors of most interest to anesthesiologists are the G protein–coupled receptors, ligand-gated ion channels, and voltage gated ion channels on the cell membrane. G protein–coupled receptors are the most abundant receptors known. Opioids, serotonin, all vasoactive amines, prostaglandins, and histamine are examples of drugs whose effects are mediated through G protein receptors. Ligand-gated ion channels regulate neural conduction by affecting the flux of sodium, potassium, chloride, or calcium into the cell. Hypnotics (e.g., propofol, midazolam, thiopental), ketamine, and muscle relaxants exert their effects on the ligand-gated ion channel. Voltage-gated ion channels are responsible for transmission of the action potential down a nerve, and are the target of local anesthetic action.

Clinical Evaluation of Drug Effects

Figure 5-11 shows the common relationship between exposure to a drug and the drug effect. This is described with the sigmoidal relationship:

$$Effect = E_0 + (E_{max} - E_0) \frac{C^\gamma}{C_{50}{}^\gamma + C^\gamma}.$$

In this equation E_0 is the baseline effect in the absence of drug, and E_{max} is the maximum possible drug effect. C is concentration, dose, or another measure of drug exposure. C_{50} is the concentration associated with 50% of peak drug effect and is a measure of drug potency. A drug with a left-shifted concentration versus response curve (i.e., lower C_{50}) is more potent, and a right-shifted concentration versus response curve is less potent. The exponent γ, also called the Hill coefficient, relates to the sigmoidicity (steepness) of the relationship.

The ED_{50} is the dose of a drug required to produce a specific effect in 50% of individuals. The LD_{50} is the dose of a drug required to produce death in 50% of patients (or, more often, animals). The therapeutic index of a drug is the ratio between the LD_{50} and the ED_{50} (LD_{50}/ED_{50}), as shown in Figure 5-12. The larger the therapeutic index, the safer the drug.

DRUG-DRUG INTERACTIONS

There are numerous types of mechanisms by which drugs can interact pharmacodynamically. The nature of pharmacodynamic drug-drug interactions is so diverse that an anesthesiologist can safely assume there will be some interaction between anesthetic drugs and virtually all drugs that have action on either the central nervous system (CNS) or the cardiovascular system.

Some of these drug interactions, such as the interaction between hypnotics and opioids, are fundamental to the practice of anesthesia. Figure 5-13 shows the interaction between fentanyl and isoflurane MAC (upper graph),[12] and between propofol and alfentanil (lower graph).[13] Typically a small amount of opioid can provide a huge reduction in the concentration of hypnotic necessary to block responsiveness, but some hypnotic is necessary to assure nonresponsiveness.

Drug-drug pharmacodynamic interactions are frequently approached using response surfaces.[14] The response surface

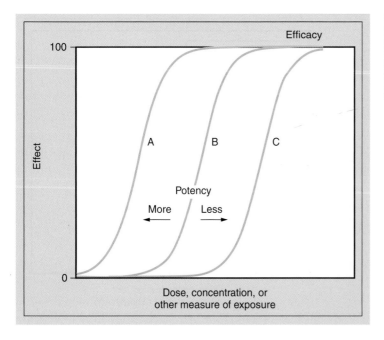

Figure 5-11 Relationship among efficacy, potency, and individual variability as they relate to a typical sigmoidal dose or concentration vs. response curve. (From Miller RD [ed]. Miller's Anesthesia, 7th ed. Philadelphia, Churchill Livingstone Elsevier, 2010, pp 479-513.)

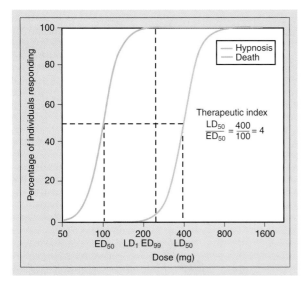

Figure 5-12 Relationship among median effective dose (ED$_{50}$), median lethal dose (LD$_{50}$), and therapeutic index. (Adapted from Shafer SL, Flood P, Schwinn DA. (From Miller RD [ed]. Miller's Anesthesia, 7th ed. Philadelphia, Churchill Livingstone Elsevier, 2010, pp 479-513.)

is the three-dimensional surface that shows the expected effect of any combination of two drugs. Figure 5-14 shows typical response surfaces for drugs with additive interactions, supra-additive interactions (e.g., synergy), and infra-additive interactions.

QUESTIONS OF THE DAY

1. How are most anesthetic drugs (e.g., opiates and benzodiazepines) removed from the body?
2. What are the differences in clearance of a drug that is flow limited versus a drug that is capacity limited?
3. What is the context-sensitive half-time and how does it compare to the half-life of an anesthetic drug?
4. What is the relationship between a drug's affinity and its efficacy?
5. How is the therapeutic index of a drug defined?

ACKNOWLEDGMENT

The editors and publisher would like to thank Dr. Pankaj K. Sikka for contributing a chapter on this topic to the prior edition of this work. It has served as the foundation for the current chapter.

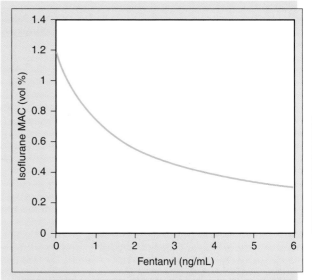

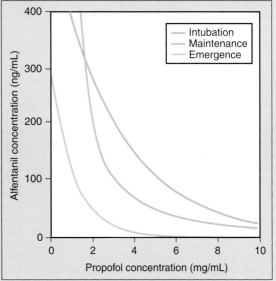

Figure 5-13 The top graph shows the influence of fentanyl on the minimum alveolar concentration of isoflurane associated with 50% probability of movement on incision.(Adapted from McEwan AI, Smith C, Dyar O, et al. Isoflurane minimum alveolar concentration reduction by fentanyl. Anesthesiology 1993;78:864-869.) The lower graph shows the influence of alfentanil on the concentration of propofol associated with a 50% probability of response to intubation and incision, as well as a 50% probability of awakening at the end of surgery. (Adapted from Vuyk J, Lim T, Engbers FH, et al. The pharmacodynamic interaction of propofol and alfentanil during lower abdominal surgery in women. Anesthesiology 1995;83:8-22.)

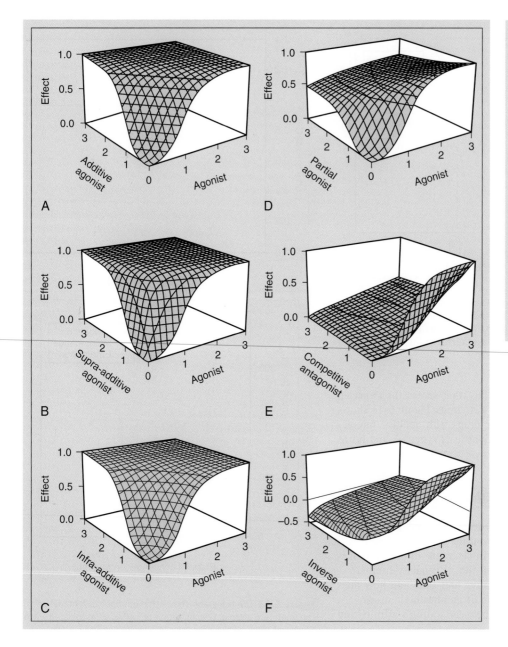

Figure 5-14 Response surfaces for potential pharmacodynamic interactions of anesthetic drugs. **A,** Additive interaction between two agonists that have the same mechanism of action (e.g., fentanyl and alfentanil interaction). **B,** Supra-additive interaction between two agonists (e.g., isoflurane and fentanyl). **C,** Infra-additive interaction between two agonists (reported for cyclopropane and nitrous oxide). (Adapted from Minto CF, Schnider TW, Short TG, et al. Response surface model for anesthetic drug interactions. *Anesthesiology* 2000;92:1603-1616.)

REFERENCES

1. Björkman S, Stanski DR, Verotta D, et al: Comparative tissue concentration profiles of fentanyl and alfentanil in humans predicted from tissue/blood partition data obtained in rats, *Anesthesiology* 72:865–873, 1990.
2. Kanazawa H, Okada A, Igarashi E, et al: Determination of midazolam and its metabolite as a probe for cytochrome P450 3A4 phenotype by liquid chromatography-mass spectrometry, *J Chromatogr A* 1031:213–218, 2004.
3. Bailey DG, Malcolm J, Arnold O, et al: Grapefruit juice-drug interactions, *Br J Clin Pharmacol* 46:101–110, 1998.
4. Wagner JG: *Pharmacokinetics for the Pharmaceutical Scientist*, Lancaster, PA, Technomic Publishing, 1993.
5. Cockcroft DW, Gault MH: Prediction of creatinine clearance from serum creatinine, *Nephron* 16:31–41, 1976.
6. Takizawa D, Hiraoka H, Goto F, et al: Human kidneys play an important role in the elimination of propofol, *Anesthesiology* 102:327–330, 2005.
7. Egan TD, Shafer SL: Target-controlled infusions for intravenous anesthetics: Surfing USA not!, *Anesthesiology* 99:1039–1041, 2003.
8. Scott JC, Ponganis KV, Stanski DR: EEG quantitation of narcotic effect: The comparative pharmacodynamics of

fentanyl and alfentanil, *Anesthesiology* 62:234–241, 1985.

9. Hughes MA, Glass PS, Jacobs JR: Context-sensitive half-time in multicompartment pharmacokinetic models for intravenous anesthetic drugs, *Anesthesiology* 76:334–341, 1992.

10. Shafer SL, Varvel JR: Pharmacokinetics, pharmacodynamics, and rational opioid selection, *Anesthesiology* 74:53–63, 1991.

11. Youngs EJ, Shafer SL: Pharmacokinetic parameters relevant to recovery from opioids, *Anesthesiology* 81:833–842, 1994.

12. McEwan AI, Smith C, Dyar O, et al: Isoflurane minimum alveolar concentration reduction by fentanyl, *Anesthesiology* 78:864–869, 1993.

13. Vuyk J, Lim T, Engbers FH, et al: The pharmacodynamic interaction of propofol and alfentanil during lower abdominal surgery in women, *Anesthesiology* 83:8–22, 1995.

14. Minto CF, Schnider TW, Short TG, et al: Response surface model for anesthetic drug interactions, *Anesthesiology* 92:1603–1616, 2000.

6 CLINICAL CARDIAC AND PULMONARY PHYSIOLOGY

John Feiner

No specialty in medicine manages cardiac and pulmonary physiology as directly on a daily basis as anesthesiology.[1-3] An understanding of cardiorespiratory physiology prepares the anesthesia team to manage critical and common situations in anesthesia, including hypotension, arterial hypoxemia, hypercapnia, and high peak airway pressures.

HEMODYNAMICS

Arterial Blood Pressure

Systemic blood pressure and mean arterial pressure (MAP) are commonly monitored by anesthesia providers with a blood pressure cuff or an indwelling arterial cannula. Although treatment of chronic systemic hypertension is sometimes necessary, acute hypotension is a problem during many anesthetics. Hypotension varies from mild clinically insignificant reductions in MAP from general anesthesia or regional anesthesia to life-threatening emergencies. Hypotension can be severe enough to jeopardize organ perfusion, causing injury and an adverse outcome. Organs of most immediate concern are the heart and brain, followed by the kidneys, liver, and lungs. All have typical injury patterns associated with prolonged "shock." Understanding the physiology behind hypotension is critical for diagnosis and treatment.

Physiologic Approach to Hypotension

The logical treatment of acute hypotension categorizes MAP into its physiologic components:

$$MAP = SVR \times CO$$

In the equation, SVR is the systemic vascular resistance, and CO is cardiac output.

Although most of our focus is on understanding MAP, systolic blood pressure (SBP), diastolic blood pressure (DBP), and pulse pressure (SBP – DBP) also require attention.

The pulse pressure is created by the addition of stroke volume (SV) on top of a DBP within the compliant vascular tree. The aorta is responsible for most of this compliance. Increased pulse pressure can occur with an increased SV, but it most often occurs because of the poor aortic compliance that accompanies aging. Decreasing DBP can have more dramatic effects on SBP if vascular compliance is poor.

SYSTEMIC VASCULAR RESISTANCE

Most drugs administered during general anesthesia and neuraxial regional anesthesia decrease SVR. Many pathologic causes can produce profound reductions in SVR, including sepsis, anaphylaxis, spinal shock, and reperfusion of ischemic organs. The calculation for SVR follows:

$$SVR = 80 \cdot \frac{MAP - CVP}{CO}$$

In the equation, MAP is the mean arterial pressure, CVP is the central venous pressure, CO is cardiac output, and the factor 80 converts units into dyne/sec/cm^5 from pressure in millimeters of mercury (mm Hg) and CO given in liters per minute (L/min).

Pulmonary artery (PA) catheterization can be used to obtain the measurements necessary for calculating SVR, but this monitor is not usually immediately available. Signs of adequate perfusion (e.g., warm extremities, good pulse oximeter signal) may sometimes be present when hypotension is caused by low SVR. On the other hand, hypertension nearly always involves excessive vasoconstriction.

Resistance is inversely proportional to the fourth power of the radius. Individually, small vessels offer a very high resistance to flow. However, total SVR is decreased when there are many vessels arranged in parallel. Capillaries, despite being the smallest blood vessels, are not responsible for most of the SVR because there are so many in parallel. Most of the resistance to blood flow in the arterial side of the circulation is in the arterioles.

CARDIAC OUTPUT

As a cause of hypotension, decreased CO may be more difficult to treat than decreased SVR. Increased CO is not usually associated with systemic hypertension, and most hyperdynamic states, such as sepsis and liver failure, are associated with decreased systemic blood pressure.

CO is defined as the amount of blood (L/min) pumped by the heart. Although the amount of blood pumped by the right side and left side of the heart can differ in the presence of certain congenital heart malformations, these amounts are usually the same. CO is the product of heart rate (HR) and stroke volume (SV), the net amount of blood ejected by the heart in one cycle:

$$CO = HR \times SV$$

CO can be measured clinically by thermodilution via a pulmonary artery (PA) catheter and by transesophageal echocardiography (TEE). Less invasive devices to measure CO are being developed. Because the normal CO changes according to body size, cardiac index (CO divided by body surface area) often is used.

HEART RATE

Tachycardia and bradycardia can cause hypotension when CO is small. The electrocardiogram (ECG), pulse oximetry, or physical examination can identify bradycardia or tachycardia. The identification of a P wave on the ECG is essential for analyzing HR. Loss of sinus rhythm and atrial contraction results in decreased ventricular filling. Atrial contraction is responsible for a significant percentage of preload, even more so in patients with a poorly compliant ventricle. A slow HR may result in enhanced ventricular filling and an increased SV, but an excessively slow HR results in an inadequate CO. Tachycardia may result in insufficient time for the left ventricle to fill and result in low CO and hypotension.

EJECTION FRACTION

Ejection fraction (EF) is the percentage of ventricular blood volume that is pumped by the heart in a single contraction (SV/end-diastolic volume [EDV]). Unlike SV, the EF does not differ on the basis of body size, and an EF of 60% to 70% is considered normal. Because CO can be maintained by increasing HR, the SV should be calculated to better assess cardiac function.

PRELOAD

Preload refers to the amount the cardiac muscle is "stretched" before contraction. Preload is best defined clinically as the EDV of the heart. EDV can be measured directly with TEE. Filling pressures (e.g., left atrial pressure [LA], pulmonary capillary wedge pressure [PCWP], pulmonary artery diastolic pressure [PAD]) can also be used to assess preload. Central venous pressure (CVP) measures filling pressures on the right side of the heart, which correlates with filling pressures on the left side of the heart in the absence of pulmonary disease and when cardiac function is normal. The relationship between pressure and volume of the heart in diastole is depicted by ventricular compliance curves (Fig. 6-1). With a poorly compliant heart, normal filling pressures may not produce an adequate EDV. Likewise, trying to fill a "stiff" left ventricle to a normal volume may increase intracardiac and pulmonary capillary pressures excessively.

Frank-Starling Mechanism

The Frank-Starling mechanism is a physiologic description of the increased pumping action of the heart with increased filling. A larger preload results in increased contraction necessary to eject the added ventricular volume, resulting in a larger SV and similar EF. Reduced ventricular filling, as in hypovolemia, results in reduced SV. Small increases in preload may have dramatic effects ("volume responsiveness") on SV and CO (Fig. 6-2).

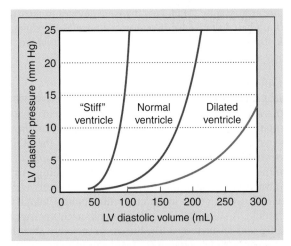

Figure 6-1 The pressure-volume relationship of the heart in diastole is shown in the compliance curves plotting left ventricular (LV) diastolic volume versus pressure. The "stiff" heart shows a steeper rise of pressure with increased volume than the normal heart. The dilated ventricle shows a much more compliant curve.

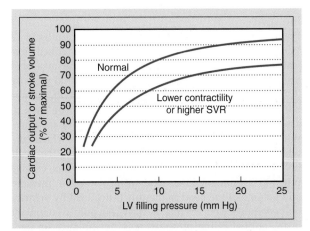

Figure 6-2 The cardiac function curve shows the typical relationship between preload, represented by left ventricular (LV) filling pressure, and cardiac function, reflected in cardiac output or stroke volume. Filling pressure can be measured as left atrial pressure or pulmonary capillary wedge pressure. At low preload, augmentation of filling results in significantly increased cardiac output. This is the steeper portion of the curve. At higher LV filling pressures, little improvement in function occurs with increased preload, and with overfilling, a decrement in function can occur because of impaired perfusion (not shown). Lower contractility or higher systemic vascular resistance (SVR) shifts the normal curve to the right and downward.

At higher points on the curve, little additional benefit is derived from increases in preload.

Causes of Low Preload

Causes of low preload include hypovolemia and venodilation. Hypovolemia may result from hemorrhage or fluid losses. Venodilation occurs with general anesthesia and may be even more prominent in the presence of neuraxial anesthesia. Additional causes of decreased preload include tension pneumothorax and pericardial tamponade, which prevent ventricular filling due to increased pressure around the heart, even though blood volume and filling pressures are adequate.[4] Such conditions may manifest with a systolic pressure variation (i.e., change in SBP with tidal breathing) that can be observed on an arterial blood pressure tracing.[5] The extreme form of this is pulsus paradoxus, a pulse that changes markedly during tidal breathing. In the setting of normal or increased CVP, the presence of cardiac tamponade may exist. Systolic pressure variation is also useful in identifying hypovolemia, and is a more sensitive and specific indicator of intravascular volume responsiveness than CVP.

Pathologic problems on the right side of the heart may prevent filling of the left ventricle. Pulmonary embolism and other causes of pulmonary hypertension prevent the right side of the heart from pumping a sufficient volume to fill the left side of the heart. The interventricular septum may be shifted, further constricting filling of the left side of the heart.

CONTRACTILITY

Contractility, or the inotropic state of the heart, is a measure of the force of contraction independent of loading conditions (preload or afterload). It can be measured for research purposes by the rate at which pressure develops in the cardiac ventricles (dP/dT) or by systolic pressure-volume relationships (Fig. 6-3). Decreased myocardial contractility may be a cause of hypotension (Table 6-1).[6]

AFTERLOAD

Afterload is the resistance to ejection of blood from the left ventricle with each contraction. Clinically, afterload is largely determined by SVR. When SVR is increased, the heart does not empty as completely, resulting in a lower SV, EF, and CO (see Fig. 6-2). High SVR also increases cardiac filling pressures. Low SVR improves SV and increases CO such that a low SVR is often associated with a higher CO (Fig. 6-4).

Low SVR decreases cardiac filling pressures. This finding may suggest that preload rather than afterload is the cause of hypotension. Low SVR allows more extensive emptying and a lower end-systolic volume (ESV), one of the hallmarks of low SVR on TEE. With the same venous return, the heart does not fill to the same EDV, resulting in lower left ventricular filling pressures (see Fig. 6-4). A similar process occurs when the SVR is increased.

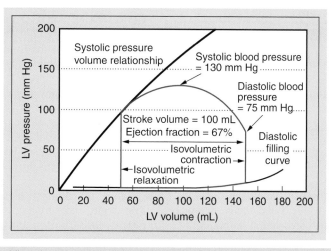

Figure 6-3 The closed loop *(red line)* shows a typical cardiac cycle. Diastolic filling occurs along the typical diastolic curve from a volume of 50 mL to an end-diastolic volume (EDV) of 150 mL. Isovolumetric contraction increases the pressure in the left ventricle (LV) until it reaches the pressure in the aorta (at diastolic blood pressure) and the aortic valve opens. The LV then ejects blood, and volume decreases. Pressure in the LV and aorta reaches a peak at some point during ejection (systolic blood pressure), and the pressure then drops until the point at which the aortic valve closes (roughly the dicrotic notch). The LV relaxes, without changing volume (isovolumetric relaxation). When the pressure decreases below left atrial pressure, the mitral valve opens, and diastolic filling begins. The plot shows a normal cycle, and the stroke volume (SV) is 100 mL, ejection fraction (EF) is SV/EDV = 67%, and blood pressure is 130/75 mm Hg. The systolic pressure-volume relationship *(black line)* can be constructed from a family of curves under different loading conditions (i.e., different preload) and reflects the inotropic state of the heart.

Table 6-1 Conditions Associated with Decreased Myocardial Contractility as a Cause of Hypotension
Myocardial ischemia
Anesthetic drugs
Cardiomyopathy
Previous myocardial infarction
Valvular heart disease (decreased stroke volume independent of preload)

Such stress-induced increases in cardiac filling pressures are more pronounced in patients with poor cardiac function.

CARDIAC REFLEXES

The cardiovascular regulatory system consists of peripheral and central receptor systems that can detect various physiologic states, a central "integratory" system in the brainstem, and neurohumoral output to the heart and vascular system. A clinical understanding of cardiac reflexes is based on the concept that the cardiovascular system in the brainstem integrates the signal and provides a response through the autonomic nervous system.

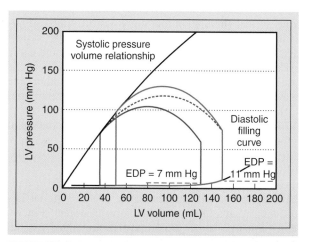

Figure 6-4 Changes in the cardiac cycle that can occur with vasodilatation are depicted. The cycle in green is the same cycle shown in Figure 6-3. The red dashed line suggests the transition to the new cardiac cycle shown in blue. The systolic blood pressure has decreased to 105 mm Hg. The end-systolic volume has decreased, as has the end-diastolic volume. End-diastolic pressure (EDP) has decreased from 11 to 7 mm Hg in this example. The ejection fraction is slightly increased; however, the stroke volume may decrease, but with restoration of left ventricular (LV) filling pressures to the same level as before, the stroke volume will be higher.

Autonomic Nervous System

The heart and vascular systems are controlled by the autonomic nervous system. Sympathetic and parasympathetic efferents innervate the sinoatrial and atrioventricular nodes. Sympathetic nervous system stimulation increases HR through activation of β_1-adrenergic receptors. Parasympathetic nervous system stimulation can profoundly slow HR through stimulation of muscarinic acetylcholine receptors in the sinoatrial and atrioventricular nodes, whereas parasympathetic nervous system suppression contributes to increased HR. Conduction through the atrioventricular node is increased and decreased by sympathetic and parasympathetic nervous system innervation, respectively. Sympathetic nervous system stimulation increases myocardial contractility. Parasympathetic nervous system stimulation may decrease myocardial contractility slightly, but it has its major effect through decreasing HR.

Baroreceptors

Baroreceptors in the carotid sinus and aortic arch are activated by increased systemic blood pressure that stimulates stretch receptors to send signals through the vagus and glossopharyngeal nerves to the central nervous system. The sensitivity of baroreceptors to systemic blood pressure changes varies and is significantly altered by long-standing essential hypertension. A typical response to acute hypertension is increased parasympathetic nervous system stimulation that decreases HR. Vagal stimulation and decreases in sympathetic nervous system activity also decrease myocardial contractility and cause reflex vasodilatation. This carotid sinus reflex can be used therapeutically to produce vagal stimulation that may be an effective treatment for supraventricular tachycardia.

The atria and ventricles are innervated by a variety of sympathetic and parasympathetic receptor systems. Atrial stretch (i.e., Bainbridge reflex) can increase HR, which may help match CO to venous return.

Stimulation of the chemoreceptors in the carotid sinus has respiratory and cardiovascular effects. Arterial hypoxemia results in sympathetic nervous system stimulation, although more profound and prolonged arterial hypoxemia can result in bradycardia, possibly through central mechanisms. A variety of other reflexes include bradycardia with ocular pressure (i.e., oculocardiac reflex) and bradycardia with stretch of abdominal viscera. The Cushing reflex includes bradycardia in response to increased intracranial pressure.

Many anesthetics blunt cardiac reflexes in a dose-dependent fashion, with the result that sympathetic nervous system responses to hypotension are reduced. The blunting of such reflexes represents an additional mechanism by which anesthetic drugs contribute to hypotension.

CORONARY BLOOD FLOW

The coronary circulation is unique in that a larger percentage of oxygen is extracted by the heart than in any other vascular bed, up to 60% to 70%, compared with the 25% extraction for the body as a whole. The consequence of this physiology is that the heart cannot use increased oxygen extraction as a reserve mechanism. In cases of threatened oxygen supply, vasodilatation to increase blood flow is the primary compensatory mechanism of the heart.

Coronary reserve is the ability of the coronary circulation to increase flow over the baseline state. Endogenous regulators of coronary blood flow include adenosine, nitric oxide, and adrenergic stimulation. With coronary artery stenosis, compensatory vasodilatation downstream can maintain coronary blood flow until about 90% stenosis, when coronary reserve begins to become exhausted.

The perfusion pressure of a vascular bed is usually calculated as the difference between MAP and venous pressure. Instantaneous flow through the coronary arteries varies throughout the cardiac cycle, peaking during systole. The heart is fundamentally different from other organs, because the myocardial wall tension developed during systole can completely stop blood flow in the subendocardium. The left ventricle is therefore perfused predominantly during diastole. The end-diastolic pressure in the left ventricle (LVEDP) may exceed CVP and represents the effective downstream pressure. Perfusion pressure to most of the left ventricle is therefore DBP minus LVEDP. The right ventricle, with its lower intramural pressure, is perfused during diastole and systole.

PULMONARY CIRCULATION

The pulmonary circulation includes the right ventricle, pulmonary arteries, pulmonary capillary bed, and pulmonary veins, ending in the left atrium. The bronchial circulation supplies nutrients to lung tissue, and empties into the pulmonary veins and left atrium. The pulmonary circulation differs substantially from the systemic circulation in its regulation, normal pressures (Table 6-2), and responses to drugs. Use of a pulmonary artery catheter to measure pressures in the pulmonary circulation requires a fundamental understanding of their normal values and their meaning. Pulmonary hypertension has idiopathic causes and may accompany several common diseases (e.g., cirrhosis of the liver, sleep apnea). It is associated with significant anesthetic-related morbidity and mortality rates.

Pulmonary Artery Pressure

PAP is much lower than systemic pressure because of low pulmonary vascular resistance (PVR). Like the systemic

Table 6-2 Normal Values for Pressures in the Venous and Pulmonary Arterial System

Value	CVP (mm Hg)	PAS (mm Hg)	PAD (mm Hg)	PAM (mm Hg)	PCWP (mm Hg)
Normal	2-8	15-30	4-12	9-16	4-12
High	>12	>30	>12	>25	>12
Pathologic	>18	>40	>20	>35	>20

CVP, central venous pressure; PAD, pulmonary artery diastolic pressure; PAM, pulmonary artery mean pressure; PAS, pulmonary artery systolic pressure, PCWP, pulmonary capillary wedge pressure.

circulation, the pulmonary circulation accepts the entire CO and must adapt its resistance to meet different conditions.

Pulmonary Vascular Resistance

Determinants of PVR are different from SVR in the systemic circulation. During blood flow through the pulmonary circulation, resistance is thought to occur in the larger vessels, small arteries, and capillary bed. Vessels within the alveoli and the extra-alveolar vessels respond differently to forces within the lung.

The most useful physiologic model for describing changes in the pulmonary circulation is the "distention" of capillaries and the "recruitment" of new capillaries. This distention and recruitment of capillaries explains the changes in PVR in a variety of circumstances. Increased PAP causes distention and recruitment of capillaries, increasing the cross-sectional area and lowering PVR. Increased CO also decreases PVR through distention and recruitment. The reciprocal changes between CO and PVR maintain pulmonary pressures fairly constant over a wide range of CO.

Lung volumes have different effects on intra-alveolar and extra-alveolar vessels. At high lung volumes, intra-alveolar vessels can be compressed, whereas extra-alveolar vessels have lower resistance. The opposite is true at low lung volumes. Therefore, higher PVR occurs at high and low lung volumes. Increased PVR at low lung volumes helps to divert blood flow from collapsed alveoli, such as during one-lung ventilation.

Sympathetic nervous system stimulation can cause pulmonary vasoconstriction, but the effect is not large, in contrast to the systemic circulation, in which neurohumoral influence is the primary regulator of vascular tone. The pulmonary circulation has therefore been very difficult to treat with drugs. Nitric oxide is an important regulator of vascular tone and can be given by inhalation. Prostaglandins and phosphodiesterase inhibitors (e.g., sildenafil) are pulmonary vasodilators, but the pharmacologic responses that can be achieved in pulmonary hypertension are limited.

HYPOXIC PULMONARY VASOCONSTRICTION
Hypoxic pulmonary vasoconstriction (HPV) is the pulmonary vascular response to a low PA_{O_2} (partial pressure of oxygen in alveolar blood). In many patients, HPV is an important adaptive response that improves gas exchange by diverting blood away from poorly ventilated areas, decreasing shunt fraction. Normal regions of the lung can easily accommodate the additional blood flow without increasing PAP. Global alveolar hypoxia, such as occurs with apnea or at high altitude, can cause significant HPV and increased PAP.

PULMONARY EMBOLI
Pulmonary emboli obstruct blood vessels, increasing the overall resistance to blood through the pulmonary vascular system. Common forms of emboli are blood clots and air, but they also include amniotic fluid, carbon dioxide, and fat emboli.

ARTERIAL THICKENING
Arteriolar thickening occurs in several clinical circumstances. It is associated with certain types of long-standing congenital heart disease. Primary pulmonary hypertension is an idiopathic disease associated with arteriolar hyperplasia. Similar changes are associated with cirrhosis of the liver (i.e., portopulmonary hypertension).

Zones of the Lung

A useful concept in pulmonary hemodynamics is West's zones of the lung. Gravity determines the way pressures change in the vascular system relative to the measurement at the level of the heart. These differences are small compared with arterial pressures, but for venous pressure and PAP, these differences are clinically significant. Every 20 cm of change in height produces a 15-mm Hg pressure difference. This can create significant positional differences in PAP that affects blood flow in the lung in various positions, such as upright and lateral positions.

In zone 1, airway pressures exceed PAP and pulmonary venous pressures. Zone 1 therefore has no blood flow despite ventilation. Normally, zone 1 does not exist, but with positive-pressure ventilation or low PAP, as may occur under anesthesia or with blood loss, zone 1 may develop. In zone 2, airway pressure is greater than pulmonary venous pressure, but it is not greater than PAP. In zone 2, flow is proportional to the difference between PAP and airway pressure. In zone 3, PAP and venous pressure exceed airway pressure, and a normal blood flow pattern results (i.e., flow is proportional to the difference between PAP and venous pressure). Position can also be used therapeutically to decrease blood flow to abnormal areas of the lung, such as unilateral pneumonia, and thereby improve gas exchange. Blood flow through the collapsed lung during one-lung ventilation is also reduced by this physiologic effect.

Pulmonary Edema

Fluid balance in the lung depends on hydrostatic driving forces. Excessive pulmonary capillary pressures cause fluid to leak into the interstitium and then into alveoli. The pulmonary lymphatic system is very effective in clearing fluid, but it can be overwhelmed. Hydrostatic pulmonary edema is expected with high left ventricular filling pressures, and patients become at risk of pulmonary edema as PCWP exceeds 20 mm Hg. Pulmonary edema can also occur with "capillary leak" from lung injury, such as acid aspiration or sepsis.

PULMONARY GAS EXCHANGE

Oxygen

Oxygen must pass from the environment to the tissues, where it is consumed during aerobic metabolism. Arterial hypoxemia is most often defined as a low Pa_{O_2} (partial pressure of oxygen in arterial blood). An arbitrary definition of arterial hypoxemia ($Pa_{O_2} < 60$ mm Hg) is commonly used but not necessary. Occasionally, arterial hypoxemia is used to describe a Pa_{O_2} that is low relative to what might be expected based on the inspired oxygen concentration ($F_{I_{O_2}}$). Arterial hypoxemia (which reflects pulmonary gas exchange) is distinguished from hypoxia, a more general term including tissue hypoxia, which also reflects circulatory factors.

Mild and even moderate arterial hypoxemia (e.g., at high altitude) can be well tolerated and is not usually associated with substantial injury or adverse outcomes. Anoxia, a complete lack of oxygen, is potentially fatal and is often associated with permanent neurologic injury, depending on its duration. Arterial hypoxemia is most significant when anoxia is threatened, and the difference between the two may be less than 1 minute.

MEASUREMENTS OF OXYGENATION

Measurements of arterial blood oxygen levels include Pa_{O_2}, arterial oxygen content (Ca_{O_2}), and oxyhemoglobin saturation (Sa_{O_2}). Pa_{O_2} and Sa_{O_2} are related through the oxyhemoglobin dissociation curve (Fig. 6-5). Understanding the oxyhemoglobin dissociation curve is facilitated by the ability to measure continuous oxyhemoglobin saturation with pulse oximetry (Sp_{O_2}) and measurement of Pa_{O_2} with arterial blood gas analysis.

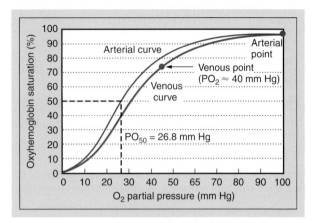

Figure 6-5 The oxyhemoglobin dissociation curve is S shaped and relates oxygen partial pressure to the oxyhemoglobin saturation. A typical arterial curve is shown in red. The higher P_{CO_2} and the lower pH of venous blood cause a rightward shift of the curve and facilitate unloading of oxygen in the tissues (blue). Normal adult P_{50}, the P_{O_2} at which hemoglobin is 50% saturated, is shown (26.8 mm Hg). Normal Pa_{O_2} of about 100 mm Hg results in a Sa_{O_2} of about 98%. Normal Pv_{O_2} is about 40 mm Hg, resulting in a saturation of about 75%.

Oxyhemoglobin Dissociation Curve

Rightward and leftward shifts of the oxyhemoglobin dissociation curve provide significant homeostatic adaptations to changing oxygen availability. P_{50}, the P_{O_2} at which hemoglobin is 50% saturated with oxygen, is a measurement of the position of the oxyhemoglobin dissociation curve (see Fig. 6-5, Table 6-3). The normal P_{50} value of adult hemoglobin is 26.8 mm Hg.

A rightward shift causes little change in loading conditions (essentially the same Sa_{O_2} at P_{O_2} of 100 mm Hg), but it allows larger amounts of oxygen to dissociate from hemoglobin in the tissues. This improves tissue oxygenation. Carbon dioxide and metabolic acid shift the oxyhemoglobin dissociation curve rightward, whereas alkalosis shifts it leftward. Fetal hemoglobin is left shifted, an adaptation uniquely suited to placental physiology. Oxygen in arterial blood is bound to hemoglobin and dissolved in the

Table 6-3 Events That Shift the Oxyhemoglobin Dissociation Curve

Left Shift	Right Shift
($P_{50} < 26.8$ mm Hg)	($P_{50} > 26.8$ mm Hg)
Alkalosis	Acidosis
Hypothermia	Hyperthermia
Decreased 2,3-diphosphoglycerate (stored blood)	Increased 2,3-diphosphoglycerate (chronic arterial hypoxemia or anemia)

P_{50}, P_{O_2} value at which hemoglobin is 50% saturated with oxygen.

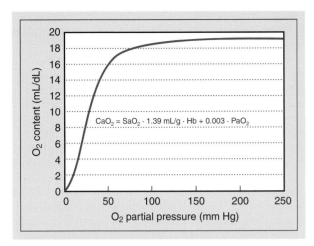

Figure 6-6 The relationship between Pa_{O_2} and oxygen content is also sigmoidal, because most of the oxygen is bound to hemoglobin. Oxygen content at the plateau of the curve ($P_{O_2} >$ 100 mm Hg) continues to rise because dissolved oxygen still contributes a small, but not negligible, quantity.

plasma. The blood oxygen content is the sum of the two forms. Although amounts of dissolved oxygen are fairly trivial at normal P_{O_2} levels, at high $F_{I_{O_2}}$ dissolved oxygen can be physiologically and clinically important. Although under normal conditions only a fraction of the oxygen on hemoglobin (25%) can be used, all of the dissolved oxygen added while giving supplemental oxygen is used.

Arterial Oxygen Content

Ca_{O_2} is calculated based on Sa_{O_2} and partial pressure plus the hemoglobin concentration (Fig. 6-6).

$$Ca_{O_2} = Sa_{O_2} \, (Hb \times 1.39) + 0.003 \, (Pa_{O_2})$$

In the equation, Hb is the hemoglobin level, 1.39 is the capacity of hemoglobin for oxygen (1.39 mL of O_2/g of Hb fully saturated), and 0.003 mL O_2/dL/mm Hg is the solubility of oxygen. For example, if Hb = 15 g/dL and Pa_{O_2} = 100 mm Hg, resulting in nearly 100% saturation, the value of Ca_{O_2} is calculated as follows:

$$
\begin{aligned}
Ca_{O_2} &= 1.00 \, (15 \times 1.39) + 100 \, (0.003) \\
&= 20.85 + 0.3 \\
Ca_{O_2} &= 21.15 \text{ mL/dL}
\end{aligned}
$$

Dissolved oxygen can continue to provide additional Ca_{O_2}, which can be clinically significant with $F_{I_{O_2}}$ of 1.0 and with hyperbaric oxygen. The oxygen cascade depicts the passage of oxygen from the atmosphere to the tissues (Fig. 6-7).

DETERMINANTS OF ALVEOLAR OXYGEN PARTIAL PRESSURE

The alveolar gas equation describes transfer of oxygen from the environment into the alveoli:

$$PA_{O_2} = F_{I_{O_2}} \bullet (P_B - P_{H_2O}) - \frac{P_{CO_2}}{RQ}$$

In the previous equation, P_B is the barometric pressure, P_{H_2O}, is the vapor pressure of water (47 mm Hg at normal body temperature of 37° C), and RQ is the respiratory quotient (the ratio of carbon dioxide production to oxygen consumption). For example, while breathing 100% oxygen ($F_{I_{O_2}}$ = 1.0) at sea level (P_B = 760 mm Hg) and the P_{H_2O} = 47 mm Hg with Pa_{CO_2} = 40 mm Hg, the alveolar P_{O_2} (PA_{O_2}) difference in the partial pressure of

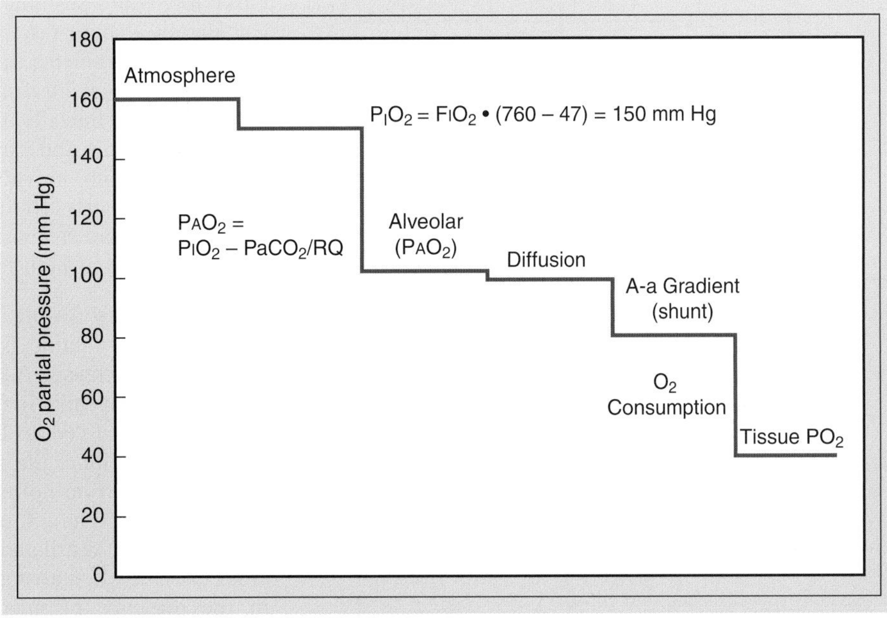

Figure 6-7 The oxygen cascade depicts the physiologic steps as oxygen travels from the atmosphere to the tissues. Oxygen starts at 21% in the atmosphere and is initially diluted with water vapor to about 150 mm Hg, $P_{I_{O_2}}$. Alveolar P_{O_2} (PA_{O_2}) is determined by the alveolar gas equation. Diffusion equilibrates P_{O_2} between the alveolus and the capillary. The A-a (alveolar-to-arterial) gradient occurs with intrapulmonary shunt and ventilation to perfusion ($\dot{V}/\dot{Q}$) mismatch. Oxygen consumption then reduces P_{O_2} to tissue levels (about 40 mm Hg).

oxygen ($P_{AO_2} - P_{aO_2}$) is calculated as follows. RQ is usually assumed to be 0.8 on a normal diet.

$$P_{AO_2} = 1.0\,(760 - 47) - 40/0.8$$
$$= 713 - 50$$
$$P_{AO_2} = 663 \text{ mm Hg}$$

The alveolar gas equation describes the way in which inspired oxygen and ventilation determine P_{aO_2}. It also describes the way in which supplemental oxygen improves oxygenation. One clinical consequence of this relationship is that supplemental oxygen can easily compensate for the adverse effects of hypoventilation (Fig. 6-8).

Low barometric pressure is a cause of arterial hypoxemia at high altitude. Modern anesthesia machines have safety mechanisms to prevent delivery of hypoxic gas mixtures. Nevertheless, death from delivery of gases other than oxygen is still occasionally reported because of errors in pipe connections made during construction or remodeling of operating rooms. Current anesthesia machines have multiple safety features to prevent delivery of hypoxic gas mixtures. Delivery of an inadequate F_{IO_2} may occur when oxygen tanks run dry, or failure to recognize accidental disconnection of a self-inflating bag (Ambu) from its oxygen source.

Apnea is an important cause of arterial hypoxemia, and storage of oxygen in the lung is of prime importance in delaying the appearance of arterial hypoxemia in humans. Storage of oxygen on hemoglobin is secondary, because use of this oxygen requires significant oxyhemoglobin desaturation. In contrast to voluntary breath-holding, apnea during anesthesia occurs at functional residual capacity (FRC). This substantially reduces the time to oxyhemoglobin desaturation compared with a breath-hold at total lung capacity.

The time can be estimated for S_{aO_2} to reach 90% when the FRC is 2.5 L and the P_{aO_2} is 100 mm Hg. Normal oxygen consumption is about 300 mL/min, although this is somewhat lower during anesthesia. It would take only about 30 seconds under these room air conditions to develop arterial hypoxemia. After breathing 100% oxygen, it might take 7 minutes to reach an S_{aO_2} of 90%. In reality, the time it takes to develop arterial hypoxemia after breathing 100% oxygen varies. Desaturation begins when sufficient numbers of alveoli have collapsed and intrapulmonary shunt develops, not simply when oxygen stores have become exhausted. In particular, obese patients develop arterial hypoxemia with apnea substantially faster than lean patients.

VENOUS ADMIXTURE

Venous admixture describes physiologic causes of arterial hypoxemia for which P_{AO_2} is normal. The alveolar-to-arterial oxygen (A-a) gradient reflects venous admixture. Normal A-a gradients are 5 to 10 mm Hg, but they increase with age. For example, if the arterial P_{O_2} while breathing 100% oxygen were measured as 310 mm Hg, the A-a gradient can be calculated from the previous example.

$$\text{A-a gradient} = P_{AO_2} - P_{aO_2}$$
$$= 663 \text{ mm Hg} - 310 \text{ mm Hg}$$
$$= 353 \text{ mm Hg}$$

A picture of gas exchange can be accomplished mathematically by integrating all the effects of shunting, supplemental oxygen, and the oxyhemoglobin dissociation curve to create "isoshunt" diagrams (Fig. 6-9). Although calculating a shunt fraction may be the most exact way to quantitate problems in oxygenation, it requires information only available from a PA catheter, and therefore is not always clinically useful. A-a gradients are clinically more simple and useful to derive, but do not represent a constant measurement of oxygenation with different F_{IO_2} levels. The P/F ratio (P_{aO_2}/F_{IO_2}) is a simple and useful measurement of oxygenation that remains more consistent at high F_{IO_2} (Fig. 6-10).

Intrapulmonary Shunt

Intrapulmonary shunt is one of the most important causes of an increased A-a gradient and the development of arterial hypoxemia. In the presence of an intrapulmonary shunt, mixed venous blood is not exposed to alveolar gas, and it continues through the lungs to mix with oxygenated blood from normal areas of the lung. This mixing lowers the P_{aO_2}. Clinically, shunting occurs when alveoli are not ventilated, as occurs in the presence of atelectasis, or when alveoli are filled with fluid, as occurs in the presence of pneumonia or pulmonary edema.

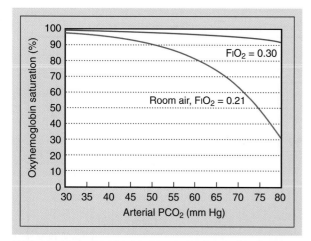

Figure 6-8 Hypoventilation decreases oxygenation, as determined by the alveolar gas equation. The blue curve shows what is expected for room air ($F_{IO_2} = 0.21$). High Pa_{CO_2} further shifts the oxyhemoglobin dissociation curve to the right. However, as little as 30% oxygen can completely negate the effects of hypoventilation (red curve).

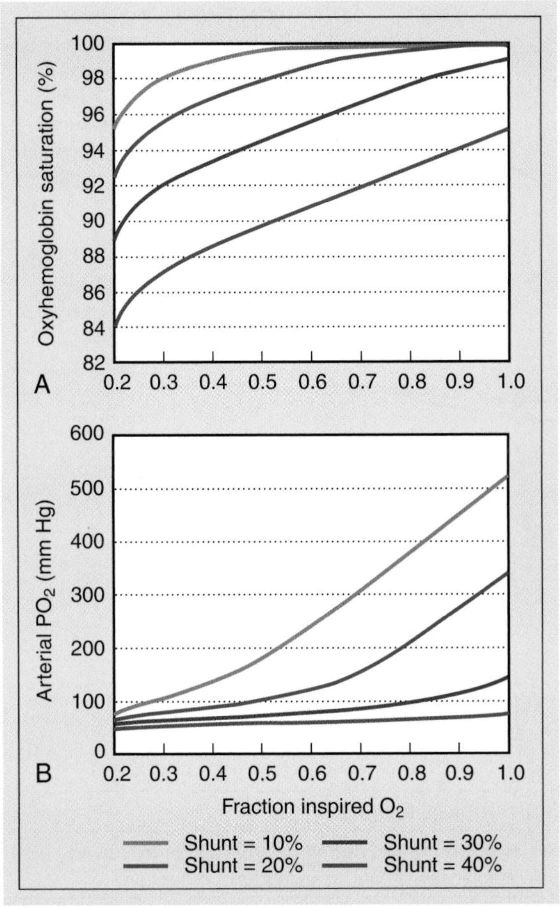

Figure 6-9 The effect of intrapulmonary shunting and F_{IO_2} on Pa_{O_2} (*top*) and Sa_{O_2} (*bottom*) is shown graphically at shunt fractions from 10% (mild) to 40% (severe). Assumed values for these calculations are hemoglobin, 14 g/dL; Pa_{CO_2}, 40 mm Hg; arterial-to-venous oxygen content difference, 4 mL O_2/dL; and sea level atmospheric pressure, 760 mm Hg. Increased F_{IO_2} still substantially improves oxygenation at high shunt fractions, but is unable to fully correct it.

The quantitative effect of an intrapulmonary shunt is described by the shunt equation:

$$\frac{\dot{Q}_S}{\dot{Q}_t} = \frac{Cc'O_2 - CaO_2}{Cc'O_2 - C\bar{v}O_2}$$

In the equation, $\dot{Q}_S/\dot{Q}_t$ is the shunt flow relative to total flow (i.e., shunt fraction), C is the oxygen content, c′ is end-capillary blood (for a theoretical normal alveolus), a is arterial blood, and $\bar{v}$ is mixed venous blood.

Ventilation–Perfusion Mismatch

Ventilation-perfusion ($\dot{V}/\dot{Q}$) mismatch is similar to intrapulmonary shunt ($\dot{V}/\dot{Q}=0$), with some important distinctions. In $\dot{V}/\dot{Q}$ mismatch, disparity between the amount of ventilation and perfusion in various alveoli leads to areas of high $\dot{V}/\dot{Q}$ (i.e., well-ventilated alveoli) and areas of low $\dot{V}/\dot{Q}$ (i.e., poorly ventilated alveoli). Because of the shape of the oxyhemoglobin dissociation curve, the improved oxygenation in well-ventilated areas cannot compensate for the low P_{O_2} in the poorly ventilated areas, resulting in arterial hypoxemia.

Clinically, in $\dot{V}/\dot{Q}$ mismatch, administering 100% oxygen can achieve a P_{O_2} on the plateau of the oxyhemoglobin dissociation curve even in poorly ventilated alveoli. Conversely, administering 100% oxygen in the presence of an intrapulmonary shunt only adds more dissolved oxygen in the normally perfused alveoli. Arterial hypoxemia remaining despite administration of 100% oxygen is always caused by the presence of an intrapulmonary shunt.

Diffusion Impairment

Diffusion impairment is not equivalent to low diffusing capacity. For diffusion impairment to cause an A-a gradient, equilibrium has not occurred between the P_{O_2} in the alveolus and the P_{O_2} in pulmonary capillary blood. This rarely occurs, even in patients with limited diffusing capacity. The small A-a gradient that can result from diffusion impairment is easily eliminated with supplemental oxygen, making this a clinically unimportant problem.

Venous Oxygen Saturation

Low $S\bar{v}_{O_2}$ causes a subtle but important effect when intrapulmonary shunt is already present.[7] Shunt is a mixture of venous blood and blood from normal regions of the lungs. If the $S\bar{v}_{O_2}$ is lower, the resulting mixture must have a lower Pa_{O_2}. Low CO may lower $S\bar{v}_{O_2}$ significantly.

Carbon Dioxide

Carbon dioxide is produced in the tissues and removed from the lungs by ventilation. Carbon dioxide is carried in the blood as dissolved gas, as bicarbonate, and as a small amount bound to hemoglobin as carbaminohemoglobin. Unlike the oxyhemoglobin dissociation curve, the dissociation curve for carbon dioxide is essentially linear.

HYPERCAPNIA

Hypercapnia (i.e., high Pa_{CO_2}) may be a sign of respiratory difficulty or oversedation with opioids. Although hypercapnia itself may not be dangerous, Pa_{CO_2} value greater than 80 mm Hg may cause CO_2 narcosis, possibly contributing to delayed awakening in the postanesthesia care unit. The greatest concern of hypercapnia is that it may indicate a risk of impending respiratory failure and apnea, in which arterial hypoxemia and anoxia can rapidly ensue. Although the presence of hypercapnia may be obvious if capnography is used, this monitor is not always available, and substantial hypercapnia may go unnoticed. Supplemental oxygen can prevent arterial

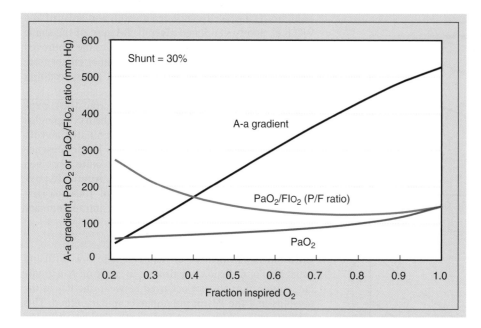

Figure 6-10 Despite a constant shunt fraction of 0.3 (30%), the A-a gradient is much higher at high F_{IO_2}, indicating problems in its usefulness as a measurement of oxygenation with different F_{IO_2} values. The ratio of P_{aO_2} to F_{IO_2} (the P/F ratio) is remarkably constant at high F_{IO_2}, making it a useful measurement of oxygenation when the gold standard, shunt fraction, is not available.

hypoxemia despite severe hypercapnia, and an arterial blood gas analysis would not necessarily be performed if hypercapnia were not suspected (see Fig. 6-8).

DETERMINANTS OF ARTERIAL CARBON DIOXIDE PARTIAL PRESSURE

P_{aCO_2} is a balance of production and removal. If removal exceeds production, P_{aCO_2} decreases. If production exceeds removal, P_{aCO_2} increases. The resulting P_{aCO_2} is expressed by the alveolar carbon dioxide equation:

$$P_{aCO_2} = k \cdot \frac{\dot{V}_{CO_2}}{\dot{V}_A}$$

In the equation, k is a constant (0.863) that corrects units, $\dot{V}_{CO_2}$ is carbon dioxide production, and $\dot{V}_A$ is alveolar ventilation.

Rebreathing
Because breathing circuits with rebreathing properties are frequently used in anesthesia, elevated inspired P_{CO_2} is a potential cause of hypercapnia. Exhausted carbon dioxide absorbents and malfunctioning expiratory valves on the anesthesia delivery circuit are possible causes of rebreathing in the operating room that are easily detected with capnography. Use of certain transport breathing circuits may be the most common cause of clinically significant rebreathing, which may be unrecognized because capnography is not routinely used during patient transport from the operating room.

Increased Carbon Dioxide Production
Several important physiologic causes of increased carbon dioxide production may cause hypercapnia under

Table 6-4 Causes of Increased Carbon Dioxide Production

Fever
Malignant hyperthermia
Systemic absorption during laparoscopy procedures (physiologically similar to increased production)
Thyroid storm

anesthesia (Table 6-4). Other brief increases in CO_2 production may occur when administering sodium bicarbonate, which is converted into CO_2, or when releasing a tourniquet, where carbon dioxide has accumulated in the tissues of the leg and then returns to the circulation.

Increased Dead Space
Dead space, or "wasted ventilation," refers to areas receiving ventilation that do not participate in gas exchange. Dead space is further categorized as anatomic, alveolar, and physiologic (total) dead space. Anatomic dead space represents areas of the tracheobronchial tree that are not involved in gas exchange. This includes equipment dead space, such as the endotracheal tube and tubing distal to the Y-connector of the anesthesia delivery circuit. Alveolar dead space represents alveoli that do not participate in gas exchange due to lack of blood flow. Physiologic or total dead space represents the sum of anatomic and alveolar dead space. Most pathologically significant changes in dead space represent increases in alveolar dead space.

Dead space is increased in many clinical conditions. Emphysema and other end-stage lung diseases, such as cystic fibrosis, are often characterized by substantial dead space. Pulmonary embolism is a potential cause of significant increases in dead space. Physiologic processes that decrease PAP, such as hemorrhagic shock, can be expected to increase dead space (increased zone 1). Increased airway pressure and positive end-expiratory pressure (PEEP) can also increase dead space.

Quantitative estimates of dead space are described by the Bohr equation, which expresses the ratio of dead space ventilation ($\dot{V}_D$) relative to tidal ventilation ($\dot{V}_T$).

$$\frac{\dot{V}_D}{\dot{V}_T} = \frac{Pa_{CO_2} - P\bar{E}_{CO_2}}{Pa_{CO_2}}$$

In the equation, $P\bar{E}_{CO_2}$ is the mixed-expired carbon dioxide.

For example, if the $Pa_{CO_2} = 40$ mm Hg and the $P\bar{E}_{CO_2} = 20$ mm Hg during controlled ventilation of the lungs, the $\dot{V}_D/\dot{V}_T$ can be calculated as follows:

$$\begin{aligned}
\dot{V}_D/\dot{V}_T &= (40 - 20)/40 \\
&= 20/40 \\
\dot{V}_D/\dot{V}_T &= 0.5
\end{aligned}$$

Some physiologic dead space (25% to 30%) is considered normal because some anatomic dead space is always present. The Pa_{CO_2}-$P_{ET_{CO_2}}$ gradient is a useful indication of the presence of alveolar dead space.

Hypoventilation

Decreased minute ventilation is the most important and common cause of hypercapnia (Fig. 6-11). This may be due to decreased tidal volume, breathing frequency, or both. Alveolar ventilation ($\dot{V}_A$) combines minute ventilation and dead space ($\dot{V}_A = \dot{V}_T - \dot{V}_D$). Ventilatory depressant effects of anesthetic drugs are a common cause of hypoventilation. Although increased minute ventilation can often completely compensate for elevated carbon dioxide production, rebreathing, or dead space, there is no physiologically useful compensation for inadequate minute ventilation.

If alveolar ventilation decreases by one half, Pa_{CO_2} is expected to double (see Fig. 6-11). This change occurs over several minutes as a new steady state develops. CO_2 changes during apnea are more complicated. During the first 30 to 60 seconds of apnea, Pa_{CO_2} increases to mixed venous levels, a fairly rapid increase. The 6 mm Hg increase from a normal Pa_{CO_2} of 40 mm Hg to the normal Pv_{CO_2} of 46 mm Hg occurs within 1 minute, but this jump can be higher and faster in patients with lower lung volumes or high arterial-to-venous carbon dioxide differences. After the first minute, Pa_{CO_2} increases more slowly as carbon dioxide production adds carbon dioxide to the blood, at about 3 mm Hg per minute.

DIFFERENTIAL DIAGNOSIS OF INCREASED ARTERIAL CARBON DIOXIDE PARTIAL PRESSURE

Increased Pa_{CO_2} values can be analyzed by assessing minute ventilation, capnography, and measuring an arterial blood gas value. Capnography can easily detect rebreathing. A clinical assessment of minute ventilation by physical examination and as measured by most mechanical ventilators should be adequate. Comparison of end-tidal P_{CO_2} with Pa_{CO_2} can identify abnormal alveolar dead space. Abnormal carbon dioxide production can be inferred. However, significant abnormalities of carbon dioxide physiology often are unrecognized when Pa_{CO_2} is normal, because increased minute ventilation can compensate for substantial increases in dead space and carbon dioxide production. Noticing the presence of increased dead space when minute ventilation is high and Pa_{CO_2} is 40 mm Hg is just as important as noticing abnormal dead space when the Pa_{CO_2} is 80 mm Hg and minute ventilation is normal.

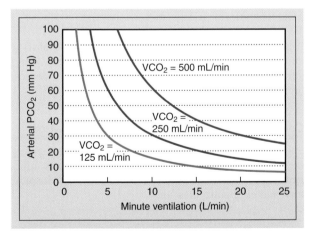

Figure 6-11 Carbon dioxide has a hyperbolic relationship with ventilation. The depicted curves are simulated with a normal resting carbon dioxide production (250 mL/min), low carbon dioxide production (125 mL/min, as during anesthesia), and increased carbon dioxide production (500 mL/min, as during moderate exercise). The value of physiologic dead space is assumed to be 30% in these calculations.

PULMONARY MECHANICS

Pulmonary mechanics concerns pressure, volume, and flow relationships in the lung and bronchial tree (Fig. 6-12). An understanding of pulmonary mechanics is essential for managing the ventilated patient. Pressures in the airway are routinely measured or sensed by the anesthesia provider delivering positive-pressure ventilation.

Static Properties

The lung is made of elastic tissue that stretches under pressure (Fig. 6-13). Surface tension has a significant role in the compliance of the lung due to the air-fluid

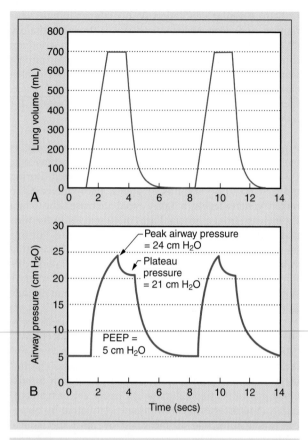

Figure 6-12 Lung volume is shown as a function of time (*top*) in a typical volume-controlled ventilator with constant flow rates. Lung volume increases at a constant rate during inspiration because of constant flow. Exhalation occurs with a passive relaxation curve. The lower panel shows the development of pressure over time. Pressure is produced from a static compliance component (see Fig. 6-13) and a resistance component. If flow is held at the plateau, a plateau pressure is reached, where there is no resistive pressure component. In this example, peak airway pressure (PAP) is 24 cm H_2O, and positive end-expiratory pressure (PEEP) is 5 cm H_2O. Dynamic compliance is tidal volume: $(V_T)/(PAP - PEEP) = 37$ mL/cm H_2O. Plateau pressure (Pplat) is 21 cm H_2O, and static compliance is $V_T/(Pplat - PEEP) = 44$ mL/cm H_2O.

interface in the alveoli. Surfactant decreases surface tension and stabilizes small alveoli, which would otherwise tend to collapse.

The chest wall has its own compliance curve. At FRC, the chest wall tends to expand, but negative (subatmospheric) intrapleural pressure keeps the chest wall collapsed. The lungs tend to collapse, but they are held expanded due to the pressure difference from the airways to the intrapleural pressure. FRC is the natural balance point between the lungs tending to collapse and chest wall tending to expand.

Dynamic Properties and Airway Resistance

Airway resistance is mainly determined by the radius of the airway, but turbulent gas flow may make resistance worse. A number of clinical processes can affect airway resistance (Table 6-5). Resistance in small airways is physiologically different, because they have no cartilaginous structure or smooth muscle. Unlike capillaries, which have positive pressure inside to keep them open, small airways have zero (atmospheric) pressure during spontaneous ventilation. However, these airways are kept open by the same forces (i.e., pressure inside is greater than the pressure outside) that keep capillaries open. Negative pressure is transmitted from the intrapleural pressure, and this pressure difference keeps small airways open. When a disease process, such as emphysema, makes pleural pressure less negative, resistance in the small airways is increased, and dynamic compression occurs during exhalation.

During positive-pressure ventilation, resistance in anesthesia breathing equipment or airways manifests as elevated airway pressures, because flow through resistance causes a pressure change. Distinguishing airway resistance effects from static compliant components is a useful first step in the differential diagnosis of high peak airway pressures. This is facilitated by anesthesia machines that are equipped to provide an inspiratory pause. During ventilation, airway pressure reaches a peak inspiratory pressure, but when ventilation is paused, the pressure component from gas flow and resistance disappears, and the airway pressure decreases toward a plateau pressure (see Fig. 6-12).

CONTROL OF BREATHING

Anesthesia providers are in a unique position to observe ventilatory control mechanisms because most drugs administered for sedation and anesthesia depress breathing.

Central Integration and Rhythm Generation

Specific areas of the brainstem are involved in generating the respiratory rhythm, processing afferent signal information, and changing the efferent output to the inspiratory and expiratory muscles.

Central Chemoreceptors

Superficial areas on the ventrolateral medullary surface respond to pH and P_{CO_2}. Carbon dioxide is in rapid equilibrium with carbonic acid and therefore immediately affects the local pH surrounding the central chemoreceptors. Although the signal is transduced by protons, not carbon dioxide directly, it is acceptable to describe these

Figure 6-13 A static compliance curve of a normal lung has a slight S shape. Slightly higher pressure can be required to open alveoli at low lung volumes (i.e., beginning of the curve), whereas higher distending pressures are needed as the lung is overdistended. Static compliance is measured as the change (Δ) in volume divided by the change in pressure (inspiratory pressure [PIP] − positive end-expiratory pressure [PEEP]), which is 46 mL/cm H_2O in this example.

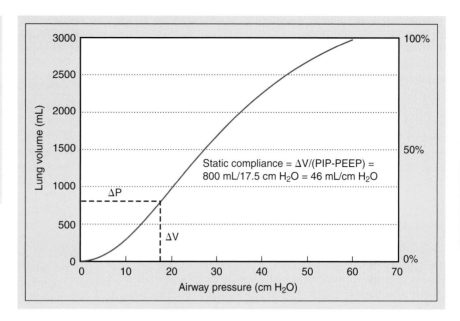

Static compliance = $\Delta V/(PIP\text{-}PEEP)$ = 800 mL/17.5 cm H_2O = 46 mL/cm H_2O

Table 6-5 Determinants of Airway Resistance
Radius of the airways

Smooth muscle tone
    Bronchospasm
    Inflammation of the airways (asthma, chronic bronchitis)

Foreign bodies
Compression of airways
Turbulent gas flow (helium a temporizing measure)
Anesthesia equipment

chemoreceptors clinically as carbon dioxide responsive. The central chemoreceptors are protected from rapid changes in metabolic pH by the blood-brain barrier.

Peripheral Chemoreceptors

Carotid bodies are the primary peripheral chemoreceptors in humans; aortic bodies have no significant role. Low Po_2, high Pco_2, and low pH stimulate the carotid bodies.[8] Unlike the central chemoreceptors, metabolic acids immediately affect peripheral chemoreceptors. Because of high blood flow, peripheral chemoreceptors are effectively at arterial, not venous, blood values.

Hypercapnic Ventilatory Response

Ventilation increases dramatically as $Paco_2$ is increased. In the presence of high Po_2 values, most of this ventilatory response results from the central chemoreceptors,

whereas in the presence of room air, about one third of the response results from peripheral chemoreceptor stimulation. The ventilatory response to carbon dioxide is fairly linear, although at $Paco_2$ levels below resting values, minute ventilation does not tend to go to zero because of an "awake" drive to breathe (Fig. 6-14). At a high $Paco_2$ value, minute ventilation is eventually limited by maximal minute ventilation.

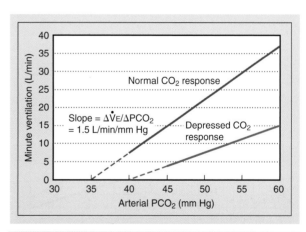

Figure 6-14 The hypercapnic ventilatory response (HCVR) is measured as the slope of the plot of Pco_2 versus minute ventilation ($\dot{V}E$). End-tidal Pco_2 is usually substituted for $Paco_2$ for clinical studies. The apneic threshold is the Pco_2 at which ventilation is zero. It can be extrapolated from the curve, but it is difficult to measure in awake volunteers, although it is easy to observe in patients under general anesthesia. A depressed carbon dioxide response results from opioids, which lower the slope and raise the apneic threshold.

Lowering $Paco_2$ during anesthesia, as produced by assisted ventilation, results in a point at which ventilation ceases, called the apneic threshold. As CO_2 rises, ventilation returns at the apneic threshold, then stabilizes at a $Paco_2$ set-point that is about 5 mm Hg higher.

The brainstem response to carbon dioxide is slow, with 90% of steady-state ventilation being reached in about 5 minutes. When allowing the $Paco_2$ to rise in an apneic patient, it may take a noticeably long time to stabilize minute ventilation, which is a direct consequence of the dynamics of the central ventilatory drive.

Hypoxic Ventilatory Response

Ventilation increases as Pao_2 and Sao_2 decrease, reflecting stimulation of the peripheral chemoreceptors. The central response to hypoxia actually results in decreased minute ventilation, called hypoxic ventilatory decline (HVD). The timing and combination of these effects means that in prolonged arterial hypoxemia, ventilation rises to an initial peak, reflecting the rapid response of the peripheral chemoreceptors, then falls to an intermediate plateau in 15 to 20 minutes reflecting the slower addition of HVD.

Although it is Po_2 that affects the carotid body, it is easier to consider the hypoxic ventilatory response in terms of oxyhemoglobin desaturation because minute ventilation changes linearly with Sao_2 (Fig. 6-15). The effects of hypoxia and hypercapnia on the carotid body are synergistic. At high $Paco_2$ levels, the response to hypoxia is much larger, whereas low $Paco_2$ levels can dramatically

decrease responsiveness. Unlike the hypercapnic ventilatory response, the response to hypoxia is rapid and takes only seconds to appear.

Effects of Anesthesia

Opioids, sedative-hypnotics, and volatile anesthetics have profound depressant effects on ventilation and ventilatory control. Opioid receptors are present on neurons considered responsible for respiratory rhythm generation. Sedative-hypnotics work primarily on γ-aminobutyric acid A receptors ($GABA_A$), which provide inhibitory input in multiple neurons of the respiratory system. Volatile anesthetics decrease excitatory neurotransmission. All of these drugs exert most of their depressant effects in the central integratory area and therefore clinically appear to decrease the hypoxic and hypercapnic ventilatory responses similarly. Specific effects of drugs on peripheral chemoreceptors include the inhibitory effects of dopamine and the slight excitatory effects of dopaminergic blockers such as droperidol.

Disorders of Ventilatory Control

Neonates of low postconceptual age (<60 weeks) may have episodes of apnea after anesthesia. Likewise, sudden infant death syndrome may be a result of immature ventilatory control systems. Ondine's curse, originally described after surgery near the upper cervical spinal cord, results in profound hypoventilation during sleep and anesthesia due to abnormalities in the central integratory system that seem to blunt the hypoxic and hypercapnic ventilatory responses. Idiopathic varieties of Ondine's curse have been found in children and are referred to as primary central alveolar hypoventilation syndromes. Morbidly obese patients and those with sleep apnea may exhibit abnormalities of ventilatory control.

Periodic breathing is commonly observed during drug-induced sedation. Mechanistically, this is most likely when peripheral chemoreceptors are activated by mild arterial hypoxemia. Continual overcorrection and undercorrection of the Pao_2 leads to oscillations of $Paco_2$ and Sao_2. Periodic breathing is also common during sleep at higher altitudes.

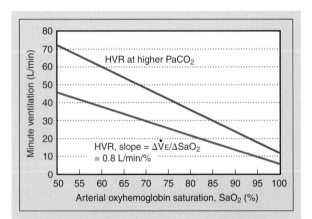

Figure 6-15 Hypoxic ventilatory response (HVR) expressed relative to Sao_2 is approximately linear, which is simpler than the curvilinear response expressed as a function of Pao_2. HVR is the slope of the linear plot. HVR is higher at higher carbon dioxide concentrations. Both absolute ventilation and the slope are shifted. Low $Paco_2$ likewise lowers HVR.

INTEGRATION OF THE HEART AND LUNGS

The interrelationship between the heart and lungs is suggested by the Fick equation, which relates oxygen consumption and oxygen needs at the tissue level.

$$\dot{V}_{O_2} = CO \cdot (Cao_2 - C\bar{v}o_2)$$

In the equation, $\dot{V}_{O_2}$ is oxygen consumption, CO is cardiac output, Cao_2 is the arterial oxygen content, and $C\bar{v}o_2$ is the mixed venous oxygen content.

Oxygen Delivery

Oxygen delivery (DO_2) is the total amount of oxygen supplied to tissues and is a function of CO and CaO_2:

$$DO_2 = CO \cdot CaO_2$$

DO_2 can be limited by decreases in CO or CaO_2. CaO_2 can be limited by anemia or hypoxemia.

Oxygen Extraction

Different indices can be used to assess how much oxygen is removed from blood by tissues to meet their metabolic demand. Mixed venous oxygen saturation ($S\bar{v}O_2$) is normally about 75%. If tissues extract more oxygen, $S\bar{v}O_2$ decreases. However, with high FIO_2, $S\bar{v}O_2$ may increase because of the added amount of dissolved oxygen, even though true extraction has not changed. The arterial-venous oxygen content difference ($CaO_2 - C\bar{v}O_2$) is independent of changes in FIO_2 and is therefore a useful measurement of the balance of oxygen supply and demand. On the other hand, the arterial-venous oxygen content difference decreases in anemia because extracting the same percentage of oxygen means extracting less total oxygen because of the lower hemoglobin concentration. The most reliable figure is the calculated oxygen extraction ratio:

$$O_2 \text{ extraction} = \frac{CaO_2 - C\bar{v}O_2}{CaO_2}$$

ANEMIA

An example of threatened oxygen supply is anemia. To adapt to anemia, the body can increase CO or extract more oxygen. The normal physiologic response is to increase CO and maintain oxygen delivery. Increased HR and SV are responsible for this compensation. However, under anesthesia with a near-absent HR response, increased oxygen extraction is a more important mechanism of compensation.

METABOLIC DEMAND

Increased oxygen consumption is usually met with a combination of increased CO and increased oxygen extraction. Whereas oxygen consumption is usually constant and relatively low under anesthesia, recovery from anesthesia may be associated with significant increases in metabolic demands. Shivering and early ambulation after outpatient surgery are stresses that may affect patients still recovering from anesthesia or after significant blood loss. Increased minute ventilation is required to meet increased oxygen needs and to eliminate the extra carbon dioxide produced.

QUESTIONS OF THE DAY

1. What are common causes of inadequate preload in a patient receiving anesthesia?
2. How do the determinants of pulmonary vascular resistance differ from systemic vascular resistance?
3. What shift of the oxyhemoglobin dissociation curve (leftward or rightward) improves tissue oxygenation? What conditions are associated with this shift?
4. What are the physiologic causes of an increased A-a gradient?
5. What is the relationship between minute ventilation and carbon dioxide in the awake patient?

REFERENCES

1. Berne RM, Levy MN: *Cardiovascular Physiology*, ed 8, St. Louis, 2001, Mosby.
2. Nunn JF: *Nunn's Applied Respiratory Physiology*, ed 5, Boston, 2000, Butterworth-Heinemann.
3. West JB: *Respiratory Physiology: The Essentials*, ed 8, Philadelphia, 2007, Lippincott Williams & Wilkins.
4. Gelman S: Venous function and central venous pressure. A physiologic story, *Anesthesiology* 108:735–748, 2008.
5. Michard F: Changes in arterial pressure during mechanical ventilation, *Anesthesiology* 103:419–428, 2005; quiz 449–445.
6. Topalian S, Ginsberg F, Parrillo JE: Cardiogenic shock, *Crit Care Med* 36: S66–S74, 2008.
7. Shepherd SJ, Pearse RM: Role of central and mixed venous oxygen saturation measurement in perioperative care, *Anesthesiology* 111:649–656, 2009.
8. Weir EK, Lopez-Barneo J, Buckler KJ, et al: Acute oxygen-sensing mechanisms, *N Engl J Med* 353:2042–2055, 2005.

II

7 AUTONOMIC NERVOUS SYSTEM

David Glick

The autonomic nervous system (ANS) is responsible for the body's involuntary activities (including cardiovascular, gastrointestinal, and thermoregulatory homeostasis). The ANS is divided into two major branches: the sympathetic nervous system (SNS), which controls the "fight or flight" responses, and the parasympathetic nervous system (PNS), which oversees the body's maintenance functions including digestion and genitourinary function. The activities of both the SNS and PNS are essential to survival, and both disease states and the stress of surgery can lead to changes in the ANS that can have potentially deleterious effects on the body. Thus, the object during anesthetic management is to modify the body's normal autonomic responses to keep the patient safe. Contemporary anesthesiologists have many pharmacologic drugs at their disposal that can profoundly alter autonomic activity; however, to use these drugs most effectively, a thorough understanding of the anatomy and physiology of the ANS is essential.

ANATOMY OF THE AUTONOMIC NERVOUS SYSTEM

The Sympathetic Nervous System

The preganglionic fibers of the SNS originate from the thoracolumbar region of the spinal cord (Fig. 7-1). The cell bodies of these neurons lie in the spinal gray matter, and the nerve fibers extend to paired ganglia along the sympathetic chains, immediately lateral to the vertebral column, or to unpaired distal plexuses (e.g., the celiac or mesenteric plexuses). Preganglionic sympathetic fibers not only synapse at the ganglion of the level of their origin in the spinal cord but can also course up and down the paired ganglia. A sympathetic response, therefore, is not confined to the segment from which the stimulus originates, as discharge can be amplified and diffuse. The postganglionic neurons of the SNS then travel to the target organ. Thus, the sympathetic preganglionic fibers are relatively

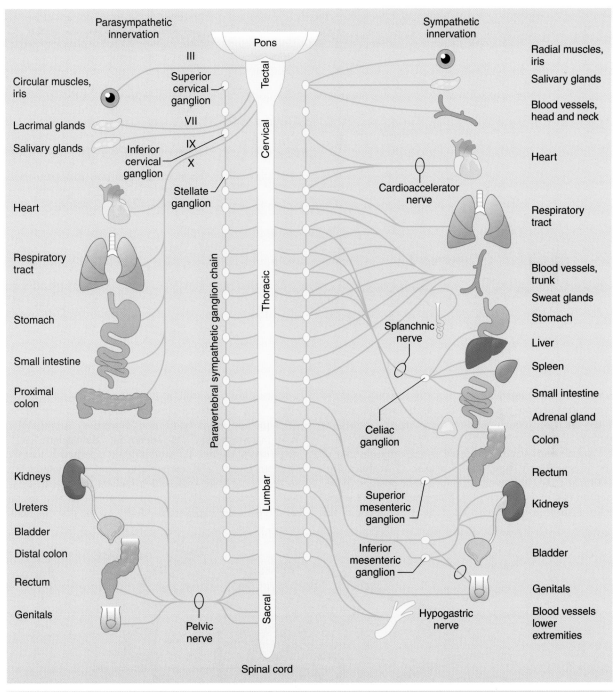

Figure 7-1 Schematic representation of the autonomic nervous system depicting the functional innervation of peripheral effector organs and the anatomic origin of peripheral autonomic nerves from the spinal cord. Although both paravertebral sympathetic ganglia chains are presented, the sympathetic innervation to the peripheral effector organs is shown only on the right part of the figure, whereas the parasympathetic innervation of peripheral effector organs is depicted on the left. The roman numerals on nerves originating in the tectal region of the brainstem refer to the cranial nerves that provide parasympathetic outflow to the effector organs of the head, neck, and trunk. (From Ruffolo R. Physiology and biochemistry of the peripheral autonomic nervous system. In Wingard L, Brody T, Larner J, et al [eds]. Human Pharmacology: Molecular to Clinical. St. Louis, Mosby-Year Book, 1991, p 77.)

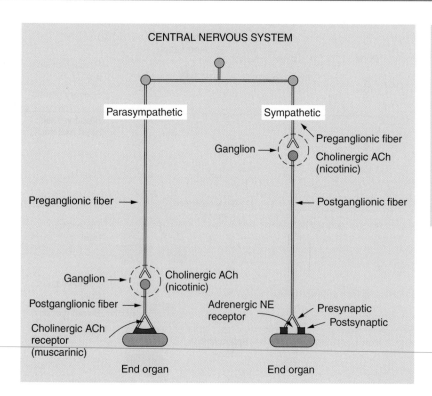

CENTRAL NERVOUS SYSTEM

Figure 7-2 Schematic diagram of the peripheral autonomic nervous system. Preganglionic fibers and postganglionic fibers of the parasympathetic nervous system release acetylcholine (ACh) as the neurotransmitter. Postganglionic fibers of the sympathetic nervous system release norepinephrine (NE) as the neurotransmitter (exceptions are fibers to sweat glands, which release ACh). (From Lawson NW, Wallfisch HK. Cardiovascular pharmacology: A new look at the pressors. In Stoelting RK, Barash J [eds]. Advances in Anesthesia. Chicago, Year Book Medical Publishers, 1986, pp 195-270.)

short because sympathetic ganglia are generally close to the central nervous system (CNS), and the postganglionic fibers run a long course before innervating effector organs (Fig. 7-2).

The neurotransmitter released at the terminal end of the preganglionic sympathetic neuron is acetylcholine (ACh), and the cholinergic receptor on the postganglionic neuron is a nicotinic receptor. Norepinephrine is the primary neurotransmitter released at the terminal end of the

postganglionic neuron at the synapse with the target organ (Fig. 7-3). Other classical neurotransmitters of the SNS include epinephrine and dopamine. Additionally, co-transmitters, such as adenosine triphosphate (ATP) and neuropeptide Y, modulate sympathetic activity. Norepinephrine and epinephrine bind postsynaptically to adrenergic receptors, which include the α_1-, β_1-, β_2-, and β_3-receptors. When norepinephrine binds to the α_2-receptors, located presynaptically on the postganglionic

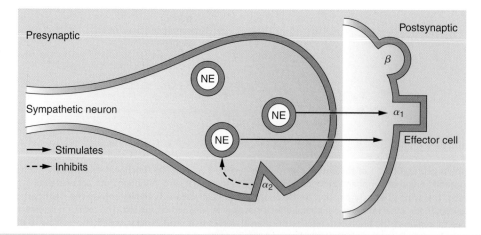

Figure 7-3 Schematic depiction of the postganglionic sympathetic nerve ending. Release of the neurotransmitter norepinephrine (NE) from the nerve ending results in stimulation of postsynaptic receptors, which are classified as α_1, β_1, and β_2. Stimulation of presynaptic α_2-receptors results in inhibition of NE release from the nerve ending. (Adapted from Ram CVS, Kaplan NM: Alpha- and beta-receptor blocking drugs in the treatment of hypertension. In Harvey WP [ed]. Current Problems in Cardiology. Chicago, Year Book Medical Publishers, 1970.)

Figure 7-4 Biosynthesis of norepinephrine and epinephrine in sympathetic nerve terminal (and adrenal medulla). **A,** Perspective view of molecules. **B,** Enzymatic processes. (From Tollenaeré JP. Atlas of the Three-Dimensional Structure of Drugs. Amsterdam, Elsevier North-Holland, 1979, as modified by Vanhoutte PM. Adrenergic neuroeffector interaction in the blood vessel wall. Fed Proc 37:181, 1978.)

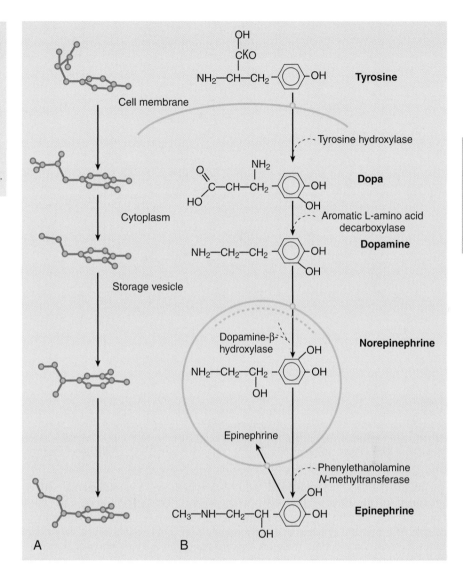

sympathetic nerve terminal, subsequent norepinephrine release is decreased (negative feedback). Dopamine (D) binds to D_1 receptors postsynaptically or D_2 receptors presynaptically.

Sympathetic neurotransmitters are synthesized from tyrosine in the postganglionic sympathetic nerve ending (Fig. 7-4). The rate-limiting step is the transformation of tyrosine to dihydroxyphenylalanine (DOPA), which is catalyzed by the enzyme tyrosine hydroxylase. DOPA is then converted to dopamine and, once inside the storage vesicle at the nerve terminal, is beta-hydroxylated to norepinephrine. In the adrenal medulla, norepinephrine is methylated to epinephrine. The neurotransmitters are stored in vesicles until the postganglionic nerve is stimulated. Then the vesicles merge with the cell membrane and release their contents into the synapse (Fig. 7-5). In general 1% of the total stored norepinephrine is released

with each depolarization, so there is a tremendous functional reserve. The norepinephrine then binds to the pre- and postsynaptic adrenergic receptors. The postsynaptic receptors then activate second messenger systems in the postsynaptic cell via G protein–linked activity. Once norepinephrine is released from the receptor, most of it is actively taken up at the presynaptic nerve terminal and transported to storage vesicles for reuse. Norepinephrine that escapes the reuptake process and makes its way into the circulation is metabolized by either the monoamine oxidase (MAO) or catechol-O-methyltransferase (COMT) enzyme in the blood, liver, or kidney.

The Parasympathetic Nervous System

The PNS arises from cranial nerves III, VII, IX, and X, as well as from sacral segments (see Fig. 7-1). Unlike the

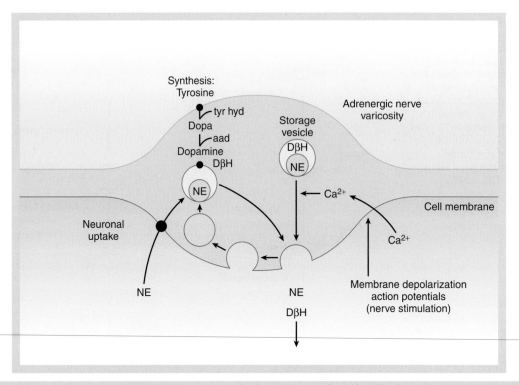

Figure 7-5 Release and reuptake of norepinephrine at sympathetic nerve terminals. aad, aromatic L-amino decarboxylase; DβH, dopamine β-hydroxylase; dopa, L-dihydroxyphenyalanine; NE, norepinephrine; tyr hyd, tyrosine hydroxylase; solid circle, active carrier. (From Vanhoutte PM. Adrenergic neuroeffector interaction in the blood vessel wall. Fed Proc 37:181, 1978, as modified by Shepherd J, Vanhoutte P. Neurohumoral regulation. In Shepherd S, Vanhoutte P [eds]. The Human Cardiovascular System: Facts and Concepts. New York, Raven Press, 1979, p 107.)

ganglia of the SNS, the ganglia of the PNS are in close proximity to (or even within) their target organs (see Fig. 7-2). Like the SNS, the preganglionic nerve terminals release ACh into the synapse, and the postganglionic cell binds the ACh via nicotinic receptors. The postganglionic nerve terminal then releases ACh into the synapse it shares with the target organ cell. The ACh receptors of the target organ are muscarinic receptors. Like the adrenergic receptors, muscarinic receptors are coupled to G proteins and second messenger systems. ACh is rapidly inactivated within the synapse by the cholinesterase enzyme.

The effects of stimulating adrenergic and cholinergic receptors throughout the body are listed in Table 7-1.

ADRENERGIC PHARMACOLOGY

Endogenous Catecholamines

Table 7-2 summarizes the pharmacologic effects and therapeutic doses of catecholamines.

NOREPINEPHRINE
Norepinephrine, the primary adrenergic neurotransmitter, binds to α- and β-receptors. It is used primarily for its

α_1-adrenergic effects that increase systemic vascular resistance. Like all the endogenous catecholamines, the half-life of norepinephrine is short (2.5 minutes), so it is usually given as a continuous infusion at rates of 3 μg/min or more and titrated to the desired effect. The increase in systemic resistance can lead to reflex bradycardia. Additionally, because norepinephrine vasoconstricts the pulmonary, renal, and mesenteric circulations, infusions must be monitored to prevent injury to vital organs. Prolonged infusion of norepinephrine can also cause ischemia in the fingers because of the marked peripheral vasoconstriction.

EPINEPHRINE
Like norepinephrine, epinephrine binds to α- and β-adrenergic receptors. Exogenous epinephrine is used intravenously in life-threatening circumstances to treat cardiac arrest, circulatory collapse, and anaphylaxis. It is also commonly used locally to decrease the spread of local anesthetics and to reduce surgical blood loss. Among the therapeutic effects of epinephrine are positive inotropy, chronotropy, and enhanced conduction in the heart (β_1); smooth muscle relaxation in the vasculature and bronchial tree (β_2); and vasoconstriction (α_1). The effects that predominate depend on the dose of epinephrine administered.

Table 7-1 Responses Elicited in Effector Organs by Stimulation of Sympathetic and Parasympathetic Nerves

Effector Organ	Adrenergic (A) Response	Receptor Involved	Cholinergic (C) Response	Dominant Response (A or C)
Heart				
Rate of contraction	Increase	β1	Decrease	C
Force of contraction	Increase	β1	Decrease	C
Blood vessels				
Arteries (most)	Vasoconstriction	α1		A
Skeletal muscle	Vasodilation	β2		A
Veins	Vasoconstriction	α2		A
Bronchial tree	Bronchodilation	β2	Bronchoconstriction	C
Splenic capsule	Contraction	α1		A
Uterus	Contraction	α1	Variable	A
Vas deferens	Contraction	α1		A
Prostatic capsule	Contraction	α1		A
Gastrointestinal tract	Relaxation	α2	Contraction	C
Eye				
Radial muscle, iris	Contraction (mydriasis)	α1		A
Circular muscle, iris			Contraction (miosis)	C
Ciliary muscle	Relaxation	β	Contraction (accommodation)	C
Kidney	Renin secretion	β1		A
Urinary bladder				
Detrusor	Relaxation	β	Contraction	C
Trigone and sphincter	Contraction	α1	Relaxation	A, C
Ureter	Contraction	α1	Relaxation	A
Insulin release from pancreas	Decrease	α2		A
Fat cells	Lipolysis	β1		A
Liver glycogenolysis	Increase	α1		A
Hair follicles, smooth muscle	Contraction (piloerection)	α1		A
Nasal secretion			Increase	C
Salivary glands	Increase secretion	α1	Increase secretion	C
Sweat glands	Increase secretion	α1	Increase secretion	C

From Ruffolo R. Physiology and biochemistry of the peripheral autonomic nervous system. In Wingard L, Brody T, Lamer J, et al (eds). Human Pharmacology: Molecular to Clinical. St. Louis, Mosby-Year Book, 1991, p 77.

Table 7-2 Pharmacologic Effects and Therapeutic Doses of Catecholamines

Catecholamine	Mean Arterial Pressure	Heart Rate	Cardiac Output	Systemic Vascular Resistance	Renal Blood Flow	Cardiac Dysrhythmias	Preparation (mg/250 mL)	Intravenous Dose (µg/kg/min)
Dopamine	+	+	+ + +	+	+ + +	+	200 (800 µg/mL)	2-20
Norepinephrine	+++	−	−	+++	---	+	4 (16 µg/mL)	0.01-0.1
Epinephrine	+	++	++	+ +	--	+++	1 (4 µg/mL)	0.03-0.15
Isoproterenol	−	+++	+++	--	−	+++	1 (4 µg/mL)	0.03-0.15
Dobutamine	+	+	+++	−	++	−	250 (1000 µg/mL)	2-20

+, mild increase; + +, moderate increase; +++, marked increase; −, mild decrease; --, moderate decrease; ---, marked decrease.

Epinephrine also has endocrine and metabolic effects that include increasing the levels of blood glucose, lactate, and free fatty acids.

An intravenous dose of 1.0 mg is given for cardiovascular collapse, asystole, ventricular fibrillation, electromechanical dissociation, or anaphylactic shock to constrict the peripheral vasculature and maintain myocardial and cerebral perfusion. In less acute circumstances, epinephrine is given as a continuous infusion. The response of individual patients to epinephrine varies, so the infusion must be titrated to effect while the patient is monitored for signs of compromised renal, cerebral, or myocardial perfusion. In general, an infusion rate of 1 to 2 μg/min should primarily stimulate β_2-receptors and decrease airway resistance and vascular tone. A rate of 2 to 10 μg/min increases heart rate, contractility, and conduction through the atrioventricular node. At doses larger than 10 μg/min the α_1-adrenergic effects predominate, and the resulting generalized vasoconstriction can lead to reflex bradycardia.

Epinephrine also can be administered as an aerosol to treat severe croup or airway edema. Bronchospasm is treated with epinephrine administered subcutaneously in doses of 300 μg every 20 minutes with a maximum of three doses. Epinephrine treats bronchospasms both via its direct effect as a bronchodilator and because it decreases antigen-induced release of bronchospastic substances (as may occur during anaphylaxis) by stabilizing the mast cells that release these substances.

Because epinephrine decreases the refractory period of the myocardium, the risk of arrhythmias during halothane anesthesia is increased when epinephrine is given. The risk of arrhythmias seems to be less in children but increases with hypocapnia.

DOPAMINE

In addition to binding to α- and β-receptors, dopamine also binds to dopaminergic receptors. Besides its direct effects, dopamine acts indirectly by stimulating the release of norepinephrine from storage vesicles. Dopamine is unique in its ability to improve blood flow through the renal and mesenteric beds in shock-like states by binding to postjunctional D_1 receptors. Dopamine is rapidly metabolized by MAO and COMT and has a half-life of 1 minute, so it must be given as a continuous infusion. At doses between 0.5 and 2.0 μg/kg/min, D_1 receptors are stimulated and renal and mesenteric beds are dilated. When the infusion is increased to 2 to 10 μg/kg/min, the β_1-receptors are stimulated and cardiac contractility and output are increased. At doses of 10 μg/kg/min and higher, α_1-receptor binding predominates, and there is marked generalized constriction of the vasculature, negating any benefit to renal perfusion.

In the past, dopamine was frequently used to treat patients in shock. The concept was that infusions of dopamine, by improving renal blood flow, could protect the kidney and aid in diuresis. Recent studies have found that dopamine does not have a beneficial effect on renal function in shock states, and its routine use for patients in shock has been called into question.[1]

Synthetic Catecholamines

ISOPROTERENOL

Isoproterenol (Isuprel) provides relatively pure and nonselective β-adrenergic stimulation. Its β_1-adrenergic stimulation is greater than its β_2-adrenergic effects. Its popularity has declined because of adverse effects such as tachycardia and arrhythmias. It is no longer part of the Advanced Cardiac Life Support protocols (also see Chapter 44), and its principal use now is as a chronotropic agent after cardiac transplantation. Because isoproterenol is not taken up into the adrenergic nerve endings, its half-life is longer than that of the endogenous catecholamines.

DOBUTAMINE

Dobutamine, a synthetic analog of dopamine, has predominantly β_1-adrenergic effects. When compared with isoproterenol, inotropy is more affected than chronotropy. It exerts less of a β_2-type effect than isoproterenol does and less of an α_1-type effect than does norepinephrine. Unlike dopamine, endogenous norepinephrine is not released nor does it act at dopaminergic receptors.

Dobutamine is particularly useful in patients with congestive heart failure (CHF) or myocardial infarction complicated by low cardiac output. Doses smaller than 20 μg/kg/min usually do not produce tachycardia. Because dobutamine directly stimulates β_1-receptors, it does not rely on endogenous norepinephrine stores for its effects and may still be useful in catecholamine-depleted states such as chronic CHF. Prolonged treatment with dobutamine causes downregulation of β-receptors, and tolerance to its hemodynamic effects is significant after 3 days. To avoid this problem of tachyphylaxis, intermittent infusions of dobutamine have been used in the long-term treatment of heart failure. These treatments have improved exercise tolerance but not survival.[2]

FENOLDOPAM

Fenoldopam is a selective D_1 agonist and potent vasodilator that enhances renal blood flow and diuresis. Because of mixed results in clinical trials, fenoldopam is no longer used for treatment of chronic hypertension or CHF. Instead, intravenous fenoldopam, at infusion rates of 0.1 to 0.8 μg/kg/min, has been approved to treat severe hypertension. Fenoldopam is an alternative to sodium nitroprusside with fewer side effects (e.g., no thiocyanate toxicity, rebound effect, or coronary steal) and improved renal function. Its peak effects take 15 minutes.

Noncatecholamine Sympathomimetic Amines

Most noncatecholamine sympathomimetic amines act at α- and β-receptors through both direct (binding of the drug by adrenergic receptors) and indirect (release of endogenous norepinephrine stores) activity. Mephentermine and metaraminol are rarely used anymore, so the only widely used noncatecholamine sympathomimetic amine at this time is ephedrine.

EPHEDRINE

Ephedrine increases arterial blood pressure and has a positive inotropic effect. Because it does not have detrimental effects on uterine blood flow in animal models, ephedrine became widely used as a pressor in hypotensive pregnant patients. However, phenylephrine is now preferred due to a decreased risk of fetal acidosis (also see Chapter 33). As a result of its β_1-adrenergic stimulating effects, ephedrine is helpful in treating moderate hypotension, particularly if accompanied by bradycardia. The usual dose is 2.5 to 25 mg given intravenously or 25 to 50 mg administered intramuscularly.

Tachyphylaxis to the indirect effects of ephedrine may develop as norepinephrine stores are depleted. In addition, although drugs with indirect activity are widely used as a first-line therapy for intraoperative hypotension, epidemiologic studies of adverse events during anesthesia suggest that dependence on ephedrine in life-threatening events may contribute to morbidity.[3]

SELECTIVE α-ADRENERGIC RECEPTOR AGONISTS

α_1-Adrenergic Agonists

PHENYLEPHRINE

Phenylephrine (Neo-Synephrine), a selective α_1-agonist, is frequently used for peripheral vasoconstriction when cardiac output is adequate (e.g., in the hypotension that may accompany spinal anesthesia). It is also used to maintain afterload in patients with aortic stenosis whose coronary perfusion is compromised by a decline in systemic vascular resistance. Given intravenously, phenylephrine has a rapid onset and relatively short duration of action (5 to 10 minutes). It may be given as a bolus of 40 to 100 μg or as an infusion starting at a rate of 10 to 20 μg/min. Larger doses of up to 1 mg slow supraventricular tachycardia through reflex action. Phenylephrine is also a mydriatic and nasal decongestant. Applied topically, alone or in combination with local anesthetics, phenylephrine is used to prepare the nostril for nasotracheal intubation.

α_2-Adrenergic Agonists

α_2-Agonists are assuming greater importance as anesthetic adjuvants and analgesics. Their primary effect is sympatholytic. They reduce peripheral norepinephrine release by stimulation of prejunctional inhibitory α_2-receptors. Traditionally, they have been used as antihypertensive drugs, but applications based on their sedative, anxiolytic, and analgesic properties are becoming increasingly common.

CLONIDINE

Clonidine, the prototypical drug of this class, is a selective agonist for α_2-adrenoreceptors. Its antihypertensive effects result from central and peripheral attenuation of sympathetic outflow. Clonidine withdrawal may precipitate hypertensive crises, so it should be continued throughout the perioperative period. A transdermal patch is available if a patient cannot take clonidine orally. If it is not continued perioperatively blood pressure should be monitored closely with ready ability to treat hypertension. Labetalol is used to treat clonidine withdrawal syndrome.

Although experience with α_2-agonists as a sole anesthetic is limited, these drugs reduce the requirements for other intravenous or inhaled anesthetics as part of a general or regional anesthetic technique.[4] Perioperative use of clonidine and the other α_2-agonists dexmedetomidine and mivazerol also decreased myocardial infarction and perioperative mortality rates in patients who had vascular surgery.[5]

In addition to their use in the operative setting, α_2-agonists provide effective analgesia for acute and chronic pain, particularly as adjuncts to local anesthetics and opioids. Epidural clonidine is indicated for the treatment of intractable pain, which is the basis for approval of parenteral clonidine in the United States as an orphan drug. Clonidine also is used to treat patients with reflex sympathetic dystrophy and other neuropathic pain syndromes.

DEXMEDETOMIDINE

Like clonidine, dexmedetomidine is highly selective for the α_2-receptors. Its half-life of 2.3 hours and distribution half-life of less than 5 minutes make its clinical effect quite short. Unlike clonidine, dexmedetomidine is available as an intravenous solution in the United States. The usual dosing is an infusion of 0.3 to 0.7 μg/kg/hour either with or without a 1 μg/kg loading dose given over 10 minutes.

In healthy volunteers, dexmedetomidine increases sedation, analgesia, and amnesia; it decreases heart rate, cardiac output, and circulating catecholamines in a dose-dependent fashion. The MAC-sparing sedative and analgesic effects demonstrated in preclinical and volunteer studies have been borne out in clinical practice. The relatively minor impact of α_2-induced sedation on respiratory function combined with the short duration of action of dexmedetomidine has led to its use for awake fiberoptic intubation.[6] Dexmedetomidine infusions for the perioperative management of obese patients with obstructive sleep apnea minimized the need for narcotics while providing adequate analgesia.[7]

β_2-ADRENERGIC RECEPTOR AGONISTS

β_2-Agonists are used to treat reactive airway disease. With large doses the β_2-receptor selectivity can be lost, and severe side effects related to β_1-adrenergic stimulation are possible. Commonly used agents include metaproterenol (Alupent, Metaprel), terbutaline (Brethine, Bricanyl), and albuterol (Proventil, Ventolin).

β_2-Agonists are also used to interrupt premature labor. Ritodrine (Yutopar) has been marketed for this purpose. Unfortunately, β_1-adrenergic adverse effects are common, particularly when the drug is given intravenously.

α-ADRENERGIC RECEPTOR ANTAGONISTS

α_1-Antagonists have long been used as antihypertensive drugs, but their side effects, which include marked orthostatic hypotension and fluid retention, have made them less popular as other medications for controlling arterial blood pressure have become available.

Phenoxybenzamine

Phenoxybenzamine (Dibenzyline) is the prototypical α_1-adrenergic antagonist (though it also has α_2-antagonist effects). Because it irreversibly binds α_1-receptors, new receptors must be synthesized before complete recovery. Phenoxybenzamine decreases peripheral resistance and increases cardiac output. Its primary adverse effect is orthostatic hypotension that can lead to syncope with rapid changes from lying to standing positions. Nasal stuffiness is another effect. Phenoxybenzamine is most commonly used in the treatment of pheochromocytomas. It establishes a "chemical sympathectomy" preoperatively that makes arterial blood pressure less labile during surgical resection of these catecholamine-secreting tumors. When exogenous sympathomimetics are given after α_1-blockade their vasoconstrictive effects are inhibited. Despite its irreversible binding to the receptor, the recommended treatment for a phenoxybenzamine overdose is an infusion of norepinephrine because some receptors remain free of the drug.

Prazosin

Prazosin (Minipress) is a potent selective α_1-blocker that antagonizes the vasoconstrictor effects of norepinephrine and epinephrine. Orthostatic hypotension is a major problem with prazosin. Unlike other antihypertensive drugs, prazosin improves lipid profiles by lowering low-density lipid levels and raising the level of high-density lipids. The usual starting dose of prazosin is 0.5 to 1 mg given at bedtime because of orthostatic hypotension.

Yohimbine

α_2-Antagonists such as yohimbine increase the release of norepinephrine but they have found little clinical utility in anesthesia.

β-ADRENERGIC ANTAGONISTS

β-Adrenergic antagonists (i.e., β-blockers) are frequently taken by patients about to undergo surgery. Clinical indications for β-adrenergic blockade include ischemic heart disease, postinfarction management, arrhythmias, hypertrophic cardiomyopathy, hypertension, heart failure, migraine prophylaxis, thyrotoxicosis, and glaucoma. In the 1990s, a study by the Perioperative Ischemia Research Group demonstrated the value of initiating β-blockade perioperatively in patients at risk for coronary artery disease.[8] Study subjects given perioperative β-blockers had a markedly reduced all-cause 2-year mortality rate (68% survival in placebo group vs. 83% in atenolol-treated group). The presumed mechanism for this improved survival was a diminution of the surgical stress response by the β-blockers. These and other confirmatory findings led to tremendous political and administrative pressure to increase the use of β-blockers perioperatively. Recent studies, however, have questioned the value of perioperative β-blockade. The POBBLE study showed no reduction in 30-day mortality risk in patients who had vascular surgery (one of the "at-risk" groups from previous studies),[9] and the DIPOM study showed no benefit in diabetics (another "at-risk" group).[10] Finally, in a large retrospective study, there were negative effects of β-blockade in patients without clear-cut coronary artery disease.[11] So, at this point, the only strong indication for initiating β-blockade perioperatively is for patients who need vascular surgery and are at high cardiac risk because of a finding of ischemia on preoperative testing.[12] β-Blockers should be continued in patients who are already taking them for angina, arrhythmias, or hypertension because acute β-blocker withdrawal can lead to life-threatening events.

The most widely used β-adrenergic blockers in anesthetic practice are propranolol, metoprolol, labetalol, and esmolol because they are available as intravenous formulations and have well-characterized effects. The most important differences among these agents are in cardioselectivity and duration of action. Nonselective β-blockers act at the β_1- and β_2-receptors. Cardioselective β-blockers have stronger affinity for β_1-adrenergic receptors than for β_2-adrenergic receptors. With β_1 selective blockade, velocity of atrioventricular conduction, heart rate, and cardiac contractility decrease. The release of renin by the juxtaglomerular apparatus and lipolysis at adipocytes also decrease. At higher doses, the relative selectivity for β_1-receptors is lost and β_2-receptors are also blocked, with the potential for bronchoconstriction, peripheral vasoconstriction, and decreased glycogenolysis.

Adverse Effects of β-Adrenergic Blockade

Life-threatening bradycardia, even asystole, may occur with β-blockade, and decreased contractility may precipitate CHF in patients with compromised cardiac function. In patients with bronchospastic lung disease, β_2-blockade may be fatal. Diabetes mellitus is a relative contraindication to the long-term use of β-adrenergic antagonists because warning signs of hypoglycemia (tachycardia and tremor) can be masked and because compensatory glycogenolysis is blunted. To avoid worsening of hypertension, use of β-blockers in patients with pheochromocytomas should be avoided unless α-receptors have already been blocked. Overdose of β-blocking drugs may be treated with atropine, but isoproterenol, dobutamine, or glucagon also may be required along with cardiac pacing to maintain an adequate rate of contraction.

Undesirable drug interactions are possible with β-blockers. The rate and contractility effects of verapamil are additive to those of β-blockers, so care must be taken when combining these drugs. Similarly, the combination of digoxin and β-blockers can have powerful effects on heart rate and conduction and should be used with special care.

Specific β-Adrenergic Blockers

PROPRANOLOL

Propranolol (Inderal, Ipran), the prototypical β-blocker, is a nonselective β-blocking drug. Because of its high lipid solubility, it is extensively metabolized in the liver, but metabolism varies greatly from patient to patient. Clearance of the drug can be affected by liver disease or altered hepatic blood flow. Propranolol is available in an intravenous form and was initially given as either a bolus or an infusion. Infusions of propranolol have largely been supplanted by the shorter-acting esmolol. For bolus administration, doses of 0.1 mg/kg may be given, but most practitioners initiate therapy with much smaller doses, typically 0.25 to 0.5 mg, and titrate to effect. Propranolol shifts the oxyhemoglobin dissociation curve to the right, which might account for its efficacy in vasospastic disorders.[13]

METOPROLOL

Metoprolol (Lopressor), a cardioselective β-adrenergic blocker, is approved for the treatment of angina pectoris and acute myocardial infarction. No dosing adjustments are necessary in patients with liver failure. The usual oral dose is 100 to 200 mg/day taken once or twice daily for hypertension and twice daily for angina pectoris. Intravenous doses of 2.5 to 5 mg may be administered every 2 to 5 minutes up to a total dose of 15 mg, with titration to heart rate and blood pressure.

LABETALOL

Labetalol (Trandate, Normodyne) acts as a competitive antagonist at the α_1- and β-adrenergic receptors. Metabolized by the liver, its clearance is affected by hepatic perfusion. Labetalol may be given intravenously every 5 minutes in 5- to 10-mg doses or as an infusion of up to 2 mg/min. It can be effective in the treatment of patients with aortic dissection,[14] or hypertensive emergencies. Because vasodilation is not accompanied by tachycardia, labetalol has been given to cardiac patients postoperatively. It may be used to treat hypertension in pregnancy both on a long-term basis and in more acute situations.[15] Uterine blood flow is not affected, even with significant reductions in blood pressure.[16]

ESMOLOL

Because it is hydrolyzed by blood-borne esterases, esmolol (Brevibloc) has a uniquely short half-life of 9 to 10 minutes, which makes it particularly useful in anesthetic practice. It can be used when β-blockade of short duration is desired or in critically ill patients in whom the adverse effects of bradycardia, heart failure, or hypotension may require rapid withdrawal of the drug. Esmolol is cardioselective, and the peak effects of a loading dose are seen within 5 to 10 minutes and diminish within 20 to 30 minutes. It may be given as a bolus of 0.5 mg/kg or as an infusion. When used to treat supraventricular tachycardia a bolus of 500 µg/kg is given over 1 minute, followed by an infusion of 50 µg/kg/min for 4 minutes. If the heart rate is not controlled, a repeat loading dose followed by a 4-minute infusion of 100 µg/kg/min is given. If needed, this sequence is repeated with the infusion increased in 50 µg/kg/min increments up to 200 or 300 µg/kg/min. Esmolol is safe and effective for the treatment of intraoperative and postoperative hypertension and tachycardia. If continuous use is required, it may be replaced by a longer-lasting cardioselective β-blocker such as metoprolol.

CHOLINERGIC PHARMACOLOGY

In contrast to the rich selection of drugs to manipulate adrenergic responses, there is a relative paucity of drugs that affect cholinergic transmission. A small number of direct cholinergic agents are used topically for the treatment of glaucoma or to restore gastrointestinal or urinary function. The classes of drugs with relevance to the anesthesiologist are the anticholinergic agents (muscarinic antagonists) and the anticholinesterases.

Muscarinic Antagonists

The muscarinic antagonists compete with neurally released acetylcholine for access to muscarinic cholinoceptors and block acetylcholine's effects. The results are faster heart rate, sedation, and dry mouth. With the exception of the quaternary ammonium compounds that

Table 7-3 Comparative Effects of Anticholinergics Administered Intramuscularly as Pharmacologic Premedication

Effect	Atropine	Scopolamine	Glycopyrrolate
Antisialogogue effect	+	+++	++
Sedative and amnesic effects	+	+++	0
Increased gastric fluid pH	0	0	0/+
Central nervous system toxicity	+	++	0
Relaxation of lower esophageal sphincter	++	++	++
Mydriasis and cycloplegia	+	+++	0
Heart rate	++	0/+	+

0, none; +, mild; ++, moderate; +++, marked.

do not readily cross the blood-brain barrier and have few actions on the CNS, there is no significant specificity of action among these drugs; they block all muscarinic effects with equal efficacy, although there are some quantitative differences in effect (Table 7-3).

In the era of ether anesthetics, a muscarinic antagonist was added to anesthetic premedication to decrease secretions and to prevent harmful vagal reflexes. This addition is less important with modern inhaled anesthetics. Preoperative use of these drugs continues in some pediatric and otorhinolaryngologic cases or when fiberoptic intubation is planned.

Atropine with its tertiary structure can cross the blood-brain barrier. Thus, large doses (1 to 2 mg) can affect the CNS. In contrast, because of the quaternary structure of the synthetic antimuscarinic drug glycopyrrolate (Robinul) it does not cross the blood-brain barrier. Glycopyrrolate has a longer duration of action than atropine and has largely replaced atropine for blocking the adverse muscarinic effects (bradycardia) of the anticholinesterase drugs that reverse neuromuscular blockade. Scopolamine also crosses the blood-brain barrier and can have profound CNS effects. The patch preparation of scopolamine is used prophylactically for postoperative nausea and vomiting, but it may be associated with adverse eye, bladder, skin, and psychological effects. The distortions of mentation (e.g., delusions or delirium) that can follow treatment with atropine or scopolamine are treated with physostigmine, an anticholinesterase that is able to cross the blood-brain barrier.

Cholinesterase Inhibitors

Anticholinesterase drugs impair the inactivation of acetylcholine by the cholinesterase enzyme and sustain cholinergic agonism at nicotinic and muscarinic receptors. These drugs are used to reverse neuromuscular blockade (see Chapter 12) and to treat myasthenia gravis. The most prominent side effect of these drugs is bradycardia. The commonly used cholinesterase inhibitors are physostigmine, neostigmine, pyridostigmine, and edrophonium. In addition to reversing the effects of neuromuscular blocking agents by increasing the concentration of acetylcholine at the neuromuscular junction, cholinesterase inhibitors stimulate intestinal function or are applied topically to the eye as a miotic. One topical drug (echothiophate iodide) irreversibly binds cholinesterase and can interfere with the metabolism of succinylcholine (as the anticholinesterases impair the function of the pseudocholinesterase enzyme as well).

QUESTIONS OF THE DAY

1. What are the potential indications for epinephrine administration (by any route) during the perioperative period?
2. What is the mechanism of ephedrine's cardiovascular effects?
3. Why is phenoxybenzamine administered to patients with pheochromocytoma? What is the mechanism of action?
4. What are the potential adverse effects of β-blocker administration?
5. What are the most significant differences in the pharmacokinetics of esmolol versus propranolol?

ACKNOWLEDGMENT

The editors and publisher would like to thank Dr. Muhammad Iqbal Shaikh for contributing a chapter on this topic to the prior edition of this work. It has served as the foundation for the current chapter.

REFERENCES

1. Holmes CL, Walley KR: Bad medicine: Low-dose dopamine in the ICU, *Chest* 123:1266–1275, 2003.

2. Krell MJ, Kline EM, Bates ER, et al: Intermittent, ambulatory dobutamine infusions in patients with severe congestive heart failure, *Am Heart J* 112:787–791, 1986.

3. Caplan RA, Ward RJ, Posner K, et al: Unexpected cardiac arrest during spinal anesthesia: A closed claims analysis of predisposing factors, *Anesthesiology* 68:5–11, 1988.

4. Maze M, Tranquilli W: Alpha-2 adrenergic agonists: Defining the role in clinical anesthesia, *Anesthesiology* 74:581–605, 1991.

5. Wijeysundera DN, Naik JS, Beattie WS: Alpha-2 adrenergic agonists to prevent perioperative cardiovascular complications—A meta-analysis, *Am J Med* 114:742–752, 2003.

6. Bergese SD, Khabiri B, Roberts WD, et al: Dexmedetomidine for conscious sedation in difficult awake fiberoptic intubation cases, *J Clin Anesth* 19:141–144, 2007.

7. Ramsay MA, Saha D, Hebeler RF: Tracheal resection in the morbidly obese patient: The role of dexmedetomidine, *J Clin Anesth* 18:452–454, 2006.

8. Mangano DT, Layug EL, Wallace A, et al: Effect of atenolol on mortality and cardiovascular morbidity after noncardiac surgery. Multicenter Study of Perioperative Ischemia Research Group, *N Engl J Med* 335:1713–1720, 1996.

9. Brady AR, Gibbs JS, Greenhalgh RM, et al: Perioperative beta-blockade (POBBLE) for patients undergoing infrarenal vascular surgery: Results of a randomized double-blind controlled trial, *J Vasc Surg* 41:602–609, 2005.

10. Juul AB, Wetterslev J, Gluud C, et al: Effect of perioperative beta blockade in patients with diabetes undergoing major non-cardiac surgery: Randomized placebo controlled, blinded multicentre trial, *BMJ* 332:1482–1488, 2006.

11. Lindenauer PK, Pekow P, Wang K, et al: Perioperative beta-blocker therapy and mortality after major noncardiac surgery, *N Engl J Med* 353:349–361, 2005.

12. Fleisher L, Beckman JA, Brown KA, et al: ACCF/AHA focused update on perioperative beta blockade incorporated into the ACC/AHA 2007 guidelines on perioperative cardiovascular evaluation and care for noncardiac surgery: A report of the American College of Cardiology Foundation/American Heart Association Task Force on Practice Guidelines, *Circulation* 120:e169–e276, 2009.

13. Pendleton RG, Newman DJ, Sherman SS, et al: Effect of propranolol upon the hemoglobin-oxygen dissociation curve, *J Pharmacol Exp Ther* 180:647–656, 1972.

14. DeSanctis RW, Doroghazi RM, Austen WG, et al: Aortic dissection, *N Engl J Med* 317:1060–1067, 1987.

15. Lavies NG, Meiklejohn BH, May AE, et al: Hypertensive and catecholamine response to tracheal intubations in patients with pregnancy-induced hypertension, *Br J Anaesth* 63:429–434, 1989.

16. Jouppila P, Kirkinen P, Koivula A, et al: Labetalol does not alter the placental and fetal blood flow or maternal prostanoids in pre-eclampsia, *Br J Obstet Gynaecol* 93:543–547, 1986.

8 INHALED ANESTHETICS

Rachel Eshima McKay

HISTORY (Also See Chapter 1)

The discovery of inhaled anesthesia reflects the contributions of clinicians and scientists in the United States and England (Fig. 8-1).[1] The most commonly used inhaled anesthetics in modern anesthesia include volatile liquids (i.e., halothane, enflurane, isoflurane, desflurane, and sevoflurane) and a single gas (i.e., nitrous oxide) (Figs. 8-2 and 8-3). None of these inhaled anesthetics meets all the criteria of an "ideal" inhaled anesthetic, and the chemical characteristics differ among the drugs (see Table 8-1).

THE FIRST INHALED ANESTHETICS

Nitrous Oxide

Nitrous oxide gas was first synthesized in 1772 by the English chemist, author, and Unitarian minister Joseph Priestley. Twenty-seven years later, Sir Humphry Davy observed nitrous oxide's capability to produce analgesia. Davy, suffering from a toothache, administered nitrous oxide to himself and found that it relieved his pain. Davy administered nitrous oxide to numerous visitors at the Pneumatic Institute in Bristol and observed its euphoric effect. Davy eventually published a book on nitrous oxide in 1800, making the following observation: "As nitrous oxide in its extensive operation appears capable of destroying physical pain, it may probably be used with advantage during surgical operations in which no great effusion of blood takes place." It was not until 42 years later that nitrous oxide was administered prospectively to patients for relief of pain associated with surgical procedures.

Horace Wells, a 29-year-old Boston dentist, noticed the hypnotic and analgesic effects of nitrous oxide at a public exhibition in Hartford, Connecticut, in 1842. At the exhibition, Wells saw a young man painlessly

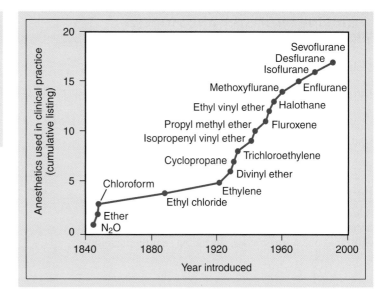

Figure 8-1 Anesthetics used in clinical practice. The history of anesthesia began with the introduction of nitrous oxide, ether, and chloroform. After 1950, all introduced drugs, with the exception of ethyl vinyl ether, have contained fluorine. All anesthetics introduced beginning with halothane have been nonflammable. (From Eger EI: Desflurane (Suprane): A Compendium and Reference. Nutley, NJ, Anaquest, 1993, pp 1-11, used with permission.)

sustain an accidental cut to his shin after inhalation of nitrous oxide. The next day, Wells himself underwent a dental extraction by a fellow dentist. Wells felt only minimal pain with the extraction, and he subsequently learned the method of nitrous oxide synthesis to make it available to his own patients. Soon thereafter, Wells began applying nitrous oxide to his practice to produce "painless dentistry." Two years later, he arranged to demonstrate painless surgery using nitrous oxide administration at the Massachusetts General Hospital. During administration of nitrous oxide to a young male student for a wisdom tooth extraction, the patient groaned and moved even though stating that he felt little pain during the procedure. Wells was discredited as a result of this demonstration.

Diethyl Ether

William Morton, a Boston dentist and contemporary of Wells, had observed Wells' use of nitrous oxide in his painless dentistry practice. Morton noticed parallels between nitrous oxide's effects and those obtained with diethyl ether during "ether frolics," in which ether was breathed for its inebriating effects. Like Wells, Morton applied ether in his dental practice and then asked to demonstrate its anesthetic properties at the Massachusetts General Hospital on October 16, 1846 ("ether day"). In contrast to Wells' debacle, Morton's demonstration was received with great enthusiasm. The results of successful ether anesthetics were soon published in the Boston Medical and Surgical Journal. Although Crawford Long administered diethyl ether to a patient in 1842, four years earlier than Morton, he did not publicize his work, and Morton therefore

has traditionally been credited with the discovery of diethyl ether's capability to produce anesthesia.

Chloroform

James Simpson, an obstetrician from Edinburgh, Scotland, sought to develop an anesthetic that did not share the protracted induction, flammability, and postoperative nausea seen with diethyl ether. After considerable self-experimentation with several liquids obtained from his apothecary, he discovered the anesthetic effects of chloroform. He began to use chloroform inhalation for relief of pain during labor and delivery in 1846. Chloroform soon became popular as an inhaled anesthetic in England, although diethyl ether dominated practice in North America. Over the next few decades, chloroform was associated with several unexplained intraoperative deaths of otherwise healthy patients and with numerous cases of hepatotoxicity.

INHALED ANESTHETICS BETWEEN 1920 AND 1940

Between 1920 and 1940, ethylene, cyclopropane, and divinyl ether were introduced into use as anesthetics, gaining acceptance over the older inhaled anesthetics (with the exception of nitrous oxide) by producing a faster, more pleasant induction of anesthesia and by allowing faster awakening at the conclusion of surgery. Although these anesthetics produced anesthesia, each had serious drawbacks. Many were flammable (i.e., diethyl ether, divinyl ether, ethylene, and cyclopropane), whereas others, halogenated entirely with chlorine, were toxic (i.e., chloroform, ethyl chloride, and trichloroethylene).

FLUORINE CHEMISTRY AND MODERN INHALED ANESTHETICS

Techniques of fluorine chemistry, developed from efforts to produce the first atomic weapons, found a fortuitous, socially beneficial purpose in providing a method of synthesizing modern inhaled anesthetics.[2,3] Modern inhaled anesthetics are halogenated partly or entirely with fluorine (see Fig. 8-2). Fluorination provides greater stability and lesser toxicity.

Halothane

Halothane was introduced into clinical practice in 1956 and became widely used. It had several advantages compared with the older anesthetics, including nonflammability,

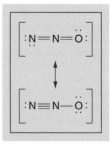

Figure 8-3 Molecular structure of nitrous oxide. Nitrous oxide is a linear molecule existing in two resonance structures. Dots denote nonbonding electrons.

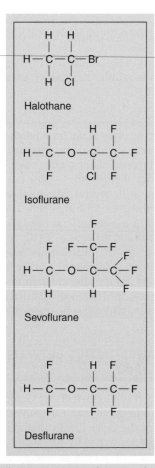

Figure 8-2 Molecular structures of potent volatile anesthetics. Halogenated volatile anesthetics are liquids at room temperature. Among the volatile anesthetics, halothane is an alkane derivative, whereas all the others are derivatives of methyl ethyl ether. Isoflurane is the chemical isomer of enflurane.

a pleasant odor, lesser organ toxicity, and pharmacokinetic properties allowing a much faster induction of anesthesia and emergence compared with ether. Unfortunately after 4 years of commercial use, reports of fulminant hepatic necrosis after halothane anesthesia began to appear in patients in which other causes of liver damage were not evident. The issue of unpredictable liver damage stimulated the search for other volatile anesthetics. Halothane also sensitizes the myocardium to the dysrhymogenic effects of catecholamines.

Methoxyflurane

Methoxyflurane was first introduced into clinical practice in 1960. Within the first decade of its introduction, reports of renal failure with methoxyflurane anesthesia appeared, leading to studies confirming a dose-related nephrotoxicity because of the inorganic fluoride that resulted from the metabolism of this anesthetic.

Enflurane

Enflurane was introduced to clinical practice in 1972. Unlike halothane, it did not sensitize the heart to catecholamines, and it was not associated with hepatotoxicity. However, enflurane was metabolized to inorganic fluoride and could cause evidence of seizure activity on the electroencephalogram (EEG), especially when administered at high concentrations and in the presence of hypocapnia.

Isoflurane

Isoflurane was introduced into clinical practice in 1980 and was widely used clinically. It was not associated with cardiac dysrhythmias. Because it is not metabolized as readily as halothane and enflurane, isoflurane should be associated with less toxicity. Isofurane allowed a more rapid onset of surgical anesthesia and faster awakening compared with its predecessors.

Table 8-1 Comparative Characteristics of Inhaled Anesthetics

Characteristic	Isoflurane	Enflurane	Halothane	Desflurane	Sevoflurane	Nitrous Oxide
Partition coefficient						
Blood-gas	1.46	1.9	2.54	0.45	0.65	0.46
Brain-blood	1.6	1.5	1.9	1.3	1.7	1.1
Muscle-blood	2.9	1.7	3.4	2.0	3.1	1.2
Fat-blood	45	36	51	27	48	2.3
MAC (age 30-55 years)	1.15	1.63	0.76	6.0	1.85	104
Vapor pressure at 20° C (mm Hg)	240	172	244	669	160	
Molecular weight (g)	184.5	184.5	197.4	168	200	44
Stable in hydrated CO_2 absorbent	Yes	Yes	No*	Yes	No*	Yes
Stable in dehydrated CO_2 absorbent	No		No*†	No†	No*†‡	Yes
Percent metabolized	0-0.2		15-40	0-0.2	5-8	

*Compound A.
†Carbon monoxide.
‡Severe exothermic reactions reported. MAC, minimum alveolar concentration.

Sevoflurane and Desflurane

Sevoflurane and desflurane are halogenated exclusively with fluorine and were first synthesized during the late 1960s and 1970s, respectively.[2,3] Both were expensive and difficult to synthesize, and were therefore not immediately considered for commercial use. In the 1980s, their development was reconsidered in light of a new appreciation that a growing proportion of anesthetic practice was taking place in the outpatient setting and that drugs halogenated exclusively with fluorine were less soluble in blood and tissues, allowing faster awakening and recovery (see Fig. 8-1 and Tables 8-1 and 8-2).

MECHANISM OF ACTION

The question of how inhaled anesthetics produce the anesthetic state may be addressed at many levels of biologic organization, including their location of action within the central nervous system, the molecules with which they interact, and the nature of this biologic interaction. Answering these questions requires an ability to measure anesthetic effects.[4] Although inhaled anesthetics have been used to provide surgical anesthesia for almost 160 years, there is no single, accepted definition of what constitutes the anesthetic state. For experimental purposes, an operational definition of immobility in response to surgical stimulation and amnesia for intraoperative events has proved useful.

Measurable Characteristics

Measurable and universal characteristics of all inhaled anesthetics include production of *immobility* and *amnestic effects*. Immobility is measured by the minimum alveolar concentration (MAC) of anesthetic required to suppress movement to a surgical incision in 50% of patients (see Table 8-2).[2,5] However, the presence of amnesia or awareness is difficult to assure (also see Chapters 20 and 46). Although *analgesia* is part of the anesthetic state, it also cannot be measured in an immobile patient who cannot remember. Surrogate measures of pain (i.e., increased heart rate or systemic blood pressure) suggest that inhaled anesthetics do not suppress the perception of painful stimuli. Some inhaled anesthetics have hyperalgesic (pain-enhancing) effects in low concentrations. *Skeletal muscle relaxation* is a common, but not universal, central effect of inhaled anesthetics, as evidenced by nitrous oxide, which increases skeletal muscle tone.

IMMOBILITY

Potent inhaled anesthetics produce immobility in large part by their actions on the spinal cord, as evidenced by determination of MAC in decerebrate animals.[6] Studies in rodents suggest that nitrous oxide activates descending noradrenergic pathways originating in the periaqueductal gray matter brainstem, which in turn inhibit nociceptive input in the dorsal horn of the spinal cord.[7,8]

AMNESTIC EFFECTS (Also See Chapter 46)

Supraspinal structures such as the amygdala, hippocampus, and cortex are considered highly probable targets for the amnestic effects of anesthetics.

CENTRAL NERVOUS SYSTEM DEPRESSION AND ION CHANNELS

Inhaled anesthetics produce central nervous system depression by their actions on ion channels, which govern the electrical behavior of the nervous system.[4] Inhaled anesthetics probably produce anesthesia by enhancing the function of inhibitory ion channels and

Table 8-2   Factors That Increase or Decrease Anesthetic Requirements

Factors Increasing MAC

Drugs
  Amphetamine (acute use)
  Cocaine
  Ephedrine
  Ethanol (chronic use)

Age
  Highest at age 6 months

Electrolytes
  Hypernatremia
  Hyperthermia
Red hair

Factors Decreasing MAC

Drugs
  Propofol
  Etomidate
  Barbiturates
  Benzodiazepines
  Ketamine
  α_2-Agonists (clonidine, dexmedetomidine)
  Ethanol (acute use)
  Local anesthetics
  Opioids
  Amphetamines (chronic use)
  Lithium
  Verapamil

Age
  Elderly patients

Electrolyte disturbance
  Hyponatremia

Other factors
  Anemia (hemoglobin <5 g/dL)
  Hypercarbia
  Hypothermia
  Hypoxia
Pregnancy

MAC, minimum alveolar concentration.

by blocking the function of excitatory ion channels. Enhancing the function of inhibitory ion channels leads to hyperpolarization of the neuron. Hyperpolarization results when chloride anions enter neurons through γ-aminobutyric acid A receptors (GABA$_A$) or glycine receptors or when there is an efflux of potassium cations out of neurons through potassium ion channels. Blocking the function of excitatory ion channels prevents depolarization of the neuron by preventing the passage of positive charges into the neuron (i.e., passage of sodium ions through N-methyl-D-aspartate [NMDA] receptors or sodium channels). Anesthetics may also affect the release of neurotransmitters, and this effect may be mediated in part by ion channels that regulate the release of neurotransmitters.

PHYSICAL PROPERTIES

Molecular Structure

Modern inhaled anesthetics, with the exception of nitrous oxide, are halogenated hydrocarbons (see Figs. 8-2 and 8-3). Halothane lacks the ether moiety present on isoflurane, sevoflurane, and desflurane, accounting for its capability to produce ventricular cardiac dysrhythmias. Isoflurane and desflurane differ only by the substitution of one chlorine atom for fluorine. Fluorine substitution confers greater stability and resistance to metabolism.

Vapor Pressure and Delivery

Nitrous oxide exists as a gas at ambient temperature, although it becomes a liquid at higher pressures. The remaining inhaled anesthetics are liquids at ambient temperatures.

VARIABLE-BYPASS VAPORIZERS
(Also See Chapter 15)

Halothane, sevoflurane, and isoflurane are delivered by variable-bypass vaporizers (Tec 4, 5, and 7; North American Draeger 19.n and 20.n). The variable-bypass vaporizer contains two streams of inflowing fresh gas, one contacting a reservoir (sump) of liquid anesthetic and the other bypassing the sump. Concentration of anesthetic in the gas leaving the vaporizer is determined by the relative flow of fresh gas through the sump channel versus the bypass channel, and control of concentration occurs by adjustment of the dial on the vaporizer. Each variable-bypass vaporizer is temperature compensated, maintaining constant output over a wide range of temperatures, and is calibrated for an individual anesthetic because vapor pressures differ (see Table 8-1). Tilting or overfilling of a vaporizer can potentially lead to delivery of an overdose of anesthetic if anesthetic vapor gets into the bypass channel.

  The Datex-Ohmeda Aladin Cassette Vaporizer, used in the Datex-Ohmeda Anesthesia Delivery Unit (ADU) machines, is a single electronically controlled vaporizer with its bypass housed within the ADU and the sump located within interchangable, magnetically coded cassettes for delivery of halothane, enflurane, isoflurane, sevoflurane, and desflurane. The Aladin utilizes variable bypass as a means of regulating output concentration, doing so via activity of a central processing unit (CPU). The CPU receives input from multiple sources, including the concentration setting, flowmeters, and internal pressure and temperature sensors, and in turn regulates a flow control valve at the outlet of the vaporizing chamber. If pressure in the cassette (sump) exceeds that in the bypass chamber, which would occur if room temperature exceeds 22.8° C during desflurane administration, a one-way check valve is designed to close, preventing retrograde flow of anesthetic saturated gas back into the ADU with subsequent anesthetic overdose.

HEATED VAPORIZER

The vapor pressure of desflurane at sea level is 700 mm Hg at 20° C (near boiling state at room temperature), and delivery by a variable-bypass vaporizer can produce unpredictable concentrations. For this reason, a specially designed vaporizer (Tec 6, Datex-Ohmeda) that heats desflurane gas to 2 atmospheres of pressure is used to accurately meter and deliver desflurane vapor corresponding to adjustments of the concentration dial by the anesthesiologist. In contrast to the variable-bypass vaporizers, the output concentration of desflurane from the Tec 6 is constant across a range of barometric pressures.[9] Therefore, at high altitudes, the partial pressure of desflurane will be lower at a given Tec 6 vaporizer setting and output (volume percent) concentration than at sea level, leading to underdosing of the anesthetic unless an adjustment is made that accounts for the higher altitude: required vaporizer setting = (desired vaporizer setting at sea level × 760 mm Hg) / local barometric pressure (in mm Hg).[10] The converse (a greater output) can occur with variable bypass vaporizers.

Stability

Anesthetic degradation by metabolism or by an interaction with carbon dioxide absorbents (especially when desiccated) produces several potentially toxic compounds.[11]

METABOLISM AND DEGRADATION

Methoxyflurane produces inorganic fluoride, which is responsible for the sporadic incidence of nephrotoxicity (i.e., high-output renal failure) after prolonged anesthesia. Compound A (i.e., trifluoroethyl vinyl ether), produced from the breakdown of sevoflurane, and a similar compound produced from halothane, are nephrotoxic in animals after prolonged exposure. In humans, prolonged anesthesia with sevoflurane and low fresh gas flows (1 L/min) results in compound A exposure adequate to produce transient proteinuria, enzymuria, and glycosuria, but there is no evidence of increased serum creatinine concentrations or long-term deleterious effects on renal function. Nevertheless, the package insert for sevoflurane recommends low fresh gas flow (<2 L/min) be restricted to less than 2 MAC hours (i.e., MAC concentration × duration of administration) of sevoflurane anesthesia.

CARBON DIOXIDE ABSORBENTS AND EXOTHERMIC REACTIONS

Variables influencing the amount of volatile anesthetic degradation on exposure to carbon dioxide absorbents include the condition (i.e., hydration and temperature) and chemical makeup of the absorbent, fresh gas flow rates, minute ventilation, and most important, the anesthetic itself.[12] Although desflurane and isoflurane are very stable in hydrated carbon dioxide absorbents up to temperatures of more than 60° C, full desiccation of conventional carbon dioxide absorbents containing sodium and potassium hydroxide causes degradation and carbon monoxide production from all volatile anesthetics regardless of temperatures (see Table 8-1). High fresh gas flow rates (especially those exceeding normal minute ventilation) accelerate the desiccation of absorbent, and the desiccation leads to accelerated degradation. Because degradation is an exothermic process, the absorbent temperature may increase dramatically.

The exothermic reaction that results from interaction of desiccated carbon dioxide absorbent and volatile anesthetics (especially sevoflurane) can produce extremely high temperatures inside the absorbent canister.[13,14] The temperature increase may lead to explosion and fire in the canister or anesthetic circuit. The remote risk of fire and explosion from exothermic reactions can be avoided entirely by employing measures that ensure maintenance of adequate hydration in the carbon dioxide absorbent (i.e., changing the absorbent regularly, turning fresh gas flow down or off on unattended anesthesia machines, limiting fresh gas flow rates during anesthesia, and when in doubt about the hydration of the absorbent, changing it). Commercially available carbon dioxide absorbents with decreased or absent monovalent bases (i.e., sodium hydroxide and potassium hydroxide) do not result in extensive degradation on exposure to volatile anesthetics, regardless of the absorbent hydration status.

RELATIVE POTENCY OF INHALED ANESTHETICS

The relative potency between inhaled anesthetics is most commonly described by the dose required to suppress movement in 50% of patients in response to surgical incision.[5] This dose (a single point on a dose-response curve) is designated the MAC. Because the standard deviation in the MAC is approximately 10%, 95% of patients should not move in response to incision at 1.2 MAC of the inhaled anesthetic, and 99% of patients should not move in response to incision at 1.3 MAC of the inhaled anesthetic. MAC is affected by several variables but is unaffected by gender or duration of surgery and anesthesia (see Table 8-2).[5]

MAC allows potencies to be compared among anesthetics (see Table 8-1); 1.15% isoflurane is equipotent with 6% desflurane in preventing movement in response to a surgical incision in patients of a similar age and body temperature. Remarkably, MAC values for different inhaled anesthetics are additive. For example, 0.5 MAC of nitrous oxide administered with 0.5 MAC of isoflurane has the same effect as 1 MAC of any inhaled anesthetic in preventing movement in response to incision (reflecting anesthetic-induced inhibition of reflex responses at the level of the spinal cord.[6] The concentration of anesthetic at the brain needed to prevent movement in response to a surgical incision is likely to be larger than the MAC.

The anesthetic dose required to produce amnesia probably has more variability than the MAC. The alveolar concentration of isoflurane preventing recall of a verbal stimulus was 0.20 MAC in 50% and 0.40 MAC in 95% of volunteers.[15] Assuming a standard normal distribution of dose response, the standard deviation in minimum concentration preventing recall is therefore approximately half the mean value (0.1 MAC). Referring to standard normal curves, we can calculate that the concentration needed by 1 in 100,000 subjects with the highest anesthetic requirement would be 4.27 standard deviations (SD) above the mean (i.e., greater than 0.627 MAC) to prevent recall of verbal stimulus. Extrapolation of this value to the context of surgery must be made with caution, however, because the dose required to prevent recall of painful as opposed to verbal stimulation may be considerably larger.[16] The ratio of concentration needed to prevent motor response to surgical incision (reflected in MAC) to that required to suppress consciousness and prevent recall differs slightly between individual potent inhaled anesthetics, and differs substantially between potent inhaled as anesthetic collectively versus nitrous oxide. Volunteers given isoflurane did not exhibit recall given 0.45 MAC isoflurane, whereas recall did occur with as much as 0.6 MAC of nitrous oxide.[17]

PHARMACOKINETICS OF INHALED ANESTHETICS

Pharmacokinetics of inhaled anesthetics describes their uptake (absorption) from alveoli into the systemic circulation, distribution in the body, and eventual elimination by the lungs or metabolism principally in the liver (Table 8-3).[18] By controlling the inspired partial pressure (PI) (same as the concentration [%] when referring to the gas phase) of an inhaled anesthetic, a gradient is created such that the anesthetic is delivered from the anesthetic machine to its site of action, the brain. The primary objective of inhalation anesthesia is to achieve a constant and optimal brain partial pressure (Pbr) of the anesthetic.

The brain and all other tissues equilibrate with the partial pressure of the inhaled anesthetic delivered to them by the arterial blood (Pa). Likewise, the blood equilibrates with the alveolar partial pressure (PA) of the anesthetic:

$$P_A \rightleftharpoons Pa \rightleftharpoons Pbr$$

Maintaining a constant and optimal PA becomes an indirect but useful method for controlling the Pbr. The PA of an inhaled anesthetic mirrors its Pbr and is the reason the PA is used as an index of anesthetic depth, a reflection of the rate of induction and recovery from anesthesia,

Table 8-3 Factors Determining Partial Pressure Gradients Necessary for Establishment of Anesthesia

Transfer of inhaled anesthetic from anesthetic machine to alveoli
  Inspired partial pressure
  Alveolar ventilation
  Characteristics of anesthetic breathing system

Transfer of inhaled anesthetic from alveoli to arterial blood
  Blood-gas partition coefficient
  Cardiac output
  Alveolar-to-venous partial pressure difference

Transfer of inhaled anesthetic from arterial blood to brain
  Brain-blood partition coefficient
  Cerebral blood flow
  Arterial-to-venous partial pressure difference

and a measure of equal potency (see earlier discussion under "Relative Potency of Inhaled Anesthetics"). Understanding the factors that determine the PA and the Pbr allows the anesthesiologist to skillfully control and adjust the dose of inhaled anesthetic delivered to the brain.

Factors That Determine the Alveolar Partial Pressure

The PA and ultimately the Pbr of an inhaled anesthetic are determined by input (delivery) into the alveoli minus uptake (loss) of the drug from the alveoli into the pulmonary arterial blood. Input of the inhaled anesthetic depends on the PI, alveolar ventilation ($\dot{V}_A$), and characteristics of the anesthetic breathing system. Uptake of the inhaled anesthetic depends on the solubility, cardiac output (CO), and alveolar-to-venous partial pressure difference (PA − Pv). These six factors act simultaneously to determine the PA. Metabolism and percutaneous loss of inhaled anesthetics do not significantly influence PA during induction and maintenance of anesthesia.

INSPIRED ANESTHETIC PARTIAL PRESSURE

A high PI is necessary during initial administration of an inhaled anesthetic. This initial high PI (i.e., input) offsets the impact of uptake into the blood and accelerates induction of anesthesia as reflected by the rate of increase in the PA. This effect of the PI is known as the concentration effect. Clinically, the range of concentrations necessary to produce a concentration effect is probably possible only with nitrous oxide (Fig. 8-4).[19]

With time, as uptake into the blood decreases, the PI should be decreased to match the decreased anesthetic uptake. Decreasing the PI to match decreasing uptake with time is critical if the anesthesiologist is to achieve the goal of maintaining a constant and optimal Pbr. For example, if the PI were maintained constant with time

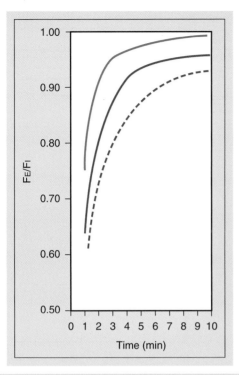

Figure 8-4 The impact of the inspired concentration (%) (FI) on the rate of increase of the alveolar (end-tidal) concentration (FE) is known as the concentration effect. The lines indicate concentrations of 85% (*green*), 50% (*blue*), and 10% (*dashed red*). (From Eger EI: Effect of inspired anesthetic concentration on the rate of rise of alveolar concentration. Anesthesiology 1963;24:153-157, used with permission.)

(input constant), the PA (and depth of anesthesia as reflected by the Pbr) would progressively increase as uptake of the anesthetic into the blood diminished with time.

SECOND GAS EFFECT

The second gas effect is a distinct phenomenon that occurs independently of the concentration effect. The ability of the large-volume uptake of one gas (first gas) to accelerate the rate of increase of the PA of a concurrently administered companion gas (second gas) is known as the second gas effect. For example, the initial large volume uptake of nitrous oxide accelerates the uptake of companion gases such as volatile anesthetics and oxygen. The transient increase (about 10%) in PaO₂ that accompanies the early phase of nitrous oxide administration reflects the second gas effect of nitrous oxide on oxygen. This increase in PaO₂ has been designated alveolar hyperoxygenation. Increased tracheal inflow of all inhaled gases (i.e., first and second gases) and concentration of the second gases in a smaller lung volume (i.e., concentrating effect) because of the high-volume uptake of the first gas are the explanations for the second gas

effect. Although the second gas effect is based on proven pharmacokinetic principles, its clinical importance is doubtful.

ALVEOLAR VENTILATION

Increased V̇A, like PI, promotes input of inhaled anesthetics to offset uptake into the blood. The net effect is a more rapid rate of increase in the PA and induction of anesthesia. Predictably, hypoventilation has the opposite effect, acting to slow the induction of anesthesia.

Controlled ventilation of the lungs that results in hyperventilation and decreased venous return accelerates the rate of increase of the PA by virtue of increased input (i.e., increased V̇A) and decreased uptake (i.e., decreased CO). As a result, the risk of anesthetic overdose may be increased during controlled ventilation of the lungs, and it may be appropriate to decrease the PI of volatile anesthetics when ventilation of the lungs is changed from spontaneous to controlled to maintain the PA similar to that present during spontaneous ventilation.

Another effect of hyperventilation is decreased cerebral blood flow because of any associated decrease in the PaCO₂. Conceivably, the impact of increased anesthetic input on the rate of increase of the PA would be offset by decreased delivery of anesthetic to the brain. Theoretically, coronary blood flow may remain unchanged, such that increased anesthetic input produces myocardial depression, and decreased cerebral blood flow prevents a concomitant onset of central nervous system depression.

ANESTHETIC BREATHING SYSTEM
(Also See Chapter 14)

Characteristics of the anesthetic breathing system that influence the rate of increase of the PA include the volume of the system, solubility of inhaled anesthetics in the rubber or plastic components of the system, and gas inflow from the anesthetic machine. The volume of the anesthetic breathing system acts as a buffer to slow attainment of the PA. High gas inflow from the anesthetic machine negates this buffer effect. Solubility of inhaled anesthetics in the components of the anesthetic breathing system initially slows the rate at which the PA increases. At the conclusion of an anesthetic, reversal of the partial pressure gradient in the anesthetic breathing system results in elution of the anesthetics that slows the rate at which the PA decreases.

SOLUBILITY

The solubility of inhaled anesthetics in blood and tissues is denoted by partition coefficients (see Table 8-1). A partition coefficient is a distribution ratio describing how the inhaled anesthetic distributes itself between two phases at equilibrium (when the partial pressures are identical). For example, a blood-gas partition coefficient of 10 means that the concentration of the inhaled anesthetic is 10 in the blood and 1 in the alveolar gas when the partial pressures of that anesthetic in these two phases are identical. Partition coefficients are temperature dependent. For example, the solubility of a gas in a liquid is increased when the temperature of the liquid decreases. Unless otherwise stated, partition coefficients are given for 37° C.

Blood-Gas Partition Coefficient

High blood solubility means that a large amount of inhaled anesthetic must be dissolved (i.e., undergo uptake) in the blood before equilibrium with the gas phase is reached. The blood can be considered a pharmacologically inactive reservoir, the size of which is determined by the solubility of the anesthetic in the blood. When the blood-gas partition coefficient is high, a large amount of anesthetic must be dissolved in the blood before the P_A equilibrates with the P_A (Fig. 8-5).[18] Clinically, the impact of high blood solubility on the rate of increase of the P_A can be offset to some extent by increasing the P_I. When blood solubility is low, minimal amounts of the anesthetic have to be dissolved in the blood before equilibrium is reached such that the rate of increase of the P_A and that of the P_A and P_{br} are rapid (see Fig. 8-5).[20]

Tissue-Blood Partition Coefficients

Tissue-blood partition coefficients determine the time necessary for equilibration of the tissue with the P_A (see Table 8-1). This time can be predicted by calculating a time constant (i.e., amount of inhaled anesthetic that can be dissolved in the tissue divided by tissue blood flow) for each tissue. Brain-blood partition coefficients for a volatile anesthetic such as isoflurane result in time constants of about 3 to 4 minutes. Complete equilibration of any tissue, including the brain, with the P_A requires at least three time constants. This is the rationale for maintaining the P_A of this volatile anesthetic constant for 10 to 15 minutes before assuming that the P_{br} is similar. Time constants for less soluble anesthetics such as nitrous oxide, desflurane, and sevoflurane are about 2 minutes, and complete equilibration is achieved in approximately 6 minutes (i.e., three time constants).

Anesthetic Transfer by Intertissue Diffusion

There is growing evidence that a portion of anesthetic uptake may occur not by blood flow to various tissues, but by direct transfer from tissues with lower to higher affinity for the anesthetic (i.e., from lean to adipose tissues), such as the interface between viscera and omental fat (see "Context-Sensitive Half-Time"). Larger people[21] and animals[22] with presumably greater lean-fat surface area interface, show greater uptake of sevoflurane and isoflurane. Transfer to bulk fat by blood flow during an anesthetic of clinically realistic duration (less than 12 to 24 hours) is unlikely to explain these differences, given the relatively small blood flow received by the bulk fat compartment and its relatively large size.

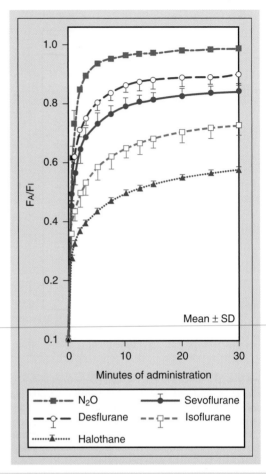

Figure 8-5 The blood-gas partition coefficient is the principal determinant of the rate at which the alveolar concentration (F_A) increases toward a constant inspired concentration (F_I). The rate of induction of anesthesia is paralleled by the rate of increase in the F_A. Despite similar blood solubility (see Table 8-1), the rate of increase of F_A is more rapid for nitrous oxide (*dashed gold line*) than for desflurane (*dashed purple line*) or sevoflurane (*solid blue line*), reflecting the impact of the concentration effect on nitrous oxide (see Fig. 8-4). Greater tissue solubility of desflurane and sevoflurane may also contribute to a slower rate of increase in the F_A of these drugs compared with nitrous oxide. (From Yasuda N, Lockhart SH, Eger EI II, et al. Comparison of kinetics of sevoflurane and isoflurane in humans. Anesth Analg 1991;72:316-324, used with permission.)

Nitrous Oxide and Methionine Synthase Inactivation

Nitrous oxide is unique among anesthetics by its inactivation of methionine synthase, the enzyme regulating vitamin B_{12} and folate metabolism. Although impact of the enzyme inactivation may be subtle or subclinical in many patients, those with underlying critical illness or preexisting vitamin B_{12} deficiency may suffer neurologic or hematologic sequelae. Homocysteine, which requires functional methionine synthase for conversion to methionine, is associated with increased risk of adverse coronary events when present in elevated concentration in the blood.[23] Patients receiving nitrous oxide during carotid endarterectomy showed significantly elevated homocysteine levels and frequency of myocardial ischemic episodes compared to patients not receiving nitrous oxide.[24]

Nitrous Oxide Transfer to Closed Gas Spaces

The blood-gas partition coefficient of nitrous oxide (0.46) is 34 times greater than that of nitrogen (0.014). This differential solubility means that nitrous oxide can leave the blood to enter an air-filled cavity 34 times more rapidly than nitrogen can leave the cavity to enter the blood. As a result of this preferential transfer of nitrous oxide, the volume or pressure of the air-filled cavity increases. The entrance of nitrous oxide into an air-filled cavity surrounded by a compliant wall (e.g., intestinal gas, pneumothorax, pulmonary blebs, air embolism) causes the gas space to expand. Conversely, entrance of nitrous oxide into an air-filled cavity surrounded by a noncompliant wall (e.g., middle ear, cerebral ventricles, supratentorial subdural space) causes an increase in pressure.

The magnitude of volume or pressure increase in the air-filled cavity is influenced by the P_A of nitrous oxide, blood flow to the air-filled cavity, and duration of nitrous oxide administration. In an animal model, inhalation of 75% nitrous oxide doubles the volume of a pneumothorax in 10 minutes.[25] The presence of a closed pneumothorax is a contraindication to the administration of nitrous oxide. Decreasing pulmonary compliance during administration of nitrous oxide to a patient with a history of chest trauma (i.e., rib fractures) may reflect nitrous oxide–induced expansion of a previously unrecognized pneumothorax. Likewise, air bubbles associated with venous air embolism expand rapidly when exposed to nitrous oxide. In contrast to the rapid expansion of a pneumothorax or air bubbles (i.e., venous air embolism), the increase in bowel gas volume produced by nitrous oxide is slow. The question of whether to administer nitrous oxide to patients undergoing intra-abdominal surgery is of little importance if the operation is short. Limiting the inhaled concentration of nitrous oxide to 50%, however, may be a prudent recommendation when bowel gas volume is increased (e.g., bowel obstruction) preoperatively. Following this guideline, bowel gas volume at most would double, even during prolonged operations.[25]

CARDIAC OUTPUT

The CO influences uptake into the pulmonary arterial blood and therefore P_A by carrying away more or less anesthetic from the alveoli. A high CO (e.g., fear) results in more rapid uptake, such that the rate of increase in the P_A and the induction of anesthesia are slowed. A low CO (e.g., shock) speeds the rate of increase of the P_A because there is less uptake into the blood to oppose input. A common clinical impression is that induction of anesthesia in patients in shock is rapid.

Shunt

A right-to-left intracardiac or intrapulmonary shunt slows the rate of induction of anesthesia. This slowing reflects the dilutional effect of shunted blood containing no anesthetic on the partial pressure of anesthetic in blood coming from ventilated alveoli. A similar mechanism is responsible for the decrease in Pa_{O_2} in the presence of a right-to-left shunt.

A left-to-right shunt (e.g., arteriovenous fistula, volatile anesthetic-induced increases in cutaneous blood flow) results in delivery to the lungs of venous blood containing a higher partial pressure of anesthetic than that present in venous blood that has passed through the tissues. As a result, a left-to-right tissue shunt offsets the dilutional effect of a right-to-left shunt on the Pa. The effect of a left-to-right shunt on the rate of increase in the Pa is detectable only if there is the concomitant presence of a right-to-left shunt. Likewise, the dilutional effect of a right-to-left shunt is greatest in the absence of a left-to-right shunt. All factors considered, it seems unlikely that the impact of a right-to-left shunt would be clinically apparent.

Wasted Ventilation

Ventilation of nonperfused alveoli does not influence the rate of induction of anesthesia because a dilutional effect on the Pa is not produced. The principal effect of wasted ventilation is the production of a difference between the P_A and Pa of the inhaled anesthetic. A similar mechanism is responsible for the difference often observed between the end-tidal P_{CO_2} and Pa_{CO_2}.

ALVEOLAR-TO-VENOUS PARTIAL PRESSURE DIFFERENCES

The $P_A - Pv$ reflects tissue uptake of inhaled anesthetics. Highly perfused tissues (i.e., brain, heart, kidneys, and liver) account for less than 10% of body mass but receive about 75% of the CO (Table 8-4). As a result, these highly perfused tissues equilibrate rapidly with the Pa. After three time constants (6 to 12 minutes for inhaled

Table 8-4 Body Tissue Compartments

Compartment	Body Mass (% of 70-kg Adult Male)	Blood Flow (% Cardiac Output, 70-kg Adult Male)
Vessel-rich group	10	75
Muscle group	50	19
Fat group	20	5
Vessel-poor group	20	1

Table 8-5 Proposed Mechanisms of Circulatory Effects Produced by Inhaled Anesthetics

Direct myocardial depression
Inhibition of central nervous system and sympathetic nervous system outflow
Depression of transmission of impulses through autonomic ganglia
Attenuated carotid sinus reflex activity
Decreased formation of cyclic adenosine monophosphate
Inhibition of calcium reuptake by myocardial sarcoplasmic reticulum
Decreased influx of calcium ions through slow channels

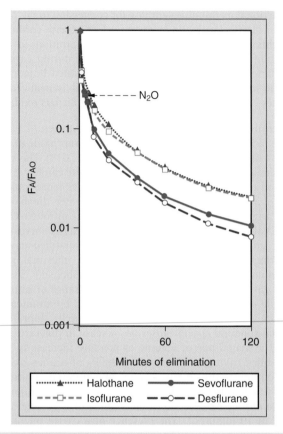

Figure 8-6 Elimination of inhaled anesthetics is reflected by the decrease in the alveolar concentration (F_A) compared with the concentration present at the conclusion of anesthesia (F_{AO}). Awakening from anesthesia is paralleled by these curves. (From Yasuda N, Lockhart SH, Eger El II, et al. Comparison of kinetics of sevoflurane and isoflurane in humans. Anesth Analg 1991;72:316-324, used with permission.)

anesthetics), about 75% of the returning venous blood is at the same partial pressure as the P_A (i.e., narrow $P_A - P_V$). For this reason, uptake of volatile anesthetics from the alveoli is greatly decreased after 6 to 12 minutes, as reflected by a narrowing of the $P_I - P_A$ difference. After this time, the inhaled concentrations of volatile anesthetics should be decreased to maintain a constant P_A in the presence of decreased uptake.

Skeletal muscle and fat represent about 70% of the body mass but receive less than 25% of the CO (Table 8-5). These tissues continue to act as inactive reservoirs for anesthetic uptake for several hours. Equilibration of fat with inhaled anesthetics in the arterial blood is probably never achieved.

Recovery from Anesthesia

Recovery from anesthesia can be defined as the rate at which the P_A decreases with time (Fig. 8-6).[20] In many respects, recovery is the inverse of induction of anesthesia. For example, $\dot{V}_A$, solubility, and CO determine the rate at which the P_A decreases. After discontinuation of anesthetic administration, elimination of anesthetic occurs by ventilation of the lungs. As the alveolar partial pressure decreases, anesthetic is subsequently transferred from the tissues (including the brain) into the alveoli. Hypoventilation or use of fresh gas flows low enough to permit rebreathing of anesthetic will lead to transfer of anesthetic back into the tissues (including the brain), delaying patient recovery.

HOW DOES RECOVERY DIFFER FROM INDUCTION OF ANESTHESIA?

Recovery from anesthesia differs from induction of anesthesia with respect to the absence of a concentration effect on recovery (the P_I cannot be less than zero), the variable tissue concentrations of anesthetics at the start

of recovery, and the potential importance of metabolism on the rate of decrease in the P_A.

Tissue Concentrations

Tissue concentrations of inhaled anesthetics serve as a reservoir to maintain the P_A when the partial pressure gradient is reversed by decreasing the P_I to or near zero at the conclusion of anesthesia. The impact of tissue storage depends on the duration of anesthesia and solubility of the anesthetics in various tissue compartments. For example, time to recovery is prolonged in proportion to the duration of anesthesia for a soluble anesthetic (e.g., isoflurane), whereas the impact of duration of administration on time to recovery is minimal with poorly soluble anesthetics (e.g., sevoflurane, desflurane) (Fig 8-7).[1] The variable concentrations of anesthetics in different tissues at the conclusion of anesthesia contrasts with induction of anesthesia, when all tissues initially have the same zero concentration of anesthetic.

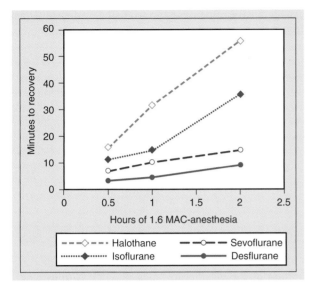

Figure 8-7 An increase in the duration of anesthesia during a constant dose of anesthetic (1.6 MAC) is associated with increases in the time to recovery (i.e., motor coordination in an animal model), with the greatest increases occurring with the most blood-soluble anesthetics. MAC, minimum alveolar concentration. (From Eger EI II: Desflurane (Suprane): A Compendium and Reference. Nutley, NJ, Anaquest, 1993, pp 1-11, used with permission.)

Metabolism

An important difference between induction of anesthesia and recovery from anesthesia is the potential impact of metabolism on the rate of decrease in the P_A at the conclusion of anesthesia. In this regard, metabolism is a principal determinant of the rate of decrease in the P_A of the highly lipid-soluble methoxyflurane. Metabolism and $\dot{V}_A$ are equally important in the rate of decrease in the P_A of halothane, whereas the rate of decrease in the P_A of less lipid-soluble isoflurane, desflurane, and sevoflurane principally results from $\dot{V}_A$.[11]

CONTEXT-SENSITIVE HALF-TIME

The pharmacokinetics of the elimination of inhaled anesthetics depends on the length of administration (the "context") and the solubility of the inhaled anesthetic in blood and tissues. As with injected anesthetics, it is possible to use computer simulations to determine context-sensitive decrement times for volatile anesthetics (the time required to decrease in anesthetic concentrations in the central nervous system to a fraction of that given from a starting point of interest). The kinetic modeling is based upon presence of each tissue compartment within the body (i.e., blood, vessel-rich group, muscle, fat), the relative size of each compartment, the proportional blood flow received by each compartment, and the solubility of each specific anesthetic in the tissue composing the compartment. During anesthetic administration, equilibration

implies continued uptake of anesthetic until tissue concentration becomes almost as great as alveolar concentration. Equilibration of anesthetic concentration between the alveoli and a small (less than 10% body mass) compartment with high blood flow (i.e., heart, kidneys, brain) occurs within a relatively short period of time (10 to 15 minutes). Conversely, anesthetic equilibration in larger compartments with lesser proportional blood flow (i.e., skeletal muscle and bulk fat) occurs over a longer period of time (hours), as anesthetic uptake continues. The time needed for a 50% decrease in anesthetic concentrations of isoflurane, desflurane, and sevoflurane is less than 5 minutes and does not increase significantly with increasing duration of anesthesia.[26] Presumably, this is a reflection of the initial phase of elimination, which is primarily a function of $\dot{V}_A$. Determination of other decrement times ($\geq$80%) reveals larger differences between various inhaled anesthetics, especially as anesthetic duration becomes longer (Fig. 8-8). Simulation may underestimate the uptake of anesthesia, especially with more soluble anesthetics, since it does not account for anesthetic transferred from lean to fatty tissues by intertissue diffusion.

Elimination of all but small amounts of anesthetics (smaller than need for patients to follow commands) must take place before a patient regains coordinated protective

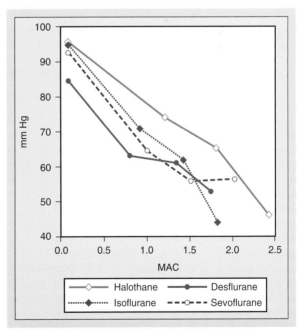

Figure 8-8 The effects of increasing concentrations (MAC) of halothane, isoflurane, desflurane, and sevoflurane on mean arterial pressure (mm Hg) when administered to healthy volunteers. MAC, minimum alveolar concentration. (From Cahalan MK: Hemodynamic Effects of Inhaled Anesthetics. Review Courses. Cleveland, International Anesthesia Research Society, 1996, pp 14-18, used with permission.)

functions, such as the ability to swallow and breathe effectively. Surgical patients given longer anesthesia, and a more soluble anesthetic (sevoflurane compared to desflurane) required a longer time interval between awakening and regaining the ability to swallow effectively.[21] Awake subjects given small concentrations of sevoflurane and isoflurane demonstrate pharyngeal discoordination[27] and diminished chemical ventilatory drive.[28]

DIFFUSION HYPOXIA

Diffusion hypoxia may occur at the conclusion of nitrous oxide administration if patients are allowed to inhale room air. The initial high-volume outpouring of nitrous oxide from the blood into the alveoli when inhalation of this gas is discontinued can so dilute the P_{AO_2} that the Pa_{O_2} decreases. The occurrence of diffusion hypoxia is prevented by filling the patient's lungs with oxygen at the conclusion of nitrous oxide administration.

EFFECTS ON ORGAN SYSTEMS

Circulatory Effects

Equipotent concentrations of inhaled anesthetics have similar circulatory effects, especially during the maintenance of anesthesia in human volunteers (see Table 8-5).[29] However, patients undergoing surgery may respond differently from healthy volunteers. For example, factors such as coexisting disease, extremes of age, nonoptimal intravascular volume status, presence of surgical stimulation, and concurrent drugs may alter, attenuate, or exaggerate the responses expected based on data obtained from healthy volunteers.

RESPONSES DURING MAINTENANCE OF ANESTHESIA
Mean Arterial Pressure

Mean arterial pressure (MAP) decreases with increasing concentrations of desflurane, sevoflurane, isoflurane, halothane, and enflurane in a dose-dependent manner (see Fig. 8-8).[16,17] With the exception of halothane, the decrease in MAP primarily reflects a decrease in systemic vascular resistance (SVR) versus a decrease in CO (Figs. 8-9 and 8-10).[29,30] In contrast, halothane decreases MAP partly or entirely by decreasing CO, whereas SVR is relatively unchanged. These findings are supported by measurements of SVR in patients receiving desflurane, sevoflurane, and isoflurane while undergoing cardiopulmonary bypass perfusion. The dose-related decrease in SVR is minimized by substitution of nitrous oxide for a portion of the volatile drug (Fig. 8-11).[31] Nitrous oxide, in contrast to the other inhaled anesthetics, causes unchanged or mildly increased MAP (Table 8-6).

Heart Rate

Stepwise increases in the delivered concentrations of isoflurane, desflurane, and sevoflurane increase heart rates in patients and volunteers, although at different concentrations (Fig. 8-12).[30] At concentrations as low as 0.25 MAC, isoflurane causes a linear, dose-dependent heart rate increase. Heart rate increases minimally with desflurane concentrations of less than 1 MAC. When desflurane concentrations are increased above 1 MAC, the heart rate accelerates in a linear, dose-dependent manner.

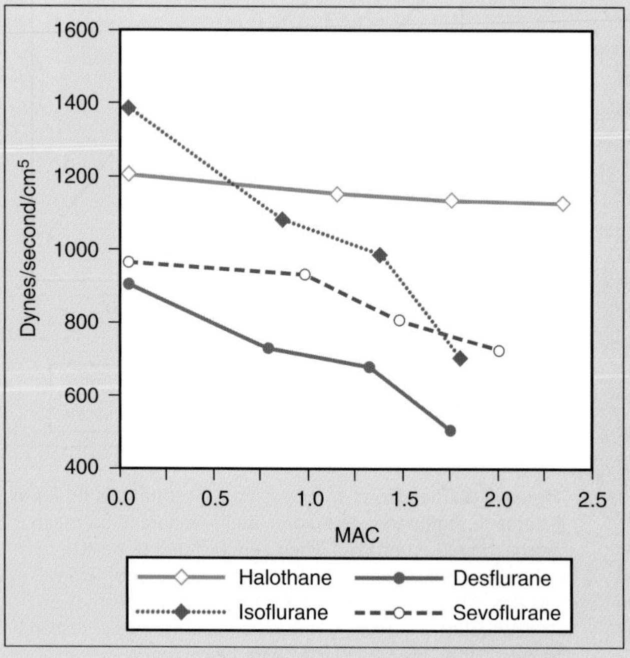

Figure 8-9 The effects of increasing concentrations (MAC) of halothane, isoflurane, desflurane, and sevoflurane on systemic vascular resistance (dynes/sec/cm^5) when administered to healthy volunteers. (From Cahalan MK: Hemodynamic Effects of Inhaled Anesthetics. Review Courses. Cleveland, International Anesthesia Research Society, 1996, pp 14-18, used with permission.)

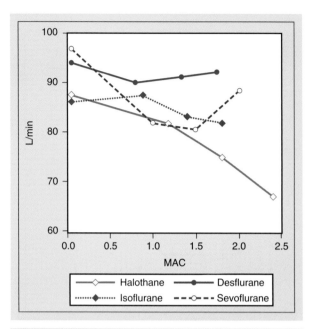

Figure 8-10 The effects of increasing concentrations (MAC) of halothane, isoflurane, desflurane, and sevoflurane on cardiac index (L/min) when administered to healthy volunteers. MAC, minimum alveolar concentration. (From Cahalan MK: Hemodynamic Effects of Inhaled Anesthetics. Review Courses. Cleveland, International Anesthesia Research Society, 1996, pp 14-18, used with permission.)

Table 8-6 Evidence of a Sympathomimetic Effect of Nitrous Oxide Administered Alone or Added to Unchanging Concentrations of Volatile Anesthetics

Diaphoresis
Increased body temperature
Increased plasma concentrations of catecholamines
Increased right atrial pressure
Mydriasis
Vasoconstriction in the systemic and pulmonary circulations

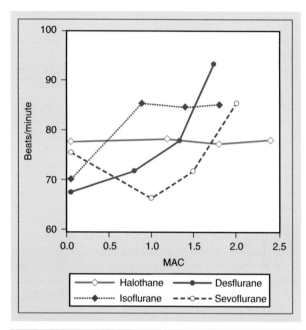

Figure 8-12 The effects of increasing concentrations (MAC) of halothane, isoflurane, desflurane, and sevoflurane on heart rate (beats/min) when administered to healthy volunteers. MAC, minimum alveolar concentration. (From Cahalan MK: Hemodynamic Effects of Inhaled Anesthetics. Review Courses. Cleveland, International Anesthesia Research Society, 1996, pp 14-18, used with permission.)

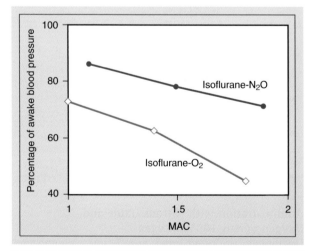

Figure 8-11 The substitution of nitrous oxide for a portion of isoflurane produces less decrease in systemic blood pressure than the same dose of volatile anesthetic alone. (From Eger EI II: Isoflurane (Forane): A Compendium and Reference. Madison, WI, Ohio Medical Products, 1985, pp 1-110, used with permission.)

In contrast to desflurane and isoflurane, heart rate in the presence of sevoflurane does not increase until the concentration exceeds 1.5 MAC.[32] However, induction with 8% sevoflurane (i.e., single-breath induction) causes tachycardia in both children and adult patients undergoing controlled hyperventilation. This tachycardia may result from sympathetic nervous system stimulation associated with epileptiform brain activity.[33]

The tendency for desflurane to stimulate the circulation (i.e., increase MAP and heart rate) is attenuated with administration of β-adrenergic blocker (esmolol), opioid (fentanyl), and passage of time (10 to 15 minutes) during maintenance of anesthesia (see also "Circulatory Effects with Rapid Concentration Increase"). The dose-related increase in heart rate seen with desflurane concentrations more than 1 MAC is not attenuated by substitution of some of the desflurane by nitrous oxide. Isoflurane, sevoflurane, and desflurane, like halothane, diminish baroreceptor responses in a concentration-dependent manner. The transient increase in heart rate above 1 MAC seen with desflurane results from sympathetic nervous system stimulation rather than a reflex baroreceptor activity response to decreased MAP.[34]

Cardiac Index

The cardiac index is minimally influenced by administration of desflurane, sevoflurane, or isoflurane over a wide range of concentrations in healthy young adults (see Fig. 8-10).[29] Transesophageal echocardiography data show that desflurane produces minor increases in the ejection fraction and left ventricular velocity of circumferential shortening compared with awake measurements.

Circulatory Effects with Rapid Concentration Increase

At concentrations of less than 1 MAC, desflurane does not increase heart rate or MAP. However, abrupt increases in inspired desflurane concentrations above 1 MAC cause transient circulatory stimulation in the absence of opioids, adrenergic blockers, or other analgesic adjuncts (Fig. 8-13).[35] To a lesser extent, isoflurane has a similar capability to evoke increases in heart rate and blood pressure. Accompanying the hemodynamic stimulation seen with abrupt increased concentrations of desflurane and isoflurane are increases in plasma epinephrine and norepinephrine concentrations and sympathetic nervous system activity. An abrupt increase in the inspired sevoflurane concentration from 1 MAC to 1.5 MAC is associated with a slight decrease in heart rate.

A stepwise increase in end-tidal desflurane concentration from 4% to 8% within 1 minute may result in a doubling of the heart rate and blood pressure above baseline. Administration of small doses of opioids, clonidine, or esmolol profoundly attenuates the heart rate and blood pressure responses to the stepwise increase in desflurane concentration. Repetition of the rapid increase in end-tidal desflurane concentration from 4% to 8% after 30 minutes results in minimal changes of the heart rate and MAP, suggesting that the receptors mediating these circulatory changes adapt to repeated stimulation. Circulatory stimulation is not seen with abrupt increases in the concentrations of sevoflurane, halothane, or enflurane up to 2 MAC (see Fig. 8-13).[35]

Sevoflurane and halothane are frequently used for inhalation induction because of their lack of pungency. Induction of anesthesia in children with halothane, but not sevoflurane, depresses myocardial contractility. In adults, maintenance of anesthesia with 1 MAC of sevoflurane or halothane in 67% nitrous oxide decreases myocardial contractility. In adults, sevoflurane can transiently increase heart rate when controlled ventilation is used.

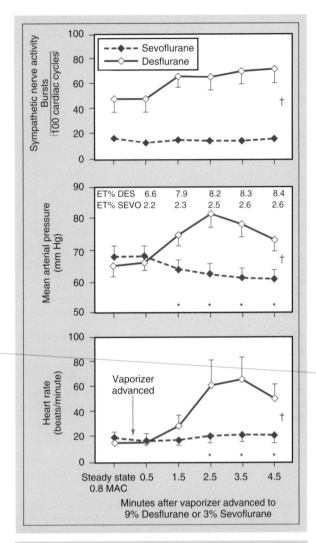

Figure 8-13 A rapid increase in the inspired concentration of sevoflurane from 0.8 MAC to 3% did not alter sympathetic nerve activity, mean arterial pressure, or heart rate. Conversely, a rapid increase in the inspired concentration of desflurane from 0.8 MAC to 9% significantly increased sympathetic nerve activity, mean arterial pressure, and heart rate (mean $\pm$ SE; *$P < 0.05$). ET, end-tidal; MAC, minimum alveolar concentration. (From Ebert TJ, Muzi M, Lopatka CW: Neurocirculatory responses to sevoflurane in humans: A comparison to desflurane. Anesthesiology 1995;83:88-95, used with permission.)

Administration with Nitrous Oxide and Oxygen versus 100% Oxygen

Desflurane, isoflurane, and sevoflurane, administered with nitrous oxide and oxygen, decrease the MAP, SVR, cardiac index, and left ventricular stroke work index (LVSWI) in a dose-dependent manner, whereas heart rate, pulmonary artery pressure, and central venous pressure increase, consistent with the findings in which each volatile anesthetic is administered in oxygen alone (see Fig. 8-11).[29,30] Direct comparison reveals a more pronounced diminution of MAP, SVR, cardiac index, and LVSWI and a more rapid heart rate and larger CO when desflurane is administered in oxygen rather than in nitrous oxide at roughly equivalent MAC multiples.[31]

MYOCARDIAL CONDUCTION AND DYSRHYTHMOGENICITY

Isoflurane, sevoflurane, and desflurane do not predispose the heart to premature ventricular extrasystoles.[36] In contrast, halothane does sensitize the myocardium to premature ventricular extrasystoles, especially in the presence of catecholamines; this relationship is exaggerated with hypercarbia. Inhaled anesthetics probably suppress ventricular dysrhythmias during myocardial ischemia by prolonging the effective refractory period.

The choice of inhaled anesthetic influences the occurrence of reflex bradydysrhythmias that may result from vagal stimulation. Children anesthetized with sevoflurane, compared with halothane, exhibit fewer episodes of decreased heart rate or sinus node arrest in response to surgical traction on the ocular muscles (also see Chapters 31 and 34).

QT Interval

Inhaled anesthetics prolong the QT interval on the electrocardiogram.[37] Although each anesthetic's relative tendency to prolong the QT interval has not been compared systematically, sevoflurane should be avoided in patients with known congenital long QT syndrome (LQTS). Although sevoflurane and propofol anesthetics cause QT interval prolongation in children, neither anesthetic increases transmural dispersion of repolarization, a measure of the heterogeneous rates of repolarization of myocardial cells during phases 2 and 3 of the action potential.[38] The clinical significance of QT prolongation with sevoflurane and other inhaled anesthetics in susceptible patients is unclear. In patients with LQTS, β-adrenergic blockade is the mainstay of therapy. Patients with known LQTS have been safely anesthetized with all modern inhaled anesthetics when concurrently on β-blocking drugs. Numerous malignant intraoperative arrhythmias have been reported in patients undergoing anesthesia with halothane that were subsequently attributed to undiagnosed LQTS, and none of the patients had received β-blocking drugs.[37]

PATIENTS WITH CORONARY ARTERY DISEASE

Numerous studies in patients undergoing coronary artery bypass surgery or at risk for coronary artery disease have failed to demonstrate a difference in outcome between groups receiving inhalation (i.e., desflurane) versus intravenous (i.e., fentanyl or sufentanil) anesthetic techniques or between groups receiving one inhaled anesthetic versus another (i.e., desflurane versus isoflurane or sevoflurane versus isoflurane).[39] Concerns that isoflurane's capacity to dilate small-diameter coronary arteries might cause coronary steal, in which a patient with susceptible anatomy might develop regional myocardial ischemia as a result of coronary vasodilatation, were not valid. Volatile anesthetics instead exert a protective effect on the heart, limiting the area of myocardial injury and preserving function after exposure to ischemic insult.

Anesthetic Preconditioning

The explanation for the protective benefits of volatile anesthetics against myocardial ischemia is called anesthetic preconditioning, and it is not explained by favorable alteration of myocardial oxygen supply-demand ratio. Evidence suggests that volatile anesthetics exert protective effects on the myocardium in the setting of compromised regional perfusion. In patients undergoing coronary artery bypass graft (CABG) surgery, maintenance with 0.2 to 1 MAC of desflurane or sevoflurane decreased the incidence of abnormally elevated troponin levels compared with patients receiving propofol.[40] Sevoflurane administered for the entire duration of CABG surgery versus prebypass or postbypass administration resulted in a less frequent rate of postoperative myocardial infarction compared with sevoflurane administered only in the prebypass or postbypass period, and prebypass or postbypass administration resulted in a lower risk of myocardial infarction compared with propofol anesthesia.[41]

Mechanisms of Ischemic Preconditioning

Ischemic preconditioning is a fundamental protective mechanism present in all tissues in all species. In ischemic preconditioning, exposure to single or multiple brief episodes of ischemia can confer a protective effect on the myocardium against reversible or irreversible injury with a subsequent prolonged ischemic insult. There are two distinct periods after a brief ischemic episode during which the myocardium is protected. The first period occurs for 1 to 2 hours after the conditioning episode and then dissipates. In the second period, the benefit reappears 24 hours later and can last as long as 3 days. The opening of mitochondrial adenosine triphosphate (ATP)-sensitive potassium channels (K_{ATP}) is the crucial event that confers the protective activity, resulting from binding of various ligands to G protein–coupled receptors. Volatile anesthetics have been shown to enhance ischemic preconditioning or provide direct myocardial protection, and the K_{ATP} channels play a central role in their protective effects.[42]

Ventilation Effects

Inhaled anesthetics increase the frequency of breathing and decrease tidal volume as anesthetic concentration increases. Although minute ventilation is relatively preserved, the decreased tidal volume leads to a relatively greater proportion of dead space ventilation relative to alveolar ventilation. Gas exchange becomes progressively less efficient at deeper levels of anesthesia, and Pa_{CO_2} increases proportionally with anesthetic concentration (Fig. 8-14).[1] Effects are similar among potent anesthetics at given MAC multiples.

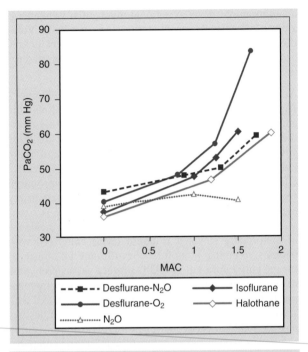

Figure 8-14 Inhaled anesthetics produce drug-specific and dose-dependent increases in Pa_{CO_2}. (From Eger EI II: Desflurane (Suprane): A Compendium and Reference. Nutley, NJ, Anaquest, 1993, pp 1-119, used with permission.)

Substitution of nitrous oxide (60%) for an equivalent portion of volatile anesthetic may attenuate the increase in Pa_{CO_2} at deeper levels of anesthesia.

Volunteers and patients breathing desflurane (and other volatile anesthetics) show a dose-related blunting of carbon dioxide responsiveness, which leads to apnea in subjects receiving 1.7 MAC of desflurane in oxygen (Fig 8-15).[1] Compared with volunteers, the blunting of ventilation with inhaled anesthetics may be less pronounced in patients undergoing surgery, reflecting the stimulatory effect of surgery on breathing (Fig. 8-16).[1] Volatile anesthetics all blunt the ventilatory stimulation evoked by arterial hypoxemia.[43]

CHEST WALL CHANGES

Inhaled anesthetics contribute to conformational changes in the chest wall that may influence ventilatory mechanics. Cephalad displacement of the diaphragm and inward displacement of the rib cage occur from enhanced expiratory muscle activity, and the net result contributes to reduction in functional residual capacity. Atelectasis occurs preferentially in the dependent areas of the lung and occurs to a greater extent when spontaneous ventilation is permitted.

HYPOXIC PULMONARY VASOCONSTRICTION

Inhaled anesthetics alter pulmonary blood flow, but inhibition of hypoxic pulmonary vasoconstriction is minimal. For example, arterial oxygenation is similar in

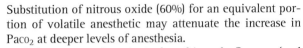

Figure 8-15 All inhaled anesthetics produce similar dose-dependent decreases in the ventilatory responses to carbon dioxide. (From Eger EI II: Desflurane (Suprane): A Compendium and Reference. Nutley, NJ, Anaquest, 1993, pp 1-119, used with permission.)

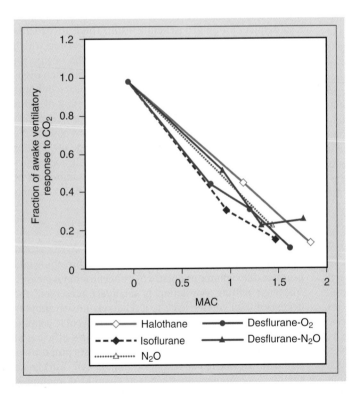

Figure 8-16 Impact of surgical stimulation on the resting Pa_{CO_2} (mm Hg) during administration of isoflurane or halothane. (From Eger EI II: Desflurane (Suprane): A Compendium and Reference. Nutley, NJ, Anaquest, 1993, pp 1-119, used with permission.)

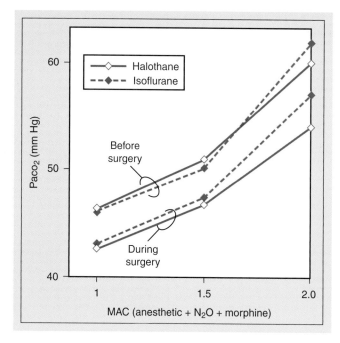

patients undergoing one-lung ventilation with isoflurane versus desflurane anesthesia and sevoflurane versus propofol anesthesia.[44]

AIRWAY RESISTANCE

In the absence of bronchoconstriction, bronchodilating effects of inhaled anesthetics are small. In volunteers, isoflurane, halothane, and sevoflurane, but not nitrous oxide and thiopental, decrease respiratory systemic resistance after tracheal intubation. In nonsmokers, airway resistance shows no change after tracheal intubation and desflurane anesthesia compared with a modest decrease with sevoflurane, whereas smokers show a mild, transient increase in airway resistance after tracheal intubation and desflurane anesthesia.[45] Some or all of the changes in airway resistance may be mediated by changes in gas density.

AIRWAY IRRITANT EFFECTS

Inhaled anesthetics differ in their capacity to irritate airways (i.e., pungency). Sevoflurane, halothane, and nitrous oxide are nonpungent and cause minimal or no irritation over a broad range of concentrations. Desflurane and isoflurane are pungent, and they can irritate the airways in concentrations exceeding 1 MAC, particularly in the absence of intravenous medications (e.g., opioids, sedative-hypnotics) that decrease the perception of pungency.

Sevoflurane or halothane is selected most frequently when an inhaled induction of anesthesia is desired. However, desflurane and isoflurane may be administered to surgical patients by means of a laryngeal mask airway without a greater incidence of airway irritation (e.g., coughing, breath-holding, laryngospasm, arterial oxygen desaturation)

compared with sevoflurane or propofol, because maintenance usually does not require a concentration in excess of 1 MAC (i.e., nonirritating concentrations).[46]

Central Nervous System Effects (Also See Chapter 30)

CEREBRAL BLOOD FLOW

Nitrous oxide administered without volatile anesthetics causes cerebral vasodilatation and increases cerebral blood flow. The cerebral metabolic rate for oxygen ($CMRO_2$) increases modestly. Coadministration of opioids, barbiturates, or propofol (but not ketamine) counteracts these effects.[47] Inhaled anesthetics do not abolish cerebral vascular responsiveness to changes in Pa_{CO_2}.[48]

Halothane, isoflurane, sevoflurane, and desflurane decrease $CMRO_2$. In normocapnic humans, these volatile anesthetics cause cerebral vasodilatation at concentrations above 0.6 MAC. There is a biphasic dose-dependent effect on cerebral blood flow. At 0.5 MAC, the decrease in $CMRO_2$ counteracts the vasodilatation such that cerebral blood flow does not change significantly. At concentrations in excess of 1 MAC, vasodilating effects predominate and cerebral blood flow increases, especially if systemic blood pressure is maintained at awake levels. The cerebral blood flow increase is relatively greater with halothane compared with isoflurane, sevoflurane, or desflurane.

INTRACRANIAL PRESSURE (Also See Chapter 30)

Intracranial pressure increases with all of the volatile anesthetics at doses higher than 1 MAC, and autoregulation (i.e., adaptive mechanism normalizing cerebral blood flow over a wide range of systemic arterial pressures in awake patients) is impaired at concentrations of less than 1 MAC. Patients undergoing craniotomy for supratentorial tumors who receive 1 MAC of isoflurane or desflurane show decreased cerebral perfusion pressure and an arterial-venous oxygen difference for oxygen but no change in intracranial pressure.[49] However, patients undergoing pituitary tumor resection who receive 1 MAC of desflurane, isoflurane, or sevoflurane show small increases in intracranial pressure and decreased cerebral blood flow. Neurosurgical patients receiving 50% nitrous oxide plus 0.5 MAC of desflurane or isoflurane apparently have greater brain relaxation than those receiving 1 MAC of desflurane or isoflurane without nitrous oxide. Inhaled anesthetics do not abolish cerebral vascular responsiveness to changes in Pa_{CO_2}.[48]

EVOKED POTENTIALS

All volatile anesthetics and nitrous oxide depress the amplitude and increase the latency of somatosensory evoked potentials in a dose-dependent manner. Evoked potentials may be abolished at 1 MAC of volatile anesthetic alone or above 0.5 MAC administered with 50% nitrous oxide. Low concentrations of volatile anesthetics (0.2 to 0.3 MAC) decrease the reliability of motor evoked potential monitoring.[50]

ELECTROENCEPHALOGRAPHIC EFFECTS

Volatile anesthetics cause characteristic, dose-dependent changes in the EEG. Increasing depth of anesthesia from the awake state is characterized by increased amplitude and synchrony. Periods of electrical silence begin to occupy a greater proportion of the time as depth increases (i.e., burst suppression). This isoelectric pattern predominates on the EEG within the range of 1.5 to 2.0 MAC.

Sevoflurane and enflurane may be associated with epileptiform activity on the EEG, especially at higher concentrations or when controlled hyperventilation is instituted. Seizure-like activity has been reported in children during sevoflurane induction, but the clinical implications of these observations are not clear.[51]

Neuromuscular Effects

Volatile anesthetics produce dose-related skeletal muscle relaxation and enhance the activity of neuromuscular blocking drugs. Enhancement of the relaxant effect of rocuronium is greater with desflurane than with sevoflurane or isoflurane, although all volatile anesthetics enhance skeletal muscle relaxation compared with intravenous anesthetics (e.g., propofol plus fentanyl). Elimination of volatile anesthetic enhances recovery from neuromuscular blockade. A decrease in the desflurane concentration to 0.25 MAC has a greater effect on reversal of neuromuscular block after vecuronium administration than an equipotent decrease in isoflurane concentration.

Malignant Hyperthermia

Although all potent inhaled anesthetics have the potential to trigger malignant hyperthermia, studies on humans and animals suggest less risk with desflurane, sevoflurane, and possibly isoflurane compared with halothane.

Hepatic Effects

Hepatic injury after anesthesia may be categorized as severe (immune mediated) or mild.[52]

IMMUNE-MEDIATED LIVER INJURY

Severe hepatic injury may follow anesthesia with halothane, isoflurane, sevoflurane, or desflurane. This severe form involves massive hepatic necrosis that can lead to death or necessitate liver transplantation. The mechanism for this severe injury is immunologic, requiring prior exposure to a volatile anesthetic. Halothane, isoflurane, and desflurane all undergo oxidative metabolism by cytochrome P-450 enzymes to produce trifluoroacetate. The trifluoroacetate can bind covalently to hepatocyte proteins. The trifluoroacetyl-hepatocyte moieties can act as haptens, which the body recognizes as foreign and to which the immune system forms antibodies. Subsequent exposure to any anesthetic capable of producing trifluoroacetate may provoke an immune response, leading to severe hepatic necrosis.[53] Sevoflurane is metabolized to hexafluoroisopropanol, a compound that does not appear to have the equivalent antigenic behavior as trifluoroacetate.[54]

MILD LIVER INJURY

A clinically mild form of liver injury may follow administration of halothane. The main characteristic of this more common entity is modest elevation of serum transaminase levels. This mild form of liver injury is thought to be mediated by reductive metabolism of halothane and may be more likely to occur after concomitant decreases in hepatic blood flow and associated reductions in oxygen delivery to the liver.

HISTORY OF PRIOR ANESTHESIA-RELATED HEPATIC DYSFUNCTION

Although volatile anesthetics are frequently not given in patients who have experienced unexplained symptoms of hepatic dysfunction after inhaled anesthesia on a previous occasion, volatile anesthetics are probably not harmful to patients with preexisting hepatic disease unrelated to anesthesia.

QUESTIONS OF THE DAY

1. What conditions increase or decrease the minimum alveolar concentration (MAC) of inhaled anesthetics?
2. What are the six factors that determine the alveolar partial pressure of an inhaled anesthetic?

3. During inhaled anesthetic induction, what is the relationship between the blood-gas partition coefficient and the rate of increase of anesthetic partial pressure?

4. Why does nitrous oxide administration lead to expansion (or increased pressure) of air-filled cavities?

5. What is the mechanism for the decrease in mean arterial pressure with administration of desflurane, sevoflurane, isoflurane, and halothane?

6. What electroencephalographic (EEG) changes occur with increasing concentrations of inhaled anesthetics?

ACKNOWLEDGMENT

The editors and publisher would like to thank Drs. James Sonner and Warren R. McKay for contributing a chapter on this topic to the prior edition of this work. It has served as the foundation for the current chapter.

REFERENCES

1. Eger EI: *Desflurane (Suprane): A compendium and reference*, Nutley, NJ, 1993, Anaquest.

2. Eger EI II: *History of Modern Inhaled Anesthetics: The Pharmacology of Inhaled Anesthetics*, ed 1, San Antonio, TX, 2000, Dannemiller Memorial Educational Foundation.

3. Eger EI II: New inhaled anesthetics, *Anesthesiology* 80:906–922, 1994.

4. Eger EI II, Koblin DD, Harris RA, et al: Hypothesis: Inhaled anesthetics produce immobility and amnesia by different mechanisms at different sites, *Anesth Analg* 84:915–918, 1997.

5. Quasha AL, Eger EI II, et al: Determination and application of MAC, *Anesthesiology* 53:315–334, 1980.

6. Rampil IJ: Anesthetic potency is not altered after hypothermic spinal cord transection in rats, *Anesthesiology* 80:606–610, 1994.

7. Guo TZ, Poree L, Golden W, et al: Antinociceptive response to nitrous oxide is mediated by supraspinal opiate and spinal alpha 2 adrenergic receptors in the rat, *Anesthesiology* 85(4):846–852, 1996.

8. Sawamura S, Kingery WS, Davies MF, et al: Antinociceptive action of nitrous oxide is mediated by stimulation of noradrenergic neurons in the brainstem and activation of [alpha]2B adrenoceptors, *J Neurosci* 20(24):9242–9251, 2000.

9. Weiskopf RB, Sampson D, Moore MA: The desflurane (Tec 6) vaporizer: Design, design considerations and performance evaluation, *Br J Anaesth* 72(4):474–479, 1994.

10. Brockwell RC, Andrews JJ: Vaporizers (in delivery systems for inhaled anesthetics). In Barash PG, Cullen BF, Stoelting RK, Cahallan M, editors: *Clinical Anesthesia*, ed 6, Philadelphia, 2009, Lippincott Williams & Wilkins, pp 667–669.

11. Carpenter RL, Eger EI II, Johnson BH, et al: The extent of metabolism of inhaled anesthetics in humans, *Anesthesiology* 65:201–205, 1986.

12. Wissing H, Kuhn I, Warnken U, et al: Carbon monoxide production from desflurane, enflurane, halothane, isoflurane, and sevoflurane with dry soda lime, *Anesthesiology* 95:1205–1212, 2001.

13. Laster MJ, Roth P, Eger EI II: Fires from the interaction of anesthetics with desiccated absorbent, *Anesth Analg* 99:769–774, 2004.

14. Wu J, Previte JP, Adler E, et al: Spontaneous ignition, explosion, and fire with sevoflurane and barium hydroxide lime, *Anesthesiology* 101:534–537, 2004.

15. Chortkoff BS, Bennett HL, Eger EI II: Subanesthetic concentrations of isoflurane suppress learning as defined by the category-example task, *Anesthesiology* 79(1):16–22, 1993.

16. Sonner JM, Gong D, Eger EI II: Naturally occurring variability in anesthetic potency among inbred mouse strains, *Anesth Analg* 91(3):720–726, 2000.

17. Dwyer R, Bennett HL, Eger EI II, et al: Effects of isoflurane and nitrous oxide in subanesthetic concentrations on memory and responsiveness in volunteers, *Anesthesiology* 77(5):888–898, 1992.

18. Eger EI II: Uptake of inhaled anesthetics: The alveolar to inspired anesthetic difference. In Eger EI II, editor: *Anesthetic Uptake and Action*, Baltimore, 1974, Williams & Wilkins, pp 77–96.

19. Eger EI: Effect of inspired anesthetic concentration on the rate of rise of alveolar concentration, *Anesthesiology* 24:153–157, 1963.

20. Yasuda N, Lockhart SH, Eger EI II, et al: Comparison of kinetics of sevoflurane and isoflurane in humans, *Anesth Analg* 72:316–324, 1992.

21. McKay RE, Malhotra A, Cakmakkaya OS, et al: Effect of increased body mass index and anaesthetic duration on recovery of protective airway reflexes after sevoflurane vs desflurane, *Br J Anaesth* 104:175–182, 2010.

22. Wahrenbrock EA, Eger EI II, Laravuso RB, et al: Anesthetic uptake—Of mice and men (and whales), *Anesthesiology* 40(1):19–23, 1974.

23. Aronow WS, Ahn C: Increased plasma homocysteine is an independent predictor of new coronary events in older persons, *Am J Cardiol* 86(3):346–347, 2000.

24. Badner NH, Beattie WS, Freeman D, et al: Nitrous oxide-induced increased homocysteine concentrations are associated with increased postoperative myocardial ischemia in patients undergoing carotid endarterectomy, *Anesth Analg* 91(5):1073–1079, 2000.

25. Eger EI II, Saidman JL: Hazards of nitrous oxide anesthesia in bowel obstruction and pneumothorax, *Anesthesiology* 26:61–66, 1965.

26. Bailey JM: Context-sensitive half-times and other decrement times of inhaled anesthetics, *Anesth Analg* 85:681–686, 1997.

27. Sundman E, Witt H, Sandin R, et al: Pharyngeal function and airway protection during subhypnotic concentrations of propofol, isoflurane, and sevoflurane: Volunteers examined by pharyngeal videoradiography and simultaneous manometry, *Anesthesiology* 95(5):1125–1132, 2001.

28. Dahan A, Teppema LJ: Influence of anaesthesia and analgesia on the control of breathing, *Br J Anaesth* 91:40–49, 2003.

29. Cahalan MK: *Hemodynamic Effects of Inhaled Anesthetics. Review Courses*, Cleveland, 1996, International Anesthesia Research Society.

30. Cahalan MK, Weiskopf RB, Eger EI II, et al: Hemodynamic effects of desflurane/nitrous oxide anesthesia in volunteers, *Anesth Analg* 73:157–164, 1991.

31. Eger EI: *Isoflurane (Forane): A Compendium and Reference*, Madison, WI, 1985, Ohio Medical Products.

32. Malan TP Jr., DiNardo JA, Isner RJ, et al: Cardiovascular effects of sevoflurane compared with those of

isoflurane in volunteers, *Anesthesiology* 83:918–928, 1995.

33. Yli-Hankala A, Vakkuri AP, Sarkela M, et al: Epileptiform electroencephalogram during mask induction of anesthesia with sevoflurane, *Anesthesiology* 91:1596, 1999.

34. Ebert TJ, Perez F, Uhrich TD, et al: Desflurane-mediated sympathetic activation occurs in humans despite preventing hypotension and baroreceptor unloading, *Anesthesiology* 88:1227–1232, 1998.

35. Ebert TJ, Muzi M, Lopatka CW: Neurocirculatory responses to sevoflurane in humans: A comparison to desflurane, *Anesthesiology* 83:88–95, 1995.

36. Navarro R, Weiskopf RB, Moore MA, et al: Humans anesthetized with sevoflurane or isoflurane have similar arrhythmic response to epinephrine, *Anesthesiology* 80:545–549, 1994.

37. Booker PD, Whyte SD, Ladusans EJ: Long QT syndrome and anaesthesia, *Br J Anaesth* 90:349–366, 2003.

38. Whyte SD, Booker PD, Buckley DG: The effects of propofol and sevoflurane on the QT interval and transmural dispersion of repolarization in children, *Anesth Analg* 100:71–77, 2005.

39. Grundmann U, Muler M, Kleinschmidt S, et al: Cardiovascular effects of desflurane and isoflurane in patients with coronary artery disease, *Acta Anaesthesiol Scand* 40:1101–1107, 1996.

40. DeHert SG, Cromheecke S, ten Broecke PW, et al: Effects of propofol, desflurane, and sevoflurane on recovery of myocardial function after coronary surgery in elderly high-risk patients, *Anesthesiology* 99:314–323, 2003.

41. DeHert SG, Van der Linden PJ, Cromheecke S, et al: Cardioprotective properties of sevoflurane in patients undergoing coronary surgery and cardiopulmonary bypass are related to the modalities of its administration, *Anesthesiology* 101:299–310, 2004.

42. Zaugg M, Lucchinetti E, Spahn D, et al: Volatile anesthetics mimic cardiac preconditioning by priming the activation of the mitoK$_{ATP}$ channels via multiple signaling pathways, *Anesthesiology* 97:4–14, 2002.

43. Sjögren D, Lindahl SG, Sollevi A: Ventilatory responses to acute and sustained hypoxia during isoflurane anesthesia, *Anesth Analg* 86:403–409, 1998.

44. Beck DH, Doepfmer UR, Sinemus C, et al: Effects of sevoflurane and propofol on pulmonary shunt fraction during one-lung ventilation for thoracic surgery, *Br J Anaesth* 86:38–43, 2001.

45. Goff MJ, Arain SR, Ficke DJ, et al: Absence of bronchodilation during desflurane anesthesia: A comparison to sevoflurane and thiopental, *Anesthesiology* 93:404–408, 2000.

46. Eshima R, Maurer A, King T, et al: A comparison of upper airway responses during desflurane and sevoflurane administration via a laryngeal mask airway, *Anesth Analg* 96:701–705, 2003.

47. Petersen KD, Landsfeldt U, Cold GE, et al: Intracranial pressure and cerebral hemodynamics in patients with cerebral tumors: A randomized prospective study of patients subjected to craniotomy in propofol-fentanyl, isoflurane-fentanyl, or sevoflurane-fentanyl anesthesia, *Anesthesiology* 98:329–336, 2003.

48. Mielck F, Stephen H, Buhre W, et al: Effects of 1 MAC desflurane on cerebral metabolism, blood flow and carbon dioxide reactivity in humans, *Br J Anaesth* 81:155–160, 1998.

49. Fraga M, Rama-Maceiras P, Rodino S, et al: The effects of isoflurane and desflurane on intracranial pressure, cerebral perfusion pressure, and cerebral arteriovenous oxygen content difference in normocapnic patients with supratentorial brain tumors, *Anesthesiology* 98:1085–1090, 2003.

50. Lotto ML, Banoub M, Schubert A: Effects of anesthetic agents and physiologic changes on intraoperative motor evoked potentials, *J Neurosurg Anesthesiol* 16:32–42, 2004.

51. Akeson J, Didricksson I: Convulsions on anaesthetic induction with sevoflurane in young children, *Acta Anaesthesiol Scand* 48:405–407, 2004.

52. Martin JL: Volatile anesthetics and liver injury: A clinical update or what every anesthesiologist should know, *Can J Anesth* 52:125–129, 2005.

53. Njoku D, Laster MJ, Gong DH, et al: Biotransformation of halothane, enflurane, isoflurane and desflurane to trifluoroacetylated liver proteins: Association between protein acetylation and hepatic injury, *Anesth Analg* 84:173–178, 1997.

54. Frink EJ, Ghantous H, Malan TP, et al: Plasma inorganic fluoride with sevoflurane anesthesia: correlation with indices of hepatic and renal function, *Anesth Analg* 74:231–235, 1992.

9 INTRAVENOUS ANESTHETICS

Helge Eilers

Intravenous nonopioid anesthetics have an important role in modern anesthesia practice (Table 9-1).[1-7] They are widely used to facilitate rapid induction of anesthesia or to provide sedation during monitored anesthesia care and for patients in intensive care settings. With the introduction of propofol, intravenous anesthesia also became a more common component for maintenance of anesthesia. However, similar to inhaled anesthetics, the currently available intravenous anesthetics do not produce only desired effects (hypnosis, amnesia, analgesia, immobility). Therefore, "balanced anesthesia" evolved by using smaller doses of multiple drugs rather than using larger doses with one or two drugs. The fundamental drugs used with "balanced anesthesia" include inhaled anesthetics, sedative/hypnotics, opioids, and neuromuscular blocking drugs.

The intravenous anesthetics used for induction of general anesthesia are lipophilic and preferentially partition into highly perfused lipophilic tissues (brain, spinal cord), which accounts for their rapid onset of action. Regardless of the extent and speed of their metabolism, termination of the effect of a single bolus dose is a result of redistribution of the drug into less perfused and inactive tissues such as skeletal muscles and fat. Thus, all drugs used for induction of anesthesia have a similar duration of action for a single dose despite significant differences in their metabolism.

PROPOFOL

Propofol is probably the most frequently administered anesthetic drug for induction of anesthesia.[2,3,6] In addition, propofol is used during maintenance of anesthesia and is a common selection for sedation in the operating room as well as in the intensive care unit. Increasingly, propofol is also utilized for conscious sedation and short duration general anesthesia in locations outside the operating room such as interventional radiology suites and the emergency room (also see Chapter 38).

Table 9-1 Drugs Classified as Intravenous Anesthetics

Isopropylphenols
 Propofol
 Fospropofol

Barbiturates
 Thiopental
 Methohexital

Benzodiazepines
 Diazepam
 Midazolam
 Lorazepam

Phencyclidine
 Ketamine

Carboxylated imidazole
 Etomidate

α_2-Adrenergic agonist
 Dexmedetomidine

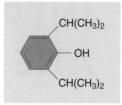

Figure 9-1 Chemical structure of 2,6-diisopropylphenol (propofol).

important. Although either ethylenediaminetetraacetic acid (0.05 mg/mL), metabisulfite (0.25 mg/mL), or benzyl alcohol (1 mg/mL) is added to the emulsions by the different manufacturers as retardants of bacterial growth, solutions should be used as soon as possible or at least within 6 hours after opening the propofol vial. The solutions appear milky white and slightly viscous, their pH is approximately 7, and the propofol concentration is 1% (10 mg/mL). In some countries, a 2% formulation is available. Because the emulsion contains egg yolk lecithin, susceptible patients may experience allergic reactions. The addition of metabisulfite in one of the formulations has raised concern regarding its use in patients with reactive airways (asthma) or sulfite allergies.

Physicochemical Characteristics

Propofol (2,6-diisopropylphenol) is an alkylphenol with hypnotic properties that is chemically distinct from other groups of intravenous anesthetics (Fig. 9-1). It is insoluble in aqueous solutions and is therefore formulated as an emulsion containing 10% soybean oil, 2.25% glycerol, and 1.2% lecithin, the major component of the egg yolk phosphatide fraction. Because the available formulations support bacterial growth, good sterile technique is

Pharmacokinetics

Propofol is rapidly metabolized in the liver, and the resulting water-soluble compounds are presumed to be inactive and excreted through the kidneys (Table 9-2). Plasma clearance is high and exceeds hepatic blood flow,

Table 9-2 Pharmacokinetic Data for Intravenous Anesthetics

Drug	Induction Dose (mg/kg IV)	Duration of Action (min)	Vd_{ss} (min)	$T_{1/2}\alpha$ (min)	Protein Binding (%)	Clearance (mL/kg/min)	$T_{1/2}\beta$ (hr)
Propofol	1-2.5	3-8	2-10	2-4	97	20-30	4-23
Thiopental	3-5	5-10	2.5	2-4	83	3.4	11
Methohexital	1-1.5	4-7	2.2	5-6	73	11	4
Midazolam	0.1-0.3	15-20	1.1-1.7	7-15	94	6.4-11	1.7-2.6
Diazepam	0.3-0.6	15-30	0.7-1.7	10-15	98	0.2-0.5	20-50
Lorazepam	0.03-0.1	60-120	0.8-1.3	3-10	98	0.8-1.8	11-22
Ketamine	1-2	5-10	3.1	11-16	12	12-17	2-4
Etomidate	0.2-0.3	3-8	2.5-4.5	2-4	77	18-25	2.9-5.3
Dexmedetomidine	N/A	N/A	2-3	6	94	10-30	2-3

Data are for average adult patients. The duration of action reflects the duration after an average single IV dose.
IV, intravenous; N/A, not applicable; $T_{1/2}\alpha$, distribution half-time; $T_{1/2}\beta$, elimination half-time; Vd_{ss}, volume of distribution at steady state.

thus indicating the importance of extrahepatic metabolism, which has been confirmed during the anhepatic phase of liver transplantation. The lungs probably play a major role in this extrahepatic metabolism and may account for the elimination of up to 30% of a bolus dose of propofol. The rapid plasma clearance of propofol explains the more complete recovery from propofol with less "hangover" than observed with thiopental. However, as with other intravenous drugs, transfer of propofol from the plasma (central) compartment and the associated termination of drug effect after a single bolus dose are mainly the result of redistribution from highly perfused (brain) to poorly perfused (skeletal muscles) compartments. Wake-up after an induction dose of propofol usually occurs within 8 to 10 minutes, as evident from the time course of the decline in plasma concentration after a single bolus dose (Fig. 9-2).[2,6]

CONTINUOUS INTRAVENOUS INFUSION

Rapid metabolism of propofol resulting in efficient plasma clearance in conjunction with slow redistribution from poorly perfused compartments back into the central compartment makes propofol suitable for use as a continuous intravenous infusion. The context-sensitive half-time describes the elimination half-time after a continuous infusion as a function of the duration of the infusion (Fig. 9-3).[8,9] The context-sensitive half-time of propofol is brief, even after a prolonged infusion, and recovery remains relatively prompt.

COMPARTMENTAL MODEL

The kinetics of propofol (and other intravenous anesthetics) after a single bolus and after continuous infusion is best described by a three-compartment model. These mathematical models have been used as the basis for the development of systems for target-controlled infusions.

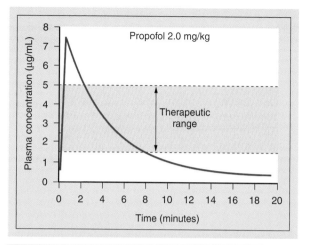

Figure 9-2 Time course of the propofol plasma concentration after a simulated single bolus injection of 2.0 mg/kg. The shape of this curve is similar for other induction drugs, although the slope and the absolute concentrations are different. (From Reves JG, Glass PSA, Lubarsky DA, McEvoy MD. Intravenous nonopioid anesthetics. In Miller RD [ed]: Miller's Anesthesia, 6th ed. Philadelphia, Churchill Livingstone, 2005.)

Pharmacodynamics

The presumed mechanism of action of propofol is through potentiation of the chloride current mediated through the γ-aminobutyric acid type A (GABA$_A$) receptor complex.[10]

CENTRAL NERVOUS SYSTEM

In the central nervous system (CNS), propofol primarily acts as a hypnotic and does not have any analgesic properties. It produces a decrease in cerebral blood flow (CBF) and the cerebral metabolic rate for oxygen

Figure 9-3 Context-sensitive half-time for the most commonly used intravenous anesthetics. Propofol, etomidate, and ketamine have the smallest increase in context-sensitive half-times, with prolonged infusions making these drugs more suitable for use as continuous infusions. (From Reves JG, Glass PSA, Lubarsky DA, McEvoy MD. Intravenous nonopioid anesthetics. In Miller RD [ed]: Miller's Anesthesia, 6th ed. Philadelphia. Churchill Livingstone, 2005.)

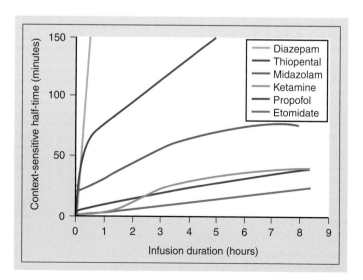

($CMRO_2$), which results in decreases in intracranial pressure (ICP) and intraocular pressure. The magnitude of these changes is comparable to those produced by thiopental. Although propofol can produce a desired decrease in ICP, the reduced CBF combined with the reduced mean arterial pressure caused by peripheral vasodilatation can critically decrease cerebral perfusion pressure (also see Chapter 30).

Propofol probably is neuroprotective during focal ischemia to the same extent as thiopental or isoflurane. When administered in large doses, propofol produces burst suppression in the electroencephalogram (EEG), an end point that has been used for the administration of intravenous anesthetics for neuroprotection during neurosurgical procedures. Occasionally, excitatory effects such as twitching or spontaneous movement can be observed during induction of anesthesia with propofol. Although these effects may resemble seizure activity, propofol is actually an anticonvulsant and may be safely administered to patients with seizure disorders.[6]

CARDIOVASCULAR SYSTEM

Propofol produces a larger decrease in systemic arterial blood pressure than any other drug used for induction of anesthesia. Propofol causes profound vasodilatation, whereas its direct myocardial depressant effect is not clear. Vasodilation occurs in both the arterial and venous circulation and leads to reductions in preload and afterload. The effect on systemic blood pressure is more pronounced in elderly patients, especially those with reduced intravascular fluid volume. Also a rapid injection can facilitate the development of hypotension. Propofol markedly inhibits the normal baroreflex response and produces only a small increase in heart rate, thus further exacerbating its hypotensive effect. Profound bradycardia and asystole after the administration of propofol can occur in healthy adults despite prophylactic anticholinergics.[11]

RESPIRATORY SYSTEM

Propofol is a respiratory depressant and often produces apnea following a dose used to induce anesthesia. A maintenance infusion will reduce minute ventilation through reductions in tidal volume and respiratory rate, with the effect on tidal volume being more pronounced. The ventilatory response to hypoxia and hypercapnia is also reduced. Propofol causes a greater reduction in upper airway reflexes than thiopental does, which makes it well suited for instrumentation of the airway, such as placement of a laryngeal mask airway. When compared with thiopental, propofol decreases the incidence of wheezing after induction of anesthesia and tracheal intubation in healthy and asthmatic patients.[12]

OTHER EFFECTS

Unlike many other anesthetics, propofol has antiemetic activity. Similar to thiopental and unlike volatile anesthetics, propofol probably does not enhance neuromuscular blockade from neuromuscular blocking drugs. Yet, propofol often provides excellent clinical conditions for endotracheal intubation without the use of neuromuscular blocking drugs. Unexpected tachycardia occurring during propofol anesthesia should prompt laboratory evaluation for possible metabolic acidosis (propofol infusion syndrome).[13]

Clinical Uses

Pain on injection is a common complaint and can be reduced by premedication with an opioid or coadministration with lidocaine, 50 to 100 mg intravenously. Dilution of propofol and the use of larger veins for injection can reduce the incidence and severity of injection pain.

INDUCTION AND MAINTENANCE OF ANESTHESIA

Propofol (1 to 2.5 mg/kg IV) is most commonly administered for induction of general anesthesia. Increasing age, reduced cardiovascular reserve, or premedication with benzodiazepines or opioids reduces the required induction dose, whereas children need larger doses (2.5 to 3.5 mg/kg IV). Generally, titration of the induction dose (i.e., rather than an arbitrary bolus dose) helps prevent severe hemodynamic changes. Propofol is also often used for maintenance of anesthesia either as part of a balanced anesthesia regimen in combination with volatile anesthetics, nitrous oxide, sedative-hypnotics, and opioids or as part of a total intravenous anesthetic technique, usually in combination with opioids. Therapeutic plasma concentrations for maintenance of anesthesia normally range between 3 and 8 μg/mL (typically requiring a continuous infusion rate between 100 and 200 μg/kg/min) when combined with nitrous oxide or opioids.

SEDATION

Propofol is a popular choice for sedation of mechanically ventilated patients in the intensive care unit and for sedation during procedures in or outside the operating room. The required plasma concentration is 1 to 2 μg/mL, which will normally necessitate a continuous infusion rate between 25 and 75 μg/kg/min. Because of its pronounced respiratory depressant effect and its narrow therapeutic range, propofol should be administered only by individuals trained in airway management.

ANTIEMETIC

Subanesthetic bolus doses of propofol or a subanesthetic infusion can be used to treat postoperative nausea and vomiting (10 to 20 mg IV, 10 μg/kg/min as an infusion).

FOSPROPOFOL

Propofol is the most commonly used intravenous anesthetic for induction and maintenance of anesthesia and probably also during monitored anesthesia care and conscious sedation. As mentioned earlier, injection pain during administration of propofol can often be perceived as severe and the lipid emulsion has several disadvantages. Intense research has focused on finding alternative formulations or alternative related drugs that would address some of the problems. Fospropofol is a water-soluble prodrug of propofol and in 2008 was licensed by the Food and Drug Administration (FDA) as a sedating agent for use during monitored anesthesia care.[14]

Physicochemical Characteristics

Fospropofol, initially known under the name GPI 15715, is a water-soluble phosphate ester prodrug of propofol and is chemically described as 2,6-diisopropylphenoxymethyl phosphate disodium salt (Fig. 9-4). It is metabolized by alkaline phosphatase in a reaction producing propofol, phosphate, and formaldehyde. Aldehyde dehydrogenase in the liver and in erythrocytes rapidly metabolizes formaldehyde to produce formate, which is further metabolized by 10-formyltetrahydrofolate dehydrogenase.[14] The available fospropofol formulation is a sterile, aqueous, colorless, and clear solution that is supplied in a single-dose vial at a concentration of 35 mg/mL under the trade name Lusedra.

Pharmacokinetics

Because the active compound is propofol and fospropofol is a prodrug that requires metabolism to form propofol, the pharmacokinetics are more complex than for propofol itself. Multicompartment models with two compartments for fospropofol and three for propofol have been used to describe the kinetics. However, previous studies on pharmacokinetics/pharmacodynamics and tolerability of fospropofol have been based on an inaccurate analytical assay, and therefore, reliable data on the kinetics are lacking.[14] Six previously published studies have recently been retracted.[15]

Pharmacodynamics

The effect profile is similar to that of propofol, but onset and recovery are prolonged compared to propofol because the prodrug has to be converted into an active form first.

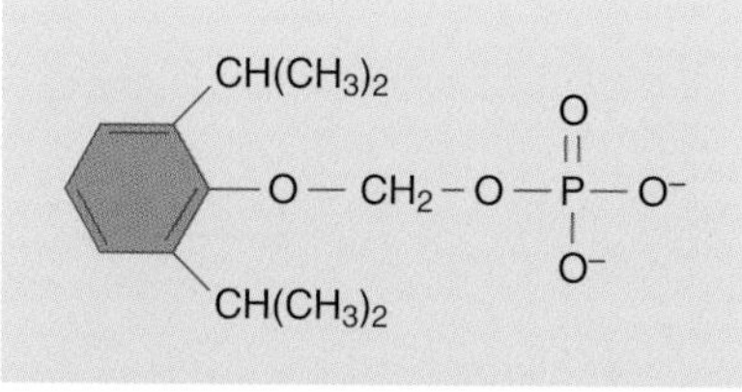

Figure 9-4 Structure of fospropofol.

Clinical Uses

Fospropofol is currently approved for sedation during monitored anesthesia care. Similar to propofol, the active metabolic product of fospropofol, airway compromise is a major concern during the use of fospropofol. Hence, it is recommended that fospropofol be administered only by personnel trained in airway management.

BARBITURATES

Before the introduction of propofol and its increasing use for induction of anesthesia, the intravenous anesthetics most commonly used for induction were barbiturates (thiopental, methohexital).[2,4]

Physicochemical Characteristics

Barbiturates are derived from barbituric acid (lacks hypnotic properties) through substitutions at the N1, C2, and C5 positions (Fig. 9-5). Based on their substitution at position 2, barbiturates used for induction of anesthesia can be grouped into thiobarbiturates, substituted with a sulfur (thiopental), or oxybarbiturates, substituted with an oxygen (methohexital). Hypnotic, sedative, and anticonvulsant effects, as well as lipid solubility and onset time, are determined by the type and position of substitution.

Thiopental and methohexital are formulated as sodium salts mixed with anhydrous sodium carbonate. After reconstitution with water or normal saline, the solutions (2.5% thiopental and 1% methohexital) are alkaline with a pH higher than 10. Although this property prevents bacterial growth and helps increase the shelf life of the solution after reconstitution, it will lead to precipitation when mixed with acidic drug preparations such as neuromuscular blocking drugs. These precipitates can irreversibly block intravenous delivery lines if mixing occurs during administration. Furthermore, accidental injection into an artery or infiltration into paravenous tissue will cause extreme pain and may lead to severe tissue injury.

Several barbiturates, including thiopental and methohexital, have optical isomers with different potencies. However, the available formulations are racemic mixtures, and their potencies reflect the summation of the potencies of the individual isomers.

Pharmacokinetics

Barbiturates, except for phenobarbital, undergo hepatic metabolism most importantly by oxidation, but also by N-dealkylation, desulfuration, and destruction of the barbituric acid ring structure. The resulting metabolites are inactive and excreted through urine and, after conjugation, through bile. In contrast, phenobarbital is mainly

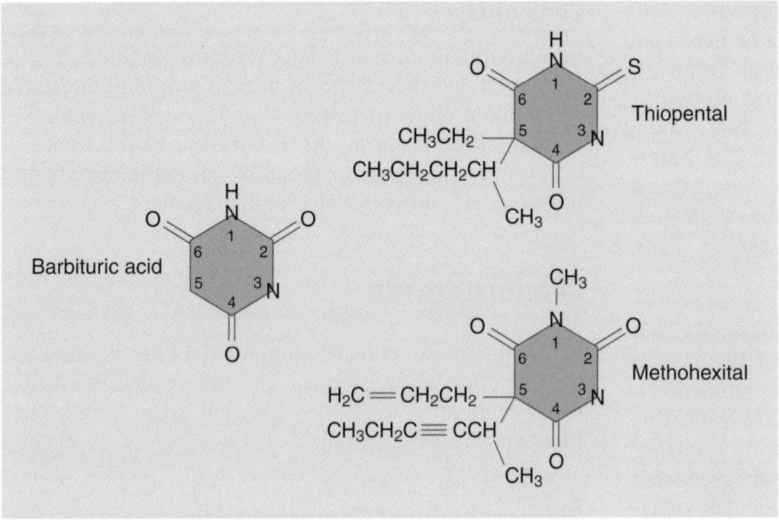

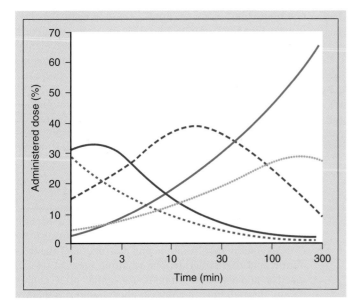

Figure 9-5 Structure of barbituric acid and its derivatives.

eliminated unchanged through renal excretion. Chronic administration of barbiturates or the administration of other drugs that induce oxidative microsomal enzymes (enzyme induction) enhances barbiturate metabolism. Through stimulation of aminolevulinic acid synthetase, the production of porphyrins is increased. Therefore, barbiturates should not be administered to patients with acute intermittent porphyria.

Methohexital is cleared more rapidly by the liver than thiopental is and thus has a shorter elimination half-time. This accounts for faster and more complete recovery after methohexital administration. Although thiopental is metabolized slowly and has a long elimination half-time, recovery after a single bolus administration is comparable to methohexital and propofol because it depends on redistribution to inactive tissue sites rather than

metabolism (Fig. 9-6).[16] However, even single-bolus induction doses of thiopental can, in some cases, lead to psychomotor impairment that lasts up to several hours. If administered as repeated boluses or as a continuous infusion, especially when using larger doses to produce burst suppression on the EEG, recovery from the effects of thiopental will be markedly prolonged because of the long context-sensitive half-time (see Fig. 9-3).

Pharmacodynamics

The mechanism of action for the effect of barbiturates in the CNS presumably involves both enhancement of inhibitory neurotransmission and inhibition of excitatory transmission. Although the effects on inhibitory transmission probably result from activation of the $GABA_A$

Figure 9-6 After rapid intravenous injection of thiopental, the percentage of the administered dose remaining in blood (*gold line*) rapidly decreases as the drug moves from blood to highly perfused vessel-rich tissues (*blue line*), especially the brain. Subsequently, thiopental is redistributed to skeletal muscles (*red line*) and, to a lesser extent, to fat (*pink line*). Ultimately, most of the administered dose of thiopental undergoes metabolism (*green line*). (From Saidman LJ. Uptake, distribution, and elimination of barbiturates. In Eger EI [ed]: Anesthetic Uptake and Action. Baltimore, Williams & Wilkins, 1974, pp 264-284, used with permission.)

receptor complex, the effects on excitatory transmission are less well understood.

CENTRAL NERVOUS SYSTEM

Barbiturates produce dose-dependent CNS depression ranging from sedation to general anesthesia when administered in induction doses.[4] They do not have analgesic properties may even reduce pain threshold, and thus could be classified as an antianalgesic. Barbiturates are potent cerebral vasoconstrictors and produce predictable decreases in CBF, cerebral blood volume, and ICP. As a result, they decrease $CMRO_2$ in a dose-dependent manner up to a maximum dose at which the EEG becomes flat-line. The ability of barbiturates to decrease ICP and $CMRO_2$ makes these drugs useful in the management of patients with space-occupying intracranial lesions (also see Chapter 30). Furthermore, they may provide neuroprotection from focal cerebral ischemia (stroke, surgical retraction, temporary clips during aneurysm surgery), but probably not from global cerebral ischemia (cardiac arrest). An exception to the generalization that barbiturates decrease electrical activity on the EEG is methohexital, which activates epileptic foci, thus facilitating their identification during surgery designed to ablate these sites. For the same reason, methohexital is also a popular choice for anesthesia to facilitate electroconvulsive therapy.

CARDIOVASCULAR SYSTEM

Administration of barbiturates for induction of anesthesia typically produces modest decreases in systemic blood pressure that are smaller than those produced by propofol. This decrease in systemic blood pressure is principally due to peripheral vasodilation and reflects barbiturate-induced depression of the medullary vasomotor center and decreased sympathetic nervous system outflow from the CNS. Although barbiturates blunt the baroreceptor reflex, compensatory increases in heart rate limit the decrease in blood pressure and make it transient. Moreover, dilation of peripheral capacitance vessels leads to pooling of blood and decreased venous return, thus resulting in the potential for reduced cardiac output and systemic blood pressure. Indeed, exaggerated decreases in systemic blood pressure are likely to follow the administration of barbiturates to patients with hypovolemia, cardiac tamponade, cardiomyopathy, coronary artery disease, or cardiac valvular disease because such patients are less able to compensate for the effects of peripheral vasodilation. Hemodynamic effects are also more pronounced with larger doses and rapid injection. The negative inotropic effects of barbiturates, which are readily demonstrated in isolated heart preparations, are usually masked in vivo by baroreceptor reflex-mediated responses.

RESPIRATORY SYSTEM

Barbiturates are respiratory depressants and lead to decreased minute ventilation through reduced tidal volumes and respiratory rate. Anesthetic induction doses of thiopental and methohexital typically induce transient apnea, which will be more pronounced if other respiratory depressants are also administered. Barbiturates also decrease the ventilatory responses to hypercapnia and hypoxia. Resumption of spontaneous breathing after an anesthetic induction dose of a barbiturate is characterized by a slow breathing rate and decreased tidal volume. Suppression of laryngeal reflexes and cough reflexes is not as profound as after propofol administration, which makes barbiturates an inferior choice for airway instrumentation in the absence of neuromuscular blocking drugs. Furthermore, stimulation of the upper airway or trachea (secretions, laryngeal mask airway, direct laryngoscopy, tracheal intubation) during inadequate depression of airway reflexes may result in laryngospasm or bronchospasm. This phenomenon is not unique to barbiturates but is true in general when the drug dose is inadequate to suppress the airway reflexes.

Side Effects

Accidental intra-arterial injection of barbiturates results in excruciating pain and intense vasoconstriction, often leading to severe tissue injury involving gangrene.[4] Aggressive therapy is directed at reversing the vasoconstriction to maintain perfusion and reduce the drug concentration mainly by dilution. Approaches to treatment include blockade of the sympathetic nervous system (stellate ganglion block) in the involved extremity. Barbiturate crystal formation probably results in the occlusion of more distal and small-diameter arteries and arterioles. Barbiturate crystal formation in veins is less hazardous because of the ever-increasing diameter of veins. Accidental subcutaneous injection (extravasation) of barbiturates results in local tissue irritation, thus emphasizing the importance of using dilute concentrations of barbiturates (2.5% thiopental, 1% methohexital). If extravasation occurs, some recommend local injection of the tissues with 0.5% lidocaine (5 to 10 mL) in an attempt to dilute the barbiturate concentration.

Life-threatening allergic reactions to barbiturates are rare, with an estimated occurrence of 1 in 30,000 patients. However, barbiturate-induced histamine release can occasionally be seen.

Clinical Uses

The principal clinical uses of barbiturates are rapid intravenous induction of anesthesia and treatment of increased ICP or to provide neuroprotection from focal cerebral ischemia.[4] A continuous intravenous infusion of a barbiturate such as thiopental is seldom used to maintain anesthesia because of its long context-sensitive half-time and prolonged recovery period (see Fig. 9-3).[9]

INDUCTION OF ANESTHESIA

Administration of thiopental (3 to 5 mg/kg IV) or methohexital (1 to 1.5 mg/kg IV) produces induction of anesthesia (unconsciousness) in less than 30 seconds. Patients may experience a garlic or onion taste during induction of anesthesia.

Succinylcholine or a nondepolarizing neuromuscular blocking drug is often administered shortly after the barbiturate to produce skeletal muscle relaxation and facilitate tracheal intubation. The combination of a barbiturate, usually thiopental, and succinylcholine administered intravenously in rapid succession is the classic drug regimen used for "rapid-sequence induction of anesthesia." An important advantage of rapid-sequence induction of anesthesia is avoidance of facemask ventilation and early tracheal intubation with a cuffed tube (provides protection against aspiration in at-risk patients). Although thiopental is the drug that has traditionally been used in this setting, propofol is also a frequent choice.

For patients who are not at increased risk for aspiration of gastric contents, an alternative approach to the rapid intravenous induction of anesthesia is the administration of small doses of barbiturates (thiopental, 0.5 to 1.0 mg/kg IV), followed by placement of the facemask on the patient's face and delivery of an inhaled anesthetic such as sevoflurane to complete the induction of anesthesia. The small dose of barbiturate improves patient acceptance of the facemask and negates any unpleasant memory of the pungency of the volatile anesthetic. This slow induction of anesthesia helps titrate the anesthetic effect more carefully and thereby avoids exaggerated hemodynamic responses. A slower induction with careful titration can also be accomplished by using only intravenous anesthetics, but propofol would probably be a more logical choice for this application because it has a shorter context-sensitive half-time (see Fig. 9-3).[9] Rectal administration of a barbiturate such as methohexital (20 to 30 mg/kg) may be used to facilitate induction of anesthesia in mentally challenged and uncooperative pediatric patients.

NEUROPROTECTION (Also See Chapter 30)

Traditionally, an isoelectric EEG indicating maximal reduction of $CMRO_2$ has been used as the end point for barbiturate administration with the goal of neuroprotection. More recent data demonstrating equal protection after smaller doses have challenged this practice.[4] One risk of the use of high-dose barbiturate therapy to decrease ICP or to provide protection against focal cerebral ischemia (cardiopulmonary bypass, carotid endarterectomy, thoracic aneurysm resection) is the associated hypotension, which could lead to critically reduced cerebral perfusion pressure and may require the administration of vasoconstrictors to maintain adequate perfusion pressure.

BENZODIAZEPINES

Benzodiazepines commonly used in the perioperative period include diazepam, midazolam, and lorazepam, as well as the selective benzodiazepine antagonist flumazenil.[1,5] Benzodiazepines are unique among the group of intravenous anesthetics in that their action can readily be terminated by administration of their selective antagonist flumazenil. Their most desired effects are anxiolysis and anterograde amnesia, which are extremely useful for premedication.

Physicochemical Characteristics

The chemical structure of the benzodiazepines contains a benzene ring fused to a seven-member diazepine ring, hence their name (Fig. 9-7). The three commonly used benzodiazepines in the perioperative setting are all highly lipophilic, with midazolam having the highest lipid solubility. All three drugs are highly protein bound, mainly to serum albumin. Although they are used as parenteral formulations, all three drugs are absorbed after oral administration. Other possible routes of administration include intramuscular, intranasal, and sublingual. Exposure of the acidic midazolam preparation to the physiologic pH

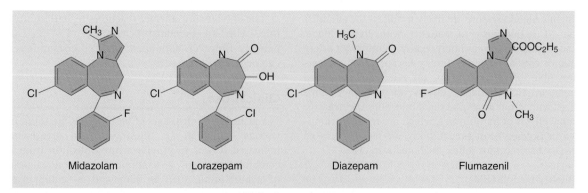

Figure 9-7 Chemical structure of the most commonly used benzodiazepines and their antagonist flumazenil.

of blood causes a change in the ring structure that renders the drug more lipid soluble, thus speeding its passage across the blood-brain barrier and its onset of action.

Pharmacokinetics

The highly lipid-soluble benzodiazepines rapidly enter the CNS, which accounts for their rapid onset of action, followed by redistribution to inactive tissue sites and subsequent termination of the drug effect (see Table 9-2). Metabolism of benzodiazepines occurs in the liver through microsomal oxidation (*N*-dealkylation and aliphatic hydroxylation) or glucuronide conjugation. Microsomal oxidation, the primary pathway for metabolism of midazolam and diazepam, is more susceptible to external factors such as age, diseases (hepatic cirrhosis), and the administration of other drugs that modulate the efficiency of the enzyme systems.

Diazepam undergoes hepatic metabolism to active metabolites (desmethyldiazepam and oxazepam) that may contribute to the prolonged effects of this drug. By contrast, midazolam is selectively metabolized by hepatic CYP4503A4 to a single dominant and inactive metabolite, 1-hydroxymidazolam. Furthermore, the short duration of action of a single dose of midazolam is due to its lipid solubility, which leads to rapid redistribution from the brain to inactive tissue sites. Despite its prompt passage into the brain, midazolam is considered to have a slower effect-site equilibration time than propofol and thiopental. In this regard, intravenous doses of midazolam should be sufficiently spaced to permit the peak clinical effect to be recognized before a repeat dose is considered.

The elimination half-time of diazepam greatly exceeds that of midazolam, thus suggesting that the CNS effects of diazepam are probably prolonged in comparison to midazolam, especially in elderly patients. Midazolam has the shortest context-sensitive half-time, which makes it the only one of the three benzodiazepine drugs suitable for continuous infusion (see Fig. 9-6).[9]

Pharmacodynamics

Benzodiazepines work through activation of the $GABA_A$ receptor complex and enhancement of GABA-mediated chloride currents, thereby leading to hyperpolarization of neurons and reduced excitability (Fig. 9-8).[17] There are specific binding sites for benzodiazepines on the γ-subunits of $GABA_A$ receptors, which explains why they were initially termed benzodiazepine receptors. Consistent with its greater potency, midazolam has an affinity for benzodiazepine receptors that is approximately twice that of diazepam.

GABA receptors that are responsive to benzodiazepines occur almost exclusively on postsynaptic nerve endings in the CNS, with the greatest density being in the cerebral cortex. The anatomic distribution of $GABA_A$ receptors (restricted to the CNS) is consistent with the

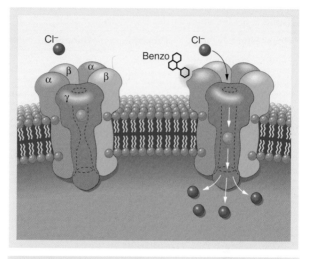

Figure 9-8 Schematic depiction of the γ-aminobutyric acid (GABA) receptor forming a chloride ion channel. Benzodiazepines (Benzo) attach selectively to α-subunits and are presumed to facilitate the action of the inhibitory neurotransmitter GABA on the α-subunits. (From Mohler H, Richards JG. The benzodiazepine receptor: A pharmacological control element of brain function. Eur J Anesthesiol Suppl 1988;2:15-24, used with permission.)

minimal effects of these drugs outside the CNS. Indeed, the magnitude of depression of ventilation and the development of hypotension after the administration of benzodiazepines are lower than that observed when barbiturates are used for induction of anesthesia (Table 9-3).

SPECTRUM OF EFFECTS

The wide spectrum of effects of benzodiazepines is similar for all drugs in this class, although potencies for individual effects may vary between drugs.[5] The most important effects of benzodiazepines are their sedative-hypnotic action and their amnestic properties (anterograde amnesia). In addition, benzodiazepines function as anticonvulsants and are used to treat seizures. These effects are mediated through the α_1-subunits of the GABA receptor, whereas anxiolysis and muscle relaxation are mediated through the γ-subunits. The site of action for muscle relaxation is in the spinal cord, and it requires much higher doses than the other effects do.

SAFETY PROFILE

Benzodiazepines have a very favorable side effect profile and, when administered alone, cause only minimal depression of ventilation and the cardiovascular system, which makes them relatively safe even in larger doses. Furthermore, the CNS effects of benzodiazepines can be antagonized by the selective benzodiazepine antagonist, flumazenil.

CENTRAL NERVOUS SYSTEM (Also See Chapter 30)

Like propofol and barbiturates, benzodiazepines decrease $CMRO_2$ and CBF, but to a smaller extent. In contrast to

Table 9-3 Summary of the Pharmacodynamic Effects of Commonly Used Intravenous Anesthetics

Dose/Effect	Propofol	Thiopental	Midazolam	Ketamine	Etomidate	Dexmedetomidine
Dose for induction of anesthesia (mg/kg IV)	1.5-2.5	3-5	0.1-0.3	1-2	0.2-0.3	
Systemic blood pressure	Decreased	Decreased	Unchanged to decreased	Increased	Decreased	Decreased
Heart rate	Unchanged to decreased	Increased	Unchanged	Increased	Unchanged to increased	Decreased
Systemic vascular resistance	Decreased	Decreased	Unchanged to decreased	Increased	Unchanged to decreased	Decreased
Ventilation	Decreased	Decreased	Unchanged	Unchanged	Unchanged to decreased	Unchanged
Respiratory rate	Decreased	Decreased	Unchanged	Unchanged	Unchanged to decreased	Unchanged
Response to carbon dioxide	Decreased	Decreased	Unchanged	Unchanged	Decreased	Unchanged
Cerebral blood flow	Decreased	Decreased	Unchanged	Increased to unchanged	Decreased	Unchanged
Cerebral metabolic requirements for oxygen	Decreased	Decreased	Unchanged	Increased to unchanged	Decreased	Unchanged to decreased
Intracranial pressure	Decreased	Decreased	Unchanged	Unchanged to increased	Decreased	Unchanged
Anticonvulsant	Unclear	Yes	Yes	Unclear	No	
Anxiolysis	No	No	Yes	No	No	Yes?
Analgesia	No	No	No	Yes	No	No?
Emergence delirium	No?	No	No	Yes	No	No
Nausea and vomiting	Decreased	Unchanged	Unchanged to decreased	Unchanged	Increased	Unchanged
Adrenocortical suppression	No	No	Yes?	No	Yes	No
Pain on injection	Yes	No	No	No	No	No

IV, intravenous.

propofol and thiopental, midazolam is unable to produce an isoelectric EEG, thus emphasizing that there is a ceiling effect on benzodiazepine-induced decreases in $CMRO_2$. Patients with decreased intracranial compliance demonstrate little or no change in ICP after the administration of midazolam. Benzodiazepines have not been shown to possess neuroprotective properties. They are potent anticonvulsants for the treatment of status epilepticus, alcohol withdrawal, and local anesthetic-induced seizures.

CARDIOVASCULAR SYSTEM
Midazolam, as used for induction of anesthesia, produces a larger decrease in arterial blood pressure than that of diazepam. These changes are most likely due to peripheral vasodilatation in as much as cardiac output is not changed. Midazolam-induced hypotension is more likely in hypovolemic patients.

RESPIRATORY SYSTEM
Benzodiazepines produce minimal depression of ventilation, although transient apnea may follow rapid intravenous administration of midazolam for induction of anesthesia, especially in the presence of opioid premedication. Benzodiazepines decrease the ventilatory response to carbon dioxide, but this effect is not usually significant if they are administered alone. More severe respiratory depression can occur when benzodiazepines are administered together with opioids.[1,18]

Side Effects

Allergic reactions to benzodiazepines are extremely rare to nonexistent. Pain during intravenous injection and subsequent thrombophlebitis are most pronounced with diazepam and reflect the poor water solubility of this benzodiazepine. It is the organic solvent, propylene glycol, required to dissolve diazepam that is most likely responsible for pain during intramuscular or intravenous administration, as well as for the unpredictable absorption after intramuscular injection. Midazolam is more water soluble (but only at low pH), thus obviating the need for an organic solvent and decreasing the likelihood of exaggerated pain or erratic absorption after intramuscular injection or pain during intravenous administration.

Clinical Uses

Benzodiazepines are used for (1) preoperative medication, (2) intravenous sedation, (3) intravenous induction of anesthesia, and (4) suppression of seizure activity. The slow onset and prolonged duration of action of lorazepam limit its usefulness for preoperative medication or induction of anesthesia, especially when rapid and sustained awakening at the end of surgery is desirable. Flumazenil (8 to 15 µg/kg IV) may be useful for treating patients experiencing delayed awakening, but its duration of action is brief (about 20 minutes) and resedation may occur.

PREOPERATIVE MEDICATION AND SEDATION (Also See Chapter 13)

The amnestic, anxiolytic, and sedative effects of benzodiazepines are the basis for the use of these drugs for preoperative medication. Midazolam (1 to 2 mg IV) is effective for premedication, sedation during regional anesthesia, and brief therapeutic procedures.[5,19] When compared with diazepam, midazolam produces a more rapid onset, with more intense amnesia and less postoperative sedation. Midazolam is commonly used for oral premedication for children. For example, 0.5 mg/kg administered orally 30 minutes before induction of anesthesia provides reliable sedation and anxiolysis in children without producing delayed awakening.[20]

The synergistic effects between benzodiazepines and other drugs, especially opioids and propofol, facilitate better sedation and analgesia. However, the combination of these drugs also enhances their respiratory depression and may lead to airway obstruction or apnea.[18] Benzodiazepine effects, as well as its synergistic effects, are more pronounced in the elderly (see Chapter 35) so smaller doses and careful titration may be necessary.

INDUCTION OF ANESTHESIA

Although rarely used for this purpose, general anesthesia can be induced by the administration of midazolam (0.1 to 0.3 mg/kg IV). The onset of unconsciousness, however, is slower than after the administration of thiopental, propofol, or etomidate. Onset of unconsciousness is facilitated when a small dose of opioid (fentanyl, 50 to 100 µg IV) is injected 1 to 3 minutes before midazolam is administered. Despite the possible production of lesser circulatory effects, it is unlikely that the use of midazolam or diazepam for induction of anesthesia offers any advantages over barbiturates or propofol. Delayed awakening is a potential disadvantage of administering a benzodiazepine for induction of anesthesia.

SUPPRESSION OF SEIZURE ACTIVITY

The efficacy of benzodiazepines, especially diazepam, as anticonvulsants is consistent with the ability of these drugs to enhance the inhibitory effects of GABA, particularly in the limbic system. Indeed, diazepam (0.1 mg/kg IV) is often effective in abolishing seizure activity produced by local anesthetics, alcohol withdrawal, and status epilepticus.

KETAMINE

Ketamine, a phencyclidine derivative introduced into clinical use in 1965, is different from most other intravenous anesthetics in that it produces significant analgesia.[2,3] The characteristic cataleptic state observed after an induction dose of ketamine is known as "dissociative anesthesia," wherein the patient's eyes remain open with a slow nystagmic gaze (cataleptic state).

Physicochemical Characteristics

Ketamine is a partially water-soluble and highly lipid-soluble derivative of phencyclidine (Fig. 9-9). It is between 5 and 10 times more lipid soluble than thiopental. Of the two stereoisomers the S-(+) form is more potent than the R-(−) isomer. Only the racemic mixture of ketamine (10, 50, 100 mg/mL) is available in the United States.

The use of ketamine has always been limited by its unpleasant psychomimetic side effects, but its unique features make it a very valuable alternative in certain settings, mostly because of the potent analgesia with minimal respiratory depression. Most recently it has become popular as an adjunct administered at subanalgesic doses to limit or reverse opioid tolerance.

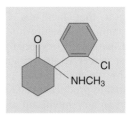

Figure 9-9 Chemical structure of ketamine.

Pharmacokinetics

The high lipid solubility of ketamine ensures a rapid onset of the drug's effect. Like other intravenous induction drugs, the effect of a single bolus injection is terminated by redistribution to inactive tissue sites. Metabolism occurs primarily in the liver and involves N-demethylation by the cytochrome P-450 system. Norketamine, the primary active metabolite, is less potent (one third to one fifth the potency of ketamine) and is subsequently hydroxylated and conjugated into water-soluble inactive metabolites that are excreted in urine. Ketamine is the only intravenous anesthetic that has low protein binding (12%) (see Table 9-2).

Pharmacodynamics

The mechanism of action of ketamine is complex, but the major effect is probably produced through inhibition of the N-methyl-D-aspartate receptor complex.[21] If ketamine is administered as the sole anesthetic, amnesia is not as complete as with the administration of a benzodiazepine. Reflexes are often preserved, but it cannot be assumed that patients are able to protect their upper airway. The eyes remain open and the pupils are moderately dilated with a nystagmic gaze. Frequently, lacrimation and salivation are increased, and premedication with an anticholinergic drug may be indicated to limit this effect (see Table 9-3).

EMERGENCE REACTIONS

The unpleasant emergence reactions after ketamine administration are the main factor limiting its use. Such reactions may include vivid colorful dreams, hallucinations, out-of-body experiences, and increased and distorted visual, tactile, and auditory sensitivity. These reactions can be associated with fear and confusion, but a euphoric state may also be induced, which explains the potential for abuse of the drug. Children usually have a lesser incidence of severe emergence reactions. Combination with a benzodiazepine may be indicated to limit the unpleasant emergence reactions and also increase amnesia.

CENTRAL NERVOUS SYSTEM (Also See Chapter 30)

In contrast to the intravenous anesthetics, ketamine is a cerebral vasodilator that increases CBF, as well as $CMRO_2$. Thus, ketamine is usually not used in patients with intracranial pathology, especially increased ICP. Nevertheless, these perceived undesirable effects on CBF may be blunted by the maintenance of normocapnia.[22] Despite the potential to produce myoclonic activity, ketamine is considered an anticonvulsant and may be recommended as treatment of status epilepticus when more conventional drugs are ineffective.

CARDIOVASCULAR SYSTEM

Ketamine can produce significant, but transient increases in systemic blood pressure, heart rate, and cardiac output, presumably by centrally mediated sympathetic stimulation. These effects, which are associated with increased cardiac work and myocardial oxygen consumption, are not always desirable and can be blunted by coadministration of benzodiazepines, opioids, or inhaled anesthetics. Though more controversial, ketamine is a direct myocardial depressant. This property is usually masked by its stimulation of the sympathetic nervous system, but it may become apparent in critically ill patients with limited ability to increase their sympathetic nervous system activity.

RESPIRATORY SYSTEM

Ketamine does not produce significant respiratory depression. When used as a single drug, the respiratory response to hypercapnia is preserved and analysis of arterial blood gases remain stable. Transient hypoventilation and, in rare cases, a short period of apnea can follow rapid administration of large intravenous doses for induction of anesthesia. The ability to protect the upper airway in the presence of ketamine cannot be assumed despite the presence of active airway reflexes. Especially in children, the risk for laryngospasm because of increased salivation is increased and can be reduced by premedication with an anticholinergic drug. Ketamine relaxes bronchial smooth muscles and may be helpful in patients with reactive airways and in the management of patients experiencing bronchoconstriction.

Clinical Uses

The unpleasant emergence reactions after the administration of ketamine have restricted its use in the perioperative period.[23] Nevertheless, ketamine's unique properties, including profound analgesia, stimulation of the sympathetic nervous system, bronchodilation, and minimal respiratory depression, make it an important alternative to the other intravenous anesthetics and a desirable adjunct in many cases. Moreover, ketamine can be administered by multiple routes (intravenous, intramuscular, oral, rectal, epidural), thus making it a useful option for premedication in mentally challenged and uncooperative pediatric patients (also see Chapter 34).

INDUCTION AND MAINTENANCE OF ANESTHESIA

Induction of anesthesia can be achieved with ketamine, 1 to 2 mg/kg intravenously or 4 to 6 mg/kg intramuscularly. Though not commonly used for maintenance of anesthesia, the short context-sensitive half-time makes ketamine a consideration for this purpose (see Fig. 9-3).[9] For example, general anesthesia can be achieved with the infusion of ketamine, 15 to 45 µg/kg/min, plus 50% to 70% nitrous oxide or by ketamine alone, 30 to 90 µg/kg/min.

ANALGESIA

Small bolus doses of ketamine (0.2 to 0.8 mg/kg IV) may be useful during regional anesthesia when additional analgesia is needed (cesarean section under neuraxial anesthesia with an insufficient regional block). Ketamine provides effective analgesia without compromise of the airway. An infusion of a subanalgesic dose of ketamine (3 to 5 µg/kg/min) during general anesthesia and in the early postoperative period may be useful to produce analgesia or reduce opioid tolerance and opioid-induced hyperalgesia.[24]

ETOMIDATE

Etomidate is an intravenous anesthetic with hypnotic but not analgesic properties and with minimal hemodynamic effects.[2,3,7] The pharmacokinetics of etomidate makes it suitable for use as a continuous infusion, but mainly because of its endocrine side effects it is not more widely used.

Physicochemical Characteristics

Etomidate is a carboxylated imidazole derivative that has two optical isomers (Fig. 9-10). The available preparation contains only the active D-(+) isomer, which has hypnotic properties. The drug is poorly soluble in water and is therefore supplied as a 2-mg/mL solution in 35% propylene glycol. The solution has a pH of 6.9 and thus does not cause problems with precipitation like thiopental does.

Pharmacokinetics

An induction dose of etomidate produces rapid onset of anesthesia, and recovery depends on redistribution to inactive tissue sites, comparable to thiopental and propofol. Metabolism is primarily by ester hydrolysis to inactive metabolites, which are then excreted in urine (78%) and bile (22%). Less than 3% of an administered dose of etomidate is excreted as unchanged drug in urine.

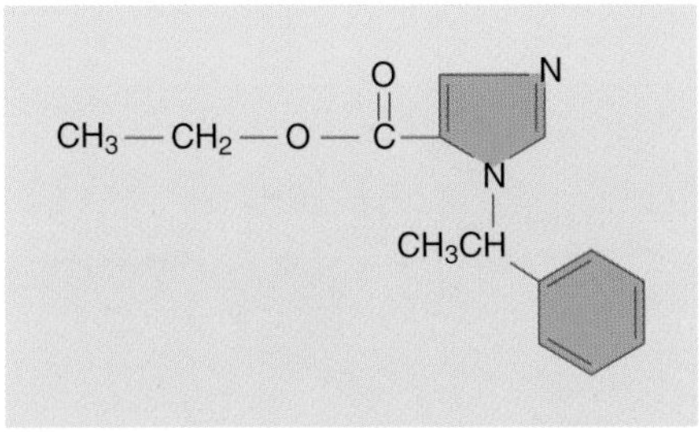

Figure 9-10 Chemical structure of etomidate.

Clearance of etomidate is about five times that for thiopental, as reflected by a shorter elimination half-time (see Table 9-2). The duration of action is linearly related to the dose, with each 0.1 mg/kg providing about 100 seconds of unconsciousness. Because of its minimal effects on hemodynamics and short context-sensitive half-time, larger doses, repeated boluses, or continuous infusions can safely be administered (see Fig. 9-3).[9] Etomidate, like most other intravenous anesthetics, is highly protein bound (77%), primarily to albumin.

Pharmacodynamics

Etomidate has GABA-like effects and seems to primarily act through potentiation of $GABA_A$-mediated chloride currents, like most other intravenous anesthetics.[7]

CENTRAL NERVOUS SYSTEM (Also See Chapter 30)

Etomidate is a potent cerebral vasoconstrictor, as reflected by decreases in CBF and ICP. These effects of etomidate are similar to those produced by comparable doses of thiopental. Despite its reduction of $CMRO_2$, etomidate failed to show neuroprotective properties in animal studies, and human studies are lacking. Excitatory spikes on the EEG are more frequent after etomidate than from thiopental. Similar to methohexital, etomidate may activate seizure foci, manifested as fast activity on the EEG. In addition, spontaneous movements characterized as myoclonus occur in more than 50% of patients receiving etomidate, and this myoclonic activity may be associated with seizure-like activity on the EEG.

CARDIOVASCULAR SYSTEM

A characteristic and desired feature of induction of anesthesia with etomidate is cardiovascular stability after bolus injection.[7] In this regard, arterial blood pressure decreases are modest or absent and principally reflect decreases in systemic vascular resistance. Therefore, the systemic blood pressure-lowering effects of etomidate are probably exaggerated in the presence of hypovolemia. Etomidate produces minimal changes in heart rate and cardiac output. The depressive effects of etomidate on myocardial contractility are minimal at concentrations used for induction of anesthesia.

RESPIRATORY SYSTEM

The depressant effects of etomidate on ventilation are less pronounced than those of barbiturates, although apnea may occasionally follow rapid intravenous injection of the drug. Depression of ventilation may be exaggerated when etomidate is combined with inhaled anesthetics or opioids.

ENDOCRINE SYSTEM

Etomidate causes adrenocortical suppression by producing a dose-dependent inhibition of 11β-hydroxylase, an enzyme necessary for the conversion of cholesterol to

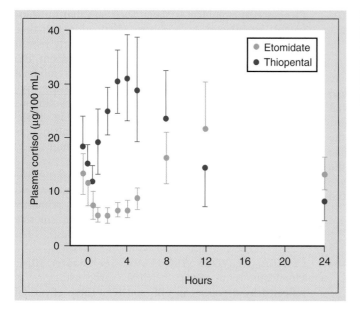

Figure 9-11 Etomidate, but not thiopental, is associated with decreases in the plasma concentrations of cortisol. *$P < 0.005$ versus thiopental, mean ± SD. (From Fragen RT, Shanks CA, Molteni A, et al. Effects of etomidate on hormonal responses to surgical stress. Anesthesiology 1984;61:652-656, used with permission.)

cortisol (Fig. 9-11).[25] This suppression lasts 4 to 8 hours after an induction dose of etomidate. Yet, no adverse effect on outcome has been described.

Clinical Uses

Etomidate is an alternative to propofol and barbiturates for the rapid intravenous induction of anesthesia, especially in patients with compromised myocardial contractility. After a standard induction dose (0.2 to 0.3 mg/kg IV), the onset of unconsciousness is comparable to that achieved by thiopental and propofol. There is a frequent incidence of pain during intravenous injection of etomidate, which may be followed by venous irritation. Involuntary myoclonic movements are common but may be masked by the concomitant administration of neuromuscular blocking drugs. Awakening after a single intravenous dose of etomidate is rapid, with little evidence of any residual depressant effects. Etomidate does not produce analgesia, and postoperative nausea and vomiting may be more common than after the administration of thiopental or propofol. The principal limiting factor in the clinical use of etomidate for induction of anesthesia is its ability to transiently depress adrenocortical function.[25] Theoretically, this suppression may be either desirable for stress-free anesthesia or undesirable if it prevents useful protective responses against stresses that accompany the perioperative period.

DEXMEDETOMIDINE

Dexmedetomidine is a highly selective α_2-adrenergic agonist.[26] Recognition of the usefulness of α_2-agonists is based on observations of decreased anesthetic requirements in patients receiving chronic clonidine therapy. The effects of dexmedetomidine can be antagonized with α_2-antagonist drugs.

Physicochemical Characteristics

Dexmedetomidine is the active S-enantiomer of medetomidine, a highly selective α_2-adrenergic agonist and imidazole derivative that is used in veterinary medicine. Dexmedetomidine is water soluble and available as a parenteral formulation (Fig. 9-12).

Pharmacokinetics

Dexmedetomidine undergoes rapid hepatic metabolism involving conjugation, N-methylation, and hydroxylation, followed by conjugation. Metabolites are excreted through urine and bile. Clearance is high, and the elimination half-time is short (see Table 9-2). However, there is a significant increase in the context-sensitive half-time from 4 minutes after a 10-minute infusion to 250 minutes after an 8-hour infusion.

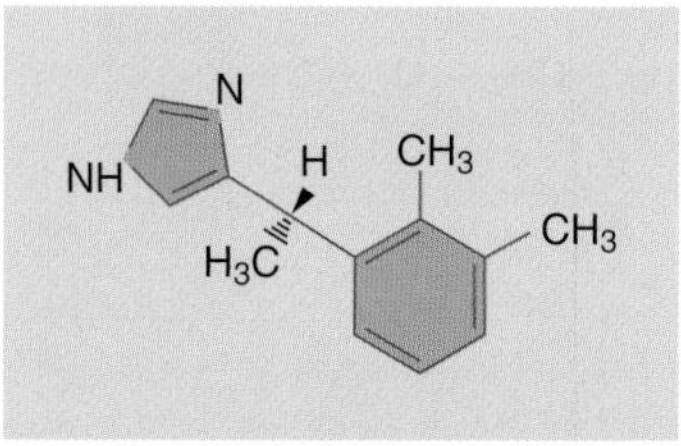

Figure 9-12 Chemical structure of dexmedetomidine.

Pharmacodynamics

Dexmedetomidine produces its selective α_2-agonist effects through activation of CNS α_2-receptors. Hypnosis presumably results from stimulation of α_2-receptors in the locus ceruleus, and the analgesic effect originates at the level of the spinal cord. The sedative effect produced by dexmedetomidine has a different quality than that produced by other intravenous anesthetics in that it more resembles a physiologic sleep state through activation of endogenous sleep pathways. Dexmedetomidine decreases in CBF without significant changes in ICP and $CMRO_2$ (see Table 9-3). Tolerance and dependence can occur.

CARDIOVASCULAR SYSTEM

Dexmedetomidine infusion produces moderate decreases in heart rate and systemic vascular resistance and, consequently, decreases in systemic blood pressure. A bolus injection may produce transient increases in systemic blood pressure and pronounced decreases in heart rate, an effect that is probably mediated through activation of peripheral α_2-adrenergic receptors. Bradycardia associated with dexmedetomidine infusion may require treatment. Heart block, severe bradycardia, or asystole may result from unopposed vagal stimulation. The response to anticholinergic drugs is unchanged.

RESPIRATORY SYSTEM

The effects of dexmedetomidine on the respiratory system are a small to moderate decrease in tidal volume and very little change in the respiratory rate. The ventilatory response to carbon dioxide is unchanged. Although the respiratory effects are mild, upper airway obstruction as a result of sedation is possible. In addition, dexmedetomidine has a synergistic sedative effect when combined with other sedative-hypnotics.

Clinical Uses

Dexmedetomidine is principally used for the short-term sedation of tracheally intubated and mechanically ventilated patients in an intensive care setting.[26] In the operating room, dexmedetomidine may be used as an adjunct to general anesthesia or to provide sedation as during awake fiberoptic tracheal intubation or during regional anesthesia. When administered during general anesthesia, dexmedetomidine (0.5- to 1-µg/kg initial dose over a period of 10 to 15 minutes, followed by an infusion of 0.2 to 0.7 µg/kg/hour) decreases the dose requirements for inhaled and injected anesthetics. Awakening and the transition to the postoperative setting may benefit from dexmedetomidine-produced sedative and analgesic effects without respiratory depression.

QUESTIONS OF THE DAY

1. What are the effects of propofol on the cardiovascular system?
2. What are the major differences in the pharmacology of fospropofol versus propofol?
3. How do barbiturates affect cerebral blood flow (CBF) and cerebral metabolic rate for oxygen ($CMRO_2$)
4. What is the effect of benzodiazepines on minute ventilation and the ventilatory response to carbon dioxide?
5. How does ketamine affect CBF and $CMRO_2$?
6. What are the hemodynamic effects of dexmedetomidine when given by bolus or continuous infusion?

REFERENCES

1. Olkkola KT, Ahonen J: Midazolam and other benzodiazepines, *Handb Exp Pharmacol* 182:335–360, 2008.
2. Reves JG, Glass PSA, Lubarsky DA, et al: Intravenous nonopioid anesthetics. In Miller RD, editor: *Miller's Anesthesia*, ed 6, Philadelphia, 2005, Churchill Livingstone, pp 317–378.
3. Stoelting RK, Hillier SC: Nonbarbiturate intravenous anesthetic drugs. In Stoelting RK, Hillier SC, editors: *Pharmacology and Physiology in Anesthetic Practice*, ed 4, Philadelphia, 2006, Lippincott Williams & Wilkins, pp 155–178.
4. Stoelting RK, Hillier SC: Barbiturates. In Stoelting RK, Hillier SC, editors: *Pharmacology and Physiology in Anesthetic Practice*, ed 4, Philadelphia, 2006, Lippincott Williams & Wilkins, pp 127–139.
5. Stoelting RK, Hillier SC: Benzodiazepines. In Stoelting RK, Hillier SC, editors: *Pharmacology and Physiology in Anesthetic Practice*, ed 4, Philadelphia, 2006, Lippincott Williams & Wilkins, pp 140–154.
6. Vanlersberghe C, Camu F: Propofol, *Handb Exp Pharmacol* 182:227–252, 2008.
7. Vanlersberghe C, Camu F: Etomidate and other non-barbiturates, *Handb Exp Pharmacol* 182:267–282, 2008.
8. Glass PS: Half-time or half-life: What matters for recovery from intravenous anesthesia? *Anesthesiology* 112:1266–1269, 2010.
9. Hughes MA, Glass PS, Jacobs JR: Context-sensitive half-time in multicompartment pharmacokinetic models for intravenous anesthetic drugs, *Anesthesiology* 76:334–341, 1992.
10. Franks NP: Molecular targets underlying general anaesthesia, *Br J Pharmacol* 147(Suppl 1):S72–S81, 2006.
11. Tramer MR, Moore RA, McQuay HJ: Propofol and bradycardia: causation, frequency and severity, *Br J Anaesth* 78:642–651, 1997.
12. Eames WO, Rooke GA, Wu RS, et al: Comparison of the effects of etomidate, propofol, and thiopental on respiratory resistance after tracheal intubation, *Anesthesiology* 84:1307–1311, 1996.
13. Burow BK, Johnson ME, Packer DL: Metabolic acidosis associated with propofol in the absence of other causative factors, *Anesthesiology* 101:239–241, 2004.
14. Fechner J, Ihmsen H, Jeleazcov C, et al: Fospropofol disodium, a water-soluble prodrug of the intravenous anesthetic propofol (2,6-diisopropylphenol),

Expert Opin Investig Drugs 18:1565–1571, 2009.

15. Struys MM, Fechner J, Schuttler J, et al: Erroneously published fospropofol pharmacokinetic-pharmacodynamic data and retraction of the affected publications, *Anesthesiology* 112:1056–1057, 2010.

16. Saidman L: Uptake, distribution, and elimination of barbiturates. In Eger EI, editor: *Anesthetic uptake and action*, Baltimore, 1974, Williams & Wilkins, pp 264–284.

17. Mohler H, Richards JG: The benzodiazepine receptor: A pharmacological control element of brain function, *Eur J Anaesthesiol Suppl* 2:15–24, 1988.

18. Bailey PL, Pace NL, Ashburn MA, et al: Frequent hypoxemia and apnea after sedation with midazolam and fentanyl, *Anesthesiology* 73:826–830, 1990.

19. Reves JG, Fragen RJ, Vinik HR, et al: Midazolam: Pharmacology and uses, *Anesthesiology* 62:310–324, 1985.

20. Cote CJ, Cohen IT, Suresh S, et al: A comparison of three doses of a commercially prepared oral midazolam syrup in children, *Anesth Analg* 94:37–43, 2002.

21. Franks NP: General anaesthesia: from molecular targets to neuronal pathways of sleep and arousal, *Nat Rev Neurosci* 9:370–386, 2008.

22. Albanese J, Arnaud S, Rey M, et al: Ketamine decreases intracranial pressure and electroencephalographic activity in traumatic brain injury patients during propofol sedation, *Anesthesiology* 87:1328–1334, 1997.

23. Kohrs R, Durieux ME: Ketamine: Teaching an old drug new tricks, *Anesth Analg* 87:1186–1193, 1998.

24. Himmelseher S, Durieux ME: Ketamine for perioperative pain management, *Anesthesiology* 102:211–220, 2005.

25. Fragen RJ, Shanks CA, Molteni A, et al: Effects of etomidate on hormonal responses to surgical stress, *Anesthesiology* 61:652–656, 1984.

26. Kamibayashi T, Maze M: Clinical uses of alpha$_2$-adrenergic agonists, *Anesthesiology* 93:1345–1349, 2000.

10 OPIOIDS

Talmage D. Egan

Opioids play an indispensible role in the practice of anesthesiology, critical care, and pain management. A sound understanding of opioid pharmacology, including both basic science and clinical aspects, is critical for the safe and effective use of these important drugs. This chapter will focus almost exclusively on intravenous opioid receptor agonists used perioperatively.

BASIC PHARMACOLOGY

Structure-Activity

The opioids of clinical interest in anesthesiology share many structural features. Morphine is a benzylisoquinoline alkaloid (Fig. 10-1). Many commonly used semisynthetic opioids are created by simple modification of the morphine molecule. Codeine, for example, is the 3-methyl derivative of morphine. Similarly, hydromorphone, hydrocodone, and oxycodone are also synthesized by relatively simple modifications of morphine. More complex alteration of the morphine molecular skeleton results in mixed agonist-antagonists such as nalbuphine and even complete antagonists such as naloxone.

The fentanyl series of opioids are chemically related to meperidine. Meperidine is the first completely synthetic opioid and can be regarded as the prototype clinical phenylpiperidine (see Fig 10-1). Fentanyl is a simple modification of the basic phenylpiperidine structure. Other commonly used fentanyl congeners such as alfentanil and sufentanil are somewhat more complex versions of the same phenylpiperidine skeleton.

Opioids share many physicochemical features in common, although some individual drugs have unique features (Table 10-1). In general, opioids are highly soluble weak bases that are highly protein bound and largely ionized at physiologic pH. Opioid physicochemical properties influence their clinical behavior. For example, relatively unbound, un-ionized molecules such as alfentanil and remifentanil have a shorter latency to peak effect after bolus injection.

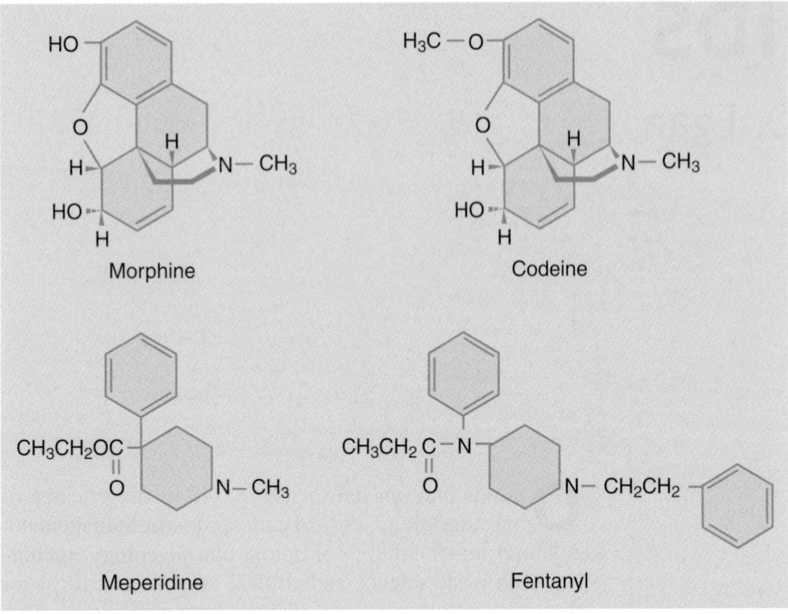

Figure 10-1 The molecular structures of morphine, codeine, meperidine and fentanyl. Note that codeine is a simple modification of morphine (as are many other opiates); fentanyl and its congeners are more complex modifications of meperidine, a phenylpiperidine derivative.

Table 10-1 Selected Opioid Physicochemical and Pharmacokinetic Parameters

	Morphine	Fentanyl	Sufentanil	Alfentanil	Remifentanil
pKa	8.0	8.4	8.0	6.5	7.1
% un-ionized at pH 7.4	23	<10	20	90	67?
Octanol-H_2O partition coefficient	1.4	813	1778	145	17.9
% bound to plasma protein	20-40	84	93	92	80
Diffusible fraction (%)	16.8	1.5	1.6	8.0	13.3
Vdc (L/kg)	0.1-0.4	0.4-1.0	0.2	0.1-0.3	0.06-0.08
Vdss (L/kg)	3-5	3-5	2.5-3.0	0.4-1.0	0.2-0.3
Clearance (mL/min/kg)	15-30	10-20	10-15	4-9	30-40
Hepatic extraction ratio	0.6-0.8	0.8-1.0	0.7-0.9	0.3-0.5	NA

NA, not applicable; Vdc, volume of distribution of central compartment; Vdss, volume of distribution at steady state.
From Bailey PL. Egan TD. Stanley TH. Intravenous opioid anesthetics. In Miller RD (ed). Anesthesia. 7th ed. Philadelphia, Churchill Livingstone, 2010, p. 791.

Mechanism

Opioids produce their main pharmacologic effects by interacting with opioid receptors, which are typical of the G protein–coupled family of receptors widely found in biology (e.g., β-adrenergic, dopaminergic, among others). Expression of cloned opioid receptors in cultured cells has facilitated analysis of the intracellular signal transduction mechanisms activated by the opioid receptors.[1] Binding of opioid agonists with the receptors leads to activation of the G protein, producing effects that are primarily inhibitory (Fig. 10-2); these effects ultimately culminate in hyperpolarization of the cell and reduction of neuronal excitability.

Three classical opioid receptors have been identified using molecular biology techniques: mu, kappa, and delta. More recently, a fourth opioid receptor, ORL1 (also known as NOP), has also been identified, although its function is quite different from that of the classical opioid receptors. Each of these opioid receptors has a commonly employed experimental bioassay, associated endogenous ligand(s), a set of agonists and antagonists and a spectrum of physiologic effects when the receptor is agonized (Table 10-2). Although the existence of opioid receptor subtypes (e.g., mu-1, mu-2, etc.) has been proposed, it is not clear from molecular biology techniques that distinct genes code for them. Post-translational

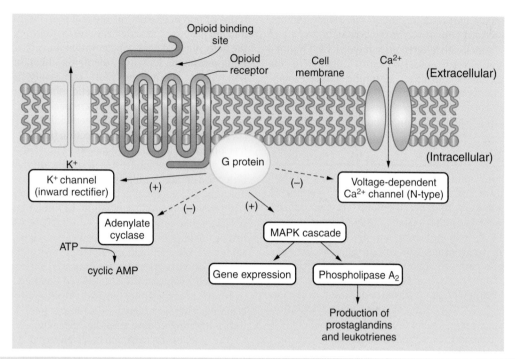

Figure 10-2 Opioid mechanisms of action. The endogenous ligand or drug binds to the opioid receptor and activates the G protein, resulting in multiple effects that are primarily inhibitory. The activities of adenylate cyclase and the voltage dependent Ca^{2+} channels are depressed. The inwardly rectifying K^+ channels and mitogen activated protein kinase (MAPK) cascade are activated. AMP, adenosine monophosphate; ATP, adenosine triphosphate.

Table 10-2 A Summary of Selected Features of Opioid Receptors

	Mu (μ)	Delta (δ)	Kappa (κ)
Tissue bioassay*	Guinea pig ileum	Mouse vas deferens	Rabbit vas deferens
Endogenous ligand	β-Endorphin Endomorphin	Leu-enkephalin Met-enkephalin	Dynorphin
Agonist prototype	Morphine Fentanyl	Deltorphin	Buprenorphine Pentazocine
Antagonist prototype	Naloxone	Naloxone	Naloxone
Supraspinal analgesia	Yes	Yes	Yes
Spinal analgesia	Yes	Yes	Yes
Ventilatory depression	Yes	No	No
Gastrointestinal effects	Yes	No	Yes
Sedation	Yes	No	Yes

*Traditional experimental method to assess opioid receptor activity in vivo.
From Bailey PL. Egan TD. Stanley TH. Intravenous opioid anesthetics. In Miller RD (ed). Anesthesia. 5th ed. New York, Churchill Livingstone, 2000, p 312.

modification of opioid receptors certainly occurs and may be responsible for conflicting data regarding opioid receptor subtypes.[2]

Opioids exert their therapeutic effects at multiple sites. They inhibit the release of substance P from primary sensory neurons in the dorsal horn of the spinal cord, mitigating the transfer of painful sensations to the brain. Opioid actions in the brainstem modulate nociceptive transmission in the dorsal horn of the spinal cord through descending inhibitory pathways. Opioids probably change the affective response to pain through actions in the forebrain; decerebration prevents opioid analgesic efficacy in rats.[3] Furthermore, morphine induces signal changes in "reward structures" in the human brain.[4]

Studies in genetically altered mice have yielded important information about opioid receptor function. In mu opioid receptor knockout mice, morphine-induced analgesia, reward effect, and withdrawal effect are absent.[5,6] Importantly, mu receptor knockout mice also fail to exhibit respiratory depression in response to morphine.[7]

Metabolism

The intravenous opioids in common perioperative clinical use are transformed and excreted by a wide variety of metabolic pathways. In general, opioids are metabolized by the hepatic microsomal system, although hepatic conjugation and subsequent excretion by the kidney are important for some drugs. For certain opioids, the specific metabolic pathway involved has important clinical implications in terms of active metabolites (e.g., morphine, meperidine) or an ultrashort duration of action (e.g., remifentanil). For other opioids, genetic variation in the metabolic pathway can drastically alter the clinical effects (e.g., codeine). These nuances are addressed in a subsequent section focused on individual drugs.

CLINICAL PHARMACOLOGY

Pharmacokinetics

Pharmacokinetic differences are the primary basis for the rational selection and administration of opioids in perioperative anesthesia practice. Key pharmacokinetic behaviors are (1) the latency to peak effect site concentration after bolus injection (i.e., bolus front-end kinetics), (2) the time to clinically relevant decay of concentration after bolus injection (i.e., bolus back-end kinetics), (3) the time to steady-state concentration after starting a continuous infusion (i.e., infusion front-end kinetics), and (4) the time to clinically relevant decay in concentration after stopping a continuous infusion (i.e., infusion back-end kinetics).

Applying opioid pharmacokinetic concepts to clinical anesthesiology requires recognition of several fundamental principles. First, a table of pharmacokinetic parameters has limited clinical value (see Table 10-1). Understanding pharmacokinetic behavior is best achieved through computer simulation. Second, the pharmacokinetic implications of opioids administered by bolus injection or continuous infusion, must be considered separately.[8] Third, pharmacokinetic information must be integrated with knowledge about the concentration-effect relationship and drug interactions (i.e., pharmacodynamics) in order to be clinically useful.

The latency to peak effect and the offset of effect after bolus injection (i.e., bolus front-end kinetics and bolus back-end kinetics) of intraveous opioids can be explored by predicting the time course of effect-site concentrations after a bolus is administered. Because the opioids differ in terms of potency (and thus the required dosages), for comparison purposes, the effect site concentrations must reflect the percentage of peak concentration for each drug. Considering morphine, fentanyl, sufentanil, alfentanil, and remifentanil as among the most commonly used opioids intraoperatively, pharmacokinetic simulation illustrates opioids differ in terms of latency to peak effect after a bolus is administered (i.e., bolus front-end kinetics) (Fig. 10-3).

The simulation of a bolus injection (Fig. 10-3, top panel) has obvious clinical implications. For example, when a rapid onset of opioid effect is desirable, morphine may not be a good choice. Similarly, when the clinical goal is a brief duration of opioid effect followed by rapid dissipation, remifentanil or alfentanil might be preferred. Note how remifentanil's concentration has declined very substantially before fentanyl's peak concentration has even been achieved. The simulation illustrates why the front-end kinetics of fentanyl make it a drug well suited for patient-controlled analgesia (PCA) (also see Chapters 39 and 40). In contrast to morphine, the peak effect of a fentanyl bolus is manifest before a typical PCA lockout period has elapsed, thus mitigating a "dose stacking" problem.

The latency to peak effect is governed by the speed with which the plasma and effect site come to equilibrium (i.e., the ke0 parameter). Drugs with a more rapid equilibration have a higher "diffusible fraction" (i.e., the proportion of drug that is un-ionized and unbound) and high lipid solubility (see Table 10-1). However, a very large dose of even a slow onset opioid can produce a rapid onset (because a supratherapeutic drug level in the effect site is reached even though the peak concentration comes later).

The time to steady state after beginning a continuous infusion is also best examined by pharmacokinetic simulation. Using the same prototypes as with bolus administration, pharmacokinetic simulation (Fig. 10-3, middle panel) shows the time required to achieve steady-state effect site concentrations (i.e., infusion front-end kinetics).

This simulation of simple, constant rate infusions has obvious clinical implications. First, the time required to reach a substantial fraction of the ultimate steady-state concentration is very long in the context of intraoperative use. To reach a near steady state more quickly requires a bolus be administered before the infusion is commenced (or increased). Remifentanil perhaps represents a partial exception to this general rule. Also, opioid concentrations will increase for many hours after an infusion is commenced; in other words, concentrations are typically increasing even though the infusion rate may have been the same for hours! That remifentanil achieves a near steady state relatively quickly is certainly part of why it has emerged as a popular drug for total intravenous anesthesia (TIVA).

The time to offset of effect after stopping a steady-state infusion is best expressed by the context-sensitive half-time simulation (CSHT).[9] Defined as the time required to achieve a 50% decrease in concentration after stopping a

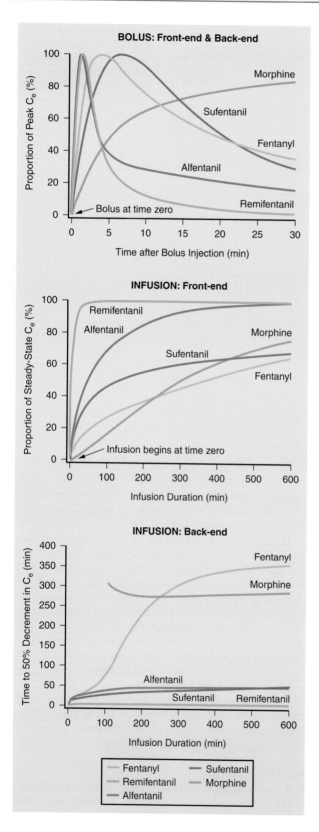

BOLUS: Front-end & Back-end

Morphine

Sufentanil

Fentanyl

Alfentanil

Bolus at time zero

Remifentanil

Proportion of Peak C$_e$ (%)

Time after Bolus Injection (min)

INFUSION: Front-end

Remifentanil

Alfentanil

Morphine

Sufentanil

Fentanyl

Infusion begins at time zero

Proportion of Steady-State C$_e$ (%)

Infusion Duration (min)

INFUSION: Back-end

Fentanyl

Morphine

Alfentanil

Sufentanil   Remifentanil

Time to 50% Decrement in C$_e$ (min)

Infusion Duration (min)

Fentanyl	Sufentanil
Remifentanil	Morphine
Alfentanil	

continuous, steady-state infusion, the CSHT is a means of normalizing the pharmacokinetic behavior of drugs so that rational comparisons can be made regarding the predicted offset of drug effect. The CSHT is thus focused on "infusion back-end" kinetics.

The bottom panel of Figure 10-3 is a CSHT simulation for commonly used intravenous opioids. Several clinically important points are apparent. First, for most drugs, the CSHT changes with time. Thus, for brief infusions, the predicted back-end kinetics for the various drugs do not differ much (remifentanil is a notable exception to this general rule). As the infusion time lengthens, the CSHTs begin to differentiate, providing a rational basis for drug selection. Second, depending on the desired duration of opioid effect, either the shorter-acting or longer-acting drugs can be chosen. Finally, the shapes of these curves differ depending on the degree of concentration decline required. In other words, the curves representing the time required to achieve a 20% or an 80% decrease in concentration (e.g., the 20% or 80% decrement time simulations) are quite different.[8] Thus, depending on the anesthesia technique applied, the CSHT simulations are not necessarily the clinically relevant simulations (i.e., a 50% decrease may not be the clinical goal). Also, CSHT simulation for morphine does not account for active metabolites (see later discussion of individual drugs under "Unique Features of Individual Opioids").

Pharmacodynamics

In most respects, the mu agonist opioids can be considered pharmacodynamic equals with important pharmacokinetic differences; that is, in terms of pharmacodynamics, both the therapeutic and adverse effects are essentially the same. Their efficacy as analgesics and their propensity to produce ventilatory depression are indistinguishable from each other. Pharmacodynamic differences do exist with nonopioid receptor mechanisms such as histamine release.

Because the nervous system profoundly influences the function of the entire body, mu opioid agonist pharmacodynamic effects are observed in many organ systems. Figure 10-4 summarizes the major pharmacodynamic effects of the fentanyl congeners. Depending on the clinical circumstances and clinical goals of treatment, some of these widespread effects can be viewed as therapeutic or adverse. For example, in some clinical settings the sedation produced by mu agonists might be viewed as a

Figure 10-3 Opioid pharmacokinetics. Simulations illustrating front-end and back-end pharmacokinetic behavior after administration by bolus injection or continuous infusions of morphine, fentanyl, alfentanil, sufentanil, and remifentanil using pharmacokinetic parameters from the literature (see text for details).[41,51-54]

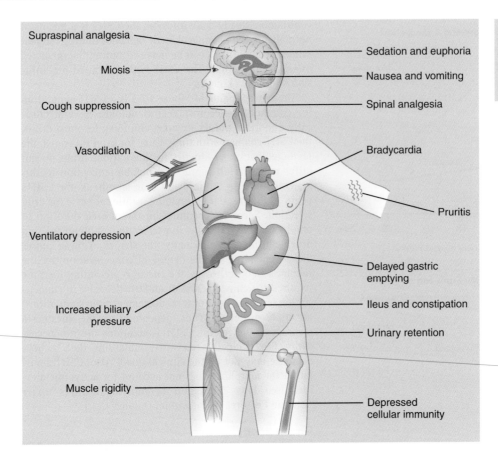

Supraspinal analgesia

Miosis

Cough suppression

Vasodilation

Ventilatory depression

Increased biliary pressure

Muscle rigidity

Sedation and euphoria

Nausea and vomiting

Spinal analgesia

Bradycardia

Pruritis

Delayed gastric emptying

Ileus and constipation

Urinary retention

Depressed cellular immunity

Figure 10-4 Opioid pharmacodynamics. A summary chart of selected effects of the fentanyl congeners (see text for details).

goal of therapy. In others, drowsiness would clearly be thought of as an adverse effect.

THERAPEUTIC EFFECTS

The relief of pain is the primary therapeutic effect of opioid analgesics. Acting at spinal and brain mu receptors, opioids provide analgesia both by attenuating the nociceptive traffic from the periphery and also by altering the affective response to painful stimulation centrally. Mu agonists are most effective in treating "second pain" sensations carried by slowly conducting, unmyelinated C fibers; they are less effective in treating "first pain" sensations (carried by small, myelinated A-delta fibers) and neuropathic pain. A unique aspect of opioid-induced analgesia (in contrast to drugs like local anesthetics) is that other sensory modalities are not affected (e.g., touch, temperature, among others).

Perioperatively (certainly intraoperatively), the drowsiness produced by mu agonists is also one of the targeted effects. The brain is the anatomic substrate for the sedative action of mu agonists. With increasing doses, mu agonists eventually produce drowsiness and sleep (the relief of pain no doubt contributes to the promotion of sleep in uncomfortable patients both pre- and postoperatively). With

sufficient doses, the mu agonists produce pronounced delta wave activity on the electroencephalogram, which resembles the pattern observed during natural sleep.

Mu agonists can of course produce significant pain relief at doses that do not produce sleep. This action is the basis of their clinical utility in the treatment of pain in ambulatory patients. On the other hand, the fact that increasing doses eventually produce drowsiness (and therefore the inability to request additional doses) is the essential scientific foundation for the safety of patient-controlled analgesia devices. However, even large doses of opioids do not reliably produce unresponsiveness and amnesia and thus opioids cannot be viewed as complete anesthetics when used alone.

Opioids also suppress the cough reflex via the cough centers in the medulla. Attenuation of the cough reflex presumably makes coughing and "bucking" against the indwelling endotracheal tube less likely.

ADVERSE EFFECTS

Respiratory depression is the primary adverse effect associated with mu agonist drugs. When the airway is secured and ventilation is controlled intraoperatively, opioid-induced depression of ventilation is of little consequence.

However, opioid-induced respiratory depression in the postoperative period can lead to brain injury and death.

Mu agonists alter the ventilatory response to arterial carbon dioxide at the ventilatory control center in the medulla. The depression of ventilation is mediated by the mu receptor; mu receptor knockout mice do not exhibit respiratory depression from morphine.[10]

In unmedicated humans, increases in arterial carbon dioxide partial pressure markedly increase minute volume (Fig. 10-5). Under the influence of opioid analgesics, the curve is flattened and shifted to the right; for a given carbon dioxide partial pressure the minute volume is lower.[11] More importantly, the "hockey stick" shape of the normal curve is lost; there may be a partial pressure of carbon dioxide below which the patient will not breathe (i.e., the "apneic threshold") in the presence of opioids.

The clinical signs of depressed ventilation are quite subtle with moderate opioid doses. Postoperative patients receiving opioid analgesic therapy can be awake and alert and yet have a significantly decreased minute volume. Respiratory rate (often associated with a slightly increased tidal volume) also decreases. As the opioid concentration is increased, the respiratory rate and tidal volume progressively decrease, eventually culminating in an irregular ventilatory rhythm and then complete apnea.

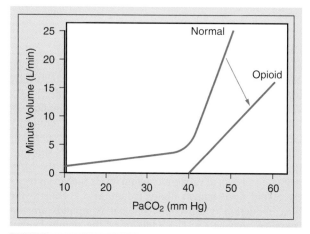

Figure 10-5 Opioid-induced ventilatory depression study methodology. The method characterizes the relationship between PaCO₂ and minute volume. The curve labeled "Normal" represents the expected response of minute volume to rising PaCO₂ levels in an awake human. Note the dramatic increase in minute volume as CO₂ tension rises. The curve labeled "Opioid" represents the blunted response of minute volume to rising CO₂ levels following administration of an opioid. Note that the slope of the curve decreases and the curve no longer has a "hockey-stick" shape; this means that at physiologic PaCO₂ levels, the patient receiving sufficient opioid may be apneic or severely hypoventilatory. (Adapted with permission from Gross JB. When you breathe IN you inspire, when you DON'T breathe, you...expire: New insights regarding opioid-induced ventilatory depression. Anesthesiology 2003;99:767-770.)

A variety of factors can increase the risk of opioid-induced ventilatory depression. Clear risk factors include large opioid dose, advanced age, concomitant use of other central nervous system depressants, and renal insufficiency (for morphine). Natural sleep also increases the ventilatory depressant effect of opioids.[12]

Opioids can alter cardiovascular physiology by a variety of different mechanisms. Compared to many other anesthetic drugs (e.g., propofol, volatile anesthetics), however, the cardiovascular effects of opioids, particularly the fentanyl congeners, are relatively minimal (morphine and meperidine are exceptions—see the following section on individual drugs).

The fentanyl congeners cause bradycardia by increasing vagal nerve tone in the brainstem, which experimentally can be blocked by microinjection of naloxone into the vagal nerve nucleus or by peripheral vagotomy.[13,14]

Opioids also produce vasodilation by depressing vasomotor centers in the brainstem and to a lesser extent by a direct effect on vessels. This action decreases both preload and afterload. Decreases in arterial blood pressure are more pronounced in patients with increased sympathetic tone such as patients with congestive heart failure or hypertension. Clinical doses of opioids do not appreciably alter myocardial contractility.

Opioids can induce muscle rigidity, usually from the rapid administration of large bolus doses of the fentanyl congeners. This rigidity can even make bag and mask ventilation during induction of anesthesia nearly impossible because of vocal cord rigidity and closure.[15] The rigidity tends to coincide with the onset of unresponsiveness.[16] Although the mechanism of opioid-induced muscle rigidity is unknown, it is not a direct action on muscle because it can be eliminated by neuromuscular blocking drugs.

Opioids also cause nausea and vomiting. Opioids stimulate the chemoreceptor trigger zone in the area postrema on the floor of the fourth ventricle in the brain. This can lead to nausea and vomiting, which are exacerbated by movement (this is perhaps why ambulatory surgery patients are more likely to be troubled by postoperative nausea and vomiting, PONV) (also see Chapter 37).

Pupillary constriction induced by mu agonists can be a useful diagnostic sign indicating some ongoing opioid effect. Opioids stimulate the Edinger-Westphal nucleus of the oculomotor nerve to produce miosis. Even small doses of opioid elicit this response and very little tolerance to the effect develops. Thus, miosis is a useful, albeit nonspecific, indicator of opioid exposure even in opioid-tolerant patients. Opioid-induced pupillary constriction is naloxone reversible.

Opioids have important effects on gastrointestinal physiology. Opioid receptors exist throughout the enteric plexus of the bowel. Stimulation of these receptors by opioids causes tonic contraction of gastrointestinal smooth muscle, thereby decreasing coordinated, peristaltic contractions. Clinically, this results in delayed gastric emptying and presumably larger gastric volumes in patients receiving opioid therapy preoperatively. Postoperatively, patients can develop opioid-induced ileus that can potentially delay the resumption of proper nutrition and discharge from the hospital. An extension of this acute problem is chronic gastrointestinal constipation associated with long-term opioid therapy.

Similar effects are observed in the biliary system, which also has an abundance of mu receptors. Mu agonists can produce contraction of the gallbladder smooth muscle and spasm of the sphincter of Oddi, potentially causing a falsely positive cholangiogram during gallbladder and bile duct surgery. These effects are completely naloxone reversible and can be partially reversed by glucagon treatment.

Although the urologic effects are minimal, opioids can sometimes cause urinary retention by decreasing bladder detrusor tone and by increasing the tone of the urinary sphincter. These effects are in part centrally mediated, although peripheral effects are also likely given the widespread presence of opioid receptors in the genitourinary tract.[17,18] Although the urinary retention associated with opioid therapy is not typically pronounced, it can be troublesome in males, particularly when the opioid is administered intrathecally or epidurally.

Opioids depress cellular immunity. Morphine and the endogenous opioid beta-endorphin, for example, inhibit the transcription of Interleukin 2 in activated T cells, among other immunologic effects.[19] Individual opioids (and perhaps classes of opioids) may differ in terms of the exact nature and extent of their immunomodulatory effects. Although opioid-induced impairment of cellular immunity is not well understood, impaired wound healing, perioperative infections, and cancer recurrence are possible adverse outcomes.

Drug Interactions

Drug interactions can be based on two mechanisms: pharmacokinetic (i.e., where one drug influences the concentration of the other) or pharmacodynamic (i.e., where one drug influences the effect of the other). In anesthesia practice, although unintended pharmacokinetic interactions sometimes occur, pharmacodynamic interactions occur with virtually every anesthetic and are produced by design.

The most common pharmacokinetic interaction in opioid clinical pharmacology is observed when intravenous opioids are combined with propofol. Perhaps because of the hemodynamic changes induced by propofol and their impact on pharmacokinetic processes, opioid concentrations may be higher when given in combination with a continuous propofol infusion.[20]

The most important pharmacodynamic drug interaction involving opioids is the synergistic interaction that

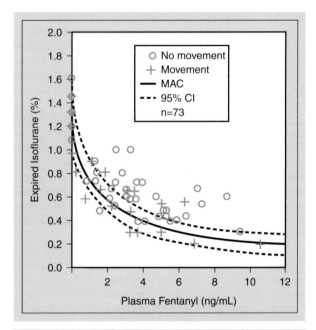

Figure 10-6 Volatile anesthetic minimum alveolar concentration (MAC) reduction by opioids: the prototype example of isoflurane and fentanyl. The solid curve is MAC; the dotted curves are the 95% confidence intervals (see text for details). (Adapted with permission from McEwan AI, Smith C, Dyar O, et al. Isoflurane minimum alveolar concentration reduction by fentanyl. Anesthesiology 1993;78:864-869.)

occurs when opioids are combined with sedatives.[21] When combined with volatile anesthetics, opioids dramatically reduce the minimum alveolar concentration (MAC) of a volatile anesthetic (Fig. 10-6). Careful examination of "opioid-MAC reduction" data reveals several clinically critical concepts (see Fig. 10-6). First, opioids synergistically reduce MAC. Second, the MAC reduction is substantial (as much as 75% or more). Third, most of the MAC reduction occurs at moderate opioid levels (i.e., even modest opioid doses substantially reduce MAC). Fourth, the MAC reduction is not complete; that is, opioids are not complete anesthetics. The addition of the opioid cannot completely eliminate the need for the other anesthetic. And fifth, there are an infinite number of hypnotic-opioid combinations that will achieve MAC (this implies that clinicians must choose the optimal combination based on the goals of the anesthetic and operation). All of these concepts also apply when opioids are used in combination with propofol for TIVA.[22]

Special Populations

HEPATIC FAILURE

Even though the liver is the metabolic organ primarily responsible for the biotransformation of most opioids, liver failure is usually not severe enough to have a major impact on opioid pharmacokinetics. Of course, the anhepatic phase of orthotopic liver transplantation is a notable exception to this general rule (also see Chapter 36). With ongoing drug administration, concentrations of opioids that rely on hepatic metabolism increase when the patient has no liver. Even after partial liver resection, an increase in the ratio of morphine glucuronides to morphine occurs, indicating a decrease in the rate of morphine metabolism.[23] Because remifentanil's metabolism is completely unrelated to hepatic clearance mechanisms, its disposition is not affected during liver transplantation.[24]

Pharmacodynamic considerations can be important for opioid therapy in patients with severe liver disease. Patients with ongoing hepatic encephalopathy are especially vulnerable to the sedative effects of opioids. As a consequence, this drug class must be used with caution in this patient population.

KIDNEY FAILURE

Renal failure has implications of major clinical importance with respect to morphine and meperidine (see the following section on individual drugs). For the fentanyl congeners, the clinical importance of kidney failure is much less marked. Remifentanil's metabolism is not affected by kidney disease.[25]

Morphine is principally metabolized by conjugation in the liver; the resulting water-soluble glucuronides (i.e., morphine 3-glucuronide and morphine 6-glucuronide – M3G and M6G) are excreted via the kidney. The kidney also plays a role in the conjugation of morphine and may account for as much as half of its conversion to M3G and M6G.

M3G is inactive, but M6G is an analgesic with a potency rivaling morphine. Very high levels of M6G and life-threatening respiratory depression can develop in patients with renal failure (Fig. 10-7).[26] Consequently, morphine may not be a good choice in patients with severely altered renal clearance mechanisms.

The clinical pharmacology of meperidine is also significantly altered by renal failure. Normeperidine, the main metabolite, has analgesic and excitatory central nervous system (CNS) effects that range from anxiety and tremulousness to myoclonus and frank seizures. Because the active metabolites are subject to renal excretion, CNS toxicity secondary to accumulation of normeperidine is especially a concern in patients with renal failure. This shortcoming of meperidine has caused many hospital formularies to restrict its use or to remove it from the formulary altogether.

GENDER

Gender may have an important influence on opioid pharmacology. Morphine is more potent in women than in men and has a slower onset of action in women.[27] Some of these differences may be related to cyclic gonadal hormones and psychosocial factors.

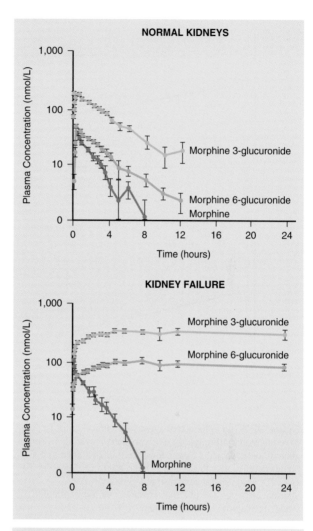

Figure 10-7 The pharmacokinetics of morphine and its metabolites in normal volunteers versus kidney failure patients. Note the significant accumulation of the metabolites in renal failure. (Adapted with permission from Osborne R, Joel S, Grebenik K, et al. The pharmacokinetics of morphine and morphine glucuronides in kidney failure. Clin Pharmacol Ther 1993;54:158-167.)

AGE (Also See Chapter 35)

Advancing age is clearly an important factor influencing the clinical pharmacology of opioids. For example, fentanyl congeners are more potent in the older patient (Fig. 10-8).[28,29] Decreases in clearance and central distribution volume also occur in older patients.

With advanced age, although pharmacokinetic changes also play a role, pharmacodynamic differences are primarily responsible for the decreased dose requirement in older patients (>65 years of age). Remifentanil doses should be decreased by at least 50% or more in elderly patients. Similar dosage reductions are also prudent for the other opioids as well.

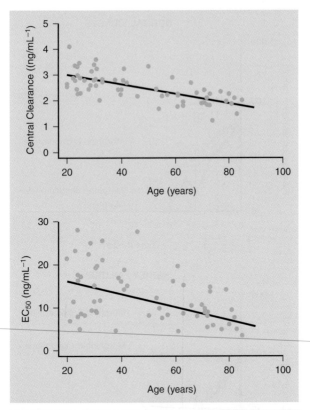

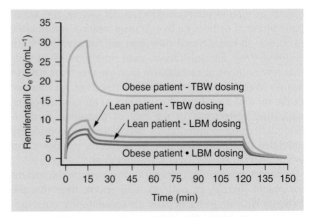

Figure 10-9 A pharmacokinetic simulation illustrating the consequences of calculating the remifentanil dosage based on total body weight (TBW) or lean body mass (LBM) in obese and lean patients (1 μg/kg bolus injection followed by an infusion of 0.5 μg/kg/min for 15 min and 0.25 μg/kg/min for an additional 105 min). Note that TBW-based dosing in an obese patient results in dramatically higher concentrations. (Adapted with permission from Egan TD, Huizinga B, Gupta SK, et al. Remifentanil pharmacokinetics in obese versus lean patients. Anesthesiology 1998;89:562-573.)

Figure 10-8 The influence of age on the clinical pharmacology of remifentanil. Although there is considerable variability, in general, older subjects have a lower central clearance and a higher potency (i.e., lower EC_{50}). (From Minto CF, Schnider TW, Egan TD, et al. Influence of age and gender on the pharmacokinetics and pharmacodynamics of remifentanil. I. Model development. Anesthesiology 1997;86:10-23.)

OBESITY

Opioid pharmacokinetic parameters, especially clearance, appear to be more closely related to lean body mass rather than to total body weight. In practical terms, this means that morbidly obese patients do indeed require a larger dosage than lean patients in order to achieve the same target concentration, but the very obese patients do not need nearly as much as would be suggested by their total body weight.[30]

For example, a total body weight (TBW) based dosing scheme results in much higher remifentanil effect-site concentrations than a dosing calculation based on lean body mass (LBM).[31] In contrast, TBW and LBM dosing schemes result in similar concentrations for lean patients (Fig.10-9). These concepts likely apply to other opioids as well.

Unique Features of Individual Opioids

CODEINE

Codeine, while not commonly used intraoperatively, has special importance among opioids because of the well-characterized pharmacogenomic nuance associated with it. Codeine is actually a prodrug; morphine is the active compound. Codeine is metabolized (in part) by O-demethylation into morphine, a metabolic process mediated by the liver microsomal isoform CYP2D6.[32] Patients who lack CYP2D6 because of deletions, frame shift, or splice mutations (i.e., approximately 10% of the white population) or whose CYP2D6 is inhibited (e.g., patients taking quinidine) would not be expected to benefit from codeine even though they exhibit a normal response to morphine.[33,34]

MORPHINE

Morphine is the prototype opioid against which all newcomers are compared. There is no evidence that any synthetic opioid is more effective in controlling pain than nature's morphine. Were it not for the histamine release and the resulting hypotension associated with morphine, fentanyl may not have replaced morphine as the most commonly used opioid intraoperatively.

Morphine has a slow onset time. Morphine's pKa renders it almost completely ionized at physiologic pH. This property, along with its low lipid solubility, accounts for morphine's prolonged latency to peak effect; morphine penetrates the central nervous system slowly. This feature has both advantages and disadvantages associated with it. The prolonged latency to peak effect means that morphine is perhaps less likely to cause acute respiratory depression after bolus injection of typical analgesic doses compared to the more rapid acting opioids. On the other hand, the slow onset time means that clinicians are perhaps more likely to inappropriately "stack" multiple morphine doses in a patient experiencing severe pain, thus creating the potential for a toxic "overshoot."[35]

Morphine's active metabolite, M6G, has important clinical implications. Although conversion to M6G accounts for only 10% of morphine's metabolism, M6G may contribute to morphine's analgesic effects even in patients with normal renal function, particularly with longer term use. Because of morphine's high hepatic extraction ratio, the bioavailability of orally administered morphine is significantly lower than after parenteral injection. The hepatic first pass effect on orally administered morphine results in high M6G levels. In fact, M6G may be the primary active compound when morphine is administered orally.[36] As noted in the section "Kidney Failure," M6G's accumulation to potentially toxic levels in dialysis patients is another important implication of this active metabolite.

FENTANYL

Fentanyl may be the most important opioid used in modern anesthesia practice. A unique aspect of fentanyl's clinical application is that it can be delivered in numerous ways. In addition to the intravenous route, fentanyl can also be delivered by transdermal, transmucosal, transnasal, and transpulmonary routes.

Oral transmucosal delivery of fentanyl citrate (OTFC) results in the faster achievement of higher peak levels than when the same dose is swallowed.[37] Avoidance of the first pass effect results in substantially greater bioavailability. That OTFC is noninvasive and rapid in onset has made it a successful therapy for breakthrough pain in opioid-tolerant cancer patients, often in combination with a transdermal fentanyl patch.

ALFENTANIL

Alfentanil was the first opioid to be administered almost exclusively by continuous infusion. Because of its relatively short terminal half-life, alfentanil was originally predicted to have a rapid offset of effect after termination of a continuous infusion.[38] Subsequent advances in pharmacokinetic theory (i.e., the CSHT) proved this assertion to be false.[8] However, alfentanil is in fact a short-acting drug after a single bolus injection because of its high "diffusible fraction"; it reaches peak effect site concentrations quickly and then begins to decline (see the previous discussion of "Pharmacokinetics"). Alfentanil illustrates how a drug can exhibit different pharmacokinetic profiles depending upon the method of administration (i.e., bolus versus continuous infusion). More so than fentanyl and sufentanil, alfentanil's metabolism by the liver may be more unpredictable because of the significant interindividual variability of hepatic CYP3A4, the primary enzyme responsible for alfentanil biotransformation.

SUFENTANIL

Sufentanil's distinguishing feature is that it is the most potent opioid commonly used in anesthesia practice. Because it is more intrinsically efficacious at the opioid receptor, the absolute doses used are much smaller compared to the other less potent drugs (e.g., a 1000-fold less than morphine doses).

REMIFENTANIL

Remifentanil is a prototype example of how specific clinical goals can be achieved by designing molecules with specialized structure-activity (or structure-metabolism) relationships. By losing its mu receptor agonist activity upon ester hydrolysis, a very short-acting opioid results (Fig. 10-10).[39] The perceived unmet need driving remifentanil's development was having an opioid with a rapid onset and offset so that the drug could be titrated up and down as necessary to meet the dynamic needs of the patient during the rapidly changing conditions of anesthesia and surgery.

Compared to the currently marketed fentanyl congeners, remifentanil's context-sensitive half-time is short, on the order of about 5 minutes.[40] Pharmacodynamically, remifentanil exhibits a short latency to peak effect similar to alfentanil and a potency slightly less than that of fentanyl.[41]

Remifentanil's role in modern anesthesia practice is now relatively well established. Remifentanil is perhaps

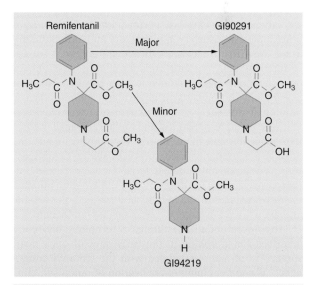

Figure 10-10 Remifentanil's metabolic pathway. De-esterification (i.e., ester hydrolysis) by nonspecific plasma and tissue esterases to an inactive acid metabolite (GI-190291) accounts for the vast majority of remifentanil's metabolism. (Adapted with permission from Egan TD, Lemmens HJ, Fiset P, et al. The pharmacokinetics of the new short-acting opioid remifentanil (GI87084B) in healthy adult male volunteers. Anesthesiology 1993;79:881-892.)

best suited for situations in which its responsive pharmacokinetic profile can be exploited to advantage (e.g., when rapid recovery is desirable, when the anesthetic requirement rapidly fluctuates, when opioid titration is unpredictable or difficult, when there is a substantial danger to opioid overdose, or when a "high dose" opioid technique is advantageous but the patient is not going to be mechanically ventilated postoperatively).[42] Remifentanil's most common clinical application is the provision of TIVA in combination with propofol. It is also commonly given by bolus when only a very brief pulse of opioid effect followed by rapid recovery is desired (e.g., in preparation for local anesthetic injection during monitored anesthesia care) (see Chapter 37).

CLINICAL APPLICATION

Opioids play a vital role in virtually every area of anesthesia practice. In the treatment of postoperative pain (also see Chapter 40), opioids are of prime importance, whereas in most other settings in perioperative medicine opioids are therapeutic adjuncts used in combination with other drugs.

Common Clinical Indications

Postoperative analgesia is the longest standing indication for opioid therapy in anesthesia practice. In the modern era, opioid administration via patient-controlled analgesia (PCA) devices is perhaps the most common mode of delivery (also see Chapter 40). In recent years, opioids are increasingly combined postoperatively with various other analgesics, such as nonsteroidal anti-inflammatory drugs (NSAIDs) to increase efficacy and safety.

Internationally, the most common clinical indication for opioids in anesthesia practice is their use for "balanced anesthesia." This perhaps misguided term connotes the use of multiple drugs (e.g., volatile anesthetics, neuromuscular blockers, sedative-hypnotics, and opioids) in smaller doses to produce the state of anesthesia. With this technique, the opioids are primarily used for their ability to decrease MAC. A basic assumption underlying this balanced anesthesia approach is that the drugs used in combination mitigate the disadvantages of the individual drugs (i.e., the volatile anesthetics) used in larger doses as single drug therapy.

"High-dose opioid anesthesia," a technique originally described for morphine in the early days of open heart surgery[43] and later associated with the fentanyl congeners,[44] is another common application of opioids in clinical anesthesia. The original scientific underpinning of this approach was that high doses of opioids enabled the clinician to reduce the concentration of volatile anesthetic to a minimum, thereby avoiding the direct myocardial depression and other untoward hemodynamic effects in patients whose cardiovascular systems were already compromised. In addition, that fentanyl often produces a relative bradycardia could be helpful in patients with myocardial ischemia. Currently, while the general concept is still applied, the opioid doses used are smaller. Opioids are also administered for their possible beneficial effects in terms of cardioprotection (i.e., preconditioning).

Total intravenous anesthesia (TIVA) is a more recently developed and increasingly popular indication for opioids in anesthesia practice. This technique relies entirely upon intravenous agents for the provision of general anesthesia. Most commonly, continuous infusions of remifentanil or alfentanil are combined with a propofol infusion. Both the opioid and the sedative are often delivered by target-controlled infusion (TCI) enabled pumps. A clear advantage of this technique, perhaps among others, is the enhanced patient well-being in the early postoperative period, including less nausea and vomiting and often a feeling of euphoria.[45]

Rational Drug Selection and Administration

In articulating a scientific foundation for rational opioid selection, pharmacokinetic considerations are extremely important. Indeed, the mu agonists (opioids) can be considered pharmacodynamic equals with important pharmacokinetic differences.[46] In other words, all mu agonists are essentially equally efficacious when equipotent concentrations are achieved, but they differ in terms of their pharmacokinetic behavior. Thus, rational selection of one mu opioid agonist over another requires the clinician to identify the desired temporal profile of drug effect and then choose an opioid that best enables the clinician to achieve it (within obvious constraints such as pharmacoeconomic concerns).

In selecting the appropriate opioid, among the key questions to address are: How quickly must the desired opioid effect be achieved? How long must the opioid effect be maintained? How critical is it that the opioid-induced ventilatory depression or sedation dissipate quickly (e.g., will the patient be mechanically ventilated postoperatively)? Is the capability to raise and lower the level of opioid effect quickly during the anesthetic critical? Will there be significant pain postoperatively that will require opioid treatment? All of these questions relate to the optimal temporal profile of opioid effect. The answers to these questions are addressed through the application of pharmacokinetic concepts.

For example, when a brief pulse of opioid effect followed by rapid recovery is desired (e.g., to provide analgesia for a retrobulbar block), a bolus of remifentanil or alfentanil might be preferred. When long-lasting opioid effect is desired, such as when there will be significant postoperative pain or when the trachea will remain intubated, a fentanyl infusion is a prudent choice. If the patient should be awake and alert shortly after the procedure is finished (e.g., a craniotomy in which the surgeons hope to perform a neurologic examination in the operating room immediately postoperatively), a remifentanil infusion might be advantageous.

The formulation of a rational administration strategy also requires the proper application of pharmacokinetic principles. An important goal of any dosing scheme is to reach and maintain a steady-state level of opioid effect. Nowadays, in order to achieve a steady-state concentration in the site of action, opioids are frequently administered by continuous infusion. This is increasingly accomplished through the use of TCI technology, which requires that the clinician be familiar with the appropriate pharmacokinetic model for the opioid of interest. When these systems are not available, the clinician must remember that infusions must be preceded by a bolus in order to come to a near steady state in a timely fashion.

EMERGING DEVELOPMENTS

Opioids and Cancer Recurrence

Do opioids administered as part of a general anesthetic for cancer surgery have an adverse impact on cancer recurrence rates? The immunosuppressive effects of opioids (particularly morphine) and their influence on angiogenesis have been shown in animal studies and in vitro. Retrospective human studies also provide some support for this hypothesis. For example, a retrospective study comparing prostate cancer recurrence rates in patients who received standard postoperative opioid analgesia versus patients who received postoperative epidural analgesia documented a more frequent cancer recurrence rate in the standard opioid analgesia cohort.[47]

Surgical treatment often represents the best chance for curing cancer, but an operation is presumably associated with systemic release of tumor cells. Moreover, micrometastatic disease often exists despite surgery. The body's natural anticancer defenses, in combination with adjunctive chemotherapy or radiation therapy, are relied upon to prevent the residual microscopic disease from proliferating into a frank cancer recurrence. In addition to opioid analgesia, the stress response to surgery and an independent effect of general anesthesia may also contribute to the impairment of cellular immunity that is responsible for the increased cancer recurrence risk. If this hypothesis is confirmed through prospective trials, it would presumably have a major impact on the anesthesia techniques applied to cancer surgery patients, including a more prominent role for regional postoperative analgesia techniques to reduce the overall opioid dose given to patients. At this stage, this hypothesis is unproved and the data must be interpreted with caution until more definitive information is available.[48]

QUESTIONS OF THE DAY

1. What is the mechanism of the pharmacologic effect of opioids?
2. What is the definition of "context-sensitive half-time" (CSHT)? How does the CSHT differ among the commonly used intravenous opioids?
3. How are intravenous opioids metabolized? Which opioids have clinically significant active metabolites?
4. How do opioids affect gastrointestinal physiology? What is the mechanism?
5. What are the issues to address when selecting a specific opioid for use during anesthesia?

ACKNOWLEDGMENT

The editors and publisher would like to thank Dr. Robert K. Stoelting for contributing a chapter on this topic to the prior edition of this work. It has served as the foundation for the current chapter.

REFERENCES

1. Minami M, Satoh M: Molecular biology of the opioid receptors: Structures, functions and distributions, *Neurosci Res* 23:121–145, 1995.
2. Pan L, Xu J, Yu R, et al: Identification and characterization of six new alternatively spliced variants of the human mu opioid receptor gene, Oprm, *Neuroscience* 133:209–220, 2005.
3. Matthies BK, Franklin KB: Formalin pain is expressed in decerebrate rats but not attenuated by morphine, *Pain* 51:199–206, 1992.
4. Becerra L, Harter K, Gonzalez RG, et al: Functional magnetic resonance imaging measures of the effects of morphine on central nervous system circuitry in opioid-naive healthy volunteers, *Anesth Analg* 103:208–216, 2006.
5. Matthes HW, Maldonado R, Simonin F, et al: Loss of morphine-induced analgesia, reward effect and withdrawal symptoms in mice lacking the mu-opioid-receptor gene, *Nature* 383:819–823, 1996.
6. Sora I, Takahashi N, Funada M, et al: Opiate receptor knockout mice define mu receptor roles in endogenous nociceptive responses and morphine-induced analgesia, *Proc Natl Acad Sci U S A* 94:1544–1549, 1997.
7. Dahan A, Sarton E, Teppema L, et al: Anesthetic potency and influence of morphine and sevoflurane on respiration in mu-opioid receptor knockout mice, *Anesthesiology* 94:824–832, 2001.
8. Shafer SL, Varvel JR: Pharmacokinetics, pharmacodynamics, and rational opioid selection, *Anesthesiology* 74:53–63, 1991.
9. Hughes MA, Glass PS, Jacobs JR: Context-sensitive half-time in multicompartment pharmacokinetic models for intravenous anesthetic drugs, *Anesthesiology* 76:334–341, 1992.
10. Romberg R, Sarton E, Teppema L, et al: Comparison of morphine-6-glucuronide and morphine on respiratory depressant and antinociceptive responses in wild type and mu-opioid receptor deficient mice, *Br J Anaesth* 91:862–870, 2003.
11. Gross JB: When you breathe IN: you inspire, when you DON'T breathe, you…expire: New insights regarding opioid-induced ventilatory depression, *Anesthesiology* 99:767–770, 2003.

12. Forrest WH Jr, Bellville JW: The effect of sleep plus morphine on the respiratory response to carbon dioxide, *Anesthesiology* 25:137–141, 1964.

13. Laubie M, Schmitt H, Vincent M: Vagal bradycardia produced by microinjections of morphine-like drugs into the nucleus ambiguus in anaesthetized dogs, *Eur J Pharmacol* 59:287–291, 1979.

14. Reitan JA, Stengert KB, Wymore ML, et al: Central vagal control of fentanyl-induced bradycardia during halothane anesthesia, *Anesth Analg* 57:31–36, 1978.

15. Bennett JA, Abrams JT, Van Riper DF, et al: Difficult or impossible ventilation after sufentanil-induced anesthesia is caused primarily by vocal cord closure, *Anesthesiology* 87:1070–1074, 1997.

16. Streisand JB, Bailey PL, LeMaire L, et al: Fentanyl-induced rigidity and unconsciousness in human volunteers. Incidence, duration, and plasma concentrations, *Anesthesiology* 78:629–634, 1993.

17. Dray A, Metsch R: Inhibition of urinary bladder contractions by a spinal action of morphine and other opioids, *J Pharmacol Exp Ther* 231:254–260, 1984.

18. Dray A, Metsch R: Spinal opioid receptors and inhibition of urinary bladder motility in vivo, *Neurosci Lett* 47:81–84, 1984.

19. Borner C, Warnick B, Smida M, et al: Mechanisms of opioid-mediated inhibition of human T cell receptor signaling, *J Immunol* 183:882–889, 2009.

20. Bouillon T, Bruhn J, Radu-Radulescu L, et al: Non-steady state analysis of the pharmacokinetic interaction between propofol and remifentanil, *Anesthesiology* 97:1350–1362, 2002.

21. McEwan AI, Smith C, Dyar O, et al: Isoflurane minimum alveolar concentration reduction by fentanyl, *Anesthesiology* 78:864–869, 1993.

22. Vuyk J, Lim T, Engbers FH, et al: The pharmacodynamic interaction of propofol and alfentanil during lower abdominal surgery in women, *Anesthesiology* 83:8–22, 1995.

23. Rudin A, Lundberg JF, Hammarlund-Udenaes M, et al: Morphine metabolism after major liver surgery, *Anesth Analg* 104:1409–1414, 2007.

24. Dershwitz M, Hoke JF, Rosow CE, et al: Pharmacokinetics and pharmacodynamics of remifentanil in volunteer subjects with severe liver disease, *Anesthesiology* 84:812–820, 1996.

25. Hoke JF, Shluman D, Dershwitz M, et al: Pharmacokinetics and pharmacodynamics of remifentanil in persons with renal failure compared with healthy volunteers, *Anesthesiology* 87:533–541, 1997.

26. Osborne R, Joel S, Grebenik K, et al: The pharmacokinetics of morphine and morphine glucuronides in kidney failure, *Clin Pharmacol Ther* 54:158–167, 1993.

27. Sarton E, Olofsen E, Romberg R, et al: Sex differences in morphine analgesia: An experimental study in healthy volunteers, *Anesthesiology* 93:1245–1254, 2000.

28. Minto CF, Schnider TW, Egan TD, et al: Influence of age and gender on the pharmacokinetics and pharmacodynamics of remifentanil. I. Model development, *Anesthesiology* 86:10–23, 1997.

29. Scott JC, Stanski DR: Decreased fentanyl and alfentanil dose requirements with age. A simultaneous pharmacokinetic and pharmacodynamic evaluation, *J Pharmacol Exp Ther* 240:159–166, 1987.

30. Bouillon T, Shafer SL: Does size matter? *Anesthesiology* 89:557–560, 1998.

31. Egan TD, Huizinga B, Gupta SK, et al: Remifentanil pharmacokinetics in obese versus lean patients, *Anesthesiology* 89:562–573, 1998.

32. Poulsen L, Brosen K, Arendt-Nielsen L, et al: Codeine and morphine in extensive and poor metabolizers of sparteine: Pharmacokinetics, analgesic effect and side effects, *Eur J Clin Pharmacol* 51:289–295, 1996.

33. Caraco Y, Sheller J, Wood AJ: Pharmacogenetic determination of the effects of codeine and prediction of drug interactions, *J Pharmacol Exp Ther* 278:1165–1174, 1996.

34. Eckhardt K, Li S, Ammon S, et al: Same incidence of adverse drug events after codeine administration irrespective of the genetically determined differences in morphine formation, *Pain* 76:27–33, 1998.

35. Lotsch J, Dudziak R, Freynhagen R, et al: Fatal respiratory depression after multiple intravenous morphine injections, *Clin Pharmacokinet* 45:1051–1060, 2006.

36. Osborne R, Joel S, Trew D, et al: Morphine and metabolite behavior after different routes of morphine administration: Demonstration of the importance of the active metabolite morphine-6-glucuronide, *Clin Pharmacol Ther* 47:12–19, 1990.

37. Streisand JB, Varvel JR, Stanski DR, et al: Absorption and bioavailability of oral transmucosal fentanyl citrate, *Anesthesiology* 75:223–229, 1991.

38. Stanski DR, Hug CC Jr: Alfentanil—A kinetically predictable narcotic analgesic, *Anesthesiology* 57:435–438, 1982.

39. Egan TD: Remifentanil pharmacokinetics and pharmacodynamics. A preliminary appraisal, *Clin Pharmacokinet* 29:80–94, 1995.

40. Egan TD, Lemmens HJ, Fiset P, et al: The pharmacokinetics of the new short-acting opioid remifentanil (GI87084B) in healthy adult male volunteers, *Anesthesiology* 79:881–892, 1993.

41. Egan TD, Minto CF, Hermann DJ, et al: Remifentanil versus alfentanil: Comparative pharmacokinetics and pharmacodynamics in healthy adult male volunteers [published erratum appears in *Anesthesiology* 1996;85(3):695], *Anesthesiology* 84:821–833, 1996.

42. Egan TD: The clinical pharmacology of remifentanil: A brief review, *J Anesth* 12:195–204, 1998.

43. Lowenstein E, Hallowell P, Levine FH, et al: Cardiovascular response to large doses of intravenous morphine in man, *N Engl J Med* 281:1389–1393, 1969.

44. Lunn JK, Stanley TH, Eisele J, et al: High dose fentanyl anesthesia for coronary artery surgery: Plasma fentanyl concentrations and influence of nitrous oxide on cardiovascular responses, *Anesth Analg* 58:390–395, 1979.

45. Hofer CK, Zollinger A, Buchi S, et al: Patient well-being after general anaesthesia: A prospective, randomized, controlled multi-centre trial comparing intravenous and inhalation anaesthesia, *Br J Anaesth* 91:631–637, 2003.

46. Mather LE: Pharmacokinetic and pharmacodynamic profiles of opioid analgesics: A sameness amongst equals? *Pain* 43:3–6, 1990.

47. Biki B, Mascha E, Moriarty DC, et al: Anesthetic technique for radical prostatectomy surgery affects cancer recurrence: A retrospective analysis, *Anesthesiology* 109:180–187, 2008.

48. Bovill JG: Surgery for cancer: Does anesthesia matter? *Anesth Analg* 110:1524–1526, 2009.

49. Egan TD: Target-controlled drug delivery: progress toward an intravenous "vaporizer" and automated anesthetic administration, *Anesthesiology* 99:1214–1219, 2003.

50. Egan TD, Shafer SL: Target-controlled infusions for intravenous anesthetics: Surfing USA not!, *Anesthesiology* 99:1039–1041, 2003.

51. Lotsch J, Skarke C, Schmidt H, et al: Pharmacokinetic modeling to predict morphine and morphine-6-glucuronide

plasma concentrations in healthy young volunteers, *Clin Pharmacol Ther* 72:151–162, 2002.

52. Lotsch J, Skarke C, Schmidt H, et al: The transfer half-life of morphine-6-glucuronide from plasma to effect site assessed by pupil size measurement in healthy volunteers, *Anesthesiology* 95:1329–1338, 2001.

53. Gepts E, Shafer SL, Camu F, et al: Linearity of pharmacokinetics and model estimation of sufentanil, *Anesthesiology* 83:1194–1204, 1995.

54. Scott JC, Cooke JE, Stanski DR: Electroencephalographic quantitation of opioid effect: Comparative pharmacodynamics of fentanyl and sufentanil, *Anesthesiology* 74:34–42, 1991.

II

11 LOCAL ANESTHETICS

Kenneth Drasner

Local anesthesia can be defined as loss of sensation in a discrete region of the body caused by disruption of impulse generation or propagation. Local anesthesia can be produced by various chemical and physical means. However, in routine clinical practice, local anesthesia is produced by a narrow class of compounds, and recovery is normally spontaneous, predictable, and complete.

HISTORY

Cocaine's systemic toxicity, its irritant properties when placed topically or around nerves, and its substantial potential for physical and psychological dependence generated interest in identification of an alternative local anesthetic.[1] Because cocaine was known to be a benzoic acid ester (Fig. 11-1), developmental strategies focused on this class of chemical compounds. Although benzocaine was identified before the turn of the century, its poor water solubility restricted its use to topical anesthesia, for which it still finds some limited application in modern clinical practice. The first useful injectable local anesthetic, procaine, can be considered the prototype on which all commonly used local anesthetics are based. The procaine molecule is derived from an aromatic acid (para-aminobenzoic acid) and an amino alcohol, yielding a structure with three distinct regions: an aromatic head, which imparts lipophilicity; a terminal amine tail, a proton acceptor that imparts hydrophobicity; and a hydrocarbon chain attached to the aromatic acid by an ester linkage (Fig. 11-2). Several other derivatives of para-aminobenzoic acid were developed as local anesthetics during the first half of the past century, most notably tetracaine and chloroprocaine, both embodying modifications of the aromatic ring (Fig. 11-3).

In 1948, lidocaine was introduced, and it was the first departure from the amino-ester series. Being derived from an aromatic amine (i.e., xylidine) and an amino acid, the hydrocarbon chain and the aromatic head of

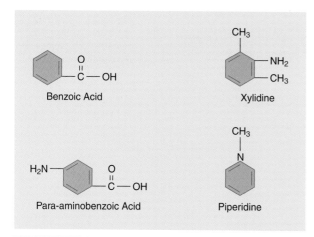

Figure 11-1 Important components of local anesthetics: benzoic acids, xylidine, para-aminobenzoic acid, and piperidine.

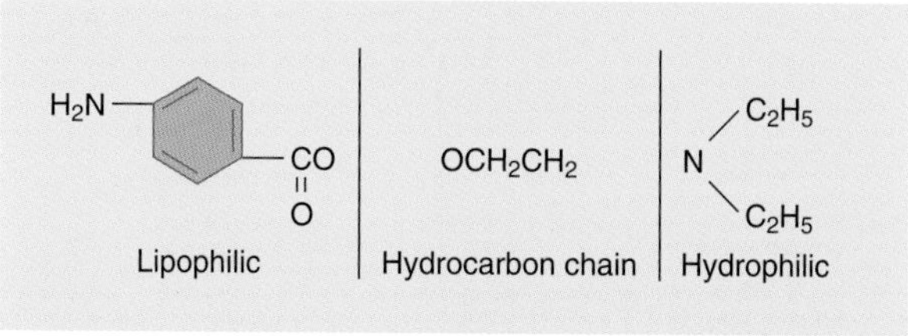

Figure 11-2 Local anesthetics consist of a lipophilic and hydrophilic portion separated by a connecting hydrocarbon chain.

biotransformation in the liver rather than undergoing ester hydrolysis in plasma, as is the case for the amino-esters.

MECHANISMS OF ACTION AND FACTORS AFFECTING BLOCK

Nerve Conduction

Local anesthetics block the transmission of the action potential by inhibition of voltage-gated sodium ion channels. Under normal or resting circumstances, the neural membrane is characterized by a negative potential of roughly −90 mV (the potential inside the nerve fiber is negative relative to the extracellular fluid). This negative potential is created by active outward transport of sodium and inward transport of potassium ions, combined with a membrane that is relatively permeable to potassium and relatively impermeable to sodium ions. With excitation of the nerve, there is an increase in the membrane permeability to sodium ions, causing a decrease in the transmembrane potential. If a critical potential is reached (i.e., threshold potential), there is a rapid and self-sustaining influx of sodium ions resulting in depolarization, after which the resting membrane potential is reestablished. From an electrophysiologic standpoint, local anesthetics block conduction of neural transmission by decreasing the rate of depolarization in response to excitation, preventing achievement of the threshold potential. They do not alter the resting trans-membrane potential, and they have little effect on the threshold potential.

Anesthetic Effect and the Active Form of the Local Anesthetic

Local anesthetics exert their electrophysiologic effects by blocking sodium ion conductance. This effect is primarily mediated by interaction with specific receptors that are within the inner vestibule of the sodium ion channel. The commonly used injectable local anesthetics exist in two forms that are in dynamic equilibrium, an uncharged base or a protonated quaternary amine. Most likely, the charged form of the local anesthetic molecule binds to the receptor and is responsible for the predominant action of these drugs. However, the pharmacology is a bit more complex, as the charged structure is highly hydrophilic, and relatively incapable of penetrating the nerve membrane to reach its site of action. The neutral base plays a critical role in the local anesthetic effect by permitting the anesthetic to penetrate the nerve membrane to gain access to the receptor (Fig. 11-4).[2] After penetration, re-equilibration occurs, permitting the charged form of the local anesthetic to bind. These drugs also may reach the sodium channel laterally

the lidocaine molecule are linked by an amide bond (rather than an ester), imparting greater stability. This molecular structure also averts the allergic reactions commonly associated with ester anesthetics (which result from sensitivity to the cleaved aromatic acid). Because of these favorable properties, lidocaine became the template for the development of a series of amino-amide anesthetics (see Fig. 11-3).

Most amino-amide local anesthetics are derived from xylidine, including mepivacaine, bupivacaine, ropivacaine, and levobupivacaine (see Fig. 11-1). In contrast to lidocaine, the terminal amino portion of these newer compounds is contained within a piperidine ring (see Fig. 11-1), and the series is commonly referred to as pipecholyl xylidines. Ropivacaine and levobupivacaine share an additional distinctive characteristic: they are single enantiomers rather than racemic mixtures. They are products of a developmental strategy that takes advantage of the differential stereoselectivity of neuronal and cardiac sodium ion channels in an effort to reduce the potential for cardiac toxicity (see "Adverse Effects"). Because they are amides, all of the newer local anesthetics require

131

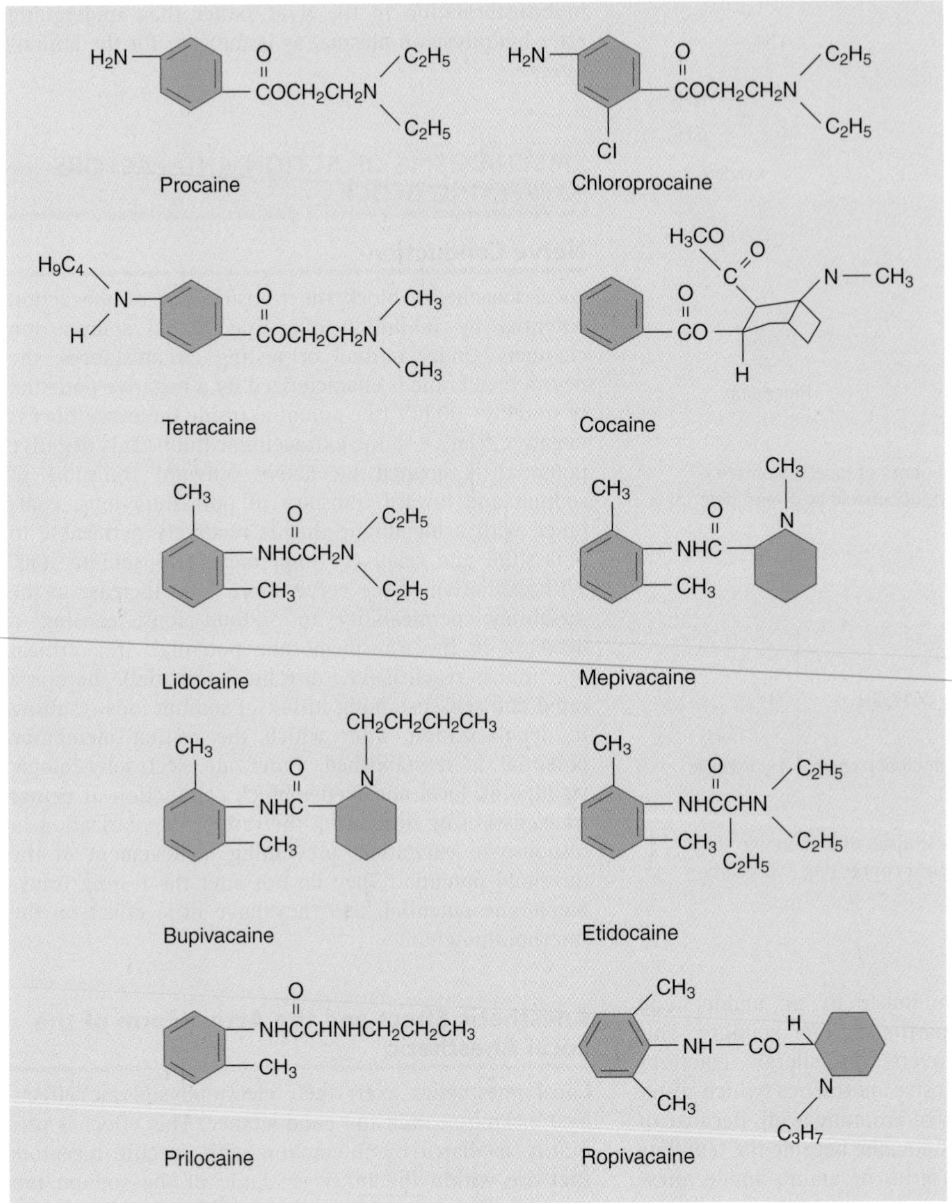

Figure 11-3 Chemical structures of ester (i.e., procaine, chloroprocaine, tetracaine, and cocaine) and amide (i.e., lidocaine, mepivacaine, bupivacaine, etidocaine, prilocaine, and ropivacaine) local anesthetics.

(i.e., hydrophobic pathway). Yet this mechanism cannot completely account for all of the local anesthetic effect. For example, benzocaine exists only in an uncharged form, and it is not affected by pH, but it still possesses local anesthetic activity.

Sodium Ion Channel State, Anesthetic Binding, and Use-Dependent Block

According to the modulated receptor model, sodium ion channels alternate between several conformational states, and local anesthetics bind to these different conformational states with different affinities. During excitation, the sodium channel moves from a resting-closed state to an activated-open state, with passage of sodium ions and consequent depolarization. After depolarization, the channel assumes an inactivated-closed conformational state. Local anesthetics bind to the activated and inactivated states more readily than the resting state, attenuating conformational change. Drug dissociation from the inactivated conformational state is slower than from the resting state. Thus, repeated depolarization produces more effective anesthetic binding. The electrophysiologic consequence of this effect is progressive

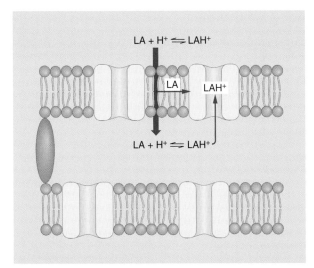

$$LA + H^+ \rightleftharpoons LAH^+$$

$$LA \quad LAH^+$$

$$LA + H^+ \rightleftharpoons LAH^+$$

Figure 11-4 During diffusion of local anesthetic across the nerve sheath and membrane to receptor sites within the inner vestibule of the sodium channel, only the uncharged base (LA) can penetrate the lipid membrane. After reaching the axoplasm, ionization occurs, and the charged cationic form (LAH^+) attaches to the receptor. Anesthetic may also reach the channel laterally (i.e., hydrophobic pathway). (From Covino BG, Scott DB, Lambert DH. Handbook of Spinal Anesthesia and Analgesia. Philadelphia, WB Saunders, 1994, p 7, used with permission.)

enhancement of conduction blockade with repetitive stimulation, an effect referred to as *use-dependent* or *frequency-dependent* block. For this reason, selective conduction blockade of nerve fibers by local anesthetics may in part be related to the characteristic frequency of activity of the nerve.

Critical Role of pH

The relative proportion of charged and uncharged local anesthetic molecules is a function of the dissociation constant of the drug and the environmental pH. Recalling the Henderson-Hasselbalch equation, the dissociation constant (K_a) can be expressed as follows:

$$pK_a = pH - \log[\text{base}]/[\text{conjugate acid}]$$

If the concentration of the base and conjugate acid are equal, the latter component of the equation cancels (because $\log 1 = 0$). Thus, the pK_a provides a useful way to describe the propensity of a local anesthetic to exist in a charged or an uncharged state. The lower the pK_a, the greater is the percent of un-ionized fraction at a given pH. For example, the highly lipophilic compound benzocaine has a pK_a of 3.5, and the molecule exists solely as the neutral base under physiologic conditions. In contrast, because the pK_a values of the commonly used

injectable anesthetics are between 7.6 and 8.9, less than one half of the molecules are un-ionized at physiologic pH (Table 11-1). Because local anesthetics are poorly soluble in water, they are generally marketed as water-soluble hydrochloride salts. These hydrochloride salt solutions are acidic, contributing to the stability of local anesthetics but potentially impairing the onset of a block. Bicarbonate is sometimes added to local anesthetic solutions to increase the un-ionized fraction in an effort to hasten the onset of anesthesia. Other conditions that lower pH, such as tissue acidosis produced by infection, may likewise have a negative impact on the onset and quality of local anesthesia.

Lipid Solubility

Lipid solubility of a local anesthetic affects its tissue penetration and its uptake in the nerve membrane. This physiochemical property impacts the fundamental characteristics of local anesthetics. Lipid solubility is ordinarily expressed as a partition coefficient, which is determined by comparing the solubility of the drug in a nonpolar solvent, such as *n*-heptane or octanol, with the solubility in an aqueous phase, generally water or buffered solution. Although results may vary depending on the specific methodology, lipid solubility generally correlates with local anesthetic potency and duration of action, and to a lesser extent, it varies inversely with latency or the time to onset of local anesthetic effect. Duration of the local anesthetic effect also correlates with protein binding, which likely serves to retain anesthetic within the nerve.

When considering physiochemical characteristics as they relate to the local anesthetic effect, it is important to appreciate that measures of anesthetic activity may also be impacted by the in vitro or in vivo system in which these effects are determined. For example, tetracaine is approximately 20 times more potent than bupivacaine when assessed in isolated nerve, but these drugs are generally equipotent when assessed in intact in vivo systems. Even within in vivo systems, comparisons among local anesthetics may vary based on the model or the specific site of application (spinal versus peripheral block) because of secondary effects such as the inherent vasoactive properties of the anesthetic.

Differential Local Anesthetic Blockade

Nerve fibers can be classified according to fiber diameter, presence (type A and B) or absence (type C) of myelin, and function (Table 11-2). Nerve fiber diameter influences conduction velocity; a larger diameter correlates with more rapid nerve conduction. The presence of myelin also increases conduction velocity. This effect results from insulation of the axolemma from the surrounding media, forcing current to flow through periodic

II

Table 11-1 Comparative Pharmacology and Common Current Use of Local Anesthetics

Classification and Compounds	pKₐ	% Nonionized at pH 7.4	Potency*	Max. Dose (mg) for Infiltration†	Duration after Infiltration (min)	Topical	Local	IV	Periph	Epi	Spinal
Esters											
Procaine	8.9	3	1	500	45–60	No	Yes	No	Yes	No	Yes
Chloroprocaine	8.7	5	2	600	30–60	No	Yes	Yes	Yes	Yes	Yes‡
Tetracaine	8.5	7	8			Yes	Yes§	No	No	No	Yes
Amides											
Lidocaine	7.9	24	2	300	60–120	Yes	Yes	Yes	Yes	Yes	Yes‡
Mepivacaine	7.6	39	2	300	90–180	No	Yes	No	Yes	Yes	Yes‡
Prilocaine	7.9	24	2	400	60–120	Yes¶	Yes	Yes	Yes	Yes	Yes‡
Bupivacaine, levobupivacaine	8.1	17	8	150	240–480	No	Yes	No	Yes	Yes	Yes
Ropivacaine	8.1	17	6	200	240–480	No	Yes	No	Yes	Yes	Yes

*Relative potencies vary based on experimental model or route of administration.
†Dosage should take into account the site of injection, use of a vasoconstrictor, and patient-related factors.
‡Use of procaine, lidocaine, mepivacaine, prilocaine, and chloroprocaine for spinal anesthesia is somewhat controversial; indications are evolving (see text).
§Used in combination with another local anesthetic to increase duration.
¶Formulated with lidocaine as eutectic mixture.
Epi, epidural; IV, intravenous; Periph, peripheral.

Table 11-2 Classification of Nerve Fibers

Type	Fiber Subtype	Diameter (μm)	Conduction Velocity (m/sec)	Function
A (myelinated)	Alpha	12-20	80-120	Proprioception, large motor
	Beta	5-15	35-80	Small motor, touch, pressure
	Gamma	3-8	10-35	Muscle tone
	Delta	2-5	5-25	Pain, temperature, touch
B (myelinated)		3	5-15	Preganglionic autonomic
C (unmyelinated)		0.3-1.5	0.5-2.5	Dull pain, temperature, touch

interruptions in the myelin sheath (i.e., nodes of Ranvier). With respect to local anesthetic effect, conduction blockade is predictably absent if at least three successive nodes of Ranvier are exposed to adequate concentrations of local anesthetics. However, the observation that sensitivity to local anesthetic blockade is inversely related to nerve fiber diameter probably does not reflect cause and effect. There is actually evidence to suggest that large, myelinated nerve fibers are more sensitive to local anesthetic blockade than smaller, unmyelinated fibers.[3] Nonetheless, in clinical practice, incremental increases in the concentrations of local anesthetics result in progressive interruption of transmission of autonomic, sensory, and motor neural impulses and therefore production of autonomic nervous system blockade, sensory anesthesia, and skeletal muscle paralysis. The mechanisms underlying this divergence between clinical experience and experimental data are poorly understood, but they may be related to the anatomic and geographic arrangement of nerve fibers, variability in the longitudinal spread required for neural blockade, effects on other ion channels, and inherent impulse activity.

PROPENSITY TO INDUCE DIFFERENTIAL BLOCKADE

Local anesthetics are not equivalent in their propensity to induce differential blockade. For example, for equivalent analgesic or local anesthetic effect, etidocaine produces more profound motor block than bupivacaine. This characteristic makes bupivacaine a more valuable drug, particularly for use in labor or for postoperative pain management, and it accounts for etidocaine's limited use in clinical anesthesia. Attempts to identify local anesthetics with far greater sensory selectivity have been largely unsuccessful, although such effects can be achieved with alternative compounds under certain circumstances, such as that achieved with spinal administration of opioids.

Spread of Local Anesthesia after Injection

When local anesthetics are deposited around a peripheral nerve, they diffuse from the outer surface (mantle) toward the center (core) of the nerve along a concentration gradient (Fig. 11-5).[4] As a result, nerve fibers located in the mantle of the mixed nerve are blocked first. These

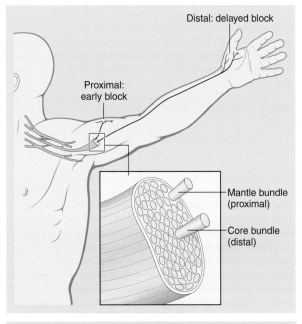

Figure 11-5 Local anesthetics deposited around a peripheral nerve diffuse along a concentration gradient to block nerve fibers on the outer surface (mantle) before more centrally located (core) fibers. This accounts for early manifestations of anesthesia in more proximal areas of the extremity.

mantle fibers are generally distributed to more proximal anatomic structures, whereas distal structures are innervated by fibers near the core. This anatomic arrangement accounts for the initial development of proximal anesthesia with subsequent distal involvement as local anesthetic diffuses to reach more central core nerve fibers. Consequently, skeletal muscle paralysis may precede the onset of sensory blockade if the motor nerve fibers are more superficial. The sequence of onset and recovery from conduction blockade of sympathetic, sensory, and motor nerve fibers in a mixed peripheral nerve depends as much or more on the anatomic location of the nerve fibers within the mixed nerve as on their intrinsic sensitivity to local anesthetics.

PHARMACOKINETICS

Local anesthetics differ from most drugs used in medicine because they are deposited at the target site, and systemic absorption and circulation attenuate or curtail the drug's effect rather than deliver the drug to its intended site of action. High plasma concentrations of local anesthetics after absorption from injection sites (or unintended intravascular injection) are undesirable and are the origin of their potential toxicity. Peak plasma concentrations achieved are determined by the rate of systemic uptake and, to a lesser extent, the rate of clearance of the local anesthetic. Uptake is affected by several factors related to the physiochemical properties of the local anesthetic and local tissue blood flow. Uptake tends to be delayed for local anesthetics with high lipophilicity and protein binding.

Local Anesthetic Vasoactivity

Anesthetics differ somewhat in their vasoactivity, but most are vasodilators at clinically relevant concentrations, although this effect varies with site of injection. Such differences may be clinically important. For example, the lower systemic toxicity of S (–) ropivacaine compared with the R (+) enantiomer in part may result from its vasoconstrictive activity (see "Adverse Effects"). The variable effect of vasoconstrictors added to local anesthetic solutions used for spinal anesthesia is another example. In contrast to lidocaine or bupivacaine, there is some evidence that tetracaine produces a significant increase in spinal cord blood flow. Consequently, prolongation of spinal anesthesia by epinephrine or other vasoconstrictors is more pronounced with tetracaine than with other commonly used spinal anesthetics.

Metabolism

The amino-ester local anesthetics undergo hydrolysis, whereas the amino-amide local anesthetics undergo metabolism by hepatic microsomal enzymes. The lungs are also capable of extracting local anesthetics such as lidocaine, bupivacaine, and prilocaine from the circulation. The rate of this metabolism and first-pass pulmonary extraction may influence toxicity (see "Systemic Toxicity"). In this regard, the relatively rapid hydrolysis of the ester local anesthetic chloroprocaine makes it less likely to produce sustained plasma concentrations than other local anesthetics, particularly the amino-amides. However, patients with atypical plasma cholinesterase levels may be at increased risk of developing excessive plasma concentrations of chloroprocaine or other ester local anesthetics due to absent or limited plasma hydrolysis. Hepatic metabolism of lidocaine is extensive, and clearance of this local anesthetic from plasma parallels hepatic blood flow. Liver disease or decreases in hepatic blood flow, as occur with congestive heart failure or general anesthesia, can decrease the rate of metabolism of lidocaine. Low water solubility of local anesthetics usually limits renal excretion of the parent compound to less than 5% of the injected dose.

Vasoconstrictors

Addition of a vasoconstrictor (e.g., 1:200,000 or 5 μg/mL of epinephrine) to local anesthetic solutions used for infiltration, peripheral block, and epidural or spinal anesthesia produces local vasoconstriction, which limits systemic absorption of local anesthetic and prolongs the duration of action while having little effect on the onset of anesthesia. Decreased systemic absorption of local anesthetic increases the likelihood that the rate of metabolism will match the rate of absorption, decreasing the possibility of systemic toxicity. Epinephrine may also decrease the likelihood of a systemic reaction by serving as a marker for detection of intravascular injection. However, systemic absorption of epinephrine may contribute to cardiac dysrhythmias or accentuate systemic hypertension in vulnerable patients. Epinephrine should be avoided when performing peripheral nerve blocks in areas that may lack collateral flow (e.g., digital blocks). In contrast, epinephrine-induced vasoconstriction decreases local bleeding and may provide added benefit when combined with local anesthetics used for infiltration anesthesia.

ADVERSE EFFECTS

Important adverse effects of local anesthetics, although rare, may occur from systemic absorption, local tissue toxicity, allergic reactions, and drug-specific effects.

Systemic Toxicity

Systemic toxicity of local anesthetics results from excessive plasma concentrations of these drugs, most often from accidental intravascular injection during performance of peripheral nerve blocks. Less often, excessive plasma concentrations result from absorption of local anesthetics from tissue injection sites. The magnitude of local anesthetic systemic absorption depends on the dose injected, the specific site of injection, and the inclusion of a vasoconstrictor in the local anesthetic solution. Systemic absorption of local anesthetic is greatest after injection for intercostal nerve blocks and caudal anesthesia, intermediate after epidural anesthesia, and least after brachial plexus blocks (Fig. 11-6).[5]

Clinically significant systemic toxicity results from effects on the central nervous system and cardiovascular system. Establishment of maximal acceptable local

Figure 11-6 Peak plasma concentrations of local anesthetics resulting during performance of various types of regional anesthetic procedures. (From Covino BD, Vassals HG. Local Anesthetics: Mechanism of Action in Clinical Use. Orlando, FL, Grune & Stratton, 1976, p 97, used with permission.)

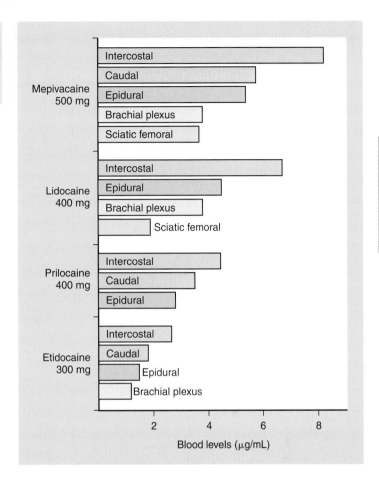

anesthetic doses for performance of regional anesthesia is an attempt to limit plasma concentrations that can result from systemic absorption of these drugs (see Table 11-1). However, standard dosage recommendations are not evidence-based, are inconsistent, and they fail to take into account the specific injection site and patient-related factors.[6] Nonetheless, dosage recommendations represent guidelines for providing a starting point from which adjustments based on clinical circumstances and evolving evidence can be made.

CENTRAL NERVOUS SYSTEM TOXICITY

Increasing plasma concentrations of local anesthetics classically produce circumoral numbness, facial tingling, restlessness, vertigo, tinnitus, and slurred speech, culminating in tonic-clonic seizures, though marked variation from this pattern is quite common.[7] Local anesthetics are neuronal depressants, and onset of seizures is thought to reflect selective depression of cortical inhibitory neurons, leaving excitatory pathways unopposed. However, larger doses may affect inhibitory and excitatory pathways, resulting in central nervous system depression and even coma. These effects generally parallel anesthetic

potency. Arterial hypoxemia and metabolic acidosis can occur rapidly during seizure activity, and acidosis potentiates the central nervous system toxicity of the local anesthetics.

Early tracheal intubation to facilitate ventilation and maintenance of oxygenation may be prudent, and is essential in patients at risk for aspiration. Neuromuscular blocking drugs can stop the peripheral manifestations of seizure activity but not the underlying central nervous system activity. Accordingly, treatment must include administration of drugs to stop the central nervous system seizure activity. Benzodiazepines have been generally considered the drugs of first choice because of their efficacy and relative hemodynamic stability. However, propofol is usually more immediately accessible, and it would seem preferable to administer small doses of propofol for seizure suppression when reliance on a benzodiazepine would engender a significant delay in treatment, particularly when there is no evidence of cardiac compromise. Moreover, propofol attenuates anesthetic-induced dysrrhythmias and depression of mean arterial blood pressure during continuous infusion of bupivacaine in rats.[8]

CARDIOVASCULAR SYSTEM TOXICITY

The cardiovascular system is generally more resistant to the toxic effects of local anesthetics than the central nervous system. Nevertheless, high plasma concentrations of local anesthetics can produce profound hypotension due to relaxation of arteriolar vascular smooth muscle and direct myocardial depression. The cardiac toxicity, in part, reflects the ability of local anesthetics to block cardiac sodium ion channels. As a result, cardiac automaticity and conduction of cardiac impulses are impaired, manifesting on the electrocardiogram as prolongation of the PR interval and widening of the QRS complex. Local anesthetics may also produce profound direct cardiac toxicity, and they are not all equivalent in this regard. For example, the ratio of the dose required to produce cardiovascular collapse compared with that producing seizures for lidocaine is about twice that for bupivacaine.[9] Such findings support the concept that bupivacaine has greater cardiac toxicity, which has been the driving force for development of single-enantiomer anesthetics, such as ropivacaine and levobupivacaine.

LIPID RESUSCITATION

Recently, a series of systematic experimentation and clinical events have identified a practical and apparently effective therapy for systemic anesthetic toxicity.[1] Based on experiments in rats[10] and dogs,[11] which demonstrated that administration of a lipid emulsion could attenuate bupivacaine cardiotoxicity, intralipid was given to a patient who sustained a cardiac arrest following an interscalene block performed with bupivacaine and mepivacaine.[12] Administration of lipid occurred after a prolonged but unsuccessful attempt at resuscitation using standard Advanced Cardiac Life Support (ACLS) algorithms (also see Chapter 44). The patient subsequently responded to defibrillation, ultimately making a complete recovery. The numerous reports which soon followed provided further support for the efficacy of lipid resuscitation for bupivacaine carditoxicity and extended the potential use of lipid rescue for treatment of ropivacaine cardiotoxicity, as well as local anesthetic CNS toxicity.[13] Moreover, experimental work and anecdotal clinical reports also provided evidence that lipid may have utility for treatment of toxicity induced by a wide variety of compounds, such as verapamil, clomipramine, haloperidol, and buproprion.[14] The mechanism by which lipid is effective is incompletely understood, but its predominant action is most likely related to its ability to extract bupivacaine (or other lipophilic drugs) from aqueous plasma or tissue targets, thus reducing their effective concentration ("lipid sink"). Accordingly, solutions of lipid emulsion should be stocked and readily accessible in any area where local anesthetics are administered, as well as locations where overdoses from any lipophilic drug might be treated. A more detailed discussion of this topic and guidelines for administration can be found in a publication by the American Society of

Regional Anesthesia Task Force on Local Anesthetic Systemic Toxicity[6] (asra.com), and at lipidrescue.org. Importantly, *propofol should not be administered for this purpose*, as the relatively enormous volume of this solution required for lipid therapy would deliver potentially lethal quantities of propofol.

Allergic Reactions

Allergic reactions to local anesthetics are rare, despite the frequent use of these drugs. It is estimated that less than 1% of all adverse reactions to local anesthetics are caused by allergic mechanisms. Most adverse responses attributed to allergic reactions are instead due to additives or manifestations of systemic toxicity from excessive plasma concentrations of the local anesthetic. Hypotension associated with syncope may be psychogenic or vagally mediated, whereas tachycardia and palpitations may occur from systemic absorption of epinephrine.

CROSS-SENSITIVITY

The amino-ester local anesthetics, which produce metabolites related to para-aminobenzoic acid, are more likely to evoke hypersensitivity reactions than the amino-amides. Although cross-sensitivity does not exist between classes of local anesthetics, allergic reactions may also be caused by methylparaben or similar compounds that resemble para-aminobenzoic acid, which are used as preservatives in commercial formulations of ester and amide local anesthetics. Although patients known to be allergic to ester local anesthetics can receive amide local anesthetics, this recommendation assumes that the local anesthetic was responsible for evoking the initial allergic reaction, rather than a common preservative.

DOCUMENTATION

Documentation of allergy to local anesthetics is based principally on clinical history (e.g., rash, laryngeal edema, hypotension, bronchospasm). However, elevations of serum tryptase, a marker of mast cell degranulation, may have some value with respect to confirmation, and intradermal testing may help establish the local anesthetic as the offending antigen if other drugs (e.g., sedative-hypnotics, opioids) have been administered concurrently.

SPECIFIC LOCAL ANESTHETICS

Amino-Esters

PROCAINE

The earliest injectable local anesthetic, procaine, enjoyed extensive use during the first half of the past century, primarily as a spinal anesthetic. Its instability and the considerable potential for hypersensitivity reactions resulted in limited use after the introduction of lidocaine. Concerns regarding transient neurologic symptoms (TNS) associated with spinal lidocaine (see "Lidocaine") have renewed interest in procaine as a spinal anesthetic. However, limited data suggest that procaine offers only small advantage with respect to TNS, and spinal procaine is associated with a significantly higher incidence of nausea.[15]

TETRACAINE

Tetracaine is still commonly used for spinal anesthesia. As such, it has a long duration of action, particularly if used with a vasoconstrictor, although this combination results in a surprisingly high risk of TNS.[16] Tetracaine is available as a 1% solution or as Niphanoid crystals; the crystal form is preferable because of the relative instability of the anesthetic in solution. Tetracaine is rarely used for epidural anesthesia or peripheral nerve blocks because of its slow onset, profound motor blockade, and potential toxicity when administered at high doses. Although it is an ester, its rate of metabolism is one fourth that of procaine and one tenth that of chloroprocaine.

CHLOROPROCAINE

Chloroprocaine initially gained popularity as an epidural anesthetic, particularly in obstetrics because its rapid hydrolysis virtually eliminated concern about systemic toxicity and fetal exposure to the local anesthetic. Unfortunately, neurotoxic injury, presumed to occur from accidental intrathecal injection of high doses intended for the epidural space, tempered enthusiasm for neuraxial administration of chloroprocaine. Some early experimental studies attributed this toxicity to the preservative, sodium bisulfite, contained in the commercial formulation.[17] However, more recent studies do not demonstrate neurotoxicity from intrathecal bisulfite and even suggest a neuroprotective effect for this compound.[18] In any event, a formulation of chloroprocaine devoid of preservatives and antioxidants is available.

Chloroprocaine produces epidural anesthesia of a relatively short duration. Epidural administration of chloroprocaine is sometimes avoided because it impairs the anesthetic or analgesic action of epidural bupivacaine and of opioids used concurrently or sequentially.[19] Chloroprocaine has been recently reevaluated as a spinal anesthetic,[20–22] reflecting clinical concerns related to the possible toxicity of lidocaine placed in the subarachnoid space,[23] and the low doses required for spinal anesthesia would not be predicted to produce toxicity. These initial reports have been encouraging, and the off-label use of chloroprocaine for this purpose is now fairly extensive, though published experience to date remains limited. Of note, despite the controversy, chloroprocaine solutions used for spinal anesthesia should be bisulfite-free, and the intrathecal dose should not exceed 60 mg.

Amino-Amide Local Anesthetics

LIDOCAINE

Lidocaine is the most commonly used local anesthetic. It is used for local topical and regional intravenous applications, peripheral nerve block, and spinal and epidural anesthesia. Although recent issues have led to restricted use of lidocaine for spinal anesthesia, this local anesthetic remains popular for all other applications, including epidural anesthesia.

Potential neurotoxicity (i.e., cauda equina syndrome) when lidocaine is administered for spinal anesthesia has emerged as a concern, especially when used with a continuous spinal technique.[24] Most of the initial injuries resulted from neurotoxic concentrations of anesthetic in the caudal region of the subarachnoid space achieved by the combination of maldistribution and relatively high doses of anesthetic administered through small-gauge spinal catheters.[25] However, even doses of lidocaine routinely used for single-injection spinal anesthesia (75 to 100 mg) have been associated with neurotoxicity.[23]

TNS is a syndrome of pain and dysesthesia that may occur in up to one third of patients receiving intrathecal doses of lidocaine (but rarely occurs with bupivacaine).[16,26,27] These symptoms were initially called transient radicular irritation, but this term was later abandoned in favor of TNS because of the lack of certainty regarding their cause. In addition to the use of intrathecal lidocaine, cofactors that contribute to the occurrence of TNS include the lithotomy position,[16,26] positioning for knee arthroscopy,[26] and outpatient status.[16] In contrast, local anesthetic concentration, the presence of glucose, concomitant administration of epinephrine, and technique-related factors such as the size or type of needle do not alter the incidence of TNS with lidocaine.[16]

Symptoms of TNS generally manifest within the first 12 to 24 hours after surgery, most often resolve within 3 days, and rarely persist beyond a week. Although self-limited, the pain can be quite severe, often exceeding that induced by the surgical procedure, and on rare occasions requiring rehospitalization for pain control. Nonsteroidal anti-inflammatory drugs are often fairly effective and should be used as first-line treatment. TNS is not associated with sensory loss, motor weakness, or bowel and bladder dysfunction. The etiology and significance of these symptoms remain to be established, but discrepancies between factors affecting TNS and experimental animal toxicity cast doubt that TNS and persistent neurologic deficits (e.g., cauda equina syndrome) are mediated by the same mechanism.

MEPIVACAINE

Mepivacaine was the first in the series of pipecholyl xylidines, combining the piperidine ring of cocaine with the xylidine ring of lidocaine (see Figs. 11-1 and 11-3). This resulted in an anesthetic with characteristics very similar to lidocaine, although with less vasodilation, and a slightly longer duration of action. The clinical use of mepivacaine parallels lidocaine, with the exception that it is relatively ineffective as a topical local anesthetic. As a spinal anesthetic, it appears to have a low, although not insignificant, incidence of TNS.

PRILOCAINE

Prilocaine was introduced into clinical practice with the anticipation that its rapid metabolism and low acute toxicity (central nervous system toxicity about 40% less than lidocaine) would make it a useful drug. Unfortunately, administration of high doses (>600 mg) may result in clinically significant accumulation of the metabolite, ortho-toluidine, an oxidizing compound capable of converting hemoglobin to methemoglobin. Prilocaine-induced methemoglobinemia spontaneously subsides and can be reversed by the administration of methylene blue (1 to 2 mg/kg IV over 5 minutes). Nevertheless, the capacity to induce dose-related methemoglobinemia has limited the clinical acceptance of this local anesthetic.

Similar to other anesthetics, prilocaine has recently received attention as a spinal anesthetic, owing to dissatisfaction with spinal lidocaine. Available data, albeit limited, suggest prilocaine has a duration of action similar to lidocaine with a much lower incidence of transient neurologic symptoms. Although prilocaine is not currently approved for use in the United States, nor is there any formulation available that would be appropriate for intrathecal administration, regulatory approval appears to be forthcoming in Europe.

BUPIVACAINE

Bupivacaine is a congener of mepivacaine, with a butyl rather than a methyl group on the piperidine ring, a modification that imparts a longer duration of action. This characteristic, combined with its high-quality sensory anesthesia relative to motor blockade, has established bupivacaine as the most commonly used local anesthetic for epidural anesthesia during labor and for postoperative pain management. Bupivacaine is also commonly used for peripheral nerve block, and it has a relatively unblemished record as a spinal anesthetic.

Refractory cardiac arrest has been associated with the use of 0.75% bupivacaine when accidentally injected intravenously during attempted epidural anesthesia,[28] and this concentration is no longer recommended for epidural anesthesia. The most likely mechanism for bupivacaine's cardiotoxicity relates to the nature of its interaction with cardiac sodium ion channels.[29] When electrophysiologic differences between anesthetics are compared, lidocaine is found to enter the sodium ion channel quickly and to leave quickly. In contrast, recovery from bupivacaine blockade during diastole is relatively prolonged, making it far more potent with respect to depressing the maximum upstroke velocity of the

cardiac action potential (V_{max}) in ventricular cardiac muscle. As a result, bupivacaine has been labeled a "fast-in, slow-out" local anesthetic. This characteristic likely creates conditions favorable for unidirectional block and reentry. Other mechanisms may contribute to bupivacaine's cardiotoxicity, including disruption of atrioventricular nodal conduction, depression of myocardial contractility, and indirect effects mediated by the central nervous system.[30] This potential for cardiotoxicity places important limitations on the total dose of bupivacaine, and it underscores the vital role of fractional dosing and methods to detect inadvertent intravascular injection during high-volume regional block. The recent identification of lipid emulsion as a therapeutic intervention for bupivacaine cardiotoxicity does not diminish the critical importance of these preventive measures. Of note, cardiotoxicity is of no concern when small doses are administered for spinal anesthesia.

Single-Enantiomer Local Anesthetics

Concerns for bupivacaine cardiotoxicity have focused attention on the stereoisomers of bupivacaine and on its homolog, ropivacaine.

STEREOCHEMISTRY

Isomers are different compounds that have the same molecular formula. Subsets of isomers that have atoms connected by the same sequence of bonds but that have different spatial orientations are called stereoisomers. Enantiomers are a particular class of stereoisomers that exist as mirror images. The term chiral is derived from the Greek cheir for "hand," because the forms can be considered nonsuperimposable mirror images. Enantiomers have identical physical properties except for the direction of the rotation of the plane of polarized light. This property is used to classify the enantiomer as dextrorotatory (+) if the rotation is to the right or clockwise and as levorotatory (–) if it is to the left or counterclockwise. A racemic mixture is a mixture of equal parts of enantiomers and is optically inactive because the rotation caused by the molecules of one isomer is canceled by the opposite rotation of its enantiomer. Chiral compounds can also be classified on the basis of absolute configuration, generally designated as R (rectus) or S (sinister). Enantiomers may differ with respect to specific biologic activity. For example, the S (–) enantiomer of bupivacaine has inherently less cardiotoxicity than its R (+) mirror image.

ROPIVACAINE

Ropivacaine (levopropivacaine) is the S (–) enantiomer of the homolog of mepivacaine and bupivacaine with a propyl tail on the piperidine ring. In addition to a more favorable interaction with cardiac sodium ion channels, ropivacaine has a greater propensity to produce vasoconstriction, which may contribute to its reduced cardiotoxicity. In vitro and in vivo studies provide some support for the reduced cardiotoxicity of ropivacaine compared with bupivacaine.

Motor blockade is less pronounced, and electrophysiologic studies raise the possibility that C fibers are preferentially blocked, together suggesting that ropivacaine may produce greater differential block. However, as expected from its lower lipid solubility, ropivacaine was found to be less potent than bupivacaine. The question of potency is critical to any comparison of these anesthetics; if more drug needs to be administered to achieve a desired effect, the apparent benefits with respect to cardiotoxicity (or differential block) may not exist when more appropriate equipotent comparisons are made. It appears that ropivacaine offers some advantage with respect to cardiotoxicity, but any benefit over bupivacaine with respect to differential block is marginal, at best.

LEVOBUPIVACAINE

Levobupivacaine is the single S (–) enantiomer of bupivacaine. Similar to ropivacaine, cardiotoxicity is reduced, but there is no advantage over bupivacaine with respect to differential blockade. As with ropivacaine, the clinically significant advantage of this compound over the racemic mixture is restricted to situations in which relatively high doses of anesthetic are administered.

Eutectic Mixture of Local Anesthetics

The keratinized layer of the skin provides an effective barrier to diffusion of topical anesthetics, making it difficult to achieve anesthesia of intact skin by topical application. However, a combination of 2.5% lidocaine and 2.5% prilocaine cream (i.e., eutectic mixture of local anesthetics [EMLA]) is available for this purpose. This mixture has a lower melting point than either component, and it exists as an oil at room temperature that is capable of overcoming the barrier of the skin. EMLA cream is particularly useful in children for the prevention or attentuation of pain associated with venipuncture or placement of an intravenous catheter, although it may take up to an hour before adequate topical anesthesia is produced.

FUTURE LOCAL ANESTHETICS

Local anesthetics play a central role in modern anesthetic practice. However, despite major advances in pharmacology and techniques for administration over the past century, this class of compounds has a relatively narrow therapeutic index with respect to their potential for neurotoxicity and for adverse cardiovascular and central nervous system effects. Toxicity has been the prominent force behind the evolution of these compounds and the manner in which they are used. Data demonstrate that the neurotoxicity of these compounds does not result from blockade of the voltage-gated sodium channel, indicating that local anesthetic effect and toxicity are not mediated by a common mechanism.[31] Local anesthetic binding to alternative sites at the sodium ion channel may display far greater affinity for neuronal over cardiac channels. The future may see the development of anesthetics with far better therapeutic advantage.

QUESTIONS OF THE DAY

1. What is the mechanism of local anesthetic blockade of nerve conduction?
2. Will the addition of sodium bicarbonate hasten the onset of local anesthetic action? Under what circumstances?
3. How does the metabolism of amino-amide local anesthetics differ from amino-ester local anesthetics?
4. What are the manifestations of systemic local anesthetic toxicity? What are the initial steps in management?
5. Why is bupivacaine associated with greater cardiotoxicity than lidocaine? What is the mechanism?

REFERENCES

1. Drasner K: Local anesthetic systemic toxicity: A historical perspective, *Reg Anesth Pain Med* 35:162–166, 2010.
2. Covino BG, Scott DB, Lambert DH: *Handbook of Spinal Anaesthesia and Analgesia*, Philadelphia, 1994, WB Saunders.
3. Gissen AJ, Covino BG, Gregus J: Differential sensitivities of mammalian nerve fibers to local anesthetic agents, *Anesthesiology* 53:467–474, 1980.
4. Winnie AP, Tay CH, Patel KP, et al: Pharmacokinetics of local anesthetics during plexus blocks, *Anesth Analg* 56:852–861, 1977.
5. Covino BG, Vassallo HG: *Local Anesthetics: Mechanisms of Action and Clnical Use*, Philadelphia, 1976, Grune & Stratton.
6. Rosenberg PH, Veering BT, Urmey WF: Maximum recommended doses of local anesthetics: a multifactorial concept, *Reg Anesth Pain Med* 29:564–575, 2004.
7. Neal JM, Bernards CM, Butterworth JF, et al: ASRA Practice Advisory on Local Anesthetic Systemic Toxicity, *Reg Anesth Pain Med* 35:152–161, 2010.
8. Ohmura S, Kawada M, Ohta T: Systemic toxicity and resuscitation in bupivacaine-, levobupivacaine-, or ropivacaine-infused rats, *Anesth Analg* 93:743–748, 2001.
9. de Jong RH, Ronfeld RA, DeRosa RA: Cardiovascular effects of convulsant and supraconvulsant doses of amide local anesthetics, *Anesth Analg* 61:3–9, 1982.
10. Weinberg GL, VadeBoncouer T, Ramaraju GA, et al: Pretreatment or resuscitation with a lipid infusion shifts the dose-response to bupivacaine-induced asystole in rats, *Anesthesiology* 88:1071–1075, 1998.
11. Weinberg G, Ripper R, Feinstein DL, et al: Lipid emulsion infusion rescues dogs from bupivacaine-induced cardiac toxicity, *Reg Anesth Pain Med* 28:198–202, 2003.
12. Rosenblatt MA, Abel M, Fischer GW: Successful use of a 20% lipid emulsion

to resuscitate a patient after a presumed bupivacaine-related cardiac arrest, *Anesthesiology* 105:217–218, 2006.

13. Spence AG: Lipid reversal of central nervous system symptoms of bupivacaine toxicity, *Anesthesiology* 107:516–517, 2007.

14. Sirianni AJ, Osterhoudt KC, Calello DP, et al: Use of lipid emulsion in the resuscitation of a patient with prolonged cardiovascular collapse after overdose of bupropion and lamotrigine, *Ann Emerg Med* 51:412–415, 2008.

15. Hodgson PS, Liu SS, Batra MS: Procaine compared with lidocaine for incidence of transient neurologic symptoms, *Reg Anesth Pain Med* 25:218–222, 2000.

16. Freedman JM, Li DK, Drasner K, et al: Transient neurologic symptoms after spinal anesthesia: An epidemiologic study of 1,863 patients, *Anesthesiology* 89:633–641, 1998.

17. Gissen AJ, Datta S, Lambert DH: The chloroprocaine controversy. Is chloroprocaine neurotoxic? *Reg Anesth* 9:135–144, 1984.

18. Taniguchi M, Bollen AW, Drasner K: Sodium bisulfite: Scapegoat for chloroprocaine neurotoxicity? *Anesthesiology* 100:85–91, 2004.

19. Eisenach JC, Schlairet TJ, Dobson CE 2nd, et al: Effect of prior anesthetic solution on epidural morphine analgesia, *Anesth Analg* 73:119–123, 1991.

20. Casati A, Fanelli G, Danelli G, et al: Spinal anesthesia with lidocaine or preservative-free 2-chlorprocaine for outpatient knee arthroscopy: A prospective, randomized, double-blind comparison, *Anesth Analg* 104:959–964, 2007.

21. Drasner K: Chloroprocaine spinal anesthesia: Back to the future? *Anesth Analg* 100(2):549–552, 2005.

22. Kouri ME, Kopacz DJ: Spinal 2-chloroprocaine: A comparison with lidocaine in volunteers, *Anesth Analg* 98:75–80, 2004.

23. Drasner K: Lidocaine spinal anesthesia: A vanishing therapeutic index? *Anesthesiology* 87:469–472, 1997.

24. Drasner K: Local anesthetic neurotoxicity: Clinical injury and strategies that may minimize risk, *Reg Anesth Pain Med* 27:576–580, 2002.

25. Rigler ML, Drasner K: Distribution of catheter-injected local anesthetic in a model of the subarachnoid space, *Anesthesiology* 75:684–692, 1991.

26. Hampl KF, Schneider MC, Ummenhofer W, et al: Transient neurologic symptoms after spinal anesthesia, *Anesth Analg* 81:1148–1153, 1995.

27. Pollock JE, Neal JM, Stephenson CA, et al: Prospective study of the incidence of transient radicular irritation in patients undergoing spinal anesthesia, *Anesthesiology* 84:1361–1367, 1996.

28. Albright GA: Cardiac arrest following regional anesthesia with etidocaine or bupivacaine, *Anesthesiology* 51:285–287, 1979.

29. Clarkson CW, Hondeghem LM: Mechanism for bupivacaine depression of cardiac conduction: Fast block of sodium channels during the action potential with slow recovery from block during diastole, *Anesthesiology* 62:396–405, 1985.

30. Bernards CM, Artu AA: Hexamethonium and midazolam terminate dysrhythmias and hypertension caused by intracerebroventricular bupivacaine in rabbits, *Anesthesiology* 74:89–96, 1991.

31. Sakura S, Bollen AW, Ciriales R, et al: Local anesthetic neurotoxicity does not result from blockade of voltage-gated sodium channels, *Anesth Analg* 81:338–346, 1995.

12 NEUROMUSCULAR BLOCKING DRUGS

Ronald D. Miller

Neuromuscular blocking drugs (NMBDs) interrupt transmission of nerve impulses at the neuromuscular junction (NMJ) and thereby produce paresis or paralysis of skeletal muscles. On the basis of electrophysiologic differences in their mechanisms of action and duration of action, these drugs can be classified as depolarizing NMBDs (mimic the actions of acetylcholine [ACh]) and nondepolarizing NMBDs (interfere with the actions of ACh), the latter of which are further subdivided into long-, intermediate-, and short-acting drugs (Table 12-1). Succinylcholine (SCh) is the only depolarizing NMBD used clinically. It is also the only NMBD that has both a rapid onset and ultrashort duration of action. Among the nondepolarizing NMBDs, rocuronium's onset time most closely resembles that of SCh.

CLINICAL USES

The principal clinical uses of NMBDs are to produce skeletal muscle relaxation for facilitation of tracheal intubation and to provide optimal surgical working conditions. NMBDs may also be administered during cardiopulmonary resuscitation and to patients in emergency departments, and intensive care units to facilitate mechanical ventilation of the patient's lungs. Of prime importance is to recognize that NMBDs lack analgesic or anesthetic effects and should not be used to render an inadequately anesthetized patient paralyzed. An inadequately anesthetized, but paralyzed patient is a major risk for awareness during general anesthesia (see Chapter 46). Ventilation of the lungs must be mechanically provided whenever significant skeletal muscle weakness is produced by these drugs. Clinically, intraoperative evaluation of neuromuscular blockade is typically provided by visually monitoring the mechanical response (twitch response) produced by electrical stimulation of a peripheral nerve (usually a branch of the ulnar or facial nerve) delivered from a peripheral nerve

stimulator (see the section "Monitoring the Effects of Nondepolarizing Neuromuscular Blocking Drugs").

Choice of Neuromuscular Blocking Drug

The choice of NMBD is influenced by its speed of onset, duration of action, route of elimination, and associated side effects, such as drug-induced changes in systemic arterial blood pressure or heart rate, or both. Rapid onset and brief duration of skeletal muscle paralysis, characteristic of SCh, are useful when tracheal intubation is the reason for administering an NMBD. Because of its rapid onset time, rocuronium is often used to facilitate tracheal intubation, but its duration of action is much longer than that of SCh. Although SCh can be given intermittantly, nondepolarizing NMBDs are usually selected when longer periods of neuromuscular blockade (e.g., more than 15 to 45 minutes) are needed. When rapid onset of skeletal muscle paralysis is not necessary, skeletal muscle relaxation can be induced by the administration of long- or intermediate-acting nondepolarizing NMBDs to facilitate tracheal intubation.

Hypersensitivity Reactions

The overall incidence of anesthetic-related hypersensitivity reactions ranges between 1/5000 and 1/20,000 procedures.[1] NMBDs are the triggering drugs for more than 35% of these reactions. SCh is the most common offender. Even though it does not release histamine, rocuronium was identified as producing an increased risk for hypersensitivity reactions in France and Norway, with no confirmation from other countries. More recently, a follow-up study from Norway of 83 cases of anaphylaxis during general anesthesia revealed that 77% of these reactions were mediated by immunoglobulin E and 93% were associated with NMBDs, again with SCh being the most common drug.[2] There may be cross-sensitivity between all NMBDs because of the presence of a common antigenic component, the quaternary ammonium group. Anaphylactic reactions after the first exposure to an NMBD may reflect sensitization from previous contact with cosmetics or soaps that also contain antigenic quaternary ammonium groups. Sugammadex (see "Antagonism of Nondepolarizing Neuromuscular Blocking Drugs" later in this chapter) was not approved by the Food and Drug Administration (FDA) because of hypersensitivity concerns. It is approved in Europe and other countries.

NEUROMUSCULAR JUNCTION

The anatomy of the NMJ consists of a prejunctional motor nerve ending separated from the highly folded postjunctional membrane of the skeletal muscle by a synaptic cleft (Fig. 12-1).[3,4] Nicotinic acetylcholine receptors

Table 12-1 Classification of Neuromuscular Blocking Drugs
Depolarizing (Rapid Onset and Ultrashort-Acting)   Succinylcholine
Nondepolarizing
Long-Acting   Pancuronium
Intermediate-Acting   Vecuronium   Rocuronium   Atracurium   Cisatracurium
Short-Acting   Mivacurium

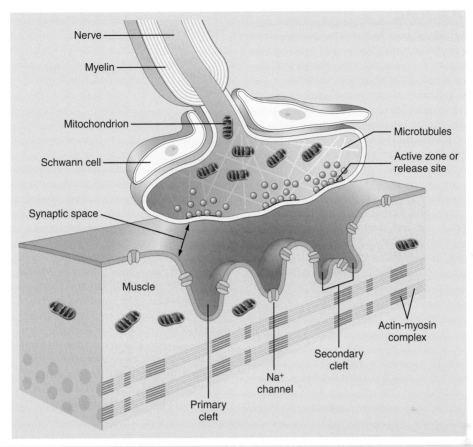

Figure 12-1 Adult neuromuscular junction with the three cells that constitute the synapse: the motor neuron (i.e., nerve terminal), muscle fiber, and Schwann cell. The motor neuron from the ventral horn of the spinal cord innervates the muscle. Each fiber receives only one synapse. The motor nerve loses its myelin and terminates on the muscle fiber. The nerve terminal, covered by a Schwann cell, has vesicles clustered about the membrane thickenings, which are the active zones, toward its synaptic side and mitochondria and microtubules toward its other side. A synaptic gutter, made up of a primary and many secondary clefts, separates the nerve from the muscle. The muscle surface is corrugated, and dense areas on the shoulders of each fold contain acetylcholine receptors. Sodium channels are present at the clefts and throughout the muscle membrane. (From Martyn JAJ. Neuromuscular physiology and pharmacology. In Miller RD [ed]. Miller's Anesthesia, 6th ed. Philadelphia, Churchill Livingstone, 2005.)

(nAChR) are located at pre- and postjunctional sites.[4] Neuromuscular transmission is initiated by arrival of an impulse at the motor nerve terminal with an associated influx of calcium ions and resultant release of the ligand ACh. ACh binds to AChRs (the ligand-gated channel) on postjunctional membranes and thereby causes a change in membrane permeability to ions, principally potassium and sodium. This change in permeability and movement of ions causes a decrease in the transmembrane potential from about -90 mV to -45 mV (threshold potential), at which point a propagated action potential spreads over the surfaces of skeletal muscle fibers and leads to muscular contraction. ACh is rapidly hydrolyzed (within 15 msec) by the enzyme acetylcholinesterase (true cholinesterase), thus restoring membrane permeability (repolarization) and preventing sustained depolarization. Acetylcholinesterase is primarily located in the folds of

the end-plate region, which places it in close proximity to the site of action of ACh.

Prejunctional Receptors and Release of Acetylcholine

ACh is synthesized in the motor nerve terminal, and the protein synapsin anchors the ACh vesicle to the release site of the terminal. Some of the ACh is then released and the rest is held in reserve for response to a stimulus. Presynaptic receptors, aided by calcium, facilitate replenishment of the motor nerve terminal, which can be stimulated by SCh and neostigmine and depressed by small doses of nondepolarizing NMBDs. Inhibition of these presynaptic nAChRs explains the fade in response to high frequency repetitive stimulation such as tetanic or even train-of-four stimulation.[4]

Postjunctional Receptors

Postjunctional receptors are glycoproteins consisting of five subunits (Fig. 12-2).[4] The subunits of the receptor are arranged such that a channel is formed that allows the flow of ions along a concentration gradient across cell membranes. This flow of ions is the basis of normal neuromuscular transmission. Extrajunctional receptors retain the two α-subunits but may have an altered γ- or δ-subunit by the substitution of an ε-unit.

The two α-subunits are the binding sites for ACh and the sites occupied by NMBDs. For example, occupation of one or both α-subunits by a nondepolarizing NMBD causes the ion channel to remain closed, and ion flow to produce depolarization cannot occur. SCh attaches to α-sites and causes the ion channel to remain open (mimics ACh), thereby resulting in prolonged depolarization. Large doses of nondepolarizing NMBDs (large molecules) may also act to occlude the channel and in this way prevent the normal flow of ions. Neuromuscular blockade secondary to occlusion of the channels is resistant to drug-enhanced antagonism with anticholinesterase drugs. The lipid environment around cholinergic receptors can be altered by drugs such as volatile anesthetics, thus changing the properties of the ion channels. This probably accounts for the augmentation of neuromuscular blockade by volatile anesthetics.

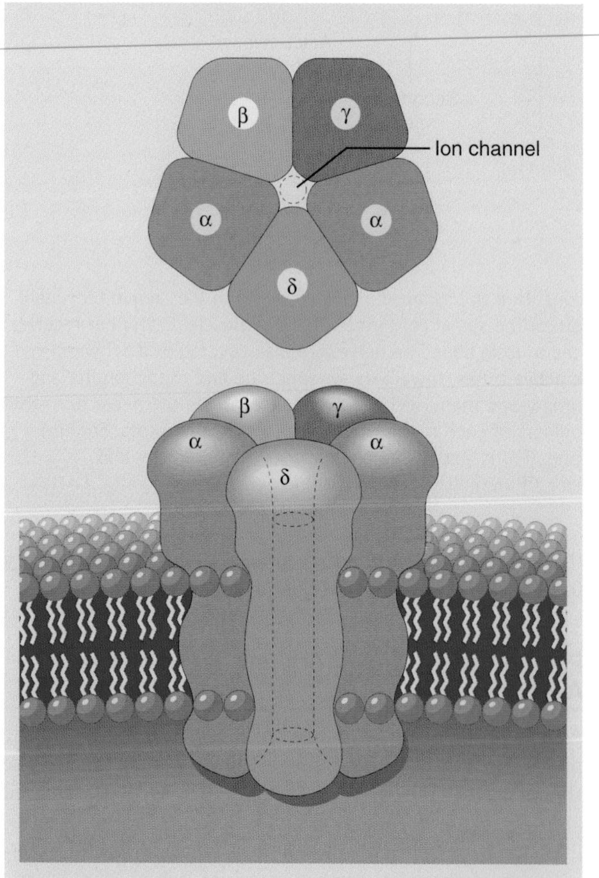

Extrajunctional Receptors

Postjunctional receptors are confined to the area of the end plate precisely opposite the prejunctional receptors, whereas extrajunctional receptors (the ε-unit is replaced by γ-subunits) are present throughout skeletal muscles. Extrajunctional receptor synthesis is normally suppressed by neural activity. Prolonged inactivity, sepsis, and denervation or trauma (burn injury) to skeletal muscles may be associated with a proliferation of extrajunctional receptors. When activated, extrajunctional receptors stay open longer and permit more ions to flow, which in part explains the exaggerated hyperkalemic response when SCh is administered to patients with denervation or burn injury. Proliferation of these receptors also accounts for the resistance or tolerance to nondepolarizing NMBDs, as can occur with burns or prolonged (several days) mechanical ventilation of the lungs (also see discussion under "Hyperkalemia").[5,6]

Figure 12-2 The postjunctional nicotinic cholinergic receptor consists of five subunits (α, α, β, γ, δ) arranged to form an ion channel. (From Taylor P. Are neuromuscular blocking agents more efficacious in pairs? Anesthesiology 1985;63:1-3, used with permission.)

STRUCTURE-ACTIVITY RELATIONSHIPS

NMBDs are quaternary ammonium compounds that have at least one positively charged nitrogen atom that binds to the α-subunit of postsynaptic cholinergic receptors (Fig. 12-3). In addition, these drugs have structural similarities to the endogenous neurotransmitter ACh. For example, SCh is two molecules of ACh linked by methyl groups. The long, slender, flexible structure of ACh allows it to bind to and activate cholinergic receptors. The bulky rigid molecules that are characteristic of nondepolarizing NMBDs, though containing portions similar to ACh, do not activate cholinergic receptors.

Nondepolarizing NMBDs are either aminosteroid compounds (pancuronium, vecuronium, rocuronium) or benzylisoquinolinium compounds (atracurium, cisatracurium, mivacurium). Pancuronium is the bisquaternary aminosteroid NMBD most closely related to ACh structurally. The ACh-like fragments of pancuronium give the steroidal molecule its high degree of neuromuscular blocking activity. Vecuronium and rocuronium are monoquaternary analogs of pancuronium. Aminosteroid NMBDs lack hormonal activity. Benzylisoquinolinium derivatives are more likely than aminosteroid derivatives to evoke the release of histamine, presumably reflecting the presence of a tertiary amine.

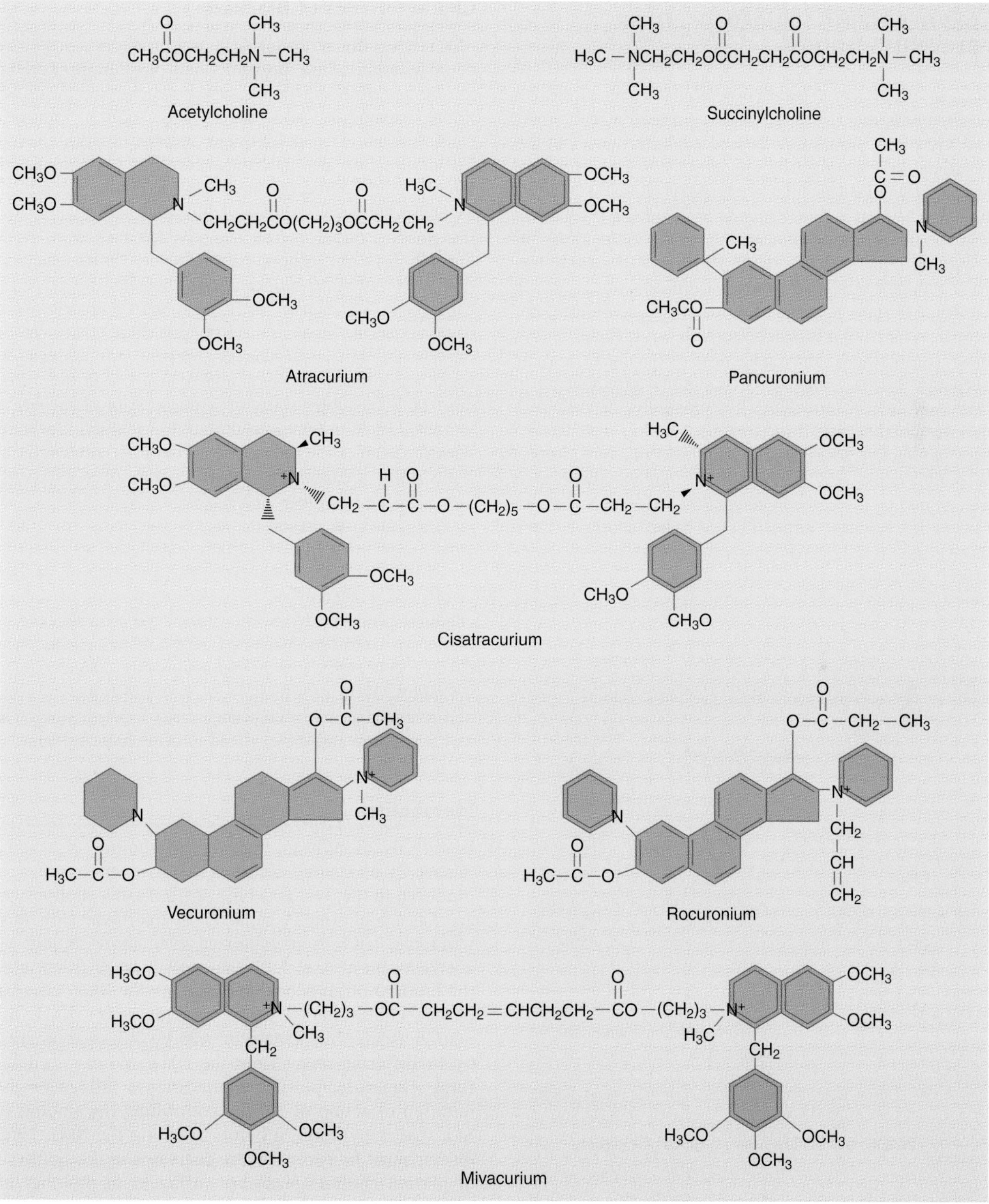

Figure 12-3 Chemical structure of acetylcholine and neuromuscular blocking drugs.

DEPOLARIZING NEUROMUSCULAR BLOCKING DRUGS

SCh is the only depolarizing NMBD used clinically. Furthermore, it is the only NMBD with both a rapid onset and ultrashort duration of action. Typically, doses of 0.5 to 1.5 mg/kg intravenously are administered and produce a rapid onset of skeletal muscle paralysis (30 to 60 seconds) that lasts 5 to 10 minutes because of its unique breakdown (Fig. 12-4). These characteristics make SCh ideal for providing rapid skeletal muscle paralysis to facilitate tracheal intubation. SCh has been used clinically for more than 50 years. Despite consistent industrial efforts, no drug has been developed that is better than SCh for tracheal intubation.[7] Although an intravenous dose of 0.5 mg/kg may be adequate, 1.0 to 1.5 mg/kg is commonly administered to facilitate tracheal intubation. If a subparalyzing dose of a nondepolarizing NMBD (pretreatment with 5% to 10% of its 95% effective dose [ED_{95}]) is administered 2 to 4 minutes before injection of SCh to blunt fasciculations, the dose of SCh should be increased by about 70%. Although ideal for facilitating tracheal intubation, SCh has many adverse effects (see Table 12-4). As an alternative, the intermediate-acting nondepolarizing NMBD rocuronium has an onset time as rapid as SCh in doses ranging from 1.0 to 1.2 mg/kg.

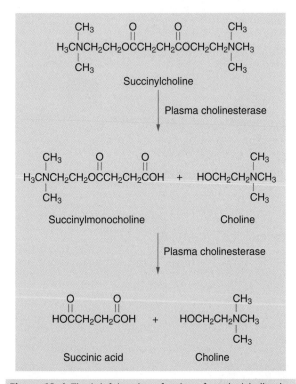

Figure 12-4 The brief duration of action of succinylcholine is due to its rapid hydrolysis in plasma by cholinesterase enzyme to inactive metabolites (succinylmonocholine has 1/20 to 1/80 the activity of succinylcholine at the neuromuscular junction.)

Characteristics of Blockade

SCh mimics the action of ACh and produces a sustained depolarization of the postjunctional membrane. Skeletal muscle paralysis occurs because a depolarized postjunctional membrane and inactivated sodium channels cannot respond to subsequent release of ACh (hence, the designation depolarizing neuromuscular blockade). Depolarizing neuromuscular blockade is also referred to as phase I blockade. Phase II blockade is present when the postjunctional membrane has become repolarized but still does not respond normally to ACh (desensitization neuromuscular blockade). The mechanism of phase II blockade is unknown but may reflect the development of nonexcitable areas around the end plates that become repolarized but nevertheless prevent the spread of impulses initiated by the action of ACh. With the initial dose of SCh, subtle signs of a phase II blockade begin to appear (fade to tetanic stimulation).[8] Phase II blockade, which resembles the blockade produced by nondepolarizing NMBDs, predominates when the dose of SCh exceeds 3 to 5 mg/kg IV (Table 12-2).

The sustained depolarization produced by the initial administration of SCh is initially manifested as transient generalized skeletal muscle contractions known as fasciculations. Furthermore, the sustained opening of sodium channels produced by SCh is associated with leakage of potassium from the interior of cells sufficient to increase plasma concentrations of potassium by about 0.1 to 0.4 mEq/L. With proliferation of extrajunctional nAChRs and damaged muscle membranes, many more channels will leak potassium and thereby lead to acute hyperkalemia.

Metabolism

Hydrolysis of SCh to inactive metabolites is accomplished by plasma cholinesterase (pseudocholinesterase) produced in the liver (see Fig. 12-4). Plasma cholinesterase has an enormous capacity to hydrolyze SCh at a rapid rate (ACh is metabolized even more rapidly by acetylcholinesterase) such that only a small fraction of the original intravenous dose reaches the NMJ. Because plasma cholinesterase is not present at the NMJ, the neuromuscular blockade produced by SCh is terminated by its diffusion away from the NMJ into extracellular fluid. Therefore, plasma cholinesterase influences the duration of action of SCh by controlling the amount of SCh that is hydrolyzed before reaching the NMJ. Liver disease must be severe before decreases in the synthesis of plasma cholinesterase are sufficient to prolong the effects of SCh. Potent anticholinesterases, as used in the treatment of myasthenia gravis, and certain chemotherapeutic drugs (nitrogen mustard, cyclophosphamide) may so decrease plasma cholinesterase activity that prolonged skeletal muscle paralysis follows the administration of SCh.

Table 12-2 Comparison of Depolarizing (Succinylcholine) and Nondepolarizing (Rocuronium) Neuromuscular Blocking Drugs

	Succinylcholine		Rocuronium
	Phase I	*Phase II*	
Administration of rocuronium	Antagonize	Augment	Augment
Administration of succinylcholine	Augment	Augment	Antagonize
Administration of neostigmine	Augment	Antagonize	Antagonize
Fasciculations	Yes		No
Response to single electrical stimulation (single twitch)	Decreased	Decreased	Decreased
Train-of-four ratio	>0.7	<0.3	<0.3
Response to continuous (tetanus) electrical stimulation	Sustained	Unsustained	Unsustained
Post-tetanic facilitation	No	Yes	Yes

Table 12-3 Variants of Plasma Cholinesterase and Duration of Action of Succinylcholine

Variants of Plasma Cholinesterase	Type of Butylcholinesterase	Incidence	Dibucaine Number (% Inhibition of Enzyme Activity)	Duration of Succinylcholine-Induced Neuromuscular Blockade (min)
Homozygous, typical	UU	Normal	70-80	5-10
Heterozygous	UA	1/480	50-60	20
Homozygous, atypical	AA	1/3200	20-30	60-180

ATYPICAL PLASMA CHOLINESTERASE

Atypical plasma cholinesterase lacks the ability to hydrolyze ester bonds in drugs such as SCh and mivacurium. The presence of this atypical enzyme is often recognized only after an otherwise healthy patient experiences prolonged skeletal muscle paralysis (>1 hour) after the administration of a conventional dose of SCh or mivacurium. Subsequent determination of the dibucaine number permits diagnosis of the presence of atypical plasma cholinesterase. Dibucaine is an amide local anesthetic that inhibits normal plasma activity by about 80%, whereas the activity of atypical enzyme is inhibited by about 20% (Table 12-3). The dibucaine number reflects the quality of plasma cholinesterase (ability to metabolize SCh and mivacurium) and not the quantity of enzyme that is circulating in plasma. For example, decreases in plasma cholinesterase activity because of liver disease or anticholinesterases are often associated with a normal dibucaine number.

Adverse Side Effects

Adverse side effects after the administration of SCh are numerous and may limit or even contraindicate the use of this NMBD in certain patients (Table 12-4). After 50 years of use, SCh continues to cause serious complications.[9,10] SCh usually should not be given to patients 24 to 72 hours after major burns, trauma, and extensive denervation of

Table 12-4 Adverse Side Effects of Succinylcholine

Cardiac dysrhythmias
Sinus bradycardia
Junctional rhythm
Sinus arrest
Fasciculations
Hyperkalemia
Myalgia
Myoglobinuria
Increased intraocular pressure
Increased intragastric pressure
Trismus

skeletal muscles because it may result in acute hyperkalemia and cardiac arrest.[5,6] Administration of SCh to apparently healthy boys with unrecognized muscular dystrophy has resulted in acute hyperkalemia and cardiac arrest. For this reason, the FDA has issued a warning against the use of SCh in children, except for emergency control of the airway.

CARDIAC DYSRHYTHMIAS

Sinus bradycardia, junctional rhythm, and even sinus arrest may follow the administration of SCh. These

Table 12-5 Autonomic Nervous System and Histamine-Releasing Effects of Neuromuscular Blocking Drugs

Drug*	Nicotinic Receptors at Autonomic Ganglia	Cardiac Postganglionic Muscarinic Receptors	Histamine Release
Succinylcholine	Modest stimulation	Modest stimulation	Minimal
Pancuronium	None	Modest blockade	None
Vecuronium	None	None	None
Rocuronium	None	None	None
Atracurium	None	None	Slight†
Cisatracurium	None	None	None
Mivacurium	None	None	Slight†

*ED$_{95}$, 95% effective dose.
†Occurs only with doses estimated to be 2 to 3 × ED$_{95}$.

responses reflect the action of SCh at cardiac postganglionic muscarinic receptors, where this drug mimics the normal effects of ACh (Table 12-5). Cardiac dysrhythmias are most likely to occur when a second intravenous dose of SCh is administered about 5 minutes after the first dose. Intravenous administration of atropine 1 to 3 minutes before SCh decreases the likelihood of these cardiac responses. Yet, atropine administered intramuscularly with the preoperative medication does not reliably protect against SCh-induced decreases in heart rate. The effects of SCh at autonomic nervous system ganglia also mimic the actions of the neurotransmitter ACh and may be manifested as ganglionic stimulation with associated increases in systemic blood pressure and heart rate (see Table 12-5).

HYPERKALEMIA
Administration of SCh can rapidly result in massive hyperkalemia, serious cardiac arrythmias, and even cardiac arrest.[5,6] In some patients, potassium levels can exceed 10 mEq/L. The classic conditions that lead to hyperkalemia after SCh include burns, trauma, and spinal cord or other major neurologic damage. Any time prolonged skeletal muscle inactivity (critical care) or extensive muscle damage exists, patients may be susceptible to hyperkalemia 48 hours after injury and is dependent on the development of extrajunctional, atypical receptors as described above.[4-6] When muscle has returned to its normal state, hyperkalemia will not occur. However, the judgment as to the "normal" state of the muscle is a clinically difficult estimation. In addition, extrajunctional receptors and hyperkalemia will develop in any patient who is immobile (critical care patients) for several days if SCh is given. For example, cardiac arrest has occurred when SCh has been used for emergency endotracheal intubation in the intensive care unit. The use of SCh for urgent tracheal intubation is contraindicated or not allowed in many intensive care units. The duration of susceptibility to the hyperkalemic effects of SCh is

unknown, but the risk is probably decreased 3 to 6 months after denervation injury. All factors considered, it might be prudent to avoid administration of SCh to any patient more than 24 hours after a burn injury, extensive trauma, or spinal cord transection or who may become an intensive care patient.

Even though they may have increased potassium levels, patients with renal failure are not susceptible to exaggerated release of potassium, and SCh can be safely administered to these patients, assuming that they do not have uremic neuropathy.

MYALGIA
Postoperative skeletal muscle myalgia, manifested particularly in the muscles of the neck, back, and abdomen, may follow the administration of SCh. Myalgia localized to neck muscles may be described as a "sore throat" by the patient and incorrectly attributed to the previous presence of a tracheal tube. Young adults undergoing minor surgical procedures that permit early ambulation seem most likely to complain of myalgia. Unsynchronized contractions of skeletal muscle fibers (fasciculations) associated with generalized depolarization lead to myalgia. Prevention of fasciculations by prior administration of subparalyzing doses of a nondepolarizing NMBD (pretreatment) or lidocaine will decrease the incidence but not totally prevent myalgia.[11] Magnesium will prevent fasciculations, but not myalgia. Nonsteroidal anti-inflammatory drugs are effective in treating the myalgia.

INCREASED INTRAOCULAR PRESSURE
SCh causes a maximum increase in intraocular pressure 2 to 4 minutes after its administration. This increase in intraocular pressure is transient and lasts only 5 to 10 minutes. The mechanism by which SCh increases intraocular pressure is unknown, although contraction of extraocular muscles with associated compression of the globe may be involved. The concern that contraction of

extraocular muscles could cause extrusion of intraocular contents in the presence of an open eye injury has resulted in the common clinical practice of avoiding the administration of SCh to these patients. This theory has never been substantiated and is challenged by the report of patients with an open eye injury in whom intravenous administration of SCh did not cause extrusion of global contents.[12] Furthermore, there is evidence that contraction of extraocular muscles does not contribute to the increase in intraocular pressure that accompanies the administration of SCh.[13]

INCREASED INTRACRANIAL PRESSURE

Increases in intracranial pressure after the administration of SCh can occur but are of little or no concern.

INCREASED INTRAGASTRIC PRESSURE

SCh causes unpredictable increases in intragastric pressure. When intragastric pressure does increase, it seems to be related to the intensity of fasciculations, thus emphasizing the potential value of preventing this skeletal muscle activity by prior administration of a subparalyzing dose of a nondepolarizing NMBD. An unproven hypothesis is that this increased intragastric pressure may cause passage of gastric fluid and contents into the esophagus and pharynx with a subsequent risk for pulmonary aspiration.

TRISMUS

Incomplete jaw relaxation with masseter jaw rigidity after a halothane-SCh sequence is not uncommon in children (occurs in about 4.4% of patients) and is considered a normal response. In extreme cases this response may be so severe that the ability to mechanically open the patient's mouth is limited. The difficulty lies in separating the normal response to SCh from the masseter rigidity that may be associated with malignant hyperthermia.

Because SCh is not recommended for use in children, except for emergency airway control, trismus is less of an issue.

NONDEPOLARIZING NEUROMUSCULAR BLOCKING DRUGS

Nondepolarizing NMBDs are classified clinically as long-, intermediate-, and short-acting (see Table 12-1). These drugs act by competing with ACh for α-subunits at the postjunctional nicotinic cholinergic receptors and preventing changes in ion permeability (see Fig. 12-2). As a result, depolarization cannot occur (hence, the designation nondepolarizing neuromuscular blockade), and skeletal muscle paralysis develops. Unlike SCh, skeletal muscle fasciculations do not accompany the onset of nondepolarizing neuromuscular blockade. Differences in onset, duration of action, rate of recovery, metabolism, and clearance influence the clinical decision to select one drug versus another (Table 12-6). For example, rocuronium has the most rapid onset time and minimal cardiovascular effects; cisatracurium is not dependent on the kidney for its elimination. Do these characteristics make rocuronium choice for facilitating endotracheal intubation and cisatracurium for kidney transplantation? Yet, only vecuronium and rocuronium are antagonized by sugammadex. These are a few of the variables that influence the choice of NMBD to be used for individual clinical situations.

Pharmacokinetics

Nondepolarizing NMBDs, because of their quaternary ammonium groups, are highly ionized, water-soluble compounds at physiologic pH and possess limited lipid solubility. As a result, these drugs cannot easily cross lipid membrane barriers, such as the blood-brain barrier,

Table 12-6 Comparative Pharmacology of Nondepolarizing Neuromuscular Blocking Drugs

Drug	ED$_{95}$ (mg/kg)	Onset to Maximum Twitch Depression (min)	Duration to Return to ≥25%* (min)	Intubating Dose (mg/kg)	Continuous Infusion (mg/kg/ min)	Renal Excretion (% Unchanged)	Hepatic Degradation (%)	Biliary Excretion (% Unchanged)	Hydrolysis in Plasma
Pancuronium	0.07	3-5	60-90	0.1		80	10	5-10	No
Vecuronium	0.05	3-5	20-35	0.08-0.1	1	15-25	20-30	40-75	No
Rocuronium	0.3	1-2	20-35	0.6-1.2		10-25	10-20	50-70	No
Atracurium	0.2	3-5	20-35	0.4-0.5	6-8	NS	NS	NA	Enzymatic, spontaneous
Cisatracurium	0.05	3-5	20-35	0.1	1-1.5	NS	NS	NS	Spontaneous
Mivacurium	0.08	2-3	12-20	0.25	5-6	NS	NS	NS	Enzymatic

NS, not significant.
*Control twitch height (minutes).

renal tubular epithelium, gastrointestinal epithelium, or placenta. Therefore, nondepolarizing NMBDs do not produce central nervous system effects, renal tubular reabsorption is minimal, oral administration is ineffective, and maternal administration does not adversely affect the fetus. Redistribution of nondepolarizing NMBDs also exerts a role in the pharmacokinetics of these drugs.

Many of the variable pharmacologic responses of patients to nondepolarizing NMBDs can be explained by differences in pharmacokinetics, which can be changed by many factors, such as hypovolemia, hypothermia, and the presence of hepatic or renal disease (or both). Renal and hepatic elimination is aided by access to a large fraction of the administered drug because of the high degree of ionization, which maintains high plasma concentrations of nondepolarizing NMBDs and also prevents renal reabsorption of excreted drug.

Renal disease markedly alters the pharmacokinetics of only the long-acting nondepolarizing NMBDs, such as pancuronium. The intermediate-acting NMBDs are eliminated by the liver (rocuronium), by metabolism by plasma cholinesterase (mivacurium), by Hofmann elimination (atracurium or cisatracurium), or by a combination of these mechanisms.

Pharmacodynamic Responses

Enhancement of neuromuscular blockade by volatile anesthetics reflects a pharmacodynamic action as manifested by decreased plasma concentrations of nondepolarizing NMBDs required to produce a given degree of neuromuscular blockade in the presence of volatile anesthetics. In addition to volatile anesthetics, other drugs, such as aminoglycoside antibiotics, local anesthetics, cardiac antiarrhythmic drugs, dantrolene, magnesium, lithium, and tamoxifen (an antiestrogenic drug), may enhance the neuromuscular blockade produced by nondepolarizing NMBDs. A few drugs may diminish the effects of a nondepolarizing NMBD, including calcium, corticosteroids, and anticonvulsant (phenytoin) drugs. Some neuromuscular diseases can be associated with altered pharmacodynamic responses (myasthenia gravis, Duchenne muscular dystrophy). Burn injury causes resistance to the effects of nondepolarizing NMBDs, as reflected by the need to establish a higher plasma concentration of drug to achieve the same pharmacologic effect as in patients without a burn injury. There is resistance to the effects of nondepolarizing NMBDs in skeletal muscles affected by a cerebral vascular accident, perhaps reflecting proliferation of extrajunctional receptors that respond to ACh.

Cardiovascular Effects

Nondepolarizing NMBDs may exert minor cardiovascular effects through drug-induced release of histamine, effects on cardiac muscarinic receptors, or effects on nicotinic receptors at autonomic ganglia (see Table 12-5). Transient hypotension can occur with atracurium and mivacurium, but usually with large doses (>0.4 and 0.15 mg/kg, respectively). The relative magnitude of the circulatory effects varies from patient to patient and depends on factors such as underlying autonomic nervous system activity, blood volume status, preoperative medication, drugs administered for maintenance of anesthesia, and concurrent drug therapy.

Critical Care Medicine and Critical Illness Myopathy and Polyneuropathy[3,4]

Currently, NMBDs are not used as often as in the past. Yet, a small fraction of patients with asthma (receiving corticosteroids) or acutely injured patients with multiple organ system failure (including sepsis) who require mechanical ventilation of the lungs for prolonged periods (usually more than 6 days) may manifest prolonged skeletal muscle weakness on recovery that is augmented by the skeletal muscle paralysis produced by NMBDs. These patients exhibit moderate to severe quadriparesis with or without areflexia, but they usually retain normal sensory function. The time course of the weakness is unpredictable, and in some patients the weakness may progress and persist for weeks or months. The pathophysiology of this myopathy is not well understood. Therefore, NMBDs should be given for 2 days or less and only after the use of analgesics, sedatives, and adjustments to ventilator settings have been maximally used. Although myopathy occurs autonomously, administration of NMBDs can augment the severity of this condition. SCh probably should not be used to facilitate endotracheal intubation in critically ill patients because of reports of cardiac arrest, presumably caused by acute hyperkalemia. In fact, SCh is not allowed for use in many critical care units.

LONG-ACTING NONDEPOLARIZING NEUROMUSCULAR BLOCKING DRUGS

Pancuronium

Pancuronium is a bisquaternary aminosteroid nondepolarizing NMBD with an ED_{95} of 70 μg/kg; it has an onset of action of 3 to 5 minutes and a duration of action of 60 to 90 minutes (see Table 12-6 and Fig. 12-3). An estimated 80% of a single dose of pancuronium is eliminated unchanged in urine. In the presence of renal failure, plasma clearance of pancuronium is decreased 30% to 50%, thus resulting in a prolonged duration of action. An estimated 10% to 40% of pancuronium undergoes hepatic deacetylation to inactive metabolites, with the exception of 3-desacetylpancuronium, which is approximately 50% as potent as pancuronium at the NMJ.

CARDIOVASCULAR EFFECTS

Pancuronium typically produces a modest 10% to 15% increase in heart rate, mean arterial pressure, and cardiac output. The increase in heart rate reflects pancuronium-induced selective blockade of cardiac muscarinic receptors (atropine-like effect), principally in the sinoatrial node. Histamine release and autonomic ganglion blockade are not produced by pancuronium.

INTERMEDIATE-ACTING NONDEPOLARIZING NEUROMUSCULAR BLOCKING DRUGS

Rocuronium, vecuronium, atracurium, and cisatracurium are classified as intermediate-acting nondepolarizing NMBDs. In contrast to the long-acting nondepolarizing NMBD pancuronium, these drugs possess efficient clearance mechanisms that create a shorter duration of action.

When compared with pancuronium, these drugs have (1) a similar onset of maximum neuromuscular blockade, with the exception of rocuronium, which is unique because of its rapid onset, which can (with large doses) parallel that of SCh; (2) approximately one third the duration of action (hence the designation intermediate acting); (3) a 30% to 50% more rapid rate of recovery; and (4) minimal to absent cardiovascular effects except for atracurium. Neostigmine or sugammadex antagonism of the neuromuscular blockade produced by intermediate-acting nondepolarizing NMBDs is facilitated by the concomitant spontaneous recovery that occurs after rapid clearance of the drug.

Vecuronium

Vecuronium is a monoquaternary aminosteroid nondepolarizing NMBD with an ED_{95} of 50 µg/kg that produces an onset of action of 3 to 5 minutes and a duration of action of 20 to 35 minutes (see Fig. 12-3 and Table 12-6). This drug undergoes both hepatic and renal excretion. Metabolites are pharmacologically inactive, with the exception of 3-desacetylvecuronium, which is approximately 50% to 70% as potent as the parent compound. The increased lipid solubility of vecuronium as compared with pancuronium also facilitates biliary excretion of vecuronium. The effect of renal failure on the duration of action of vecuronium is small, but repeated or large doses may result in prolonged neuromuscular blockade. Vecuronium is typically devoid of circulatory effects, emphasizing its lack of vagolytic effects (pancuronium) or histamine release (atracurium).

Rocuronium

Rocuronium is a monoquaternary aminosteroid nondepolarizing NMBD with an ED_{95} of 0.3 mg/kg that has an onset of action of 1 to 2 minutes and a duration of action of 20 to 35 minutes (see Table 12-6 and Fig. 12-3). The lack of potency of rocuronium in comparison to vecuronium is an important factor in determining the rapid onset of neuromuscular blockade produced by this NMBD. Conceptually, when a large number of molecules are administered, the result is a larger number of molecules that are available to diffuse to the NMJ. Thus, a rapid onset of action is more likely to be achieved with a less potent drug such as rocuronium. The onset of maximum single twitch depression after the intravenous administration of rocuronium at 3 to 4 × ED_{95} (1.2 mg/kg) resembles the onset of action of SCh after the intravenous administration of 1 mg/kg (Fig. 12-5).[14] However, the large doses of rocuronium (3 to 4 × ED_{95}) needed to mimic the onset time of SCh produce a duration of action resembling that of pancuronium.[15]

Clearance of rocuronium is largely as unchanged drug in bile, with deacetylation not occurring. Renal excretion

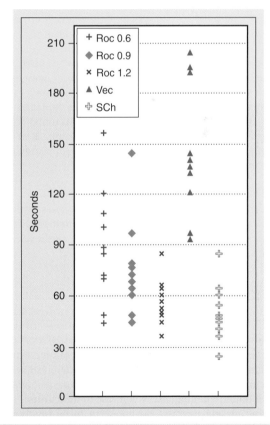

Figure 12-5 The onset to maximum twitch depression is similar after the intravenous administration of rocuronium (Roc) at doses of 0.9 mg/kg and 1.2 mg/kg and succinylcholine (SCh), 1 mg/kg. Vec, vecuronium. (From Magorian TT, Flannery KB, Miller RD. Comparison of rocuronium, succinylcholine and vecuronium for rapid sequence induction of anesthesia. Anesthesiology 1993;79:913-918, used with permission.)

of the drug may account for as much as 30% of a dose, and administration of this drug to patients in renal failure could result in a longer duration of action, especially with repeated doses or prolonged intravenous infusion.

Atracurium

Atracurium is a bisquaternary benzylisoquinolinium nondepolarizing NMBD (mixture of 10 stereoisomers) with an ED_{95} of 0.2 mg/kg that produces an onset of action of 3 to 5 minutes and a duration of action of 20 to 35 minutes (see Table 12-6 and Fig. 12-3). Clearance of this drug is by a chemical mechanism (spontaneous nonenzymatic degradation at normal body temperature and pH known as Hofmann elimination) and a biologic mechanism (ester hydrolysis by nonspecific plasma esterases). Laudanosine is the major metabolite of both pathways. This metabolite is not active at the NMJ but may, in high, nonclinical concentrations, cause central nervous system stimulation. The two routes of metabolism occur simultaneously and are independent of hepatic and renal function, as well as plasma cholinesterase activity. As such, the duration of atracurium-induced neuromuscular blockade is similar in normal patients and those with absent or impaired renal or hepatic function or those with atypical plasma cholinesterase (emphasizes that ester hydrolysis of atracurium is unrelated to the plasma cholinesterase responsible for the hydrolysis of SCh and mivacurium). Ester hydrolysis accounts for an estimated two thirds of degraded atracurium. Hofmann elimination accounts for the remaining breakdown of atracurium.

CARDIOVASCULAR EFFECTS

Because of histamine release with larger doses, atracurium can cause hypotension and tachycardia. However, doses smaller than $2 \times ED_{95}$ rarely cause cardiovascular effects.

Cisatracurium

Cisatracurium is a benzylisoquinolinium nondepolarizing NMBD with an ED_{95} of 50 µg/kg that has an onset of action of 3 to 5 minutes and a duration of action of 20 to 35 minutes (see Table 12-6 and Fig. 12-3).[16] Structurally, cisatracurium is an isolated form of 1 of the 10 stereoisomers of atracurium. This drug principally undergoes degradation by Hofmann elimination. In contrast to atracurium, nonspecific plasma esterases do not seem to be involved in the clearance of cisatracurium. The organ-independent clearance of cisatracurium means that this nondepolarizing NMBD, like atracurium, can be administered to patients with renal or hepatic failure without a change in its duration of action. Cisatracurium is often used in patients undergoing renal transportation. Cisatracurium, in contrast to atracurium, is devoid of histamine-releasing effects, so

cardiovascular changes do not accompany the rapid intravenous administration of even large doses of cisatracurium.

SHORT-ACTING NONDEPOLARIZING NEUROMUSCULAR BLOCKING DRUGS

Mivacurium

Mivacurium is a benzylisoquinolinium nondepolarizing NMBD with an ED_{95} of 80 µg/kg that has an onset of action of 2 to 3 minutes and a duration of action of 12 to 20 minutes (see Table 12-6 and Fig. 12-3). As such, the duration of action of mivacurium is approximately twice that of SCh and 30% to 40% that of the intermediate-acting nondepolarizing NMBDs. Mivacurium consists of three stereoisomers, with the two most active isomers undergoing hydrolysis by plasma cholinesterase at a rate equivalent to 88% that of SCh. Hydrolysis of these two isomers is responsible for the short duration of action of mivacurium. As with SCh, hydrolysis of mivacurium is decreased and its duration of action increased in patients with atypical plasma cholinesterase (see Table 12-3). Mivacurium is currently not being marketed in the United States and therefore is not available for use by Americans delivering anesthetic care.

MONITORING THE EFFECTS OF NONDEPOLARIZING NEUROMUSCULAR BLOCKING DRUGS

Evaluation of the mechanically evoked responses produced by electrical stimulation delivered from a peripheral nerve stimulator is the most reliable method to monitor the pharmacologic effects of NMBDs. Use of a peripheral nerve stimulator permits titration of the NMBD to produce the desired pharmacologic effect, and at the conclusion of surgery the responses evoked by the nerve stimulator are used to judge spontaneous recovery from an NMBD-induced neuromuscular blockade, which is facilitated by the administration of anticholinesterase drugs (e.g., neostigmine) (see the discussion under "Antagonism of Nondepolarizing Neuromuscular Blocking Drugs").

Monitoring of the neuromuscular blockade from NMBDs surprisingly is not routinely used during administration of anesthesia. Most surveys have found that only 30% to 70% of anesthesiologists in the United States and Europe use perpherial nerve stimulation as a monitor. Yet, such monitoring allows NMBDs to be given in a more efficacious manner. Such monitoring provides a more precise guide for NMBD requirements intraoperatively and effective antagonism by neostigmine. More recently, complications in the postanesthesia care unit (PACU) are less frequent when monitoring is used.

Even though they are not consistently used, monitoring the effects of NMBDs should be routinely performed.[17] As with many other monitors (e.g., pulse oximetry, see Chapter 20), perhaps using objective monitoring (i.e., peripheral nerve stimulation) will become mandatory when NMBDs are given. No matter which pattern of peripheral nerve stimulation is used, clinical care will be improved if any type of such monitoring is used. Of prime importance is using anesthetic monitoring. Despite the presence of studies designed to establish the relative efficacy of different types of stimulation,[18] the type of stimulation being used is of secondary importance. Nevertheless, the well-informed clinician should have some basic knowledge of the various types of stimulation proposed and used. Furthermore, the various types of stimulation have varying sensitivity with the degree of neuromuscular blockade detected (see Table 12-7). Conceptually, the question that can be asked is, "How many receptors can be still occupied and have a normal response to that particular pattern of stimulation?" When the pattern of stimulation requires more receptors to be unoccupied in order to have a normal response, then that approach will be more sensitive in detecting residual neuromuscular blockades. Now the technical aspects of monitoring of neuromuscular blockade will be described.

Most often, superficial electrodes or subcutaneous needles (must have a metal hub) are placed over the ulnar nerve at the wrist or elbow or the facial nerve on the lateral aspect of the face, and a supramaximal electrical stimulus is delivered from the peripheral nerve stimulator.[19,20] The adductor pollicis muscle is innervated solely by the ulnar nerve, which accounts for the popularity of placing stimulating electrodes from the peripheral nerve stimulator over the ulnar nerve. Facial nerve stimulation and observation of the orbicularis oculi muscle, though difficult to quantitate, may be a consideration when

mechanically evoked responses to stimulation of the ulnar nerve are not visible because of positioning of the upper extremities.[21] Another consideration is the observation that monitoring the response of the orbicularis oculi muscle to facial nerve stimulation more closely reflects the onset of neuromuscular blockade at the larynx than does the response of the adductor pollicis to ulnar nerve stimulation (Fig. 12-6).[22] Moreover, the onset of neuromuscular blockade after the administration of nondepolarizing NMBDs is more rapid, but less intense at the laryngeal muscles (vocal cords) than at the peripheral muscles (adductor pollicis) (see Fig. 12-5).[21] In this regard, the period of laryngeal paralysis may be dissipating before a maximum effect is reached at the adductor pollicis. In contrast, the onset of neuromuscular blockade at the laryngeal muscles and at the muscles innervated by the ulnar nerve is similar when SCh is administered. Thus, monitoring the twitch response at the adductor pollicis is more likely to parallel the intensity of the drug-induced effect at the laryngeal adductors when SCh is administered.

Patterns of Stimulation

Mechanically evoked responses used for monitoring the effects of NMBDs include the single twitch response, train-of-four (TOF) ratio, double burst suppression, tetanus, and post-tetanic stimulation (Figs. 12-6 to 12-10).[19,20] These mechanically evoked responses are evaluated visually, manually by touch (tactile), or by recording. The depth of neuromuscular blockade may be defined as the percentage of a predetermined inhibition of twitch response from control height (ED_{95}, dose necessary to depress the twitch response 95%) and the duration of drug effect as the time from drug administration until the twitch response recovers to a percentage of control height (see Table 12-6).

Figure 12-6 The effects of rocuronium (in terms of maximum depression of the single twitch response) are less intense and the duration of action is less at the adductor muscles of the larynx than at the adductor pollicis. (From Meistelman C, Plaud B, Donati F. Rocuronium [ORG 9426] neuromuscular blockade at the adductor muscles of the larynx and adductor pollicis in humans. Can J Anaesth 1992;39:665-669, used with permission.)

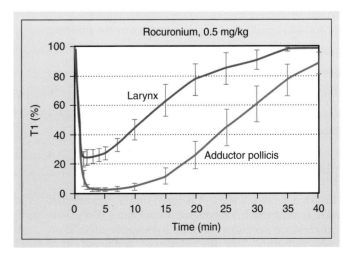

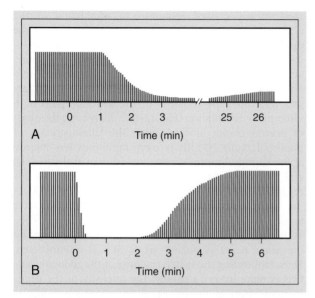

Figure 12-7 Schematic illustration of the onset and recovery from the neuromuscular blocking effects of a nondepolarizing (**A**) or a depolarizing (**B**) neuromuscular blocking drug ("0 time" indicates injection of the neuromuscular blocking drug) as depicted by the mechanically evoked single twitch response to repeated electrical stimulation of the nerve. (Modified from Viby-Mogensen J. Clinical assessment of neuromuscular transmission. Br J Anaesth 1982;54:209-223, used with permission.)

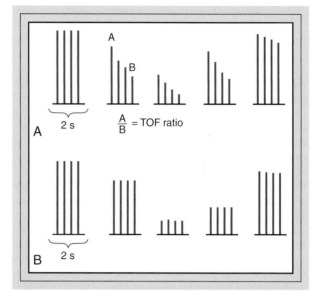

Figure 12-8 Schematic illustration of the mechanically evoked response to train-of-four (TOF) electrical stimulation of the nerve after injection of a nondepolarizing neuromuscular blocking drug (**A**) or a depolarizing (succinylcholine) neuromuscular blocking drug (**B**). The TOF ratio is less than 1 (fades) only in the presence of effects at the neuromuscular junction produced by a nondepolarizing neuromuscular blocking drug. (Modified from Viby-Mogensen J. Clinical assessment of neuromuscular transmission. Br J Anaesth 1982;54:209-223, used with permission.)

The response to peripheral nerve stimulation can be used to answer the following questions:

1. Is the neuromuscular blockade adequate for surgery?
2. Is the neuromuscular blockade excessive?
3. Can this neuromuscular blockade be antagonized?

Depression of the twitch response greater than 90% or elimination of two to three twitches of the TOF correlates with acceptable skeletal muscle relaxation for performance of intra-abdominal surgery in the presence of an adequate concentration of volatile anesthetic. If all twitches from TOF stimulation are absent, more NMBD should not be given until some twitch is present. If some of the twitches from TOF stimulation are present, antagonism is likely to be successful (see the section, "Antagonism of Nondepolarizing Neuromuscular Blocking Drugs").

TRAIN-OF-FOUR STIMULATION

TOF stimulation (four electrical stimulations at 2 Hz delivered every 0.5 second) is based on the concept that ACh is depleted by successive stimulations. Only four twitches are necessary because subsequent stimulation fails to further alter the release of additional ACh.

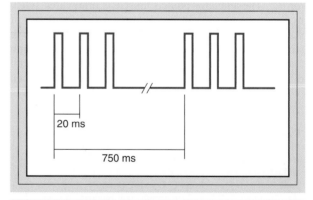

Figure 12-9 Schematic illustration of the stimulation pattern of double burst stimulation (three electrical impulses at 50 Hz separated by 750 msec). (From Bevan DR, Donati F, Kopman AF. Reversal of neuromuscular blockade. Anesthesiology 1992;77:785-792, used with permission.)

In the presence of effects produced at the neuromuscular junction by nondepolarizing NMBDs, the height of the fourth twitch is lower than that of the first twitch, thereby allowing calculation of a TOF ratio (fade) (see Fig. 12-8).[19] Recovery of the TOF ratio to greater than

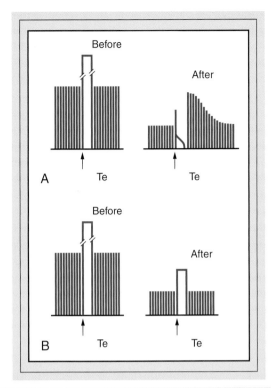

Figure 12-10 Schematic illustration of the evoked response to tetanic (Te) stimulation (50 Hz for 5 seconds) before and after the intravenous injection of a nondepolarizing neuromuscular blocking drug (**A**) or a depolarizing (succinylcholine) neuromuscular blocking drug (**B**). (Modified from Viby-Mogensen J. Clinical assessment of neuromuscular transmission. Br J Anaesth 1982;54:209-223, used with permission.)

0.7 correlates with complete return to control height of a single twitch response. In the presence of effects produced at the neuromuscular junction by SCh, the TOF ratio remains near 1.0 because the height of all four twitch responses is decreased by a similar amount (phase I blockade) (see Fig. 12-8).[19] A TOF ratio of less than 0.3 in the presence of SCh reflects phase II blockade (see Table 12-2).

DOUBLE BURST SUPPRESSION

Accurate estimation of the TOF ratio is not reliable clinically by either visual or manual assessment. Difficulty in estimating the TOF ratio may be due to the fact that the two middle twitch responses interfere with comparison of the first and last twitch response. In this regard, double burst suppression (two bursts of three electrical stimulations separated by 750 msec) is perceived by the observer as two separate twitches (see Fig. 12-9).[20] The observer's ability to detect a TOF ratio less than 0.3 is improved with double burst suppression, but the ability to conclude that the TOF ratio is greater than 0.7 is still not ensured.[23] In contrast to the difficulty in quantifying the TOF ratio, determination of the number of electrically evoked twitch responses to TOF stimulation is more likely to be reproducible. For example, the fourth twitch can be observed when the first twitch is equivalent to 30% to 40% of control twitch height, which corresponds to a TOF ratio of about 0.35. Counting the number of visible TOF responses may be helpful in predicting the ease with which neuromuscular blockade can be antagonized with an anticholinesterase drug (Table 12-8) (see the section "Antagonism of Nondepolarizing Neuromuscular Blocking Drugs").[20]

TETANUS

Tetanus (continuous or tetanic electrical stimulation for 5 seconds at about 50 Hz) is an intense stimulus for the release of ACh at the NMJ. In the presence of effects produced at the NMJ by nondepolarizing NMBDs, the response to tetanus is not sustained (fades), whereas in the presence of SCh-induced effects at the NMJ, the response to tetanus is greatly decreased but does not fade with a phase I blockade (Fig. 12-10).[19] A sustained response to tetanus is present when the TOF ratio is greater than 0.7. At the cessation of tetanus, there is an

Table 12-7	Choice of Anticholinesterase Drug			
TOF Visible Twitches	**Estimated TOF Fade**	**Anticholinesterase Drug and Dose (mg/kg IV)**	**Anticholinergic Drug and Dose (μg/kg IV)***
None†		Not recommended	Not recommended
≤2	++++	Neostigmine 0.07	Glycopyrrolate, 7, or atropine, 15
3-4	+++	Neostigmine 0.04	Glycopyrrolate, 7, or atropine, 15
4	++	Edrophonium 0.5	Atropine 7
4	0	Edrophonium 0.25	Atropine 7

++++, marked; +++, moderate; ++, minimal; 0, none; TOF, train-of-four.
*Administered simultaneously with an anticholinesterase drug.
†Postpone drug-assisted antagonism until some evoked response is visible.
Adapted from Bevan DR, Donati F, Kopman AF. Reversal of neuromuscular blockade. Anesthesiology 1992;77:785-792, used with permission.

increase in the immediately available stores of ACh such that the subsequent twitch responses are transiently enhanced (post-tetanic facilitation) (see Fig. 12-10).[19]

ANTAGONISM OF NONDEPOLARIZING NEUROMUSCULAR BLOCKING DRUGS

Antagonism of the effects of nondepolarizing NMBDs as achieved by the intravenous administration of an anticholinesterase drug (usually neostigmine, but possibly and rarely edrophonium or pyridostigmine) may be recommended on a routine basis. Even if all tests of the adequacy of normal neuromuscular function are normal, 50% of the receptors at the NMJ may still be occupied by an NMBD. Patients will likely need more available receptors for adequate skeletal muscle strength. An excellent rule to follow is: "when in doubt, it is better to have as many receptors free of the effects of NMBDs as possible" (see Tables 12-7 and 12-8).[19,20] Unequivocal clinical confirmation (sustained head lift or leg lift, or both, for 5 seconds, tongue depressor test or a TOF > 0.9) provides assurance of adequate recovery (spontaneous and drug assisted) from the effects of NMBDs.

ADVERSE OUTCOMES FROM INADEQUATE ANTAGONISM OF NEUROMUSCULAR BLOCKADE

The time starting with the extubation of the trachea, transport to the PACU, and the first 30 minutes in the PACU can be one of the most dangerous times in the perioperative period. Inadequately antagonized or residual neuromuscular blockade can impair the integrity of the airway[24] and cause critical respiratory events in the PACU.[25] Analysis of large numbers of patients indicate that residual neuromuscular blockade is usually a component of adverse outcomes and even death. Specifically, residual neuromuscular blockade contributes to airway obstruction, inadequate ventilation, and hypoxia and has an incidence of 0.8% to 6.9%.[25] Other factors contributing to adverse effects in the PACU include obesity, opioids, emergency surgery, long duration of surgery, and abdominal surgery.[25] Clearly, clinicians should do everything possible to assure that residual neuromuscular blockade does not persist into the postoperative period by careful monitoring,[26,27] close observation, and alertness that such a blockade might exist.[28] The importance of residual neuromuscular blockade is increasingly recognized by scholarly analysis of this topic.[27–29]

Anticholinesterase Drugs (Neostigmine)

Anticholinesterase drugs are typically administered during the time when spontaneous recovery from the neuromuscular blockade is occurring so that the effect of the pharmacologic antagonist adds to the rate of spontaneous recovery from the nondepolarizing NMBD. Neostigmine is the most common anticholinesterase drug currently used. The rapid spontaneous recovery rate characteristic of intermediate-acting NMBDs is an advantage over a long-acting NMBD such as pancuronium. For example, the incidence of weakness in the postoperative period despite administration of neostigmine is more frequent in patients receiving pancuronium than an intermediate- or short-acting NMBD.

Anticholinesterase drugs, such as neostigmine, accelerate the already established pattern of spontaneous recovery at the neuromuscular junction by inhibiting the activity of acetylcholinesterase and thereby leading to the accumulation of ACh at nicotinic neuromuscular and muscarinic sites. Increased amounts of ACh in the region of the neuromuscular junction improve the chance that two ACh molecules will bind to the α-subunits of the nicotinic cholinergic receptors (see Fig. 12-2). This action

Table 12-8 Clinical Tests of Neuromuscular Transmission

Test	Normal Function	% of Receptors Occupied*	Comment
Tidal volume	5 mL/kg	80	Insensitive
Train-of-four	No fade	70	Somewhat uncomfortable
Vital capacity	At least 20 mL/kg	70	Requires patient cooperation
Sustained tetanus (50 Hz)	No fade	60	Uncomfortable
Double burst suppression	No fade	60	Uncomfortable
Head lift	180 Degrees for 5 sec	50	Requires patient cooperation
Handgrips	Sustained for 5 sec	50	Requires patient cooperation

*Approximate percentage of receptors occupied when the response returns to its normal value.
Adapted from Naguib M, Lien CA. Pharmacology of muscle relaxants and their antagonists. In Miller RD (ed). Miller's Anesthesia, 6th ed. Philadelphia, Churchill Livingstone, 2005.

alters the balance of the competition between ACh and a nondepolarizing NMBD in favor of the neurotransmitter (ACh) and restores neuromuscular transmission. In addition, neostigmine may generate antidromic action potentials and repetitive firing of motor nerve endings (presynaptic effects).

The quaternary ammonium structure of anticholinesterase drugs greatly limits their entrance into the central nervous system such that selective antagonism of the peripheral nicotinic effects of nondepolarizing NMBDs at the NMJ is possible. For example, the peripheral cardiac muscarinic effects of neostigmine (bradycardia) are prevented by the prior or simultaneous intravenous administration of atropine or glycopyrrolate. In fact, either atropine or glycopyrrolate must be given when neostigmine is given.

Factors Influencing the Success of Antagonism of Neuromuscular Blocking Drugs

Factors influencing the success of antagonism of NMBDs include (1) the intensity of the neuromuscular blockade at the time that the pharmacologic antagonist is administered, (2) the choice of antagonist drug, (3) the dose of antagonist drug, (4) the rate of spontaneous recovery from the NMBD, and (5) the concentration of the inhaled anesthetic.

Neostigmine is the most commonly administered antagonist. The greater the spontaneous recovery, as judged by the response to peripheral nerve stimulation, the more rapidly that complete recovery will occur from neostigmine administration. Although large doses of neostigmine will result in more rapid antagonism, the maximum dose should be limited to 60 to 70 µg/kg. Antagonism will be more rapid in the presence of an NMBD with rapid elimination (atracurium instead of pancuronium). The rate of antagonism can also be hastened by reducing the concentration of the volatile anesthetic.

Evaluation of the Adequacy of Antagonism

Adequacy of recovery (spontaneous and drug assisted) from the neuromuscular blocking effects produced by nondepolarizing NMBDs should be determined by the result of multiple tests of skeletal muscle strength (see Table 12-8).[26–29] Even though a TOF ratio of at least 0.9 has been recommended, visual estimation of the TOF is neither accurate nor reliable. In the absence of an accurately measured TOF ratio, a sustained response to tetanus or the ability to maintain head lift for 5 to 10 seconds usually indicates a TOF ratio greater than 0.9. Grip strength is also a useful indicator of recovery from the effects of NMBDs. Although a TOF ratio higher than 0.7 or its equivalent provides evidence of the patient's ability to sustain adequate ventilation, the pharyngeal musculature may still be weak and upper airway obstruction remains a risk. Furthermore, diplopia, dysphagia, an increased risk of aspiration, and a decreased ventilatory response to hypoxia in the presence of a TOF ratio greater than 0.9 emphasize the value of more sensitive clinical methods for assessing neuromuscular function, such as sustained head lift or leg lift (or both) for 5 seconds or an evaluation of masseter muscle strength (tongue depressor test).[29]

Allowing spontaneous recovery from NMBDs without the aid of drug-assisted antagonism (administration of an anticholinesterase drug) is not recommended unless there is compelling clinical evidence that significant residual neuromuscular blockade does not persist. Avoidance of drug-assisted antagonism (neostigmine) for fear of increasing the incidence of postoperative nausea and vomiting is not warranted.

When the initial response to an anticholinesterase drug seems inadequate, the following questions should be answered before additional antagonist drug is administered:

1. Has sufficient time elapsed for the anticholinesterase drug to antagonize the nondepolarizing NMBD (15 to 30 minutes)?
2. Is the neuromuscular block too intense to be antagonized?
3. Is acid-base and electrolyte status normal?
4. Is body temperature normal?
5. Is the patient taking any drugs that could interfere with antagonism?
6. Has clearance of the nondepolarizing NMBD from plasma been decreased by renal or hepatic dysfunction (or by both)?

Answers to these questions will often provide the reason for failure of anticholinesterase drugs, such as neostigmine, to adequately antagonize nondepolarizing neuromuscular blockade.

A New Antagonist of Neuromuscular Blocking Drugs[30]

A γ-cyclodextrin (sugammadex) is under development that antagonizes steroidal NMBDs, especially rocuronium, by encapsulating and inactivating them. This mechanism of action is totally different from that of neostigmine in that no action on any cholinesterase takes place. Sugammadex has no action itself at the neuromuscular junction. The rate that it reliably reverses even a profound neuromuscular block is rapid (2 to 3 minutes) and complete. Furthermore, no cardiovascular effects occur; therefore, no other drug such as atropine is needed. Large doses of sugammadex can be given alone without cardiovascular effects. It could have major impact in three major ways. First, a rocuronium-sugammadex combination can be used for a rapid sequence induction of anesthesia and recovery more rapid than with SCh. Second, it can allow more profound neuromuscular blocks to be induced intraoperatively without fear of inadequate reversal. Lastly, as indicated earlier, the incidence of residual neuromuscular blockade should be reduced or eliminated.

Sugammadex has been approved for use in Europe and successfully used in thousands of patients. It will be approved in many other countries in 2010. It is hoped that sugammadex will eventually be approved in the United States.

SUMMARY

Neuromuscular blocking drugs are vital components of anesthetic care and airway management. When these drugs were introduced over 50 years ago, we were taught to either give small doses or even avoid paralysis if possible. We now have much safer drugs, better antagonist drugs and monitoring devices, and more knowledge. We even have evidence that proper use of neuromuscular blocking drugs can add safety if properly used.[31] The principles in this chapter represent contemporary use of neuromuscular blocking drugs and their antagonists.[32]

QUESTIONS OF THE DAY

1. What are the characteristics of succinylcholine phase I and phase II blockade?
2. What conditions can lead to life-threatening hyperkalemia with succinylcholine administration?
3. Which medications commonly administered in the perioperative period can lead to enhanced action of nondepolarizing neuromuscular blocking drugs (NMBDs)?
4. What are the potential adverse outcomes from residual neuromuscular blockade that may present in the post-anesthesia care unit (PACU)?
5. What clinical and peripheral nerve stimulation tests most accurately predict adequate reversal of nondepolarizing NMBDs?
6. How does the mechanism of action of sugammadex differ from neostigmine, when used to antagonize nondepolarizing NMBD activity?

REFERENCES

1. McNeill O, Kerridge RK, Boyle MJ: Review of procedures for investigation of anaesthesia-associated anaphylaxis in Newcastle, Australia, *Anaesth Intensive Care* 36:201–207, 2008.
2. Harboe T, Guttormsen AB, Irgens A, et al: Anaphylaxis during anesthesia in Norway: a 6-year single-center follow-up study, *Anesthesiology* 102:897–903, 2005.
3. Martyn JAJ: Neuromuscular physiology and pharmacology. In Miller RD, editor: *Miller's Anesthesia*, ed 6, Philadelphia, 2005, Churchill Livingstone.
4. Fagerlund MJ, Eriksson LI: Current concepts in neuromuscular transmission, *Br J Anaesth* 103:108–114, 2009.
5. Gronert GA: Succinylcholine-induced hyperkalemia and beyond, 1975, *Anesthesiology* 111:1372–1377, 2009.
6. Martyn JAJ, Richtsfeld M: Succinylcholine-induced hyperkalemia in acquired pathologic states: etiologic factors and molecular mechanisms, *Anesthesiology* 104:158–169, 2006.
7. Miller R: Will succinylcholine ever disappear? *Anesth Analg* 98:1674–1675, 2004.
8. Naguib M, Lien CA, Aker J, et al: Posttetanic potentiation and fade in the response to tetanic and train-of-four stimulation during succinylcholine-induced block, *Anesth Analg* 98:1686–1691, 2004.
9. Baumann A, Studnicska D, Audibert G, et al: Refractory anaphylactic cardiac arrest after succinylcholine administration, *Anesth Analg* 109:137–140, 2009.
10. Holak EJ, Connelly JF, Pagel PS: Suxamethonium-induced hyperkalaemia 6 weeks after chemoradiotherapy in a patient with rectal carcinoma, *Br J Anaesth* 98:766–768, 2007.
11. Schreiber JU, Lysakowski C, Fuchs-Buder T, et al: Prevention of succinylcholine-induced fasciculation and myalgia: a meta-analysis of randomized trials, *Anesthesiology* 103:877–884, 2005.
12. Libonati MM, Leahy JJ, Ellison N: The use of succinylcholine in open eye surgery, *Anesthesiology* 62:637–640, 1985.
13. Kelly RE, Dinner M, Turner LS, et al: Succinylcholine increases intraocular pressure in the human eye with the extraocular muscles detached, *Anesthesiology* 79:948–952, 1993.
14. Magorian T, Flannery KB, Miller RD: Comparison of rocuronium, succinylcholine and vecuronium for rapid sequence induction of anesthesia, *Anesthesiology* 79:913–918, 1993.
15. Sluga M, Ummenhofer W, Studer W, et al: Rocuronium versus succinylcholine for rapid sequence induction of anesthesia and endotracheal intubation: a prospective, randomized trial in emergent cases, *Anesth Analg* 101:1356–1361, 2005.
16. Mellinghoff H, Radbruch L, Diefenbach C, et al: A comparison of cisatracurium and atracurium: Onset of neuromuscular block after bolus injection and recovery after subsequent infusion, *Anesth Analg* 83:1072–1075, 1996.
17. Eriksson LI: Evidence-based practice and neuromuscular monitoring: it's time for routine quantitative assessment, *Anesthesiology* 98:1037–1039, 2003.
18. Claudius C, Skovgaard LT, Viby-Mogensen J: Is the performance of acceleromyography improved with preload and normalization? *Anesthesiology* 110:1261–1270, 2009.
19. Viby-Mogensen J: Clinical assessment of neuromuscular transmission, *Br J Anaesth* 54:209–223, 1982.
20. Bevan DR, Donati F, Kopman AF: Reversal of neuromuscular blockade, *Anesthesiology* 77:785–792, 1992.
21. Sayson SC, Mongan PD: Onset of action of mivacurium chloride: A comparison of neuromuscular blockade monitoring at the adductor pollicis and the orbicularis oculi, *Anesthesiology* 81:35–42, 1994.
22. Meistelman C, Plaud B, Donati F: Rocuronium (ORG 9426) neuromuscular blockade at the adductor muscles of the larynx and adductor pollicis in humans, *Can J Anaesth* 39:665–669, 1992.
23. Kopman AF, Yee PS, Neuman GG: Relationship of the train-of-four fade to the clinical signs and symptoms of residual paralysis in awake volunteers, *Anesthesiology* 86:765–771, 1997.
24. Herbstreit F, Peters J, Eikermann M: Impaired upper airway integrity by residual neuromuscular blockade: increased airway collapsibility and blunted genioglossus muscle activity in

response to negative pharyngeal pressure, *Anesthesiology* 110:1253–1260, 2009.

25. Murphy GS, Szokol JW, Marymont JH, et al: Residual neuromuscular blockade and critical respiratory events in the postanesthesia care unit, *Anesth Analg* 107:130–137, 2008.

26. Brull SJ, Naguib M, Miller RD: Residual neuromuscular block: Rediscovering the obvious, *Anesth Analg* 107:11–14, 2008.

27. Murphy GS, Szokol JW, Marymont JH, et al: Intraoperative acceleromyographic monitoring reduces the risk of residual neuromuscular blockade and adverse respiratory events in the postanesthesia care unit, *Anesthesiology* 109:389–398, 2008.

28. Kopman AF: Residual neuromuscular block and adverse respiratory events, *Anesth Analg* 107:1756, 2008.

29. Srivastava A, Hunter JM: Reversal of neuromuscular block, *Br J Anaesth* 103:115–129, 2009.

30. Caldwell JE, Miller RD: Clinical implications of sugammadex, *Anaesthesia* 64:66–72, 2009.

31. Lundstrom LH, Moller AM, Rosenstock C, et al: Avoidance of neuromuscular blocking agents may increase the risk of difficult tracheal intubation: A cohort study of 103,812 consecutive adult patients recorded in the Danish Anaesthesia Database, *Br J Anaesth* 103:283–290, 2009.

32. Naguib M, Lien CA: Pharmacology of muscle relaxants and their antagonists. In Miller RD, editor: *Miller's Anesthesia*, ed 6, Philadelphia, 2005, Churchill Livingstone.

II

PREOPERATIVE PREPARATION AND INTRAOPERATIVE MANAGEMENT

13 PREOPERATIVE EVALUATION AND MEDICATION

Bobbie Jean Sweitzer

OVERVIEW

The American Society of Anesthesiologists (ASA) has published a practice advisory that suggests a preanesthesia visit should include the following:[1]

- An interview with the patient or guardian to establish a medical, anesthesia and medication history
- An appropriate physical examination
- Indicated diagnostic testing
- Review of diagnostic data (laboratory, electrocardiogram, radiographs, consultations)
- Assignment of an ASA physical status score (ASA-PS) (Table 13-1).
- A formulation and discussion of anesthesia plans with the patient or a responsible adult before obtaining informed consent

A battery of tests is commonly used when evaluating patients. This practice may be based on institutional policies or on the mistaken belief that tests can substitute for taking a history or performing a physical examination. Preoperative tests without specific indications lack utility and may lead to patient injury because they prompt further testing to evaluate abnormal results, unnecessary interventions, delay of surgery, anxiety, and even inappropriate therapies. Complete and thorough histories are necessary to plan appropriate and safe anesthesia care; they are more accurate and cost effective in establishing diagnoses than screening laboratory tests.[2] Gathering the necessary information and sharing that information among the various providers can be challenging.

History and Physical Examination

The important components of the anesthesia history are shown in Figure 13-1. The patient or surrogate can provide the information on paper, via Internet-based programs, during a telephone interview, or in person. The patient's medical conditions, medications, allergies, past operations,

Table 13-1 American Society of Anesthesiologists Physical Status Classification*

ASA 1	Healthy patient without organic, biochemical, or psychiatric disease.
ASA 2	A patient with mild systemic disease, e.g., mild asthma or well-controlled hypertension. No significant impact on daily activity. Unlikely impact on anesthesia and surgery.
ASA 3	Significant or severe systemic disease that limits normal activity, e.g., renal failure on dialysis or class 2 congestive heart failure. Significant impact on daily activity. Likely impact on anesthesia and surgery.
ASA 4	Severe disease that is a constant threat to life or requires intensive therapy, e.g., acute myocardial infarction, respiratory failure requiring mechanical ventilation. Serious limitation of daily activity. Major impact on anesthesia and surgery.
ASA 5	Moribund patient who is likely to die in the next 24 hours with or without surgery.
ASA 6	Brain-dead organ donor.

*"E" added to the above classifications indicates emergency surgery, Available at www.asahq.org.

and use of tobacco, alcohol, or illicit drugs are documented. Cardiovascular, pulmonary, and neurologic symptoms are noted. The presence of disease is identified as well as its severity, stability, current or recent exacerbations, treatment, and planned interventions. Cardiorespiratory fitness or functional capacity not only predicts outcome and perioperative complications, but also indicates a need for further evaluation.[3,4] Better fitness improves cardiorespiratory reserve and decreases morbidity through improved lipid and glucose profiles and reductions in arterial blood pressure and obesity. Conversely, an inability to exercise may be a result of cardiopulmonary disease. Patients unable to attain average levels of exercise (4 to 5 metabolic equivalents or METs, such as walking four blocks or up two flights of stairs) are at increased risk of perioperative complications (Table 13-2).[4] A personal or family history of adverse events with anesthesia such as severe postoperative nausea or vomiting (PONV), prolonged emergence or delirium, or susceptibility to malignant hyperthermia or pseudocholinesterase deficiency should be noted and considered in planning the anesthetic.

At a minimum, the preanesthetic examination includes an airway, heart, and lung examination; review of vital signs, including oxygen saturation; and measurement of height and weight. Figure 13-2 illustrates the Mallampati classification and Table 13-3 lists the key components of the airway examination (also see Chapter 16). When airways which are difficult to manage are identified, necessary equipment and skilled personnel must be made available. Auscultation of the heart and inspection of the

pulses, peripheral veins, and extremities for the presence of edema are important diagnostically and may affect care plans. The pulmonary examination includes auscultation for wheezing, listening for decreased or abnormal breath sounds, and notation of cyanosis or clubbing and effort of breathing. For patients with functional deficits or disease, or planning neurologic procedures or regional anesthesia, a neurologic examination is performed to document abnormalities that may aid in diagnosis or interfere with positioning and to establish a baseline. The following section discusses selected co-morbidities that may impact the administration of anesthesia.

Co-Morbidities Impacting Administration of Anesthesia

Coronary artery disease (CAD) varies from mild, stable disease with little impact on perioperative outcome to severe disease accounting for significant complications during anesthesia and surgery. The history and the physical examination form the foundation for the cardiac assessment. Medical records and previous diagnostic studies are reviewed, especially noninvasive stress tests and catheterization results. Often a phone call to the primary care physician or cardiologist will yield important information and obviate the need for further testing or consultation.

The most recent American College of Cardiology/ American Heart Association (ACC/AHA) guidelines for cardiovascular evaluation for noncardiac surgery have decreased recommendations for testing or revascularization.[4] An algorithm for patients with perioperative cardiac risk is followed in stepwise fashion, stopping at the first point that applies to the patient (Fig. 13-3). Step 1 considers the urgency of surgery. For emergency surgery, the focus is perioperative surveillance (e.g., serial electrocardiograms, enzymes, monitoring) and risk reduction (e.g., β-adrenergic blockers, statins, pain management). Step 2 focuses on active cardiac conditions such as acute myocardial infarction (MI), unstable or severe angina, decompensated heart failure, severe valvular disease, and significant arrhythmias. Active cardiac conditions warrant postponement for all except life-saving emergency procedures. Step 3 considers the surgical risk or severity. Patients without active cardiac conditions (see Step 2) who will undergo low-risk surgery can proceed without further cardiac testing. Step 4 assesses functional capacity as defined by METs (see Table 13-2).[3] Asymptomatic patients with average functional capacity can proceed to surgery. Step 5 considers patients with poor or indeterminate functional capacity who need intermediate-risk or vascular surgery. The number of clinical predictors (CAD, compensated heart failure, cerebrovascular disease, diabetes, and renal insufficiency) determines the likely benefit of further cardiac testing. Patients with no clinical predictors proceed to surgery. Those patients with risk predictors

Patient's Name_____ Age _____ Sex _____ Date of Surgery_____
Proposed Operation_____
Primary care physician name/phone # _____ Cardiologist/phone # _____

1. Please list **all previous operations** (and approximate dates)

a.	d.
b.	e.
c.	f.

2. Please list any **allergies** to medications, latex, food or other (and your reactions to them)

a.	c.
b.	d.

3. Circle <u>TESTS</u> that you have already completed, list where and when you had them. Please bring all existing reports for your visit. We are NOT suggesting that you require (or need to have) these tests.

a. **ECG** Date:	d. **BLOOD WORK** Date:
LOCATION:	LOCATION:
b. **STRESS TEST** Date:	e. **SLEEP STUDY** Date:
LOCATION:	LOCATION:
c. **ECHO/ultrasound of heart** Date:	f. Other: Date:
LOCATION:	LOCATION:

4. Please list **all medications** you have taken in the last month (include over-the-counter drugs, inhalers, herbals, dietary supplements and aspirin)

Name of Drug	Dose and how often	Name of Drug	Dose and how often
a.		f.	
b.		g.	
c.		h.	
d.		i.	
e.		j.	

(Please check YES or NO and circle specific problems) YES NO

4. Have you taken steroids (prednisone or cortisone) in the last year?............... ☐ ☐
5. Have you ever smoked?   (Quantify in ____ packs/day for ____ years)............ ☐ ☐
   Do you still smoke?   (Quantify in ____ packs/day)................................. ☐ ☐
   Do you drink alcohol? (If so, how much?)_____.................. ☐ ☐
   Do you use or have you ever used any illegal drugs? (we need to know for your safety) ☐ ☐
6. Can you walk up one flight of stairs without stopping?............................. ☐ ☐
7. Have you had any problems with your heart? **(circle all that apply)**............. ☐ ☐
   (chest pain or pressure, heart attack, abnormal ECG, skipped beats, murmur, palpitations, heart failure)
8. Do you have high blood pressure?... ☐ ☐
9. Do you have diabetes?... ☐ ☐
10. Have you had any problems with your lungs or your chest? **(circle all that apply)** ☐ ☐
    (shortness of breath, emphysema, bronchitis, asthma, TB, abnormal chest x-ray)
11. Are you ill now or were you recently ill with a cold, fever, chills, flu or productive cough? ☐ ☐
    Describe recent changes _____
12. Have you or anyone in your family had serious bleeding problems? **(circle all that apply)** ☐ ☐
    (prolonged bleeding from nose, gums, tooth extractions, or surgery)
13. Have you had any problems with your blood? **(circle all that apply)**............. ☐ ☐
    (anemia, leukemia, lymphoma, sickle cell disease, blood clots, transfusions)
14. Have you ever had problems with your: **(circle all that apply)**
    Liver (cirrhosis; hepatitis A, B, C; jaundice)? .... ☐ ☐
    Kidney (stones, failure, dialysis)?... ☐ ☐
    Digestive system (frequent heartburn, hiatus hernia, stomach ulcer)?......... ☐ ☐
    Back, Neck or Jaws (TMJ, rheumatoid arthritis, herniation)?................... ☐ ☐
    Thyroid gland (underactive or overactive)?..................................... ☐ ☐
15. Have you ever had: **(circle all that apply)**
    Seizures?... ☐ ☐
    Stroke, facial, leg or arm weakness, difficulty speaking?.................... ☐ ☐
    Cramping pain in your legs with walking?..................................... ☐ ☐
    Problems with hearing, vision or memory?.................................... ☐ ☐
16. Have you ever been treated with chemotherapy or radiation therapy? **(circle all that apply)**
    List indication and dates of treatment: _____
17. Women: Could you be pregnant? Last menstrual period began: _____ ☐ ☐

Figure 13-1 The important components of patient history for preoperative evaluation.

Continued

18. Have you ever had problems with anesthesia or surgery? **(circle all that apply)** .... ☐ ☐
    (severe nausea or vomiting, malignant hyperthermia [in blood relatives or self], breathing
    difficulties, or problems with placement of a breathing tube)
19. Do you have any chipped or loose teeth, dentures, caps, bridgework, braces, problems ☐ ☐
    opening your mouth or swallowing, or choking while eating? **(circle all that apply)**
20. Do your physical abilities limit your daily activities? .... ☐ ☐
21. Do you snore? .... ☐ ☐
22. Do you have sleep apnea? .... ☐ ☐
23. Please list any medical illnesses not noted above:
    _____
    _____

24. Additional comments or questions for the anesthesiologist?
    _____
    _____

THANK YOU FOR YOUR HELP!

Figure 13-1, cont'd. For legend see p. 167

Table 13-2 Metabolic Equivalents of Functional Capacity

MET	Functional Levels of Exercise
1	Eating, working at computer, dressing
2	Walking down stairs or in your house, cooking
3	Walking 1-2 blocks
4	Raking leaves, gardening
5	Climbing 1-2 flights of stairs, dancing, bicycling
6	Playing golf, carrying clubs
7	Playing singles tennis
8	Rapidly climbing stairs, jogging slowly
9	Jumping rope slowly, moderate cycling
10	Swimming quickly, running or jogging briskly
11	Skiing cross country, playing full-court basketball
12	Running rapidly for moderate to long distances

MET, metabolic equivalent. 1 MET = consumption of 3.5 mL O_2/min/kg of body weight.
From Jette M, Sidney K, Blumchen G. Metabolic equivalents (METS) in exercise testing, exercise prescription, and evaluation of functional capacity. Clin Cardiol 1990;13:555-565.

may benefit from further testing but only if the results will alter management. Many traditional risk factors for CAD such as smoking, hypertension, older age, male gender, hypercholesterolemia, and family history may not actually increase perioperative risk.

The benefits versus the risks of coronary revascularization before noncardiac surgery are controversial. The only randomized prospective study of preoperative revascularization versus medical management failed to show a difference in outcome.[5] Noncardiac surgery soon after revascularization is associated with frequent rates of morbidity and mortality.[6] Patients who have had a percutaneous coronary intervention (PCI), especially with a drug-eluting stent (DES), require months, if not a lifetime, of antiplatelet therapy to prevent restenosis or acute thromboses. The type of stent, DES or bare metal stent (BMS), must be identified and managed in collaboration with a cardiologist. A scientific advisory with recommendations for managing patients with coronary stents

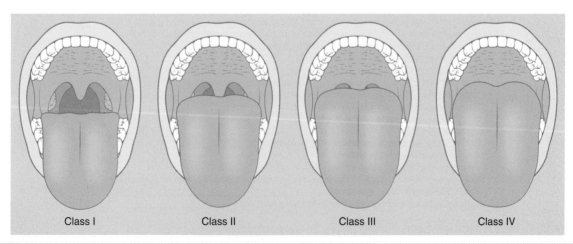

Class I   Class II   Class III   Class IV

Figure 13-2 The Mallampati Airway Classification.

Table 13-3 Components of the Airway Examination

Length of upper incisors
Condition of the teeth
Relationship of upper (maxillary) incisors to lower (mandibular) incisors
Ability to protrude or advance lower (mandibular) incisors in front of upper (maxillary) incisors
Interincisor or intergum (if edentulous) distance
Tongue size
Visibility of the uvula
Presence of heavy facial hair
Compliance of the mandibular space
Thyromental distance with head in maximum extension
Length of the neck
Thickness or circumference of the neck
Range of motion of the head and neck

appears in Table 13-4.[7] Taking antiplatelet drugs should not be stopped without consultation with a cardiologist familiar with coronary stents and an in-depth discussion with the patient regarding the risks of terminating these drugs.[7] Elective procedures that necessitate interrupting dual antiplatelet therapy should be delayed during the high-risk period (see Table 13-4). If at all possible, aspirin is continued throughout the perioperative period, and the thienopyridine (typically clopidogrel) restarted as soon as possible. Evidence supports the small risk of bleeding complications with continued aspirin during most procedures (Fig. 13-4).[8] Premature discontinuation of dual antiplatelet therapy can cause catastrophic stent thrombosis, MI, or death. Noncardiac surgery and most invasive procedures increase the risk of stent thrombosis, which is associated with high mortality rate.[7,9,10] Stent thrombosis is best treated with PCI, which can be performed safely even

Figure 13-3 Simplified algorithm for cardiovascular evaluation of patients for noncardiac surgery. (From Fleisher LA, Beckman JA, Brown KA, et al: ACC/AHA 2007 guidelines on perioperative cardiovascular evaluation and care for noncardiac surgery, J Am Coll Cardiol 50:1707-1732, 2007.)

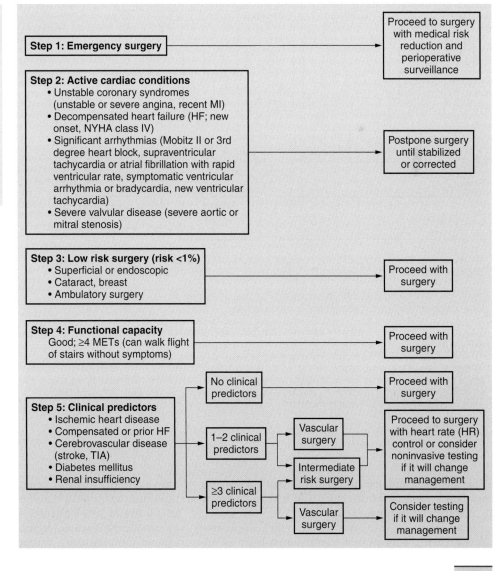

Table 13-4 Recommendations for Perioperative Management of Antiplatelet Drugs in Patients with Coronary Stents

- Health care providers who perform invasive procedures must be aware of the potentially catastrophic risks of premature discontinuation of thienopyridine (e.g., clopidogrel or ticlopidine) therapy. Such professionals should contact the patient's cardiologist to discuss optimal strategies if issues regarding antiplatelet therapy are unclear.
- Elective procedures involving risk of bleeding should be deferred until an appropriate course of thienopyridine therapy (12 months after placement of drug-eluting stent [DES] and 1 month after placement of bare-metal stent [BMS]) has been completed.
- Patients with DES who must undergo procedures after the 12-month waiting period that mandate discontinuing thienopyridine therapy should continue aspirin if at all possible and have the thienopyridine restarted as soon as possible.

Adapted from Grines CL, Bonow RO, Casey DE, et al. Prevention of premature discontinuation of dual antiplatelet therapy in patients with coronary artery stents: A science advisory from the American Heart Association, American College of Cardiology, Society for Cardiovascular Angiography and Interventions, American College of Surgeons, and American Dental Association, with Representation from the American College of Physicians. J Am Coll Cardiol 2007;49:734-739.

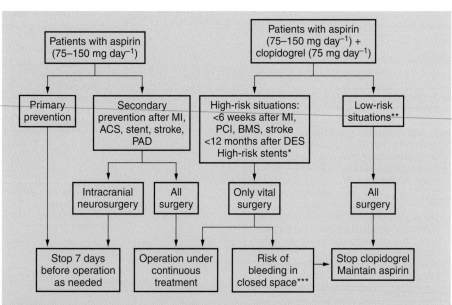

Figure 13-4 Algorithm for perioperative management of patients taking antiplatelet therapy. (From Chassot PG. Perioperative antiplatelet therapy: The case for continuing therapy in patients at risk of myocardial infarction. Br J Anaesth 2007;99:316-328.)

MI, myocardial infarction; ACS, acute coronary syndrome; PAD, peripheral arterial disease; PCI, percutaneous coronary intervention; BMS, bare metal stent; DES, drug eluting stent.

*High-risk stents: long (>36 mm), proximal, overlapping, or multiple stents, stents in chronic total occlusions, or in small vessels or bifurcated lesions.

**Examples of low-risk situations: >3 months after BMS, stroke, uncomplicated MI, PCI without stenting.

***Risk of bleeding in closed space: intracranial neurosurgery, intra-medullary canal surgery, posterior eye chamber ophthalmic surgery. In these situations, the risk/benefit ratio of upholding vs withdrawing aspirin must be evaluated for each case individually; in case of aspirin upholding, early postoperative re-institution is important.

in the immediate postoperative period.[11] High-risk patients may best be managed in facilities with immediate access to interventional cardiology.[9]

Heart failure is a significant risk factor for perioperative adverse events. Patients with compensated heart failure have a 5% to 7% risk of perioperative cardiac complications, and those with decompensation have an even higher rate—a 20% to 30% incidence. Heart failure may be caused by systolic dysfunction (decreased ejection fraction from abnormal contractility), diastolic dysfunction (increased filling pressures with abnormal relaxation but normal contractility and ejection fraction), or a combination of the two. Diastolic dysfunction accounts for almost half of all cases of heart failure, but there is little science to guide care in the perioperative period. Hypertension can cause diastolic dysfunction, and left ventricular hypertrophy on an electrocardiogram (ECG) raises suspicion of dysfunction. Ischemic heart disease is a common cause of systolic dysfunction (50% to 75% of cases). Recent weight gain, complaints of shortness of breath, fatigue, orthopnea, paroxysmal nocturnal dyspnea, nocturnal cough, peripheral edema, hospitalizations, and recent changes in management are significant. Because decompensated heart failure is a high-risk cardiac condition elective surgery should be postponed (see Fig. 13-3).[4] Left ventricular and diastolic function may be evaluated with echocardiography (Table 13-5). Patients with class IV failure (symptoms at rest) need evaluation by a cardiologist before undergoing anesthesia. Minor procedures with conscious sedation may proceed as long as the patient's condition is stable.

Cardiac murmurs can be clinically unimportant or a sign of valvular abnormalities. Functional murmurs from turbulent flow across the aortic or pulmonary outflow tracts are found with high output states (hyperthyroidism, pregnancy, anemia). Elderly patients and those with risk factors for CAD, a history of rheumatic fever, excessive intravascular volume, pulmonary disease, cardiomegaly, or an abnormal ECG and a murmur are likely to have valvular disease. Evaluation with echocardiography is beneficial if general or spinal anesthesia is planned (Table 13-6). Diastolic murmurs are always pathologic and require evaluation.

Table 13-5 Recommendations for Preoperative Noninvasive Evaluation of Left Ventricular (LV) Function

Class IIa
(Reasonable to perform)
1. It is reasonable for patients with dyspnea of unknown origin to undergo preoperative evaluation of LV function.
2. It is reasonable for patients with current or previous heart failure with worsening dyspnea or other change in clinical status to undergo preoperative evaluation of LV function if not performed within 12 months.

Class IIb
(May be considered)
1. Reassessment of LV function in clinically stable patients with previously documented cardiomyopathy is not well established.

Class III
(Should NOT be performed because it is not helpful)
1. Routine perioperative evaluation of LV function in patients is not recommended.

Adapted from Fleisher LA, Beckman JA, Brown KA, et al. ACC/AHA 2007 Guidelines on perioperative cardiovascular evaluation and care for noncardiac surgery. J Am Coll Cardiol 2007;50:3159-3241.

Table 13-6 ACC/AHA Guideline Summary: Echocardiography in Asymptomatic Patients with Cardiac Murmurs

Class I
There is evidence and/or general agreement that echocardiography is useful in asymptomatic patients with the following cardiac murmurs:
- Diastolic murmurs
- Continuous murmurs
- Late systolic murmurs
- Murmurs associated with ejection clicks
- Murmurs that radiate to the neck or back
- Grade 3 or louder systolic murmurs

Class IIa
The weight of evidence or opinion is in favor of usefulness of echocardiography in asymptomatic patients with the following cardiac murmurs:
- Murmurs associated with other abnormal physical findings on cardiac examination
- Murmurs associated with an abnormal electrocardiogram or chest radiograph

Class III
There is evidence and/or general agreement that echocardiography is not useful in asymptomatic patients with the following murmurs:
- Grade 2 or softer midsystolic murmurs considered innocent or functional by an experienced observer

From Bonow, RO, Carabello, BA, Chatterjee, K, et al. ACC/AHA 2006 guidelines for the management of patients with valvular heart disease. A report of the American College of Cardiology/American Heart Association Task Force on Practice Guidelines (Writing committee to revise the 1998 guidelines for the management of patients with valvular heart disease). J Am Coll Cardiol 2006;48:e1.

Regurgitant heart disease is better tolerated perioperatively than stenotic disease. Aortic stenosis is the most common valvular lesion in the United States (2% to 4% of adults older than 65 years). Severe stenosis is associated with a high risk for perioperative complications. Aortic sclerosis, present in 25% of people 65 to 74 years old and 50% of those more than 84 years old, causes a systolic ejection murmur similar to that heard with stenosis but does not compromise hemodynamics.[12] Patients with severe or critical stenosis should undergo only emergency and life-saving procedures without cardiology evaluation.[13] Antibiotic prophylaxis to prevent infective endocarditis is no longer recommended for patients with valvular abnormalities in native hearts (Tables 13-7 and 13-8).[14]

Pacemakers and implantable cardioverter-defibrillators (ICDs) can be affected by electrical or magnetic interference. Consultation with the device manufacturer or cardiologist may be needed. Patients usually have a wallet card with important designations and phone numbers. Patients with ICDs invariably have heart failure, ischemic or valvular disease, cardiomyopathies, or potentially lethal

Table 13-7 Summary of Major Changes in American Heart Association Infective Endocarditis Prophylaxis Guidelines

- Bacteremia from daily activities is much more likely to cause infective endocarditis (IE) than bacteremia from a dental procedure.
- An extremely small number of cases of IE may potentially be prevented by antibiotic prophylaxis.
- Prophylaxis is not recommended solely on the basis of an increased lifetime risk of IE.
- Recommendations for IE prophylaxis apply only to those conditions listed in Table 13-8.
- Prophylaxis is recommended for all dental procedures that involve manipulation of gingival tissues or periapical region of teeth or perforation of oral mucosa only for patients with conditions listed in Table 13-8.
- Prophylaxis is recommended for procedures on respiratory tract or infected skin, skin structures, or musculoskeletal tissue only for patients with conditions listed in Table 13-8.
- Prophylaxis is not recommended for GU or GI tract procedures.

GI, gastrointestinal; GU, genitourinary.
From Wilson W, Taubert KA, Gewitz M, et al. Prevention of infective endocarditis: Guidelines from the American Heart Association, Rheumatic Fever, Endocarditis, and Kawasaki Disease Committee, Council on Cardiovascular Disease in the Young, and the Council on Clinical Cardiology, Council on Cardiovascular Surgery and Anesthesia, and the Quality of Care and Outcomes Research Interdisciplinary Working Group. Circulation 2007;116:1736-1754.

Table 13-8 Cardiac Conditions Associated with the Highest Risk of Adverse Outcome from Endocarditis

Prosthetic cardiac valve
Previous infective endocarditis

Congenital heart disease (CHD)*
   Unrepaired cyanotic CHD, including palliative shunts and conduits
   Completely repaired congenital heart defect with prosthetic material or device, whether placed by surgery or by catheter intervention, during the first 6 months after the procedure†
   Repaired CHD with residual defects at the site or adjacent to the site of a prosthetic patch or prosthetic device (which inhibit endothelialization)

Cardiac valvulopathy developing in a cardiac transplant recipient

*Except for the conditions listed, antibiotic prophylaxis is no longer recommended for any other form of CHD.
†Prophylaxis is recommended because endothelialization of prosthetic material occurs within 6 months after the procedure.
From Wilson W, Taubert KA, Gewitz M, et al. Prevention of infective endocarditis: Guidelines from the American Heart Association, Rheumatic Fever, Endocarditis, and Kawasaki Disease Committee, Council on Cardiovascular Disease in the Young, and the Council on Clinical Cardiology, Council on Cardiovascular Surgery and Anesthesia, and the Quality of Care and Outcomes Research Interdisciplinary Working Group. Circulation 2007;116:1736-1754.

arrhythmias. Some monitors, ventilators, vibrations, or chest prepping may fool the sensors into increasing pacing, leading to ischemia or inappropriate treatment. Special features such as rate adaptive mechanisms in some pacemakers are disabled, or the device is reprogrammed to asynchronous pacing to prevent interference.[15] Antitachyarrhythmia functions are disabled before procedures if interference or unexpected patient movement is undesirable.[15] An unexpected discharge with patient movement can be catastrophic during delicate intracranial, spinal, or ocular procedures. Central line placement can trigger cardioversion. Typically ICDs are deactivated only after arrival to a facility with devices for monitoring and cardioversion. Many ICDs are complex and reliance on a magnet to disable them, except in emergencies, is not recommended. Some devices are programmed to ignore magnet placement, or magnets may permanently disable anti-tachyarrhythmic therapy. Magnets only suspend antishock therapies in some ICDs while they are in place. Magnets affect only the anti-tachycardia function, not the pacing function of an ICD. If a pacemaker or ICD is reprogrammed, or if a magnet is used at any time, the device must be re-interrogated and re-enabled before the patient leaves a monitored setting.

Hypertension severity and duration correlate with the degree of end-organ damage, morbidity, and mortality.

Ischemic heart disease, heart failure, renal insufficiency, and cerebrovascular disease are common in hypertensive patients. Yet mild hypertension with a preoperative blood pressure (BP) less than 180/110 mm Hg is not clearly associated with perioperative cardiac risk. Elective surgery probably should be delayed for patients with severe hypertension (DBP > 115 mm Hg; SBP > 200 mm Hg) until BP is less than 180/110 mm Hg. If significant end-organ damage is present, or intraoperative hypotensive techniques are planned, the goal is to restore BP to normal levels as much as possible before surgery.[16] Decreased risk may require weeks of therapy for regression of vascular changes. Actually, rapid decreasing of BP may increase the chance of cerebral or coronary ischemia. Intraoperative hypotension is probably far more dangerous than hypertension.[16] Patients being evaluated preopertively ideally should have their BP controlled in an optimal state.

Pulmonary disease increases risk for both pulmonary and nonpulmonary perioperative complications. Postoperative pulmonary complications (PPC) are common and increase costs, morbidity rate, and mortality risk. Some predictors are advanced age, heart failure, chronic obstructive pulmonary disease (COPD), smoking, general health status (including impaired sensorium and functional dependency), and obstructive sleep apnea (Table 13-9).[17,18] Well-controlled asthma does not increase perioperative complications.[19] Patients with poorly controlled asthma,

Table 13-9 Risk Factors for Postoperative Pulmonary Complications, with Summary Strength of the Evidence for Association of Patient, Procedure, and Laboratory Factors with Specific Complications*

Factor	Strength of Recommendation[†]	Odds Ratios[‡]
Potential Patient-Related Risk Factor		
Advanced age	A	2.09-3.04
ASA class ≥II	>A	2.55-4.87
CHF	A	2.93
Functionally dependent	A	1.65-2.51
COPD	A	1.79
Weight loss	B	1.62
Impaired sensorium	B	1.39
Cigarette use	B	1.26
Alcohol use	B	1.21
Abnormal findings on chest examination	B	NA
Diabetes	C	
Obesity	D	
Asthma	D	
Obstructive sleep apnea	I	
Corticosteroid use	I	
HIV infection	I	
Arrhythmia	I	
Poor exercise capacity	I	
Potential Procedure-Related Risk Factor		
Aortic aneurysm repair	A	6.90
Thoracic surgery	A	4.24
Abdominal surgery	A	3.01
Upper abdominal surgery	A	2.91
Neurosurgery	A	2.53
Prolonged surgery	A	2.26
Head and neck surgery	A	2.21
Emergency surgery	A	2.21
Vascular surgery	A	2.10
General anesthesia	A	1.83
Perioperative transfusion	B	1.47
Hip surgery	D	
Gynecologic or urologic surgery	D	
Esophageal surgery	I	
Laboratory Tests		
Albumin level <35 g/L	A	2.53
Chest radiography	B	4.81
BUN level >7.5 mmol/L (>21 mg/dL)	B	NA
Spirometry	I	

*ASA, American Society of Anesthesiologists; BUN, blood urea nitrogen; CHF, congestive heart failure; COPD, chronic obstructive pulmonary disease; HIV, human immunodeficiency virus; NA, not available.
[†]Recommendations: A = good evidence to support the particular risk factor or laboratory predictor; B = at least fair evidence to suggest a particular risk factor or laboratory predictor; C = at least fair evidence to suggest that the particular factor is not a risk factor or that the laboratory test does not predict risk; D = good evidence to suggest that the particular factor is not a risk factor or that the laboratory test does not predict risk; I = insufficient evidence to determine whether factor increases risk or whether the laboratory test predicts risk, and evidence is lacking, is of poor quality, or is conflicting.
[‡]For factors with A or B rating. Odds ratios are trim-and-fill estimates. When these estimates were not possible, we provide the pooled estimate. Reproduced from: Smetana GV, Lawrence VA, Cornell JE. Preoperative pulmonary risk stratification for noncardiothoracic surgery: Systematic review for the American College of Physicians. Ann Intern Med 2006;144:158-595.

as evidenced by wheezing at the time of anesthetic induction, are at a higher risk for complications.[19] Unlike asthma, COPD increases the risk of pulmonary complications; the more severe the COPD, the greater the risk. However, there is no degree of severity that absolutely precludes surgery.

Surprisingly the risks with COPD are less than those with heart failure, advanced age, or poor general health.

Administering corticosteroids and inhaled β-adrenergic agonists preoperatively markedly decreases the incidence of bronchospasm after tracheal intubation and may shorten hospital and intensive care unit stays.[17] Brief preoperative administration of preoperative steroids (up to 1 week) are safe and do not appear to increase postoperative infections or delay wound healing. Prednisone 0.5 to 1 mg/kg orally for 1 to 4 days before surgery for patients who are likely to require endotracheal intubation and who have persistent airway obstruction despite use of inhaled medications is recommended.

Recovery time, pain, and reduction in lung volumes are less after laparoscopic procedures, but whether pulmonary complications are affected is unclear. PPC risk is less frequent after percutaneous interventions. In a study of endovascular versus open abdominal aortic aneurysm repair, PPC rates were 3% and 16%, respectively.[17] General anesthesia is associated with more risk for PPC than with peripheral nerve blocks. Two large meta-analyses and retrospective and randomized trials suggest that PPC rates are less frequent for patients who have spinal or epidural anesthesia or epidural analgesia postoperatively compared to general anesthesia.[20] Routine pulmonary function tests, chest radiography, or arterial blood gases do not predict PPC risk and offer little more information than can be determined by clinical evaluation. PPC rates are reduced by maximizing airflow in obstructive disease, treating infections and heart failure, and using lung expansion maneuvers such as coughing, deep breathing, incentive spirometry, positive end-expiratory pressure (PEEP), and continuous positive airway pressure (CPAP).

Obstructive sleep apnea (OSA), which is caused by intermittent airway obstruction, affects up to 9% of women and 24% of men. Most of them are unaware of the diagnosis.[21] Snoring, daytime sleepiness, hypertension, obesity, and a family history of OSA are risk factors for OSA.[22] A large neck circumference predicts an increased chance of OSA. The STOP-Bang questionnaire was developed and validated in an anesthesia preoperative clinic to screen for OSA (Fig. 13-5).[23] Patients with OSA have increased rates of diabetes, hypertension, atrial fibrillation, bradyarrhythmias, ventricular ectopy, stroke, heart failure, pulmonary hypertension, dilated cardiomyopathy, and CAD.[24] Ventilation via a mask, direct laryngoscopy, endotracheal intubation, and fiberoptic visualization of the airway are more difficult in patients with OSA. Such patients are likely to have perioperative airway obstruction, hypoxemia, atelectasis, ischemia, pneumonia, and prolonged hospitalizations.[18] Patients who use CPAP devices should bring them on the day of their procedures. The ASA has published recommendations for the perioperative care of

---

Have you been diagnosed with sleep apnea by a sleep study? Yes ☐ No ☐

Have you received treatment for sleep apnea, such as CPAP or Bi-PAP? Yes ☐ No ☐

Please answer the following four questions with a *yes* or *no* answer:

1) Do you snore loudly (louder than talking or loud enough to be heard through closed doors)?
   Yes ☐ No ☐

2) Do you often feel tired, fatigued, or sleepy during the daytime?
   Yes ☐ No ☐

3) Has anyone observed you stop breathing during your sleep?
   Yes ☐ No ☐

4) Do you have or are you being treated for high blood pressure?
   Yes ☐ No ☐

FOR STAFF USE ONLY, DO NOT WRITE BELOW THIS LINE

---

5) Is the BMI ≥35 kg/m^2?
   Yes ☐ No ☐

6) Is the patient ≥50 years of age?
   Yes ☐ No ☐

7) Is the neck circumference greater than 15.7 inches (40 cm)?
   Yes ☐ No ☐

8) Is the patient male?
   Yes ☐ No ☐

Total number of questions answered YES: _____ Is the patient at high risk for OSA?
Yes ☐ No ☐

High risk of OSA: Yes to >3 items

Figure 13-5 STOP-Bang screening questionnaire for obstructive sleep apnea. (From Chung F, Yegneswaran B, Liao P, et al. STOP Questionnaire. A tool to screen patients for obstructive sleep apnea. Anesthesiology 108:812-821, 2008.)

patients with OSA, which includes preoperative diagnosis and treatment of OSA if possible, and appropriateness of ambulatory surgery.[25]

Dyspnea is caused by an increased respiratory drive or a respiratory system subject to an increased mechanical load. The most common causes of acute dyspnea are COPD, asthma, and heart failure (Fig. 13-6). Specific preoperative tests for patients with dyspnea are indicated by the results of the history and physical examination. Most of the conditions that cause dyspnea, except for the psychogenic ones, increase the risk of perioperative complications, especially if the condition is poorly controlled or unknown to the anesthesiologist. When preoperative evaluation yields a proper diagnosis, effective treatment can improve the patient's medical condition.

Renal disease is associated with hypertension, cardiovascular disease, excessive intravascular volume, electrolyte disturbances, metabolic acidosis, and often a need to alter the type and amount of anesthetic drugs administered. Renal insufficiency is a risk factor probably equal to CAD. In elective cases, dialysis is performed within 24 hours of surgery, but not immediately before, to avoid acute volume depletion and electrolyte alterations. Chronic hyperkalemia may not need treatment if potassium blood concentrations are less than 6 mEq/dL and within the range of a patient's established levels. Radiocontrast medium transiently decreases glomerular filtration rate (GFR) in almost all patients, but patients with diabetes or renal insufficiency are at highest risk. For patients with a GFR less than 60 mL·kg^{-1}·min^{-1} alkalinizing renal tubular fluid with sodium bicarbonate or simple hydration may reduce injury.

Diabetic patients are at risk for multiorgan dysfunction, with renal insufficiency, strokes, peripheral neuropathies, visual impairment, and cardiovascular disease most prevalent. Tight glucose control in stroke, coronary bypass surgery, or critically ill individuals may improve outcomes but is controversial.[26] Whether tight control perioperatively for noncardiac surgery confers benefit or simply increases the risk of hypoglycemia is not clear. Chronically poor control increases co-morbid conditions such as vascular disease, heart failure, and infections and likely increases the risk of surgery. Chronically poor control predicts higher blood glucose levels perioperatively.[27] Targeting control in the immediate perioperative period likely will not have a substantial impact on

Figure 13-6 Guideline for the evaluation of dyspnea.

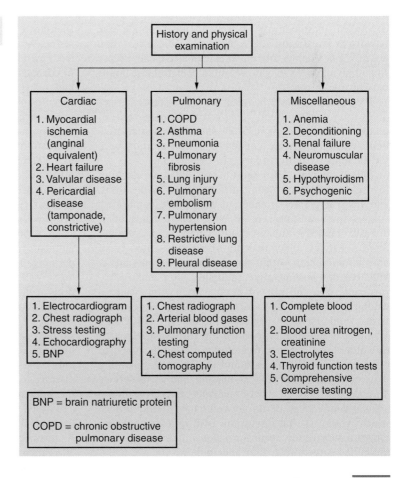

outcomes in diabetics having surgery. Increased levels of blood glucose or even treatment of high levels for non-cardiac surgery. Diabetic ketoacidosis and hypoglycemia (glucose <50 g/dL) are the only conditions that absolutely warrant perioperative intervention. The goals of glucose control are to prevent hypoglycemia during fasting, extreme hyperglycemia, and ketosis.

Extreme obesity is defined by a body mass index (BMI) of 40 or more. Obese patients may have OSA, heart failure, diabetes, hypertension, pulmonary hypertension, difficult airways, decreased arterial oxygenation, and increased gastric volume. Special equipment is needed to care for obese patients: oversized blood pressure cuffs, airway management devices, and large procedure tables and gurneys to support excessive weight.

Anemia, common preoperatively, is a marker for increased risk of perioperative death, and a predictor of short- and long-term outcomes in the general population. Preoperative anemia is the strongest predictor of the need for transfusions, which increase morbidity and mortality rates.[28] If the cause of anemia is unknown, an evaluation is generally indicated before elective procedures, especially if blood loss or anticoagulation is anticipated. For asymptomatic patients with chronic anemia and no history of CAD who will undergo a low-risk procedure, the minimal physiologic perturbations during a well-conducted anesthetic are unlikely to pose enough risk to warrant transfusion unless the hemoglobin is less than 6 g/dL[29] (see Chapter 24). Patients with sickle cell disease should be managed in concert with a hematologist familiar with the disease.

Pregnant patients scheduled for nonobstetric procedures may require fetal monitoring. Management of preterm labor or even delivery should be anticipated. Perioperative plans are confirmed in consultation with the patient's obstetrician (also see Chapter 33).

Elderly patients (also see Chapter 35) have declines in organ function, respond differently to medications, and have a greater number of co-morbid conditions. Among the conditions are arthritis, hypertension, heart disease, diabetes, renal insufficiency, and vascular disease. Patients older than 85 years with a history of hospital admission within the previous 6 months are at high risk for postoperative admission after ambulatory surgery.[30] Yet, the rate of perioperative complications among the very elderly (>85 years old) does not exclude them from having surgical procedures.[31] Discharge planning in advance may lessen the costs of perioperative elder care. Preoperative clinics can be designed to offer multidisciplinary care and postdischarge planning that coordinates with surgical, nursing, and social service departments. Many elderly patients have or desire advanced directives or do-not-resuscitate (DNR) orders, which require special discussion. DNR orders should no longer automatically occur for patients undergoing anesthesia and surgery (Fig. 13-7 and Table 13-10).

CONSULTATIONS

Collaborative care of patients is often necessary and beneficial. Consultation initiated by the preoperative physician should seek specific advice regarding diagnosis and status of the patient's condition(s). Letters or notes stating "cleared for surgery" or "low risk" are not sufficient to help the anesthesia provider design a safe anesthetic. A summation of the patient's medical problems and condition and the results of diagnostic tests are necessary. Preoperative consultations should be sought for the following:

- Diagnosis, evaluation, and improvement of a new or poorly controlled condition
- Creation of a clinical risk profile that the patient, anesthesiologist, and surgeon use to make management decisions

Close coordination and good communication among the preoperative anesthesiologist, surgeon and consultant are vitally important.

TESTING

Diagnostic testing and the benefits of disease-indicated testing versus a screening battery of tests have been studied. Few abnormalities detected by routine testing result in changes in management and rarely have such changes had a beneficial effect.[32,33] Preoperative tests without specific indications lack utility and may lead to patient injury because of unnecessary interventions, delay of surgery, anxiety, and even inappropriate therapies. The evaluation of abnormal results is costly. On average, 1 in 2000 preoperative tests result in patient harm from pursuit of abnormalities detected by those tests.[2] Perhaps not following up on an abnormal result is a greater medicolegal risk than not identifying the abnormality to begin with.

In a pilot study of over 1000 patients undergoing ambulatory surgery, there was no increase in adverse perioperative events in patients who had no preoperative tests.[34] There was no increase in OR delays or cancellations or differences in outcome from lack of testing. Several other studies have shown that the information from resting 12-lead ECGs does not add value to the care of surgical patients.[4,35] The specificity of an ECG abnormality in predicting postoperative cardiac adverse events is only 26%, and a normal ECG does not exclude cardiac disease.[33] An ECG should not be done simply because the patient is of advanced age. Recommendations for age-based testing were derived from the frequent incidence of abnormalities found on ECGs of elderly patients. A prospective observational study in patients aged 50 years or older having major noncardiac surgery found

_____ Option 1 - Full Resuscitation

I, _____ , desire that full resuscitation measures be employed during my anesthesia and in the postanesthesia care unit, regardless of the situation.

_____ Option 2 - Limited Resuscitation: Procedure-directed

During my anesthesia and in the postanesthesia care unit, I, _____ , refuse the following procedures:

_____

_____

_____ Option 3 - Limited Resuscitation: Goal-directed

I, _____ , desire attempts to resuscitate me during my anesthesia and in the postanesthesia care unit only if, in the clinical judgement of the attending anesthesiologist and surgeon, the adverse clinical events are believed to be both temporary and reversible.

_____ Option 4 - Limited Resuscitation: Goal-directed

I, _____ , desire attempts to resuscitate me during my anesthesia and in the postanesthesia care unit only if, in the clinical judgement of the attending anesthesiologist and surgeon, such resuscitation efforts will support the following goals and values of mine: _____

Patient or surrogate signature	Date
Physician signature	Date
Witness signature	Date

Figure 13-7 Anesthesia care for the patient with an existing do-not-resuscitate (DNR) order. (From Truog RD, Waisel DB. Do-not-resuscitate orders: From the ward to the operating room; from procedures to goals. Int Anesthesiol Clin 2001;39:53-65.)

Table 13-10 Do Not Resuscitate (DNR) Orders in the Perioperative Period

Policies automatically suspending DNR orders or other directives that limit treatment before procedures involving anesthetic care may not sufficiently address a patient's rights to self-determination in a responsible and ethical manner. Such policies, if they exist, should be reviewed and revised, as necessary, to reflect the content of these guidelines.

A. *Full Attempt at Resuscitation:* The patient or designated surrogate may request the full suspension of existing directives during the anesthetic and immediate postoperative period, thereby consenting to the use of any resuscitation procedures that may be appropriate to treat clinical events that occur during this time.

B. *Limited Attempt at Resuscitation Defined With Regard to Specific Procedures:* The patient or designated surrogate may elect to continue to refuse certain specific resuscitation procedures (for example, chest compressions, defibrillation, or tracheal intubation). The anesthesiologist should inform the patient or designated surrogate about (1) which procedures are essential to the success of the anesthesia and the proposed procedure and (2) which procedures are not essential and may be refused.

C. *Limited Attempt at Resuscitation Defined With Regard to the Patient's Goals and Values:* The patient or designated surrogate may allow the anesthesiologist and surgical team to use clinical judgment in determining which resuscitation procedures are appropriate in the context of the situation and the patient's stated goals and values. For example, some patients may want full resuscitation procedures to be used to manage adverse clinical events that are believed to be quickly and easily reversible, but to refrain from treatment for conditions that are likely to result in permanent sequelae, such as neurologic impairment or unwanted dependence upon life-sustaining technology.

From Ethical Guidelines for the Anesthesia Care of Patients with Do-Not-Resuscitate Orders or other Directives that Limit Treatment Committee of Origin: Ethics (Approved by the ASA House of Delegates on October 17, 2001, and last affirmed on October 22, 2008) accessed 11/17/2010.

abnormalities in 45% of the preoperative ECGs. Bundle branch blocks, associated with postoperative MI and death, had no added predictive value over clinical risk factors.[36] The Centers for Medicare and Medicaid Services (CMS) do not reimburse for "preoperative" or age-based ECGs.[37] The ASA Preoperative Evaluation Practice Advisory recognized that ECGs did not improve prediction beyond risk factors identified by patient history.[38] Indications for preoperative ECGs are shown in Table 13-11.[4] Chest radiographs do not predict postoperative pulmonary complications.[17]

Healthy patients of any age and patients with known, stable, chronic diseases undergoing low- to intermediate-risk procedures are unlikely to benefit from any *routine* tests. A test is ordered only if the results will impact the decision to proceed with the planned procedure or alter the care plans. It is misguided to believe that discovering abnormalities on ECGs, chest radiographs, or blood work impacts care or outcomes for many patients or procedures. Studies have shown that elimination of routine testing does not increase risk.[4,17,34] However, clinical evaluation of patients preoperatively is still necessary. Eliciting a history of increased dyspnea on exertion, new onset chest pain, or syncope, and providing patients with appropriate preoperative medication instructions is of greater benefit than ordering ECGs or blood tests. Tests to establish a diagnosis, evaluate a worsening condition, or aid in preoperative decisions and management for patients with severe co-morbidities are shown in Table 13-12. Tests for selected patients may be indicated simply because of planned anesthesia or surgery (Table 13-13).

The ASA Preoperative Evaluation Practice Advisory recognized that the literature "... *is insufficient to inform patients or physicians whether anesthesia causes harmful effects on early pregnancy,*" and suggests that pregnancy testing be offered to women if the test result will alter management.[38] Some practices and facilities provide patients with information about the potential risks of anesthesia and surgery on pregnancy but allow them to decline testing. Other practices mandate that all females of childbearing age undergo a urine pregnancy test on the day of surgery. Perhaps in facilities with a mandatory testing policy, patients should be informed that consent for surgery and anesthesia includes consent for pregnancy testing.

Table 13-11 Recommendations for Preoperative Resting 12-Lead Electrocardiogram (ECG)

Class I
(Procedure is indicated)
1. Preoperative resting 12-lead ECG is recommended for patients with at least one clinical risk factor* who are undergoing vascular surgical procedures.
2. Preoperative resting 12-lead ECG is recommended for patients with known CHD, peripheral arterial disease, or cerebrovascular disease who are undergoing intermediate-risk surgical procedures.

Class IIa
(Procedure is reasonable to perform)
1. Preoperative resting 12-lead ECG is reasonable in persons with no clinical risk factors who are undergoing vascular surgical procedures.

Class IIb
(Procedure may be considered)
1. Preoperative resting 12-lead ECG may be reasonable in patients with at least one clinical risk factor who are undergoing intermediate-risk operative procedures.

Class III
(Procedure should NOT be performed because it is not helpful)
1. Preoperative and postoperative resting 12-lead ECGs are not indicated in asymptomatic persons undergoing low-risk surgical procedures.

*Clinical risk factors are ischemic heart disease, heart failure, cerebrovascular disease, diabetes, and renal insufficiency.
CHD, coronary heart disease.
Adapted from Fleisher LA, Beckman JA, Brown KA, et al. ACC/AHA 2007 Guidelines on perioperative cardiovascular evaluation and care for noncardiac surgery. J Am Coll Cardiol 2007;50:e159-e241.

MEDICATIONS

Instructions to patients to continue or discontinue drugs will likely improve outcomes more than testing will. The co-morbidities and the nature of the procedure are considered when managing medications preoperatively. Some medications have beneficial effects during anesthesia and surgery, others are detrimental, and in still other cases, suddenly stopping therapy has a negative effect. A summary of recommendations for perioperative administration of medications is in Table 13-14. Several drug classes and emerging controversies deserve special mention.

Generally, cardiac medications and antihypertensive drugs are continued preoperatively. Angiotensin-converting enzyme inhibitors (ACEIs), angiotensin receptor blockers (ARBs), diuretics, and anticoagulants may be beneficial even on the day of surgery. Continuing or discontinuing these drugs depends on the intravascular volume and hemodynamic status of the patient, the degree of cardiac dysfunction, the adequacy of arterial blood pressure control, and the anticipated anesthetic and intravascular volume concerns. Continuing all medications for patients with severe disease, or those undergoing low- to intermediate-risk procedures, sedation or centroneuraxial anesthesia is likely best. If ACEIs and ARBs are continued, doses of induction and other anesthetic drugs may be altered. Vasopressin should be available to prevent or mitigate hypotension.[39] The potential for refractory hypotension must be balanced against the positive therapeutic impact of continuing these drugs perioperatively on a case-by-case basis.

Table 13-12 Preoperative Diagnostic Testing Recommendations

Albumin	Anasarca; liver disease; malnutrition; malabsorption
β-hCG	Suspected pregnancy
CBC	Alcohol abuse; anemia; dyspnea; hepatic or renal disease; malignancy; malnutrition; personal history of bleeding; poor exercise tolerance; recent chemotherapy or radiation therapy
Creatinine	Renal disease; poorly controlled diabetes
Chest radiograph	Active, acute or chronic significant pulmonary symptoms such as cough or dyspnea; abnormal unexplained physical findings on chest examination; decompensated heart failure; malignancy within the thorax; radiation therapy*
Electrocardiogram	Alcohol abuse; active cardiac condition (new or worsening chest pain or dyspnea, palpitations, tachycardia, irregular heart beat, unexplained bradycardia, undiagnosed murmur, S_3, decompensated heart failure); implanted cardioverter-defibrillator (ICD); obstructive sleep apnea; pacemaker; pulmonary hypertension; radiation therapy*; severe obesity; syncope; use of amiodarone or digoxin
Electrolytes	Alcohol abuse; cardiovascular, hepatic, renal or thyroid disease; diabetes; malnutrition; use of digoxin or diuretics
Glucose	Diabetes; severe obesity; use of steroids
LFTs	Alcohol abuse; hepatic disease; recent hepatitis exposure; undiagnosed bleeding disorder
Platelet count	Alcohol abuse; hepatic disease; bleeding disorder (personal or family history); hematologic malignancy; recent chemotherapy or radiation therapy; thrombocytopenia
PT	Alcohol abuse; hepatic disease; malnutrition; bleeding disorder (personal or family history); use of warfarin
PTT	Bleeding disorder (personal or family history); undiagnosed hypercoagulable state; use of unfractionated heparin
TSH, T_3, T_4	Goiter; thyroid disease; unexplained dyspnea, fatigue, palpitations, tachycardia
Urinalysis	Urinary tract infection (suspected)

*Only with radiation therapy to chest, breasts, lungs, thorax.
CBC, complete blood count; β-hCG, β-human chorionic gonadotropin [assay] (pregnancy test); LFTs, liver function tests (albumin, bilirubin, alanine and aspartate aminotransferases); PT, prothrombin time; PTT, partial thromboplastin time; T_3, triiodothyronine; T_4, thyroxine; TSH, thyroid-stimulating hormone.

Furosemide can always be administered intravenously after induction of anesthesia. It is recommended (class I indications) that β-blockers be continued in patients who take them to treat angina, symptomatic arrhythmias, or hypertension (Table 13-15).[40] Minimizing risk for high-risk patients scheduled for elective surgery may entail postponing surgery to optimize β-adrenergic blockers and statin therapy. Statins reduce length of hospital stay and risk of stroke, renal dysfunction, MI, and even death.[41-43] No study of perioperative statin therapy has reported serious risks with the use of these drugs.[42] Abruptly terminating statin administration may be associated with an increased risk, including death.[44] Statins should be continued in the perioperative period, and serious consideration should be given to starting them in patients with known, or risk factors for, atherosclerotic disease.

Aspirin is commonly used to decrease risk of events in patients with known, or risk factors for, vascular disease, diabetes, renal insufficiency, or simply advanced age. Traditionally aspirin has been withdrawn in the perioperative period because of concern of bleeding. However, this practice has come under scrutiny. A meta-analysis of almost 50,000 patients undergoing a variety of noncardiac surgeries (30% taking aspirin perioperatively) found that aspirin increased bleeding complications by a factor of 1.5, but not the severity, except in patients undergoing intracranial surgery and possibly transurethral resection of the prostate.[8] Surgeons blinded to aspirin administration could not identify patients taking or not taking aspirin based on bleeding.[11] There is an increased risk of vascular events when aspirin taken regularly is stopped perioperatively.[45] There may be a rebound hypercoagulable state when aspirin is withdrawn.[46] Acute coronary syndromes occurred 8.5 ± 3.6 days and acute cerebral events 14.3 ± 11.3 days after aspirin cessation, the typical duration of interruption for surgery, and events were twice as common in patients who had stopped taking aspirin in the previous 3 weeks when compared to those who continued aspirin.[8] Stopping aspirin for 3 to 4 days is usually sufficient, if aspirin is stopped at all, and dosing should be resumed as soon as possible. New platelets formed after aspirin (half-life of approximately 15 minutes) is stopped will not be affected. Normally functioning platelets at a concentration of more than $50,000/mm^3$ are adequate to control surgical bleeding. For many minor, superficial procedures such as cataract extraction, endoscopies, and peripheral procedures, the risk of withdrawing aspirin in at-risk patients is greater than the risk of

Table 13-13 Recommendations for Patient-Specific Baseline Testing before Anesthesia*

Procedure/Patient Type	Test
Injection of contrast dye	Creatinine[†]
Potential for significant blood loss	Hemoglobin/hematocrit[†]
Likelihood of transfusion requirement	Type and screen
Possibility of pregnancy	Pregnancy test[‡]
End-stage renal disease	Potassium level[§]
Diabetes	Glucose level determination on day of surgery[§]
Active cardiac condition (e.g., decompensated heart failure, arrhythmia, chest pain, murmur)	Electrocardiogram

*Not to establish a diagnosis or to guide *preoperative* management.
[†]Results from laboratory tests within 3 months of surgery are acceptable unless major abnormalities are present or the patient's condition has changed.
[‡]A routine pregnancy test before surgery is not recommended before the day of surgery. A careful history and local practice determine whether a pregnancy test is indicated.
[§]No absolute level of either potassium or glucose has been determined to preclude surgery and anesthesia. The benefits of the procedure must be balanced against the risk of proceeding in a patient with abnormal results.

bleeding.[47] Aspirin should be discontinued if taken only for primary prevention (no history of stents, strokes, MI) (see Fig. 13-4 and Table 13-14).[48] Aspirin administration should be continued if taken for secondary prevention (history of stents or vascular disease), except for procedures with a risk of bleeding in closed spaces (e.g., intracranial, posterior chamber of the eye). Neuraxial and peripheral anesthesia in patients taking aspirin is safe and endorsed by the American Society of Regional Anesthesia (ASRA).[49] The risk of spinal hematoma with clopidogrel is unknown. Based on labeling and ASRA guidelines clopidogrel is discontinued 7 days before planned neuraxial blockade.

Low-molecular-weight heparin (LMWH) is discontinued 12 to 24 hours before procedures with a risk of bleeding or a planned neuraxial block (Table 13-16).[49] Warfarin may increase bleeding except during minor procedures such as cataract surgery without bulbar blocks. The usual recommendation is to withhold five doses of warfarin before operation (if the international normalized ratio [INR] is 2 to 3) to allow the INR to decrease to within reference limits (see Table 13-16).[49] If the INR is greater than 3.0, warfarin should be withheld longer. If the INR is measured the day before surgery and is greater than 1.8, a small dose of vitamin K (1 to 5 mg orally or subcutaneously) can reverse anticoagulation.[50] Substitution with shorter-acting anticoagulants such as unfractionated or LMWH, referred to as bridging, is controversial (see Table 13-16). Bridging is usually reserved for patients who have had an acute arterial or venous thromboembolism within 1 month before surgery, if surgery cannot be postponed, for patients with certain mechanical heart valves, or for patients with high-risk hypercoagulable states.[50]

Type 1 diabetics have an absolute insulin deficiency and require insulin to prevent ketoacidosis even if they are not hyperglycemic. Type 2 diabetics are often insulin-resistant

Table 13-14 Preanesthesia Medication Instructions

Continue on Day of Surgery	Discontinue on Day of Surgery Unless Otherwise Indicated
Antidepressant, antianxiety, and psychiatric medications (including monoamine oxidase inhibitors*)	
Antihypertensives ■ Generally to be continued	Antihypertensives ■ Consider discontinuing angiotensin-converting enzyme inhibitors or angiotensin receptor blockers 12-24 hr before surgery if taken only for hypertension; especially with lengthy procedures, significant blood loss or fluid shifts, use of general anesthesia, multiple antihypertensive medications, well-controlled blood pressure; hypotension is particularly dangerous

Aspirin[†]
■ Patients with known vascular disease
■ Patients with drug-eluting stents for <12 months
■ Patients with bare metal stents for <1 month
■ Before cataract surgery (if no bulbar block)
■ Before vascular surgery
■ Taken for secondary prophylaxis
	Aspirin[†]
	■ Discontinue 5-7 days before surgery:
	  • If risk of bleeding > risk of thrombosis
	  • For surgeries with serious consequences from bleeding
	  • Taken only for primary prophylaxis (no known vascular disease)

Table 13-14 Preanesthesia Medication Instructions—cont'd

Continue on Day of Surgery	Discontinue on Day of Surgery Unless Otherwise Indicated
Asthma medications	
Autoimmune medications ■ Methotrexate (if no risk of renal failure)	Autoimmune medications ■ Methotrexate (if risk of renal failure) ■ Entanercept (Enbrel), infliximab (Remicade), adalimumab (Humira): check with prescriber
Birth control pills	
Cardiac medications	
Clopidogrel (Plavix)* ■ Patients with drug-eluting stents for <12 months ■ Patients with bare metal stents for <1 month ■ Before cataract surgery (if no bulbar block)	Clopidogrel (Plavix)* ■ Patients not included in group recommended for continuation
COX-2 inhibitors	COX-2 inhibitors ■ If surgeon is concerned about bone healing
Diuretics ■ Triamterene, hydrochlorothiazide	Diuretics ■ Potent loop diuretics
Eye drops	
Estrogen compounds ■ When used for birth control or cancer therapy	Estrogen compounds ■ When used to control menopause symptoms or for osteoporosis
Gastrointestinal reflux medications	Gastrointestinal reflux medications (Tums)
	Herbals and nonvitamin supplements ■ 7-14 days before surgery
	Hypoglycemic agents, oral
Insulin ■ *Type 1 diabetes*: take ~ 1/3 of intermediate to long-acting (NPH, lente) ■ *Type 2 diabetes*: take up to 1/2 long-acting (NPH) or combination (70/30) preparations ■ Glargine (Lantus): decrease if dose is ≥1 unit/kg ■ With insulin pump delivery, continue lowest night-time basal rate	Insulin ■ Regular insulin (*exception*: with insulin pump, continue lowest basal rate—generally nighttime dose) ■ Discontinue if blood sugar level <100
Narcotics for pain or addiction Seizure medications	Nonsteroidal anti-inflammatory drugs ■ 48 hr before day of surgery
Statins	Topical creams and ointments
Steroids (oral or inhaled)	Viagra or similar medications ■ Discontinue 24 hr before surgery
Thyroid medications	Vitamins, minerals, iron
Warfarin ■ Cataract surgery, no bulbar block	Warfarin‡ ■ Discontinue 5 days before surgery

*See text for details.
†Except when the risk or consequences of bleeding are severe (generally only with intracranial or posterior eye procedures).
‡Bridging may be necessary; see text for details.
COX-2, cyclooxygenase-2.

and prone to extreme hyperglycemia. Both type 1 and 2 diabetics should discontinue intermittent short-acting insulin. Patients with insulin pumps continue with their lowest basal rate, which is typically a nighttime rate. Type 1 diabetics take a small amount (usually 1/3 to 1/2) of their usual intermediate- to long-acting morning insulin (e.g., lente or NPH) the day of surgery to avoid ketoacidosis. Type 2 diabetics take none or up to half a dose of

Table 13-15 American College of Cardiology Foundation (ACCF)/American Heart Association (AHA) Perioperative Beta Blocker Recommendations

Class I

1. Beta blockers should be continued in patients undergoing surgery who are receiving beta blockers for treatment of conditions with ACCF/AHA Class I guideline indications for the drugs. *(Level of Evidence: C)*

Class IIa

1. Beta blockers titrated to heart rate and blood pressure are probably recommended for patients undergoing vascular surgery who are at high cardiac risk owing to coronary artery disease or the finding of cardiac ischemia on preoperative testing *(Level of Evidence: B)*
2. Beta blockers titrated to heart rate and blood pressure are reasonable for patients in whom preoperative assessment for vascular surgery identifies high cardiac risk, as defined by the presence of more than 1 clinical risk factor.* *(Level of Evidence: C)*
3. Beta blockers titrated to heart rate and blood pressure are reasonable for patients in whom preoperative assessment identifies coronary artery disease or high cardiac risk, as defined by the presence of more than 1 clinical risk factor,* who are undergoing intermediate-risk surgery *(Level of Evidence: B)*

Class IIb

1. The usefulness of beta blockers is uncertain for patients who are undergoing either intermediate-risk procedures or vascular surgery in whom preoperative assessment identifies a single clinical risk factor in the absence of coronary artery disease.* *(Level of Evidence: C)*
2. The usefulness of beta blockers is uncertain in patients undergoing vascular surgery with no clinical risk factors* who are not currently taking beta blockers. *(Level of Evidence: B)*

Class III

1. Beta blockers should not be given to patients undergoing surgery who have absolute contraindications to beta blockade. *(Level of Evidence: C)*
2. Routine administration of high-dose beta blockers in the absence of dose titration is not useful and may be harmful to patients not currently taking beta blockers who are undergoing noncardiac surgery *(Level of Evidence: B)*

*Clinical risk factors include history of ischemic heart disease, history of compensated or previous heart failure, history of cerebrovascular disease, diabetes mellitus, and renal insufficiency (defined in the Revised Cardiac Risk Index as preoperative serum creatinine concentration of >2 mg/dL.[40]

Table 13-16 Outpatient Periprocedural Bridging Protocol

Enoxaparin or Low-Molecular-Weight Heparin (LMWH)

Do not use enoxaparin if $CrCl_{est} < 40$ mL/min, body weight > 150 kg, or patient has history of bleeding complications on enoxaparin, pork allergy, or heparin-induced thrombocytopenia.

Special consideration is needed for patients undergoing centroneuraxial anesthesia and for timing of catheter placement and removal. Enoxaparin dosing must be coordinated with the anesthesia service based on American Society of Regional Anesthesia (ASRA) guidelines.[49]

The first enoxaparin dose depends on how quickly the INR becomes subtherapeutic after cessation of warfarin. Obtain an INR determination before enoxaparin administration.

Day −7: Last dose of warfarin is given if INR is 3.0-3.5. Repeat INR on day-5 and begin enoxaparin when INR is subtherapeutic.
Day −6: Last dose of warfarin is given if INR is 2.5-3.0 Repeat INR on day-4 and begin enoxaparin when INR is subtherapeutic.
Day −5: Last dose of warfarin is given if INR is 2.0-2.5. Repeat INR on day-4 and begin enoxaparin when INR is subtherapeutic.
Days −4, −3 and −2: Continue enoxaparin—no warfarin.
Day −1: Last dose of enoxaparin is given at 0700.
Day 0: Day of surgery.

Alternative Management Using Administration of Oral Vitamin K

If enoxaparin is contraindicated (i.e., $CrCl_{est} < 40$ mL/min, body weight > 150 kg, or patient has history of bleeding complications on enoxaparin, pork allergy, or heparin-induced thrombocytopenia), the following procedure using orally administered vitamin K is recommended:

Day −3: Last dose of warfarin is given.
Day −2: Hold warfarin and administer vitamin K in a single oral dose of 5 mg.
Day −1: Obtain INR and repeat dose of vitamin K if INR ≥ 1.5.
Day 0: Obtain STAT INR 1 hour before the scheduled arrival time for the procedure

$CrCl_{est}$, estimated rate of creatinine clearance; INR, international normalized ratio.

intermediate- to long-acting (e.g., lente or NPH) or a combination (70/30 preparations) insulin on the day of operation. Taking half the usual dose of intermediate-, long-acting, or combination insulin on the day of surgery improves perioperative glycemic levels compared to taking no insulin.[51] Ultra-long-acting insulin such as glargine insulin can be taken as scheduled.

Metformin does not need to be discontinued before the day of surgery and will not cause hypoglycemia during fasting periods of 1 to 2 days. There is no risk of lactic acidosis with metformin in patients with a functioning liver and kidneys. Therefore, for patients who continue metformin, procedures are not canceled, but metformin is not administered postoperatively until the risk of lactic acidosis has passed. There are no data to support the recommendation to stop metformin 24 to 48 hours before surgery, which increases the risk of hyperglycemia.[52] Sulfonylurea drugs with very long half-lives (e.g., chlorpropamide) can cause hypoglycemia in fasting patients. Newer oral drugs (acarbose, pioglitazone) used as single-agent therapy do not cause hypoglycemia during fasting. However, to avoid confusion oral hypoglycemic drugs are generally withheld on the day of surgery. Patients taking steroids regularly take their usual dose on the day of surgery. Stress-associated adrenal insufficiency in some patients may require additional steroids perioperatively. A normal daily adrenal output of cortisol (30 mg) is equivalent to 5 to 7.5 mg of prednisone. The hypothalamic-pituitary axis (HPA) is not suppressed with less than 5 mg/day of prednisone or its equivalent. In patients taking 5 to 20 mg/day of prednisone or its equivalent for more than 3 weeks, the HPA may be suppressed. The HPA is suppressed with more than 20 mg/day of prednisone or its equivalent when taken for more than 3 weeks. The risk of adrenal insufficiency remains for up to 1 year after the cessation of high-dose steroids. During the stress of surgery, trauma, or infection an intact HPA will respond by increasing output of glucocorticoids. Supplementation with steroids depends on the amount of stress, duration and severity of the procedure, and the regular daily dose of steroid (Table 13-17). Infections, psychosis, poor wound healing, and hyperglycemia increase with high doses of perioperative steroids, which are rarely necessary.[53]

Herbals and supplements should be discontinued 7 to 14 days before surgery. The exception is valerian, a central nervous system depressant, which may cause a benzodiazepine-like withdrawal when discontinued; if possible, intake of valerian should be tapered before a planned anesthetic. Mandatory discontinuation of these medications, or cancellation of anesthesia when these medications have been continued, is not supported by available data. Herbal therapy alone is not a contraindication to neuraxial anesthesia. ASRA specifically advises against mandatory discontinuation of herbals or forgoing regional anesthesia in patients taking herbal drugs.[49]

Historically, monoamine oxidase inhibitors (MAOIs) were discontinued before surgery, but because of their long duration of action, they must be discontinued at least 3 weeks before surgery. Discontinuation of MAOIs may produce severe depression or result in suicide. The safest alternative is to continue MAOIs and adjust the anesthetic plan. Patients also continue any narcotic pain medications to prevent withdrawal symptoms and discomfort. Anxiolytics are continued as well. Drugs used to treat addiction such as methadone or nicotine-replacement therapies also are continued.[54] Inhalers and long-term medications for asthma or chronic obstructive pulmonary disease are continued on the day of surgery.[55]

Patients who are particularly anxious should be given pharmacologic premedication. Outpatients benefit from a prescription for a short course of benzodiazepines such as lorazepam to be taken in the days preceding surgery as well as on the day of operation. Opioids are useful in those patients experiencing preoperative pain, discomfort associated with placement of a regional

Table 13-17 Recommendations for Perioperative Glucocorticoid Coverage

Surgical Stress	Target Hydrocortisone Equivalent	Steroid Dosing				
		Preoperative	Intraoperative	Postoperative		
				Immediately	Day 1	Day 2
Minor (e.g., inguinal herniorrhaphy)	25 mg/day for 1 day	Usual daily dose of steroid	None[†]	None[†]	Usual daily dose*[†]	
Moderate (e.g., colon resection, total joint replacement, lower extremity revascularization)	50-75 mg/day for 1-2 days	Usual daily dose of steroid	50 mg[†] hydrocortisone	20 mg[†] hydrocortisone every 8 hr	20 mg[†] hydrocortisone every 8 hr	
Major (e.g., pancreatoduodenectomy, esophagectomy)	100-150 mg/day for 2-3 days	Usual daily dose of steroid	50 mg[†] hydrocortisone	50 mg[†] hydrocortisone every 8 hr	50 mg[†] hydrocortisone every 8 hr	50 mg[†] hydrocortisone every 8 hr

*If the postoperative course is uncomplicated, the patient can resume the usual steroid dose on postoperative day 1.
[†]If postoperative complications occur, continued glucocorticoid administration will be necessary commiserate with the level of stress.
Dosages from Salem M, Tainsh RE, Bromberg J, et al. Perioperative glucocorticoid coverage. A reassessment 42 years after emergence of a problem. Ann Surg 1994;219:416-425.

anesthetic, or insertion of invasive monitors before induction of anesthesia. Patients with a history of protracted severe PONV can be offered a prescription for a scopolamine patch to be placed 2 to 4 hours preoperatively. Patients with closed angle glaucoma should not be prescribed scopolamine. Patients at increased risk for pulmonary aspiration (parturients, nonfasting individuals, significant symptoms of esophageal reflux, anticipated difficult airway management) benefit from attempts to alter gastric contents. H_2 antagonists (ranitidine, famotidine), proton pump inhibitors (omeprazole), and antacids (sodium citrate) increase gastric fluid pH. Prokinetics (metoclopramide) stimulate gastric emptying. Table 13-18 outlines commonly used preoperative medications.

FASTING

Current guidelines (Table 13-19) for preoperative fasting for the adult patient recommend that "fasting from solids (and) nonhuman milk should exceed a period of 6 hours before procedures requiring general anesthesia, regional anesthesia, or sedation/analgesia." Liberalization of preoperative fasting rules to include clear liquids up to 2 hours before anesthesia is acceptable for patients without conditions that may increase the risk of aspiration, such as an incompetent lower esophageal sphincter with reflux, hiatal hernia, diabetes mellitus, gastric motility disorders, intra-abdominal masses (including the gravid uterus), and bowel obstruction.[56]

Table 13-19 Guidelines for Food and Fluid Intake before Elective Surgery

Time Before Surgery	Food or Fluid Intake
Up to 8 hours	Food and fluids as desired
Up to 6 hours*	Light meal (e.g., toast and clear liquids†); infant formula; nonhuman milk
Up to 4 hours*	Breast milk
Up to 2 hours*	Clear liquids† only; no solids or foods containing fat in any form
During the 2 hours	No solids, no liquids

*This guideline applies only to patients who *are not* at risk for delayed gastric emptying. Patients with the following conditions *are* at risk for delayed gastric emptying: morbid obesity; diabetes mellitus; pregnancy; a history of gastroesophageal reflux; a surgery-limited stomach capacity; a potential difficult airway; opiate analgesic therapy.
†Clear liquids are water, carbonated beverages, sports drinks, coffee or tea (without milk). The following are *not* clear liquids: juice with pulp; milk; coffee or tea with milk; infant formula; any beverage with alcohol.
From Practice guidelines for preoperative fasting and the use of pharmacologic agents to reduce the risk of pulmonary aspiration: Application to healthy patients undergoing elective procedures: A report by the American Society of Anesthesiologists Task Force on Preoperative Fasting, Anesthesiology 90:896–905, 1999.

Table 13-18 Drugs for Pharmacologic Premedication before Anesthesia

Classification	Drug	Typical Adult Dose (mg)	Route of Administration
Benzodiazepines	Midazolam	1-2.5	IV
	Lorazepam	0.5-2	Oral, IV
Opioids	Hydromorphone	0.5-1	IV
	Fentanyl	25-100 µg	IV
Antihistamines	Diphenhydramine	12.5-50	Oral, IV
Antiemetics	Scopolamine	1.5	Topical
	Dexamethasone	4	IV
	Dolasetron	12.5	IV
	Ondansetron	4	IV
H_2 antagonists	Ranitidine	150	Oral
	Famotidine	20-40	IV, oral
Antacids	Nonparticulate sodium citrate	15-30 mL	Oral
Proton pump inhibitors	Omeprazole	20	Oral
	Pantoprazole	40	IV
Gastrointestinal stimulants	Metoclopramide*	10	Oral, IV

*Rare incidence of prolonged QT interval.
IV, Intravenous.

FORMULATION OF ANESTHETIC PLAN, ASSESSMENT OF RISK, AND INFORMED CONSENT

The choice of anesthesia (general, regional or sedation), monitors, or specific anesthetic drugs rarely alters outcome or risk. However, impressions from clinical experience continue to influence beliefs and recommendations when devising a plan of anesthesia care. Factors to consider when formulating a planned anesthetic are shown in Table 13-20.

Risk assessment is useful to compare outcomes, control costs, allocate compensation, and assist in the difficult decision of canceling or recommending a procedure not be done when the risks are too high. Yet risk assessment, at its best, is hampered by individual patient variability. Risks have traditionally been attributed to the patient's co-morbid conditions, general health status, age, anesthetic technique, and the planned procedure (Fig. 13-8 and Tables 13-3, 13-9, and 13-21). Nevertheless, some assessment of risk is important in order to inform patients during the consent process (Table 13-22).

Table 13-20 Considerations That Influence the Choice of Anesthetic Technique

Coexisting diseases
Site of the surgery
Position of the patient during surgery
Risk of aspiration
Age of the patient
Patient cooperation
Anticipated ease of airway management
Coagulation status
Previous response to anesthesia
Preference of the patient

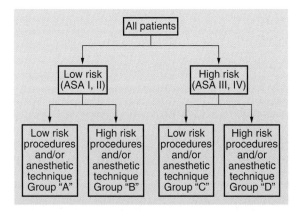

Figure 13-8 Example of a risk classification incorporating both patient co-morbidity and surgical severity. (From Pasternak LR: Risk assessment in ambulatory surgery: challenges and new trends. Can J Anaesth 51(S1):R1–R5, 2004.)

Table 13-21 Cardiac Risk* Stratification for Noncardiac Surgical Procedures

Risk Stratification	Example Procedures
Vascular (reported cardiac risk often more than 5%)	Aortic and other major vascular surgery Peripheral vascular surgery
Intermediate (reported cardiac risk generally 1% to 5%)	Intraperitoneal and intrathoracic surgery Carotid endarterectomy Head and neck surgery Orthopedic surgery Prostate surgery
Low† (reported cardiac risk generally less than1%)	Endoscopic procedures Superficial procedure Cataract surgery Breast surgery Ambulatory surgery

*Combined incidence of cardiac death and nonfatal myocardial infarction.
†These procedures generally do not require further preoperative cardiac testing.
From Fleisher LA, Beckman JA, Brown KA, et al: ACC/AHA 2007 guidelines on perioperative cardiovascular evaluation and care for noncardiac surgery, J Am Coll Cardiol 50:1707–1732, 2007.

Informed consent must be obtained for all nonemergency procedures and is a legal requirement in all jurisdictions of the United States. At a minimum, informed consent involves the indications for the treatment in terms a layperson can understand, and elucidation of alternatives. Many anesthesiologists perform preoperative evaluations, and obtain informed consent moments before a patient will undergo a major, potentially life-threatening or disfiguring procedure. This is often an awkward and unpleasant situation for the anesthesiologist, patient, and family. The effects of extensive disclosure are stressful at a time when patients and families may be ill-prepared to rationally consider the implications. An increase in preoperative anxiety may adversely affect postoperative outcomes because increased anxiety correlates with increased postoperative analgesic requirements and prolonged recovery and hospital stay. Anxiety impairs retention of information. However, anxiety is lower in patients seen by the anesthesiologist in advance of surgery compared to those receiving only premedication.

CONCLUSION

Preoperative preparation can decrease the risk of complications and improve outcomes during and after procedures requiring anesthesia. Innovation in preoperative preparation needs to continue if patients are to receive the best preoperative services. Identification and modification of risk require fundamentally good medicine; systems of care; clinical assessment; and experienced, knowledgeable, and dedicated health care providers.

Table 13-22 Commonly Disclosed Risks of Anesthesia

With General Anesthesia

Frequently Occurring, Minimal Impact
- Oral or dental damage
- Sore throat
- Hoarseness
- Postoperative nausea/vomiting
- Drowsiness/confusion
- Urinary retention

Infrequently Occurring, Severe
- Awareness
- Visual loss
- Aspiration
- Organ failure
- Malignant hyperthermia
- Drug reactions
- Failure to wake up/recover
- Death

With Regional Anesthesia

Frequently Occurring, Minimal Impact
- Prolonged numbness/weakness
- Post-dural puncture headache
- Failure of technique

Infrequently Occurring, Severe
- Bleeding
- Infection
- Nerve damage/paralysis
- Persistent numbness/weakness
- Seizures
- Coma
- Death

Adapted from O'Leary CE. American Society of Anesthesiologists Newsletter 2010;74:20-21.

QUESTIONS OF THE DAY

1. What components of the preanesthetic physical examination should be performed on every patient? What additional examination should be performed on a patient scheduled for a regional anesthetic?
2. A patient with recent percutaneous coronary intervention with a drug eluting stent requires surgery. How should elective surgery be managed with respect to cessation of antiplatelet therapy? How should urgent or emergent surgery be managed?
3. What are the risk factors for development of postoperative pulmonary complications? Is asthma a risk factor?
4. What routine preoperative tests should be ordered prior to low- or intermediate-risk surgery in ASA Physical Status 1 or 2 patients?
5. What factors determine whether angiotensin-converting enzyme inhibitors (ACEIs) or angiotensin receptor blockers (ARBs) should be stopped on the morning of surgery?
6. What anesthetic risks are commonly disclosed to patients prior to surgery?

ACKNOWLEDGMENTS

The editors and publisher would like to thank Drs. Rachel Dotson, Jeanine P. Wiener-Kronish, and Temitayo Ajayi for contributing a chapter on this topic to the prior edition of this work. It has served as the foundation for the current chapter.

REFERENCES

1. American Society of Anesthesiologists Task Force on Preanesthesia Evaluation: Practice advisory for preanesthesia evaluation: A report by the American Society of Anesthesiologists Task Force on Preanesthesia Evaluation, *Anesthesiology* 96:485–496, 2002.
2. Apfelbaum JL: Preoperative evaluation, laboratory screening, and selection of adult surgical outpatients in the 1990s, *Anesth Rev* 17(Suppl 2):4–12, 1990.
3. Hlatky MA, Boineau RE, Higginbotham MB, et al: A brief self-administered questionnaire to determine functional capacity (The Duke Activity Status Index), *Am J Cardiol* 64:651–654, 1989.
4. Fleisher LA, Beckman JA, Brown KA, et al: ACC/AHA 2007 guidelines on perioperative cardiovascular evaluation and care for noncardiac surgery, *J Am Coll Cardiol* 50:1707–1732, 2007.
5. McFalls EO, Ward HB, Moritz TE, et al: Coronary-artery revascularization before elective major vascular surgery, *N Engl J Med* 351:2795–2804, 2004.
6. Breen P, Lee JW, Pomposelli F, et al: Timing of high-risk vascular surgery following coronary artery bypass surgery: A 10-year experience from an academic medical centre, *Anaesthesia* 59:422–427, 2004.
7. Grines CL, Bonow RD, Casey DE Jr, et al: Prevention of premature discontinuation of dual antiplatelet therapy in patients with coronary artery stents: A science advisory from the American Heart Association American College of Cardiology, Society for Cardiovascular Angiography and Interventions, American College of Surgeons, and American Dental Association with representation from the American College of Physicians, *J Am Coll Cardiol* 49:734–739, 2007.
8. Burger W, Chemnitius JM, Kneissl GD, et al: Low-dose aspirin for secondary cardiovascular prevention—Cardiovascular risks after its perioperative withdrawal versus bleeding risks with its continuation—

Review and meta-analysis, *J Intern Med* 257:399–414, 2005.

9. Newsome LT, Weller RS, Gerancher JC, et al: Coronary artery stents: II. Perioperative considerations and management, *Anesth Analg* 107:570–590, 2008.

10. Rabbitts JA, Nuttall GA, Brown MJ, et al: Cardiac risk of noncardiac surgery after percutaneous coronary intervention with drug-eluting stents, *Anesthesiology* 109:596–604, 2008.

11. Berger PB, Bellot V, Bell MR, et al: An immediate invasive strategy for the treatment of acute myocardial infarction early after noncardiac surgery, *Am J Cardiol* 87:1100–1102, 2001.

12. Otto CM, Lind BK, Kitzman DW, et al: Association of aortic-valve sclerosis with cardiovascular mortality and morbidity in the elderly, *N Engl J Med* 341:142–147, 1999.

13. American College of Cardiology/American Heart Association Task Force on Practice Guidelines, Society of Cardiovascular Anesthesiologists, Society for Cardiovascular Angiography and Interventions, et al: ACC/AHA 2006 guidelines for the management of patients with valvular heart disease, *J Am Coll Cardiol* 48:598–675, 2006.

14. Wilson W, Taubert KA, Gewitz M, et al: Prevention of infective endocarditis: Guidelines from the American Heart Association, Rheumatic Fever, Endocarditis, and Kawasaki Disease Committee, Council on Cardiovascular Disease in the Young, Council on Clinical Cardiology, Council on Cardiovascular Surgery and Anesthesia, and the Quality of Care and Outcomes Research Interdisciplinary Working Group, *Circulation* 116:1736–1754, 2007.

15. American Society of Anesthesiologists Task Force on Perioperative Management of Patients with Cardiac Rhythm Management Devices: Practice advisory for the perioperative management of patients with cardiac rhythm management devices: Pacemakers and implantable cardioverter-defibrillators, *Anesthesiology* 103:186–198, 2005.

16. Howell SJ, Sear JW, Foex P: Hypertension, hypertensive heart disease and perioperative cardiac risk, *Br J Anaesth* 92:570–583, 2004.

17. Smetana GW, Lawrence VA, Cornell JE: Preoperative pulmonary risk stratification for noncardiothoracic surgery: Systematic review for the American College of Physicians, *Ann Intern Med* 144:581–595, 2006.

18. Hwang D, Shakir N, Limann B, et al: Association of sleep-disordered breathing with postoperative complications, *Chest* 133:1128–1134, 2008.

19. Warner DO, Warner MA, Barnes RD, et al: Perioperative respiratory complications in patients with asthma, *Anesthesiology* 85:460–467, 1996.

20. Lawrence VA, Cornell JE, Smetana GW: Strategies to reduce postoperative complications after noncardiothoracic surgery: Systematic review for the American College of Physicians, *Ann Intern Med* 144:596–608, 2006.

21. Young T, Palta M, Dempsey J, et al: The occurrence of sleep-disordered breathing among middle-aged adults, *N Engl J Med* 328:1230–1235, 1993.

22. Young T, Skatrud J, Peppard PE: Risk factors for obstructive sleep apnea in adults, *JAMA* 291:2013–2016, 2004.

23. Chung F, Yegneswaran B, Liao P, et al: STOP questionnaire: a tool to screen patients for obstructive sleep apnea, *Anesthesiology* 108:812–821, 2008.

24. Caples SM, Gami AS, Somers VK: Obstructive sleep apnea, *Ann Intern Med* 142:187–197, 2005.

25. American Society of Anesthesiologists Task Force on Perioperative Management of Patients with Obstructive Sleep Apnea: Practice guidelines for the perioperative management of patients with obstructive sleep apnea, *Anesthesiology* 104:1081–1093, 2006.

26. Lipshutz AK, Gropper MA: Perioperative glycemic control, *Anesthesiology* 110:408–421, 2009.

27. Moitra VK, Greenberg J, Arunajadai S, et al: The relationship between glycosylated hemoglobin and perioperative glucose control in patients with diabetes, *Can J Anaesth* 57:322–329, 2010.

28. Beattie WS, Karkouti K, Wijeysundera DN, et al: Risk associated with preoperative anemia in noncardiac surgery, *Anesthesiology* 110:574–581, 2009.

29. Practice guidelines for perioperative blood transfusion and adjuvant therapies, *Anesthesiology* 105:198–208, 2004.

30. Fleisher LA, Pasternak LR, Herbert R, et al: Inpatient hospital admission and death after outpatient surgery in elderly patients: Importance of patient and system characteristics and location of care, *Arch Surg* 139:67–72, 2004.

31. Polanczyk CA, Marcantonio E, Goldman L, et al: Impact of age on perioperative complications and length of stay in patients undergoing noncardiac surgery, *Ann Intern Med* 134:637–643, 2001.

32. Narr BJ, Hansen TR, Warner MA: Preoperative laboratory screening in healthy Mayo patients: Cost-effective elimination of tests and unchanged outcomes, *Mayo Clin Proc* 66:155–159, 1991.

33. Liu LL, Dzankic S, Leung JM: Preoperative electrocardiogram abnormalities do not predict postoperative cardiac complications in geriatric surgical patients, *J Am Geriatr Soc* 50:1186–1191, 2002.

34. Chung F, Yuan H, Yin L, et al: Elimination of preoperative testing in ambulatory surgery, *Anesth Analg* 108:467–475, 2009.

35. Gold BS, Young ML, Kinman JL, et al: The utility of preoperative electrocardiograms in the ambulatory surgical patient, *Arch Intern Med* 152:301–305, 1991.

36. van Klei WA, Bryson GL, Yang H, et al: The value of routine preoperative electrocardiography in predicting myocardial infarction after noncardiac surgery, *Ann Surg* 246:165–170, 2007.

37. Centers for Medicare and Medicaid Services: Available at http://www.cms.hhs.org. Accessed February 9, 2009.

38. American Society of Anesthesiologists Task Force on Preanesthesia Evaluation: Practice advisory for preanesthesia evaluation: A report by the American Society of Anesthesiologists Task Force on Preanesthesia Evaluation, *Anesthesiology* 96:485–496, 2002.

39. Comfere T, Sprung J, Kumar MM, et al: Angiotensin system inhibitors in a general surgical population, *Anesth Analg* 100:636–644, 2005.

40. Fleischmann KE, Beckman JA, Buller CE, et al: 2009 ACCF/AHA focused update on perioperative beta blockade incorporated into the ACC/AHA 2007 guidelines on perioperative cardiovascular evaluation and care for noncardiac surgery, *J Am Coll Cardiol* 54:2102–2128, 2009.

41. van de Pol MA, van Houdenhoven M, Hans EW, et al: Influence of cardiac risk factors and medication on length of hospitalization in patients undergoing major vascular surgery, *Am J Cardiol* 97:1423–1426, 2006.

42. Kapoor AS, Kanji H, Buckingham J, et al: Strength of evidence of preoperative use of statins to reduce cardiovascular risk: Systemic review of controlled studies, *BMJ* 333:1149–1155, 2006.

43. Le Manach Y, Coriat P, Collard CD, et al: Statin therapy within the perioperative period, *Anesthesiology* 108:1141–1146, 2008.

44. Le Manach Y, Godet G, Coriat P, et al: The impact of postoperative discontinuation or continuation of chronic statin therapy on postoperative outcome after major vascular surgery, *Anesth Analg* 104:1326–1333, 2007.

III

45. Albaladejo P, Geeraerts T, Francis F, et al: Aspirin withdrawal and acute lower limb ischemia, *Anesth Analg* 99:440–443, 2004.

46. Senior K: Aspirin withdrawal increases risk of heart problems, *Lancet* 362:1558, 2003.

47. Eisen GM, Baron TH, Dominitz JA, et al: Guideline on the management of anticoagulation and antiplatelet therapy for endoscopic procedures, *Gastrointest Endosc* 55:775–779, 2002.

48. Chassot PG, Delabays A, Spahn DR: Perioperative antiplatelet therapy: The case for continuing therapy in patients at risk of myocardial infarction, *Br J Anaesth* 99:316–328, 2007.

49. Horlocker TT, Wedel DJ, Rowlingson JC, et al: Regional anesthesia in the patient receiving antithrombotic or thrombolytic therapy. American Society of Regional Anesthesia and Pain Medicine Evidence-Based Guidelines, *Reg Anesth Pain Med* 35:64–101, 2010.

50. Douketis JD, Berger PB, Dunn AS, et al: The perioperative management of antithrombotic therapy: American College of Chest Physicians Evidence-Based Clinical Practice Guidelines (8th edition), *Chest* 133:299S–339S, 2008.

51. Likavec A, Moitra V, Greenberg J, et al: Comparison of preoperative blood glucose levels in patients receiving different insulin regimens, *Anesthesiology* 105:A567, 2006.

52. Salpeter SR, Greyber E, Pasternak GA, et al: Risk of fatal and nonfatal lactic acidosis with metformin use in type 2 diabetes mellitus (review): *Cochrane Database Syst Rev* http://www.thecochranelibrary.com. Accessed January 17, 2010.

53. Salem M, Tainsh RE, Bromberg J, et al: Perioperative glucocorticoid coverage. A reassessment 42 years after emergence of a problem, *Ann Surg* 219:416–425, 1994.

54. Spell NO III: Stopping and restarting medications in the perioperative period, *Med Clin North Am* 85:1117–1128, 2001.

55. Qaseem A, Snow V, Fitterman N, et al: Risk assessment for and strategies to reduce perioperative pulmonary complications for patients undergoing noncardiothoracic surgery: A guideline from the American College of Physicians, *Ann Intern Med* 144:575–580, 2006.

56. Practice guidelines for preoperative fasting and the use of pharmacologic agents to reduce the risk of pulmonary aspiration: Application to healthy patients undergoing elective procedures: A report by the American Society of Anesthesiologists Task Force on Preoperative Fasting, *Anesthesiology* 90:896–905, 1999.

A BASIC STANDARDS FOR PREANESTHESIA CARE*

Committee of Origin: Standards and Practice Parameters (Approved by the House of Delegates on October 14, 1987, and last affirmed on October 20, 2010)

These standards apply to all patients who receive anesthesia care. In exceptional circumstances, these standards may be modified. When such is the case, the circumstances shall be documented in the patient's record.

An anesthesiologist shall be responsible for determining the medical status of the patient and developing a plan of anesthesia care.

The anesthesiologist, before the delivery of anesthesia care, is responsible for the following:

1. Reviewing the available medical record
2. Interviewing and performing a focused examination of the patient to:
   a. Discuss the medical history, including previous anesthetic experiences and medical therapy
   b. Assess aspects of the patient's physical condition that might affect decisions regarding perioperative risk and management
3. Ordering and reviewing pertinent available tests and consultations as necessary for the delivery of anesthesia care
4. Ordering appropriate preoperative medications
5. Ensuring that consent has been obtained for the anesthesia care
6. Documenting in the chart that the above has been performed

---

*Basic Standards for Preanesthesia Care is reprinted with permission of the American Society of Anesthesiologists, 520 N. Northwest Highway, Park Ridge, IL 60068-2573.www.asahq.org. Accessed 11/19/2010.

III

14 CHOICE OF ANESTHETIC TECHNIQUE

Ronald D. Miller

The preoperative anesthetic evaluation (see Chapter 13) provides a database with which to make decisions regarding risk assessment and perioperative management. Regardless of the site (dedicated preanesthesia clinic, inpatient hospital visit, or primary care clinic) and health care provider performing the preoperative evaluation, the final assessment is the responsibility of the anesthesia provider rendering the anesthetic care for the patient.[1] The anesthesiologist is ultimately responsible for (1) determining the medical status of the patient, (2) developing a plan of anesthesia care, and (3) reviewing with the patient or a responsible adult the proposed care plan. After review of the patient's medical history and laboratory and other test results from the patient's medical record, confirmation by a focused physical examination, and review of the patient's fasting status, the anesthesia care provider can then select the anesthetic technique. This chapter provides a broad view of the decision-making process necessary for deciding which anesthetic technique to select. The reader of this chapter will be directed to other chapters for details regarding many of the factors involved with selection of an anesthetic technique.

ANESTHETIC TECHNIQUE

The anesthesia care provider has several options available including (1) general anesthetic, (2) regional anesthetic (see Chapter 17), (3) peripheral nerve block (see Chapter 18), or (4) monitored anesthetic care (MAC). The choice of anesthetic technique (or combination of techniques) should be based on surgical and patient considerations; frequently, more than one anesthetic technique is appropriate (Table 14-1). Patient safety (see Chapter 47), the ability of the surgeon to perform the procedure, and patient comfort during and after the procedure are important issues. Intraoperative and postoperative monitoring (see Chapter 20) considerations may influence the choice of anesthetic technique. For example, if a rapid

Table 14-1 Considerations That Influence the Choice of Anesthetic Technique

Preference of patient, anesthesiologist, and surgeon
Coexisting diseases that may or may not be related to the reason for surgery (e.g., gastroesophageal reflux, diabetes mellitus, asthma)
Site of surgery
Body position of the patient during surgery
Elective or emergency surgery
Likelihood of increased amounts of gastric contents at the time of induction of anesthesia
Suspected difficult airway management and tracheal intubation
Duration of surgery or procedure
Patient age
Anticipated recovery time
Postanesthesia care unit discharge criteria

postoperative neurologic evaluation is needed, a general anesthetic with short-acting anesthetic drugs or a regional anesthetic may be selected. Conversely, if intraoperative transesophageal echocardiography is required, a general endotracheal anesthetic will probably be preferred. There are few circumstances in which a specific anesthetic technique may be safer or more efficacious than another technique.[2,3] The anesthesia care provider may perform better with techniques with which they are more experienced. During anesthesia training, learning as many anesthetic techniques as possible adds to the ability of anesthesia providers to be as flexible as possible to unique patient needs.

Unpleasant side effects associated with anesthesia may influence the choice of anesthetic technique. Because the relative levels of safety for different anesthetic techniques are frequently similar, patient satisfaction may become the principal determinant of the anesthetic technique selected. Assuming equivalent safety (also see Chapter 47), both the anesthesia provider and patient are likely to place prime importance on analgesia, followed by vomiting, nausea, and to a lesser extent, urinary retention, myalgia, and pruritus. For some patients, avoiding being awake (see Chapter 46) is the predominant concern, perhaps because of anxiety. For these patients, even in the absence of pain, the sights, sounds, and smells of the operating or procedure room are an experience to be avoided.[4,5]

An ideal anesthetic technique would incorporate optimal patient safety and satisfaction, provide excellent operating conditions for the surgeon, allow rapid recovery, and avoid postoperative side effects. In addition, the chosen technique would be low in cost, allow early transfer or discharge from the postanesthesia care unit (see Chapter 39), optimize postoperative pain control (see Chapter 40), and permit optimal operating room efficiency, including turnover times. The anesthesia provider must evaluate the medical condition and unique needs of each patient, select an acceptable anesthetic technique, and make this recommendation to the patient.

An informed patient who has an understanding of the anesthetic techniques available and the needs for accomplishing the surgery is likely to be comfortable with the anesthetic technique recommended by the anesthesia provider. Consent for anesthesia requires an informed patient, and "coercion" by the anesthesiologist should not be used to obtain consent for an anesthetic technique that the patient does not desire. On reaching this decision, the anesthesiologist should document the relevant findings, American Society of Anesthesiologists (ASA) classification, anesthetic technique, and a statement noting that the patient understands and accepts the plan and accompanying risks.

General Anesthetic

General anesthesia may be initiated by the administration of intravenous drugs or inhalation of a volatile anesthetic with or without nitrous oxide. The usual handwritten anesthetic record is progressively being replaced by electronic anesthetic records, which sometimes are connected to a hospital computer system. Paperless, computerized medical records are being adopted by increasing numbers of medical centers.[6]

INTRAVENOUS INDUCTION OF ANESTHESIA

General anesthesia is usually induced in adult patients by the intravenous administration of an anesthetic (propofol, thiopental, or etomidate) that produces rapid onset of unconsciousness (see Chapter 9). Then, ventilation can be sustained via a face mask or a laryngeal mask airway (LMA) may be inserted or a neuromuscular blocking drug may be given intravenously to facilitate direct laryngoscopy before tracheal intubation (see Chapter 16). Although a face mask and LMA are important components of airway management, they do present challenges. For example, in some patients with anatomically difficult oral cavities (e.g., edentulous patients), a leak around the mouth or nose can occur.[7] Also the LMA should not have cuff pressure exceeding 44 mm Hg.[8] The intravenous injection of an anesthetic to produce unconsciousness followed immediately by a neuromuscular blocking drug that produces a rapid onset of skeletal muscle paralysis (succinylcholine, rocuronium) is referred to as "rapid-sequence" induction of anesthesia (see later discussion for details). Frequently, the patient is breathing oxygen (3 to 5 L/min) via a face mask (preoxygenation) before rapid-sequence induction of anesthesia. Administration of oxygen (preoxygenation) is intended to replace nitrogen (denitrogenation) in the patient's functional residual capacity (about 2500 mL of 21% oxygen) with oxygen. This practice should increase the margin of safety during periods of upper airway obstruction or apnea that may accompany induction of anesthesia. In healthy awake patients, the increase in arterial hemoglobin oxygen saturation achieved with eight vital capacity breaths of 100% oxygen over a period of 60 seconds is similar to that achieved by breathing 100% oxygen for 3 minutes at normal tidal volumes.[9] Four vital capacity breaths over a 30-second period also increases arterial oxygenation, but the time until hemoglobin desaturation is shorter than in patients breathing oxygen for 3 minutes or taking eight deep breaths.

Rapid-Sequence Induction of Anesthesia[10]

Before inducing anesthesia of any type, the equipment must be checked to ascertain lack of any defects.[11,12] This evaluation especially includes use of equipment that facilitates effective airway management (also see Chapter 16).[13]

A typical rapid-sequence induction of anesthesia includes preoxygenation and subsequently cricoid pressure may be applied by an assistant just before the onset of drug-induced unconsciousness and loss of protective upper airway reflexes. An opioid (e.g., fentanyl, 1 to 2 µg/kg IV or its equivalent) is often given 1 to 3 minutes before administration of a drug to induce anesthesia. The opioid is intended to blunt the subsequent hypertensive and heart rate responses to direct laryngoscopy and tracheal intubation and also to initiate possible preemptive analgesia. Because remifentanil and alfentanil undergo more rapid blood-brain equilibration than fentanyl these opioids may be more reliable in blunting the sympathetic nervous system responses evoked by direct laryngoscopy and tracheal intubation.[7]

With the onset of unconsciousness, the patient's head is positioned to provide optimal patency of the upper airway. Positive-pressure inflation of the patient's lungs with oxygen is then instituted. Direct laryngoscopy for tracheal intubation is initiated only after the onset of skeletal muscle paralysis (often verified by a peripheral nerve stimulator), which is typically 45 to 120 seconds after the intravenous administration of sucinylcholine, 1.0 to 1.5 mg/kg, or rocuronium, 0.6 to 1.2 mg/kg. Rocuronium, 0.6 mg/kg, has slower onset time than succinylcholine. Increasing the dose of rocuronium to 1.0 to 1.2 mg/kg creates an onset time similar to that of succinylcholine (see Chapter 12). All other muscle relaxants have an onset time of 3 to 5 minutes. With experienced anesthesia providers, use of neuromuscular blocking drugs (e.g., succinylcholine or rocuronium) actually increases the safety of endotracheal intubation.[14] Yet once again, use of neuromuscular blocking drugs without adequate doses of anesthetic drugs is a prime cause of "awareness" during anesthesia (see Chapter 46).[15]

Table 14-2 Evidence of a Patent Upper Airway after Induction of Anesthesia
■ The upper part of the chest expands and the reservoir bag partially empties during inspiration.
■ The reservoir bag refills during exhalation.
■ Capnography reveals cyclic waveforms decreasing to zero during inhalation and a plateau peak (>20 mm Hg) during exhalation.
■ The pulse oximeter continues to read >95%.
■ Bilateral breath sounds are present.

Monitoring of arterial hemoglobin oxygen saturation with a pulse oximeter provides early warning should arterial oxygen desaturation occur during the period of apnea required for tracheal intubation. Proper placement of the tube in the trachea must be confirmed after direct laryngoscopy (Table 14-2). After tracheal intubation, a gastric tube may be inserted through the mouth to decompress the stomach and remove any easily accessible fluid. This orogastric tube should be removed at the conclusion of anesthesia. When gastric suction is needed postoperatively, normally the tube should be inserted through the nares rather than the mouth.

INHALED INDUCTION OF ANESTHESIA

An alternative to rapid-sequence induction of anesthesia is the inhalation of sevoflurane (nonpungent) with or without nitrous oxide.[16] Prior administration of a "sleep dose" of an anesthetic (e.g., propofol) may be used if an intravenous catheter is in place. Desflurane produces a rapid onset of effect but is not often selected for an inhaled induction of anesthesia because of its airway irritant effects. Inhaled or "mask induction" of anesthesia is most often selected for pediatric patients when prior insertion of a venous catheter is not practical (see Chapter 34). Sevoflurane may also be useful when difficult airway management is anticipated because of the absence of salivation and preservation of spontaneous breathing. The traditional "awake look" in a patient with a suspected difficult airway, which included titration of intravenous anesthetics until the patient tolerated direct laryngoscopy, has been modified to include spontaneous ventilation of high concentrations of sevoflurane until laryngoscopic evaluation is possible.

Characteristics of Inhaled Induction of Anesthesia with Sevoflurane

Loss of consciousness typically occurs within about 1 minute when breathing 8% sevoflurane. Insertion of a LMA can usually be achieved within 2 minutes after administering 7% sevoflurane via a face mask. The addition of nitrous oxide to the inspired gas mixture usually does not improve the induction of anesthesia sequence. Prior administration of benzodiazepines may facilitate an inhaled induction of anesthesia, whereas opioids may complicate this technique by increasing the likelihood of apnea.[10]

A technique for induction of anesthesia with sevoflurane includes priming the circuit (emptying the reservoir bag and opening the adjustable pressure-limiting ["popoff"] valve), dialing the vaporizer setting to 8% while using a fresh gas flow of 8 L/min, and maintaining this flow for 60 seconds before applying the face mask to the patient. At this point a single breath from end-expiratory volume to maximum inspiration followed by deep breathing typically produces loss of consciousness in 1 minute.

After an inhaled induction of anesthesia, a depolarizing or nondepolarizing neuromuscular blocking drug is administered intravenously to provide the skeletal muscle relaxation needed to facilitate direct laryngoscopy for tracheal intubation. If endotracheal intubation is not accomplished, anesthesia can be maintained by inhalation via a facemask or LMA.

MAINTENANCE OF ANESTHESIA

The objectives during maintenance of general anesthesia are amnesia, analgesia, skeletal muscle relaxation, and control of the sympathetic nervous system responses evoked by noxious stimulation. These objectives are achieved most often by the use of a combination of drugs that may include inhaled or intravenously administered drugs (or both), with or without neuromuscular blocking drugs. Each drug selected should be administered on the basis of a specific goal that is relevant to that drug's known pharmacologic effects at therapeutic doses. For example, it is not logical to administer high concentrations of volatile anesthetics to produce skeletal muscle relaxation when neuromuscular blocking drugs are specific for achieving this goal. Likewise, it is not acceptable to obscure skeletal muscle movement by administering excessive amounts of neuromuscular blocking drugs because of insufficient doses of anesthetics. The selective use of drugs for their specific pharmacologic effects permits the anesthesia provider to tailor the anesthetic to the patient's medical condition and any unique needs introduced by the surgery.

Despite its lack of potency, nitrous oxide is the most frequently administered inhaled anesthetic. Typically, nitrous oxide (50% to 70% inhaled concentration) is administered in combination with a volatile anesthetic or opioid, or both. The partial pressure of an inhaled anesthetic that produces its pharmacologic effect should be understood. For example, 60% inhaled nitrous oxide administered at sea level exerts a partial pressure of 456 mm Hg (60% of the total barometric pressure of 760 mm Hg). The same inhaled concentration of nitrous oxide (or a volatile anesthetic) administered at an altitude where the barometric pressure is less than 760 mm Hg exerts a decreased pharmacologic effect because the partial pressure of the anesthetic that can be achieved in the brain is lower.

Volatile anesthetics have the advantage of high potency, and their "dose" easily altered and titrated to produce a desired response, including skeletal muscle relaxation and prompt awakening. The excessive sympathetic nervous system responses evoked by noxious stimulation are predictably attenuated by volatile anesthetics. Yet, dose-dependent cardiac depression is a major disadvantage of volatile anesthetics (see Chapter 8). Indeed, a volatile anesthetic is seldom administered alone but usually in combination with nitrous oxide. Substitution of nitrous oxide for a portion of the dose of the volatile anesthetic allows a decrease in the delivered concentration of the volatile anesthetic, resulting in less cardiac depression despite the same total dose of anesthetic. Volatile anesthetics may provide an inadequate analgesic effect and be associated with postoperative hepatic dysfunction.

In certain instances, neuromuscular blocking drugs can be given to ensure lack of patient movement and permit a decrease in the delivered concentration of volatile anesthetics. This use of neuromuscular blocking drugs, however, must be in the presence of an adequate dose of anesthetic. In this regard, intraoperative awareness is a recognized risk of minimal concentrations or doses of anesthetic drugs ("light anesthesia"), especially when patient movements are obscured by drug-induced skeletal muscle paralysis (also see Chapter 46).

Opioids that generally do not depress the cardiovascular system are combined most often with nitrous oxide (see Chapter 10). In patients with normal left ventricular function, however, the lack of opioid-induced cardiovascular depression and the absence of attenuation of sympathetic nervous system reflexes may be manifested as systemic hypertension. When this occurs, the addition of low concentrations of a volatile anesthetic is often effective in returning arterial blood pressure to an acceptable level. Neuromuscular blocking drugs are often necessary, even in the absence of the need for skeletal muscle relaxation, because adequate doses of opioids administered in the presence of nitrous oxide are unlikely to prevent patient movement in response to painful stimulation. Another disadvantage of intravenously administered anesthetics versus inhaled anesthetics is an inability to accurately titrate and maintain a therapeutic concentration of the injected anesthetic. This disadvantage can be offset to some extent by continuous intravenous infusion of the intravenous anesthetic at a rate previously determined in other patients to be associated with therapeutic concentrations in blood. Brain function monitoring (bispectral index, entropy, auditory evoked potentials) may be helpful in titrating the dose of inhaled or injected anesthetic drugs to produce the desired degree of central nervous system depression (see Chapter 20).

Regional Anesthetic

A neuraxial regional anesthetic (spinal, epidural, caudal) is selected when maintenance of consciousness during surgery is desirable (see Chapter 17). Spinal anesthesia and epidural anesthesia each have advantages and disadvantages that may make one or the other technique better suited to a specific patient or surgical procedure. Spinal anesthesia (1) takes less time to perform, (2) produces a more rapid onset of better-quality sensory and motor anesthesia, and (3) is associated with less pain during surgery. Unlike epidural anesthesia, a continuous spinal technique is rarely used because of postspinal headache and concern about the proper maintenance of the catheter in the subarachnoid space.

The principal advantages of epidural anesthesia are (1) a lower risk for post–dural puncture headache, (2) less systemic hypotension if epinephrine is not added to the local anesthetic solution, (3) the ability to prolong or extend the anesthesia through an indwelling epidural catheter, and (4) the option of using the epidural catheter to provide postoperative analgesia. Skeletal muscle relaxation and contraction of the gastrointestinal tract are also produced by a regional anesthetic.

Patients may have preconceived and erroneous conceptions about regional anesthesia that will require the anesthesiologist to reassure them regarding the safety of this technique. The only absolute contraindication to spinal or epidural anesthesia is when a patient wishes another form of anesthesia. Certain preexisting conditions increase the relative risk of these techniques, and the anesthesia provider must balance the perceived benefits of this technique before proceeding (Table 14-3). Disadvantages of this anesthetic technique include the occasional failure to produce sensory levels of anesthesia that are adequate for the surgical stimulus and hypotension that may accompany the peripheral sympathetic nervous system blockade produced by the regional anesthetic, particularly in the presence of hypovolemia.

A regional anesthetic technique is most often selected for surgery that involves the lower part of the abdomen or the lower extremities in which the level of sensory anesthesia required is associated with minimal sympathetic nervous system blockade.[17,18] This should not, however, imply that a general anesthetic is an unacceptable technique for similar types of surgery.

For procedures lasting between 20 and 90 minutes, intravenous regional anesthesia (IVRA, or Bier block)

may be used.[2] IVRA provides reliable anesthesia for both the upper and lower extremities, although the latter may be more problematic because of the size of the lower extremities in adults. After the application of a tourniquet and exsanguination of the extremity, lidocaine (0.5%) is commonly administered into a catheter previously placed in the involved extremity. Double tourniquets (distal cuff inflated over the area where local anesthetic has infiltrated with time) help ameliorate tourniquet pain. Intravenous analgesics such as ketorolac may be useful for treatment of patient discomfort during IVRA. IVRA is more cost-effective than general anesthesia or brachial plexus block for outpatient hand surgery.

Peripheral Nerve Block

A peripheral nerve block is most appropriate as a technique of anesthesia for superficial operations on the extremities (see Chapter 18). Advantages of peripheral nerve blocks include maintenance of consciousness and the continued presence of protective upper airway reflexes. The isolated anesthetic effect produced by a peripheral nerve block is particularly attractive in patients with chronic pulmonary disease, severe cardiac impairment, or inadequate renal function. For example, insertion of a vascular shunt in the upper extremity for hemodialysis in a patient who may have associated pulmonary and cardiac disease is often accomplished with anesthesia provided by a peripheral nerve block of the brachial plexus. Likewise, avoidance of the need for neuromuscular blocking drugs in this type of patient circumvents the possible prolonged effect produced by these drugs in the absence of renal function.

A disadvantage of peripheral nerve block as an anesthetic technique is the unpredictable attainment of adequate sensory and motor anesthesia for performance of the surgery. The success rate of a peripheral nerve block is often related to the frequency with which the anesthesia provider uses this anesthetic technique. Patients must be cooperative for a peripheral nerve block to be effective. For example, acutely intoxicated and agitated patients are not ideal candidates for a peripheral nerve block. The use of ultrasound guidance in regional anesthesia has become a routine technique and has increased its use for perioperative care.[19]

Monitored Anesthesia Care

MAC is defined by the American Society of Anesthesiologists (ASA) as a procedure in which an anesthetic provider is requested or required to provide anesthetic services, which include preoperative evaluation, care during the procedure, and management after the procedure.[20,21] This responsibility includes (1) diagnosis and treatment of clinical problems during the procedure; (2) support of vital functions; (3) administration of sedatives,

Table 14-3 Conditions That May Increase the Risk Associated with Spinal or Epidural Anesthesia
Hypovolemia
Increased intracranial pressure
Coagulopathy (thrombocytopenia)
Sepsis
Infection at the cutaneous puncture site
Preexisting neurologic disease (e.g., multiple sclerosis)

analgesics, hypnotics, anesthetic drugs, or other medications as necessary for patient safety; (4) psychological support and physical comfort; and (5) provision of other services as needed to complete the procedure safely. The care of a patient undergoing MAC is held to the same standard as any other anesthetic technique, given that the level of sedation may progress rapidly, go beyond consciousness, and lead to an "unplanned" general anesthetic (specifically defined by the ASA as any instance in which the patient loses consciousness as defined by the ability to respond purposefully). When this occurs, extra care may be needed in monitoring to prevent airway mishaps such as upper airway obstruction and arterial hypoxemia, as reflected by the pulse oximeter reading.

While caring for a patient under MAC, the total dose of local anesthetic administered by the surgeon and the risk for local anesthetic toxicity must be monitored (see Chapter 11). In addition to monitoring the patient, supplemental oxygen (may not be necessary if pulse oximeter readings are acceptable while breathing room air), typically by nasal cannula, should be given. In addition to oxygen, anesthetic drugs can be given intravenously to provide anxiolysis (midazolam), sedation (propofol), and analgesia (remifentanil, ketorolac, ketamine). Depending on the patient and the procedure, fulfilling one or all of these goals (anxiolysis, sedation, and analgesia for arthroscopic surgery) may be needed. Opioid administration during MAC may be useful but also requires careful monitoring of oxygenation and ventilation. Inhaled anesthetics (nitrous oxide, sevoflurane) administered in concentrations below the threshold of loss of consciousness may be useful during surgical infiltration of local anesthetic solutions, especially for brief periods while patients are not tolerating the procedure because of agitation or inadequate analgesia. MAC may facilitate avoidance of side effects (sympatholysis, respiratory depression, delayed emergence) and may be particularly cost effective in comparison to general or regional anesthetics in the ambulatory care setting.

PREPARATION FOR ANESTHESIA

After the preoperative medication has been given, regional anesthesia may be administered in the preoperative area. With all other anesthetic techniques, the patient will be transported to the operating room for induction of anesthesia (Table 14-4). On arrival in the operating room, the patient is identified and the planned surgery reconfirmed. In fact, all of the checks performed in the preoperative area should be reconfirmed in the operating room. The patient's medical record, including the nurse's notes, should be consulted by the anesthesia provider to learn of any unexpected changes in the patient's medical condition, vital signs, or body temperature and to determine that the preoperative medication and, if indicated,

Table 14-4 Routine Preparation before Induction of Anesthesia Independent of the Anesthetic Technique Selected

Anesthesia Machine (see Table 15-9)
- Attach an anesthetic breathing system with a properly sized face mask
- Occlude the patient end of the anesthetic breathing system and fill with oxygen from the anesthesia machine ("flush valve") (applying manual pressure to the distended reservoir bag checks for leaks in the anesthetic breathing system and confirms the ability to provide positive-pressure ventilation of the patient's lungs with oxygen)
- Check the anesthetic breathing system valves
- Calibrate the oxygen analyzer with air and oxygen and set alarm limits
- Check the carbon dioxide absorbent for color change
- Check the liquid level of vaporizers
- Confirm proper function of the mechanical ventilator
- Confirm the availability and function of wall suction
- Check the final position of all flowmeter, vaporizer, and monitor (visual and audible alarm) settings

Monitors
- Blood pressure
- Pulse oximetry
- Electrocardiography
- Capnography

Drugs
- Local anesthetic (lidocaine)
- Induction drug (propofol, thiopental, etomidate)
- Opioid (fentanyl, sufentanil, alfentanil, remifentanil)
- Benzodiazepine (midazolam, diazepam)
- Anticholinergic (atropine, glycopyrrolate)
- Sympathomimetic (ephedrine, phenylephrine)
- Succinylcholine
- Nondepolarizing neuromuscular blocking drug (rocuronium, vecuronium, cisatracurium, pancuronium)
- Anticholinesterase (neostigmine, edrophonium)
- Opioid antagonist
- Benzodiazepine antagonist
- Catecholamine to treat an allergic reaction (epinephrine)

Equipment
- Intravenous solution and connecting tubing
- Catheter for vascular cannulation
- Suction catheter
- Oral and/or nasal airway
- Laryngeal mask airway
- Tracheal tube
- Nasogastric tube
- Temperature probe

prophylactic antibiotics have been administered. Likewise, any laboratory data that have become available since the preoperative visit should be reviewed.

Initial preparation for anesthesia, regardless of the technique of anesthesia selected, usually begins with insertion of a catheter in a peripheral vein and application of a blood pressure cuff. This initial preparation may be accomplished in a holding area or in the operating room. The use of separate rooms (anesthetic induction rooms) distinct from the operating room for induction of anesthesia is not recommended by some because of the questionable safety of routinely moving anesthetized patients with the necessary attached equipment from one area to another. An exception to this recommendation may be the performance of peripheral nerve blocks or epidural anesthesia in a holding or preoperative area so that the block is in place when the operating room becomes available. Likewise, an epidural catheter for postoperative pain management may be placed in the holding area before transport of the patient to the operating room and induction of general anesthesia. Monitors such as the pulse oximeter, electrocardiogram, and peripheral nerve stimulator are also applied while the patient is still awake. Immediately before induction of anesthesia, baseline vital signs (systemic blood pressure, heart rate, cardiac rhythm, arterial hemoglobin oxygen saturation, breathing rate) and the corresponding time are recorded.

Regardless of the anesthetic technique selected, the provider should verify that the anesthesia machine is present and functional (in certain circumstances such as anesthesia for cardioversion, a breathing circuit may suffice) and that specific drugs and equipment are always immediately available (see Table 14-4), including suctioning capability, adequate monitoring (systemic blood pressure, electrocardiography, pulse oximetry, capnography, body temperature), airway equipment (appropriately sized face mask, oral airway, nasal airway, LMA, laryngoscope with appropriate functional blades), materials for venous access, and drugs appropriate for emergency intravenous induction and resuscitation (induction drugs, neuromuscular blocking drugs, vasopressors, including ephedrine and phenylephrine).

Prime emphasis of this chapter is on induction and maintenance of anesthesia. Induction of anesthesia and

especially airway management has received considerable attention for at least 40 years. Examination of multiple reports reflects the increasing safety to patients and skills of anesthesia providers. The Institute of Medicine has complimented anesthesiology for its attention to safety (see Chapter 47). However, termination of anesthesia and transport of the patient to the postanesthetic care unit (see Chapter 39) can be associated with adverse events and also needs the same intense attention by the anesthesia provider as given during the induction of anesthesia.[22]

PHARMACOECONOMICS

The desire for cost containment often leads to recommendations that low-cost drugs (antiemetics, intravenous drugs to induce anesthesia, volatile anesthetics, neuromuscular blocking drugs) be used in preference to newer, but more expensive, drugs with desirable pharmacologic profiles.[23] The ultimate goal must be to obtain the best results (low toxicity, rapid awakening, absence of nausea and vomiting) at the most practical cost A useful method to decrease the cost of volatile anesthetics is the use of low fresh gas flow (2 L/min) during maintenance of anesthesia.

QUESTIONS OF THE DAY

1. A patient requires a thorough neurologic evaluation immediately after surgery. How does this influence the choice of anesthetic technique?
2. What are the potential advantages of inhaled induction of anesthesia compared to intravenous induction?
3. What are the responsibilities of the anesthesia provider before, during, and after monitored anesthesia care (MAC)?

ACKNOWLEDGMENT

The editors and publisher would like to thank Dr. Donald Taylor for contributing a chapter on this topic to the prior edition of this work. It has served as the foundation for the current chapter.

REFERENCES

1. Practice Advisory for Preoperative Evaluation: A report by the American Society of Anesthesiologists Task Force on Preanesthetic Evaluation, *Anesthesiology* 96:485, 2002.
2. Chan V, Peng P, Kaszas Z, et al: A comparative study of general anesthesia, intravenous regional anesthesia, and axillary block for outpatient hand surgery: Clinical outcome and cost analysis, *Anesth Analg* 93:1181–1184, 2001.
3. Arbous M, Grobbee D, van Kleef J, et al: Mortality associated with anaesthesia: A qualitative analysis to identify risk factors, *Anaesthesia* 56:1141–1153, 2001.
4. Rashiq S, Bray P: Relative value to surgical patients and anesthesia providers of selected anesthesia related outcomes, *BMC Med Inform Decis Mak* 3:3, 2003.
5. Macario A, Weinger M, Carney S, et al: Which clinical anesthesia outcomes are important to avoid? The perspective of patients, *Anesth Analg* 89:652–658, 1999.

6. Sittig DF, Classen DC: Safe electronic health record use requires a comprehensive monitoring and evaluation framework, *JAMA* 303:450–451, 2010.

7. Racine SX, Solis A, Hamou NA, et al: Face mask ventilation in edentulous patients: A comparison of mandibular groove and lower lip placement, *Anesthesiology* 112:1190–1193, 2010.

8. Seet E, Yousaf F, Gupta S, et al: Use of manometry for laryngeal mask airway reduces postoperative pharyngolaryngeal adverse events: a prospective, randomized trial, *Anesthesiology* 112:652–657, 2010.

9. Brake AS, Tara SK, Aoudad MT, et al: Preoxygenation: Comparison of maximal breathing and tidal volume breathing techniques, *Anesthesiology* 91:612–616, 1999.

10. El-Orbany M, Connolly LA: Rapid sequence induction and intubation: Current controversy, *Anesth Analg* 110:1318–1325, 2010.

11. Mudumbai SC, Fanning R, Howard SK, et al: Use of medical simulation to explore equipment failures and human-machine interactions in anesthesia machine pipeline supply crossover, *Anesth Analg* 110:1292–1296, 2010.

12. Murphy RS, Wilcox SJ: The link between intravenous multiple pump flow errors and infusion system mechanical compliance, *Anesth Analg* 110:1297–1302, 2010.

13. Amour J, Le Manach YL, Borel M, et al: Comparison of single-use and reusable metal laryngoscope blades for orotracheal intuation during rapid sequence induction of anesthesia: A multicenter cluster randomized study, *Anesthesiology* 112:325–332, 2010.

14. Lundstrom LH, Moller AM, Rosenstock C, et al: Avoidance of neuromuscular blocking agents may increase the risk of difficult tracheal intubation: A cohort study of 103,812 consecutive adult patients recorded in the Danish Anaesthesia Database, *Br J Anaesth* 103:283–290, 2009.

15. Errando CL, Sigl JC, Robles M, et al: Awareness with recall during general anaesthesia: A prospecttive observational evaluation of 4001 patients, *Br J Anaesth* 101:178–185, 2008.

16. Doi M, Ikeda K: Airway irritation produced by volatile anaesthetics during brief inhalation: Comparison of halothane, enflurane, isoflurane and sevoflurane, *Can J Anaesth* 40:122–128, 1993.

17. Rodgers A, Walker N, Schug S, et al: Reduction of postoperative morbidity and mortality with epidural or spinal anesthesia: Results from overview of randomized trials, *BMJ* 321:1493–1497, 2000.

18. Horlocker TT, Wedel DJ, Benzon H, et al: Regional anesthesia in the anticoagulated patient: Defining the risks, *Reg Anesth Pain Med* 28:172–197, 2003.

19. Marhofer P, Harrop-Griffiths W, Willschke H, et al: Fifteen years of ultrasound guidance in regional anaesthesia: Part 2—Recent developments in block techniques, *Br J Anaesth* 104:673–683, 2010.

20. Position on Monitored Anesthesia Care: *ASA House of Delegates,* amended October 2005. www.ashq.org.

21. Ghisi D, Aanelli A, Tosi M, et al: Monitored anesthesia care, *Minerva Anestesiol* 71:533–538, 2005.

22. Mhyre JM, Riesner MN, Polley LS, et al: A series of anesthesia-related maternal deaths in Michigan 1985-2003, *Anesthesiology* 106:1096–1104, 2007.

23. Eger EI, White PF, Bogetz MS: Clinical and economic factors important to anaesthetic choice for day-case surgery, *Pharmacoeconomics* 17:245–262, 2000.

III

15 ANESTHESIA DELIVERY SYSTEMS

Patricia Roth

An anesthesia delivery system consists of the anesthesia workstation (anesthesia machine) and anesthetic breathing system (circuit), which permit delivery of known concentrations of inhaled anesthetics and oxygen to the patient, as well as removal of the patient's carbon dioxide. Carbon dioxide can be removed either by washout (delivered gas flow greater than 5 L/min from the anesthesia machine) or by chemical neutralization.

ANESTHESIA WORKSTATION

The anesthesia machine has evolved from a simple pneumatic device to a complex integrated computer-controlled multicomponent workstation (Figs. 15-1 and 15-2).[1] The components within the anesthesia workstation function in harmony to deliver known concentrations of inhaled anesthetics to the patient. The multiple components of the anesthesia workstation include what was previously recognized as the anesthesia machine (the pressure-regulating and gas-mixing components), vaporizers, anesthesia breathing circuit, ventilator, scavenging system, and respiratory and physiologic monitoring systems (electrocardiogram, arterial blood pressure, temperature, pulse oximeter, and inhaled and exhaled concentrations of oxygen, carbon dioxide, anesthetic gases, and vapors) (Table 15-1).[1] Alarm systems to signal apnea or disconnection of the anesthetic breathing system from the patient are included. The alarms present on the pulse oximeter and capnograph must be audible to the anesthesiologist. Most anesthesia machines are powered by both electric and pneumatic power.

The anesthesia workstation ultimately provides delivery of medical gases and the vapors of volatile anesthetics at known concentrations to the common gas outlet. These gases enter the anesthetic breathing system to be delivered to the patient by spontaneous or

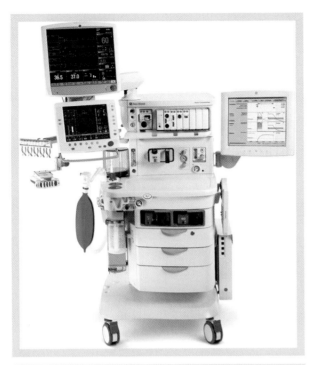

Figure 15-1 GE Aisys Anesthesia Delivery System.

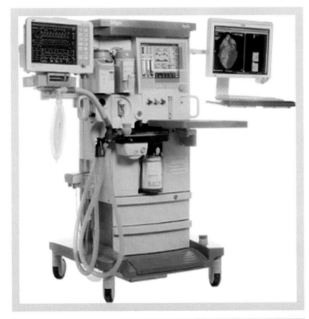

Figure 15-2 Dräger Apollo Anesthesia Workstation.

Table 15-1 Common Features of Anesthesia Machines
Inlet of hospital pipeline for compressed gases (oxygen, nitrous oxide, and air)
Inlet of compressed gas cylinders
Pressure regulators to reduce pipeline and cylinder pressure to safe and consistent levels
Fail-safe device
Flowmeters to control the amount of gases delivered to the breathing limb
Vaporizers for adding volatile anesthetic gas to the carrier gas
Common gas line through which compressed gases mixed with a volatile agent enter the breathing limb
Breathing limb, including an oxygen analyzer, inspiratory one-way valve, circle system, gas sampling line, spirometer to measure the respiratory rate and volume, expiratory one-way valve, adjustable pressure-limiting valve, carbon dioxide absorbent, reservoir bag, mechanical ventilator, and scavenging system

Fail-Safe Valve

Anesthesia machines are equipped with a fail-safe valve designed to prevent the delivery of hypoxic gas mixtures from the machine in the event of failure of the oxygen supply. This valve shuts off or proportionally decreases the flow of all gases when the pressure in the oxygen delivery line decreases to less than 30 psi. This safety measure will protect against unrecognized exhaustion of oxygen delivery from a cylinder attached to the anesthesia machine or from a central source. This valve, however, does not prevent the delivery of 100% nitrous oxide when the oxygen flow is zero but gas pressure in the circuit of the anesthesia machine is maintained. In this situation, an oxygen analyzer is necessary to detect the delivery of a hypoxic gas mixture. Far superior to the fail-safe valve or an oxygen analyzer is the continuous presence of a vigilant anesthesiologist.

Compressed Gases

Gases used in the administration of anesthesia (oxygen, nitrous oxide, air) are most often delivered to the anesthesia machine from a central supply source located in the hospital (Fig. 15-3).[2] Hospital-supplied gases enter the operating room from a central source through pipelines to color-coded wall outlets (green for oxygen, blue for nitrous oxide, and yellow for air). Color-coded pressure hoses are connected to the wall outlet by gas-specific diameter fittings that are not interchangeable (diameter index safety system [DISS], which is designed to prevent misconnections of pipeline gases). Oxygen or air from a central supply source may also be used to pneumatically drive the ventilator on the anesthesia machine.

mechanical ventilation. Exhaled gases are either returned to the patient after passing through a CO_2 absorbent or scavenged from the breathing system to the waste gas removal limb.

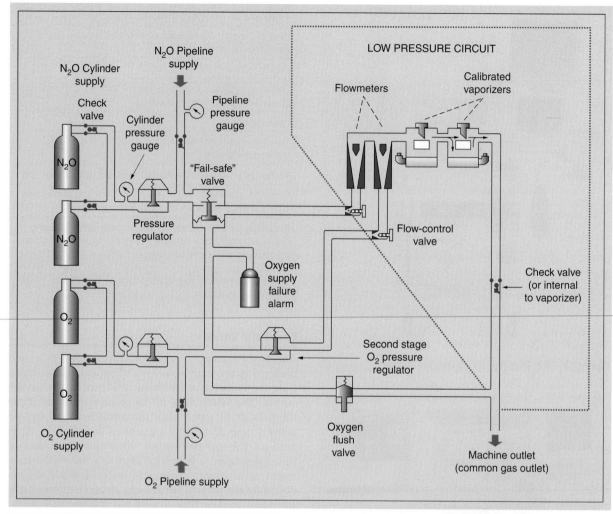

Figure 15-3 Schematic diagram of the internal circuitry of an anesthesia machine. Oxygen and nitrous oxide enter the anesthesia machine through a central supply line (most common); alternatively (infrequently), they are provided from gas cylinders attached to pin-indexed yokes on the machine. Check valves prevent transfilling of gas cylinders or flow of gas from cylinders into the central supply line. Pressure regulators decrease pressure in the tubing from the gas cylinders to about 50 psi. The fail-safe valve prevents flow of nitrous oxide if the pressure in the oxygen supply circuit decreases to less than 30 psi. Needle valves control gas flow to rotameters (flowmeters). Agent-specific vaporizers provide a reliable means to deliver preselected concentrations of a volatile anesthetic. An interlock system allows only one vaporizer to be in the "on" (delivery) setting at a time. After mixing in the manifold of the anesthesia machine, the total fresh gas flow enters the common outlet for delivery to the patient through the anesthetic breathing system (circuit). (Adapted from Check-Out. A Guide for Preoperative Inspection of an Anesthetic Machine. Park Ridge, IL, American Society of Anesthesiologists, 1987, pp 1-14, used with permission.)

Gas enters the anesthesia machine through pipeline inlet connections that are gas specific (threaded noninterchangeable connections) to minimize the possibility of a misconnection. The gas must be delivered from the central supply source at an appropriate pressure (about 50 psi) for the flowmeters on the anesthesia machine to function properly.

Anesthesia machines are also equipped with cylinders of oxygen and nitrous oxide for use should the central gas supply fail (see Fig. 15-3).[2] Color-coded cylinders are attached to the anesthesia machine by a hanger yoke assembly, which consists of two metal pins that correspond to holes in the valve casing of the gas cylinder (pin indexed safety system [PISS]) (Table 15-2). This design makes it impossible to attach an oxygen cylinder to any yoke on the anesthesia machine other than that designed for oxygen. Otherwise, a cylinder containing nitrous oxide could be attached to the oxygen yoke, which would result in the delivery of nitrous oxide when the oxygen flowmeter was activated. Color-coded pressure

Table 15-2 Characteristics of Compressed Gases Stored in E Size Cylinders Attached to the Anesthesia Machine

Characteristic	Oxygen	Nitrous Oxide	Carbon Dioxide	Air
Cylinder color	Green*	Blue	Gray	Yellow*
Physical state in cylinder	Gas	Liquid and gas	Liquid and gas	Gas
Cylinder contents (L)	625	1590	1590	625
Cylinder weight empty (kg)	5.90	5.90	5.90	5.90
Cylinder weight full (kg)	6.76	8.80	8.90	
Cylinder pressure full (psi)	2000	750	838	1800

*The World Health Organization specifies that cylinders containing oxygen for medical use be painted white, but manufacturers in the United States use green. Likewise, the international color for air is white and black, whereas cylinders in the United States are color-coded yellow.

gauges (green for oxygen, blue for nitrous oxide) on the anesthesia machine indicate the pressure of the gas in the corresponding gas cylinder (see Table 15-2).

CALCULATION OF CYLINDER CONTENTS

The pressure in an oxygen cylinder is directly proportional to the volume of oxygen in the cylinder. For example, a full E size oxygen cylinder contains about 625 L of oxygen at a pressure of 2000 psi and half this volume when the pressure is 1000 psi. Therefore, how long a given flow rate of oxygen can be maintained before the cylinder is empty can be calculated. In contrast to oxygen, the pressure gauge for nitrous oxide does not indicate the amount of gas remaining in the cylinder because the pressure in the gas cylinder remains at 750 psi as long as any liquid nitrous oxide is present. When nitrous oxide leaves the cylinder as a vapor, additional liquid is vaporized to maintain an unchanging pressure in the cylinder. After all the liquid nitrous oxide is vaporized, the pressure begins to decrease, and it can be assumed that about 75% of the contents of the gas cylinder have been exhausted. Because a full nitrous oxide cylinder (E size) contains about 1590 L, approximately 400 L of nitrous oxide remains when the pressure gauge begins to decrease from its previously constant value of 750 psi. Vaporization of a liquefied gas (nitrous oxide), as well as expansion of a compressed gas (oxygen), absorbs heat, which is extracted from the metal cylinder and the surrounding atmosphere. For this reason, atmospheric water vapor often accumulates as frost on gas cylinders and in valves, particularly during high gas flow from these tanks. Internal icing does not occur because compressed gases are free of water vapor.

Flowmeters

Flowmeters on the anesthesia machine precisely control and measure gas flow to the common gas inlet (see Fig. 15-3).[2] Measurement of the flow of gases is based

on the principle that flow past a resistance is proportional to pressure. Typically, gas flow enters the bottom of a vertically positioned and tapered (the cross-sectional area increases upward from site of gas entry) glass flow tube. Gas flow into the flowmeter tube raises a bobbin or ball-shaped float. The float comes to rest when gravity is balanced by the decrease in pressure caused by the float. The upper end of the bobbin or the equator of the ball indicates the gas flow in milliliters or liters per minute. Proportionality between pressure and flow is determined by the shape of the tube (resistance) and the physical properties (density and viscosity) of the gas. The flowmeters are initially calibrated for the indicated gas at the factory. Because few gases have the same density and viscosity, flowmeters are not interchangeable with other gases. The scale accompanying an oxygen flowmeter is green, whereas the scale for the nitrous oxide flowmeter is blue.

Gas flow exits the flowmeters and passes into a manifold (mixing chamber) located at the top of the flowmeters (see Fig. 15-3).[2] The oxygen flowmeter should be the last in the sequence of flowmeters, and thus oxygen should be the last gas added to the manifold. This arrangement reduces the possibility that leaks in the apparatus proximal to oxygen inflow can diminish the delivered oxygen concentration, whereas leaks distal to that point result in loss of volume without a qualitative change in the mixture. Nevertheless, an oxygen flowmeter tube leak can produce a hypoxic mixture regardless of the flowmeter tube arrangement (Fig. 15-4).[3] Indeed, flowmeter tube leaks are a hazard reflecting the fragile construction of this component of the anesthesia machine. Subtle cracks may be overlooked and result in errors in delivered flow.

Gases mix in the manifold and flow to an outlet port on the anesthesia machine, where they are directed into either a vaporizer or an anesthetic breathing system (see Fig. 15-3).[2] For emergency purposes, provision is made for delivery of a large volume of oxygen (35 to 75 L/min) to the outlet port through an oxygen flush valve

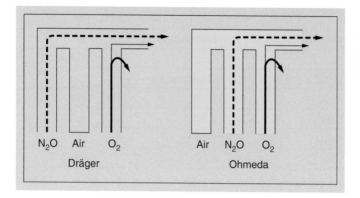

Figure 15-4 Oxygen flow tube leak. An oxygen flow tube leak can produce a hypoxic mixture regardless of the flow tube arrangement. (From Brockwell RC. Inhaled anesthetic delivery systems. In Miller RD [ed]. Miller's Anesthesia, 7th ed. Philadelphia, Churchill Livingstone, 2010, p 680, used with permission.)

that bypasses the flowmeters and manifold. The oxygen flush valve allows direct communication between the oxygen high-pressure circuit and the low-pressure circuit (see Fig. 15-3).[2] Activation of the oxygen flush valve during a mechanically delivered inspiration from the anesthesia machine ventilator permits the transmission of high airway pressure to the patient's lungs, with the possibility of barotrauma.

VAPORIZERS

Volatile anesthetics are liquids at room temperature and atmospheric pressure. Vaporization, which is the conversion of a liquid to a vapor, takes place in a closed container, referred to as a vaporizer. The vapor concentration resulting from vaporization of a volatile liquid anesthetic must be delivered to the patient with the same accuracy and predictability as other gases (oxygen, nitrous oxide).

Physics of Vaporization

The molecules that make up a liquid are in constant random motion. In a vaporizer containing a volatile liquid anesthetic, there is an asymmetrical arrangement of intermolecular forces applied to the molecules at the liquid-oxygen interface. The result of this asymmetrical arrangement is a net attractive force pulling the surface molecules into the liquid phase. This force must be overcome if surface molecules are to enter the gas phase, where their relatively sparse density constitutes a vapor. The energy necessary for molecules to escape from the liquid is supplied as heat. The heat of vaporization of a liquid is the number of calories required at a specific temperature to convert 1 g of a liquid into a vapor. The heat of vaporization necessary for molecules to leave the liquid phase is greater when the temperature of the liquid decreases.

Vaporization in the closed confines of a vaporizer ceases when equilibrium is reached between the liquid and vapor phases such that the number of molecules leaving the liquid phase is the same as the number re-entering. The molecules in the vapor phase collide with each other and the walls of the container, thereby creating pressure. This pressure is termed vapor pressure and is unique for each volatile anesthetic. Furthermore, vapor pressure is temperature dependent such that a decrease in the temperature of the liquid is associated with a lower vapor pressure and fewer molecules in the vapor phase. Cooling of the liquid anesthetic reflects a loss of heat (heat of vaporization) necessary to provide energy for vaporization. This cooling is undesirable because it lowers the vapor pressure and limits the attainable vapor concentration.

Vaporizer Classification and Design

Vaporizers are classified as agent-specific, variable-bypass, flow-over, temperature-compensated (equipped with an automatic temperature-compensating device that helps maintain a constant vaporizer output over a wide range of temperatures), and out of circuit (Fig. 15-5).[1] These contemporary vaporizers are unsuitable for the controlled vaporization of desflurane, which has a vapor pressure near 1 atm (664 mm Hg) at 20° C. For this reason, a desflurane vaporizer is electrically heated to 23° C to 25° C and pressurized with a backpressure regulator to 1500 mm Hg to create an environment in which the anesthetic has relatively lower, but predictable volatility.

Variable bypass describes dividing (splitting) the total fresh gas flow through the vaporizer into two portions. The first portion of the fresh gas flow (20% or less) passes into the vaporizing chamber of the vaporizer, where it becomes saturated (flow-over) with the vapor of the liquid anesthetic. The second portion of the fresh gas flow passes through the bypass chamber of the vaporizer. Both portions of the fresh gas flow mix at the patient outlet side of the anesthesia machine. The proportion of fresh gas flow diverted through the vaporizing chamber, and thus the concentration of volatile anesthetic delivered to the patient, is determined by the concentration control dial. The scale on the concentration control dial is in volume percent

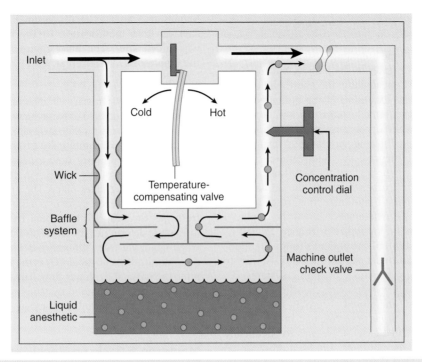

Figure 15-5 Simplified schematic of the Ohmeda Tec-type vaporizer. Rotation of the concentration control dial diverts a portion of the total fresh gas flow through the vaporizing chamber, where wicks saturated with liquid anesthetic ensure a large gas-liquid interface for efficient vaporization. A temperature-compensating valve diverts more or less fresh gas flow through the vaporizing chamber to offset the effects of changes in temperature on the vapor pressure of the liquid anesthetic (temperature-compensated vaporizer). Gases saturated with the vapor of the liquid anesthetic join gases that have passed through the bypass chamber for delivery to the machine outlet check valve. When the concentration control dial is in the off position, no fresh gas inflow enters the vaporizing chamber.

for the specific anesthetic drug. A temperature-sensitive bimetallic strip or an expansion element influences proportioning of total gas flow between the vaporizing and bypass chambers as the vaporizer temperature changes (temperature compensated) (see Fig. 15-5).[1] For example, as the temperature of the liquid anesthetic in the vaporizer chamber decreases, the temperature-sensing elements allow increased gas inflow into this chamber to offset the effect of decreased anesthetic liquid vapor pressure.

Vaporizers are often constructed of metals with high thermal conductivity (copper, bronze) to further minimize heat loss. As a result, vaporizer output is nearly linear between 20° C and 35° C.[3] Designation of vaporizers as agent specific and out of circuit emphasizes that these devices are calibrated to accommodate a single volatile anesthetic and are isolated from the anesthetic breathing system.

Tipping of vaporizers can cause liquid anesthetic to spill from the vaporizing chamber into the bypass chamber with a resultant increased vapor concentration exiting from the vaporizer. Nevertheless, the likelihood of tipping is minimized because vaporizers are secured to the anesthesia machine and there is little need to move

them. Leaks associated with vaporizers are most often due to a loose filler cap.

Commonly, two to three anesthetic-specific vaporizers are present on the anesthesia machine. A safety interlock mechanism ensures that only one vaporizer at a time can be turned on. Turning on a vaporizer requires depression of a release button on the concentration dial, followed by counterclockwise rotation of the dial. This prevents accidental movement of the dial from the off to the on position. The location of the filler port on the lower portion of the vaporizer minimizes the likelihood of overfilling of the vaporizing chamber (>125 mL) with liquid anesthetic. A window near the filler port permits visual verification of the level of liquid anesthetic in the vaporizing chamber. Use of an anesthetic-specific keyed filler device prevents placement of a liquid anesthetic into the vaporizing chamber that is different from the anesthetic for which the vaporizer was calibrated. This is uniquely important for desflurane because its vapor pressure is near 1 atm and accidental placement of desflurane in a contemporary vaporizer could result in an anesthetic overdose.[4] As with anesthesia machines, periodic maintenance (usually every 12 months) is recommended by the manufacturers of vaporizers.

ANESTHETIC BREATHING SYSTEMS

The function of anesthetic breathing systems is to deliver oxygen and anesthetic gases to the patient and to eliminate carbon dioxide. Conceptually, the anesthetic breathing system is a tubular extension of the patient's upper airway. Anesthetic breathing systems can add considerable resistance to inhalation because peak flows as high as 60 L/min are reached during spontaneous inspiration. This resistance is influenced by unidirectional valves and connectors. The components of the breathing system, particularly the tracheal tube connector, should have the largest possible lumen to minimize this resistance to breathing. Right-angle connectors should be replaced with curved connectors to minimize resistance. Substituting controlled ventilation of the patient's lungs for spontaneous breathing can offset the increased resistance to inhalation imparted by anesthetic breathing systems.

Anesthetic breathing systems are classified as open, semiopen, semiclosed, and closed according to the presence or absence of (1) a gas reservoir bag in the circuit, (2) rebreathing of exhaled gases, (3) means to chemically neutralize exhaled carbon dioxide, and (4) unidirectional valves (Table 15-3). The most commonly used anesthetic breathing systems are the (1) Mapleson F (Jackson-Rees) system, (2) Bain circuit, and (3) circle system.

Mapleson Breathing Systems

In 1954, Mapleson analyzed and described five different arrangements of fresh gas inflow tubing, reservoir tubing, facemask, reservoir bag, and an expiratory valve to administer anesthetic gases (Fig. 15-6).[5] These five different semiopen anesthetic breathing systems are designated Mapleson A to E. The Mapleson F system, which is a Jackson-Rees modification of the Mapleson D system, was added later. The Bain circuit is a modification of the Mapleson D system (Fig. 15-7).[6]

FLOW CHARACTERISTICS

The Mapleson systems are characterized by the absence of valves to direct gases to or from the patient and the absence of chemical carbon dioxide neutralization. Because of no clear separation of inspired and expired gases, rebreathing occurs when inspiratory flow exceeds the fresh gas flow. The composition of the inspired mixture depends on how much rebreathing takes place. The amount of rebreathing associated with each system is highly dependent on the fresh gas flow rate. The optimal fresh gas flow may be difficult to determine. The fresh gas flow should be adjusted when changing from spontaneous and controlled ventilation. Monitoring end-tidal CO_2 is the best method to determine the optimal fresh gas flow. The performance of these circuits is best understood by studying the gas disposition at end exhalation during spontaneous and controlled ventilation (Fig. 15-8).[7]

Mapleson F (Jackson-Rees) System

The Mapleson F (Jackson-Rees) system is a T-piece arrangement with a reservoir bag and an adjustable pressure-limiting overflow valve on the distal end of the gas reservoir bag (see Fig. 15-6).[5] The degree of rebreathing when using this anesthetic breathing system is influenced by the method of ventilation (spontaneous versus controlled) and adjustment of the pressure-limiting overflow valve (venting). Fresh gas flow equal to two to three times the patient's minute ventilation is recommended to prevent rebreathing of exhaled gases.

Table 15-3 Classification of Anesthetic Breathing Systems

System	Gas Reservoir Bag	Rebreathing of Exhaled Gases	Chemical Neutralization of Carbon Dioxide	Unidirectional Valves	Fresh Gas Inflow Rate*
Open					
Insufflation	No	No	No	None	Unknown
Open drop	No	No	No	None	Unknown
Semiopen					
Mapleson A, B, C, D	Yes	No[†]	No	One	High
Bain	Yes	No[†]	No	One	High
Mapleson E	No	No[†]	No	None	High
Mapleson F (Jackson-Rees)	Yes	No[†]	No	One	High
Semiclosed Circle	Yes	Partial	Yes	Three	Moderate
Closed Circle	Yes	Total	Yes	Three	Low

*High, greater than 6 L/min; moderate, 3 to 6 L/min; low, 0.3 to 0.5 L/min.
[†]No rebreathing of exhaled gases only when fresh gas inflow is adequate.

Figure 15-6 Anesthetic breathing systems classified as semiopen Mapleson A through F. FGF, fresh gas flow. (Modified from Willis BA, Pender JW, Mapleson WW. Rebreathing in a T-piece: Volunteer and theoretical studies of Jackson-Rees modification of Ayre's T-piece during spontaneous respiration. Br J Anaesth 1975;47:1239-1246, used with permission.)

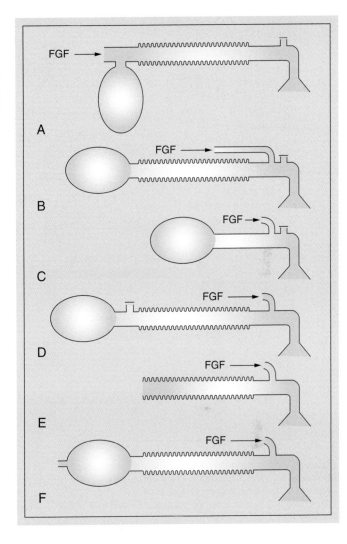

Figure 15-7 Schematic diagram of the Bain system showing fresh gas flow (FGF) entering a narrow tube within the larger corrugated expiratory limb (**A**). The only valve in the system (**B**) is an adjustable pressure-limiting (overflow) valve located near the FGF inlet and reservoir bag (**C**). (Modified from Bain JA, Spoerel WE. A streamlined anaesthetic system. Can Anaesth Soc J 1972;19:426-435, used with permission.)

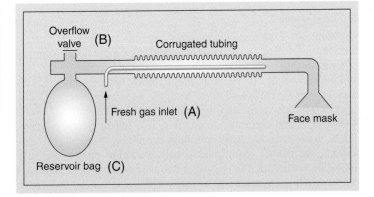

FLOW CHARACTERISTICS

During spontaneous ventilation, exhaled gases pass down the expiratory limb and mix with fresh gases (see Fig. 15-8).[7] The expiratory pause allows the fresh gas to push the exhaled gases down the expiratory limb. With the next inspiration, the inhaled gas mixture comes from the fresh gas flow and from the expiratory limb, including the reservoir bag.

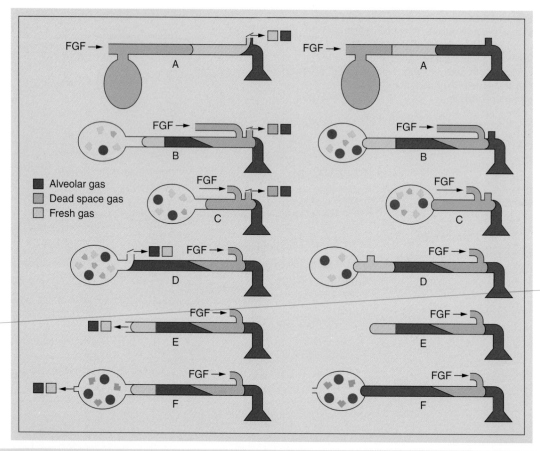

Figure 15-8 Gas disposition at end exhalation during spontaneous ventilation (*left*) or controlled ventilation (*right*) of the lungs in semiopen Mapleson A through F anesthetic breathing systems. The relative efficiency of different Mapleson systems for preventing rebreathing during spontaneous ventilation is A > DF > C > B. The relative efficiency of different Mapleson systems for preventing rebreathing during controlled ventilation is DF > B > C > A. FGF, fresh gas flow. (Modified from Sykes MK. Rebreathing circuits. A review. Br J Anaesth 1968;40:666-674, used with permission.)

CLINICAL USES

The Mapleson F system is commonly used for controlled ventilation during transport of tracheally intubated patients. Because of no moving parts except the pressure-limiting overflow valve, minimum dead space and resistence exist. This is ideal for pediatric anesthesia (see Chapter 34). The Mapleson F system may be used for both spontaneous and controlled ventilation. It is inexpensive, can be used with a facemask or endotracheal tube, is light-weight, and can be repositioned easily. Pollution of the atmosphere with anesthetic gases when using this system can be decreased by adapting it to scavenging systems.

DISADVANTAGES

Disadvantages of the Mapleson F system include (1) the need for high fresh gas inflow to prevent rebreathing, (2) the possibility of high airway pressure and barotrauma should the overflow valve become occluded,

and (3) the lack of humidification. Lack of humidification can be offset by allowing the fresh gas to pass through an in-line heated humidifier.

Bain System

The Bain circuit is a coaxial version of the Mapleson D system in which the fresh gas supply tube runs coaxially inside the corrugated expiratory tubing (see Fig. 15-7).[6] The fresh gas tube enters the circuit near the reservoir bag, but the fresh gas is actually delivered at the patient end of the circuit. The exhaled gases are vented through the overflow valve near the reservoir bag. The Bain circuit may be used for both spontaneous and controlled ventilation. Prevention of rebreathing during spontaneous ventilation requires a fresh gas flow of 200 to 300 mL/kg/min and a flow of only 70 mL/kg/min during controlled ventilation.

ADVANTAGES

Advantages of the Bain circuit include (1) warming of the fresh gas inflow by the surrounding exhaled gases in the corrugated expiratory tube, (2) conservation of moisture as a result of partial rebreathing, and (3) ease of scavenging waste anesthetic gases from the overflow valve. It is lightweight, easily sterilized, reusable, and useful when access to the patient is limited, such as during head and neck surgery.

DISADVANTAGES

Hazards of the Bain circuit include unrecognized disconnection or kinking of the inner fresh gas tube. The outer expiratory tube should be transparent to allow inspection of the inner tube.

Circle System

The circle system is the most popular anesthetic breathing system in the United States. It is so named because its essential components are arranged in a circular manner (Fig. 15-9).[3] The circle system prevents rebreathing of carbon dioxide by chemical neutralization of carbon dioxide with carbon dioxide absorbents.

CLASSIFICATION

A circle system can be classified as semiopen, semiclosed, or closed, depending on the amount of fresh gas inflow (see Table 15-3). In a semiopen system, very high fresh gas flow is used to eliminate rebreathing of gases. A semiclosed system is associated with rebreathing of gases and is the most commonly used breathing system in the United States. In a closed system, the inflow gas exactly matches that being consumed by the patient. Rebreathing of exhaled gases in the semiclosed and closed circle systems results in (1) some conservation of airway moisture and body heat and (2) decreased pollution of the surrounding atmosphere with anesthetic gases when the fresh gas inflow rate is set at less than the patient's minute ventilation.

DISADVANTAGES

Disadvantages of the circle system include (1) increased resistance to breathing because of the presence of unidirectional valves and carbon dioxide absorbent, (2) bulkiness with loss of portability, and (3) enhanced opportunity for malfunction because of the complexity of the apparatus.

IMPACT OF REBREATHING

Rebreathing of exhaled gases in a semiclosed circle system influences the inhaled anesthetic concentrations of these gases. For example, when uptake of the anesthetic gas is high, as during induction of anesthesia, rebreathing of exhaled gases depleted of anesthetic greatly dilutes the concentration of anesthetic in the fresh gas inflow. This dilutional effect of uptake is offset clinically by increasing the delivered concentration of anesthetic. As uptake of anesthetic diminishes, the impact of dilution on the inspired concentration produced by rebreathing of exhaled gases is lessened.

COMPONENTS

The circle system consists of (1) a fresh gas inlet, (2) inspiratory and expiratory unidirectional check valves, (3) inspiratory and expiratory corrugated tubing, (4) a Y-piece connector, (5) an adjustable pressure-limiting (APL) valve, also referred to as an overflow or "pop-off"

Figure 15-9 Schematic diagram of the components of a circle absorption anesthetic breathing system. Rotation of the bag/vent selector switch permits substitution of an anesthesia machine ventilator (V) for the reservoir bag (B). The volume of the reservoir bag is determined by the fresh gas inflow and adjustment of the adjustable pressure-limiting (APL) valve. (From Brockwell RC, Andrews JJ. Delivery systems for inhaled anesthetics. In Barash PG, Cullen BF, Stoelting RK [eds]. Clinical Anesthesia. Philadelphia, Lippincott Williams & Wilkins, 2006, pp 557-594, used with permission.)

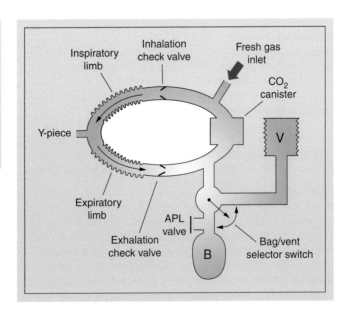

valve, (6) a reservoir bag, (7) a canister containing carbon dioxide absorbent, (8) a bag/vent selector switch, and (9) a mechanical anesthesia ventilator (see Fig. 15-9).[3]

Fresh Gas Inlet and Unidirectional Valves

Fresh gas enters the circle system through a connection from the common gas outlet of the anesthesia machine. Two unidirectional valves are situated in different limbs of the corrugated tubing such that one functions for inhalation and the other for exhalation. These valves (1) permit positive-pressure breathing and (2) prevent the rebreathing of exhaled gases until they have passed through the carbon dioxide absorbent canister and have had their oxygen content replenished. Rebreathing and hypercapnia can occur if the unidirectional valves stick in the open position, and total occlusion of the circuit can occur if they are stuck in the closed position. If the expiratory valve is stuck in the closed position, breath stacking and barotrauma can occur. If the unidirectional valves are functioning properly, the only dead space in the circle system is between the Y-piece and the patient.

Corrugated Tubing

The inspiratory and expiratory corrugated tubes serve as conduits for delivery of gases to and from the patient. Their large bore provides minimal resistance, and the corrugations provide flexibility, resist kinking, and promote turbulent instead of laminar flow. During positive-pressure ventilation, some of the delivered gas distends the corrugated tubing and some is compressed within the circuit, which leads to a smaller delivered tidal volume.

Y-Piece Connector

A Y-piece connector at the patient end of the circuit has (1) a curved elbow, (2) an outer diameter of 22 mm to fit inside a facemask, and (3) an inner diameter of 15 mm to fit onto an endotracheal tube connector.

Adjustable Pressure-Limiting Valve

When the "bag/vent" selector switch is set to "bag," the APL (overflow or "pop-off") valve (1) allows venting of excess gas from the breathing system into the waste gas scavenging system and (2) can be adjusted to allow the anesthesiologist to provide assisted or controlled ventilation of the patient's lungs by manual compression of the gas reservoir bag. The APL valve should be fully open during spontaneous ventilation so that circuit pressure remains negligible throughout inspiration and expiration.

Reservoir Bag

When the "bag/vent" selector switch is set to "bag," the gas reservoir bag maintains an available reserve volume of gas to satisfy the patient's spontaneous inspiratory flow rate (up to 60 L/min), which greatly exceeds conventional fresh gas flows (commonly 3 to 5 L/min) from the anesthesia machine. The bag also serves as a safety device because its distensibility limits pressure in the breathing circuit to less than 60 cm H_2O, even when the APL valve is closed.

Closed Anesthetic Breathing System

In a closed anesthetic breathing system, there is total rebreathing of exhaled gases after absorption of carbon dioxide, and the APL valve or relief valve of the ventilator is closed. A closed system is present when the fresh gas inflow into the circle system (150 to 500 mL/min) satisfies the patient's metabolic oxygen requirements (150 to 250 mL/min during anesthesia) and replaces anesthetic gases lost by virtue of tissue uptake. If sidestream gas analyzers are used, the analyzed gas exiting the analyzer must be returned to the breathing system to maintain a closed system.

ADVANTAGES

Advantages of a closed circle anesthetic breathing system over a semiclosed circle anesthetic breathing system include (1) maximal humidification and warming of inhaled gases, (2) less pollution of the surrounding atmosphere with anesthetic gases, and (3) economy in the use of anesthetics.

DISADVANTAGES

A disadvantage of a closed circle anesthetic breathing system is an inability to rapidly change the delivered concentration of anesthetic gases and oxygen because of the low fresh gas inflow.

DANGERS OF CLOSED ANESTHETIC BREATHING SYSTEM

The principal dangers of a closed anesthetic breathing system are delivery of (1) unpredictable and possibly insufficient concentrations of oxygen and (2) unknown and possibly excessive concentrations of potent anesthetic gases.

Unpredictable Concentrations of Oxygen

Unpredictable and possibly insufficient delivered concentrations of oxygen when using a closed anesthetic breathing system are more likely if nitrous oxide is included in the fresh gas inflow. For example, decreased tissue uptake of nitrous oxide with time in the presence of unchanged uptake of oxygen can result in a decreased concentration of oxygen in the alveoli (Table 15-4). Therefore, the use of an oxygen analyzer placed on the inspiratory or expiratory limb of the circle system is mandatory when nitrous oxide is delivered through a closed anesthetic breathing system.

Unknown Concentrations of Potent Anesthetic Gases

Exhaled gases, devoid of carbon dioxide, form a major part of the inhaled gases when a closed anesthetic breathing system is used. This means that the composition of the inhaled gases is influenced by the concentration present in the exhaled gases. The concentration of anesthetic in exhaled gases reflects tissue uptake of anesthetic. Initially, tissue uptake is maximal, and the concentration of anesthetic in the exhaled gases is minimal. Subsequent

Table 15-4 Alveolar Gas Concentration with a Closed Circle Anesthetic Breathing System

Example 1

Gas inflow is nitrous oxide, 300 mL/min, and oxygen, 300 mL/min, for 15 minutes. Nitrous oxide uptake by tissues at the time is 200 mL/min, and oxygen consumption is 250 mL/min. Alveolar gas after tissue uptake consists of 100 mL nitrous oxide and 50 mL oxygen. The alveolar concentration of oxygen (F_{AO_2}) is

$$F_{AO_2} = 50\,mL\ oxygen/(100\,mL\ nitrous\ oxide + 50\,mL\ oxygen) \times 100 = 33\%$$

Example 2

Gas inflow as in Example 1, but the duration of administration is 1 hour. At this time, tissue uptake of nitrous oxide has decreased to 100 mL/min, but oxygen consumption remains unchanged at 250 mL/min. Alveolar gas after tissue uptake consists of 200 mL nitrous oxide and 50 mL oxygen. The alveolar concentration of oxygen (F_{AO_2}) is

$$F_{AO_2} = 50\,mL\ oxygen/(200\,mL\ nitrous\ oxide + 50\,mL\ oxygen) \times 100 = 20\%$$

rebreathing of these exhaled gases dilutes the inhaled concentration of anesthetic delivered to the patient. Therefore, high inflow concentrations of anesthetic are necessary to offset maximal tissue uptake. Conversely, only small amounts of anesthetic need to be added to the inflow gases when tissue uptake has decreased. The unknown impact of tissue uptake on the concentration of anesthetic in exhaled gases makes it difficult to estimate the inhaled concentration delivered to the patient through a closed anesthetic breathing system. This disadvantage can be partially offset by administering higher fresh gas inflow (3 L/min) for about 15 minutes before instituting the use of a closed anesthetic breathing system. This approach permits elimination of nitrogen from the lungs and corresponds to the time of greatest tissue uptake of anesthetic.

ANESTHESIA MACHINE VENTILATORS

When the "bag/vent" selector switch is set to "vent," the gas reservoir bag and APL valve are eliminated from the circle anesthetic system and the patient's ventilation is delivered from the mechanical anesthesia ventilator. Anesthesia ventilators are powered by compressed gas, electricity, or both. Most conventional anesthesia machine ventilators are pneumatically driven by oxygen or air that is pressurized and, during the inspiratory phase, routed to the space inside the ventilator casing between the compressible bellows and the rigid casing. Pressurized air or oxygen entering this space forces the bellows to empty its contents into the patient's lungs through the inspiratory limb of the breathing circuit. This pressurized air or oxygen also causes the ventilator relief valve to close, thereby preventing inspiratory anesthetic gas from escaping into the scavenging system.

Oxygen is preferable to air as the ventilator driving gas because if there is a leak in the bellows, the fraction of inspired oxygen will be increased. If there is a leak in the bellows in a ventilator driven by 50 psi oxygen or air, peak inspiratory pressures will rise. During exhalation, the driving gas is either vented into the room or directed to the scavenging system, and the bellows refills as the patient exhales. Some newer anesthesia machines have mechanically driven piston-type ventilators. The piston operates much like the plunger of a syringe to deliver the desired tidal volume or airway pressure to the patient.

Bellows

Ventilators with bellows that rise during exhalation (standing or ascending bellows) are preferred because the bellows will not rise (fill) if there is a leak in the anesthesia breathing system or the system becomes accidentally disconnected (Fig. 15-10).[8] Ventilators with bellows that descend during exhalation (hanging or descending bellows) are potentially dangerous because the bellows will continue to rise and fall during a disconnection. Whenever a ventilator is used, a disconnect alarm must be activated and audible.

Humidity and Heat Exchange in the Breathing Circuit

The upper respiratory tract (especially the nose) functions as the principal heat and moisture exchanger (HME) to bring inspired gas to body temperature and 100% relative humidity in its passage to the alveoli. Water is removed from medical gases (cylinders or piped) to prevent corrosion and condensation. Tracheal intubation or the use of a laryngeal mask airway bypasses the upper airway and thus leaves the tracheobronchial mucosa the burden of heating and humidifying inspired gases. Humidification of inspired gases by the lower respiratory tract in intubated patients can lead to dehydration of the mucosa, impaired ciliary function, impaired surfactant function, inspissation of secretions, atelectasis, and a rise in the alveolar-to-arterial gradient. Breathing of dry and room-temperature gases in intubated patients is associated with water and heat loss from the patient. Heat loss is more important than water loss, and the most important reason to provide heated humidification in intubated patients is to decrease heat loss and associated decreases in body temperature, especially in infants and children, who are rendered poikilothermic by general anesthesia.

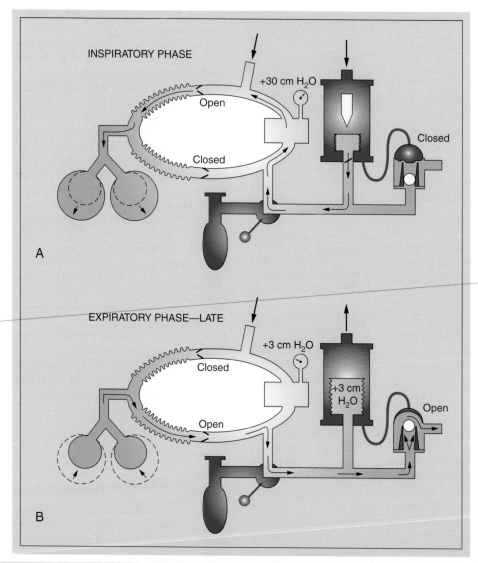

INSPIRATORY PHASE

Open

+30 cm H₂O

Closed

Closed

A

EXPIRATORY PHASE—LATE

Closed

+3 cm H₂O

+3 cm H₂O

Open

Open

B

Figure 15-10 Inspiratory (**A**) and expiratory (**B**) phases of gas flow in a traditional circle system with an ascending bellows anesthesia ventilator. The bellows physically separates the driving gas circuit from the patient's gas circuit. The driving gas circuit is located outside the bellows, and the patient's gas circuit is inside the bellows. During the inspiratory phase (**A**), the driving gas enters the bellows chamber and causes the pressure within it to increase. This increased pressure causes the ventilator's relief valve to close, thus preventing anesthetic gas from escaping into the scavenging system, and the bellows to compress, thereby delivering the anesthetic gas within the bellows to the patient's lungs. During the expiratory phase (**B**), the driving gas exits the bellows chamber. The pressure within the bellows chamber and the pilot line decline to zero, which causes the mushroom portion of the ventilator's relief valve to open. Gas exhaled by the patient fills the bellows before any scavenging occurs because a weighted ball is incorporated into the base of the ventilator's relief valve. Scavenging occurs solely during the expiratory phase because the ventilator's relief valve is open only during expiration. (From Andrews JJ. The Circle System. A Collection of 30 Color Illustrations. Washington, DC, Library of Congress, 1998, used with permission.)

Humidification

Humidification is a form of vaporization in which water vapor (moisture) is added to the gases delivered by the anesthetic breathing system to minimize water and heat loss. The water formed and the heat generated by chemical neutralization of carbon dioxide help humidify and heat the gases in the breathing circuit. Humidifiers used for anesthesia and in the intensive care unit include (1) heat and moisture exchanger (HME) humidifiers, (2) heated water vaporizers and humidifiers, and (3) nebulizers.

HEAT AND MOISTURE EXCHANGER HUMIDIFIERS

HME humidifiers are devices that when placed between the endotracheal tube and Y-piece of the circle system, conserve some of the exhaled water and heat and return it to the inspired gases. They contain a porous hydrophobic or hygroscopic membrane that traps exhaled humidified gases and returns them to the patient on inspiration. Bacterial and viral filters can be incorporated in HME humidifiers to convert them into heat and moisture exchanging filters (HMEFs).

Advantages

The advantages of HME humidifiers over other types of humidifiers are that they are (1) simple and easy to use, (2) lightweight, (3) not dependent on an external power source, (4) disposable, and (5) low cost.

Disadvantages

The disadvantages of HME humidifiers are that they (1) are not as effective as heated water vaporizers and humidifiers in maintaining patient temperature, (2) add resistance and increase the work of breathing and therefore should be used with caution in spontaneously ventilating patients, (3) can become clogged with patient secretions or blood, and (4) can increase dead space, which can cause significant rebreathing in pediatric patients. Special low-volume HMEs are available for pediatric patients.

HEATED WATER VAPORIZERS AND HUMIDIFIERS

Heated water vaporizers and humidifiers are used to deliver a relative humidity higher than that delivered by HME humidifiers. Heated water vaporizers are more frequently used in pediatric anesthesia and intensive care unit patients. Risks from heated water vaporizers and humidifiers include (1) thermal injury, (2) nosocomial infection, (3) increased work of breathing, and (4) increased risk of malfunction because of the complexity of these systems.

NEBULIZERS

Nebulizers produce a mist of microdroplets of water suspended in a gaseous medium. The quantity of water droplets delivered is not limited by the temperature of the carrier gas. In addition to water, nebulizers can deliver medications to peripheral airways.

POLLUTION OF THE ATMOSPHERE WITH ANESTHETIC GASES

Chronic exposure to low concentrations of inhaled anesthetics may pose a health hazard to operating room personnel. The Occupational Safety and Health Administration (OSHA) presently has no required exposure limits regulating nitrous oxide and volatile anesthetics. In the operating room, OSHA recommends that the concentration of nitrous oxide not exceed 25 ppm and exposure

Table 15-5 Recommendations of the American Society of Anesthesiologists Task Force on Waste Anesthetic Gases

- Waste anesthetic gases should be scavenged.
- Appropriate work practices should be used to minimize exposure to waste anesthetic gases.
- Personnel working in areas where waste anesthetic gases may be present should be educated regarding (1) current studies on the health effects of exposure to waste anesthetic gases, (2) appropriate work practices to minimize exposure, and (3) machine checkout and maintenance procedures.
- There is insufficient evidence to recommend routine monitoring of trace concentrations of waste anesthetic gases in the operating room and postanesthesia care unit.
- There is insufficient evidence to recommend routine medical surveillance of personnel exposed to trace concentrations of waste anesthetic gases, although each institution should have a mechanism for employees to report suspected work-related health problems.

From McGregor DG, Baden JM, Bannister C, et al. Waste anesthetic gases: Information for the management in anesthetizing areas and the postanesthesia care unit (PACU). Park Ridge, IL, American Society of Anesthesiologists, 1999.

concentrations of volatile anesthetics not exceed 2 ppm. Recommendations regarding waste anesthetic gases have been made by the American Society of Anesthesiologists (Table 15-5).[9]

Control of pollution of the atmosphere with anesthetic gases requires (1) scavenging of waste anesthetic gases, (2) periodic preventive maintenance of anesthesia equipment, (3) attention to the anesthetic technique, and (4) adequate ventilation of the operating rooms.

Scavenging Systems

Scavenging is the collection and subsequent removal of vented gases from the operating room. The excess gas comes from either the APL valve if the bag/vent selector switch is set to "bag" or from the ventilator relief valve if the bag/vent selector switch is set to "vent." All excess gas from the patient exits the breathing system through these valves. In addition, when the bag/vent selector switch is set to vent, some anesthetic breathing systems direct the drive gas inside the bellows canister to the scavenging system. The amount of delivered gas used to anesthetize a patient commonly far exceeds the patient's needs. The anesthesiologist must be certain that the scavenging system is operational and adjusted properly to ensure adequate scavenging. If sidestream gas analyzers are used, the analyzed gas exiting the analyzer must be directed to the scavenging system or returned to the breathing system.

Scavenging systems may be characterized as active or passive. An active system is connected to the hospital's vacuum system and gases are drawn from the machine by a vacuum. A passive system is connected to the hospital's ventilation duct and waste gases flow out of the machine on their own.

Many anesthesia machines provide scavenging with a waste gas receiver mounted on the side of the anesthesia machine. Advantages of this system include (1) a needle valve that allows the clinician to manually adjust the amount of vacuum flow through the scavenging system, (2) a needle valve that can be adjusted such that the 3-L reservoir bag will be slightly inflated and appear to "breathe" with the patient, and (3) unlike other active scavenging systems, a waste gas receiver that does not require a strong vacuum to operate.

HAZARDS

Hazards of scavenging systems include (1) obstruction of the scavenging pathways, which can result in excessive positive pressure in the breathing circuit and possible barotrauma, and (2) excessive vacuum applied to the scavenging system, which can cause negative pressures in the breathing system. Scavenging systems contain two relief valves to minimize these hazards. If gas accumulates in the scavenging system and cannot leave the anesthesia machine properly, the positive-pressure scavenge relief valve opens when the pressure reaches 10 cm H_2O to allow the gas to escape into the room. If negative pressure is applied to the scavenging system, the negative-pressure scavenge relief valve opens and allows room air to be drawn in (instead of drawing gas from the patient). Additionally, if the amount of fresh gas flow exceeds the capacity of the scavenging system, the excess waste anesthetic gas exits the scavenging system through the positive-pressure relief valve and pollutes the operating room.

Periodic Preventive Maintenance of Anesthesia Equipment

High-pressure leakage of nitrous oxide can occur as a result of faulty yokes attaching the nitrous oxide tank to the anesthesia machine or faulty connections from the central nitrous oxide gas supply to the anesthesia machine. Low-pressure leakage of anesthetic gases can occur because of leaks inside the anesthesia machine and leaks between the machine and patient. Periodic preventive maintenance of the anesthesia machine by qualified service representatives is recommended.

Anesthetic Technique

Anesthetic techniques that can lead to operating room pollution include (1) poorly fitting facemasks, (2) flushing the anesthetic delivery circuit, (3) filling anesthetic vaporizers, (4) the use of uncuffed endotracheal tubes,

(5) failure to turn off the nitrous oxide flow or vaporizers at the end of the anesthesia, and (6) the use of semiopen breathing circuits such as the Jackson-Rees, which are difficult to scavenge.

Adequate Room Ventilation

The air in the operating room should be exchanged at least 15 times per hour by the operating room ventilation system. This rate should be checked periodically by the hospital's clinical engineering department.

ELIMINATION OF CARBON DIOXIDE

Open and semiopen breathing systems eliminate carbon dioxide by venting all exhaled gases to the atmosphere. Semiclosed and closed breathing systems eliminate carbon dioxide by chemical neutralization. Chemical neutralization is accomplished by directing the exhaled gases through a carbon dioxide absorber, which consists of a canister (usually transparent) containing carbon dioxide absorbent granules. Gas flow through the absorber during exhalation is usually from top to bottom. A space at the base of the absorber allows the collection of dust and water.

Carbon Dioxide Absorbents

SODA LIME

Soda lime granules consist of water, calcium hydroxide, and small amounts of sodium and potassium hydroxide that serve as activators (Table 15-6). Soda lime granules

Table 15-6 Comparison of Carbon Dioxide Absorbents

Feature	Soda Lime	Amsorb Plus
Contents		
$Ca(OH)_2$ (%)	76-81	>80
NaOH (%)	4	0
KOH (%)	1	0
Water (%)	14-19	13-18
Remaining balance	—	$CaCl_2$
Method of hardness	Silica	Calcium sulfate and polyvinylpyrrolidine
Mesh size	4-8	4-8
Generation of compound A with sevoflurane	Yes	No
Generation of carbon monoxide with inhaled anesthetics	Yes	No
Risk of exothermic reactions and fire in the presence of sevoflurane	No	No

Table 15-7 Chemical Neutralization of Carbon Dioxide

Soda Lime
$CO_2 + H_2O \rightarrow H_2CO_3$
$H_2CO_3 + 2NaOH$ (or KOH) $\rightarrow Na_2CO_3$ (or K_2CO_3) + $2H_2O$ + Heat
Na_2CO3 (or K_2CO_3) + $Ca(OH)_2 \rightarrow CaCO_3 + 2NaOH$ (or KOH)
$H_2CO_3 + Ca(OH)_2 \rightarrow CaCO_3 + 2H_2O$ + Heat
Amsorb Plus
$CO_2 + H_2O \rightarrow H_2CO_3$
$H_2CO_3 + Ca(OH)_2 \rightarrow CaCO_3 + 2H_2O$ + Heat

fragment easily and produce alkaline dust, which can lead to bronchospasm if inhaled. Silica is added to the granules to provide hardness and minimize alkaline dust formation.

Neutralization of carbon dioxide with soda lime begins with reaction of carbon dioxide with water present in the soda lime granules and the subsequent formation of carbonic acid (Table 15-7). Carbonic acid then reacts with the hydroxides present in the soda lime granules to form carbonates (with bicarbonates as intermediates), water, and heat.

The water formed from the neutralization of carbon dioxide, the water present in the soda lime granules, and the water condensed from the patient's exhaled gases leach the alkaline bases from the soda lime granules and produce a slurry containing NaOH and KOH in the bottom of the canister. These monovalent bases can be corrosive to the skin.

AMSORB PLUS

Amsorb was introduced in the year 2000, and an improved version, Amsorb Plus, has replaced Amsorb in the United States.[10] Amsorb Plus granules consist of water, calcium hydroxide, and calcium chloride (see Table 15-6). Neutralization of carbon dioxide with Amsorb Plus begins with reaction of carbon dioxide with water present in the Amsorb Plus granules and the subsequent formation of carbonic acid (see Table 15-7). Carbonic acid then reacts with the calcium hydroxide present in the Amsorb Plus granules to form calcium bicarbonate, carbonate, water, and heat.

Unlike soda lime, Amsorb Plus does not contain the strong monovalent bases NaOH or KOH (see Table 15-6). Amsorb Plus contains $CaOH_2$, and this ingredient alone minimizes the risks associated with the degradation of inhaled anesthetics. The $CaCl_2$ contained in Amsorb Plus further minimizes these risks by acting as a humectant and thereby allowing for greater availability of water. Calcium sulfate and polyvinylpyrrolidine are added to increase hardness.

HEAT OF NEUTRALIZATION

The water formed by the neutralization of carbon dioxide with soda lime and Amsorb Plus is useful for humidifying the gases and for dissipating some of the heat generated in these exothermic reactions. The heat generated during the neutralization of carbon dioxide can be detected by warmness of the canister. Failure of the canister to become warm should alert the anesthesia provider to the possibility that chemical neutralization of carbon dioxide is not taking place.

Efficiency of Carbon Dioxide Neutralization

The efficiency of carbon dioxide neutralization is influenced by the size of the carbon dioxide granules and the presence or absence of channeling in the carbon dioxide canister.

ABSORBENT GRANULE SIZE

The optimal absorbent granule size represents a compromise between absorptive efficiency and resistance to airflow through the carbon dioxide absorbent canister. Absorbent efficiency increases as absorbent granule size decreases because the total surface area coming in contact with carbon dioxide increases. The smaller the absorbent granules, however, the smaller the interstices through which gas must flow and the greater the resistance to flow.

Absorbent granule size is designated as mesh size, which refers to the number of openings per linear inch in a sieve through which the granular particles can pass. The granular size of carbon dioxide absorbents in anesthesia practice is between 4 and 8 mesh, a size at which absorbent efficiency is maximal with minimal resistance. A 4-mesh screen means that there are four quarter-inch openings per linear inch. An 8-mesh screen has eight eighth-inch openings per linear inch.

CHANNELING

Channeling is the preferential passage of exhaled gases through the carbon dioxide absorber canister via pathways of low resistance such that the bulk of the carbon dioxide absorbent granules are bypassed. Channeling resulting from loose packing of absorbent granules can be minimized by gently shaking the canister before use to ensure firm packing of the absorbent granules. Carbon dioxide absorbent canisters are designed to facilitate uniform dispersion of exhaled gas flow through the absorbent granules.

ABSORPTIVE CAPACITY

Absorptive capacity is determined by the maximum amount of carbon dioxide that can be absorbed by 100 g of carbon dioxide absorbent. Channeling of exhaled gases through the absorbent granules can substantially decrease their efficiency. Carbon dioxide absorber canister design also influences the absorptive capacity of the carbon dioxide absorbent.

INDICATORS

Carbon dioxide absorbents contain a pH-sensitive indicator dye that changes color when the carbon dioxide absorbent granules are exhausted. When the absorptive components of the granules are exhausted, carbonic acid accumulates and produces a change in the pH and thus in the indicator dye color.

Soda lime contains the indicator dye ethyl violet, which changes granule color from white to purple when exhausted. Over time, exhausted granules may revert to their original white color even though absorptive capacity does not recover with time. On reuse, the dye quickly produces the purple color change again. Amsorb Plus contains an indicator dye that changes granule color from white to purple when exhausted and, once changed, does not revert to its original color.

Degradation of Inhaled Anesthetics

Desiccated soda lime may degrade sevoflurane, isoflurane, enflurane, and desflurane to carbon monoxide. Soda lime, either moist and containing a normal water complement or dry, degrades sevoflurane and halothane to unsaturated nephrotoxic compounds (compound A). In contrast, Amsorb Plus, either desiccated or moist, does not degrade inhaled anesthetics.

GENERATION OF CARBON MONOXIDE

Degradation of inhaled anesthetics by desiccated soda lime can lead to significant concentrations of carbon monoxide that can produce carboxyhemoglobin concentrations reaching 30% or higher.[11] Production of carbon monoxide and carboxyhemoglobin increases with (1) the inhaled anesthetic used (desflurane = enflurane > isoflurane >> halothane = sevoflurane), (2) low fresh gas flows, (3) higher concentrations of inhaled anesthetics, (4) higher absorbent temperatures, and (5) dry absorbent.

GENERATION OF COMPOUND A

Degradation of sevoflurane by soda lime can result in the production of compound A, which is a dose-dependent nephrotoxin in rats.[12] Compound A is toxic to humans exposed to the greatest concentrations clinically achievable if these concentrations are applied in excess of more than 4 to 6 hours. Production of compound A with soda lime increases with (1) low fresh gas flows, (2) higher concentrations of sevoflurane, (3) higher absorbent temperatures, and (4) absorbent desiccation.

DESICCATION

Desiccation of soda lime increases the degradation of inhaled anesthetics. The retrograde flow (from bottom to top) of fresh gas through the carbon dioxide absorber can desiccate the absorbent. This may be affected by a number of factors, including (1) the design of the anesthesia breathing system, (2) the presence or absence of a breathing reservoir bag, (3) whether the APL valve is open or closed, (4) the relative resistance through the components of the breathing circuit, (5) the fresh gas flow rate, (6) the inspiratory-to-expiratory ratio, (7) the

use of HMEs, and (8) scavenger suction. With conventional breathing system design, removing the breathing bag, opening the APL valve, and occluding the Y-piece all enhance retrograde flow and desiccation of the carbon dioxide absorbent. For example, without a patient attached to the conventional circle system, a fresh gas flow rate of 5 L/min or higher through the carbon dioxide absorbent can cause desiccation of the absorbent, particularly if a breathing bag is absent from the breathing circuit. Absence of the breathing bag facilitates retrograde flow through the circle system because the inspiratory valve produces some resistance to flow and thus causes fresh gas flow to take the retrograde path of least resistance (bottom to top) through the carbon dioxide absorbent and out the breathing bag terminal, which does not have a breathing bag attached. Desiccation requires a prolonged period (usually 48 hours) of retrograde gas flow. Accordingly, most instances of increased blood concentrations of carboxyhemoglobin occur in patients anesthetized on a Monday after continuous flow of oxygen (flowmeter accidentally left on) through the carbon dioxide absorbent over the weekend.

FIRE AND EXTREME HEAT IN THE BREATHING SYSTEM

Desiccation of the carbon dioxide absorbent Baralyme (no longer clinically available) can lead to fire within the circle system with sevoflurane use.[13] A poorly characterized chemical reaction between sevoflurane and Baralyme can produce sufficient heat and combustible degradation products to lead to the spontaneous generation of fires within the carbon dioxide absorber canister and breathing circuit. Cases of extreme heat without fire associated with desiccated soda lime have been reported in Europe. To avoid this problem, anesthesia providers should make every effort to not use desiccated carbon dioxide absorbents.

RECOMMENDATIONS REGARDING SAFE USE OF CARBON DIOXIDE ABSORBENTS

The Anesthesia Patient Safety Foundation (see Chapter 2) has published suggested steps regarding the selection of carbon dioxide absorbents and steps to take should desiccation of the carbon dioxide absorbent be a potential risk (Table 15-8).[14]

CHECKING ANESTHESIA MACHINE AND CIRCLE SYSTEM FUNCTION

Improperly checking anesthesia equipment prior to use can lead to patient injury and has also been associated with an increased risk of severe morbidity and mortality related to anesthesia care.[15,16] In 1993 a preanesthesia checkout (PAC) was developed by the Food and Drug Administration and widely accepted to be an important step in the process

Table 15-8 Consensus Statement and Recommendations of the Anesthesia Patient Safety Foundation (APSF) Task Force on Carbon Dioxide Absorbent Desiccation

The APSF recommends the use of carbon dioxide absorbents whose composition is such that exposure to volatile anesthetics does not result in significant degradation of the volatile anesthetic.
The APSF further recommends that there should be institutional, hospital, and/or departmental policies regarding steps to prevent desiccation of carbon dioxide absorbent should they choose conventional carbon dioxide absorbents that may degrade volatile anesthetics when absorbent desiccation occurs.
When absorbents are used that may degrade volatile anesthetics, conference attendees generally agreed that users could take the following steps, consistent with Emergency Care Research Institute (ECRI) recommendations: 1. Turn off all gas flow when the machine is not in use. 2. Change the absorbent regularly, on Monday morning for instance. 3. Change absorbent whenever the color change indicates exhaustion. 4. Change all absorbent, not just one canister in a two-canister system. 5. Change the absorbent when uncertain of the state of hydration, such as if fresh gas flow has been left on for an extensive or indeterminate period. 6. If compact canisters are used, consider changing them more frequently.

From Olympio MA. Carbon dioxide absorbent desiccation safety conference convened by APSF. Anesthesia Patient Safety Foundation Newsletter. Summer 2005, pp 25-29 (www.apsf.org).

of preparing to deliver anesthesia care.[17] Since that time anesthesia delivery systems have evolved to the point that one checkout procedure is not applicable to all anesthesia delivery systems currently on the market.

ASA 2008 Recommendations for Pre-Anesthesia Checkout Procedures

In 2008 the American Society of Anesthesiologists developed new Recommendations for Pre-Anesthesia Checkout Procedures in order to provide guidelines applicable to all anesthesia delivery systems so that individual departments could develop a PAC specific to the anesthesia delivery systems currently used at their facilities that could be performed consistently and expeditiously. Specifically, for newer anesthesia delivery systems that incorporate automated checkout features, items that are not evaluated by the automated checkout need to be identified, and supplemental manual checkout procedures included as needed. This information is available on the ASA website in the Clinical Information Section (Table 15-9).[18]

A complete anesthesia machine and circle system function checkout procedure should be performed each day before the first case (see Table 15-9, items 1 through 15).[18] An abbreviated checkout should be performed before each subsequent use that day (see Table 15-9, items 2, 4, 7, 11, 12, 13, 14, 15).[18] The most important preoperative checks are (1) verification that an auxiliary oxygen cylinder and self-inflating manual ventilation device (Ambu bag) are available and functioning, (2) a leak check of the machine's low-pressure system, (3) calibration of the oxygen monitor, and (4) a positive-pressure leak check of the breathing system.

VERIFICATION THAT AUXILIARY OXYGEN CYLINDER AND MANUAL VENTILATION DEVICE ARE AVAILABLE AND FUNCTIONING

Failure to ventilate is a major cause of morbidity and death related to anesthesia care. Because equipment failure with resulting inability to ventilate the patient can occur at any time, a self-inflating manual ventilation device (e.g., Ambu bag) should be present at every anesthetizing location for every case and should be checked for proper function. In addition, a source of oxygen separate from the anesthesia machine and pipeline supply, specifically an oxygen cylinder with regulator and a means to open the cylinder valve, should be immediately available and checked (see Table 15-9, item 1).[18]

LEAK CHECK OF THE MACHINE'S LOW-PRESSURE SYSTEM

A leak check of the machine's low-pressure system is performed to confirm the integrity of the anesthesia machine from the flowmeters to the common gas outlet (see Table 15-9, item 8).[18] It evaluates the portion of the anesthesia machine that is downstream from all safety devices, except the oxygen monitor. The low-pressure circuit is the most vulnerable part of the anesthesia machine because the components located within this area are the ones most subject to breakage and leaks. The machine's low-pressure system must be checked because leaks in this circuit can lead to hypoxia or patient awareness, or both.

The leak test of the low-pressure system for some anesthesia machine designs varies, and the anesthesiologist must refer to the operator's manual for instructions. Newer anesthesia machines use automated checks of the machine's low-pressure system, but internal vaporizer leaks may not be detected unless each vaporizer is turned on individually during the low-pressure system self-test.

Table 15-9 ASA 2008 Recommendations for Preanesthesia Checkout Procedures

To Be Completed Daily

Item 1: Verify that auxiliary oxygen cylinder and self-inflating manual ventilation device are available and functioning.

Item 2: Verify that patient suction is adequate to clear the airway.

Item 3: Turn on anesthesia delivery system and confirm that ac power is available.

Item 4: Verify availability of required monitors, including alarms.

Item 5: Verify that pressure is adequate on the spare oxygen cylinder mounted on the anesthesia machine.

Item 6: Verify that the piped gas pressures are $\geq$50 psi.

Item 7: Verify that vaporizers are adequately filled and, if applicable, that the filler ports are tightly closed.

Item 8: Verify that there are no leaks in the gas supply lines between the flowmeters and the common gas outlet.

Item 9: Test scavenging system function.

Item 10: Calibrate, or verify calibration of, the oxygen monitor and check the low oxygen alarm.

Item 11: Verify that carbon dioxide absorbent is not exhausted.

Item 12: Perform breathing system pressure and leak testing.

Item 13: Verify that gas flows properly through the breathing circuit during both inspiration and exhalation.

Item 14: Document completion of checkout procedures.

Item 15: Confirm ventilator settings and evaluate readiness to deliver anesthesia care. (ANESTHESIA TIME OUT)

To Be Completed before Each Procedure

Item 2: Verify that patient suction is adequate to clear the airway.

Item 4: Verify availability of required monitors, including alarms.

Item 7: Verify that vaporizers are adequately filled and if applicable that the filler ports are tightly closed.

Item 11: Verify that carbon dioxide absorbent is not exhausted.

Item 12: Perform breathing system pressure and leak testing.

Item 13: Verify that gas flows properly through the breathing circuit during both inspiration and exhalation.

Item 14: Document completion of checkout procedures.

Item 15: Confirm ventilator settings and evaluate readiness to deliver anesthesia care. (ANESTHESIA TIME OUT)

CALIBRATION OF THE OXYGEN MONITOR

The oxygen monitor is the only machine safety device that detects problems downstream from the flowmeters (see Table 15-9, item 10).[18] The other machine safety devices (the fail-safe valve, the oxygen supply failure alarm, and the proportioning system) are all upstream from the flowmeters.

POSITIVE-PRESSURE LEAK CHECK OF THE BREATHING SYSTEM

A positive-pressure leak check of the breathing system must be performed before every procedure (see Table 15-9, item 12) (Fig 15-11).[18, 19] This test does not check the integrity of the unidirectional valves inasmuch as the breathing system will pass the leak check even if the unidirectional valves are incompetent or stuck shut (see Table 15-9, item 13).[18]

QUESTIONS OF THE DAY

1. How does a variable-bypass vaporizer deliver constant inhaled anesthetic output with changes in ambient temperature?
2. What are the advantages of Amsorb Plus versus soda lime for carbon dioxide removal in a circle breathing system?
3. What are the recommended preanesthesia checkout procedures prior to each procedure performed?

ACKNOWLEDGMENT

The editors and publisher would like to thank Dr. Joan E. Howley for contributing a chapter on this topic to the prior edition of this work. It has served as the foundation for the current chapter.

Figure 15-11 A positive-pressure leak test is performed before each case by occluding the outlet of the circle anesthesia system to create a pressure of 30 cm H_2O within the anesthetic breathing system as depicted on the airway pressure gauge. The absence of a low-pressure leak in the anesthesia machine and circle system is verified by a sustained positive pressure reading on the airway pressure gauge. Should the airway pressure gauge show decreasing pressure over 10 seconds, the anesthesiologist must perform a further machine check to determine the cause of the leak. Failure to discover the cause of the leak could jeopardize the ability to provide positive-pressure ventilation of the patient's lungs during the anesthesia. (From Andrews JJ. Understanding Anesthesia Machines. Cleveland, OH, International Anesthesia Research Society Review Course Lectures, 1988, p 78, used with permission.)

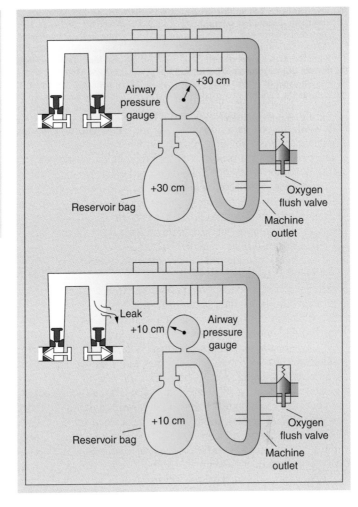

REFERENCES

1. Brockwell RC, Andrews JJ: Delivery systems for inhaled anesthetics. In Barash PG, Cullen BF, Stoelting RK, editors: *Clinical Anesthesia,* Philadelphia, 2006, Lippincott Williams & Wilkins, pp 557–594.
2. Check-Out: *A Guide for Preoperative Inspection of an Anesthetic Machine,* Park Ridge, IL, 1987, American Society of Anesthesiologists, pp 1–14.
3. Brockwell RC, Andrews JJ: Inhaled anesthetic delivery systems. In Miller RD, editor: *Miller's Anesthesia,* ed 7, Philadelphia, 2010, Churchill Livingstone, pp 667–718.
4. Andrews JJ, Johnston RV, Kramer GC: Consequences of misfilling contemporary vaporizers with desflurane, *Can J Anaesth* 40:71–74, 1993.

5. Willis BA, Pender JW, Mapleson WW: Rebreathing in a T-piece: Volunteer and theoretical studies of Jackson-Rees modification of Ayre's T-piece during spontaneous respiration, *Br J Anaesth* 47:1239–1246, 1975.
6. Bain JA, Spoerel WE: A streamlined anaesthetic system, *Can Anaesth Soc J* 19:426–435, 1972.
7. Sykes MK: Rebreathing circuits: A review, *Br J Anaesth* 40:666–674, 1968.
8. Andrews JJ: *The Circle System. A Collection of 30 Color Illustrations,* Washington, DC, 1998, Library of Congress.
9. McGregor DG, Baden JM, Bannister C, et al: *Waste Anesthetic Gases: Information for the Management in Anesthetizing Areas and the Postanesthesia Care Unit (PACU),* Park

Ridge, IL, 1999, American Society of Anesthesiologists.
10. Murray JM, Renfrew CW, Bedi A, et al: Amsorb. A new carbon dioxide absorbent for use in anesthetic breathing systems, *Anesthesiology* 91:1342–1348, 1999.
11. Baxter PJ, Garton K, Kaharasch ED: Mechanistic aspects of carbon monoxide formation from volatile anesthetics, *Anesthesiology* 89:929–941, 1998.
12. Kharasch ED, Frink EJ, Artru A, et al: Long-duration low-flow sevoflurane and isoflurane effects on postoperative renal and hepatic function, *Anesth Analg* 93:1511–1520, 2001.
13. Lester M, Roth P, Eger EI: Fires from the interaction of anesthetics with desiccated absorbent, *Anesth Analg* 99:769–774, 2004.

14. Olympio MA: Carbon dioxide absorbent desiccation safety conference convened by APSF *Anesth Patient Saf Found Newsletter* 25–29, Summer 2005. (www.apsf.org).

15. Cooper JB, Newbower RS, Kitz RJ: An Analysis of Major Errors and Equipment Failures in Anesthesia Management: Considerations for Prevention and Detection, *Anesthesiology* 60:34–42, 1984.

16. Arbous MS, Meursing AE, van Kleef JW, de Lange JJ: Impact of Anesthesia Management Characteristics on Severe Morbidity and Mortality, *Anesthesiology* 102:257–268, 2005.

17. *Anesthesia Apparatus Checkout Recommendations*, Rockville, MD, 1993, Food and Drug Administration.

18. American Society of Anesthesiologists Committee on Equipment and Facilities: *Recommendations for Pre-Anesthesia Checkout Procedures*, 2008. Accessed at http://www.asahq.org/clinical/fda.htm.

19. Andrews JJ: *Understanding Anesthesia Machines*, Cleveland, OH, 1988, International Anesthesia Research Society Review Course Lectures.

16 AIRWAY MANAGEMENT

Robin A. Stackhouse and Andrew Infosino

Competence in airway management is a critical skill for safely administering anesthesia. Difficult or failed airway management is the major factor in anesthesia-related morbidity (dental damage, pulmonary aspiration, airway trauma, unanticipated tracheostomy, anoxic brain injury, cardiopulmonary arrest) and death.[1] The incidence of difficult mask ventilation, defined as an inability to maintain oxygen saturation (SpO_2) greater than 90% or an inability to prevent or reverse the signs of inadequate ventilation, ranges from 0.07% to 5%.[2,3] Difficult tracheal intubation/laryngoscopy (defined as successful intubation requiring more than three attempts or taking longer than 10 minutes) occurs in 1.1% to 8.5% of patients.[4–7] Failed tracheal intubation occurs at an incidence of 0.01% to 0.03%.[4,5,8]

Competence in airway management requires (1) knowledge of the anatomy and physiology of the airway, (2) ability to assess the patient's airway for the anatomic features that correlate with difficult airway management, (3) skill with the many devices for airway management, and (4) appropriate application of the American Society of Anesthesiologists (ASA) algorithm for difficult airway management (Fig. 16-1).[1]

ANATOMY AND PHYSIOLOGY OF THE UPPER AIRWAY

Nose and Mouth

Air is warmed and humidified as it passes through the nares during normal breathing. Resistance to airflow through the nasal passages is twice that through the mouth and accounts for approximately two thirds of total airway resistance. The ophthalmic and maxillary divisions of the trigeminal nerve (cranial nerve V) provide innervation to the nasal mucosa as the anterior ethmoidal, nasopalatine, and sphenopalatine nerves (Fig. 16-2).[9]

The palatine nerves branch from the sphenopalatine ganglion to innervate the hard and soft palate. The mandibular division of the trigeminal nerve forms the lingual nerve, which provides sensation to the anterior two thirds of the tongue. The posterior third of the tongue, the soft palate, and the oropharynx are innervated by the glossopharyngeal nerve (cranial nerve IX) (Fig. 16-3).[10]

Pharynx

The nasal and oral cavities are connected to the larynx and esophagus by the pharynx. The pharynx is a musculofascial tube that can be divided into the nasopharynx, the oropharynx, and the hypopharynx. The nasopharynx is separated from the oropharynx by the soft palate. The epiglottis demarcates the border between the oropharynx and the hypopharynx. Innervation is by way of cranial nerves IX (glossopharyngeal) and X (vagus) (Figs. 16-4

and 16-5).[11] The vagus nerve provides sensation to the hypopharynx through the internal branches of the superior laryngeal nerves (see Fig. 16-5).[11]

Airway resistance may be increased by prominent lymphoid tissue in the nasopharynx. The tongue is the predominant cause of resistance in the oropharynx. Obstruction by the tongue is increased by relaxation of the genioglossus muscle during anesthesia.

Larynx

The adult larynx is between the third and the sixth cervical vertebrae.[12] It functions in the modulation of sound and separates the trachea from the esophagus during swallowing. This protective mechanism, when exaggerated, becomes laryngospasm. The larynx is composed of muscles, ligaments, and cartilages (thyroid, cricoid, arytenoids, corniculates, and epiglottis). The vocal cords are formed by the thyroarytenoid ligaments and are the narrowest portion of the adult airway. The anterior-posterior dimension of the vocal cords is approximately 23 mm in males and 17 mm in females. The vocal cords are 6 to 9 mm in the transverse plane but can expand to 12 mm. This calculates to a glottic aperture of 60 to 100 mm. An understanding of the motor and sensory innervation of the laryngeal structures is important for performing anesthesia of the upper airway (Table 16-1).

Trachea

The trachea begins at the sixth cervical vertebra and extends to the carina, which overlies the fifth thoracic vertebra. It is 10 to 15 cm long and supported by 16 to 20 horseshoe-shaped cartilages. The most cephalad cartilage, the cricoid, is the only one that has a full ring structure. It is shaped like a signet ring, wider in the cephalocaudal dimension posteriorly.

AIRWAY ASSESSMENT

History and Anatomic Examination

The patient's airway history should be evaluated to determine whether there are any medical, surgical, or anesthetic factors that have implications for airway management. Patients who have had a previous problem with airway management should have been informed of the problem, the apparent reasons for the difficulty, how tracheal intubation was accomplished, and the implication for future anesthetics. The previous anesthetic record should contain a description of the airway difficulties, what airway management techniques were used, and whether they were successful.[1] Patients with a history of difficult airway management can be registered with the Medic Alert system, which allows 24-hour access to the pertinent information.

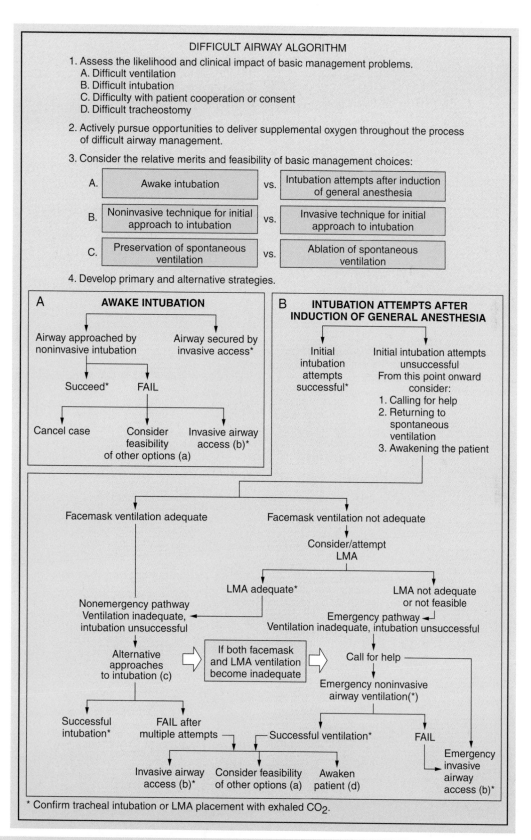

Figure 16-1 Guidelines for management of a difficult airway. LMA, laryngeal mask airway. (From Caplan RA, Benumof JL, Berry FA, et al. Practice guidelines for management of the difficult airway. Anesthesiology 2003;98:1269-1277, used with permission.)

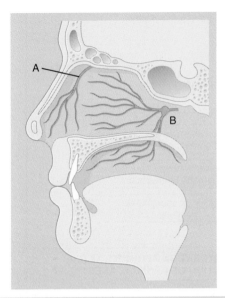

Figure 16-2 Innervation of the nasal cavity. A diagram of the lateral wall of the nasal cavity illustrates its sensory nerve supply. The anterior ethmoidal nerve, a branch of the ophthalmic division of the trigeminal nerve, supplies the anterior third of the septum and lateral wall (A). The maxillary division of the trigeminal nerve via the sphenopalatine ganglion supplies the posterior two thirds of the septum and the lateral wall (B). (From Ovassapian A. Fiberoptic Endoscopy in Anesthesia and Critical Care. New York, Raven Press, 1990, pp 57-79, used with permission.)

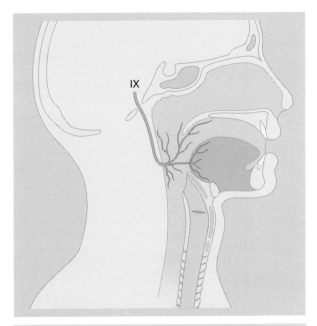

Figure 16-4 Sensory distribution of the glossopharyngeal nerve. (From Patil VU, Stehling LC, Zauder HL. Fiberoptic Endoscopy in Anesthesia. St Louis, CV Mosby, 1983.)

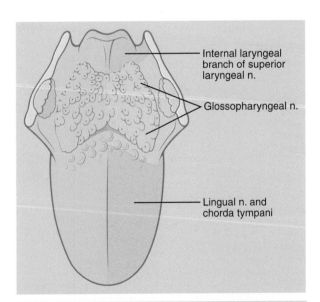

Internal laryngeal branch of superior laryngeal n.

Glossopharyngeal n.

Lingual n. and chorda tympani

Figure 16-3 Sensory innervation of the tongue. (From Stackhouse RA. Fiberoptic airway management. Anesthesiol Clin North Am 2002;20:933-951.)

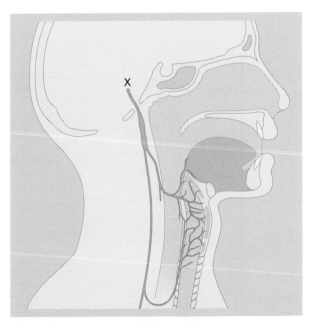

Figure 16-5 Sensory distribution of the vagus nerve. (From Patil VU, Stehling LC, Zauder HL. Fiberoptic Endoscopy in Anesthesia. St Louis, CV Mosby, 1983.)

Table 16-1 Motor and Sensory Innervation of Larynx

Nerve	Sensory	Motor
Superior laryngeal, internal division	Epiglottis Base of tongue Supraglottic mucosa Thyroepiglottic joint Cricothyroid joint	None
Superior laryngeal, external division	Anterior subglottic mucosa	Cricothyroid m.
Recurrent laryngeal	Subglottic mucosa Muscle spindles	Thyroarytenoid m. Lateral cricoarytenoid m. Interarytenoid m. Posterior cricoarytenoid m.

Table 16-2 Components of the Preoperative Airway Physical Examination

Airway Examination Component	Nonreassuring Findings
Length of upper incisors	Relatively long
Relationship of the maxillary and mandibular incisors during normal jaw closure	Prominent overbite (maxillary incisors anterior to the mandibular incisors)
Relationship of the maxillary and mandibular incisors during voluntary protrusion of the mandible	Patient cannot bring the mandibular incisors anterior to (in front of) the maxillary incisors
Interincisor distance	Less than 3 cm
Visibility of the uvula	Not visible when the tongue is protruded with the patient in a sitting position (Mallampati class higher than II)
Shape of the palate	Highly arched or very narrow
Compliance of the mandibular space	Stiff, indurated, occupied by a mass, or nonresilient
Thyromental distance	Less than three fingerbreadths
Length of the neck	Short
Thickness of the neck	Thick
Range of motion of the head and neck	Patient cannot touch the tip of the chin to the chest or cannot extend the neck

Studies of anatomic variables and their implications for difficult airway management have shown that there is low sensitivity, specificity, and positive predictive value for any single test (Table 16-2),[13] however, correlation is better with a combination of tests.[6,7] These tests are based on examination of the oropharyngeal space, neck mobility, submandibular space, and submandibular compliance. Various congenital and acquired disease states have a correlation with difficult airway management (Tables 16-3 and 16-4).

OROPHARYNGEAL SPACE

Mallampati proposed a classification system (Mallampati score) to correlate the oropharyngeal space with the ease of direct laryngoscopy and tracheal intubation.[14] With the observer at eye level, the patient holds the head in a neutral position, opens the mouth maximally, and protrudes the tongue without phonating. The airway is classified according to the visible structures (Fig. 16-6).[15]

Class I: The soft palate, fauces, uvula, and tonsillar pillars are visible.
Class II: The soft palate, fauces, and uvula are visible.
Class III: The soft palate and base of the uvula are visible.
Class IV: The soft palate is not visible.

There is a correlation between the Mallampati score, what can be seen on direct laryngoscopy, and the ease of intubation. The laryngoscopic view is classified according to the Cormack and Lehane score (Fig. 16-7).[16,17]

Grade I: Most of the glottis is visible.
Grade II: Only the posterior portion of the glottis is visible.
Grade III: The epiglottis, but no part of the glottis, can be seen.
Grade IV: No airway structures are visualized.

Table 16-3 Congenital Syndromes Associated with Difficult Endotracheal Intubation

Syndrome	Description
Trisomy 21	Large tongue, small mouth make laryngoscopy difficult Small subglottic diameter possible Laryngospasm is common
Goldenhar (oculoauriculovertebral anomalies)	Mandibular hypoplasia and cervical spine abnormality make laryngoscopy difficult
Klippel-Feil	Neck rigidity because of cervical vertebral fusion
Pierre Robin	Small mouth, large tongue, mandibular anomaly
Treacher Collins (mandibular dysostosis)	Laryngoscopy is difficult
Turner	High likelihood of difficult tracheal intubation

III

Table 16-4 Pathologic States That Influence Airway Management

Pathologic State	Difficulty
Epiglottitis (infectious)	Laryngoscopy may worsen obstruction
Abscess (submandibular retropharyngeal, Ludwig's angina)	Distortion of the airway renders facemask ventilation or tracheal intubation extremely difficult
Croup, bronchitis, pneumonia	Airway irritability with a tendency for cough, laryngospasm, bronchospasm
Papillomatosis	Airway obstruction
Tetanus	Trismus renders oral tracheal intubation impossible
Traumatic foreign body	Airway obstruction
Cervical spine injury	Neck manipulation may traumatize the spinal cord
Basilar skull fracture	Nasotracheal intubation attempts may result in intracranial tube placement
Maxillary or mandibular injury	Airway obstruction, difficult facemask ventilation and tracheal intubation Cricothyroidotomy may be necessary with combined injuries
Laryngeal fracture	Airway obstruction may worsen during instrumentation Endotracheal tube may be misplaced outside the larynx and worsen the injury
Laryngeal edema (after intubation)	Irritable airway Narrowed laryngeal inlet
Soft tissue neck injury (edema, bleeding, subcutaneous emphysema)	Anatomic distortion of the upper airway Airway obstruction
Neoplastic upper airway tumors (pharynx, larynx)	Inspiratory obstruction with spontaneous ventilation
Lower airway tumors (trachea, bronchi, mediastinum)	Airway obstruction may not be relieved by tracheal intubation Lower airway is distorted
Radiation therapy	Fibrosis may distort the airway or make manipulation difficult
Inflammatory rheumatoid arthritis	Mandibular hypoplasia, temporomandibular joint arthritis, immobile cervical vertebrae, laryngeal rotation, and cricoarytenoid arthritis make tracheal intubation difficult
Ankylosing spondylitis	Fusion of the cervical spine may render direct laryngoscopy impossible
Temporomandibular joint syndrome	Severe impairment of mouth opening
Scleroderma	Tight skin and temporomandibular joint involvement make mouth opening difficult
Sarcoidosis	Airway obstruction (lymphoid tissue)
Angioedema	Obstructive swelling renders ventilation and tracheal intubation difficult
Endocrine or metabolic acromegaly	Large tongue Bony overgrowths
Diabetes mellitus	May have decreased mobility of the atlanto-occipital joint
Hypothyroidism	Large tongue and abnormal soft tissue (myxedema) make ventilation and tracheal intubation difficult
Thyromegaly	Goiter may produce extrinsic airway compression or deviation
Obesity	Upper airway obstruction with loss of consciousness Tissue mass makes successful facemask ventilation difficult

In conjunction with the Mallampati classification, the interincisor gap, the size and position of the maxillary and mandibular teeth, and the conformation of the palate should be assessed.[1] An interincisor gap of less than 3 to 4.5 cm correlates with difficulty achieving a line of view on direct laryngoscopy.[7,18,19] Maxillary prominence or a receding mandible also correlates with a poor laryngoscopic view. Overbite results in a reduction in the effective interincisor gap when the patient's head and neck are optimally positioned for direct laryngoscopy.

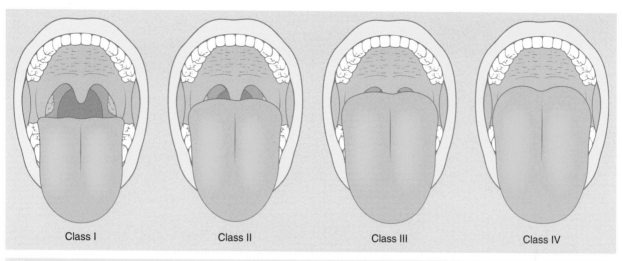

Figure 16-6 Mallampati classification. (From Samsoon GLT, Young JRB. Difficult tracheal intubation: A retrospective study. Anaesthesia 1987;42:487-490, used with permission.)

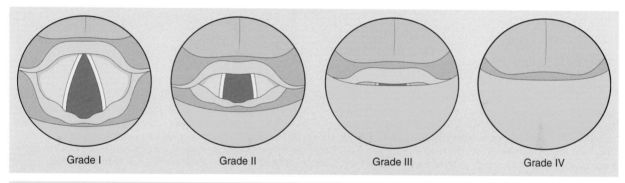

Figure 16-7 Four grades of laryngoscopic view. Grade I is visualization of the entire laryngeal aperture, grade II is visualization of just the posterior portion of the laryngeal aperture, grade III is visualization of only the epiglottis, and grade IV is visualization of just the soft palate. (From Cormack RS, Lehane J. Difficult tracheal intubation in obstetrics. Anaesthesia 1984;39:1105-1111; and Williams KN, Carli F, Cormack RS. Unexpected, difficult laryngoscopy: A prospective survey in routine general surgery. Br J Anaesth 1991;66:38-44, used with permission.)

Micrognathia limits the pharyngeal space (tongue positioned more posterior) and the space in which the soft tissues are going to be displaced during direct laryngoscopy. This causes the glottic structures to be anterior to the line of vision during direct laryngoscopy. Various genetic syndromes and acquired disease states limit the pharyngeal space and are difficult to assess on physical examination.

The extent of an individuals' ability to prognath the mandible is another correlate of the visualization of glottic structures on direct laryngoscopy. The upper lip bite test (ULBT) classification system is as follows:

Class I: Lower incisors can bite above the vermilion border of the upper lip.
Class II: Lower incisors cannot reach vermilion border.
Class III: Lower incisors cannot bite upper lip.[7,19]

ATLANTO-OCCIPITAL EXTENSION/NECK MOBILITY

Flexion of the neck, by elevating the head approximately 10 cm, aligns the laryngeal and pharyngeal axes. Extension of the head on the atlanto-occipital joint is important for aligning the oral and pharyngeal axes to obtain a line of vision during direct laryngoscopy (Fig. 16-8). These maneuvers place the head in the "sniffing" position and bring the three axes into optimal alignment. Atlanto-occipital extension is quantified by the angle traversed by the occlusal surface of the maxillary teeth when the head is fully extended from the neutral position. More than 30% limitation of atlanto-occipital joint extension from a norm of 35 degrees, or less than 80 degrees of extension/flexion, is associated with an increased incidence of difficult tracheal intubation.[19,20]

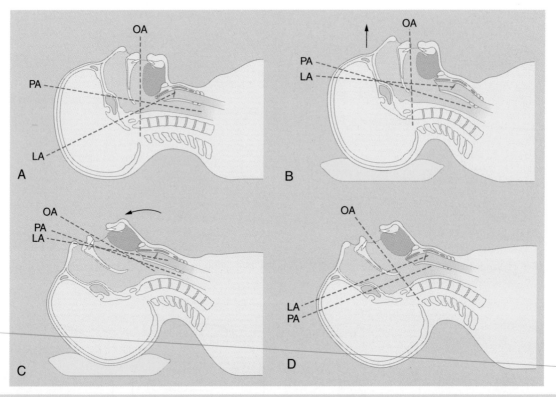

Figure 16-8 Schematic diagram showing alignment of the oral axis (OA), pharyngeal axis (PA), and laryngeal axis (LA) in four different head positions. Each head position is accompanied by an inset that magnifies the upper airway (the oral cavity, pharynx, and larynx) and superimposes, as a variously bent bold dotted line, the continuity of these three axes with the upper airway. **A,** The head is in a neutral position with a marked degree of nonalignment of the OA, PA, and LA. **B,** The head is resting on a large pad that flexes the neck on the chest and the LA with the PA. **C,** The head is resting on a pad (which flexes the neck on the chest) with concomitant extension of the head on the neck, which brings all three axes into alignment (sniffing position). **D,** Extension of the head on the neck without concomitant elevation of the head.

THYROMENTAL/STERNOMENTAL DISTANCE

A thyromental distance (mentum to thyroid cartilage) less than 6 to 7 cm correlates with a poor laryngoscopic view. This is typically seen in patients with a receding mandible or a short neck. It creates a more acute angle between the oral and pharyngeal axes and limits the ability to bring them into alignment. This distance is often estimated in fingerbreadths. Three ordinary fingerbreadths approximate this distance. If the sternomental distance is used, it should measure more than 12.5 to 13.5 cm.[4,6,7]

SUBMANDIBULAR COMPLIANCE

The submandibular space is the area into which the soft tissues of the pharynx must be displaced to obtain a line of vision during direct laryngoscopy. Anything that limits the size of this space or compliance of the tissue will decrease the amount of anterior displacement that can be achieved. Ludwig's angina, tumors, radiation scarring, burns, and previous neck surgery are conditions that can decrease submandibular compliance.[1]

BODY HABITUS

Obesity has been associated with an increased incidence of difficult airway management. Proper positioning, with a wedge-shaped bolster behind the patient's back, results in a more optimal sniffing position. However, the problem of decreased functional residual capacity (FRC) with subsequent decreased time to arterial oxygen desaturation and more difficult mask ventilation secondary to decreased compliance still persist.[1,13]

Cricothyroid Membrane and Cricothyrotomy

When routine airway management techniques have failed, the end point of the ASA difficult airway algorithm is to attain airway control by emergency invasive access (see Fig. 16-1).[1] The devices that are available for these emergency techniques are designed for accessing the airway through the cricothyroid membrane (cricothyrotomy). The cricothyroid membrane can be identified by first locating the thyroid cartilage and then sliding the fingers down the neck to the membrane, which lies just below. Alternatively, in patients who do not have a prominent thyroid cartilage, identification of the cricoid cartilage can be achieved by beginning palpation of the neck at the sternal notch and sliding the fingers up the neck until a cartilage that is wider and higher (cricoid cartilage) than those below is felt.

AIRWAY MANAGEMENT TECHNIQUES

Ventilation with a Facemask

Much attention has focused on devices to obviate the problem of difficult tracheal intubation. Failure to place an endotracheal tube is not the actual cause of the severe adverse outcomes related to difficult airway management. The primary problem is an inability to oxygenate, ventilate, prevent aspiration, or a combination of these factors. Prospectively identifying patients at risk for difficult facemask ventilation, ensuring the ability to ventilate the patient's lungs before administering longer-acting anesthetics and neuromuscular blocking drugs, and developing proficient facemask ventilation skills are critical to the practice of anesthesia.

PREDICTORS OF DIFFICULT FACEMASK VENTILATION

Independent variables associated with difficult facemask ventilation are (1) age older than 55 years, (2) a body mass index greater than 26 kg/m^2, (3) a beard, (4) lack of teeth, (5) a history of snoring, (6) repeated attempts at laryngoscopy, (7) Mallampati class III to IV, (8) neck radiation, (9) male gender, and (10) limited ability to protrude the mandible.[2-4,21,22] Advancing age, obesity, multiple laryngoscopies, Mallampati class III to IV, neck radiation, and snoring are indicators of decreased compliance and increased resistance during facemask ventilation. An appropriately sized facemask and oral or nasal airways may help mitigate these factors. A beard or lack of teeth may result in an inability to develop adequate positive pressure with the anesthesia breathing circuit. With the caveat that the patient's dentures are well adhered, allowing the teeth to be left in during induction of anesthesia may be advantageous. Alternatively, an oral airway will often give enough structure to the oral tissues to allow facemask ventilation in edentulous patients.

FACEMASK CHARACTERISTICS

Facemasks are available in a variety of sizes. Clear masks have the benefit of allowing visualization of fogging, skin color, and signs of regurgitation. The facemask should fit over the bridge of the nose with the upper border aligned with the pupils. The sides should seal just lateral to the nasolabial folds, and the bottom of the facemask should seat between the lower lip and the chin. Most facemasks come with a hooked rim around the 15- to 22-mm fitting that attaches to the anesthesia breathing circuit. This rim allows straps to be used to hold the facemask in place when a patient is breathing spontaneously or to improve the seal during mask ventilation.

TECHNIQUE

Prior to induction of anesthesia, breathing 100% O_2 allows for a prolonged duration of apnea without desaturation (DAWD). The minute ventilation for oxygen ($M\dot{V}O_2$) in an adult with an ideal body weight is approximately 3 mL/kg/min. DAWD is a function of the $M\dot{V}O_2$ and the oxygen reservoir of the function residual capacity (FRC), approximately 30 to 35 mL/kg. Several techniques of breathing oxygen at the beginning of anesthesia exist with the goal of achieving an end tidal oxygen level above 90%. Three minutes of tidal volume breathing of 100% O_2 has been found to be superior to four deep breaths in 30 seconds. Eight deep breaths in 60 seconds is equivalent to breathing 100% oxygen for 3 minutes. A patient who is not obese and has no pulmonary dysfunction can maintain a Sao_2 more than 90% for approximately 8.5 minutes. Obesity can severely decrease the DAWD. Breathing 100% oxygen in a 25- to 90-degree head-up position as well as 10 cm of continuous positive airway pressure (CPAP) followed by pressure mode ventilation (peak pressure 14 cm, positive end-expiratory pressure [PEEP] 10 cm) increase the DAWD (45 to 50 sec above a baseline of 2 to 2.5 min) in obese patients by decreasing atelectasis and improving ventilation perfusion matching.[22-24]

The facemask should be held to the patient's face with the fingers of the anesthesia provider's left hand lifting the mandible (chin lift, jaw thrust) to the facemask. Pressure on the submandibular soft tissue should be avoided because it can cause airway obstruction. The anesthesia provider's left thumb and index finger apply counter pressure on the facemask. Displacement of the mandible, atlanto-occipital joint extension, chin lift, and jaw thrust combine to maximize the pharyngeal space. Differential application of pressure with individual fingers can improve the seal attained with the facemask. The anesthesia provider's right hand is used to generate positive pressure by compressing the reservoir bag of the anesthesia breathing circuit. Ventilating pressure should be less than 20 cm H_2O to avoid insufflation of the stomach.

In instances in which the airway cannot be maintained with only one hand on the facemask, a two- or three-handed facemask technique can be used (Fig. 16-9). If not trained in airway management, the assistant can help by squeezing the reservoir bag while the anesthesia provider uses the right hand to mirror the hand position of the left and improve the facemask seal. When the second person is skilled in airway management, the primary provider maintains the standard hand position and the assistant uses both hands to generate an optimal seal.

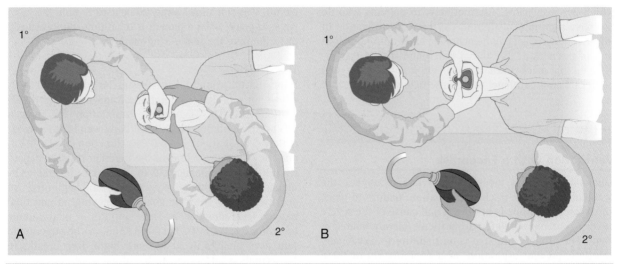

Figure 16-9 Optimal facemask ventilation. **A,** Two-person effort when the second person knows how to perform a jaw thrust. **B,** Two-person effort when the second person can only squeeze the reservoir bag. (From Benumof J. Airway Management Principles and Practice. St. Louis, Mosby-Year Book, 1996, pp 143-156.)

AIRWAY ADJUNCTS

Airway adjuncts should be used if it is difficult to generate sufficient positive pressure for adequate ventilation with the anesthesia breathing circuit. Oral and nasal airways are designed to create an air passage by displacing the tongue from the posterior pharyngeal wall. Aligning the airway with the patient's profile and approximating the anatomic path that it will take can be used to estimate the appropriate size. The distal tip of the airway should be at the angle of the mandible when the proximal end is just anterior to the mouth (oral airway) or the nose (nasal airway). An oral airway may generate a gag reflex or cause laryngospasm in an awake or lightly anesthetized patient. Nasal airways are better tolerated at lighter planes of anesthesia. However, nasal airways are relatively contraindicated in patients with coagulation or platelet abnormalities and those with basilar skull fractures.

Endotracheal Intubation

Endotracheal intubation may be considered in every patient receiving general anesthesia (Table 16-5). Orotracheal intubation by direct laryngoscopy in anesthetized patients is routinely chosen unless specific circumstances

Table 16-5 Indications for Endotracheal Intubation

- Provide a patent airway
- Prevent inhalation (aspiration) of gastric contents
- Need for frequent suctioning
- Facilitate positive-pressure ventilation of the lungs
- Operative position other than supine
- Operative site near or involving the upper airway
- Airway maintenance by mask difficult

dictate a different approach. Equipment and drugs used for tracheal intubation include a properly sized endotracheal tube, laryngoscope, functioning suction catheter, appropriate anesthetic drugs, and equipment for providing positive-pressure ventilation of the lungs with oxygen.

Elevation of the patient's head 8 to 10 cm with pads under the occiput (shoulders remaining on the table) and extension of the head at the atlanto-occipital joint serve to align the oral, pharyngeal, and laryngeal axes such that the passage and line of vision from the lips to the glottic opening are most nearly a straight line. The height of the operating table should be adjusted so that the patient's face is near the level of the standing anesthesia provider's xiphoid cartilage. If not opened by extension of the head, the patient's mouth may be manually opened by counter pressure of the right thumb on the mandibular teeth and right index finger on the maxillary teeth. Simultaneously with insertion of the laryngoscope blade, the patient's lower lip can be rolled away with the anesthesia provider's left index finger to prevent bruising by the laryngoscope blade.

CRICOID PRESSURE

Cricoid pressure (Sellick's maneuver) can be applied by an assistant exerting downward external pressure with the thumb and index finger on the cricoid cartilage to displace the cartilaginous cricothyroid ring posteriorly and thus compress the underlying esophagus against the cervical vertebrae (Fig. 16-10). Conceptually, this maneuver should prevent spillage of gastric contents into the pharynx during the period from induction of anesthesia (unconsciousness) to successful placement of a cuffed endotracheal tube. The magnitude of downward external pressure (30 newtons, approximately 3 kg, is recommended) that needs to be

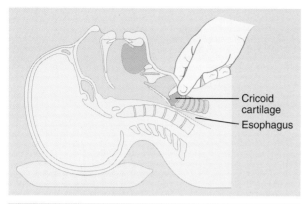

Figure 16-10 Cricoid pressure is provided by an assistant exerting downward pressure with the thumb and index finger on the cricoid cartilage (approximately 5-kg pressure) so that the cartilaginous cricothyroid ring is displaced posteriorly and the esophagus is thus compressed (occluded) against the underlying cervical vertebrae.

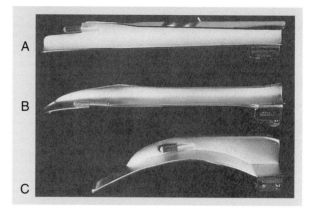

Figure 16-11 Examples of detachable laryngoscope blades that can be used interchangeably on the same handle, including a straight blade (**A**), a straight blade with a curved distal tip (**B**), and a curved blade (**C**).

exerted on the cricoid cartilage to reliably occlude the esophagus is difficult to judge. Furthermore, stimulation of the pharynx, by external pressure on the cricoid cartilage, may evoke an upper airway reflex characterized by a decrease in lower esophageal sphincter pressure, which could favor the passage of gastric contents into the esophagus.[25] For this reason, cricoid pressure probably should be applied before the induction of anesthesia in selected patients. Although the application of cricoid pressure is often performed, aspiration of gastric contents still has occurred during such application. The efficacy of cricoid pressure is not clear.[26] Furthermore, downward external pressure on the cricoid cartilage may displace the esophagus laterally rather than resulting in compression of the esophagus.[27]

USE OF THE LARYNGOSCOPE

The laryngoscope consists of a battery-containing handle to which blades with a light (bulb or fiberoptic) may be attached and removed interchangeably (Fig. 16-11). The laryngoscope is held in the anesthesia provider's left hand near the junction between the handle and blade of the laryngoscope. The blade is then inserted on the right side of the patient's mouth so that the incisor teeth are avoided and the tongue is deflected to the left, away from the lumen of the blade. Pressure on the teeth or gums must be avoided as the blade is advanced forward and centrally toward the epiglottis. The anesthesia provider's wrist is held rigid as the laryngoscope is lifted along the axis of the handle to cause anterior displacement of the soft tissues and bring the laryngeal structures into view. The handle should not be rotated as it is lifted to prevent using the patient's upper teeth or gums as a fulcrum with the blade of the laryngoscope as a lever.

Curved (Macintosh) Blade

The tip of the curved blade is advanced into the space between the base of the tongue and the pharyngeal surface of the epiglottis (Fig. 16-12A). Forward and upward movement of the blade exerted along the axis of the laryngoscope handle stretches the hyoepiglottic ligament, elevates the epiglottis, and exposes the glottic opening.

Straight (Miller) Blade

The tip of the straight blade is passed beneath the laryngeal surface of the epiglottis (see Fig. 16-12B). Forward and upward movement of the blade exerted along the axis of the laryngoscope handle directly elevates the epiglottis to expose the glottic opening. Depression or lateral movement of the patient's thyroid cartilage externally on the neck (known as optimal external laryngeal manipulation [OELM] or backward upward rightward pressure [BURP]) with the laryngoscopist's right hand may facilitate exposure of the glottic opening.[4]

Flex Tip (Heine, CLM) Blade

This blade is similar to a Macintosh blade, but it has a hinged tip that is controlled by a lever that is triggered with the thumb of the anesthesia provider's left hand during direct laryngoscopy. The laryngoscope is inserted into the vallecula, and then the lever is deployed to increase the lift on the hyoepiglottic ligament.

Choice of Laryngoscope Blade

The choice of laryngoscope blade is often based on personal preference. Advantages cited for the curved blade include less trauma to teeth with more room for passage of the endotracheal tube and less bruising of the epiglottis because the tip of the blade does not directly lift this structure. The advantage cited for the straight blade is better exposure of the glottic opening. Laryngoscope

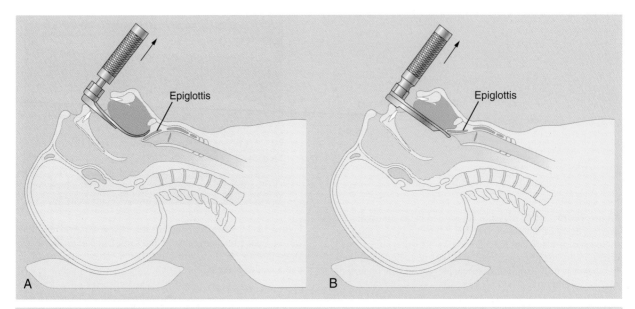

Figure 16-12 Schematic diagram depicting the proper position of the laryngoscope blade for exposure of the glottic opening. **A,** The distal end of the curved blade is advanced into the space between the base of the tongue and the pharyngeal surface of the epiglottis. **B,** The distal end of the straight blade is advanced beneath the laryngeal surface of the epiglottis. Regardless of blade design, forward and upward movement exerted along the axis of the laryngoscope handle, as denoted by the arrows, serves to elevate the epiglottis and expose the glottic opening.

blades are numbered according to their length. A Macintosh 3 or 4 blade or a Miller 2 or 3 blade is the standard intubating blade for adult patients.

ENDOTRACHEAL TUBE SIZES

Endotracheal tube sizes are specified according to their internal diameter (ID), which is marked on each tube (Table 16-6). Tracheal tubes are available in 0.5-mm ID increments. The endotracheal tube also has lengthwise centimeter markings starting at the distal tracheal end to permit accurate determination of the length inserted past the patient's lips. Tracheal tubes are most often made of clear, inert polyvinyl chloride plastic that molds to the contour of the airway after softening on exposure to body temperature. Tracheal tube material should also be radiopaque to ascertain the position of the distal tip relative to the carina and be transparent to permit visualization of secretions or airflow as evidenced by condensation of water vapor in the lumen of the tube ("breath fogging") during exhalation.

Table 16-6 Endotracheal Tube, Suction Catheter, and Stylet Size Based on Age and Weight

Age (yr)	Weight (kg)	Endotracheal Tube ID (mm)	Suction Catheter (French)	Stylet (French)
Premature	<1.5	2.5	6	6
Premature	1.5-2.5	3.0	6	6
Newborn	3.5	3.5	8	6
1	10	4.0	8	6
2-3	15	4.5	10	6
4-6	20	5.0	10	10
7-9	30	5.5	12	10
10-12	40	6.0	14	10
13-15	50	6.5	14	14
>16	>60	7.0	18	14

ID, internal diameter.

TECHNIQUE

The endotracheal tube is held in the anesthesia provider's right hand like a pencil and introduced into the right side of the patient's mouth with the natural curve directed anteriorly. It should be advanced toward the glottis from the right side of the mouth as midline insertion usually obscures visualization of the glottic opening. The tube is advanced until the proximal end of the cuff is 1 to 2 cm past the vocal cords, which should place the distal end of the tube midway between the vocal cords and carina. At this point, the laryngoscope blade is removed from the patient's mouth. The cuff of the endotracheal tube is inflated with air to create a seal against the tracheal mucosa. This seal facilitates positive-pressure ventilation of the lungs and decreases the likelihood of aspiration of pharyngeal or gastric contents. Use of the minimum volume of air in a low-pressure high-volume cuff that prevents leaks during positive ventilation pressure (20 to 30 cm H_2O) minimizes the likelihood of mucosal ischemia resulting from prolonged pressure on the tracheal wall. Nevertheless, all aspects of tracheal intubation can produce some type of laryngotracheal damage. For example, ciliary denudation has been found to occur predominantly over the tracheal rings and underlying the cuff site after only 2 hours of intubation and with tracheal wall pressure below 25 mm Hg.[28] Other serious complications attributable to endotracheal cuff pressures include tracheal stenosis, tracheal rupture, tracheoesophageal fistula, tracheocarotid fistula, and tracheoinnominate artery fistula.[29] After confirmation of correct placement (end-tidal CO_2, auscultation for bilateral breath sounds, ballottement of cuff in the suprasternal notch), the endotracheal tube is secured in position with tape.

ENDOTRACHEAL TUBE STYLETS

A variety of endotracheal tube stylets may be used in selected patients to facilitate endotracheal intubation.

Gum Elastic Bougie

A gum elastic bougie is a 60 cm long, 15-French stylet with a 40-degree curve approximately 3.5 cm from the distal tip. It has been used successfully in patients with a poor laryngoscopic view. It is passed under the epiglottis and into the airway. A characteristic bumping or clicking is felt in 90% of tracheal placements as the bougie is advanced down the tracheal cartilages, but not felt at all in esophageal placements. The bougie will typically stop at 24 to 40 cm when it enters the smaller bronchi.[4]

Schroeder Stylet

The Schroeder stylet is a disposable, plastic articulating stylet that allows the angle of the endotracheal tube to be adjusted to the correct angle while performing direct laryngoscopy and tracheal intubation. It can be used for both oral and nasal intubation.

Frova Intubating Introducer

The Frova Intubating Introducer is a 65-cm stylet with a distal angulated tip and an internal channel to accommodate a stiffening stylet or allow jet ventilation. It is available in adult and pediatric sizes (Fig. 16-13).[30]

Lighted Stylets

Lighted stylets (lightwands) consist of a malleable stylet with a light at the distal tip. The endotracheal tube is mounted on the stylet, and a "hockey stick" curve is placed in the distal third of the tube (Table 16-7, Fig. 16-14).[30] The assembled device is advanced in the midline of the airway until a well-circumscribed glow is seen through the anterior surface of the neck. As the device is advanced

III

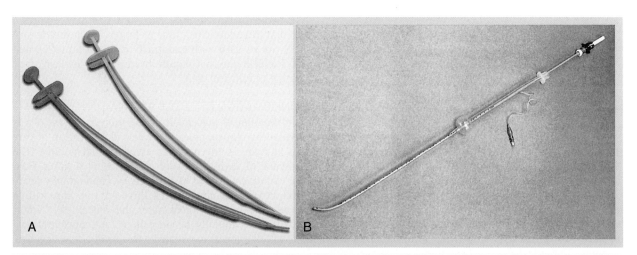

Figure 16-13 A, The Schroeder directional stylet (courtesy of Parker Medical, Englewood, CO) and **B,** the Frova Intubating Introducer (courtesy of Cook Critical Care, Bloomington, IN). (From Hagberg CA. Special devices and techniques. Anesthesiol Clin North Am 2002;20:907-932.)

Table 16-7 Lighted Stylets (Lightwands) Appropriate for Endotracheal Tube Size

Tracheal Tube Size—ID (mm)	Trachlight (Laerdal)	Intubating Fiberoptic Stylette (Sun Medical)	Fiberoptic Malleable Lighted Stylet (Anesthesia Associates)
2.5	—	—	—
3.0	Infant	—	Pediatric
3.5	Infant	—	Pediatric
4.0	Infant	Pediatric	Pediatric
4.5	Child	Pediatric	Pediatric
5.0	Child	Pediatric	Adult
5.5	Child	Adult	Adult
6.0	Adult	Adult	Adult
6.5	Adult	Adult	Adult
7.0	Adult	Adult	Adult
7.5	Adult	Adult	Adult

ID, internal diameter.

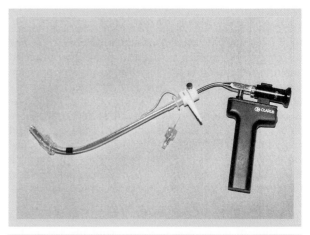

Figure 16-15 Seeing Optical Stylet system (courtesy of Clarus Medical, Minneapolis, MN).

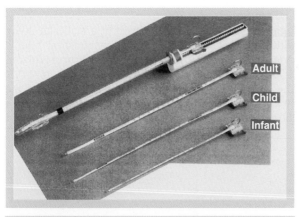

Figure 16-14 Trachlight (courtesy of Laerdal Medical Corp., Long Beach, CA). (From Hagberg CA. Special devices and techniques. Anesthesiol Clin North Am 2002;20:907-932.)

further, the light should remain distinct as it is observed to travel down the neck and until it disappears under the sternal notch. A diffuse glow indicates that there is more soft tissue being transilluminated and the device is in the esophagus rather than the trachea.

Lighted stylets do not require movement of the head or neck and can be used in patients with limited mouth opening. These devices have been useful in patients with cervical spine instability, limited interincisor gap, poor dentition, severe overbite, and facial trauma. Lighted stylets are relatively contraindicated in patients with oropharyngeal pathology (laryngeal fractures, pharyngeal masses or abscesses, foreign body) because they are passed blindly and may cause damage. There is a more frequent failure rate when lighted stylets are used in patients with thick necks and dark skin.[30]

Seeing Optical Stylet

The Seeing Optical Stylet (SOS) is a semimalleable, stainless steel high-resolution fiberoptic endoscope that is available in adult and pediatric sizes (Fig. 16-15).[30] The endotracheal tube is mounted on the SOS, and it is advanced through the upper airway just as a lighted stylet. The SOS offers the advantage of visualization of the airway structures as it is advanced. As with any fiberoptic scope, the view is dependent on the amount of space that is present. Maneuvers that increase the pharyngeal space (chin lift, jaw thrust, tongue traction) improve the field of view when using the SOS. The adult-size SOS requires a 5.5 mm ID endotracheal tube or larger. The pediatric-size SOS can be used with endotracheal tubes 3.0 to 5.0 mm ID. The SOS does not require head or neck movement or a large interincisor gap.

CONFIRMATION OF ENDOTRACHEAL INTUBATION

Confirmation of placement of the tube in the trachea is verified by clinical assessment and identification of carbon dioxide in the patient's exhaled tidal volume. The presence of carbon dioxide in the exhaled gases from the endotracheal tube as detected by capnography (end-tidal $Pco_2 > 30$ mm Hg for three to five consecutive breaths) should be immediate and sustained. Carbon dioxide may initially be present in low concentrations, but will not persist in exhaled gases from a tube accidentally placed in the esophagus.

Symmetrical bilateral movement of the chest with manual ventilation, combined with the presence of bilateral breath sounds on apical or midaxillary auscultation of the lungs is confirmed after tracheal intubation. A characteristic feel of the reservoir bag, associated with normal lung compliance during manual inflation of the lungs and the presence of expiratory refilling of the bag, is evaluated. Condensation of water in the tube lumen (breath fogging) during exhalation is evidence of tracheal placement of the tube. Progressive decreases in arterial hemoglobin oxygen saturation as evident on the pulse oximeter may alert the anesthesia provider to a previously unrecognized esophageal intubation.

FIBEROPTIC ENDOTRACHEAL INTUBATION
Indications
Fiberoptic endotracheal intubation is most frequently chosen when a difficult tracheal intubation by direct laryngoscopy is anticipated. This technique is suited to these situations because it can be performed before inducing general anesthesia, thus eliminating the risk of failed tracheal intubation and failed ventilation in anesthetized patients.

Fiberoptic endotracheal intubation is recommended for patients with unstable cervical spines. The technique does not require movement of the patient's neck and can be performed before induction of general anesthesia, thereby allowing for evaluation of the patient's neurologic function after tracheal intubation and surgical positioning.

Patients who have sustained an injury to the upper airway from either blunt or penetrating trauma are at risk for the endotracheal tube creating a false passage by exiting the airway through the disrupted tissue during direct laryngoscopy. By performing a fiberoptic intubation, not only can the injury be assessed, but the tracheal tube can also be placed beyond the level of the injury and thus eliminate the risk of causing subcutaneous emphysema, which could compress and further compromise the airway.

Contraindications
An absolute contraindication to fiberoptic endotracheal intubation is a lack of time. The technique requires time to set up the equipment and prepare the patient's airway for tracheal intubation. Therefore, if immediate airway management is required, another technique should be used.

A number of circumstances make fiberoptic endotracheal intubation relatively contraindicated because the chance of success is diminished or it poses certain risks for the patient. Because the field of vision through a fiberoptic bronchoscope (laryngoscope) depends on the presence of space around the scope, anything that impinges on upper airway size (edema of the pharynx or tongue, infection, hematoma, infiltrating masses) will make tracheal intubation more difficult. Inflating the cuff of the endotracheal tube to hold the pharyngeal walls open may be helpful. Blood and secretions easily soil the optics of a fiberoptic bronchoscope. An inability to keep the tip

clean will result in failure. Administering an antisialagogue to the patient before initiating fiberoptic intubation, suctioning, and maintaining the pharyngeal space can minimize soiling. Another relative contraindication to fiberoptic intubation is the presence of a pharyngeal abscess, which could be disrupted as the endotracheal tube is advanced and result in aspiration of purulent material.

Technique
Fiberoptic tracheal intubation may be performed through an oral or nasal approach, with the patient awake or anesthetized. In general, the nasal route is easier because the angle of curvature of the endotracheal tube naturally approximates that of the patient's upper airway. When performing an oral fiberoptic tracheal intubation, a more anterior curvature is required, which may be accomplished by using one of the commercially available intubating oral airways. Nasal fiberoptic tracheal intubation tends to be less of a stimulus for the gag reflex. The gag reflex can be overcome with adequate topical anesthesia and local anesthetic blocks. The risk of inducing bleeding is higher when the nasal route is used, however, and therefore relatively contraindicated in patients with platelet abnormalities or coagulation disorders. Oral fiberoptic tracheal intubation is preferable in patients who have a contraindication to the vasoconstrictors required for nasal intubation (pregnant women, some patients with heart disease).

The decision to perform fiberoptic tracheal intubation in an awake versus an anesthetized patient is dependent on the risk of losing airway control. It is usually safest to maintain spontaneous breathing if there is a question about the ability to manage the patient's airway.

Patient Preparation
The procedure should be explained to the patient along with assurance that the patient will be made as comfortable as possible. An antisialagogue (glycopyrrolate, 0.2 mg IV) should be administered to inhibit the formation of secretions that can obscure fiberoptic visualization. Sedation choices are numerous, but the depth of sedation should be titrated to reflect individual patient needs, with the caveat that the more tenuous the airway, the less sedation administered. Appropriate nerve blocks are then performed, and topical antibiotics are applied.

Nose and Nasopharynx
The nasal mucosa must be anesthetized and vasoconstricted, which is typically done with either a 4% cocaine solution or a combination of 3% lidocaine and 0.25% phenylephrine. Local anesthetic solutions can be applied on soaked cotton-tipped swabs or pledgets.

Tongue and Oropharynx
Topicalization may be achieved by aerosolized local anesthetic or bilateral blocks of the glossopharyngeal nerve at the base of each anterior tonsillar pillar may be performed.

Approximately 2 mL of 2% lidocaine injected at a depth of 0.5 cm is sufficient to block the glossopharyngeal nerves. Aspiration with the syringe before injecting the local anesthetic solution is necessary to ensure that the needle is not intravascular or through the tonsillar pillar.

Larynx and Trachea

Topicalization or nerve blocks may be used for the larynx and trachea. Local anesthetic may be sprayed, aerosolized, or nebulized into the airway. It should be noted that the larger particle size of a spray tends to cause it to be deposited in the pharynx, with only a small proportion reaching the trachea. Conversely, the small particle size of a nebulized spray is carried more effectively into the trachea, but also into the smaller airways, where the anesthetic is not needed and undergoes more rapid systemic absorption. Lidocaine is the preferred topical local anesthetic because of its broad therapeutic window. Benzocaine can cause methemoglobinemia even in therapeutic doses. Tetracaine has a very narrow therapeutic window, and the maximum allowable dose (1.2 mg/kg) can easily be exceeded. Cetacaine is a mixture of benzocaine and tetracaine and has the disadvantages of each local anesthetic.

Superior Laryngeal Nerve Block

Injecting local anesthetic solution bilaterally, in the vicinity of the superior laryngeal nerves where they lie between the greater cornu of the hyoid bone and the superior cornu of the thyroid cartilage as they traverse the thyrohyoid membrane to the submucosa of the piriform sinus, blocks the internal branch of the superior laryngeal nerve. The overlying skin is cleaned with alcohol or povidone-iodine (Betadine). The cornua of the hyoid bone or the thyroid cartilage may be used as a landmark. A 22- to 25-gauge needle is "walked" off the cephalad edge of the thyroid cartilage or the caudal edge of the hyoid bone, and approximately 2 mL of local anesthetic solution is injected.

Transtracheal Block

For a transtracheal block, the skin is prepared and a 20-gauge IV catheter is advanced through the cricothyroid membrane while simultaneously aspirating with an attached syringe filled with 4 mL of local anesthetic solution. When air is aspirated, the catheter is advanced into the trachea and the needle is withdrawn. The syringe is reattached to the catheter, aspiration of air is reconfirmed, and the local anesthetic solution is rapidly injected.

FLEXIBLE FIBEROPTIC LARYNGOSCOPY

Fiberoptic laryngoscopy has revolutionized the anesthesia provider's ability to safely care for patients at risk for difficult airway management and associated adverse side effects (arterial hypoxemia, hypoventilation, aspiration of gastric contents). Endotracheal tubes may be placed in the trachea with the aid of fiberoptic laryngoscopy through a nasal or oral approach in awake, sedated, or anesthetized patients.

Nasal Fiberoptic Intubation of the Trachea

Nasal fiberoptic intubation of the trachea involves the use of a lubricated endotracheal tube that is at least 1.5 mm larger than the diameter of the fiberoptic bronchoscope. Softening the endotracheal tube in warm water before use makes it less likely to cause mucosal trauma or submucosal tunneling. The endotracheal tube is advanced through the nose into the pharynx by aiming perpendicular to the plane of the patient's face just above the inferior border of the nasal alar rim. If resistance is met at the back of the nasopharynx, 90 degrees of counterclockwise rotation allows the endotracheal tube to pass less traumatically because the bevel then faces the posterior pharyngeal wall.

Secretions should be suctioned before inserting the fiberoptic bronchoscope through the endotracheal tube. It is essential that the fiberoptic bronchoscope exit the tip of the endotracheal tube and not the Murphy eye. The fiberoptic bronchoscope and the endotracheal tube are manipulated to bring the larynx into view, and the bronchoscope is advanced into the trachea.

Inflation of the endotracheal tube cuff during advancement of the fiberoptic bronchoscope in the pharynx serves to create an enlarged pharyngeal space. Because secretions tend to adhere to the pharyngeal walls, endotracheal tube cuff inflation also helps keep the optics of the fiberoptic bronchoscope from being obscured. The inflated cuff further aims the tip of the endotracheal tube anteriorly.

The target should always be kept in the center of the anesthesia provider's field of vision by flexion and rotation as the fiberoptic bronchoscope is slowly advanced. As the fiberoptic bronchoscope passes through the vocal cords, the tracheal rings will become visible. The scope is advanced to just above the carina, and then the endotracheal tube is threaded over the scope. If resistance is encountered when advancing the endotracheal tube, force should not be exerted as the fiberoptic bronchoscope can become kinked and result in diversion of the endotracheal tube into the esophagus and damage the fiberoptic bronchoscope. Resistance to advancement often means that the endotracheal tube is impacted on a vocal cord. This can be relieved by rotating the tracheal tube as it is gently advanced. The appropriate depth of endotracheal tube placement can be verified by observing the distance between the carina and the tip of the endotracheal tube as the fiberoptic bronchoscope is withdrawn. If there is any resistance when removing the fiberoptic bronchoscope, it is either through the Murphy eye or kinked in the pharynx. In both instances, the endotracheal tube and the scope must be withdrawn together to avoid damaging the fiberoptic bronchoscope.

Awake Oral Fiberoptic Tracheal Intubation

When performing awake oral fiberoptic intubation, the patient's upper airway is anesthetized (local anesthetic topicalization, superior laryngeal nerve block, or transtracheal block), with nasal topicalization omitted. Utilization of an oral intubating airway facilitates directing the bronchscope. The procedure is as described in the previous section.

Asleep Oral/Nasal Fiberoptic Tracheal Intubation

Fiberoptic intubation under general anesthesia should be considered only if adequate oxygenation and ventilation can be maintained. Both nasal intubation and oral tracheal intubation are possible, and the technique can be performed with the patient breathing spontaneously or under controlled ventilation. A nasal airway can be placed and connected to the anesthesia breathing circuit with a 15-mm connector. When providing an airway in this manner, it is preferable to use an intravenous anesthetic technique to avoid exposure of others in the room to anesthetic vapors during insufflation.

An important difference in performing fiberoptic laryngoscopy in an anesthetized patient is that the soft tissues of the pharynx, in contrast to the awake state, tend to relax and limit space for visualization with the fiberoptic bronchoscope. Using jaw thrust or a tonsil retractor, expanding the endotracheal tube cuff in the pharynx, or applying traction on the tongue may overcome this problem. It is advisable to have a second person trained in anesthesia delivery assisting when a fiberoptic intubation is performed under general anesthesia because it is difficult to maintain the patient's airway, be attentive to the monitors, and perform the fiberoptic intubation alone.

When using the nasal approach, topical anesthesia for the nasal mucosa is not required, but vasoconstriction is necessary to increase the diameter of the passage and to decrease the risk of bleeding. For the nasal or the oral approach, topical anesthesia or blocks to inhibit the reflexes of the pharynx, vocal cords, and trachea are useful because the airway reflexes are still intact and the patient may cough, develop laryngospasm, or reflux gastric contents.

The curvature of the endotracheal tube is not optimal for oral tracheal intubation, and an appropriately sized oral intubating airway serves as a more effective channel. Care must be taken to maintain the intubating airway in a midline position. Alternatively, a laryngeal mask airway (LMA) provides an excellent channel for awake oral fiberoptic intubation.

PATIL-SYRACUSE MASK

The Patil-Syracuse mask is designed with a port that will accommodate an endotracheal tube and a fiberoptic bronchoscope through a diaphragm. This device allows for spontaneous or controlled ventilation while fiberoptic nasal or oral intubation is being performed.

AINTREE AIRWAY EXCHANGE CATHETER

The Aintree catheter is an airway exchange catheter with connectors that allow ventilation with an anesthesia breathing circuit or jet ventilator. It differs from other exchange catheters by having a lumen of adequate size to accommodate a fiberoptic bronchoscope.

RIGID FIBEROPTIC LARYNGOSCOPES/ VIDEOLARYNGOSCOPES

Rigid fiberoptic laryngoscopes include the Bullard laryngoscope, UpsherScope, WuScope system, GlideScope (Fig. 16-16), McGrath Scope, and Pentax Airway Scope (AWS). The Airtraq is an optical laryngoscope but works in a similar manner as the videolaryngoscopes. These devices are all anatomically shaped, rigid fiberoptic laryngoscopes with a light source for use in patients who have conditions (limited mouth opening, inability to flex the neck) that can make traditional laryngoscopy and tracheal intubation difficult or impossible. All fiberoptic techniques are hindered if upper airway secretions obscure the optics, thus emphasizing the value of prior administration of an antisialagogue.

WuScope System

The WuScope is available in two adult sizes and consists of a three-part bivalve scope that can be disassembled for removal after tracheal intubation (see Fig. 16-16A). The laryngoscope blade is tubular, which helps generate space in the pharynx for a greater field of vision while minimizing contact of the fiberoptic system with pharyngeal secretions. It has a channel that allows instillation of medications or oxygen insufflation.

An endotracheal tube is loaded into the channel of the scope. Tracheal intubation is accomplished as with the other rigid laryngoscopes, followed by release and removal of the anterior portion of the bivalve and then removal of the posterior portion and handle by following the curvature of the airway.[30]

Bullard Laryngoscope

The Bullard laryngoscope is available in adult and pediatric sizes (see Fig. 16-16B). The fiberoptic bundles are on the posterior aspect of the blade, 26 mm from the distal tip, and create a 55-degree field of vision. This laryngoscope has an adjustable focus on the eyepiece. The laryngoscope blade contains a 3.7-mm channel for drug injection or oxygen insufflation.

The Bullard laryngoscope can be used with a battery pack handle or a fiberoptic light cable. There are several interchangeable stylets for the laryngoscope. The laryngoscope, with an endotracheal tube loaded on the stylet, is advanced in the midline of the patient's pharynx

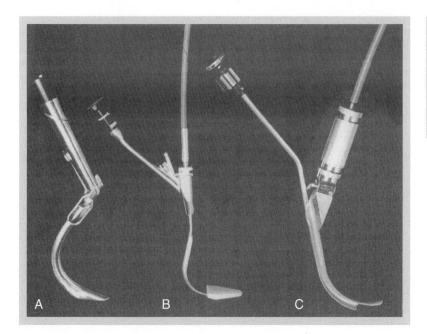

until the glottic opening is brought into view, and the endotracheal tube is then advanced under direct visualization. As a result of the stylet's position on the right side of the device, the right arytenoid cartilage may inhibit passage of the endotracheal tube. When this occurs, the laryngoscope and stylet position need to be adjusted to better align the endotracheal tube with the patient's airway.[30]

UpsherScope

The blade of the UpsherScope has a semicircular design that serves as an endotracheal tube guide and allows for easy removal of the scope after tracheal intubation (see Fig. 16-16C). It can be used with a battery-powered handle or a fiberoptic light cable. There is an adjustable-diopter eyepiece that can be immersed during cleaning. The technique for using the UpsherScope is similar to that described for the Bullard laryngoscope.[30]

GlideScope

The GlideScope is an anatomically shaped, fixed-angle (60-degree) laryngoscope blade made of medical-grade plastic. It has a miniature fog-resistant video camera embedded in the undersurface of the blade that transmits the digital image to a high-resolution, nonglare color monitor that can be mounted on a pole. Systems with reusable (GVL) and disposable (Cobalt) blades are available, as is a portable (Ranger) device. The GVL comes in sizes 2 (82 mm length, 14.5 mm thickness, for 1.8 to 10 kg patients) through 5 (102 mm length, 14 mm

thickness, for bariatric patients). Cobalt sizes range from 1 (<3.6 kg, 38 mm length, 8.7 mm thickness) to 4 (40 kg to morbidly obese, 95 mm length, 16 mm thickness). The Ranger reusable device comes in sizes 3 and 4, whereas the disposable blades come in sizes 1 to 4.

As with the other rigid laryngoscopes, it does not require line of sight and can be inserted from the side or in the midline. The tip of the laryngoscope blade may be placed in the vallecula or be used to lift the epiglottis directly. An endotracheal tube with a stylet angled to mimic that of the distal tip of the GlideScope is advanced using direct visualization until it can be seen on the monitor, after which the tube is advanced into the trachea based on the image on the monitoring screen. Although glottic visualization with the GlideScope has been shown to improve the Cormack and Lehane score by approximately 1.7 grades compared with direct visualization with a standard laryngoscope, the failed intubation rate with this device has been estimated to be 2.5% to 3%.[31,32] Moreover, failure of GlideScope intubation was correlated with poor visualization on direct laryngoscopy.[31]

Studies to evaluate the degree of cervical spine motion with the GlideScope have shown that, while using cervical spine stabilization, the greatest amount of flexion (8 to 12 degrees) was from the occiput to the third cervical vertebra (C3) (8 to 12 degrees) and the greatest flexion (8 degrees) was from C5 to T1. The greatest angulation occurred at the time that the endotracheal tube (ETT) was inserted and was equivalent to that caused by direct laryngoscopy with a Macintosh blade using the same cervical spine immobilization.[33,34]

McGrath Scope

The McGrath video laryngoscope consists of an adjustable Macintosh style blade, attached to a battery-containing handle mounted with a color display monitor that can rotate and swivel to optimize the angle of visualization. It is used with a disposable blade and the technique for intubation is as described for the GlideScope.

Pentax-AWS

The Pentax-AWS video laryngoscope is fitted with a disposable sheath that acts as a tube guide that aligns the ETT with the structures at the center of the on-screen target. One study has shown a 95% to 99% success rate with the device.[35]

Airtraq

The Airtraq is a disposable optical laryngoscope that requires a minimum oral opening of 2 cm. Intubation with this device was successful in 80% of patients after failed intubation with a Macintosh laryngoscope.[36]

RETROGRADE TRACHEAL INTUBATION

Retrograde tracheal intubation has been used in cases of difficult airway management, particularly when there is bleeding, decreased mouth opening, or limited neck movement. It should not be used when the patient's cricothyroid membrane is not identifiable or there is pathology of the anterior aspect of the neck (tumors, infection, stenosis) or coagulopathy.[37]

Technique

Placing the patient in the sniffing position optimizes the ability to identify the cricothyroid membrane. Kits for performing retrograde intubation are commercially available. The cricothyroid membrane is punctured with a needle while aspirating with an attached syringe. A change in resistance is felt as a pop when the needle enters the trachea and air can be aspirated. The syringe is detached and a wire is threaded through the needle in a cephalad direction. It is then retrieved from the mouth or nose. An endotracheal tube, with or without a fiberoptic laryngoscope, is threaded over the wire until it stops on impact with the anterior wall of the trachea. Tension on the guidewire can be relaxed to allow the endotracheal tube to pass further into the trachea before removing the wire. Commercially available kits have improved this technique by adding a guiding catheter that fits over the wire and inside the endotracheal tube.

BLIND NASOTRACHEAL INTUBATION

The use of blind nasotracheal intubation has decreased over the years with the introduction of other devices for difficult airway management. However, there are still clinical situations in which it can be lifesaving.

Technique

If time permits, the nasal mucosa should be anesthetized and vasoconstricted to minimize discomfort and bleeding. A 6.0- to 7. 0-mm ID endotracheal tube is generally chosen for an adult. An Endotrol tube, with a pulley to adjust the angle of curvature of the tube, can facilitate blind nasotracheal intubation. The endotracheal tube is advanced through the nose and into the pharynx while listening to breath sounds at the distal end of the endotracheal tube. Alternatively, the endotracheal tube can be attached to an anesthesia breathing circuit, and reservoir bag movement and carbon dioxide can be monitored to verify that the endotracheal tube is advancing into the trachea. If tugging is seen on the anterior surface of the patient's neck, the endotracheal tube is lodging in the vallecula. When this occurs, rotating the tube to free it from the epiglottis before advancing can be advantageous. If evidence of breathing through the endotracheal tube disappears, the endotracheal tube has advanced into the esophagus because it is not traversing anterior enough to enter the trachea. When this occurs, the endotracheal tube should be withdrawn back to a depth where breathing again occurs through the endotracheal tube. If a standard endotracheal tube has been used, the cuff can be inflated with air to lift it off the posterior pharyngeal wall. The endotracheal tube is then advanced until slight resistance is felt, the cuff is deflated, and then the tube is advanced further into the trachea.

SUPRAGLOTTIC AIRWAY DEVICES

Classic Laryngeal Mask Airway

The LMA has become an invaluable supraglottic airway device for routine and difficult airway management. Factors related to difficult tracheal intubation on direct laryngoscopy do not correlate with those that make LMA placement difficult. Therefore, the incidence of experiencing difficulty with both endotracheal intubation and LMA placement is very low.[38] The ASA guidelines for management of a difficult airway include the use of an LMA.[1] The difficult airway algorithm shifts back to the nonemergency pathway if an adequate airway and ventilation can be established with an LMA.

An LMA consists of a 12-mm ID flexible shaft connected to a silicone rubber mask that seals with the airway in the hypopharynx (Fig. 16-17). The distal tip of

III

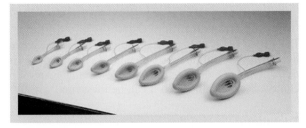

Figure 16-17 Classic laryngeal mask airways.

the cuff should be against the upper esophageal sphincter (cricopharyngeus muscle), the lateral edges rest in the piriform sinuses, and the proximal end seats under the base of the tongue. LMA size selection is determined by the patient's weight (Table 16-8).

LMA Fastrach

The LMA Fastrach (Intubating LMA, ILMA) was designed to obviate the problems encountered when attempting to blindly intubate the trachea through a classic LMA.[39] The ILMA consists of an anatomically shaped stainless steel tube connected to a laryngeal mask. It has an attached handle to aid insertion of the device and to facilitate optimization of its positioning to increase the likelihood of successful blind tracheal intubation through the device. A 15-mm connector allows for ventilation of the patient's lungs (Fig. 16-18).[38] The ILMA is designed to be used with a silicone Euromedical endotracheal tube (size 7.0 ID, 7.5 ID, or 8.0 ID). These tracheal tubes exit the laryngeal mask at a different angle than do standard endotracheal tubes and result in better alignment with the airway. The ILMA is advanced into the pharynx by following the natural curvature of the patient's upper airway.

TECHNIQUE

With the patient breathing oxygen, the Chandy maneuver (lift and posterior rotation) is used to optimize the

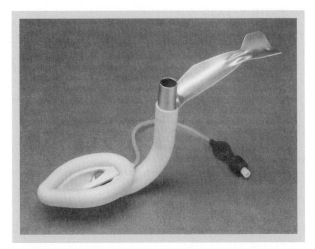

Figure 16-18 LMA Fastrach. (From Bogetz MS. Using the laryngeal mask airway to manage the difficult airway. Anesthesiol Clin North Am 2002;20:863-870.)

position of the ILMA before attempting tracheal intubation. A lubricated endotracheal tube is inserted into the ILMA. Because Euromedical tubes have low-volume, high-pressure cuffs, it is recommended that the largest size that is appropriate for the patient be used to minimize mucosal pressure from the cuff.

Slight resistance to advancing the endotracheal tube may be felt as the horizontal marking on the tube aligns with the proximal end of the ILMA. This position marks the depth at which the endotracheal tube impacts the epiglottic elevating bar in the bowl of the mask. The endotracheal tube should advance without resistance toward the glottic opening and the trachea. If resistance is felt beyond the point where the horizontal line passes into the ILMA, the cause depends on the depth that the tube has advanced. Immediate resistance indicates that the ILMA is too large. Resistance that is encountered 2 cm distal to the horizontal line may be secondary to a down-folded epiglottis. If the ILMA is too small, resistance is felt 3 cm distal. Resistance at 4 to 5 cm generally indicates that too large an ILMA has been selected. After verification of endotracheal intubation, the cuff of the ILMA is deflated, the 15-mm endotracheal tube connector is disconnected, and the ILMA is removed by using the stabilizer bar to push the endotracheal tube through the ILMA. The 15-mm connector is reattached to the tube and the anesthesia breathing circuit, and the patient's lungs are ventilated.

LMA CTrach

The LMA CTrach is a modified LMA Fastrach. It has the same anatomically curved stainless steel tube and is available in three mask sizes (3, 4, and 5). The epiglottic elevating bar has been modified to allow for visualization

Table 16-8 Appropriate-Size Laryngeal Mask Airway (LMA) Based on Patient Weight

LMA Size	Weight (kg)	Cuff Inflation Volume (mL of Air)
1	<5	4
1.5	5-10	7
2	10-20	10
2.5	20-30	14
3	30-50	20
4	50-70	30
5	70-100	40
6	>100	50

of the larynx by means of fiberoptic bundles located within the bowl of the mask. A lightweight viewer attaches magnetically after the device has been inserted.[38] Size selection, insertion (no cricoid pressure), and ventilation are as with the LMA Fastrach. The LMA Fastrach has been demonstrated to have a high first-attempt success rate for achieving ventilation; however, there have been widely disparate reports (25% to 98%) on successful first-attempt blind tracheal intubation.[39] The LMA CTrach is intended to be more rapid and less cumbersome technically than the LMA Fastrach. As with the ILMA, successful placement of the CTrach requires a minimum interincisor distance of 3 cm. Appropriate size selection is necessary to properly align the device with the airway. A recent study has shown a 4% incidence of poor visualization and failure to intubate.[40] A study to evaluate the suitability of the CTrach in patients with unstable cervical spines showed that the device exerted significant pressure and resulted in posterior displacement of the cervical spine in a C3 posterior element disruption cadaveric model.[41]

ProSeal LMA

The ProSeal LMA is a modification of the classic LMA (Fig. 16-19).[38] The cuff of the ProSeal LMA extends onto the back of the mask, which results in an improved airway seal without increasing mucosal pressure. It has a second lumen that parallels the one for the airway but opens at the distal tip of the mask to act as an esophageal vent. When optimally seated, the ProSeal LMA effectively isolates the trachea from the esophagus, thus protecting the lungs from aspiration when a minimum of 10 mL of air has been placed in the LMA cuff.[42]

Successful first-attempt placement of the ProSeal LMA varies with the insertion technique (84% with an introducer tool, 88% with digital insertion, and 100% with a

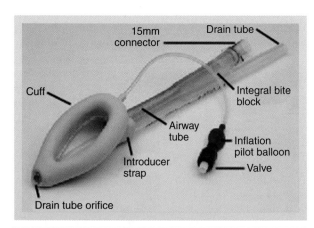

Figure 16-19 ProSeal LMA. (From Brimacombe J, Keller C: The ProSeal laryngeal mask airway. Anesthesiol Clin North Am 2002;20:871-891.)

bougie technique).[43] It is likely that cricoid pressure, as with the classic LMA, will interfere with proper placement of the ProSeal LMA. Specifically, cricoid pressure will prevent the LMA from seating distally at the cricopharyngeus muscle because the esophagus is occluded at the level of the cricoid cartilage. The ProSeal LMA protects against aspiration only if it is optimally seated.

I-Gel

The I-Gel is a supraglottic laryngeal mask airway available in sizes 1 to 5 (including 1.5 and 2.5). It has a soft noninflatable gel cuff, gastric vent tube, built-in epiglottic rest, integral bite block, and a 15-mm connector. It can be used as a primary airway, or a conduit for intubation. It is of adequate diameter to pass a 6.0 ETT through a size 3, a 7.0 ETT through a size 4, and an 8.0 ETT through a size 5. It is not recommended in patients who are at risk of aspiration, and should remain in situ for less than 4 hours.

Air-Q

The Air-Q is another laryngeal mask device that can be utilized either as a primary airway or as an intermediary channel for intubation. It is available in four sizes (1.5 to 4.5). Recommended maximum tube sizes are 5.5 ETT for the Air-Q 1.5, 6.5 ETT for the Air-Q 2.5, 7.5 ETT for the Air-Q 3.5, and an 8.5 ETT for the Air-Q 4.5.

Esophageal-Tracheal Combitube

The Esophageal-Tracheal Combitube (ETC) is a double-lumen device that can function as either an endotracheal device or an esophageal obturator (Fig. 16-20).[44] Two sizes are available. The 37-French small adult ETC can be used in patients who are between 120 and 180 cm (4-6 ft) tall, and the 41-French ETC is for patients taller than 180 cm.

TECHNIQUE

The ETC is passed blindly while lifting the patient's mandible with the other hand. Alternatively, a laryngoscope may be used to aid insertion. Whichever technique is used, the ETC should be inserted without force, because this can result in esophageal tear or rupture. The oropharyngeal cuff is inflated first with the prefilled syringe attached to the blue pilot balloon. This seats and anchors the ETC. The distal cuff is then inflated and ventilation begun through the longer (blue) lumen, which ends in fenestrations between the two cuffs. If no breath sounds are heard, ventilation should be attempted through the other lumen.[45] If ventilation is still not detected, the tube is probably placed too deeply in the esophagus and should be pulled back and ventilation attempted through the blue lumen again.

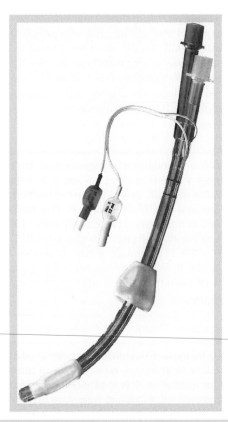

Figure 16-20 Esophageal-Tracheal Combitube. (From Gaitni LA, Vaida SJ, Agro F. The Esophageal-Tracheal Combitube. Anesthesiol Clin North Am 2002;20:893-906.)

CLINICAL USES

The ETC has been used successfully in emergency medical management and requires minimal training. Positive-pressure ventilation can be used with this device. It is recommended that airway reflexes not be intact during ETC use. The ETC protects against aspiration when properly positioned. This device is not intended for long-term airway management, however, and should be removed within a few hours to decrease the risk of ischemia of the tongue and subsequent edema formation.[45] A slowly resolving case of bilateral glossopharyngeal nerve and unilateral hypoglossal nerve dysfunction caused by high pharyngeal cuff pressures with the use of an ETC for 3 hours has been reported.[46]

Laryngeal Tube

The laryngeal tube is a multiuse single-lumen silicone tube with a dual cuff system (a pharyngeal cuff and a blind distal esophageal cuff) (Fig. 16-21).[30] Ventilation of the patient's lungs is through a fenestration between the two cuffs. The cuffs connect to a single pilot balloon. The laryngeal tube is available in sizes 1 to 5. It is passed blindly into the pharynx.

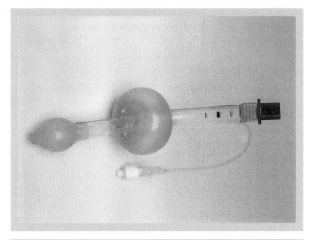

Figure 16-21 Laryngeal tube. (Courtesy of VBM Medizintechnik GmbH, Sulz.)

Pharyngeal Airway Xpress

The Pharyngeal Airway Xpress is a disposable device with a rigid curved tube and a terminal end with gills that seats at the cricopharyngeus muscle (Fig. 16-22).[30] It has a high-volume, low-pressure pharyngeal cuff and is inserted blindly. The lumen is large enough to accommodate a 7.5-mm endotracheal tube if tracheal intubation is desired.

Glottic Aperture Seal Airway

The Glottic Aperture Seal Airway is a disposable single-lumen tube that forms an airway seal with a sponge-like distal tip. A plastic insertion blade lifts the epiglottis as the tube is inserted.

Cuffed Oropharyngeal Airway

The cuffed oropharyngeal airway consists of a modified conventional oral airway with a cuff at its distal end. When the cuff is inflated, it displaces the base of the patient's tongue anteriorly and passively elevates the

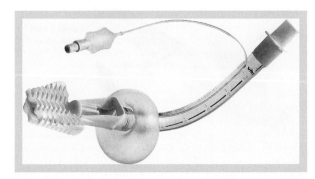

Figure 16-22 Pharyngeal Airway Xpress. (Courtesy of Vital Signs, Totowa, NJ.)

epiglottis away from the posterior pharyngeal wall. The proximal end of a cuffed oropharyngeal airway has a standard 15-mm connector that permits attachment to the anesthetic breathing circuit.

TRANSTRACHEAL TECHNIQUES

Cricothyrotomy

Cricothyrotomy can be performed in less than 30 seconds and has significant advantages over transtracheal jet ventilation because it establishes a definitive airway that can be used for up to 72 hours. After this period, the incidence of vocal cord dysfunction and subglottic stenosis increases.[47-49] The larger diameter of a cricothyrotomy tube allows both inhalation and exhalation to occur through the device, and it does not rely on a patent native airway, as does transtracheal jet ventilation. For this reason, laryngospasm during transtracheal jet ventilation can cause the patient's lungs to become rapidly overinflated and lead to pulmonary barotrauma.

The cricothyrotomy kit should require minimal or no assembly because this technique is almost always performed under emergency circumstances. The system should be designed such that if the airway is initially identified (generally by aspiration of air through a needle), the final device cannot then be forced into another tissue plane. The Seldinger technique is ideal for avoiding this problem. The final device left in the airway should be of adequate caliber (preferably > 4 mm). If the cricothyrotomy kit has a cuffed tube, pulmonary compliance is less of an issue and the airway is protected against aspiration.

Transtracheal Jet Ventilation

Commercially available products for transtracheal jet ventilation obviate the need for self-assembled products that rely on friction connections and can easily become disconnected under high-pressure (50 psi) ventilation. The risk profile for transtracheal jet ventilation is similar to that for cricothyrotomy and includes pneumothorax, pneumomediastinum, bleeding, infection, and subcutaneous emphysema. As a result of the oxygen pressure used for transtracheal jet ventilation, these complications can become life threatening very quickly. Absolute contraindications to transtracheal jet ventilation are upper airway obstruction or any disruption of the airway.[50,51]

TRACHEAL EXTUBATION

Tracheal extubation after general anesthesia requires skill and judgment learned through experience. The patient must be either deeply anesthetized or fully awake at the time of tracheal extubation. Tracheal extubation during a light level of anesthesia (disconjugate gaze, breath-holding or coughing, and not responsive to command) increases the risk for laryngospasm. A patient reaching for the endotracheal tube might indicate a localizing response to noxious stimulation in the absence of sufficient awakening from anesthesia to follow commands.

Tracheal extubation before the return of protective airway reflexes (deep tracheal extubation) is generally associated with less coughing and attenuated hemodynamic effects on emergence. This may be preferred in patients at risk from increased intracranial or intraocular pressure, bleeding into the surgical wound, or wound dehiscence. However, previous difficult facemask ventilation or endotracheal intubation, risk of aspiration, and a surgical procedure that may have resulted in airway edema or increased airway irritability are contraindications to deep tracheal extubation.

Technique

Spontaneous breathing with 100% oxygen is established before tracheal extubation. As with tracheal intubation, an FRC filled with oxygen allows for the longest safe period should breath-holding or laryngospasm occur immediately after tracheal extubation. The effects of neuromuscular blocking drugs should be fully reversed. The oropharynx is suctioned just before tracheal extubation. The endotracheal tube cuff is deflated and the tracheal tube rapidly removed from the patient's trachea and upper airway while a positive-pressure breath is delivered to help expel any secretions. The cuff should not remain deflated for any significant period before tracheal extubation because the vocal cords cannot effectively close around the endotracheal tube and supraglottic secretions can be aspirated. Timing tracheal extubation at the peak of inspiration is intended for the following exhalation or cough to eliminate any aspirated secretions from the trachea. After tracheal extubation, oxygen is delivered by facemask.

If tracheal intubation was difficult at the beginning of the procedure, awake extubation to ensure that the patient is capable of breathing spontaneously and maintaining oxygenation and ventilation is recommended. Tracheal extubation over a fiberoptic bronchoscope or an endotracheal tube exchange catheter so that immediate tracheal reintubation can be performed is also an option.

Complications

Complications of tracheal intubation are rare and should not influence the decision to place a tracheal tube. Certainly, the benefits of a properly placed tracheal tube far exceed the risks of tracheal intubation. Complications of tracheal intubation may be categorized as those

III

Table 16-9 Complications of Tracheal Intubation

During Direct Laryngoscopy and Tracheal Intubation
Dental and oral soft tissue trauma
Systemic hypertension and tachycardia
Cardiac dysrhythmias
Myocardial ischemia
Inhalation (aspiration) of gastric contents

While the Tracheal Tube Is in Place
Tracheal tube obstruction
Endobronchial intubation
Esophageal intubation
Tracheal tube cuff leak
Pulmonary barotrauma
Nasogastric distention
Accidental disconnection from the anesthesia breathing circuit
Tracheal mucosa ischemia
Accidental extubation

Immediate and Delayed Complications after Tracheal Extubation
Laryngospasm
Inhalation (aspiration) of gastric contents
Pharyngitis (sore throat)
Laryngitis
Laryngeal or subglottic edema
Laryngeal ulceration with or without granuloma formation
Tracheitis
Tracheal stenosis
Vocal cord paralysis
Arytenoid cartilage dislocation

occurring (1) during direct laryngoscopy and tracheal intubation, (2) while the tracheal tube is in place, and (3) after tracheal extubation, either immediately or after a delay of several days (Table 16-9).

COMPLICATIONS DURING DIRECT LARYNGOSCOPY AND TRACHEAL INTUBATION

Dental trauma is the most frequent type of damage related to direct laryngoscopy. It is estimated that 1 in every 4500 patients undergoing upper airway management during anesthesia sustains a dental injury that requires further treatment or extraction.[52] Patients at likely risk for dental injury include those with preexisting poor dentition and those who possess upper airway anatomy that makes direct laryngoscopy or tracheal intubation technically difficult. Use of a plastic shield placed over the upper teeth and avoidance of using the laryngoscope blade as a lever on the teeth may minimize the likelihood of dental trauma. Should injury occur, prompt consultation with a dentist is often indicated. A dislodged tooth must be recovered, but if the search is unsuccessful, appropriate radiographs of the head/neck, chest, and abdomen should be obtained to ensure that the tooth has not passed through the glottic opening into the trachea or more distal airways.[53]

Systemic hypertension and tachycardia frequently accompany direct laryngoscopy (regardless of the type of laryngoscope blade used) and tracheal intubation. These responses are usually transient and innocuous. In patients with preexisting systemic hypertension or ischemic heart disease, however, these changes may be exaggerated or may jeopardize the balance between myocardial oxygen requirements and delivery. In these patients, duration of direct laryngoscopy should be as short as possible. Serious or persistent cardiac dysrhythmias during tracheal intubation are unlikely if apneic time is minimized and adequate oxygenation and denitrogenation are performed.[53]

Direct upper airway trauma is more likely to occur with difficult tracheal intubation because of the application of more physical force to the patient's airway than is normally applied, as well as the need for multiple attempts at intubation. The most common consequence is a chipped or broken tooth. Posterior pharyngeal and lip lacerations and bruises are more likely with difficult tracheal intubation. In extreme cases, prolonged interruption of oxygenation and ventilation may result in cardiac arrest and brain damage.[53]

COMPLICATIONS WHILE THE TRACHEAL TUBE IS IN PLACE

Obstruction of the tracheal tube may occur as a result of inspissated secretions or kinking. The chance of endobronchial intubation can be minimized by calculating the proper endotracheal tube length for the patient and then noting the centimeter marking on the tube at the point of fixation at the patient's lips. In adults, taping the endotracheal tube at the patient's lips corresponding to the 21- to 23-cm markings on the tracheal tube usually places the distal end of the endotracheal tube in the midtrachea. Flexion of the patient's head may advance the tube up to 1.9 cm and convert a tracheal placement into an endobronchial intubation, especially in children. Conversely, extension of the head can withdraw the tube up to 1.9 cm and result in pharyngeal placement. Lateral rotation of the head moves the distal end of the tracheal tube approximately 0.7 cm.[53]

IMMEDIATE AND DELAYED COMPLICATIONS AFTER TRACHEAL EXTUBATION

Laryngospasm and inhalation of gastric contents are the two most serious potential immediate complications after tracheal extubation. Laryngospasm is unlikely if the depth of anesthesia is sufficient during tracheal extubation (laryngeal reflexes suppressed) or the patient is allowed to awaken before tracheal extubation (laryngeal reflexes intact). A patient who is lightly anesthetized at the time of tracheal extubation (laryngeal reflexes neither adequately suppressed nor recovered) is most at risk. If laryngospasm occurs, oxygen delivered with positive pressure through a facemask and forward displacement of the mandible with the anesthesia provider's index fingers to apply pressure at the temporomandibular joints may be sufficient treatment. Administration of succinylcholine (0.1 mg/kg IV) or an anesthetic induction agent is indicated if laryngospasm persists.[53]

Pharyngitis is the most frequent complaint after tracheal extubation, particularly in females, presumably because of thinner mucosal covering over the posterior vocal cords than in males. Skeletal muscle myalgia associated with the administration of succinylcholine may be manifested in the peripharyngeal muscles as postoperative "sore throat," which is often incorrectly attributed to tracheal intubation. Use of large (8.5 to 9.0 mm ID) versus small (6.5 to 7.0 mm ID) tracheal tubes may increase the likelihood of pharyngitis. Regardless of the mechanism, pharyngitis usually disappears spontaneously without any treatment in 48 to 72 hours. Some degree of laryngeal incompetence may be present in the first 4 to 8 hours after tracheal extubation.[53]

The major complication of prolonged tracheal intubation (>48 hours) is damage to the tracheal mucosa, which may progress to destruction of cartilaginous rings and subsequent cicatricial scar formation and tracheal stenosis. Stenosis becomes symptomatic when the adult tracheal lumen is decreased to less than 5 mm.[53]

AIRWAY MANAGEMENT IN INFANTS AND CHILDREN (Also See Chapters 33 and 34)

Airway Differences between Infants and Adults

Understanding the anatomic differences between the infant and adult airway is critical to proper airway management in pediatrics (Table 16-10). All these differences between the infant airway and the adult airway resolve as the child grows, and usually by the time the child is about 10 years old, the upper airway has taken on more adult-like characteristics.

The infant larynx is located higher in the neck at the level of C3-C4 than in adults, where the larynx is at the level of C4-C5. This causes the tongue to shift more superiorly, closer to the palate. The tongue more easily apposes the palate, which can cause airway obstruction

Table 16-10 The Infant Airway versus the Adult Airway

- Larynx positioned higher in the neck
- Tongue larger relative to mouth size
- Epiglottis larger, stiffer, and angled more posteriorly
- Head and occiput larger relative to body size
- Short neck
- Narrow nares
- Cricoid ring is the narrowest region

in situations such as the inhalation induction of anesthesia. An infant's tongue is also larger in proportion to the size of the mouth than in adults. The relatively large size of the tongue makes direct laryngoscopy more difficult and can contribute to obstruction of the upper airway during sedation, inhalation induction of anesthesia, or emergence from anesthesia. Anterior pressure on the angle of the mandible to shift the tongue to a more anterior position often solves this problem. An oral or nasal airway can also be beneficial in these situations.

The epiglottis in an infant's airway is often described as relatively larger, stiffer, and more omega shaped than an adult epiglottis. More importantly, an infant's epiglottis is typically angled in a more posterior position, thereby blocking visualization of the vocal cords during direct laryngoscopy. In infants and small children it is often necessary to lift the epiglottis with the tip of the blade of the laryngoscope to visualize the vocal cords and successfully intubate the trachea. Straight laryngoscope blades, which have a smaller profile than curved laryngoscope blades, more easily fit in the smaller infant mouth. Straight laryngoscope blades with their narrower tip also more effectively lift the epiglottis allowing better visualization of the vocal cords.

An infant's airway is often described as funnel shaped with a relatively large thyroid cartilage above and a relatively narrow cricoid cartilage below. The narrowest portion of an infant's airway is the cricoid cartilage, whereas the narrowest portion of an adult's airway is the vocal cords. The cricoid cartilage is circular in shape allowing uncuffed endotracheal tubes to successfully seal and protect the airway from aspiration. The correct size uncuffed endotracheal tube is one that results in an air leak around the endotracheal tube with the application of 20 to 25 cm H_2O positive pressure. Cuffed endotracheal tubes can be used in infants and children if the inflation of the cuff is carefully adjusted and monitored so that the leak pressure remains at 20 to 25 cm H_2O. If nitrous oxide is used during the anesthetic, the nitrous oxide will diffuse into the air-filled cuff increasing both its volume and the pressure transmitted to the underlying tracheal mucosa. If the leak pressure is too high with either an uncuffed endotracheal tube or a cuffed one, the tracheal mucosa will be compressed causing subglottic edema either at the level of the cricoid cartilage or below. This complication can result in postextubation croup or stridor in mild cases and tracheal stenosis in more severe cases involving prolonged tracheal intubation.

An infant's head and occiput are relatively larger than an adult's. The proper position for direct laryngoscopy and tracheal intubation in an adult is often described as the sniffing position with the head elevated and the neck flexed at C6-C7 and extended at C1-C2. An infant, on the other hand, requires a shoulder roll or neck roll to establish an optimal position for facemask ventilation and direct laryngoscopy. An infant's nares are relatively

III

smaller than an adult's and can offer significant resistance to airflow and increase the work of breathing, especially when secretions, edema, or bleeding narrow them.

Managing the Normal Airway in Infants and Children

A complete history plus physical examination is the first step in managing infant and pediatric airways.

HISTORY

The history should include whether there were any problems with previous anesthetics, and previous anesthetic records should be reviewed if available. A history of snoring should prompt additional questioning about whether the child has obstructive sleep apnea and should alert the anesthesia provider that respiratory obstruction may develop during the induction and emergence phases of anesthesia, as well as in the postoperative period, especially if opioids are given for pain management.

PHYSICAL EXAMINATION

It is often difficult to perform a complete physical examination on infants and children. Asking a child to look up at the sky and then down at the floor is one way of assessing neck extension and flexion, respectively. If there are any masses, tumors, or abscesses in the neck or upper airway that compromise neck flexion, extension, or breathing function, further evaluation is important and should include computed tomography to evaluate the location and degree of any airway compromise. Children will often voluntarily open their mouths to enable determination of a Mallampati classification. If an infant or child is uncooperative, external examination of the airway often reveals enough information to determine whether it is a normal or a potentially difficult airway. Examining the profile of an infant or child can indicate whether the thyromental distance is short and whether the patient has micrognathia or a hypoplastic mandible. Difficult airway management can be expected if the infant's chin is posterior to the upper lip. If the chin is neutral to the upper lip, the infant or child probably has a normal airway.

The parents and the child should be directly asked whether there are any loose teeth. If loose teeth are identified, care should be taken to avoid traumatizing the tooth during direct laryngoscopy and tracheal intubation. A very loose tooth should be removed before proceeding with direct laryngoscopy to prevent the possibility of pulmonary aspiration of the tooth.

Preanesthetic Medication

Preanesthetic medication can facilitate separation of the infant or child from the parents before the induction of anesthesia. Preanesthetic medication is often not necessary in infants younger than 6 months because stranger anxiety does not usually develop until 6 to 9 months of age. Midazolam can be administered in small doses and titrated to effect if the infant or child has an intravenous catheter in place. If the child does not have an intravenous catheter in place, midazolam syrup can be given orally (2 mg/mL) in a dose of about 0.5 mg/kg up to a maximum dose of about 20 mg. If the child is uncooperative with taking oral midazolam and preanesthetic medication is essential, midazolam can also be given intranasally, intramuscularly, or rectally. One approach to minimizing the need for preanesthetic medication is allowing the parents to be present for the induction of anesthesia. If the parents are very anxious themselves, however, their presence may make the child more anxious.

Induction of Anesthesia

If the infant or child has an intravenous catheter, induction of anesthesia with propofol or thiopental is usually safer and quicker than an inhaled induction of anesthesia. Propofol is more quickly metabolized and eliminated than thiopental, but intravenous administration of propofol can be painful, which is not routinely eliminated by the prior intravenous administration of lidocaine. Advantages of thiopental are its relatively low cost and lack of pain on intravenous administration. After the infant or child loses consciousness and the ability to ventilate with a facemask is demonstrated, an LMA can be inserted or a neuromuscular blocking drug can be given to facilitate direct laryngoscopy and tracheal intubation.

Inhaled induction of anesthesia can be performed if the infant or child does not have an intravenous catheter in place. Beginning the induction of anesthesia with the odorless mixture of nitrous oxide and oxygen through a facemask and then slowly increasing the concentration of sevoflurane is the best approach in a cooperative child. When the infant or child becomes unconscious, the nitrous oxide should be turned off to administrate 100% oxygen to the child. The increasing level of anesthesia will decrease skeletal muscle tone and may cause airway obstruction in certain infants and children. If airway obstruction does occur, it can usually be relieved by opening the mouth, extending the neck, and pushing anteriorly on the angle of the jaw. Occasionally, an oral or nasal airway may need to be inserted at this point. An intravenous catheter should be placed, and once the ability to ventilate the patient has been confirmed, either an LMA can be inserted or a neuromuscular blocking drug can be given to facilitate direct laryngoscopy and tracheal intubation.

Direct Laryngoscopy and Tracheal Intubation

When performing direct laryngoscopy and tracheal intubation in infants and children it is important to appropriately position the infant or child with a roll under the neck or shoulders. Ideally, the mouth should be viewed as being divided into three compartments, with the tongue on the left, the laryngoscope blade in the midline, and the endotracheal tube entering from the right corner of the mouth. Gentle, external posterior pressure applied with the fingers of the anesthesia provider's right hand at the level of the thyroid or cricoid cartilage is sometimes necessary to bring the vocal cords into view.

Once the trachea is intubated, correct positioning of the endotracheal tube should be confirmed by capnography, by watching the chest rise and fall, and by auscultation. Because the trachea in infants and children is short, it is easy to accidentally intubate a main stem bronchus. The correct depth of a cuffed endotracheal tube can be estimated by palpating the endotracheal tube cuff in the suprasternal notch. The correct tracheal depth of an uncuffed endotracheal tube can be estimated by placing the double line at the distal end of the endotracheal tube at the vocal cords while performing direct laryngoscopy. In infants and children it is important to reconfirm that the endotracheal tube is correctly positioned by listening for equal bilateral breath sounds after securing the endotracheal tube and at any later time when there is a change in the patient's position. It is also possible for the endotracheal tube to shift into a main stem bronchus during a laparoscopic case when the insufflation of the abdomen causes a cephalad shift of the diaphragm and the lungs.

Although it is possible to accomplish tracheal intubation without the use of neuromuscular blocking drugs, these drugs will make it easier to perform direct laryngoscopy and intubation and will decrease the incidence of laryngospasm (see Chapter 12). In nonemergency situations in infants and children, the use of a nondepolarizing neuromuscular blocking drug such as rocuronium (0.4 to 0.8 mg/kg IV) is recommended.

Airway Equipment

NASAL AND ORAL AIRWAYS
Nasal airways and oral airways can sometimes be useful in infants and pediatric patients to relieve airway obstruction, especially during facemask ventilation at the beginning or end of anesthesia. The nasal airway should be carefully placed through one of the nares after lubricating its exterior. The nasal airway must be long enough to pass through the nasopharynx, but short enough that it still remains above the glottis.

Oral airways relieve airway obstruction by displacing the tongue anteriorly. Too large an oral airway will either obstruct the glottis or may cause coughing, gagging, or laryngospasm in a patient who is not deeply anesthetized. Too small an oral airway will push the tongue posteriorly and make the airway obstruction worse. Oral airways should be placed with care to prevent trauma to the teeth and oropharynx.

LARYNGEAL MASK AIRWAYS
Laryngeal mask airways are supraglottic airway devices that can be used for both routine airway management as well as in difficult airway situations. LMAs are ideally suited for situations in which the patient is breathing spontaneously, but can also be used to deliver positive-pressure ventilation.[54] Care must be taken when using positive-pressure ventilation with an LMA to minimize peak inspiratory pressure. Patients who have lung disease or any other patient whose peak inspiratory pressures required for ventilation are higher than normal are poor candidates for an LMA because air may leak into the esophagus and result in distention of the stomach and an increased risk for emesis and aspiration. An LMA does not protect the airway from aspiration and should not be routinely used in patients with full stomachs or those at increased risk for aspiration. The LMA Classic is reusable and the LMA Unique is disposable. Both the reusable and disposable versions of the LMA are used in the same manner and are available in the same sizes.

Selection of Proper Size
Determining the appropriate size of LMA to use is most easily done by using the weight of the infant or child (see Table 16-8). An LMA that is too large will be difficult to place. An LMA that is too small will not form as good a seal, and it may be difficult to ventilate the patient's lungs with positive airway pressure. A slightly smaller LMA will seat better than a slightly larger LMA and may be beneficial in cases in which the operative site will be near or around the LMA. The LMA Flexible has a wire-reinforced airway tube that resists kinking and can be positioned in such a way that interference with surgical procedures involving the head and neck is minimized. However, the LMA Flexible in not available in size 1 and 1½.

Technique
There are numerous methods for placing an LMA in infants and children. One method is with the LMA deflated and placed in its normal orientation. Alternatively, an LMA can be both placed and removed while inflated. Placing the LMA already inflated is associated with a higher success rate and less oral trauma than placing it deflated.[55] An LMA can also be rotated 90 degrees in the lateral oropharynx to bypass the base of the tongue and then rotated 90 degrees back to its correct position. It can also be turned backward to facilitate its placement posterior to the base of the tongue and then rotated 180 degrees into its correct position.[56]

INTUBATING LARYNGEAL AIRWAYS
The Air-Q disposable intubating laryngeal airway (ILA) is a newer supraglottic airway device with several important differences than the LMA. The Air-Q disposable ILA

Table 16-11 Appropriate-Size Air-Q Disposable Intubating Laryngeal Airway (ILA) Based on Patient Weight

Air-Q Disposable ILA Size	Weight (kg)	Max ETT Size
1.5	<20	5.5
2.5	20-50	6.5
3.5	50-70	7.5
4.5	70-100	8.5

ETT, endotracheal tube.

can be used in the same situations as the LMA for both routine and difficult airways. Its major advantage is a design that facilitates endotracheal intubation with standard oral endotracheal tubes. The airway tube has a larger diameter that the LMA allowing for intubation with a larger ETT than the correspondingly sized LMA (see Table 16-11). The Air-Q ILA can be used with a specially designed ILA removal stylet that stabilizes the ETT and allows controlled removal of the ILA without dislodging the ETT from the trachea. The Air-Q ILA's major disadvantage at present is that it is only available in four sizes while the LMA is available in eight pediatric sizes. The limited number of pediatric sizes results in the possibility that the Air-Q ILA will be either too small or too large.

ENDOTRACHEAL TUBES

The appropriately sized endotracheal tube for infants and children can be estimated by using the following formula:

$$(Age + 16)/4 = \text{Endotracheal tube (ID) size}$$

It is important to remember that this formula is for uncuffed endotracheal tubes. Because the cuff is located on the outside of the endotracheal tube, to adapt this formula to cuffed endotracheal tubes it is necessary to subtract half a size from the calculated size. An endotracheal tube a half size larger and a half size smaller than calculated should always be available. Endotracheal tube size may also be based on patient age and body weight. An appropriately sized suction catheter should also always be available to suction secretions, blood, or fluid from the endotracheal tube (see Table 16-6).

Cuffed or Uncuffed Endotracheal Tubes

Historically, uncuffed endotracheal tubes were used in infants and smaller children because the appropriately sized cuffed endotracheal tube would be smaller and this would increase resistance and the work of breathing. Although concern exists that a cuffed endotracheal tube would increase the incidence of postextubation croup, that has proved not to be the case. In fact, using cuffed tubes minimizes the need for repeated

laryngoscopy and allows for lower fresh gas flows and decreased concentrations of anesthetic gases detectable in operating rooms.[57] When cuffed endotracheal tubes are used in infants and small children, the inflation pressure of the cuff must be checked and monitored during the case, especially if nitrous oxide is used. The leak pressure must also be checked when using uncuffed endotracheal tubes. If the leak pressure is too high, the endotracheal tube should be replaced with a smaller endotracheal tube, and if the leak pressure is too low, the endotracheal tube should be replaced with a larger endotracheal tube. Regardless of whether an uncuffed or cuffed endotracheal tube is chosen, it is important to maintain leak pressure around the tracheal tube no greater than 20 to 25 cm H_2O to decrease the likelihood of postextubation croup and the possibility of subsequent tracheal stenosis.

Microcuff Endotracheal Tubes

The new Microcuff pediatric endotracheal tubes appear to offer several distinct advantages over conventional pediatric cuffed endotracheal tubes. The Microcuff endotracheal tubes have a cuff that is made from a microthin polyurethane membrane that, while stronger than conventional cuffs, seals the airway at lower cuff pressures than conventional endotracheal tubes.[58] This reduces the potential for mucosal edema and postextubation croup. The cuff on the Microcuff endotracheal tube is also shorter and placed closer to the tip of the endotracheal tube, increasing the chances that the endotracheal tube is correctly placed. The Microcuff endotracheal tube also has an intubation depth mark, which indicates the correct depth for insertion and also increases the ability for correct placement.[59] The Microcuff endotracheal tubes are available in sizes down to 3.0 mm.

Stylet

Using a stylet stiffens the endotracheal tube and makes it easier to manipulate during direct laryngoscopy and tracheal intubation. The trachea of infants and small children can often be intubated without using a stylet, but a stylet may be useful for whenever a difficult tracheal intubation is anticipated. Even if intubating without a stylet, the appropriately sized stylet should always be immediately available (see Table 16-6).

Laryngoscopes

In general, a straight-blade laryngoscope is easier to use in infants and small children than a curved blade. The smaller profile of the straight blade is easier to use in the smaller mouths of infants and small children. The smaller tip of the straight blade also more effectively lifts the epiglottis than the curved blade. The disadvantage of a straight blade is that it does not retract the tongue as well to the left side of the mouth. A curved blade has a larger flange that retracts the tongue to the left more effectively and may be useful in certain patient populations in which the tongue is larger than normal (Beckwith-Wiedemann syndrome, trisomy 21).

In infants younger than 1 year, a Miller 1 straight laryngoscope blade is most useful. In children between 1 and 3 years of age, a 1½ straight laryngoscope blade, such as a Wis-Hipple, is often useful. A longer straight laryngoscope blade such as a Miller 2 is appropriate for most children between 3 and 10 years of age. The tracheas of children older than 11 years are often more easily intubated with a curved laryngoscope blade such as a Macintosh 3. Both straight and curved laryngoscope blades of various sizes should always be available.

Managing Difficult Airways in Infants and Children

The same general principles as outlined for managing a normal pediatric airway apply to managing either an unexpected or an expected difficult pediatric airway. It is unlikely that infants and children will cooperate with procedures such as awake fiberoptic tracheal intubation, so it is necessary to induce anesthesia and manage the airway with the patient asleep.

UNEXPECTED DIFFICULT AIRWAY

When an unexpected difficult airway appears in pediatric patients, the most important first step is to call for an additional anesthesia colleague to help (Fig. 16-23). It is critical to not persist with repeated attempts at direct laryngoscopy, which can result in trauma to the upper airway, edema, and bleeding. In most situations, an LMA should be inserted to provide an airway to

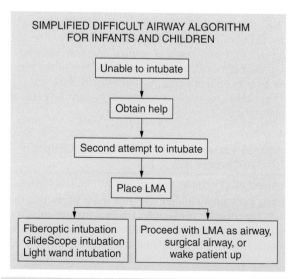

SIMPLIFIED DIFFICULT AIRWAY ALGORITHM
FOR INFANTS AND CHILDREN

Unable to intubate

Obtain help

Second attempt to intubate

Place LMA

Fiberoptic intubation
GlideScope intubation
Light wand intubation

Proceed with LMA as airway,
surgical airway, or
wake patient up

Figure 16-23 A suggested simplified algorithm for management of a difficult airway in infants and children. LMA, laryngeal mask airway.

oxygenate and ventilate the patient and allow time to obtain additional personnel and airway equipment. An LMA may be the only way to maintain an airway until the patient wakes up or a surgical airway is established. An LMA is also an excellent conduit for fiberoptic intubation.[60]

EXPECTED DIFFICULT AIRWAY

An expected difficult airway in pediatric patients should be approached with caution. Only preanesthetic medications that have minimal ventilatory depressant effects, such as midazolam, should be used. Preanesthetic medications should be administered in a location with appropriate airway equipment, including suction and a method of delivering oxygen with positive pressure. Pulse oximetry monitoring should be initiated at this time.

An additional anesthesia colleague should be available for help during the induction of anesthesia, inserting an intravenous line, and securing the airway. A surgeon capable of establishing a surgical airway and emergency airway equipment should be in the operating room before beginning the induction of anesthesia. The most difficult decision in managing an expected difficult pediatric airway is whether to attempt direct laryngoscopy or to proceed directly with an alternative strategy for managing the airway (fiberoptic, lighted stylet, surgical airway). It is often reasonable to make one attempt at direct laryngoscopy. Alternatively, the history and physical examination may indicate situations in which direct laryngoscopy will be unsuccessful such as halo traction preventing neck extension or limited mouth opening. In these cases one should proceed directly to an alternative strategy for managing the airway.

Unfortunately, a large number of difficult airway devices are effective in the adult patient, but are not currently appropriately sized for the infant and pediatric patient. The LMA CTrach and LMA Fastrach are available only in size 3 or larger and are therefore usable only in children larger than 30 kg in weight. The McGrath Video Laryngoscope is another product that can be very useful in difficult airway situations, but is not available in infant or pediatric sizes and is useful only on larger children.

LIGHTED STYLETS

A lighted stylet (lightwand) can be a useful adjunct for managing both the unexpected and the expected difficult airway in infants and children.[61] A lighted stylet can be used in patients who have limited mouth opening or limited neck flexion or extension. Tracheal intubation with the use of a lighted stylet may be much simpler and quicker than intubation with a fiberoptic bronchoscope. A lighted stylet can be used successfully in the presence of secretions or bleeding when the fiberoptic broncho-scope has failed. One disadvantage of a lighted stylet is that the operating room lights must be dimmed. A second disadvantage is that the success rate is significantly lower when the airway is deviated from midline by the presence of a mass or tumor.

Technique

The lighted stylet is placed through the endotracheal tube (smaller tubes are more likely to be successfully placed) so that the tip of the stylet is several millimeters proximal to the distal tip of the endotracheal tube (see Table 16-7). The lighted stylet with the loaded endotracheal tube is manually angled to between 90 and 120 degrees. The key to the successful use of a lighted stylet is to stay midline and anterior. The light should remain bright red as it passes from the supraglottic area into the trachea. Once the lighted stylet is in the trachea, the endotracheal tube should be advanced further into the trachea and the stylet removed. A lighted stylet can also be used for nasotracheal intubation after appropriate vasoconstriction of the nasal mucosa to minimize bleeding.

GLIDESCOPE

The GlideScope video laryngoscope (GVL) can also be useful for managing the difficult airway in infants and children. The GlideScope consists of a miniature fog-resistant high-resolution video camera embedded in a reusable laryngoscope blade. It requires a light source and the image is viewed on a color monitor. The major advantage of the GlideScope over conventional laryngoscopy is the ability to see "around a corner" and visualize the larynx even in patients with limited neck extension or very anterior airways. The GVL can facilitate teaching the difficult airway as the color monitor can be viewed by both the student and teacher at the same time and the output can be recorded to video for later review. The third major advantage of the GVL is that it is easier to learn to use than fiberoptic bronchoscopy in that it mimics the skills of direct laryngoscopy.

The major disadvantage of the GlideScope video laryngoscope is that it is available in a limited number of sizes and may be too large for some pediatric patients and too small for others. The GVL2 is 47 mm in length and is suitable for infants from 1.8 kg to 10 kg. The GVL3 is 82 mm in length and is suitable from 10 kg to adult patients. A second disadvantage is that the GVL requires a reasonable mouth opening to be used successfully.

FIBEROPTIC BRONCHOSCOPE

A flexible fiberoptic bronchoscope is another tool for managing a difficult pediatric airway. It is particularly valuable when the patient's mouth opening or neck mobility is limited. Disadvantages of a fiberoptic bronchoscope include a limited field of vision and interference from bleeding, secretions, or both. Fiberoptic bronchoscopes as small as 2.2 mm in outside diameter are available and can be used for endotracheal tubes as small as 3.0 mm ID.

These small bronchoscopes, however, do not have a suction channel and have optics that are inferior to those of larger scopes. In general, the fiberoptic bronchoscope should be at least 1 mm smaller in outside diameter than the ID of the endotracheal tube (Table 16-12).

Technique

Successful use of a fiberoptic bronchoscope as a tool to intubate the trachea in infants and children depends on several factors. Infants and children are unlikely to be able to cooperate with an awake fiberoptic intubation, and it is easier to perform an asleep fiberoptic intubation. Some anesthesia providers prefer to maintain spontaneous ventilation during fiberoptic laryngoscopy and tracheal intubation, especially if there is concern about the ability to ventilate the patient's lungs with a facemask. Frequently, it is easier to administer neuromuscular blocking drugs to a pediatric patient to provide better viewing conditions with less movement, less fogging of the bronchoscope, and less chance of laryngospasm. Using an elbow with a port that permits insertion of the fiberoptic bronchoscope allows for either continued spontaneous ventilation or assisted positive-pressure ventilation through the facemask.

For nasal fiberoptic laryngoscopy and tracheal intubation, a vasoconstrictor (phenylephrine [Neo-Synephrine]) should be administered to prevent bleeding, which will make visualization difficult. For oral fiberoptic laryngoscopy and tracheal intubation, an LMA or ILA can provide an excellent channel directly to the vocal cords while allowing for either spontaneous or controlled ventilation and oxygenation and shielding the bronchoscope from secretions and bleeding. It is useful to select the largest endotracheal tube that will easily fit through the LMA or ILA and the largest bronchoscope that will fit through the endotracheal tube (see Table 16-12). If an LMA or ILA is used as a conduit for oral fiberoptic laryngoscopy and tracheal intubation, it is simplest to leave the LMA or ILA in place until the end of the procedure while remembering to partially deflate the cuff of the LMA to prevent unnecessary pressure in the oropharynx.

Tracheal Extubation in Infants and Children
(Also See Chapter 34)

CROUP OR STRIDOR

Infants and small children are at a more likely risk than adults for croup or stridor after tracheal extubation. Croup occurs most commonly when either a cuffed or uncuffed endotracheal tube is used that is too large or when the cuff is inflated with too much air. The resulting mechanical pressure on the tracheal mucosa causes venous congestion and edema and in severe cases can even compromise the arterial blood supply and give rise to mucosal ischemia. The resulting edema can narrow the tracheal lumen,

Table 16-12 Laryngeal Mask Airway (LMA) as a Conduit for Tracheal Intubation with a Fiberoptic Bronchoscope (FOB)

LMA Size	Largest ETT Inside the LMA: ID (mm)	Largest FOB Inside the ETT: OD (mm)	Compatible FOB Models (with OD in mm)
1	3.0 uncuffed	2.2	Olympus LF-P (2.2)
1.5	4.0 uncuffed	3.0	Olympus LF-P (2.2) Pentax FI-9BS/RBS (3.0)
	3.5 cuffed	2.4	Olympus LF-P (2.2) Pentax FI-7P/BS/RBS (2.4)
2	4.5 uncuffed	3.4	Olympus LF-DP (3.1) Pentax FI-10BS/RBS (3.4)
	4.0 cuffed	3.0	Olympus LF-P (2.2) Pentax FI-9BS/RBS (3.0)
2.5	5.0 uncuffed	4.0	Olympus LF-2 (4.0) Pentax FI-10BS/RBS (3.4)
	4.5 cuffed	3.4	Olympus LF-DP (3.1) Pentax FI-10P2/BS/RBS (3.4)
3	5.5 cuffed	4.2	Olympus LF-2/GP (4.0/4.1) Pentax FI-13P/BS/RBS (4.2/4.1/4.1)
4	5.5 cuffed	4.2	Olympus LF-2/GP (4.0/4.1) Pentax FI-13P/BS/RBS (4.2/4.1/4.1)
5	6.5 cuffed	5.2	Olympus LF-TP (5.2) Pentax FI-16BS/RBS (5.1)

ETT, endotracheal tube; ID, internal diameter; OD, outside diameter.

especially in infants and small children. Because resistance to flow in an endotracheal tube is inversely proportional to the radius of the lumen to the fourth power, 1 mm of edema in an infant airway is much more significant than 1 mm of edema in an adult airway. Other risk factors for croup include multiple tracheal intubation attempts, unusual positioning of the head during surgery, increased duration of surgery, and procedures involving the upper airway, such as rigid bronchoscopy.

Manifestations

An infant or child with postextubation croup usually has respiratory distress in the postanesthesia care unit. Nasal flaring, retractions, an increased respiratory rate, audible stridor, and decreased oxygen saturation are common clinical findings.

Treatment

Treatment of postextubation croup or stridor depends on the degree of respiratory distress. Mild symptoms can be managed with humidified oxygen and prolonged observation in the postanesthesia care unit. More severe cases may require aerosolized racemic epinephrine and postoperative observation in an intensive care unit. Patients whose respiratory distress is severe and not relieved with these measures may need to be reintubated with an endotracheal tube smaller than the one previously used. Steroids administered intravenously for preventing upper airway edema are more beneficial when given before the airway is instrumented and should be administered before procedures such as rigid bronchoscopy.

OBSTRUCTIVE SLEEP APNEA

Infants and children with obstructive sleep apnea are at significant risk for airway obstruction, respiratory distress, and the potential for apnea in the postoperative period. At baseline these infants and children hypoventilate, which results in hypercapnia and often arterial hypoxemia when they are asleep. Residual inhaled anesthetics or residual neuromuscular blockade can depress airway reflexes, skeletal muscle tone and strength, and respiratory drive and result in significant airway compromise in infants and children with obstructive sleep apnea. Opioids must be very carefully titrated both intraoperatively and postoperatively because they can depress the ventilatory drive and contribute to significant hypercapnia and arterial hypoxemia in these infants and children.

Tracheal extubation in patients with obstructive sleep apnea should be considered only when these infants and children are fully awake. All infants and children with obstructive sleep apnea should be monitored postoperatively with pulse oximetry and apnea monitoring. High-risk patients should be monitored postoperatively in an intensive care unit setting.

Extubation after a Difficult Intubation

Tracheal extubation of an infant or child after a difficult intubation is considered carefully because reintubation can be more difficult than the initial intubation. The tracheas of infants and children with difficult airways should be extubated only when they are fully awake and there is no residual neuromuscular blockade.

Postoperative factors that can further compromise respiratory function must also be considered when extubating the trachea of an infant or child with a difficult airway. For example, postoperative pain, especially if there is splinting from an abdominal or thoracic incision, may compromise respiratory function. Postoperative pain requiring significant opioid use will also compromise breathing by decreasing the respiratory drive. The use of regional anesthesia, such as an epidural, may hasten the ability to extubate the trachea of these infants and children.

Edema of the airway from surgical trauma, positioning, or excessive fluid administration can significantly affect the ability to extubate the tracheas of infants and children with difficult airways and can make emergency reintubation more difficult. Infants and children with postoperative airway edema and difficult airways should remain intubated until the edema has resolved. An infant or child with a difficult airway should be extubated only when appropriate equipment and personnel are available for urgent reintubation.

QUESTIONS OF THE DAY

1. Which nerves provide sensory innervation to the oropharynx and hypopharynx?
2. What are the risk factors for difficult mask ventilation in the adult?
3. What are the contraindications to fiberoptic tracheal intubation?
4. How does the ProSeal laryngeal mask airway (LMA) differ from the classic LMA?
5. What are the most important upper airway anatomic differences in the infant compared to the adult?
6. What are the potential immediate and delayed complications after tracheal extubation? Which complications are more likely in the pediatric patient?
7. What are the advantages of cuffed versus uncuffed endotracheal tubes in the infant?

REFERENCES

1. Caplan RA, Benumof JL, Berry FA, et al: Practice guidelines for management of the difficult airway, *Anesthesiology* 98:1269–1277, 2003.
2. Langeron O, Masso E, Huraux C, et al: Prediction of difficult mask ventilation, *Anesthesiology* 92:1229–1236, 2000.
3. Langeron O, Amour J, Vivien B, et al: Clinical review: Management of difficult airways, *Crit Care* 10:243–247, 2006.
4. Crosby ET, Cooper RM, Douglas MJ, et al: The unanticipated difficult airway with recommendations for management, *Can J Anaesth* 45:757–776, 1998.
5. Hawthorne L, Wilson R, Lyons G, et al: Failed intubation revisited: 17-year experience in a teaching maternity unit, *Br J Anaesth* 76:680–684, 1996.
6. Shiga T, Wajima Z, Inoue T, et al: Predicting the difficult intubation in apparently normal patients, *Anesthesiology* 103:429–437, 2005.
7. Khan ZH, Mohammadi M, Rasouli MR, et al: The diagnostic value of the upper lip bite test combined with sternomental distance, thyromental distance and interincisor distance for the prediction of easy laryngoscopy and intubation: A prospective study, *Anesth Analg* 109:822–824, 2009.
8. Benumof JL: Management of the difficult adult airway, *Anesthesiology* 75:1087–1110, 1991.

9. Ovassapian A: *Fiberoptic Endoscopy in Anesthesia and Critical Care*, New York, 1990, Raven Press.
10. Stackhouse RA: Fiberoptic airway management, *Anesthesiol Clin North Am* 20:933–951, 2002.
11. Patil VU, Stehling LC, Zauder HL: *Fiberoptic Endoscopy in Anesthesia*, St Louis, 1983, CV Mosby.
12. Isaacs RS, Sykes JM: Anatomy and physiology of the upper airway, *Anesthesiol Clin North Am* 20:733–745, 2002.
13. Stackhouse RA, Bainton CR: Difficult airway management. In Hughes SC, Levinson G, Rosen MA, editors: *Shnider and Levinson's Anesthesia for Obstetrics*, Philadelphia, 2001, Lippincott Williams & Wilkins, pp 375–389.
14. Mallampati SR, Gatt SP, Gugino LD, et al: A clinical sign to predict difficult tracheal intubation: A prospective study, *Can Anaesth Soc J* 32:429–434, 1985.
15. Samsoon GL, Young JR: Difficult tracheal intubation: A retrospective study, *Anaesthesia* 42:487–490, 1987.
16. Cormack RS, Lehane J: Difficult tracheal intubation in obstetrics, *Anaesthesia* 39:1105–1111, 1984.
17. Williams KN, Carli F, Cormack RS: Unexpected, difficult laryngoscopy: A prospective survey in routine general surgery, *Br J Anaesth* 66:38–44, 1991.

18. Harmer M: Difficult and failed intubation in obstetrics, *Int J Obstet Anesth* 6:25–31, 1997.
19. El-Ganzouri AR, McCarthy RJ, Tuman KJ, et al: Preoperative airway assessment: Predictive value of a multivariate risk index, *Anesth Analg* 82:1197–1204, 1996.
20. Bellhouse CP, Dore C: Criteria for estimating likelihood of difficulty of endotracheal intubation with the Macintosh laryngoscope, *Anaesth Intensive Care* 16:329–337, 1988.
21. El-Orbany M, Woehlck HJ: Difficult mask ventilation, *Anesth Analg* 109:1870–1880, 2009.
22. Kheterpal S, Martin L, Shanks AM, et al: Prediction and outcomes of impossible mask ventilation. A review of 50,000 anesthetics, *Anesthesiology* 110:891–897, 2009.
23. Dixon BJ, Dixon JB, Carden JR, et al: Preoxygenation is more effective in the 25° head-up position than in the supine position in severely obese patients, *Anesthesiology* 102:1110–1115, 2005.
24. Gander S, Frascarolo P, Suter M, et al: Positive end-expiratory pressure during induction of general anesthesia increases duration of nonhypoxic apnea in morbidly obese patients, *Anesth Analg* 100:580–584, 2005.
25. Tournadre JP, Chassard D, Berrada KR, et al: Cricoid cartilage pressure decreases lower esophageal

sphincter tone, *Anesthesiology* 86:7–9, 1997.

26. Brimacombe JR, Berry AM: Cricoid pressure, *Can J Anaesth* 44:414–425, 1997.

27. Smith KJ, Dobranowski J, Yip G, et al: Cricoid pressure displaces the esophagus: An observational study using magnetic resonance imaging, *Anesthesiology* 99:60–64, 2003.

28. Klainer AS, Turndorf H, Wu WH, et al: Surface alterations due to endotracheal intubation, *Am J Med* 58:674–683, 1975.

29. Sengupta P, Sessler DI, Maglinger P, et al: Endotracheal tube cuff pressure in three hospitals, and the volume required to produce an appropriate cuff pressure, *BMC Anesthesiol* 4:8, 2004.

30. Hagberg CA: Special devices and techniques, *Anesthesiol Clin North Am* 20:907–932, 2002.

31. Cooper RM, Pacey JA, Bishop MJ, et al: Early clinical experience with a new videolaryngoscope (GlideScope) in 728 patients, *Can J Anaesth* 52:191–198, 2005.

32. Serocki G, Bein B, Scholz J, et al: Management of the predicted difficult airway: A comparison of conventional blade laryngoscopy with video-assisted blade laryngoscopy and the GlideScope, *Eur J Aneasthesiol* 27:24–30, 2010.

33. Turkstra TP, Eng M, Eng P, et al: Cervical spine motion: A fluoroscopic comparison during intubation with lighted stylet, GlideScope, and Macintosh laryngoscope, *Anesth Analg* 101:910–915, 2005.

34. Robitaille A, Williams SR, Tremblay MH, et al: Cervical spine motion during tracheal intubation with manual in-line stabilization: Direct laryngoscopy versus GlideScope® videolaryngoscopy, *Anesth Analg* 106:935–941, 2008.

35. Suzuki A, Toyama Y, Katsumi N, et al: The Pentax-AWS® rigid indirect video laryngoscope: Clinical assessment of performance in 320 cases, *Anaesthesia* 63:641–647, 2008.

36. Malin E, Montblanc Y, Ynineb Y, et al: Performance of the Airtraq laryngoscope after failed conventional tracheal intubation: a case series, *Acta Anaesthesiol Scand* 53:858–863, 2009.

37. Behringer EC: Approaches to managing the upper airway, *Anesthesiol Clin North Am* 20:813–832, 2002.

38. Bogetz MS: Using the laryngeal mask airway to manage the difficult airway, *Anesthesiol Clin North Am* 20:863–870, 2002.

39. Brain AIJ, Verghese C, Addy EV, et al: The intubating laryngeal mask. II: A preliminary clinical report of a new means of intubating the trachea, *Br J Anaesth* 79:704–709, 1997.

40. Liu EH, Wender R, Goldman AJ: The LMA CTrach™ in patients with difficult airways, *Anesthesiology* 110:941–943, 2009.

41. Brimacombe J, Keller C, Künzel KH, et al: Cervical spine motion during airway management: A cinefluoroscopic study of the posteriorly destabilized third cervical vertebrae in human cadavers, *Anesth Analg* 91:1274–1278, 2000.

42. Keller C, Brimacombe J, Kleinsasser A, et al: Does the ProSeal laryngeal mask airway prevent aspiration of regurgitated fluid? *Anesth Analg* 91:1017–1020, 2000.

43. Brimacombe J, Keller C, Judd DV: Gum elastic bougie-guided insertion of the ProSeal laryngeal mask airway is superior to the digital and introducer tool techniques, *Anesthesiology* 100:25–29, 2004.

44. Gaitni LA, Vaida SJ, Agro F: The Esophageal-Tracheal Combitube, *Anesthesiol Clin North Am* 20:894, 2002.

45. Agro F, Frass M, Benumof JL, et al: Current status of the Combitube: A review of the literature, *J Clin Anesth* 14:307–314, 2002.

46. Zamora JE, Saha TK: Combitube™ rescue for cesarean delivery followed by ninth and twelfth cranial nerve dysfunction, *Can J Anesth* 55:779–784, 2008.

47. Melker R, Florete O Jr: Percutaneous dilational cricothyrotomy and tracheostomy. In Benumof JL, editor: *Airway Management: Principles and Practice*, St Louis, 1996, Mosby Year Book.

48. Hawkins ML, Shapiro MB: Emergency cricothyrotomy: A reassessment, *Am Surg* 61:52–55, 1995.

49. Talving P, DuBose J, Inaba K, et al: Conversion of emergent cricothyrotomy to tracheotomy in trauma patients, *Arch Surg* 145(1):87–91, 2010.

50. Stackhouse RA: Transtracheal oxygenation, *Int Anesthesiol Clin* 32:85–94, 1994.

51. Slutsky AS, Watson J, Leith D, et al: Tracheal insufflation of O_2 (TRIO) at low flow rates sustains life for several hours, *Anesthesiology* 63:278–286, 1985.

52. Warner ME, Benenfeld SM, Warner MA, et al: Perianesthetic dental injuries. Frequency, outcomes, and risk factors, *Anesthesiology* 90:1302–1305, 1999.

53. Stackhouse R, Infosino A: Airway management. In Stoelting RK, Miller RD, editors: *Basics of Anesthesia*, ed 5, Philadelphia, 2007, Churchill Livingstone, pp 207–239.

54. O'Neill B, Templeton J, Camarico L, Schreiner M: The laryngeal mask airway in pediatric patients: Factors affecting ease of use during insertion and emergence, *Anesth Analg* 78:659–662, 1994.

55. Wakeling H, Butler P, Baxter P: The laryngeal mask airway: A comparison between two insertion techniques, *Anesth Analg* 85:687–690, 1997.

56. Pennant J, White P: The laryngeal mask airway: Its uses in anesthesiology, *Anesthesiology* 79:144–163, 1993.

57. Khine HH, Corddry DH, Kettrick RG, et al: Comparison of cuffed and uncuffed endotracheal tubes in young children during general anesthesia, *Anesthesiology* 86:627–631, 1997.

58. Dullenkopf A, Schmitz A, Gerber AC, et al: Tracheal sealing characteristics of pediatric cuffed tracheal tubes, *Pediatric Anesthesia* 14:825–830, 2004.

59. Weiss M, Balmer C, Dullenkopf A, et al: Intubation depth markings allow an improved positioning of endotracheal tubes in children, *Can J Anaesth* 52:721–726, 2005.

60. Benumof J: Laryngeal mask airway and the ASA difficult airway algorithm, *Anesthesiology* 84:686–699, 1996.

61. Holzman R, Nargozian C, Florence F: Lightwand intubation in children with abnormal upper airways, *Anesthesiology* 69:784–787, 1988.

III

17 SPINAL AND EPIDURAL ANESTHESIA

Kenneth Drasner and Merlin D. Larson

Collectively referred to as central neuraxial block, spinal anesthesia and epidural anesthesia represent a subcategory of regional or conduction anesthesia. In addition to their current widespread use in the operating room for surgical anesthesia and as an adjunct to general anesthesia, neuraxial techniques are effective means for controlling obstetric (see Chapter 33) and postoperative pain (see Chapter 40).

COMPARISON OF SPINAL AND EPIDURAL ANESTHESIA

Spinal anesthesia is accomplished by injecting local anesthetic solution into the cerebrospinal fluid (CSF) contained within the subarachnoid (intrathecal) space. In contrast, epidural anesthesia is achieved by injection of local anesthetic solution into the space that lies within the vertebral canal but outside or superficial to the dural sac. Caudal anesthesia represents a special type of epidural anesthesia in which local anesthetic solution is injected into the caudal epidural space through a needle introduced through the sacral hiatus. Although epidural anesthesia is routinely performed at various levels along the neuraxis, subarachnoid injections are limited to the lumbar region below the termination of the spinal cord.

When compared with epidural anesthesia, spinal anesthesia takes less time to perform, causes less discomfort during placement, requires less local anesthetic, and produces more intense sensory and motor block. In addition, correct placement of the needle in the subarachnoid space is confirmed by a clearly defined end point (appearance of CSF).

Advantages of epidural anesthesia include a decreased risk for post–dural puncture headache (assuming a negligible incidence of inadvertent dural puncture), a lower incidence of systemic hypotension, the ability to produce a segmental sensory block, and greater control over the intensity of sensory anesthesia and motor block achieved by adjustment of the local anesthetic concentration. The routine placement of catheters for epidural anesthesia imparts additional benefit by allowing titration of the block to the duration of surgery. Additionally, a catheter provides a means for long-term administration of local anesthetics or opioid-containing solutions (or both), which are highly effective for control of postoperative or obstetric pain.

Patients may remain completely awake during surgery performed under neuraxial block, but more commonly they are sedated with various combinations of intravenous drugs, including sedative-hypnotics, opioids, and anesthetics (propofol). Skeletal muscle relaxation can be profound in the presence of neuraxial anesthesia and this may obviate the need for neuromuscular blocking drugs. However, despite potential advantages, patients may be reluctant to accept neuraxial anesthesia for fear of permanent nerve damage. Although there does exist the rare possibility of neural injury as a result of neuraxial anesthesia, patient concerns generally far exceed the clinical reality and at times are based on undocumented and unfounded stories of paralysis.[1]

As with other regional techniques, central neuraxial techniques require an understanding of the underlying anatomy and physiologic principles.

ANATOMY

Vertebral Canal

The spinal cord and its nerve roots are contained within the vertebral (spinal) canal, a bony structure that extends from the foramen magnum to the sacral hiatus (Fig. 17-1).[2] On a lateral view the vertebral canal exhibits four curvatures, of which the thoracic convexity (kyphosis) and the lumbar concavity (lordosis) are of major importance to the distribution of local anesthetic solution in the subarachnoid space. In contrast, these curves have little effect on the spread of local anesthetic solutions in the epidural space.

In addition to structural support, the vertebral canal provides critical protection to vulnerable neural structures. Unfortunately, this bony canal also creates a barrier to an advancing spinal or epidural needle seeking to trespass this space. Successful neuraxial block is thus critically dependent on the anesthesia provider's appreciation of the anatomy of this structure.

ARCHITECTURE

The building blocks of the vertebral canal are the vertebrae, which are stacked to form the tubular column (Figs. 17-2 and 17-3; also see Fig. 17-1).[2,3] This complex architecture is best appreciated by examination of a skeleton or a three-dimensional model. Although the structure of the vertebrae varies considerably, depending on their location and function, each consists of an anterior vertebral body and a posterior arch. The posterior arch is created by fusion of the lateral cylindrical pedicles with the two flattened posterior laminae. A transverse process extends out laterally at each junction of the pedicle and laminae, whereas a single spinous process projects posteriorly from the junction of the two laminae. Each pedicle is notched on its superior and inferior surface, and when two adjacent vertebrae are articulated, these notches form the intervertebral foramina through which the spinal nerves emerge.

NOMENCLATURE AND FEATURES

Of the 24 true vertebrae, the first 7, located in the neck, are called cervical vertebrae, the next 12 are attached to the ribs and are called thoracic (or dorsal) vertebrae, and the remaining 5 are the lumbar vertebrae. Another five vertebrae, called false or fixed vertebrae, are fused to form the bony sacrum (Fig 17-4).[4] Thus, the sacrum and coccyx are distal extensions of the vertebral column, and the sacral canal is a continuation of the vertebral canal through the sacrum.

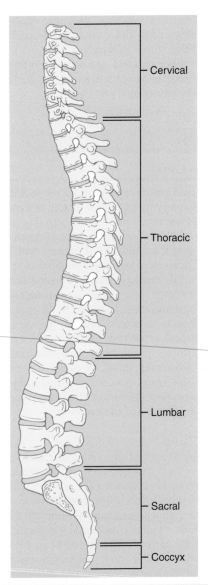

Figure 17-1 The vertebral column from a lateral view exhibits four curvatures. (From Covino BG, Scott DB, Lambert DH. Handbook of Spinal Anaesthesia and Analgesia. Philadelphia, WB Saunders, 1994, pp 12-24.)

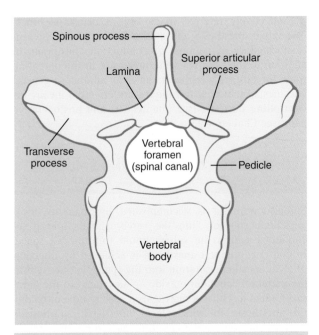

Figure 17-2 Typical thoracic vertebra. (From Covino BG, Scott DB, Lambert DH. Handbook of Spinal Anaesthesia and Analgesia. Philadelphia, WB Saunders, 1994.)

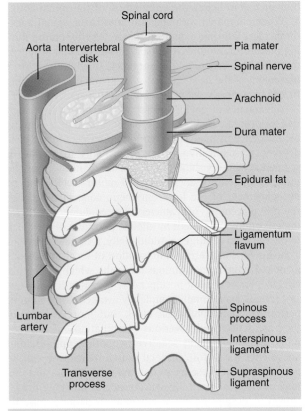

Figure 17-3 The spine in an oblique view. (From Afton-Bird G. Atlas of regional anesthesia. In Miller RD [ed]. Miller's Anesthesia. Philadelphia, Elsevier, 2005.)

The features of the midthoracic and lumbar vertebrae can ideally be represented by two articulated vertebrae (Fig. 17-5).[5] The nearly perpendicular orientation of the spinous process in the lumbar area and the downward angular orientation in the thoracic area define the angle required for placement and advancement of a needle intended to access the vertebral canal. The wide interlaminar space in the lumbar spine reflects the fact that the lamina occupies only about half the space between adjacent vertebrae. In contrast, the interlaminar space is just a few millimeters wide at the level of the thoracic vertebrae.

Figure 17-4 The sacrum in lateral and posterior view. (From Brown DL [ed]. Atlas of Regional Anesthesia. Philadelphia, WB Saunders, 1992.)

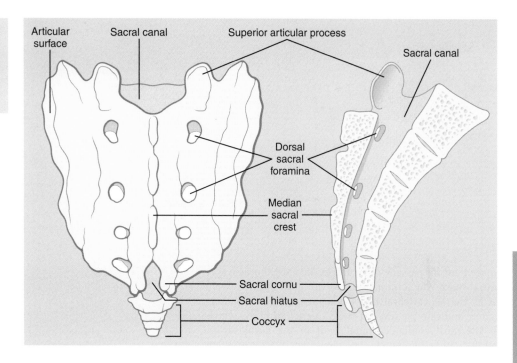

Figure 17-5 Lateral view of the thoracic and lumbar vertebrae. Note the sharp downward angulation of the thoracic spinous processes versus the nearly perpendicular angle that they assume in the lumbar vertebrae. (From Kardish K. Functional anatomy of central blockade in obstetrics. In Birnbach DJ, Gatt SP, Datta S [eds]. Textbook of Obstetric Anesthesia. Philadelphia, Churchill Livingstone, 2000, pp 121-156.)

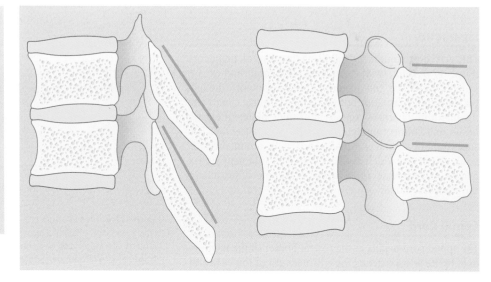

SACRUM AND SACRAL HIATUS

The sacrum is a large curved wedge-shaped bone whose dorsal surface is convex and gives rise to the powerful sacrospinalis muscle. The opening between the unfused lamina of the fourth and fifth sacral vertebrae is called the sacral hiatus. There is considerable anatomic variability in the features of the dorsal surface of the sacrum. Indeed, the sacral hiatus is absent in nearly 8% of adult subjects, thereby preventing entry through the sacrococcygeal ligament into the sacral canal and performance of caudal anesthesia.

SURFACE LANDMARKS

Surface landmarks are used to identify specific spinal interspaces (Fig. 17-6).[4] The most important of these landmarks is a line drawn between the iliac crests. This line generally traverses the body of the L4 vertebra and is the principal landmark used to determine the level for insertion of a needle intended to produce spinal anesthesia. The C7 spinous process can be appreciated as a bony knob at the lower end of the neck. The T7-T8 interspace is identified by a line drawn between the lower limits of the scapulae and is often used to guide needle

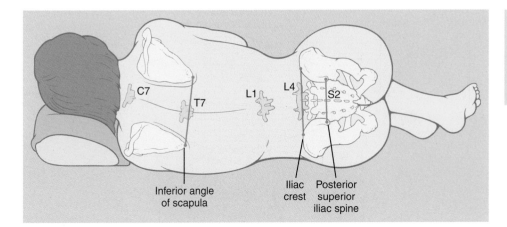

Figure 17-6 Surface landmarks are a guide to the vertebral level. (From Brown DL [ed]. Atlas of Regional Anesthesia. Philadelphia, WB Saunders, 1992.)

placement for passage of a catheter into the thoracic epidural space. The terminal portion of the twelfth rib intersects the L2 vertebral body, whereas the posterior iliac spines indicate the level of the S2 vertebral body, which is the most common caudal limit of the dural sac in adults. Other interspaces are identified by counting up or down along the spinous processes from these major landmarks.

Ligaments

The vertebral column is stabilized by several ligaments (Figs. 17-7 and 17-8).[2] Adjacent vertebral bodies are joined by anterior and posterior spinal ligaments, the latter forming the anterior border of the vertebral canal. The ligamentum flavum is composed of thick plates of elastic tissue that connect the lamina of adjacent vertebrae. The supraspinous ligament runs superficially along the spinous processes, which makes it the first ligament that a needle will traverse when using a midline approach to the vertebral canal.

Spinal Cord

The spinal cord begins at the rostral border of the medulla and, in the fetus, extends the entire length of the vertebral canal. However, because of disproportionate growth of neural tissue and the vertebral canal, the spinal cord generally terminates around the third lumbar vertebra at birth and at the lower border of the first lumbar vertebra in adults. As a further consequence of this differential growth, the spinal nerves become progressively longer and more closely aligned with the longitudinal axis of the vertebral canal. Below the conus, the roots are oriented parallel to this axis and resemble a horse's tail, from which the name cauda equina is derived (Fig. 17-9).[6] The nerve roots of the cauda equina move relatively freely within the CSF, a fortunate arrangement that permits them to be displaced rather than pierced by an advancing needle.

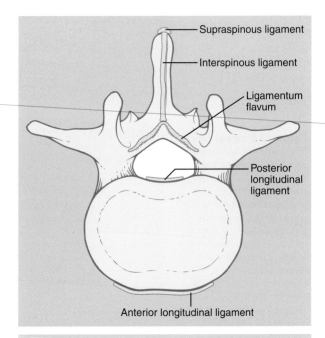

Figure 17-7 Cross section of a lumbar vertebra showing the attachment of the spinal ligaments. (From Covino BG, Scott DB, Lambert DH. Handbook of Spinal Anaesthesia and Analgesia. Philadelphia, WB Saunders, 1994, p 15.)

Meninges

In addition to the CSF, the spinal cord is surrounded and protected by three layers of connective tissue known as the meninges.

DURA MATER

The outermost layer, the dura mater, originates at the foramen magnum as an extension of the inner (meningeal) layer of cranial dura and continues caudally to

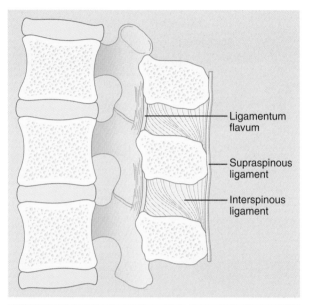

Figure 17-8 Sagittal section through adjacent lumbar vertebrae showing the attachment of the spinal ligaments. (From Covino BG, Scott DB, Lambert DH. Handbook of Spinal Anaesthesia and Analgesia. Philadelphia, WB Saunders, 1994, p 15.)

Labels in figure: Ligamentum flavum; Supraspinous ligament; Interspinous ligament

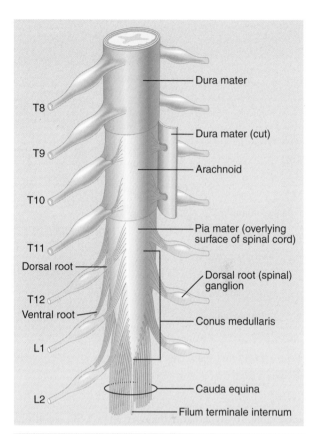

Figure 17-9 Terminal spinal cord and cauda equina. (From Bridenbaugh PO, Greene NM, Brull SJ. Spinal [subarachnoid] blockade. In Cousins MJ, Bridenbaugh PO [eds]. Neural Blockade in Clinical Anesthesia and Management of Pain. Philadelphia, Lippincott-Raven, 1998, pp 203-242.)

Labels in figure: T8; T9; T10; T11; Dorsal root; T12; Ventral root; L1; L2; Dura mater; Dura mater (cut); Arachnoid; Pia mater (overlying surface of spinal cord); Dorsal root (spinal) ganglion; Conus medullaris; Cauda equina; Filum terminale internum

terminate between S1 and S4. It is a tough fibroelastic membrane that provides structural support and a fairly impenetrable barrier that normally prevents displacement of an epidural catheter into the fluid-filled subarachnoid space. Although cases of epidural catheter migration into the subarachnoid space occur clinically, it has been well established in cadaver studies that catheters cannot penetrate an intact dura.

ARACHNOID MEMBRANE

Closely adherent to the inner surface of the dura lies the arachnoid membrane. Though far more delicate than the dura, the arachnoid serves as the major pharmacologic barrier preventing movement of drug from the epidural to the subarachnoid space. Conceptually, the dura provides support and the arachnoid membrane imparts impermeability. Because the dura and arachnoid are closely adherent, a spinal needle that penetrates the dura will generally pass through the arachnoid membrane. However, "subdural" injections can occur in clinical practice and result in a "failed spinal" because of the relative impermeability of the arachnoid membrane.

PIA

The innermost layer of the spinal meninges, the pia is a highly vascular structure closely applied to the cord that forms the inner border of the subarachnoid space. Along the lateral surface between the dorsal and ventral roots, an extension of this membrane forms the denticulate ligament—a dense serrated longitudinal projection that provides lateral suspension through its attachment to the dura. As the spinal cord tapers to form the conus medullaris, the pia continues interiorly as a thin filament, the filum terminale. Distally, the filum terminale becomes enveloped by the dura at the caudal termination of the dural sac (generally around S2) and continues inferiorly to attach to the posterior wall of the coccyx.

Spinal Nerves

Along the dorsolateral and ventrolateral aspect of the spinal cord, rootlets emerge and coalesce to form the dorsal (afferent) and ventral (efferent) spinal nerve roots (Fig. 17-10).[2] Distal to the dorsal root ganglion, these nerve roots merge to form 31 pairs of spinal nerves (8 cervical, 12 thoracic, 5 lumbar, 5 sacral, and 1 coccygeal). Because the sensory fibers traverse the posterior aspect of the subarachnoid space, they tend to lie dependent in a supine patient, thus making them particularly

III

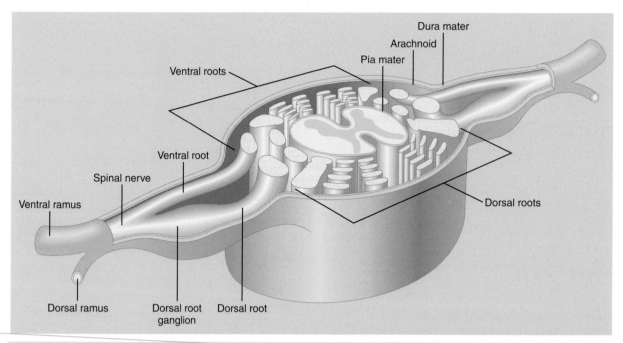

Figure 17-10 The spinal cord and nerve roots. (From Covino BG, Scott DB, Lambert DH. Handbook of Spinal Anaesthesia and Analgesia. Philadelphia, WB Saunders, 1994, p 19.)

vulnerable to hyperbaric (heavier than CSF) solutions containing local anesthetic.

As the nerves pass through the intervertebral foramen, they become encased by the dura, arachnoid, and pia, which form the epineurium, perineurium, and endoneurium, respectively. The dura becomes thinned as it traverses this area (often called the dural sleeve), thereby facilitating penetration of local anesthetic. The onset of epidural block by local anesthetics thus occurs by blockade of sodium ion conductance in this region. With time, epidural local anesthetics transfer into the subarachnoid space, and the nerve roots and spinal cord tracts are variably affected. This accounts for the observation that the onset of an epidural block spreads rostrally and caudally from the point of injection, but the pattern of recession is not a strict reversal of the onset.

PREGANGLIONIC SYMPATHETIC NERVE FIBERS

Preganglionic sympathetic nerve fibers originating in the intermediolateral gray columns of the thoracolumbar cord leave with the ventral nerve roots passing into the spinal nerve trunks (Fig. 17-11). They then leave the nerve via the white rami communicates and project to the paravertebral sympathetic ganglia or more distant sites (adrenal medulla, mesenteric and celiac plexus). After a cholinergic synapse (nicotinic) in the autonomic ganglia, the postsynaptic sympathetic nerve fibers join the spinal nerves via the gray rami communicantes and innervate diverse adrenergic effector sites.

CERVICAL NERVES

The first cervical nerve passes between the occipital bone and the posterior arch of the first cervical vertebra (atlas), and this relationship continues, with the seventh cervical nerve passing above the seventh cervical vertebra. However, because there are eight cervical nerves but only seven cervical vertebrae, the eighth cervical nerve passes between the seventh cervical vertebra and the first thoracic vertebra. Below this point, each spinal nerve passes through the inferior notch of the corresponding vertebra. For example, the T1 spinal nerve passes through the notch formed by the first and second thoracic vertebrae.

DERMATOME

The area of skin innervated by each spinal nerve is called a dermatome (Fig. 17-12).[7] Because the lower nerve roots descend before exiting the intervertebral foramen, the spinal cord terminations of the afferent fibers from each dermatome are more rostral than their corresponding vertebral level. For example, the sensory fibers from the L4 dermatome enter the spinal canal below the L4 vertebral body. However, primary afferent terminals for the L4 dermatome are located anterior to the T11-T12 interspace.

Subarachnoid Space

Between the arachnoid and the pia lies the subarachnoid space, which contains the CSF formed mainly by the choroid plexus of the lateral, third, and fourth ventricles.

Figure 17-11 Cell bodies in the thoracolumbar portion of the spinal cord (T1-L2) give rise to the peripheral sympathetic nervous system. Efferent fibers travel in the ventral root and then via the white ramus communicans to paravertebral sympathetic ganglia or more distant sites such as the celiac ganglion. Afferent fibers travel via the white ramus communicans to join somatic nerves, which pass through the dorsal root to the spinal cord.

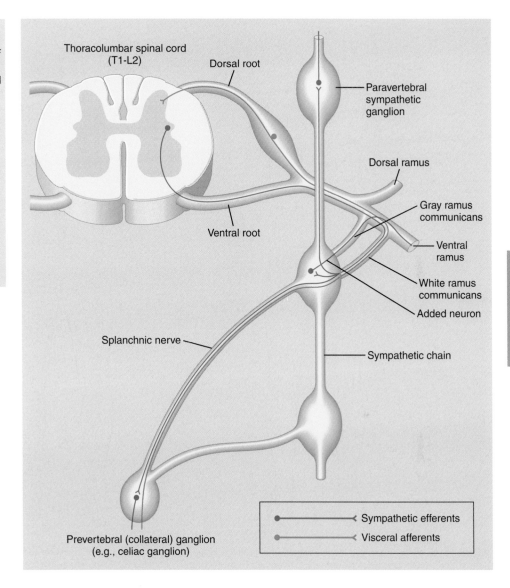

Thoracolumbar spinal cord (T1-L2)

Dorsal root

Paravertebral sympathetic ganglion

Dorsal ramus

Gray ramus communicans

Ventral ramus

Ventral root

White ramus communicans

Added neuron

Splanchnic nerve

Sympathetic chain

Prevertebral (collateral) ganglion (e.g., celiac ganglion)

⬤━━━━━ Sympathetic efferents
⬤━━━━━ Visceral afferents

III

Because the spinal and cranial arachnoid spaces are continuous, cranial nerves can be blocked by local anesthetics migrating into the CSF above the foramen magnum.

Epidural Space

The epidural space lies between the dura and the wall of the vertebral canal, an irregular column of fat, lymphatics, and blood vessels. It is bounded cranially by the foramen magnum, caudally by the sacrococcygeal ligament, anteriorly by the posterior longitudinal ligament, laterally by the vertebral pedicles, and posteriorly by both the ligamentum flavum and vertebral lamina. The epidural space is not a closed space but communicates with the paravertebral spaces by way of the intervertebral foramina. The depth of the epidural space is maximal (about 6 mm) in the midline at L2 and is 4 to 5 mm in the midthoracic region. It is minimal where the lumbar and cervical enlargements of the spinal cord (T9-T12 and C3-T2, respectively) encroach on the epidural space, with roughly 3 mm left between the ligamentum flavum and the dura. There are subcompartments in the epidural space at each vertebral level, but injected fluid generally communicates freely throughout the space from the rostral limit at the foramen magnum to the sacral hiatus caudally. There is controversy regarding the existence and clinical significance of a connective tissue band (plica mediana dorsalis) extending from the dura mater to the ligamentum flavum and hence dividing the posterior epidural space into two compartments. Anatomic studies have suggested the presence of this structure and have led to the speculation that this tissue band may be

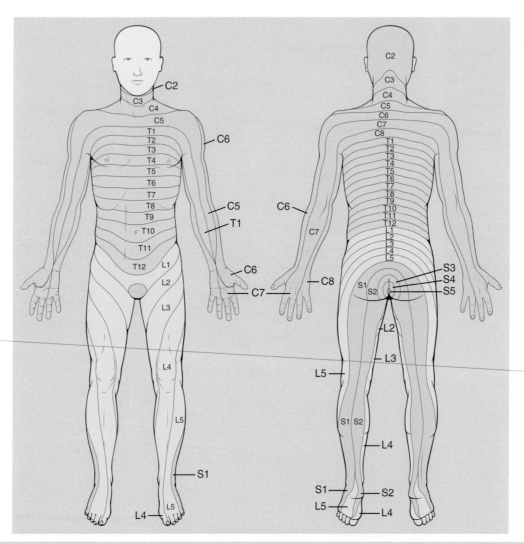

Figure 17-12 Areas of sensory innervation by spinal nerves. Note that the thoracic nerves innervate the thorax and abdomen and the lumbar and sacral nerves innervate the leg. (Modified from Veering BT, Cousins MJ. Epidural neural blockade. In Cousins MJ, Bridenbaugh PO, Carr DB, Horlocker TT [eds]. Neural Blockade in Clinical Anesthesia and Management of Pain. Philadelphia, Lippincott-Raven, 2009, pp 241-295.)

responsible for the occasional difficulty threading a catheter into the epidural space or the unexplained occurrence of a unilateral sensory block. Nevertheless, others are unable to confirm the presence of this structure.[8]

Blood Vessels

ARTERIAL

The blood supply of the spinal cord arises from a single anterior and two paired posterior spinal arteries (Fig. 17-13).[2] The posterior spinal arteries emerge from the cranial vault and supply the dorsal (sensory) portion of the spinal cord. Because they are paired and have rich collateral anastomotic links from the subclavian and intercostal arteries, this area of the spinal cord is relatively protected from ischemic damage. This is not the case with the single anterior spinal artery that originates from the vertebral artery and supplies the ventral (motor) portion of the spinal cord. The anterior spinal artery receives branches from the intercostal and iliac arteries, but these branches are variable in number and location. The largest anastomotic link, the radicularis magna (artery of Adamkiewicz), arises from the aorta in the lower thoracic or upper lumbar region.

Artery of Adamkiewicz

The vessel is highly variable but, most commonly, is on the left and enters the vertebral canal through the L1 intervertebral foramen. The artery of Adamkiewicz is

Figure 17-13 Arterial blood supply to the spinal cord. (Modified from Covino BG, Scott DB, Lambert DH. Handbook of Spinal Anaesthesia and Analgesia. Philadelphia, WB Saunders 1994, p 24.)

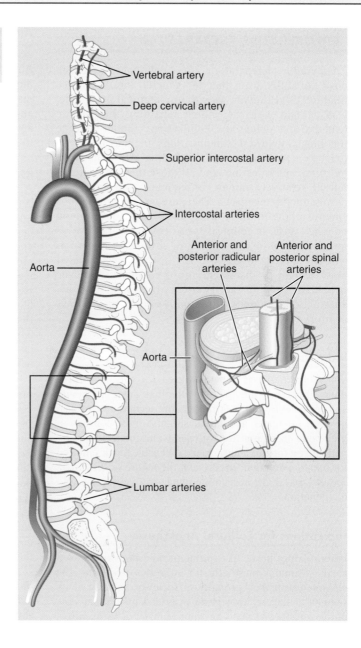

critical to the blood supply of the lower two thirds of the spinal cord, and damage to this artery during surgery on the aorta (aortic aneurysm resection) or by a stray epidural needle will produce characteristic bilateral lower extremity motor loss (anterior spinal artery syndrome).

VENOUS

The internal vertebral venous plexus drains the contents of the vertebral canal. These veins are prominent in the lateral epidural space and ultimately empty into the azygos venous system. The azygos vein enters the chest, arches over the right lung, and then empties into the superior vena cava. The internal vertebral venous plexus communicates above with the basilar sinuses of the brain and below with the pelvic connections to the inferior vena cava.

The anatomy of the venous plexus assumes additional importance in patients with increased intra-abdominal pressure or those with tumors or masses that compress the vena cava. In these patients, blood is diverted from the inferior vena cava and engorges veins in the epidural space, which increases the likelihood of accidental vascular cannulation during attempted epidural anesthesia. In addition, because the vertebral veins are enlarged, the effective volume of the epidural space is reduced, thereby resulting in greater longitudinal spread of injected local anesthetic solutions.

PREOPERATIVE PREPARATION

Preoperative preparation for regional anesthesia does not differ from that for general anesthesia (see Chapter 13). However, as with any regional anesthetic, a discussion with the patient regarding the specific benefits and potential complications should precede the block. Relevant complications include (1) those that are rare but serious, including nerve damage, bleeding, and infection, and (2) those that are common but of relatively minor consequence, such as post-dural puncture headache. There are no common serious complications (if there were, these techniques would not be used in clinical practice), and the infrequent minor problems are not of sufficient concern to warrant specific discussion. The possibility of a failed block should be discussed, and the patient should be reassured that in such circumstances, alternative anesthetic techniques will be provided to ensure their comfort.

Indications for Spinal Anesthesia

Spinal anesthesia is generally used for surgical procedures involving the lower abdominal area, perineum, and lower extremities. Although the technique can also be used for upper abdominal surgery, most consider it preferable to administer a general anesthetic to ensure patient comfort. In addition, the extensive block required for upper abdominal surgery and the nature of these procedures may have a negative impact on ventilation and oxygenation.

Indications for Epidural Anesthesia

Epidural anesthesia, like spinal anesthesia, is often used as the primary anesthetic for surgeries involving the abdomen or lower extremities. However, because of its segmental nature, anesthesia provided by lumbar epidural anesthesia may be suboptimal for procedures involving the lower sacral roots. Epidural anesthesia is also frequently used as a supplement to general anesthesia, particularly for thoracic and upper abdominal procedures. In such cases, significant benefit derives from the ability to provide continuous epidural anesthesia postoperatively to facilitate effective treatment of postoperative pain, and numerous studies confirm the superiority of epidural techniques compared to parenteral opioids.[9,10] Similarly, continuous epidural anesthesia is very effective and widely used for the control of labor pain. Cervical epidural anesthesia is very rarely used for operative surgery, but injections of solutions of corticosteroids and local anesthetics into the cervical epidural space are sometimes used to treat chronic pain.

Absolute and Relative Contraindications to Neuraxial Anesthesia

Absolute contraindications to neuraxial anesthetic techniques include patient refusal, infection at the site of planned needle puncture, elevated intracranial pressure, and bleeding diathesis. Patients should never be encouraged against their wishes to accept a regional anesthetic technique.

INFECTION
A Practice Advisory published by a task force of the American Society of Anesthesiologists addresses the issues related to infectious complications associated with neuraxial techniques, and can be reviewed for guidance.[11] Importantly, bacteremia does not necessarily mitigate against performance of a regional anesthetic technique. Although concern that an epidural abscess or meningitis might result from the introduction of infected blood during the procedure, clinical experience suggests that the risk is small and can be weighed against the potential benefit. In such cases, there is evidence to suggest that institution of appropriate antibiotic therapy before the block may decrease the risk for infection.[11]

PREEXISTING NEUROLOGIC DISEASE
The significance of any preexisting neurologic disease should be considered relative to its underlying pathophysiology. For example, patients with multiple sclerosis experience exacerbations and remissions of symptoms reflecting demyelination of peripheral nerves. Local anesthetic toxicity, when it occurs, can be associated with similar histopathology.[12] Although neuraxial anesthetic techniques have been viewed as acceptable for patients with multiple sclerosis, in the absence of compelling benefit, neuraxial techniques would be best avoided in these patients.

Chronic back pain does not represent a contraindication to neuraxial anesthetic techniques, although they may be avoided because patients may perceive a relationship between postoperative exacerbation of pain and the block, even though they are not causally related.

CARDIAC DISEASE
Patients with mitral stenosis, idiopathic hypertrophic subaortic stenosis, and aortic stenosis are intolerant of acute decreases in systemic vascular resistance. Thus, though not a contraindication, neuraxial block should be used cautiously in such cases.

ABNORMAL COAGULATION
The decision to use a neuraxial block in patients with abnormal coagulation, either endogenous or produced by the administration of anticoagulants, must be based on a risk-benefit assessment and include discussion with the patient and the surgical team. Guidelines developed

by the American Society of Regional Anesthesia and Pain Medicine (www.asra.com) are updated periodically based on evolving literature and changes in clinical practice, and can thus provide valuable guidance in the management of these patients.

SPINAL ANESTHESIA

An intravenous infusion is started before performance of the anesthetic, and all of the equipment, drugs, and monitors normally present for a general anesthetic are also required for neuraxial anesthesia. Supplemental oxygen is commonly administered. Although accurate end-tidal carbon dioxide monitoring may not always be feasible, a capnograph is often used to monitor breathing. This can be accomplished with specially designed nasal cannulae, or equipment can be easily improvised to permit sampling from nasal cannulae or face masks.

To decrease the discomfort associated with needle insertions, inclusion of an opioid in the preoperative medication should be considered. However, in selected patients premedication can be withheld, provided that there is adequate attention to infiltration of the skin and subcutaneous tissues with local anesthetic solution.

Sterile technique with hat, mask, and gloves is mandatory, and in modern practice, the required equipment is obtained from prepackaged sterile kits. Antiseptic preparation of the skin is performed, but contact with gloves and needles should be avoided because of the potential neurotoxicity of these antiseptic solutions.

Patient Positioning (Also See Chapter 19)

Spinal anesthesia can be performed with the patient in the lateral decubitus, sitting, or less commonly, the prone position. To the extent possible, the spine should be flexed by having the patient bend at the waist and bring the chin toward the chest, which will optimize the interspinous space and the interlaminar foramen.

LATERAL POSITION
The lateral decubitus position is more comfortable and more suitable for the ill or frail. It also enables the anesthesia provider to safely provide greater levels of sedation.

SITTING POSITION
The sitting position encourages flexion and facilitates recognition of the midline, which may be of increased importance in an obese patient. Because lumbar CSF is elevated in this position, the dural sac is distended, thus providing a larger target for the spinal needle. This higher pressure also facilitates recognition of the needle tip within the subarachnoid space, as heralded by the free flow of CSF. When combined with a hyperbaric anesthetic, the sitting position favors a caudal distribution, the resultant

anesthesia commonly being referred to as a "saddle block." However, in addition to being poorly suited for a heavily sedated patient, vasovagal syncope can occur.

PRONE POSITION
The prone position is rarely used except for perineal procedures performed in the "jackknife" position. Performance of spinal anesthesia in this position is more challenging because of the limited flexion, the contracted dural sac, and the low CSF pressure, which generally requires aspiration with the plunger of the syringe to achieve backflow of CSF through the spinal needle.

Selection of Interspace

Several factors influence the selection of the interspace to be used for spinal anesthesia. The most obvious is the specific anatomy of the patient's spine and the likelihood that a needle can be successfully passed into the subarachnoid space. A second and often underappreciated consideration is that the interspace selected for spinal anesthesia has considerable impact on the distribution of anesthetic within the subarachnoid space. This, in turn, will affect the success or failure of the technique. For example, the likelihood of a "failed spinal" increases as interspaces that are more caudal are used, with up to a 7% incidence occurring when the L4-L5 interspace is selected.[13]

Although more rostral interspaces are associated with higher success rates, this benefit must be balanced against the potential for traumatic injury to the spinal cord, keeping in mind that the caudal limitation of the spinal cord in an adult usually lies between the L1 and L2 vertebrae. For this reason, spinal anesthesia is not ordinarily performed above the L2-L3 interspace. Nevertheless, some risk remains because the spinal cord extends to the third lumbar vertebra in approximately 2% of adults. Furthermore, the use of a conceptual line across the iliac crests to identify the body of the L4 vertebra often results in selection of an interspace that is one or more levels higher than believed.[14]

Spinal Needles

A variety of needles are available for spinal anesthesia and are generally classified by their size (most commonly 22 to 25 gauge) and the shape of their tip (Fig. 17-14).[15] The two basic designs of spinal needles are (1) an open-ended (beveled or cutting) needle and (2) a closed tapered-tip pencil-point needle with a side port. The incidence of post–dural puncture headache varies directly with the size of the needle. The pressure is lower when a pencil-point (Whitacre or Sprotte) rather than a beveled-tip (Quincke) needle is used. Consequently, a 24- or 25-gauge pencil-point needle is usually selected when spinal anesthesia is performed on younger patients, in whom post–dural puncture headache is more likely to develop. The design of the

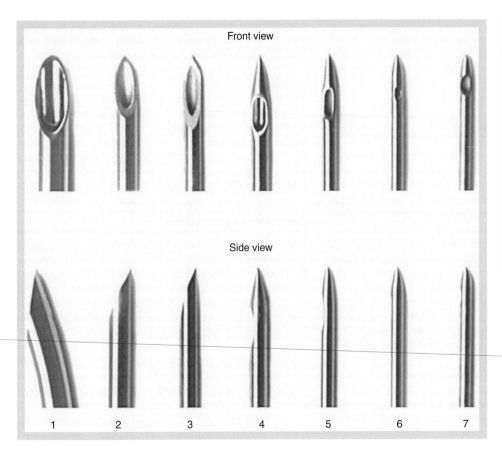

Front view

Side view

1   2   3   4   5   6   7

Figure 17-14 Comparative needle configuration for (1) 18-gauge Tuohy, (2) 20-gauge Quincke, (3) 22-gauge Quincke, (4) 24-gauge Sprotte, (5) 25-gauge Polymedic, (6) 25-gauge Whitacre, and (7) 26-gauge Gertie Marx. (From Schneider MC, Schmid M. Postdural puncture headache. In Birnbach DJ, Gatt SP, Datta S [eds]. Textbook of Obstetric Anesthesia. Philadelphia, Churchill Livingstone, 2000, pp 487-503.)

tip also affects the "feel" of the needle because a pencil-point needle requires more force to insert than a beveled-tip needle does but provides better tactile feel of the various tissues encountered as the needle is advanced.

Approach

Local anesthetic solution is infiltrated to anesthetize the skin and subcutaneous tissue at the anticipated site of cutaneous needle entry, which will be determined by the approach (midline or paramedian) to the subarachnoid space. The midline approach is technically easier, and the needle passes through less sensitive structures, thus requiring less local anesthetic infiltration to ensure patient comfort. However, the paramedian approach is better suited to challenging circumstances when there is narrowing of the interspace or difficulty in flexion of the spine. This can be readily appreciated by examination of a skeleton, which shows that the interlaminar space is largest when viewed from a slightly caudad and lateral vantage point.

MIDLINE TECHNIQUE

When using the midline approach, the needle is inserted at the top margin of the lower spinous process of the selected interspace. This point is generally easily identified by visual inspection and palpation. However, palpation of the spinous process and even identification of the midline become progressively more challenging with increasing obesity. In such circumstances, the patient should be as about perception of the needle to be midline or off to one side and adjust based on this feedback. After passage through the skin, the needle is progressively advanced with a slight cephalad orientation. Even in the lumbar area where the spinous processes are relatively straight, the interlaminar space is slightly cephalad to the interspinous space. Small needles tend to deflect or bend during insertion. Consequently, 24-gauge or smaller needles should be passed through a larger-gauge introducer needle placed in the interspinous ligament, which serves to guide and stabilize their path. This approach is particularly important when a beveled needle is used because the angle of the bevel displaces the needle from its path and causes it to veer in a direction opposite the bevel as it is being advanced.

As the spinal needle progresses toward the subarachnoid space, it passes through the skin, subcutaneous tissue, supraspinous ligament, interspinous ligament, ligamentum flavum, and the epidural space to reach and pierce the dura/arachnoid. The dural fibers appear to be largely oriented along the longitudinal axis of the dural sac. Thus, orienting the bevel of a cutting needle parallel to this axis tends to spread rather than cut the fibers, which may reduce the risk for post–dural puncture headache.

PARAMEDIAN TECHNIQUE

The point of cutaneous needle insertion for the paramedian technique is typically 1 cm lateral to the midline but varies in the rostral-caudal plane according to the patient's anatomy and the anesthesia provider's preference. Success depends on an appreciation of the anatomy and appropriate angulation of the needle and not on the precise location of needle insertion. The most common error is to underestimate the distance to the subarachnoid space and direct the needle too medially, with resultant passage across the midline. With the paramedian technique, the needle bypasses the supraspinous and interspinous ligaments, and the ligamentum flavum will be the first resistance encountered.

TAYLOR APPROACH

The Taylor approach (first described by urologist John A. Taylor) describes the paramedian technique to access the L5-S1 interspace (Fig. 17-15). Though generally the widest interspace, it is often inaccessible from the midline because of the acute downward orientation of the L5 spinous process. The spinal needle is passed from a point 1 cm caudad and 1 cm medial to the posterior superior iliac spine and advanced cephalad at a 55-degree angle with a medial orientation based on the width of the sacrum. The Taylor approach is technically challenging but very useful because it is minimally dependent on patient flexion for successful passage of the needle into the subarachnoid space.

Anesthetic Injection

After penetration of the dura by the spinal needle (can often be felt by the anesthesia provider's fingers as a rather distinct pop), the needle is further advanced a short distance to ensure that the bevel or side port rests entirely within the subarachnoid space. Free flow of CSF from the hub of the needle confirms correct placement of the distal end of the spinal needle. Occasionally, blood-tinged CSF initially appears at the hub of the needle. If clear CSF is subsequently seen, the spinal anesthetic can be completed. Conversely, if blood-tinged CSF continues to flow, the needle should be removed and reinserted at a different interspace. Should blood-tinged CSF still persist, the attempt to induce spinal anesthesia should be terminated. Similarly, spinal anesthesia should never be administered in the presence of a paresthesia. The occurrence of a paresthesia during needle placement mandates withdrawal of the needle.

If using a pencil-point needle, the side port can be positioned to encourage the desired distribution of local

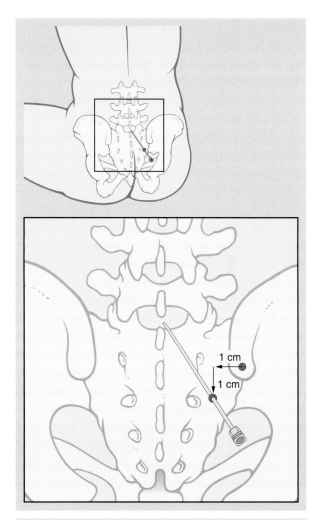

Figure 17-15 The L5-S1 paramedian (Taylor) approach. (From Brown DL [ed]. Atlas of Regional Anesthesia. Philadelphia, WB Saunders, 1992.)

anesthetic solution within the subarachnoid space, which is generally cephalad. However, the orientation of the bevel of a cutting needle has no effect on the trajectory of the anesthetic stream emerging from the tip. The needle can be secured by holding the hub between the thumb and index finger, with the dorsum of the anesthesia provider's hand resting against the patient's back; the syringe is then attached to the needle, and CSF is again aspirated to reconfirm placement. One should ensure that CSF can be easily withdrawn and flows freely into the syringe. With the syringe firmly attached to the needle to prevent loss of local anesthetic solution, the contents of the syringe are delivered into the subarachnoid space over approximately a 3 to 5 seconds. Aspiration plus reinjection of a small quantity of CSF again at the conclusion of the injection confirms the needle position and verifies subarachnoid delivery of the local anesthetic solution. Finally, the needle and syringe are withdrawn as a single unit and the antiseptic is wiped from the patient's back. The patient is then placed in a position that will encourage the desired distribution of local anesthetic solution or is positioned for surgery.

Level and Duration

The distribution of local anesthetic solution in CSF is influenced principally by (1) the baricity of the solution, (2) the contour of the spinal canal, and (3) the position of the patient in the first few minutes after injection of local anesthetic solution into the subarachnoid space. Assuming that an appropriate dose is selected, the duration of spinal anesthesia depends on the drug selected and the presence or absence of a vasoconstrictor (epinephrine or phenylephrine) in the local anesthetic solution (Table 17-1). During recovery, anesthesia regresses from the highest dermatome in a caudad direction.

BARICITY AND PATIENT POSITION

Local anesthetic solutions are classified as hypobaric, isobaric, and hyperbaric based on their density relative to the density of CSF. Baricity is an important consideration because it predicts the direction that local anesthetic solution will move after injection into CSF. Consequently, by selecting a local anesthetic solution of appropriate density relative to the position of the patient and the contour of the subarachnoid space, the anesthesia provider seeks to control both the direction and the extent of local anesthetic movement in the subarachnoid space and the resultant distribution of anesthesia.

Hyperbaric Solutions

The most commonly selected local anesthetic solutions for spinal anesthesia are hyperbaric (achieved by the addition of glucose [dextrose]), and their principal advantage is the ability to achieve greater cephalad spread of anesthesia. Commercially available hyperbaric local anesthetic solutions include 0.75% bupivacaine with 8.25% glucose and

5% lidocaine with 7.5% glucose. Tetracaine is formulated as a 1% plain solution and is most often used as a 0.5% solution with 5% glucose, which is achieved by dilution of the anesthetic with an equal volume of 10% glucose. However, the drug is also available in an ampoule containing Niphanoid crystals (20 mg), which is generally mixed with 2 mL of sterile water to produce a 1% solution.

The contour of the vertebral canal is critical to the subarachnoid distribution of hyperbaric local anesthetic solutions. For example, in the supine horizontal position, the patient's thoracic and sacral kyphosis will be dependent relative to the peak created by the lumbar lordosis (see Fig. 17-1).[2] Anesthetic delivered cephalad to this peak will thus move toward the thoracic kyphosis, which is normally around T6-T8. Placing the patient in a head-down (Trendelenburg) position will further accentuate this cephalad spread of local anesthetic solution and help ensure an adequate level of spinal anesthesia for abdominal surgery.

Hyperbaric local anesthetic solutions can also be administered caudad to the lumbosacral peak to encourage restricted sacral anesthesia (referred to as a saddle block reflecting sensory anesthesia of the area that would be in contact with a saddle). The spinal is performed with the patient seated.

Sometimes the impact of the lumbosacral lordosis should be minimized. In such cases, a pillow can be placed under the patient's knees to flatten this curve. Even more effective, the patient can be maintained in the lateral position, which will effectively eliminate the influence of the lumbosacral curvature on the distribution of local anesthetic solution in the subarachnoid space. Movement of hyperbaric local anesthetic solution will now be directly influenced by the patient's position on the operating table (the Trendelenburg position promoting cephalad spread and the reverse Trendelenburg position encouraging a restricted block).

Hypobaric Solutions

Hypobaric local anesthetic solutions find limited use in clinical practice and are generally reserved for patients

Table 17-1 Local Anesthetics Used for Spinal Anesthesia

| Drug | Concentration (%) | Dose (mg) | | Time to Onset (min) | Duration (min) | |
		T10	T4		Plain	Epinephrine (0.2 mg)
Lidocaine	5*	40-50	60-75	2-4	45-75	NR
Tetracaine	0.5	8-10	12-15	4-6	60-120	120-180
Bupivacaine	0.5-0.75	8-10	12-15	4-6	60-120	NR
Ropivacaine	0.5-0.75	10-14	15-20	4-6	60-90	NR
Chloroprocaine	2-3	40-50	60	2-4	30-60	NR

*Must be diluted to 2.5% or less before administration.
NR, not recommended.

undergoing perineal procedures in the "prone jackknife" position or undergoing hip arthroplasty where anesthetic can "float up" to the nondependent operative site. A common technique is to use a 0.1% solution (1 mg/mL) of tetracaine by diluting the commercial 10% solution with sterile water. However, although these solutions have been used in clinical practice for many years, they are extremely hypotonic, and alternative solutions prepared with third- or half-normal saline will still permit gravitational control but will present far less osmotic stress to neural tissue.

Isobaric Solutions

Isobaric local anesthetic solutions undergo limited spread in the subarachnoid space, which may be considered an advantage or disadvantage depending on the clinical circumstances. A potential advantage of isobaric local anesthetic solutions is a more profound motor block and more prolonged duration of action than that achieved with equivalent hyperbaric local anesthetic solutions. Because the distribution of local anesthetic solutions is not affected by gravity, spinal anesthesia can be performed without concern that the resultant block might be influenced by patient position. Commercially prepared "epidural" anesthetic solutions, which are generally formulated in saline, are commonly used for isobaric spinal anesthesia. However, although these solutions are considered isobaric, they actually behave clinically as though they were slightly hyperbaric, due to the effect of their low temperature relative to the cerebrospinal fluid.

Isobaric spinal anesthesia is particularly well suited for perineal or lower extremity procedures, as well as surgery involving the lower part of the trunk (hip arthroplasty, inguinal hernia repair). Although spread of local anesthetic solution may be limited caudally, subarachnoid injection does not produce segmental anesthesia because the nerves innervating more caudad structures are vulnerable to block as they pass through the region of high local anesthetic concentration.

Adjuvants

VASOCONSTRICTORS

Vasoconstrictors are frequently added to local anesthetic solutions to increase the duration of spinal anesthesia. This is most commonly achieved by the addition of epinephrine (0.1 to 0.2 mg, which is 0.1 to 0.2 mL of a 1:1000 solution) or phenylephrine (2 to 5 mg, which is 0.2 to 0.5 mL of a 1% solution). Increased duration of spinal anesthesia probably results from a reduction in spinal cord blood flow, which decreases loss of local anesthetic from the perfused areas and thus increases the duration of exposure to local anesthetic. However, with epinephrine, its α_2-adrenergic analgesic activity may contribute to the anesthetic.

The effect of vasoconstrictors is not equivalent for all local anesthetics, with tetracaine-induced spinal anesthesia exhibiting the longest prolongation. The differences in duration are partly due to the differing effects of local anesthetics on spinal cord blood flow. Tetracaine produces intense vasodilatation; the effect of lidocaine is more modest, whereas bupivacaine actually decreases both spinal cord and dural blood flow.

The addition of vasoconstrictors to local anesthetic solutions containing lidocaine has been questioned because of reports of nerve injury attributed to spinal lidocaine, and epinephrine may increase lidocaine neurotoxicity.[16] Epinephrine has been associated with significant "flulike" side effects when coadministered with spinal chloroprocaine,[17] whereas adding epinephrine or phenylephrine to tetracaine is associated with an increased risk for transient neurologic symptoms.[18]

OPIOIDS AND OTHER ANALGESIC DRUGS

Opioids may be added to local anesthetic solutions to enhance surgical anesthesia and provide postoperative analgesia. This effect is mediated at the dorsal horn of the spinal cord, where opioids mimic the effect of endogenous enkephalins. Commonly, fentanyl (25 µg) is used for short surgical procedures, and its administration does not preclude discharge home on the same day. The use of morphine (0.1 to 0.5 mg) can provide effective control of postoperative pain for roughly 24 hours, but it necessitates in-hospital monitoring for respiratory depression. Clonidine, an α_2-adrenergic drug, is not as effective as opioids, and its addition to the local anesthetic solution augments the sympatholytic and hypotensive effects of the local anesthetics.[19]

Choice of Local Anesthetic

Although there are differences among the local anesthetics with respect to the relative intensity of sensory and motor block, selection is based largely on the duration of action and potential adverse side effects.

LIDOCAINE FOR SHORT-DURATION SPINAL ANESTHESIA

For decades, lidocaine was the most commonly used short-acting local anesthetic for spinal anesthesia. It has a duration of action of 60 to 90 minutes, and it produces excellent sensory anesthesia and a fairly profound motor block. These features, in conjunction with a favorable recovery profile, make lidocaine particularly well suited for brief surgical procedures, particularly in the ambulatory setting (also see Chapter 37).

Neurotoxicity

Unfortunately, despite a long history of apparent safe use, subsequent reports of major and minor complications associated with spinal lidocaine have tarnished its reputation and jeopardize its continued clinical use. Initial reports of permanent neurologic deficits were restricted to its use for continuous spinal anesthesia, where extremely high doses were administered.[20] However, other reports suggest that injury may occur even with the administration of a dose historically recommended for single-injection spinal anesthesia.[21,22] These injuries have led to suggested modifications in practice that include a reduction in the lidocaine dose from 100 mg to 60 to 75 mg and dilution of the commercial formulation of 5% lidocaine with an equal volume of saline or CSF before subarachnoid injection.[22]

Transient Neurologic Symptoms

Lidocaine has been linked to the development of transient neurologic symptoms (pain or dysesthesia in the back, buttocks, and lower extremities) in as many as a third of patients receiving lidocaine for spinal anesthesia.[23] Factors that increase the risk for transient neurologic symptoms include patient positioning (lithotomy, knee arthroscopy) (see Chapter 19) and outpatient status (see Chapter 37).[18,24]

ALTERNATIVE LOCAL ANESTHETICS FOR SHORT-DURATION SPINAL ANESTHESIA

The etiology of transient neurologic symptoms is not established, but their occurrence has reinforced dissatisfaction with lidocaine and generated interest in alternative local anesthetics for short-duration spinal anesthesia. Mepivacaine probably has an incidence of transient neurologic symptoms less than lidocaine and may offer some benefit. Although procaine has a very short duration of action, the incidence of nausea is relatively frequent, and yet the incidence of transient neurologic symptoms is probably only marginally better.

Chloroprocaine

Chloroprocaine can be used as a spinal anesthetic.[25] Although this local anesthetic was linked to neurologic injuries in the 1980s, these injuries were due either to excessively large epidural doses that were accidentally injected into the subarachnoid space or to the preservative contained in the commercial anesthetic solution.[26] In any event, recent studies of low-dose (40 to 60 mg) preservative-free chloroprocaine suggest that chloroprocaine can produce excellent short-duration spinal anesthesia with little, if any, risk for transient neurologic symptoms.[17,27,28] The addition of epinephrine to chloroprocaine solutions for spinal anesthesia has side effects, and vasoconstrictors should not be used to prolong chloroprocaine spinal anesthesia. In contrast, both fentanyl and clonidine provide the expected enhancement of chloroprocaine spinal anesthesia without apparent side effects.

LONG-DURATION SPINAL ANESTHESIA

Bupivacaine and tetracaine are the local anesthetics most frequently used for long-duration spinal anesthesia. Although ropivacaine has been used as a spinal anesthetic, the advantages over bupivacaine are not obvious. Spinal bupivacaine is available as a 0.75% solution with 8.25% glucose for hyperbaric anesthesia. Tetracaine is prepared as 1% plain solution, which can be diluted with glucose, saline, or water to produce a hyperbaric, isobaric, or hypobaric solution, respectively. The recommended doses (5 to 20 mg) and durations of action (90 to 120 minutes) of bupivacaine and tetracaine are similar. However, bupivacaine produces slightly more intense sensory anesthesia (as evidenced by a less frequent incidence of tourniquet pain), whereas motor block with tetracaine is slightly more pronounced. The duration of tetracaine spinal anesthesia is more variable and more profoundly affected by the addition of a vasoconstrictor. Consequently, tetracaine remains the most useful spinal anesthetic in circumstances in which a prolonged block is sought. Unfortunately, the inclusion of a vasoconstrictor with tetracaine results in a significant incidence of transient neurologic symptoms.[18]

Documentation of Anesthesia

Within 30 to 60 seconds after subarachnoid injection of local anesthetic solutions, the developing level of spinal anesthesia should be determined. The desired level of spinal anesthesia is dependent on the type of surgery (Table 17-2). Nerve fibers that transmit cold sensation (C and A delta) are among the first to be blocked. Thus, an early indication of the level of a spinal anesthetic can be obtained by evaluating the patient's ability to discriminate temperature changes as produced by "wetting" the skin with an alcohol sponge. In the area blocked by the spinal anesthetic, the alcohol produces a warm or neutral sensation rather than the cold perceived in the unblocked areas. The level of sympathetic nervous system anesthesia usually exceeds the level of sensory block, which in turn exceeds the level of motor block. The level of sensory anesthesia is often evaluated by the patient's ability to discriminate sharpness as produced by a needle.

Table 17-2 Sensory Level Anesthesia Necessary for Surgical Procedures

Sensory Level	Type of Surgery
S2-S5	Hemorrhoidectomy
L2-L3 (knee)	Foot surgery
L1-L3 (inguinal ligament)	Lower extremity surgery
T10 (umbilicus)	Hip surgery Transurethral resection of the prostate Vaginal delivery
T6-T7 (xiphoid process)	Lower abdominal surgery Appendectomy
T4 (nipple)	Upper abdominal surgery Cesarean section

Table 17-3 Levels and Significance of Sensory Block

Cutaneous Level	Segmental Level	Significance
Fifth digit	C8	All cardioaccelerator fibers blocked
Inner aspect of the arm and forearm	T1-T2	Some degree of cardioaccelerator block
Apex of the axilla	T3	Easily determined landmark
Nipple	T4-T5	Possibility of cardioaccelerator block
Tip of the xiphoid	T7	Splanchnic fibers (T5-L1) may be blocked
Umbilicus	T10	Sympathetic nervous system block limited to the legs
Inguinal ligament	T12	No sympathetic nervous system block
Outer aspect of the foot	S1	Confirms block of the most difficult root to anesthetize

Table 17-4 Continuous Spinal Anesthesia: Guidelines for Anesthetic Administration

- Insert the catheter just far enough to confirm and maintain placement.
- Use the lowest effective local anesthetic concentration.
- Place a limit on the dose of local anesthetic to be used.
- Administer a test dose and assess the extent of any sensory and motor block.
- If maldistribution is suspected, use maneuvers to increase the spread of local anesthetic (change the patient's position, alter the lumbosacral curvature, switch to a solution with a different baricity).
- If well-distributed sensory anesthesia is not achieved before the dose limit is reached, abandon the technique.

Adapted from Rigler ML, Drasner K, Krejcie TC, et al. Cauda equina syndrome after continuous spinal anesthesia. Anesth Analg 1991;72:275-281.

Skeletal muscle strength is tested by asking the patient to dorsiflex the foot (S1-S2), raise the knees (L2-L3), or tense the abdominal rectus muscles (T6-T12). The first 5 to 10 minutes after the administration of hyperbaric or hypobaric local anesthetic solutions is the most critical time for adjusting the level of anesthesia (Table 17-3). The first 5 to 10 minutes are also critical for assessing cardiovascular responses (systemic arterial blood pressure and heart rate) to the evolving spinal anesthesia. Delayed bradycardia and cardiac asystole mandate continuous vigilance beyond early attainment of anesthesia.[29]

Continuous Spinal Anesthesia

Inserting a catheter into the subarachnoid space increases the utility of spinal anesthesia by permitting repeated drug administration as necessary to maintain the level and duration of sensory and motor block (Table 17-4). Anesthesia can be provided for prolonged operations without delaying recovery. An added benefit is the possibility of using lower doses of anesthetic. With the single-injection technique, relatively high doses must be administered to all patients to ensure successful anesthesia in a large percentage of cases. With a catheter in place, smaller doses can be titrated to the patient's response.

TECHNIQUE
After inserting the needle and obtaining free flow of CSF, the catheter is advanced through the needle into the subarachnoid space. Care must be exercised to limit the catheter insertion distance to 2 to 4 cm because unlike placement in the epidural space, further advancement of a subarachnoid catheter runs the risk of impaling the spinal cord. The use of large-bore epidural needles and catheters introduces a significant risk for post–dural puncture headache.

Microcatheters
Microcatheters (27 gauge and smaller) for continuous spinal anesthesia were withdrawn from clinical practice after reports of cauda equina syndrome associated with their use.[20] The injury associated with the use of microcatheters likely resulted from the combination of maldistribution and repetitive injection of local anesthetic solution. It appears that pooling of local anesthetic solution in the dependent sacral sac produced a restricted block that was inadequate for surgery. In response to inadequate anesthesia, injections were repeated and ultimately achieved adequate sensory anesthesia, but not before neurotoxic concentrations were reached in the caudal region of the subarachnoid space.[30] The microcatheter may have contributed to this problem because the long narrow-bore tubing creates resistance to injection and thereby results in a low flow rate that can encourage a restricted distribution. However, removal of microcatheters from clinical practice has not eliminated the risk. The problem of maldistribution is not restricted to microcatheters, and the same injuries have occurred with larger "epidural" catheters and other local anesthetics.[20]

Failed Spinal Anesthesia and Repetitive Subarachnoid Injections

Spinal anesthesia is not uniformly successful, and failure may derive from technical considerations such as an inability to identify the subarachnoid space or failure to inject all or part of the local anesthetic solution into the subarachnoid space. A second and generally underappreciated cause of failure is local anesthetic maldistribution. In support of this mechanism is the correlation of success rate with the vertebral interspace, the more caudad interspaces being more prone to failure.[13] This issue becomes important when considering whether to repeat a "failed" spinal and, if so, the dose of anesthetic that should be used for the second injection. In the past, a "full dose" was given. However, if failure derives from maldistribution of the local anesthetic solution, this strategy may introduce a risk of injury.[31] In essence, an overdose of local anesthesia in the subarachnoid space could occur. If a spinal anesthetic is to be repeated, one should assume that the first injection was delivered in the subarachnoid space as intended, and the combination of the two doses should not exceed that considered reasonable as a single injection for spinal anesthesia.

Physiology

Spinal anesthesia interrupts sensory, motor, and sympathetic nervous system innervation. Local anesthetic solutions injected into the subarachnoid space produce a conduction block of small-diameter, unmyelinated (sympathetic) fibers before interrupting conduction in larger myelinated (sensory and motor) fibers. The sympathetic nervous system block typically exceeds the somatic sensory block by two dermatomes. This estimate may be conservative, with sympathetic nervous system block sometimes exceeding somatic sensory block by as many as six dermatomes, which explains why systemic hypotension may accompany even low sensory levels of spinal anesthesia.

Spinal anesthesia has little, if any, effect on resting alveolar ventilation (i.e., analysis of arterial blood gases unchanged), but high levels of motor anesthesia that produce paralysis of abdominal and intercostal muscles can decrease the ability to cough and expel secretions. Additionally, patients may complain of difficulty breathing (dyspnea) despite adequate ventilation because of inadequate sensation of breathing from loss of proprioception in the abdominal and thoracic muscles.

Spinal anesthesia above T5 inhibits sympathetic nervous system innervation to the gastrointestinal tract, and the resulting unopposed parasympathetic nervous system activity results in contracted intestines and relaxed sphincters. The ureters are contracted, and the ureterovesical orifice is relaxed. Block of afferent impulses from the surgical site by spinal anesthesia is consistent with the absence of an adrenocortical response to painful stimulation. Decreased bleeding during regional anesthesia and certain types of surgery (hip surgery, transurethral resection of the prostate) may reflect a decrease in systemic blood pressure, as well as a reduction in peripheral venous pressure, whereas increased blood flow to the lower extremities after sympathetic nervous system block appears to be a major factor in the decreased incidence of thromboembolic complications after hip surgery. There does not appear to be any difference in the perioperative mortality rate between regional anesthesia and general anesthesia administered to relatively healthy patients scheduled for elective surgery.

Side Effects and Complications

Side effects associated with spinal anesthesia can usually be predicted from the physiologic effects of the block. Persistent neurologic complications are rare and can be minimized by an appreciation of the factors that can contribute to injury.

NEUROLOGIC COMPLICATIONS

Neurologic complications after spinal anesthesia may result from trauma, either directly provoked by a needle or catheter or indirectly by compression from hematoma or abscess. The occurrence of a paresthesia can, on occasion, be associated with postoperative neurologic findings, which generally resolve. Such injuries will occur with greater frequency and will be more profound if injection of anesthetic is made in the presence of a paresthesia, thus emphasizing the importance of avoiding local anesthetic injection should a paresthesia be present or halting injection should this occur during administration. Local anesthetics, if administered in sufficient quantity (particularly within restricted areas of the subarachnoid space), can induce permanent injury.[20,31] Transient neurologic symptoms are a common occurrence after the subarachnoid administration of certain local anesthetics, particularly lidocaine.[18,23,24] Despite the designation as "neurologic," the cause and significance of this self-limited condition remain to be determined.

HYPOTENSION

Hypotension (systolic arterial blood pressure <90 mm Hg) occurs in about a third of patients receiving spinal anesthesia.[32] Hypotension results from a sympathetic nervous system block that (1) decreases venous return to the heart and decreases cardiac output or (2) decreases systemic vascular resistance.

Modest hypotension (e.g., <20 mm Hg) is probably due to decreases in systemic vascular resistance, whereas more intense hypotension (>20 mm Hg) probably is the result of decreases in venous return and cardiac output. The degree of hypotension often parallels the sensory level of spinal anesthesia and the intravascular fluid volume status of the patient. Indeed, the magnitude of hypotension produced by spinal anesthesia will be more with coexisting hypovolemia.

Treatment

Spinal anesthesia-induced hypotension is treated physiologically by restoration of venous return to increase cardiac output. In this regard, the internal autotransfusion produced by a modest head-down position (5 to 10 degrees) will facilitate venous return without greatly exaggerating cephalad spread of the spinal anesthetic. Adequate intravenous hydration before the institution of spinal anesthesia is important for minimizing the effects of venodilation from sympathetic nervous system block. However, excessive amounts of intravenously administered fluids may be detrimental, particularly in a patient with limited cardiac function or ischemic heart disease, in whom excessive intravascular volume or hemodilution may be poorly tolerated.

Sympathomimetics with positive inotropic and venoconstrictor effects, such as ephedrine (5 to 10 mg IV), are often chosen as first-line drugs to maintain perfusion pressure during the first few minutes after the institution of spinal anesthesia. Phenylephrine (50 to 100 µg IV) and other sympathomimetics that increase systemic vascular resistance may decrease cardiac output and do not specifically correct the decreased venous return contributing to the spinal anesthesia-induced hypotension. Nevertheless, anesthesia providers have long used phenylephrine successfully to treat hypotension associated with spinal anesthesia. Furthermore, phenylephrine is of particular value when administration of ephedrine is associated with significant increases in heart rate. In the past, phenylephrine was contraindicated in parturients because of possible detrimental effects on uterine blood flow, which has not been confirmed (see Chapter 33).[33] In the rare instance when hypotension does not promptly respond to ephedrine or phenylephrine, epinephrine should be given to avoid progression to profound hypotension or even cardiac arrest.

BRADYCARDIA AND ASYSTOLE

The heart rate does not change significantly in most patients during spinal anesthesia. However, in an estimated 10% to 15% of patients, significant bradycardia occurs. As with hypotension, the risk for bradycardia increases with increasing sensory levels of anesthesia. Speculated mechanisms for this bradycardia include block of cardioaccelerator fibers originating from T1 through T4 and decreased venous return (Bezold-Jarisch reflex).

Although bradycardia is usually of modest (<20 bpm) severity and promptly responsive to atropine or ephedrine, precipitous bradycardia and asystole can happen in the absence of any preceding event (Fig. 17-16).[29,34] This catastrophic event can probably be prevented through maintenance of preload and reversal of bradycardia by aggressive stepwise escalation of treatment (ephedrine, 5 to 50 mg IV; atropine, 0.4 to 1.0 mg IV; epinephrine, 0.05 to 0.25 mg IV), whereas the development of profound bradycardia or asystole mandates immediate treatment with full resuscitative doses of epinephrine (1.0 mg IV).

POST-DURAL PUNCTURE HEADACHE

Post–dural puncture headache is a direct consequence of the puncture hole in the dura, which results in loss of CSF

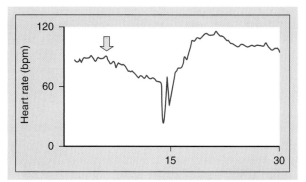

Figure 17-16 Recording of heart rate over time from a single patient who received a spinal anesthetic at the arrow, followed by a subsequent gradual decrease in heart rate that culminated in precipitous bradycardia that was unresponsive to atropine and ephedrine. Immediate institution of external cardiac compressions was promptly followed by sinus rhythm (85 beats/min). The precipitous bradycardia occurred while the patient was conversing with the anesthesia provider and in the presence of normal vital signs (oxygen saturation, 98%; systemic blood pressure, 120/50 mm Hg; heart rate, 68 beats/min). (From Mackey DC, Carpenter RL, Thompson GE, et al. Bradycardia and asystole during spinal anesthesia: A report of three cases with morbidity. Anesthesiology 1989;70:866-868, used with permission.)

at a rate exceeding production. Loss of CSF causes downward displacement of the brain and resultant stretch on sensitive supporting structures (Fig. 17-17).[35] Pain also results from distention of the blood vessels, which must compensate for the loss of CSF because of the fixed volume of the skull.

Manifestations

The pain associated with post–dural puncture headache generally begins 12 to 48 hours after transgression of the dura, but can occur immediately even up to several months after the event. The characteristic feature of post–dural puncture headache is its postural component: it appears or intensifies with sitting or standing and is partially or completely relieved by recumbency. This feature is so distinctive that it is difficult to consider the diagnosis in its absence. Post–dural puncture headache is typically occipital or frontal (or both) and is usually described as dull or throbbing. Associated symptoms such as nausea, vomiting, anorexia, and malaise are common. Ocular disturbances, manifested as diplopia, blurred vision, photophobia, or "spots," may occur and are believed to result from stretch of the cranial nerves, most commonly cranial nerve VI, as the brain descends because of the loss of CSF. Although symptomatic hearing loss is unusual, formal auditory testing will routinely reveal abnormalities.

Though generally a transient problem, loss of CSF may rarely result in significant morbidity because caudal displacement of the brain can result in tearing of

III

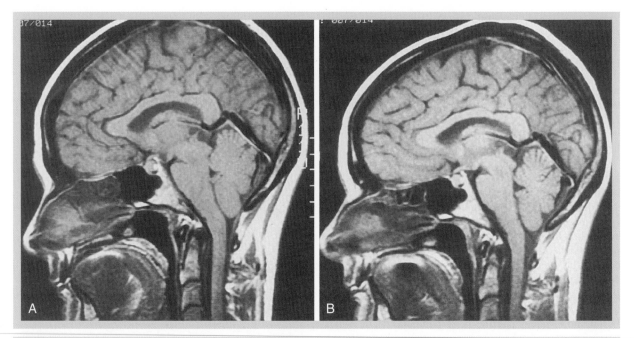

Figure 17-17 Anatomy of a "low-pressure" headache. **A,** A T1-weighted sagittal magnetic resonance image demonstrates a "ptotic brain" manifested as tonsillar herniation below the foramen magnum, forward displacement of the pons, absence of the suprasellar cistern, kinking of the chiasm, and fullness of the pituitary gland. **B,** A comparable image of the same patient after an epidural blood patch and resolution of the symptoms demonstrates normal anatomy. (From Drasner K, Swisher JL. In Brown DL [ed]. Regional Anesthesia and Analgesia. Philadelphia, WB Saunders, 1996.)

bridging veins with the development of a subdural hematoma. Concern should be raised if post–dural puncture headache is progressive or refractory or loses its postural component.

Risk Factors

Age is one of the most important factors affecting the incidence of post–dural puncture headache. Children are at low risk, but after puberty, risk increases substantially and then slowly declines with advancing age. Females are at increased risk even in the absence of pregnancy.[36] A previous history of post–dural puncture headache places a patient at increased risk for the development of this complication after a subsequent spinal anesthetic.

The incidence of post–dural puncture headache varies directly with the diameter of the needle that has pierced the dura. However, the benefit of a smaller needle with respect to post–dural puncture headache must be balanced against the technical challenge that it may impose. The common use of 24- and 25-gauge needles represents a balance between these two considerations. The shape of the hole created by the needle also has an impact on loss of CSF; this has led to the development of "pencil-point" needle tips, which appear to spread the dural and arachnoid fibers and produce less tear and a smaller hole for a given diameter needle.

Treatment

Initial treatment of post–dural puncture headache is usually conservative and consists of bed rest, intravenous fluids, analgesics, and possibly caffeine (500 mg IV). More definitively, a blood patch can be performed, in which 15 to 20 mL of the patient's blood, aseptically obtained, is injected into the epidural space. The injection should be made near or preferably below the site of initial puncture because there is preferential cephalad spread. The patient should remain supine for at least 2 hours and relief should be immediate. The immediate effect is related to the volume effect of the injected blood, whereas long-term relief is thought to occur from sealing or "patching" of the dural tear.

HIGH SPINAL ANESTHESIA

Systemic hypotension frequently accompanies high spinal anesthesia, and patients will become nauseated and agitated. Total spinal anesthesia is the term applied to excessive sensory and motor anesthesia associated with loss of consciousness. Apnea and loss of consciousness are often attributed to ischemic paralysis of the medullary ventilatory centers because of profound hypotension and associated decreases in cerebral blood flow. However, loss of consciousness may also be the direct consequence of local anesthetic effect above the foramen magnum inasmuch as patients may lose or fail to regain consciousness despite restoration of systemic arterial blood pressure. Lesser degrees of excessive spinal anesthesia may warrant conversion to a general anesthetic because of patient distress, ventilatory failure, or risk of aspiration. Total spinal anesthesia is typically manifested soon after injection of the local anesthetic solution into the subarachnoid space.

Treatment of high or total spinal anesthesia consists of maintenance of the airway and ventilation, as well as support of the circulation with sympathomimetics and intravenous fluid administration. Patients are placed in a head-down position to facilitate venous return. An attempt to limit the cephalad spread of local anesthetic solution in CSF by placing patients in a head-up position is not recommended because this position will encourage venous pooling, as well as potentially jeopardizing cerebral blood flow, which may contribute to medullary ischemia. Tracheal intubation is usually warranted and is mandated for patients at risk of aspiration of gastric contents (e.g., pregnant women). Sometimes, thiopental or propofol should be given before tracheal intubation if consciousness is retained and cardiovascular status is acceptable.

NAUSEA

Nausea occurring after the initiation of spinal anesthesia must alert the anesthesia provider to the possibility of systemic hypotension sufficient to produce cerebral ischemia. In such cases, treatment of hypotension with a sympathomimetic drug should eliminate the nausea. Alternatively, nausea may occur because of a predominance of parasympathetic activity as a result of selective block of sympathetic nervous system innervation to the gastrointestinal tract. Similar to bradycardia, the incidence of nausea and vomiting parallels the sensory level of spinal anesthesia.

URINARY RETENTION

Because spinal anesthesia interferes with innervation of the bladder, administration of large amounts of intravenous fluids can cause bladder distention, which may require catheter drainage. For this reason, excessive administration of intravenous fluids should be avoided in patients undergoing minor surgery with spinal anesthesia. However, adequate intravascular fluid replacement must be administered to maintain effective preload and reduce the degree of hypotension and possible progression to bradycardia and asystole.[29] Inclusion of epinephrine in the local anesthetic solution may be associated with a prolonged time to voiding.

BACKACHE

Minor, short-lived back pain frequently follows spinal anesthesia and is more likely with multiple attempts at correct advancement of the spinal needle. Backache may also be related to the position required for surgery. Ligament strain may occur when anesthetic-induced sensory block and skeletal muscle relaxation permit the patient to be placed in a position that would normally be uncomfortable or unobtainable. Backache can be confused with transient neurologic symptoms.

HYPOVENTILATION

Decreases in vital capacity can occur if the motor block extends into the upper thoracic and cervical dermatomes. Loss of proprioception from the intercostal musculature can produce dyspnea. Exaggerated hypoventilation may accompany the intravenous administration of drugs intended to produce a sleeplike state during spinal anesthesia. Constant vigilance of ventilatory status is enhanced by monitors, which must include pulse oximetry and may include capnography.

EPIDURAL ANESTHESIA

Epidural anesthesia, like spinal anesthesia, can be instituted with the patient in the sitting or lateral decubitus position, whereas the prone position is generally selected for caudal blocks. As with subarachnoid injection, the sitting position facilitates placement by encouraging flexion and aiding in recognition of the midline. However, the lateral position is associated with a lower incidence of venous cannulation.[37] Patients typically receive drugs to produce sedation, except when epidural catheters are placed in pregnant women.

Timing of Catheter Placement

Controversy exists regarding the wisdom of placing lumbar epidural catheters after induction of general anesthesia. Although there is concern that an inability to elicit a patient response might increase the risk for neural injury, a retrospective review challenges this assertion.[38] Nonetheless, many anesthesia providers believe that lumbar epidural anesthesia and catheter placement are best performed in a communicative patient.[39] Performance of thoracic epidural anesthesia in an anesthetized patient should be avoided.[40] However, the same considerations do not apply to pediatric anesthesia, for which a conscious patient would probably impart no benefit but instead add substantial risk (see Chapter 34). Consequently, it is standard practice to place caudal, lumbar, and even thoracic epidural catheters in children after induction of general anesthesia.

Epidural Needles

The most commonly used epidural needle (Tuohy needle) was originally designed and first used for continuous spinal anesthesia and only later adapted for epidural use. The modern Tuohy needle has a blunt tip so that it might rest against the dura without penetration, but the tip has retained its gentle curve, which serves to guide the catheter's exit obliquely from the needle. Other epidural needles represent modifications of this basic design. For example, the Weiss needle has prominent wings to help stabilize the anesthesia provider's grip, and the Crawford needle has a straighter tip that may be better suited to the steep approach of a midline thoracic epidural or to passage of a catheter into the sacral canal.

Epidural Catheters

Like needles, catheter designs vary (Fig. 17-18).[41] For example, some catheters have an inner stainless steel wire coil to impart flexibility and prevent kinking. This characteristic makes them less likely to (1) pierce an epidural vessel,[37] (2) find false passage into a fascial plane, and (3) be advanced out of the epidural space through the intervertebral foramen. However, their flexibility also makes them more difficult to thread into the epidural space. The tip of the catheter may be open or have a closed "bullet" tip with proximal ports. Bullet-tipped or multiorifice catheters tend to produce more uniform distribution of local anesthetic solution, but they have the disadvantage of requiring greater insertion depth to ensure complete delivery of local anesthetic solution into the epidural space.

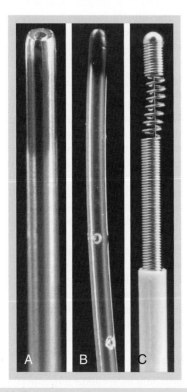

Figure 17-18 A to **C,** Epidural catheters may have an open end or several openings proximal to the tip. (From Brown DL. Spinal, epidural and caudal anesthesia. In Miller RD [ed]. Miller's Anesthesia. Philadelphia, Elsevier, 2010, pp 1611-1638.)

Epidural Kit

As with spinal anesthesia, epidural anesthesia is performed with equipment obtained from prepackaged sterile epidural kits. Most epidural kits contain a 17- or 18-gauge needle, which permits passage of a 19- or 20-gauge catheter, respectively. Both the needles and the catheters have calibrated markings so that the anesthesia provider can determine the depth of insertion from the skin, as well as the distance that the catheter has advanced past the tip of the needle.

Each epidural kit has one or two needles for infiltration of the skin and for probing the intervertebral space before insertion of the larger epidural needle. The length of this "finder needle" is usually 3.8 cm, which is sufficient to reach the subarachnoid space in some patients, although the depth of the epidural space is generally 4 to 6 cm. The distance to the epidural space will be affected by body weight and by the angulation of the needle (insertion depth is obviously greater with marked cephalic angulation).

Technique

LUMBAR AND LOW THORACIC EPIDURAL

The technique for a lumbar epidural and low thoracic epidural is similar because the anatomic features of the spine are similar at these vertebral levels. Both midline and paramedian approaches can be used successfully, but the midline is more popular. Advantages of the midline approach include (1) simpler anatomy because there is no need to determine the appropriate lateral orientation of the needle and (2) passage of the needle through less sensitive structures and less probability of contacting facet joints or large spinal nerves that innervate the leg. However, the paramedian approach is better suited when challenging circumstances such as hypertrophied bony spurs, spinal abnormalities, or failure to adequately flex create obstacles to needle advancement. Some anesthesia providers also prefer to use a paramedian approach based on the unproven concept that needle passage through the interspinous ligament increases the risk for postoperative backache.

THORACIC EPIDURAL

In contrast to procedures performed in the lumbar area, thoracic epidural anesthesia is generally accomplished through a paramedian approach. In this region the spinous processes are angulated and closely approximated, which makes it difficult to avoid bony obstruction when approaching from the midline. Identification of the lamina is the initial step. If the spinous process can be identified, a skin wheal is raised 0.5 to 1 cm off midline at the caudad tip of the spinous process. The finder needle is then directed at a right angle to the skin and the needle advanced until the lamina is contacted. Local anesthetic is deposited, the needle is withdrawn, and the longer epidural needle is positioned and advanced in a similar manner. After the lamina is contacted, the needle is repeatedly retracted and advanced in a slightly more medial and cephalad direction until it fails to make bony contact at the depth anticipated by previous insertions. If contact with bone continues to occur, the needle is retracted and positioned at a slightly different angle and the process repeated. If success is not obtained, the process is repeated at an insertion site that is slightly (about 1 cm) cephalad or caudad. The midline approach to the thoracic epidural space is similar to that described for lumbar epidurals except that the needle must be advanced cephalad at a more acute angle to pass between the steep down-sloping spinous processes (see Fig. 17-5).[5]

Identification of the Epidural Space

Firm engagement of the needle tip in the ligamentum flavum is the most critical step in identification of the epidural space when using either a paramedian or midline approach.

LOSS-OF-RESISTANCE TECHNIQUE

With the loss-of-resistance technique, a syringe containing saline, air, or both is attached to the needle, and the needle is slowly advanced while assessing resistance to injection (Fig. 17-19).[3] One method is to use a syringe containing 2 to 3 mL of saline with a small air bubble (0.1 to 0.3 mL). If the needle is properly seated in the ligamentum flavum, it will be difficult to inject the saline or the air bubble, and the plunger of the syringe will "spring back" to its original position. If the air bubble cannot be compressed without injecting the saline, the needle is most likely not in the ligamentum flavum. In this case, the needle tip may still be in the interspinous ligament, or it may be off the midline in the paraspinous muscles. After proper positioning in the ligamentum flavum, the needle is advanced while continuous pressure is exerted on the plunger of the syringe. An abrupt loss of resistance to injection signals passage through the ligamentum flavum and into the epidural space, at which point the contents of the syringe are delivered. An often-cited advantage of this method is that the dura tends to be forced away from the advancing needle by the saline ejected from the syringe. The introduction of fluid into the epidural space prior to catheter insertion also serves to reduce the incidence of epidural vein cannulation.[37]

HANGING-DROP TECHNIQUE

The "hanging-drop" technique is an alternative method for identifying the epidural space. With this technique, a small drop of saline is placed at the hub of the epidural needle. As the needle passes through the ligamentum flavum into the epidural space, the saline drop is retracted into the needle by the negative pressure in the epidural

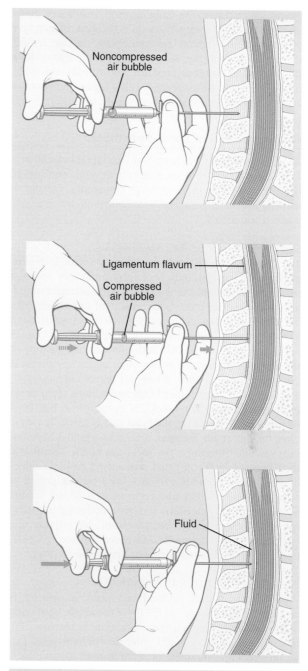

Figure 17-19 Loss-of-resistance technique. The needle is inserted into the ligamentum flavum, and a syringe containing saline and an air bubble is attached to the hub. After compression of the air bubble is obtained by applying pressure on the syringe plunger, the needle is carefully advanced until its entry into the epidural space is confirmed by the characteristic loss of resistance to syringe plunger pressure, and the fluid enters the space easily. (From Afton-Bird G. Atlas of regional anesthesia. In Miller RD [ed]. Miller's Anesthesia. Philadelphia, Elsevier, 2005.)

space. Interestingly, the hanging-drop technique can be used in the lumbar region despite the lack of negative pressure in the lumbar epidural space. In this region, the needle pushing the dura away from the ligamentum flavum creates negative pressure. Accordingly, this technique is likely to be associated with a higher incidence of accidental dura penetration (wet taps).

Administration of Local Anesthetic

As with spinal anesthesia, epidural anesthesia can be performed by injection of local anesthetic solution through the needle (single shot) or more commonly, through a catheter threaded into and maintained in the epidural space (continuous).

SINGLE-SHOT EPIDURAL ANESTHESIA

The advantage of the single-injection technique is its simplicity, and the distribution of local anesthetic solution tends to be more uniform than when administered through an indwelling catheter. Achievement of anesthesia with the single-injection technique begins with administration of a test dose of local anesthetic solution (e.g., 3 mL of 1.5% lidocaine with 1:200,000 epinephrine). Failure of the test dose to produce sensory and motor anesthesia is assessed after 3 minutes to rule out accidental subarachnoid injection (spinal anesthesia has a more rapid onset of sensory and motor block). If epinephrine has been included in the test dose, the heart rate is carefully monitored to detect an increase that may signal accidental intravascular injection. The local anesthetic solution is then injected in fractionated doses (e.g., multiple injections of 5-mL aliquots) over a 1- to 3-minute period at an appropriate volume and concentration (dose) for the planned surgical procedure. Intermittent dosing is critical because a negative test result does not conclusively rule out intravascular placement. Moreover, the needle's position may have changed during or between injections.

CONTINUOUS EPIDURAL ANESTHESIA

With the continuous epidural technique, a catheter is advanced 3 to 5 cm beyond the tip of the needle positioned in the epidural space. Further advancement increases the risk that the catheter might enter an epidural vein, exit an intervertebral foramen, or wrap around a nerve root. The epidural needle is withdrawn over the catheter, with care taken to not move the catheter. No attempt should be made to withdraw a catheter back through the needle because shearing (transection) of the catheter might result, with retention of the transected tip of the catheter in the epidural space. The catheter is taped to the patient's back, and an empty 3-mL syringe is attached to the distal end of the catheter. Negative pressure is applied to the syringe, and failure to aspirate CSF or blood helps rule out accidental subarachnoid or intravascular placement. After negative aspiration and a negative test dose, epidural anesthesia

is initiated by the administration of local anesthetic solution in fractionated doses (multiple injections of 5-mL aliquots). It is important to reconfirm negative aspiration of CSF or blood from the catheter before any subsequent dose of local anesthetic is administered. Documentation of the level of sympathetic nervous block and sensory anesthesia is determined as described for spinal anesthesia (see the earlier section "Documentation of Anesthesia").

CAUDAL ANESTHESIA

Caudal anesthesia in an adult is performed with the patient in either the prone or the lateral position. The sacral area is prepared and draped and the sacral cornu (typically 3 to 5 cm above the coccyx) identified by the anesthesia provider's palpating fingers. The depression between the cornu is the sacral hiatus, and a skin wheal is raised. The needle is introduced perpendicular to the skin through the sacrococcygeal ligament (generally felt as a rather distinct pop) and advanced until the sacrum is contacted. The needle is then slightly withdrawn, the angle is reduced, and the needle is advanced about 2 cm into the epidural caudal canal (Fig. 17-20).[3] Confirmation that the needle is properly positioned can be obtained by rapidly injecting 5 mL of air or saline through the needle

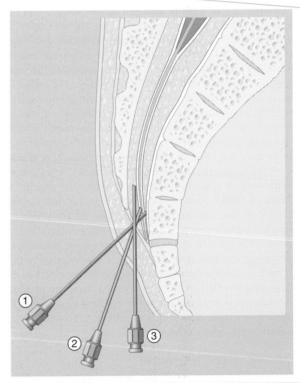

Figure 17-20 Caudal anesthesia: (1) skin penetration at a 60- to 90-degree angle, (2) redirection of the needle, and (3) slight penetration (1 to 2 mm) within the spinal canal. (From Afton-Bird G. Atlas of regional anesthesia. In Miller RD [ed]. Miller's Anesthesia. Philadelphia, Elsevier, 2005.)

while palpating the skin directly covering the caudal canal. Subcutaneous crepitus or midline swelling indicates that the needle is positioned posterior to the bony sacrum and requires replacement.

Although infection is rare, the nearness of this approach to the rectum mandates particular attention to sterile technique. Subarachnoid injection may occur if the needle is advanced too far cephalad in the sacral canal, or it may result from anatomic variation (the dural sac extends beyond S2 in approximately 10% of individuals). Anatomic variation may also hinder success inasmuch as the sacral hiatus is absent in nearly 10% of patients.

In contrast to adults, location of the sacral hiatus and performance of caudal anesthesia are technically easy in children. After induction of general anesthesia, the child is placed in the lateral position and a needle or catheter is advanced into the sacral canal. A long-acting local anesthetic will limit general anesthetic requirements and produce effective postoperative analgesia for procedures involving the perineum or lower lumbar dermatomes.

Level of Anesthesia

The principal factors affecting the spread of epidural anesthesia are dose (volume multiplied by concentration) and site of injection. However, administration of an equivalent dose (mass) at lower concentration may foster greater spread, particularly with lower concentrations of local anesthetic. Cephalad-to-caudad extension of epidural anesthesia depends on the site of administration of the local anesthetic solution into the epidural space. Lumbar epidural injections produce preferential cephalad spread because of negative intrathoracic pressure transmitted to the epidural space, whereas resistance to caudad spread of local anesthetic solution is created by narrowing of the space at the lumbosacral junction. In contrast, thoracic injections tend to produce symmetrical anesthesia and result in greater dermatomal spread for a given dose of local anesthetic. This latter effect results, at least in part, from the comparatively smaller volume of the thoracic epidural space, which is smaller in the thoracic region. The site of placement of the local anesthetic solution in the epidural space also defines the area of peak anesthetic effect, which decreases with increasing distance from the injection site.

Spread of anesthesia may vary directly with age and inversely with height, although these effects are likely to be overshadowed by interpatient variability. Achievement of anesthesia is not equivalent at all dermatomes. For example, anesthesia in the L5-S1 distribution may be relatively spared, an effect believed to result from the large diameter of these nerve roots. In contrast to spinal anesthesia, the baricity of local anesthetic solutions does not influence the level of epidural anesthesia. Likewise, patient position during performance of an epidural block is less important, but the dependent portion of the body may still manifest more intense anesthesia than the nondependent side. This effect is most noticeable in a pregnant woman who has remained in a specific lateral position for a prolonged period during labor.

Duration of Anesthesia

The duration of epidural anesthesia, as with spinal anesthesia, is principally affected by the choice of local anesthetic and whether a vasoconstrictor drug is added to the local anesthetic solution. Because achievement of epidural anesthesia is delayed relative to spinal anesthesia, onset time is an additional consideration in selection of the local anesthetic. In this regard, the local anesthetics most commonly selected for epidural anesthesia are (1) chloroprocaine (rapid onset and short duration), (2) lidocaine (intermediate onset and duration), and (3) bupivacaine, levobupivacaine, and ropivacaine (slow onset and prolonged duration of action) (Table 17-5). Tetracaine and procaine have long latency times, which makes them unsuitable for epidural use. Levobupivacaine is clinically similar to bupivacaine, whereas ropivacaine is less potent and often used at higher concentrations.

Adjuvants

EPINEPHRINE

The addition of epinephrine (generally 1:200,000; 5 μg/mL) to local anesthetic solutions decreases vascular absorption of the local anesthetic from the epidural space, thus

Table 17-5 Local Anesthetics Used for Epidural Anesthesia

Drug	Concentration (%)	Time to Onset (min)	Duration (min) Plain	Duration (min) Epinephrine (1:200,000)
Chloroprocaine	2-3	5-10	45-60	60-90
Lidocaine	1-2	10-15	60-120	90-180
Bupivacaine	0.25-0.5	15-20	120-200	150-240
Ropivacaine	0.25-1.0	10-20	120-180	150-200

maintaining effective anesthetic concentrations at the nerve roots for more prolonged periods. Decreased vascular absorption also serves to limit systemic uptake and reduce the risk for systemic toxicity from the local anesthetic. These effects are far more pronounced when epinephrine is coadministered with chloroprocaine or lidocaine than with bupivacaine. The inclusion of epinephrine also serves as a marker of intravascular injection that may occur with cannulation of an epidural vein. The use of an intravascular marker has been classified as a level IIa recommendation (level of evidence B) in a recent practice advisory published by the American Society of Regional Anesthesia.[42]

OPIOIDS

Similar to spinal anesthesia, opioids are often administered with epidural local anesthetic solutions to enhance surgical anesthesia and to provide postoperative pain control. However, in contrast to spinal administration, lipid solubility of the opioid is a critical factor in determining the selection and appropriate use of epidural opioids. For example, morphine, which is relatively hydrophilic, spreads rostrally within the CSF and can produce effective analgesia for thoracic surgery, even when administered into the lumbar epidural space. In contrast, a lipophilic opioid such as fentanyl is rapidly absorbed into the systemic circulation and exhibits little rostral spread. Consequently, the lipophilic opioids demonstrate limited selective spinal activity when administered in the lumbar epidural region because their site of action, the dorsal horn of the spinal cord, rests several segments rostral to the site of administration.

SODIUM BICARBONATE

Local anesthetic effect requires transfer across the nerve membrane. Because local anesthetics are weak bases, they exist largely in the ionic form in commercial preparations. Adding sodium bicarbonate to the solution favors the nonionized form of the local anesthetic and promotes more rapid onset of epidural anesthesia. Most commonly, 1 mL of 8.4% sodium bicarbonate is added to 10 mL of a solution containing lidocaine or chloroprocaine. Alkalinization of a bupivacaine solution is not recommended because this local anesthetic precipitates at alkaline pH.

Failed Epidural Anesthesia

Failed epidural anesthesia may occur when local anesthetic solution is not delivered into the epidural space or because spread of the local anesthetic solution is inadequate to cover the relevant dermatomes. A false loss of resistance can occur in the interspinous ligament before entry into the ligamentum flavum or as the needle passes through fascial planes. For example, the paramedian approach in the thoracic region requires the needle to pass through the latissimus dorsi and trapezius muscles as they insert onto the thoracic vertebrae. It is conceivable that a needle passing through these fascial coverings could transmit a feeling of loss of resistance to the fingers of the anesthesia provider. In some cases, failure results from advancement of the catheter through an intervertebral foramen, which generally gives rise to a limited unilateral block. Fortunately, these blocks can often be salvaged by retracting the catheter a few centimeters. Opinion varies on the presence of a midline barrier to diffusion of local anesthetics.

If epidural anesthesia is nearly adequate and there are concerns that additional local anesthetic would create a risk for systemic toxicity, small doses of chloroprocaine, which are rapidly hydrolyzed in plasma, may provide adequate extension to permit surgery.[43] At other times, failure of epidural anesthesia may be managed by replacement of the epidural catheter or abandonment of the technique in favor of a general or spinal anesthetic. However, subarachnoid injection after a failed epidural produces unpredictable and often excessive spinal anesthesia.[44] This effect probably results primarily from compression of the dural sac by the volume of anesthetic solution in the epidural space.

Physiology

The major site of action of local anesthetic solutions placed in the epidural space appears to be the spinal nerve roots, where the dura is relatively thin. A spinal nerve root site of action is consistent with the often-observed delayed onset or absence of anesthesia in the S1-S2 region, presumably reflecting the covering of these nerve roots with connective tissue. To a lesser extent, anesthesia results from diffusion of local anesthetic solutions from the epidural space into the subarachnoid space.

Because the epidural space ends at the foramen magnum, the cranial nerves cannot be blocked by epidural injection of local anesthetics. Even with very high sensory blocks there are areas of sensation that will be unaffected by local epidural anesthetics because they are innervated by afferent fibers in the cranial nerves, though it is possible to completely block the motor breathing apparatus by high epidural anesthesia despite loss of consciousness because the phrenic nerve, which innervates the diaphragm, arises from C3 to C5. The oculomotor nerve contains the pupilloconstrictor fibers that induce miosis after opioid administration. Preservation of this response may provide a potential clue to distinguish high epidural anesthesia from total spinal anesthesia in that the latter may induce pupillary dilatation and loss of the light reflex even in the presence of opioids.[45]

SYMPATHETIC NERVOUS SYSTEM BLOCK

As with spinal anesthesia, the most important physiologic alteration produced by an epidural block is sympathetic nervous system block leading to pooling of blood in the large capacitance venous system of the visceral compartment. The result is a reduction in preload and a decrease in cardiac output and systemic blood pressure. As the sympathetic nervous system block extends into the higher T1 through T4 spinal nerves, there is interruption of the cardioaccelerator fibers that control myocardial contractility and heart rate. Because of the sympatholytic effects of epidural anesthesia, patients with low blood volume or other causes of reduced venous return such as pregnancy, ascites, or vena cava obstruction are prone to exaggerated decreases in systemic blood pressure. Additionally, parasympathetic nervous system innervation of the heart is not impaired. Vagal reflexes can therefore produce significant bradycardia and even sinus arrest during epidural anesthesia.

In contrast to spinal anesthesia, the onset of sympathetic nervous system block produced by epidural anesthesia is generally slower, and the likelihood of abrupt hypotension is less. β-Agonist effects from the systemic absorption of epinephrine in the local anesthetic solution produce sufficient vasodilation to accentuate systemic blood pressure decreases when compared with those produced by local anesthetics alone.

Opinions vary regarding whether sympathetic nervous system block from epidural anesthesia is advantageous or deleterious in a normovolemic patient. Sympathetic nervous system denervation of the bowel increases mucosal blood flow and peristalsis, which may hasten the return of bowel function.[46] Thoracic epidural anesthesia with selective block of cardiac sympathetic fibers favorably alters myocardial oxygen supply, reduces cardiac ischemic events, decreases myocardial infarct size after coronary artery occlusion, and improves functional recovery from myocardial stunning in experimental animals.[47] Surgical bleeding is less for some procedures during the hypotension produced by epidural anesthesia. Disadvantages of sympathectomy include loss of the body's compensatory mechanisms in response to surgical bleeding and the risk for stroke, spinal cord ischemia, or myocardial infarction if systemic blood pressure is persistently or dangerously low. Additionally, compression of the dural sac by the large volume of epidural fluid may increase pressure in the subarachnoid space and elevate the systemic blood pressure required for adequate perfusion of the spinal cord.

MOTOR BLOCK
Motor block results in difficulty with ambulation after lumbar epidural anesthesia. This complication can impede recovery by restricting the patient to bed rest. Diaphragm function is unaffected by epidural anesthesia unless the motor block rises into the upper cervical nerve roots. With surgery in the thorax and upper abdominal region, epidural anesthesia has favorable effects on respiratory function because it prevents pain-induced splinting and permits uninhibited coughing and deep breathing.

OUTCOME
Surgery is associated with increased catabolism that results in loss of muscle protein and negative nitrogen balance. Adequate epidural anesthesia can prevent this catabolic response after surgical procedures on the lower abdominal region and lower extremity. More critically, there is evidence to suggest a reduction in morbidity when epidural analgesia is utilized for thoracic or major abdominal procedures. For example, a meta-analysis identified a less frequent incidence of cardiovascular and gastrointestinal complications, a shortened period of mechanical ventilation, and a reduction in the incidence of renal insufficiency with postoperative epidural analgesia versus systemic opioid analgesia for abdominal aortic surgery.[10]

Side Effects and Complications

Side effects of epidural anesthesia resemble those described for spinal anesthesia, with the added risks of accidental dural puncture, accidental subarachnoid injection, and local anesthetic systemic toxicity, the latter attributable to the high doses of local anesthetic required for the epidural anesthetic. Additional potential complications include epidural hematoma and epidural abscess, particularly in patients with preexisting coagulopathy or infection.

EPIDURAL HEMATOMA
Although potentially attributed to bleeding from vascular trauma during placement of the epidural needle or catheter (or both), it is recognized that both epidural hematoma and epidural abscess may occur spontaneously. If an epidural hematoma is suspected, urgent performance of magnetic resonance imaging is needed because recovery of motor function correlates inversely with the time until surgical decompression of the epidural hematoma.[48]

ACCIDENTAL DURAL PUNCTURE ("WET TAP") AND HEADACHE
Theoretically, epidural anesthesia, which avoids dural puncture, should circumvent the problem of post–dural puncture headache. Unfortunately, inadvertent trespass of the dura does occur, with the incidence greatly affected by the experience of the anesthesia provider. Moreover, if a "wet tap" does occur during attempted performance of epidural anesthesia, the risk for post–dural puncture headache is far greater than after deliberate dural puncture with a small pencil-point needle. Post–dural puncture headache that occurs in the absence of a recognized dural puncture probably reflects the fact that the CSF leak may be too small to be detectable through the epidural needle. When fluid appears at the hub of the epidural needle, it may be difficult to distinguish between CSF or saline used in the syringe to determine loss of resistance. One method to determine the source of fluid is to allow some of it to drip on the anesthesia provider's forearm. The saline, having been administered at room temperature, will be cool

and thus easily distinguished from warm CSF. However, concern for infections such as human immunodeficiency virus, which is concentrated in CSF, has largely relegated this technique to historical interest.

Management

Accidental dural puncture may be managed by converting to single-injection or continuous spinal anesthesia, or epidural anesthesia can be attempted at a different lumbar interspace. Placement of an epidural catheter at another interspace, or passage of a subarachnoid catheter, may decrease the risk for post–dural puncture headache.

SYSTEMIC HYPOTENSION

As with spinal anesthesia, systemic hypotension parallels the degree of sympathetic nervous system block. However, because the onset of sympathetic nervous system block is slower, excessive decreases in systemic blood pressure do not usually accompany epidural anesthesia administered to normovolemic patients. Treatment of hypotension is as described for spinal anesthesia.

SYSTEMIC ABSORPTION AND INTRAVASCULAR INJECTION

The large doses of local anesthetics required for epidural anesthesia plus the presence of numerous venous plexuses in the epidural space increase the likelihood of substantial systemic absorption of local anesthetic. Nevertheless, the resulting blood concentrations of local anesthetics are rarely sufficient to produce systemic toxicity, especially if epinephrine is added to the local anesthetic solution. However, accidental intravascular injection of local anesthetic will produce high blood levels and predictable toxicity ranging from mild central nervous system symptoms (restlessness, slurred speech, tinnitus) to loss of consciousness, seizures, and cardiovascular collapse. Cardiac toxicity is of particular concern with the use of bupivacaine and related anesthetic compounds (see Chapter 11).

ACCIDENTAL SUBARACHNOID INJECTION

Accidental subarachnoid injection of the large volumes of local anesthetic solution used for epidural anesthesia may produce rapid progression to total spinal anesthesia. Immediate treatment is focused on supporting ventilation and restoring or maintaining hemodynamics. However, in contrast to an excessive block produced during spinal anesthesia, the large epidural doses of local anesthetics injected into the subarachnoid space can result in permanent neurologic deficits because of the neurotoxic effects of these agents. In the past, such concerns were limited to chloroprocaine. However, reports of injury have established the potential for neurotoxic injury with the subarachnoid administration of epidural doses of lidocaine and probably any local anesthetic.[49] Consequently, consideration should be given to irrigation of the subarachnoid space with saline, particularly if CSF can be readily aspirated from the misplaced catheter. This maneuver may circumvent or minimize neurologic injury.

Although readily diagnosed in an awake patient, subarachnoid injection may go unrecognized when epidural anesthesia is used in conjunction with a general anesthetic. An unexpected dilated nonreactive pupil after local anesthetic injection into an epidural catheter may indicate migration of the catheter into the subarachnoid space.

SUBDURAL INJECTION

The subdural space is difficult to enter deliberately because the arachnoid is generally closely adherent to the overlying dura. The rare occurrence of subdural injection is difficult to detect because CSF cannot be aspirated through the catheter and the usual test dose is negative. Subdural injection of a local anesthetic solution can produce an unusual block characterized by patchy sensory anesthesia and often unilateral dominance. Subdural placement of an epidural catheter is dangerous because the catheter can abruptly pierce the thin arachnoid membrane and thereby enter the subarachnoid space.

NEURAL INJURY

Neural injury after an epidural anesthetic is very rare but seems to be more likely if a paresthesia occurs during performance of this technique. The development of paresthesia as a result of the advancing epidural needle reflects stimulation of a nerve root and is a signal to the anesthesia provider that the needle is not in the midline and needs to be redirected. As with spinal anesthesia, injection of local anesthetic solution in the presence of a paresthesia is contraindicated because nerve damage may be induced or enhanced by the injection. Nevertheless, occurrence of paresthesia is an inherent risk of epidural anesthesia, and neurologic changes attributed to the development of a paresthesia reflect injury that is almost always transient.

COMBINED SPINAL-EPIDURAL ANESTHESIA

Combined spinal-epidural anesthesia is a technique in which a spinal anesthetic and an epidural catheter are placed concurrently. This approach combines the rapid onset and intense sensory anesthesia of a spinal anesthetic with the ability to supplement and extend the duration of the block afforded by an epidural catheter. The technique is commonly used in obstetric anesthesia (see Chapter 33).

Technique

Combined spinal-epidural anesthesia is most commonly performed by placing a needle in the epidural space, followed by passage of a small spinal needle into the subarachnoid space through the lumen of the epidural

Figure 17-21 A, A spinal needle and epidural needle are used for the combined spinal-epidural technique. **B,** Tuohy needle with a "back eye" that permits placement of the spinal needle directly into the subarachnoid space (*left panel*) and subsequent threading of the epidural catheter into the epidural space after removal of the spinal needle. (Modified from Veering BT, Cousins MJ. Epidural neural blockade. In Cousins MJ, Bridenbaugh PO, Carr DB, Horlocker TT [eds]. Neural Blockade in Clinical Anesthesia and Management of Pain. Philadelphia, Lippincott-Raven, 2009, pp 241-295.)

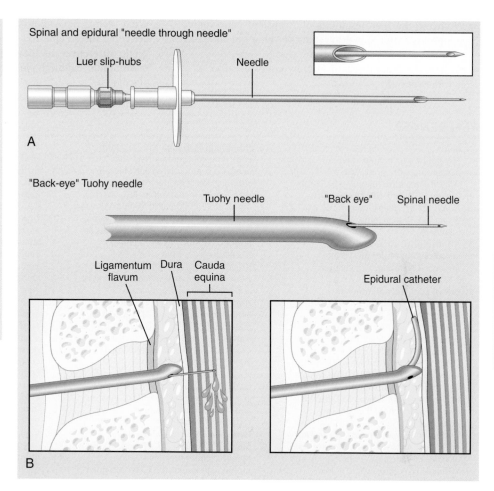

needle. After injection of the local anesthetic solution, the spinal needle is removed and a catheter is threaded into the epidural space through the epidural needle. Although standard spinal and epidural equipment may be used, there are commercially available needles specifically designed for combined spinal-epidural anesthesia (Fig. 17-21).[6]

An undocumented concern associated with combined spinal-epidural anesthesia is that the meningeal puncture site may permit high concentrations of subsequently administered epidural local anesthetics to enter the subarachnoid space or facilitate passage of the epidural catheter through the dura.

COMBINED EPIDURAL-GENERAL ANESTHESIA

Advantages of epidural block during general anesthesia include less need for opioids, pain-free emergence from anesthesia, and block of the stress response that is nearly complete for most surgical procedures performed below the umbilicus. Various modifications of the combined epidural-general anesthetic are used, but if the administration of general anesthesia is not altered by limiting the use of volatile anesthetics and opioids, there is little advantage to the technique. Combined epidural-general anesthesia requires strict attention to fluid management and blood pressure. Sympathomimetics with α-adrenergic activity, such as phenylephrine, dopamine, or epinephrine, can be used to counteract the consequences of afterload reduction, especially in patients at risk for stroke or myocardial ischemia. Excessive intravenous fluid administration to treat hypotension is discouraged because it is often not effective and can lead to intravascular fluid overload as the block recedes.

QUESTIONS OF THE DAY

1. What is the origin of the arterial blood supply to the spinal cord?
2. When inserting a spinal anesthetic, what structures are traversed by the needle during a midline approach? During a paramedian approach?

3. What are the manifestations of "transient neurologic symptoms" after spinal anesthesia? What are the risk factors?
4. What is the usual mechanism of hypotension after spinal anesthesia?

5. What factors determine the spread of local anesthesia delivered in the epidural space?
6. What differences in technique must be used during midthoracic epidural placement compared to lumbar placement?

REFERENCES

1. Matthey PW, Finegan BA, Finucane BT: The public's fears about and perceptions of regional anesthesia, *Reg Anesth Pain Med* 29(2):96–101, 2004.
2. Covino BG, Scott DB, Lambert DH: *Handbook of Spinal Anaesthesia and Analgesia*, Philadelphia, 1994, WB Saunders.
3. Afton-Bird G: Atlas of regional anesthesia. In Miller RD, editor: *Miller's Anesthesia*, Philadelphia, 2005, Elsevier.
4. Brown DL: *Atlas of Regional Anesthesia*, Philadelphia, 1992, WB Saunders.
5. Kardish K: Functional anatomy of central neuraxial blockade in obstetrics. In Birnbach DJ, Gatt SP, Datta S, editors: *Textbook of Obstetric Anesthesia*, Philadelphia, 2000, Churchill Livingstone, pp 121–126.
6. Bridenbaugh PO, Greene NM, Brull SJ: Spinal (subarachnoid) block. In Cousins MJ, Bridenbaugh PO, Carr DB, Horlocker TT, editors: *Neural Blockade in Clinical Anesthesia and Management of Pain*, Philadelphia, 1998, Lippincott, Williams & Wilkins, pp 203–242.
7. Veering BT, Cousins MJ: Epidural neural blockade. In Cousins MJ, Bridenbaugh PO, Carr DB, Horlocker TT, editors: *Neural Blockade in Clnical Anesthesia and Management of Pain*, Philadelphia, 2009, Lippincott, Williams & Wilkins, pp 241–295.
8. Harrison GR: Topographical anatomy of the lumbar epidural region: An in vivo study using computerized axial tomography, *Br J Anaesth* 83(2):229–234, 1999.
9. Block BM, Liu SS, Rowlingson AJ, et al: Efficacy of postoperative epidural analgesia: A meta-analysis, *JAMA* 290(18):2455–2463, 2003.
10. Nishimori M, Ballantyne JC, Low JH: Epidural pain relief versus systemic opioid-based pain relief for abdominal aortic surgery, *Cochrane Database Syst Rev* 3: CD005059, 2006.
11. Practice Advisory for the Prevention, Diagnosis, and Management of Infectious Complications Associated with Neuraxial Techniques: A Report by the American Society of Anesthesiologists Task Force on Infectious Complications Associated with Neuraxial Techniques, *Anesthesiology* 112:530–545, 2010.

12. Hashimoto K, Hampl KF, Nakamura Y, et al: Epinephrine increases the neurotoxic potential of intrathecally administered lidocaine in the rat, *Anesthesiology* 94(5):876–881, 2001.
13. Munhall RJ, Sukhani R, Winnie AP: Incidence and etiology of failed spinal anesthetics in a university hospital: A prospective study, *Anesth Analg* 67(9):843–848, 1988.
14. Broadbent CR, Maxwell WB, Ferrie R, et al: Ability of anaesthetists to identify a marked lumbar interspace, *Anaesthesia* 55(11):1122–1126, 2000.
15. Schneider MC, Schmid M: Post-dural puncture headache. In Birnbach DJ, Gatt SP, Datta S, editors: *Textbook of Obstetric Anesthesia*, Philadelphia, 2000, Churchill Livingstone, pp 121–126.
16. Hashimoto K, Sakura S, Bollen AW, et al: Comparative toxicity of glucose and lidocaine administered intrathecally in the rat, *Reg Anesth Pain Med* 23(5):444–450, 1998.
17. Smith KN, Kopacz DJ, McDonald SB: Spinal 2-chloroprocaine: A dose-ranging study and the effect of added epinephrine, *Anesth Analg* 98(1):81–88, 2004.
18. Freedman JM, Li DK, Drasner K, et al: Transient neurologic symptoms after spinal anesthesia: An epidemiologic study of 1,863 patients, *Anesthesiology* 89(3):633–641, 1998.
19. Elia N, Culebras X, Mazza C, et al: Clonidine as an adjuvant to intrathecal local anesthetics for surgery: Systematic review of randomized trials, *Reg Anesth Pain Med* 33(2):159–167, 2008.
20. Rigler ML, Drasner K, Krejcie TC, et al: Cauda equina syndrome after continuous spinal anesthesia, *Anesth Analg* 72(3):275–281, 1991.
21. Auroy Y, Narchi P, Messiah A, et al: Serious complications related to regional anesthesia: Results of a prospective survey in France, *Anesthesiology* 87(3):479–486, 1997.
22. Drasner K: Lidocaine spinal anesthesia: A vanishing therapeutic index? *Anesthesiology* 87(3):469–472, 1997.
23. Hampl KF, Schneider MC, Ummenhofer W, et al: Transient neurologic symptoms after spinal anesthesia, *Anesth Analg* 81(6):1148–1153, 1995.

24. Pollock JE, Neal JM, Stephenson CA, et al: Prospective study of the incidence of transient radicular irritation in patients undergoing spinal anesthesia, *Anesthesiology* 84(6):1361–1367, 1996.
25. Drasner K: Chloroprocaine spinal anesthesia: Back to the future? *Anesth Analg* 100(2):549–552, 2005.
26. Taniguchi M, Bollen AW, Drasner K: Sodium bisulfite: Scapegoat for chloroprocaine neurotoxicity? *Anesthesiology* 100(1):85–91, 2004.
27. Casati A, Fanelli G, Danelli G, et al: Spinal anesthesia with lidocaine or preservative-free 2-chlorprocaine for outpatient knee arthroscopy: A prospective, randomized, double-blind comparison, *Anesth Analg* 104(4):959–964, 2007.
28. Kouri ME, Kopacz DJ: Spinal 2-chloroprocaine: A comparison with lidocaine in volunteers, *Anesth Analg* 98(1):75–80, 2004.
29. Caplan RA, Ward RJ, Posner K, et al: Unexpected cardiac arrest during spinal anesthesia: A closed claims analysis of predisposing factors, *Anesthesiology* 68(1):5–11, 1988.
30. Rigler ML, Drasner K: Distribution of catheter-injected local anesthetic in a model of the subarachnoid space, *Anesthesiology* 75(4):684–692, 1991.
31. Drasner K, Rigler ML: Repeat injection after a "failed spinal": At times, a potentially unsafe practice, *Anesthesiology* 75(4):713–714, 1991.
32. Carpenter RL, Caplan RA, Brown DL, et al: Incidence and risk factors for side effects of spinal anesthesia, *Anesthesiology* 76(6):906–916, 1992.
33. Prakash S, Pramanik V, Chellani H, et al: Maternal and neonatal effects of bolus administration of ephedrine and phenylephrine during spinal anaesthesia for caesarean delivery: A randomised study, *Int J Obstet Anesth* 19:24–30, 2009.
34. Mackey DC, Carpenter RL, Thompson GE, et al: Bradycardia and asystole during spinal anesthesia: A report of three cases without morbidity, *Anesthesiology* 70(5):866–868, 1989.
35. Drasner K, Swisher J: Delayed complications and side effects. In Brown DL, editor: *Regional Anesthesia and Analgesia*, Philadelphia, 1996, WB Saunders.

36. Wu CL, Rowlingson AJ, Cohen SR, et al: Gender and post-dural puncture headache, *Anesthesiology* 105(3):613–618, 2006.

37. Mhyre JM, Greenfield ML, Tsen LC, et al: A systematic review of randomized controlled trials that evaluate strategies to avoid epidural vein cannulation during obstetric epidural catheter placement, *Anesth Analg* 108(4):1232–1242, 2009.

38. Horlocker TT, Abel MD, Messick JM Jr, et al: Small risk of serious neurologic complications related to lumbar epidural catheter placement in anesthetized patients, *Anesth Analg* 96(6):1547–1552, 2003 table of contents.

39. Rosenquist RW, Birnbach DJ: Epidural insertion in anesthetized adults: Will your patients thank you? *Anesth Analg* 96(6):1545–1546, 2003.

40. Drasner K: Thoracic epidural anesthesia: Asleep at the wheal? *Anesth Analg* 99(2):578–579, 2004.

41. Brown DL: Spinal, epidural and caudal anesthesia. In Miller RD, editor: *Miller's Anesthesia*, Philadelphia, 2010, Elsevier, pp 1611–1638.

42. Neal JM, Bernards CM, Butterworth JF, et al: ASRA Practice Advisory on Local Anesthetic Systemic Toxicity, *Reg Anesth Pain Med* 35:152–161, 2010.

43. Crosby E, Read D: Salvaging inadequate epidural anaesthetics: "The chloro-procaine save" *Can J Anaesth* 38(1):136–137, 1991.

44. Mets B, Broccoli E, Brown AR: Is spinal anesthesia after failed epidural anesthesia contraindicated for cesarean section? *Anesth Analg* 77(3):629–631, 1993.

45. Larson MD: Mechanism of opioid-induced pupillary effects, *Clin Neurophysiol* 119(6):1358–1364, 2008.

46. Liu SS, Carpenter RL, Mackey DC, et al: Effects of perioperative analgesic technique on rate of recovery after colon surgery, *Anesthesiology* 83(4):757–765, 1995.

47. Rolf N, Van de Velde M, Wouters PF, et al: Thoracic epidural anesthesia improves functional recovery from myocardial stunning in conscious dogs, *Anesth Analg* 83(5):935–940, 1996.

48. Groen RJ, van Alphen HA: Operative treatment of spontaneous spinal epidural hematomas: A study of the factors determining postoperative outcome, *Neurosurgery* 39(3):494–508, 1996.

49. Drasner K, Rigler ML, Sessler DI, et al: Cauda equina syndrome following intended epidural anesthesia, *Anesthesiology* 77(3):582–585, 1992.

III

18 PERIPHERAL NERVE BLOCKS

Adam B. Collins and Andrew T. Gray

Peripheral nerve blocks are used for anesthesia, postoperative analgesia, and diagnosis and treatment of chronic pain syndromes (see Chapter 43) (Table 18-1). Advantages and disadvantages of peripheral nerve blocks for anesthesia must be considered when advising patients about anesthetic options (see Chapter 14). Peripheral nerve blocks may improve acute pain management and patient disposition even when used only as adjunct techniques. Patients are often more receptive to peripheral nerve blocks when they are reassured that supplemental sedation can be administered intravenously to reduce awareness or if they become uncomfortable during surgery. During the preoperative evaluation the potential sites for peripheral nerve blocks should be examined. The presence of a skin infection in the area to be used for needle insertion must be recognized preoperatively. Confirmation of normal coagulation (history of bleeding or bruising and possibly specific coagulation tests) is generally recommended before performance of peripheral nerve blocks. The presence of a preexisting neuropathy, especially in the area involving the proposed operation, may deter the anesthesiologist from selecting peripheral nerve block anesthesia.

PREPARATION FOR NERVE BLOCKS

Patients scheduled for peripheral nerve block anesthesia are evaluated medically in the same way as patients scheduled for general or neuraxial anesthesia (see Chapter 13). Preoperative medication is useful for decreasing apprehension and providing analgesia during the needle insertions necessary to perform the block. A holding area ("block room") for performing peripheral nerve blocks may be useful for minimizing any delay once the operating room becomes available. Increasing the efficiency of block administration and operating room turnover through the use of a block room will greatly improve acceptance of regional

Table 18-1	Examples of Peripheral Nerve Blocks
Cervical plexus	
Brachial plexus	
Interscalene	
Supraclavicular	
Infraclavicular	
Axillary	
Forearm block	
Median	
Ulnar	
Radial	
Femoral	
Saphenous	
Sciatic	
Popliteal	
Ankle	
Intravenous regional anesthesia (Bier block)	

anesthesia techniques. The block room (see Chapter 20) must have appropriate monitors, equipment, and drugs available should adverse reactions to local anesthetics occur. Also for this reason, an intravenous catheter should be in place before performance of a peripheral nerve block. In the operating room, the anesthesiologist must be prepared to provide appropriate supplemental intravenous sedation or induce general anesthesia if necessary.

Prepackaged sterile trays are often used for performance of peripheral nerve blocks. Syringes may include control rings to facilitate delivery of local anesthetic solution and aspiration by the anesthesiologist with one hand. Povidone-iodine and chlorhexidine solutions are useful for skin preparation.

The choice of local anesthetic for peripheral nerve blockade depends on a number of factors, including the desired onset, duration, and degree of conduction block (see Chapter 11). Lidocaine and mepivacaine, 1% to 1.5%, produce surgical anesthesia in 10 to 20 minutes that lasts 2 to 3 hours. Ropivacaine, 0.5%, and bupivacaine, 0.375% to 0.5%, have a slower onset and produce less motor blockade, but the effect lasts for at least 6 to 8 hours. The addition of epinephrine, 1:200,000 (5 μg/mL), can serve as a marker for intravascular injection and can substantially increase the duration of a conduction block. In addition, through a decrease in the rate of systemic absorption, epinephrine can reduce peak plasma levels of local anesthetic. Considerations for the choice of local anesthetic solution for intravenous regional anesthesia are different from those for peripheral nerve blocks (see the later discussion under "Intravenous Regional Anesthesia").

SPECIFIC BLOCK TECHNIQUES

A number of methods can be used to locate peripheral nerves and guide the injection of local anesthetic solutions, including ultrasound, paresthesias, and nerve stimulation.

Ultrasound

High-resolution ultrasound imaging allows direct visualization of peripheral nerves, block needle placement, and the distribution of local anesthetic solution and thereby improves block success and minimizes local anesthetic volume (see Fig. 18-1).[1] In addition, ultrasound can also be used to visualize adjacent structures, such as blood vessels or pleurae, and may therefore reduce the risk for complications from peripheral nerve blocks. A major advantage of ultrasound imaging is that variability in surface landmarks, body habitus, and patient positioning can be appreciated.

Peripheral nerves can be round, oval, or triangular in transverse cross section (short-axis view) and can change shape along their nerve path.[2] About a third of the fascicles within a peripheral nerve can be seen with high-resolution ultrasound. Though usually considered static structures within the body, peripheral nerves can change position with external compression and extremity movement.[3] Proximal nerves such as the roots and ventral rami of the brachial plexus appear dark, or hypoechoic, in their core but bright, or hyperechoic, in their outer mantle (Fig. 18-1). This distinction occurs because incident sound waves reflect strongly off the connective tissue encasing nerve fascicles but pass through the inner portions of the

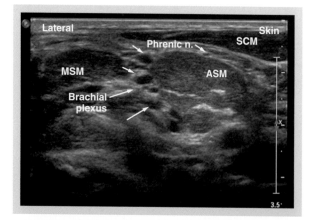

Figure 18-1 This sonogram of the right side of the neck shows the roots of the brachial plexus as they pass between the anterior and middle scalene muscles. The core of these large peripheral nerves is less echogenic than the surrounding muscle. The phrenic nerve is a small hypoechoic structure seen on the anterior surface of the anterior scalene muscle. ASM, anterior scalene muscle; MSM, middle scalene muscle; SCM, sternocleidomastoid muscle.

III

fascicles undisturbed. Ultrasound frequencies of 10 MHz or higher are required to distinguish tendons from nerves based on sonographic appearance. Fortunately, most blocks are performed in regions where this distinction is not a diagnostic issue. High-frequency ultrasound provides better resolution but poor penetration into deeper tissue because of attenuation of the sound beam. Ultrasound visibility of needles for a regional block primarily depends on the gauge and insertion angle, and larger needles parallel to the ultrasound transducer are seen most easily.[4]

Ultrasound imaging can produce transverse (short-axis) images of nerves and other structures. In short-axis imaging, cylindrical structures such as nerves appear as circles. Long-axis imaging is achieved by placing the transducer longitudinally, or parallel to the course of a nerve, such that it appears as a linear structure. Similarly, the block needle can be introduced within the plane of imaging, or in-plane, such that the entire needle and bevel are seen as a linear structure. Out-of-plane needle approach involves passing the needle from outside the plane of imaging so that it intersects the scan plane as an echogenic dot (Fig.18-2). Needles used for ultrasound-guided techniques are generally best visualized and manipulated if they are 21 gauge or larger and are long enough to take a relatively oblique tissue course under the ultrasound transducer.

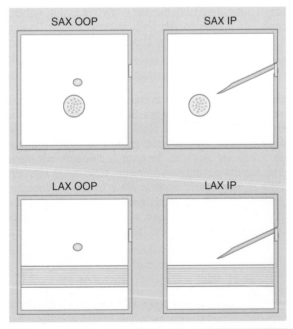

Figure 18-2 Approaches to regional block with ultrasound. SAX OOP, short-axis imaging, out-of-plane needle approach; SAX IP, short-axis imaging, in-plane needle approach; LAX OOP, long-axis imaging, out-of-plane needle approach; LAX IP, long-axis imaging, in-plane needle approach. (From Gray AT. Ultrasound-guided regional anesthesia: Current state of the art. Anesthesiology 2006;104(2):368-373.)

Paresthesias

Paresthesias are radiating electric shock-like sensations that can occur during regional anesthetic procedures. Historically, practitioners were instructed to remember the dictum "no paresthesias, no anesthesia," which indicates that paresthesias are necessary for a successful block because the needle must be in close proximity to the nerve. Today, although paresthesias remain a standard for block success, they also may increase the likelihood of nerve injury and are therefore are not usually intentionally elicited.[5] Local anesthetic solution should not be injected in the presence of a persistent paresthesia because intraneural injection accompanied by intense pain increases the likelihood of permanent nerve injury.

Nerve Stimulation

Nerve stimulation to evoke a motor response is a common way of identifying peripheral nerves that carry a mixed population of sensory and motor fibers. For nerve stimulation, the block needle is used as a stimulating cathode and another lead on the body serves as the anode to complete the electrical circuit (Fig. 18-3). Cathodal stimulation is more efficient than anodal stimulation, so it is important to not reverse the leads during nerve stimulation–guided block procedures. The location of the surface anode (usually an electrocardiographic pad) on the patient does not alter the stimulation.

A motor response evoked with currents of 0.3 to 0.5 mA indicates sufficient proximity of the block needle to the nerve for success of the block after the injection of local anesthetic solution.[6] Some authors have suggested that the threshold stimulating current (the lowest current that produces a motor response) should be greater than

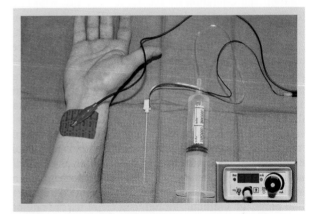

Figure 18-3 Setup for nerve stimulation. The block needle is connected to a stimulator with adjustable current (*inset*) and to extension tubing for injection of local anesthetic solution. An electrocardiographic pad can be used to complete the electrical circuit by functioning as a surface anode (shown in red). The shaft of the block needle is coated with insulation.

0.2 mA to ensure that the tip of the needle is not intraneural.[7] Injection of small amounts of local anesthetic solution (1 to 2 mL, the "Raj test") will eliminate the motor response, probably by reducing current density near the tip of the needle rather than by physical separation of the block needle and nerve.[8,9] Nerve stimulation may fail to produce a motor response in some subjects, even when paresthesias occur, suggesting direct needle to nerve contact.[10]

Nerve stimulation–based approaches may fail to produce plexus anesthesia if the nerves of the plexus are not in sufficient proximity to each other. Longer pulse widths (0.3 msec rather than 0.1 msec) can be used for the stimulation of pure sensory nerves. Nerve stimulators for monitoring neuromuscular blockade are not recommended for peripheral nerve localization because they can deliver large currents (>50 mA) and may not accurately deliver the small currents used for peripheral nerve blocks (range, 0.4 to 2.0 mA).

PERIPHERAL NERVE CATHETERS

Catheters can be placed adjacent to peripheral nerves for postoperative analgesia by infusion of dilute local anesthetic solutions. Continuous peripheral nerve blocks can be used in the hospital setting to facilitate vigorous early joint mobilization following orthopedic surgery. They can also be used to provide potent analgesia for outpatient surgery (also see Chapter 37). For placement of these catheters, the peripheral nerve should be first located in a fashion similar to that for single-injection blocks (typically nerve stimulation or ultrasound guidance with a large-bore needle), and then the catheter is threaded. Initially injecting a local anesthetic or dextrose solution to create more space adjacent to the nerve before catheter placement is useful. Catheters capable of nerve stimulation can also be used. Peripheral nerve catheters are more prone to dislodgment than epidural catheters because movement of skin near the catheter entry point is usually more likely.

CERVICAL PLEXUS BLOCK

The cervical plexus is formed by the first four cervical nerves.[11] With the patient's head turned to the opposite side, the superficial cervical plexus can be blocked by infiltration of local anesthetic solution just deep to the platysma and investing fascia of the neck along the posterior lateral border of the sternocleidomastoid muscle (Fig. 18-4). The anesthesia produced by a cervical plexus block includes the area from the inferior surface of the mandible to the level of the clavicle. A cervical plexus block is used most often to provide anesthesia in conscious patients undergoing carotid endarterectomy (see Chapter 25). Although combined superficial and deep cervical plexus blocks have traditionally been used for this surgical procedure, a superficial block alone is often sufficient.[12]

BRACHIAL PLEXUS ANATOMY

The brachial plexus arises from the ventral rami of C5 through T1 (Fig. 18-5). These rami unite to form three trunks in the space between the anterior and middle

Figure 18-4 Anatomic landmarks and method of needle placement for a superficial cervical plexus block. With the patient's head turned to the side, local anesthetic is infiltrated along the posterolateral border of the sternocleidomastoid muscle. (Adapted from Brown DL, Factor DA [eds]: Regional Anesthesia and Analgesia. Philadelphia, WB Saunders, 1996, p 245.)

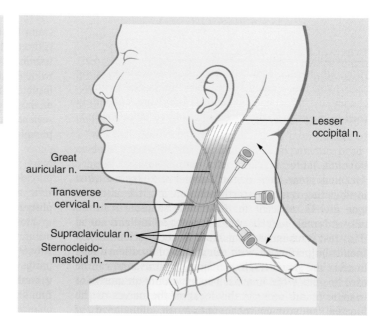

Lesser occipital n.

Great auricular n.

Transverse cervical n.

Supraclavicular n.

Sternocleidomastoid m.

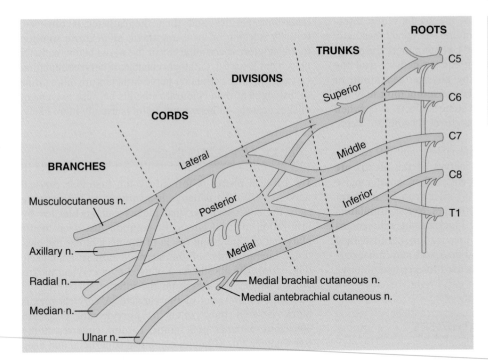

ROOTS

TRUNKS

DIVISIONS

CORDS

BRANCHES

Superior

Middle

Inferior

Lateral

Posterior

Medial

Musculocutaneous n.

Axillary n.

Radial n.

Median n.

Ulnar n.

Medial brachial cutaneous n.
Medial antebrachial cutaneous n.

C5
C6
C7
C8
T1

Figure 18-5 Roots, trunks, divisions, cords, and branches of the right brachial plexus. (Adapted from Wedel DJ, Horlocker TT. Nerve blocks. In Miller RD [ed]: Miller's Anesthesia, 7th ed. Philadelphia, Elsevier, 2010.)

scalene muscles and then pass over the first rib and under the clavicle to enter the axilla. The trunks form three anterior and three posterior divisions, which recombine to create three cords. These cords divide into terminal branches that supply all the motor and sensory innervation of the upper extremity, with the exception of the skin over the shoulders, which is supplied by the cervical plexus, and the medial aspect of the arm, which is supplied by the intercostobrachial branch of the second intercostal nerve (Fig. 18-6).

Brachial Plexus Block

Although nerves can be anesthetized anywhere along their path, four anatomic locations (interscalene, supraclavicular, infraclavicular, and axillary) are commonly used to place local anesthetic solutions to block the brachial plexus (Table 18-2).

INTERSCALENE BLOCK

An interscalene block of the brachial plexus is achieved by injecting local anesthetic solution into the interscalene groove adjacent to the transverse process of C6 (the external jugular vein often overlies this area) (Fig. 18-7). An interscalene block of the brachial plexus should be performed with the arm at the patient's side to relax the shoulder. High-frequency ultrasound can be used to image the brachial plexus within the posterior triangle of the neck. In this location the nerves of the brachial plexus do not contain an abundance of

connective tissue. Therefore, the nerves appear hypoechoic on ultrasound scans (see Fig. 18-7). Using an inplane technique, local anesthetic can be deposited adjacent to the brachial plexus between the anterior and middle scalene muscles. Injection of 20 to 30 mL of local anesthetic solution will anesthetize the cervical plexus and brachial plexus and thus permit surgery on the shoulder and more distal upper extremity, although fibers that innervate the ulnar side of the forearm and hand (C8-T1, inferior trunk) may be spared (see Fig. 18-6).

Complications

Although pneumothorax occurs infrequently, the diagnosis should be considered if cough or chest pain is produced while exploring for the location of the brachial plexus. An ipsilateral phrenic nerve block with associated hemiparesis of the diaphragm is an expected side effect of the interscalene approach to the brachial plexus. Because the phrenic nerve lies on the anterior scalene muscle, the incidence of diaphragmatic paralysis after an interscalene block is nearly 100%.[13] Although the resultant unilateral phrenic nerve block is asymptomatic in normal subjects at rest, patients with respiratory insufficiency or contralateral phrenic nerve palsy will tolerate this condition poorly.[14]

Blockade of the recurrent laryngeal nerve can also occur, but much less commonly. It can cause complete airway obstruction in patients with contralateral vocal cord palsy. A preoperative history of hoarseness or neck surgery should alert the practitioner to this possibility. Continual needle visibility under ultrasound will reduce the chance of an epidural block, subarachnoid block, and

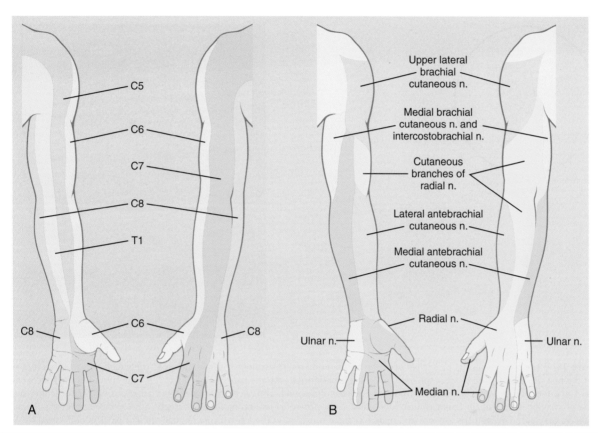

Figure 18-6 A, Cutaneous distribution of the cervical and thoracic roots of the upper extremity. **B,** Cutaneous distribution of the peripheral nerves of the upper extremity. (Adapted from Wedel DJ, Horlocker TT. Nerve blocks. In Miller RD [ed]: Miller's Anesthesia, 7th ed. Philadelphia, Elsevier, 2010.)

Table 18-2 Techniques for Brachial Plexus Block

Technique	Level	Potential Drawback
Interscalene	Roots/trunks	Spares the inferior trunk
Supraclavicular	Trunks/divisions	Risk for pneumothorax
Infraclavicular	Cords	Pectoral discomfort
Axillary	Branches	Spares the musculocutaneous nerve

injection into a vertebral artery. If local anesthetics are accidentally injected into a vertebral artery, convulsions will immediately follow. Therefore, meticulous aspiration and constant monitoring of needle position and local anesthetic spread throughout the procedure are advised.

SUPRACLAVICULAR BLOCK

Supraclavicular block of the brachial plexus is achieved by injecting 20 to 30 mL of local anesthetic solution around the brachial plexus where it is usually tightly bundled and adjacent to the subclavian artery, just cephalad to the clavicle.[15] Pneumothorax is the most common serious complication of a supraclavicular block (about a 1% incidence) and can be manifested initially as cough, dyspnea, or pleuritic chest pain. Block of the phrenic nerve occurs frequently (50% of procedures) but generally causes no clinically significant symptoms. Bilateral supraclavicular blocks are not recommended for fear of bilateral pneumothorax or phrenic nerve paralysis. Likewise, patients with chronic obstructive pulmonary disease may not be ideal candidates for a supraclavicular block. Advantages of a supraclavicular block are rapid onset and ability to perform the block with the arm in any position. The increased risk for pneumothorax may limit the use of supraclavicular block for outpatients. Because of these risks, many practitioners have advocated the use of ultrasound imaging to guide supraclavicular blocks.

The supraclavicular block can be performed with a similar technique to interscalene blocks described previously. The ultrasound probe is moved closer to the clavicle and faces caudally to facilitate imaging of the brachial plexus adjacent to the subclavian artery and over the first rib. In this location, almost all practitioners utilize in-plane technique because of the proximity of the pleura (see Fig. 18-7).

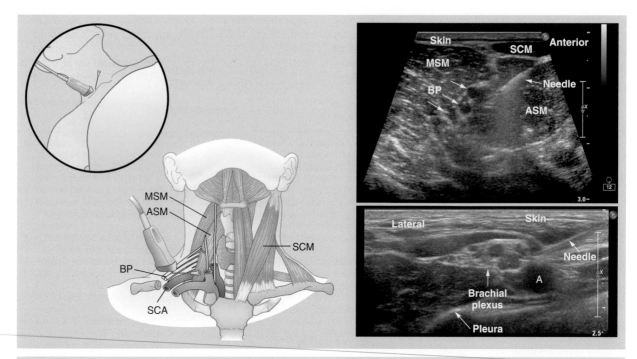

Figure 18-7 The brachial plexus passes between the anterior and middle scalene muscles and joins the subclavian artery as it passes over the first rib. Interscalene block of the brachial plexus is performed with the patient supine and the head turned to the contralateral side. The interscalene groove is imaged with high-frequency ultrasound. The needle advances from anterior to posterior within the plane of imaging. In the upper figure, interscalene block is performed by infiltrating local anesthetic around the roots of the brachial plexus as they pass between the anterior and middle scalene muscles. In the lower figure, supraclavicular block is performed by injecting local anesthetic around the divisions of the brachial plexus adjacent to the subclavian artery. In the lower sonogram, the block needle advances through the anterior scalene muscle from anterior to posterior, with the needle tip resting between the subclavian artery and the brachial plexus. ASM, anterior scalene muscle; BP, brachial plexus; MSM, middle scalene muscle; SCA, subclavian artery; SCM, sternocleidomastoid muscle.

INFRACLAVICULAR BLOCK

Infraclavicular block is a versatile procedure that can provide excellent anesthesia and analgesia for procedures on the hand, forearm, and elbow. The infraclavicular site is an excellent choice for the insertion of a continuous brachial plexus catheter because it is a secure, clean site that is comfortable for the patient.[16] Blockade of the cords of the brachial plexus occurs in the axilla, just distal to the clavicle (Fig. 18-8). The needle path is remote from the lung and neuraxis, and conduction block occurs at the point where the cords of the brachial plexus tightly surround the axillary artery. Arm abduction is not required but can facilitate assessment of the surface anatomy.

With the patient supine and the arm abducted and externally rotated, an ultrasound transducer is placed inferior to the clavicle to visualize the subclavian artery and adjacent cords of the brachial plexus. A needle is advanced caudally within the plane of imaging until its tip lies within the fascial sheath that surrounds the brachial plexus. Local anesthetic solution, 30 to 40 mL, is incrementally injected so that all three cords of the brachial plexus are surrounded by local anesthetic (see Fig. 18-8).

Disadvantages

Disadvantages of an infraclavicular block include the risk of vascular puncture and patient discomfort associated with traversing the pectoralis major and minor muscles with the block needle. Appropriate levels of sedation and adequate infiltration of local anesthetic along the needle path are required.

AXILLARY BLOCK

An axillary brachial plexus block is achieved by injecting 30 to 40 mL of local anesthetic solution around the nerves that lie in close proximity to the axillary artery (Fig. 18-9). At the level of the axilla, the terminal branches of the brachial plexus reside within the axillary sheath and in the tissue that immediately surrounds it (see Fig. 18-9). An axillary block can be used for anesthesia of the hand, forearm, and elbow.[17]

The patient is positioned supine with the arm abducted to 90 degrees and externally rotated to gain access to the axilla. A high-frequency ultrasound transducer is placed in the axilla, showing the brachial artery and the surrounding nerves of the brachial plexus. A needle is advanced from

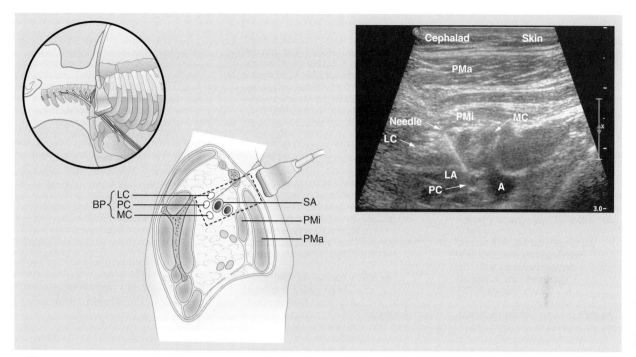

Figure 18-8 Technique of infraclavicular block. With the patient supine and the arm abducted and externally rotated, an ultrasound transducer is placed inferior to the clavicle to visualize the subclavian artery and adjacent cords of the brachial plexus. A needle is advanced caudally within the plane of imaging until its tip lies within the fascial sheath that surrounds the brachial plexus. In the sonogram the needle tip passes between the lateral and medial cords of the brachial plexus and injects local anesthetic that surrounds the three cords. A, subclavian artery; LA, local anesthetic; LC, lateral cord; MC, medial cord; PC, posterior cord; PMa, pectoralis major muscle; PMi, pectoralis minor muscle.

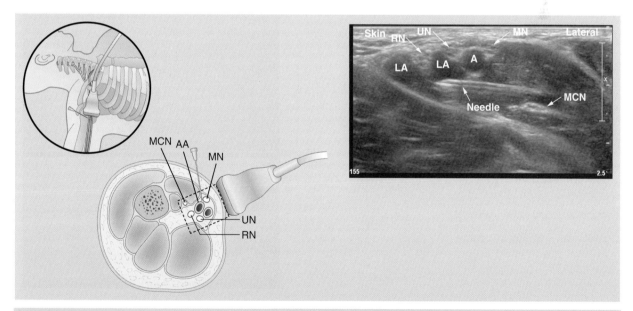

Figure 18-9 Axillary block. The arm is abducted 90 degrees. Key structures in the right axilla are visualized with a high-frequency ultrasound transducer. The arrangement of the branches of the brachial plexus around the axillary artery is shown in the inset. The sonogram shows the block needle advancing from lateral within the plane of imaging. The needle tip passes deep to the artery and injects local anesthetic that surrounds the radial nerve. Additional injections ensure local anesthetic spread around the ulnar and median nerves. AA, axillary artery; LA, local anesthetic; MCN, musculocutaneous nerve; MN, median nerve; RN, radial nerve; UN, ulnar nerve. (Adapted from Brown DL, Factor DA [eds]: Regional Anesthesia and Analgesia. Philadelphia, WB Saunders, 1996.)

superior to inferior within the plane of imaging so that the tip lies within the axillary sheath. Multiple injections of local anesthetic surround each of the nerves, including the musculocutaneous nerve, which lies lateral to the brachial plexus in the coracobrachialis muscle. A final 5 mL of local anesthetic solution is infiltrated into the subcutaneous tissue immediately superficial to the axillary artery to block the intercostobrachial, medial brachial cutaneous, and medial antebrachial cutaneous nerves (see Fig. 18-9).

Advantages and Complications

An axillary perivascular block has the advantage of being remote from the lung and neuraxis and can therefore be performed with relative safety. Potential complications include systemic local anesthetic toxicity as a result of intravascular injection and nerve injury from needle trauma, intraneural injection, or hematoma.[18]

DISTAL NERVE BLOCKS OF THE UPPER EXTREMITY—FOREARM BLOCK

Anesthesia of the hand can be achieved by injecting local anesthetic solution at the level of the forearm to block the median, ulnar, and radial nerves (Fig. 18-10). This anesthetic technique can be useful for hand surgery when a tourniquet is not used for surgical hemostasis. Nerve blocks at the forearm can also be very helpful to supplement a brachial plexus block with incomplete sensory distribution.

Median Nerve Block

The median nerve provides most of the sensory innervation to the palm of the hand. The forearm is scanned in short axis with high-frequency ultrasound showing the median nerve with a fine fascicular appearance that is distinct from the surrounding muscles and tendons. Under continuous visualization, 3 to 5 mL of local anesthetic is injected around the median nerve.

Ulnar Nerve Block

The ulnar nerve provides sensation to the dorsal and palmar sides of the ulnar aspect of the hand. The ulnar nerve is blocked by injecting 3 to 5 mL of local anesthetic solution around the ulnar nerve in the forearm, usually at a level in the forearm where the ulnar nerve is not in direct contact with the ulnar artery.

Radial Nerve Block

Most patients have radial dominance of sensation on the dorsal aspect of the hand. The superficial radial nerve is the distal sensory branch of the radial nerve that follows

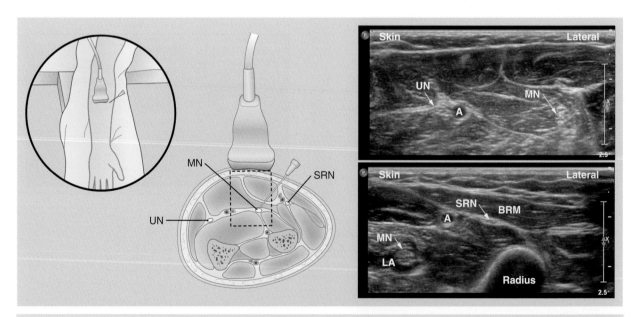

Figure 18-10 Forearm block technique: The forearm is imaged on short axis with high-frequency ultrasound. The needle is advanced within the plane of imaging to encounter each nerve. The inset shows the relevant cross-sectional anatomy at the proximal forearm. In the upper sonogram, the ulnar nerve is seen immediately medial to the ulnar artery. The median nerve lies in the middle of the forearm, has a fine echotexture similar to the ulnar nerve, and is usually hyperechoic compared to surround flexor muscles. In the lower sonogram, the superficial radial nerve lies immediately deep to the brachioradialis muscle, near the radial artery. The median nerve is surrounded by local anesthetic. LA, local anesthetic; MN, median nerve; SRN, superficial radial nerve; UN, ulnar nerve.

the radial artery along its course through the forearm. It can be blocked by ultrasound-guided infiltration of 3 to 5 mL of local anesthetic solution anywhere along its course deep to the brachioradialis muscle or in a subcutaneous ring at the level of the anatomic snuffbox.

BLOCKS OF THE LOWER EXTREMITY

Unlike the compactness of the brachial plexus, the lower extremity is supplied by nerves that are widely separated from each other as they enter the thigh. Major nerves to the lower extremity include the sciatic, posterior femoral cutaneous, femoral, lateral femoral cutaneous, and obturator nerves (Fig. 18-11). For many operations, an epidural or spinal anesthetic is easier to perform than attempting to provide the same extent of anesthesia with multiple peripheral nerve blocks. However, patient co-morbidities such as severe cardiac disease, bacteremia, and anticoagulation may make

peripheral nerve blocks the best choice for anesthesia of the lower extremity. Even when these lower extremity blocks do not serve as definitive anesthetics, they can improve patient disposition by providing superior postoperative pain relief.

Femoral Nerve Block

A femoral nerve block provides anesthesia to the anterior aspect of the thigh and knee, as well as the medial aspect of the leg, where it continues as the saphenous nerve. It is a definitive anesthetic only for superficial surgical procedures on the anterior thigh such as muscle biopsy, and is therefore typically combined with other blocks such as a sciatic nerve block to provide complete anesthesia below the knee. A femoral nerve block alone or in combination with other peripheral nerve blocks is very useful for postoperative analgesia and provides a good alternative when contraindications to neuraxial blockade are present.

III

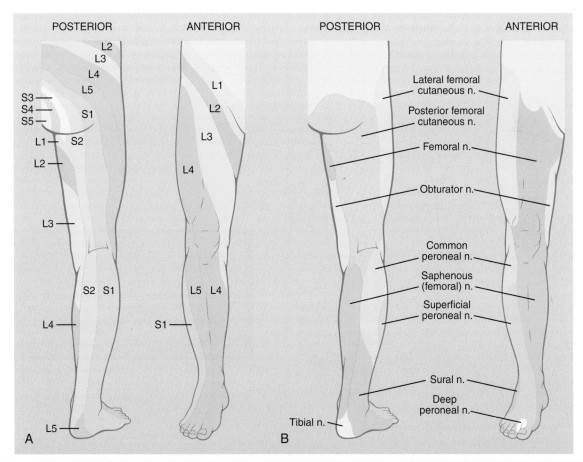

Figure 18-11 A, Cutaneous distribution of the lumbosacral nerves. **B,** Cutaneous distribution of the peripheral nerves of the lower extremity. Note that the cutaneous distribution of the obturator nerve is highly variable, but shown here on the medial aspect of the thigh. (Adapted from Wedel DJ, Horlocker TT. Nerve blocks. In Miller RD [ed]: Miller's Anesthesia, 7th ed. Philadelphia, Elsevier, 2010.)

ANATOMY

Arising from lumbar segments L2 through L4, the femoral nerve reaches the thigh by passing underneath the inguinal ligament just lateral to the femoral artery and vein and separated from them by the iliopectineal ligament. The femoral nerve lies deep to the fascia iliaca, which invests the iliopsoas muscle. Along its course, the femoral nerve divides into multiple anterior cutaneous branches of the thigh and gives rise to the saphenous nerve of the medial aspect of the leg.

PERFORMANCE OF THE BLOCK

A femoral nerve block is performed with the patient in the supine position and the thigh slightly abducted and externally rotated to improve access. The femoral nerve is appreciated on sonograms as a flattened bundle of fascicles lying between the hypoechoic subcutaneous tissue and the hyperechoic iliopsoas muscle (Fig. 18-12). The ultrasound transducer must be positioned proximally, near the femoral crease to visualize the femoral nerve before it arborizes into small terminal branches. The block needle is advanced within the plane of imaging from lateral to medial until it punctures the fascia iliaca, with a distinct pop. The needle position is optimized to create circumferential spread of 20 to 30 mL of local anesthetic around the femoral nerve (see Fig. 18-12).

Saphenous Nerve Block

The saphenous nerve is the only branch of the femoral nerve to contribute to innervation below the knee. It can be blocked at the midthigh level, where it lies anterior to the femoral artery (Fig. 18-13). The femoral artery is a landmark for the saphenous nerve, both of which lie just deep to the sartorius muscle (see Fig. 18-13). The block needle is advanced within the plane of imaging and 5 to 10 mL of local anesthetic is deposited deep to the sartorius muscle, adjacent to the femoral artery (see Fig. 18-13). This block is often combined with a popliteal nerve block for ankle anesthesia.

Sciatic Nerve Block (Classic Approach of Labat)

The sacral plexus (L4-L5, S1-S3) gives rise to the sciatic nerve, which is nearly 2 cm wide as it leaves the pelvis. The classic approach to a sciatic nerve block is with the patient lying on the side opposite the nerve to be blocked (Fig. 18-14). A line is drawn between the posterior superior iliac spine and the greater trochanter of the femur. Although ultrasound guidance can be used to perform this block, the relative depth of the nerve favors use of a low-frequency transducer that may not always be available. Using a peripheral nerve stimulator, the needle

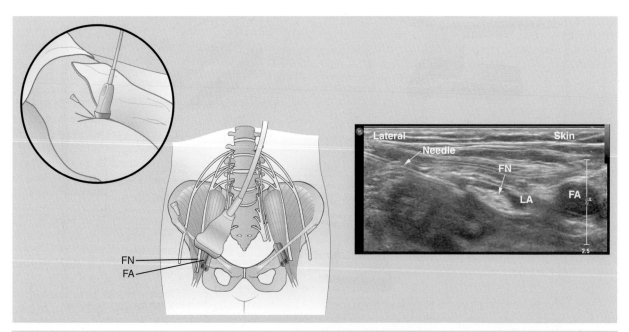

Figure 18-12 Femoral nerve block. The femoral nerve runs over the surface of the iliopsoas muscle as it passes under the inguinal ligament. The iliac fascia invests the femoral nerve and iliopsoas muscle, which is anatomically separate from the femoral sheath. Femoral nerve block is performed with short-axis imaging of femoral nerve and artery. In the sonogram, the block needle passes from lateral to medial, deep to the fascia iliaca and injects local anesthetic that surrounds the femoral nerve. FA, femoral artery; FN, femoral nerve. (Adapted from Brown DL, Factor DA [eds]: Regional Anesthesia and Analgesia. Philadelphia, WB Saunders, 1996.)

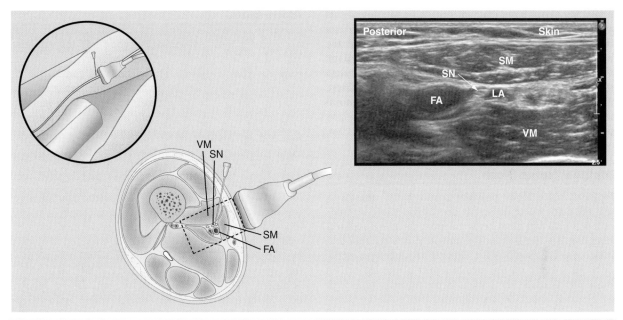

Figure 18-13 Saphenous nerve block. With the patient supine and leg externally rotated, the medial thigh is scanned in axial section with high-frequency ultrasound. The needle advances from anterior to posterior within the plane of imaging. The saphenous nerve is not always visible, but it courses with the femoral artery, just deep to the sartorius muscle. Local anesthetic surrounds the saphenous nerve. FA, femoral artery; LA, local anesthetic; SM, sartorius muscle; SN, saphenous nerve; VM, vastus medialis muscle.

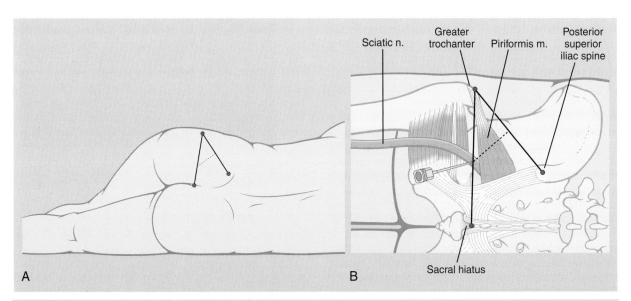

Figure 18-14 Posterior approach to a sciatic nerve block. **A,** Patient positioning. **B,** Anatomic landmarks. The sciatic nerve lies beneath a point 5 cm caudad along a perpendicular line that bisects a line joining the posterior iliac spine and the greater trochanter of the femur. This point is also usually the intersection of that perpendicular line with a line joining the greater trochanter and the sacral hiatus. (Adapted from Wedel DJ, Horlocker TT. Nerve blocks. In Miller RD [ed]: Miller's Anesthesia, 7th ed. Philadelphia, Elsevier, 2010.)

is inserted about 5 cm caudad from the midpoint of this line. Foot movement evoked by nerve stimulation is a satisfactory end point for needle placement before the injection of local anesthetic solution (about 25 to 30 mL is typically used). This block provides nearly complete anesthesia of the foot and lower part of the leg. More often, a sciatic nerve block is combined with a femoral nerve block to provide more extensive anesthesia of the lower extremity.

Popliteal Nerve Block

Popliteal nerve block provides sciatic nerve anesthesia near the point where the sciatic nerve divides into its common peroneal and tibial nerve components in the popliteal fossa (Fig. 18-15). It is most commonly used for foot and ankle surgery, usually with femoral or saphenous nerve block for surgery on the medial aspect of the leg or if a tourniquet is used. The patient is positioned supine with leg elevated about 30 cm, allowing space for an ultrasound transducer to scan the posterior thigh just proximal to the knee crease. Sliding the transducer proximally demonstrates the division of the sciatic nerve, and the needle is advanced within the plane of imaging from lateral to medial. Local anesthetic solution, 20 to 30 mL, is injected between the adjoining common peroneal and tibial nerves to surround them (see Fig. 18-15).

Ankle Block

All five peripheral nerves that supply the foot can be blocked (ankle block) at the level of the malleoli (Fig. 18-16). The tibial nerve is the major nerve to the sole of the foot. This nerve lies on the heel side of the posterior tibial artery and can be blocked by infiltrating 3 to 5 mL of local anesthetic solution in a fanning pattern around this artery. The sural nerve innervates the lateral side of the foot and can be blocked by injecting 5 mL of local anesthetic solution in the groove between the lateral malleolus and the calcaneus near the small saphenous vein. The saphenous nerve innervates the medial aspect of the foot. Infiltration of 5 mL of local anesthetic solution anterior to the medial malleolus near the great saphenous vein blocks this nerve. The deep peroneal nerve innervates the webbing between the first and second toes and is blocked by injecting 5 mL of local anesthetic solution adjacent to the anterior tibial artery. Alternatively, if arterial pulsation is absent, the deep peroneal nerve can also be blocked deep to the extensor hallucis longus tendon and extensor retinaculum. The dorsum of the foot is innervated by the superficial peroneal nerve. The superficial branches of this nerve are blocked by injecting a subcutaneous ridge of local anesthetic between the medial and lateral malleoli over the anterior surface of the foot. Because the foot does not have a generous blood supply, systemic toxicity after an ankle block is rare.

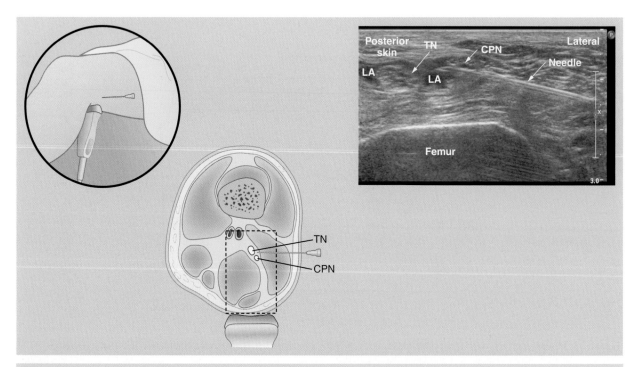

Figure 18-15 Popliteal nerve block: The patient is positioned supine with leg elevated to allow the popliteal fossa to be scanned from below with high-frequency ultrasound. The block needle passes from the lateral thigh through the biceps femoris muscle and injects local around the tibial and common peroneal nerves. CPN, common peroneal nerve; LA, local anesthetic; TN, tibial nerve.

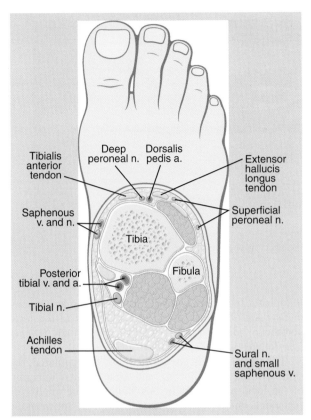

Figure 18-16 Cross-sectional anatomy for an ankle block. An ankle block is performed by injecting local anesthetic solution at five separate nerve locations. The superficial peroneal nerve, sural nerve, and saphenous nerve are usually blocked by subcutaneous infiltration because they may have already branched as they cross the ankle joint. The tibial and deep peroneal nerves require deeper injection adjacent to the accompanying blood vessels (the posterior tibial and anterior tibial arteries, respectively). Because the block needle approaches the ankle from many angles, it is convenient to elevate the foot by supporting the calf. (Adapted from Brown DL, Factor DA [eds]: Regional Anesthesia and Analgesia. Philadelphia, WB Saunders, 1996.)

INTRAVENOUS REGIONAL ANESTHESIA

Intravenous regional neural anesthesia (Bier block, named after August Bier) is a simple method of producing anesthesia of the arm or leg. This technique involves the intravenous injection of large volumes of dilute local anesthetic solutions into an extremity after occlusion of the circulation by a tourniquet. A Bier block is an alternative method of producing extremity anesthesia without blocking individual peripheral nerves. A Bier block can be used for surgical procedures with a duration of 2 hours or less. Severe tourniquet

pain and the maximum allowable tourniquet time limit the practical duration of the block. Because the duration of postoperative analgesia is also limited, this procedure is not usually performed when postoperative pain is a significant issue.

Contraindications

Contraindications to a Bier block are essentially contraindications to tourniquet application (sickle cell disease, infection, ischemic vascular disease). Pain limits the effectiveness of exsanguination of extremities with fractures. Traumatic lacerations may allow escape of local anesthetic from the extremity.

Performance of the Block

A small intravenous catheter is placed in the distal portion of the involved extremity. The arm or leg is then exsanguinated by wrapping with an Esmarch bandage (Fig. 18-17). The tourniquet is inflated to 250 to 275 mm Hg, or about 100 mm Hg above the patient's systolic blood pressure. Plain (without epinephrine) local anesthetic solution (40 to 50 mL for the upper extremity) is injected for a 70-kg adult patient. The intravenous catheter is normally removed after this injection. Beyond 45 minutes of surgery, many patients experience pain at the site of tourniquet placement. A double-tourniquet technique can be used to reduce tourniquet pain. With this technique the proximal cuff is initially inflated, and when the patient subsequently experiences pain, the more distal cuff over anesthetized skin is inflated and the proximal cuff is then deflated. Blockade of the intercostobrachial nerve by local anesthetic infiltration proximal to the tourniquet on the medial aspect of the arm can also be used to reduce pain from tourniquet inflation.

Selection of Local Anesthetic

Commonly used local anesthetic solutions for intravenous regional neural anesthesia are 0.5% lidocaine or prilocaine (plain solutions without epinephrine). Racemic bupivacaine is avoided because of potential systemic toxicity, most notably malignant ventricular cardiac dysrhythmias leading to refractory cardiac arrest. Ropivacaine (1.2 to 1.8 mg/kg in 40 mL) and levobupivacaine (40 mL of 0.125% solution) have been used for intravenous regional neural anesthesia in adult patients because they are associated with less cardiovascular and central nervous system toxicity than racemic bupivacaine is[19,20] Preservative-free solutions of local anesthetic are recommended for intravenous regional anesthesia because preservatives have been associated with thrombophlebitis.

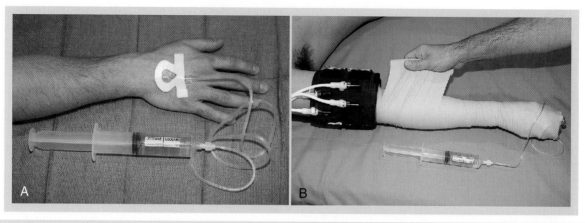

Figure 18-17 A, Placement and securing of a small intravenous catheter. **B,** Exsanguination of the arm with an Esmarch bandage before inflation of the tourniquet and injection of the local anesthetic solution through the catheter.

Characteristics of the Block

The onset of anesthesia rapidly follows the intravenous administration of local anesthetic solution into the isolated extremity. The duration of surgical anesthesia depends on the time that the tourniquet is inflated and not on the local anesthetic selected. When compared with lidocaine, the intravenous regional neural anesthesia produced by ropivacaine and levobupivacaine appears to be comparable but has slightly longer-lasting residual effects.[19,20] Technically, a regional intravenous neural block is easier and faster to perform than a brachial plexus block or lower extremity block and is readily applicable to all age groups, including pediatric patients.

Risks

The principal risk associated with intravenous regional neural anesthesia is the potential systemic toxicity that may occur when the tourniquet is deflated and large amounts of local anesthetic solution from the previously isolated part of the extremity enter the systemic circulation. Local anesthetic levels peak approximately 2 to 5 minutes after tourniquet deflation when an intravenous regional block is used. In this regard, one approach is to keep the tourniquet inflated for at least 20 minutes, even if the surgical procedure is completed in less time. If 40 minutes has elapsed, the tourniquet can be deflated in a single maneuver. Between 20 and 40 minutes, the tourniquet can be deflated, reinflated immediately, and finally deflated after 1 minute. This method will reduce the peak plasma level of local anesthetic. Limitation of extremity movement after release of the tourniquet is also useful for minimizing local anesthetic blood levels. The rapid metabolism of prilocaine is advantageous for decreasing the likelihood of systemic toxicity after deflation of the tourniquet.

Significant methemoglobinemia is unlikely to accompany metabolism of prilocaine when the total dose of this local anesthetic administered to adults is less than 600 mg (see Chapter 11).

If the extremity is not adequately exsanguinated, the skin will have a blotchy appearance after injection of the local anesthetic. In this situation, the quality of the block and surgical field will be poor. Intravenous regional sympathetic blocks with guanethidine, reserpine, or bretylium are sometimes used for chronic pain management.

QUESTIONS OF THE DAY

1. During peripheral nerve blockade aided by a nerve stimulator, what current level generally indicates sufficient proximity of the block needle to the nerve?
2. What are the potential complications of interscalene brachial plexus block?
3. Which patients may be at increased risk of complications after supraclavicular brachial plexus block?
4. What are the five peripheral nerves that supply the foot at the level of the malleoli? What are the anatomic landmarks for placement of an ankle block?
5. What are the contraindications to use of intravenous regional anesthesia (Bier block)?

ACKNOWLEDGMENT

The editors and publisher would like to thank Dr. Helge Eilers for contributing a chapter on this topic to the prior edition of this work. It has served as the foundation for the current chapter.

REFERENCES

1. Gray AT: Ultrasound-guided regional anesthesia: Current state of the art, *Anesthesiology* 104(2):368–373, 2006.

2. Schafhalter-Zoppoth I, Gray AT: The musculocutaneous nerve: Ultrasound appearance for peripheral nerve block, *Reg Anesth Pain Med* 30:385–390, 2005.

3. Schafhalter-Zoppoth I, Younger SJ, Collins AB, et al: The "seesaw" sign: Improved sonographic identification of the sciatic nerve, *Anesthesiology* 101:808–809, 2004.

4. Perlas A, Chin KJ, Chan VW, et al: Needle visualization in ultrasound-guided regional anesthesia: Challenges and solutions, *Reg Anesth Pain Med* 33:532–544, 2008.

5. Selander D, Edshage S, Wolff T: Paresthesiae or no paresthesiae? Nerve lesions after axillary blocks, *Acta Anaesthesiol Scand* 23:27–33, 1979.

6. Carles M, Pulcini A, Macchi P, et al: An evaluation of the brachial plexus block at the humeral canal using a neurostimulator (1417 patients): The efficacy, safety, and predictive criteria of failure, *Anesth Analg* 92:194–198, 2001.

7. Bigeleisen PE, Moayeri N, Groen GJ: Extraneural versus intraneural stimulation thresholds during ultrasound-guided supraclavicular block, *Anesthesiology* 110:1235–1243, 2009.

8. Hadzic A: Peripheral nerve stimulators: Cracking the code—one at a time, *Reg Anesth Pain Med* 29(3):185–188, 2004.

9. Tsui BC, Wagner A, Finucane B: Electrophysiologic effect of injectates on peripheral nerve stimulation, *Reg Anesth Pain Med* 29:189–193, 2004.

10. Mulroy MF, Mitchell B: Unsolicited paresthesias with nerve stimulator: Case reports of four patients, *Anesth Analg* 95:762–763, 2002.

11. Pandit JJ, Dutta D, Morris JF: Spread of injectate with superficial cervical plexus block in humans: An anatomical study, *Br J Anaesth* 91:733–735, 2003.

12. Pandit JJ, Bree S, Dillon P, et al: A comparison of superficial versus combined (superficial and deep) cervical plexus block for carotid endarterectomy: A prospective, randomized study, *Anesth Analg* 91:781–786, 2000.

13. Urmey WF, Talts KH, Sharrock NE: One hundred percent incidence of hemidiaphragmatic paresis associated with interscalene brachial plexus anesthesia as diagnosed by ultrasonography, *Anesth Analg* 72:498–503, 1991.

14. Hashim MS, Shevde K: Dyspnea during interscalene block after recent coronary bypass surgery, *Anesth Analg* 89:55–56, 1999.

15. Brown DL, Cahill DR, Bridenbaugh LD: Supraclavicular nerve block: Anatomic analysis of a method to prevent pneumothorax, *Anesth Analg* 76:530–534, 1993.

16. Mariano ER, Loland VJ, Bellars RH, et al: Ultrasound guidance versus electrical stimulation for infraclavicular brachial plexus perineural catheter insertion, *J Ultrasound Med* 28(9):1211–1218, 2009.

17. Schroeder LE, Horlocker TT, Schroeder DR: The efficacy of axillary block for surgical procedures about the elbow, *Anesth Analg* 83:747–751, 1996.

18. Hebl JR, Horlocker TT, Sorenson EJ, et al: Regional anesthesia does not increase the risk of postoperative neuropathy in patients undergoing ulnar nerve transposition, *Anesth Analg* 93:1606–1611, 2001.

19. Atanassoff PG, Aouad R, Hartmannsgruber MW, et al: Levobupivacaine 0.125% and lidocaine 0.5% for intravenous regional anesthesia in volunteers, *Anesthesiology* 97:325–328, 2002.

20. Chan VW, Weisbrod MJ, Kaszas Z, et al: Comparison of ropivacaine and lidocaine for intravenous regional anesthesia in volunteers: A preliminary study or anesthetic efficacy and blood level, *Anesthesiology* 90:1602–1608, 1999.

III

19 PATIENT POSITIONING AND ASSOCIATED RISKS

Jae-Woo Lee and Lydia Cassorla

Anesthesia providers share a critical responsibility for the proper positioning of patients in the operating room. Positions deemed optimal for surgery often result in undesirable physiologic changes such as hypotension from impaired venous return to the heart or oxygen desaturation due to ventilation-perfusion mismatching. In addition, peripheral nerve injuries during surgery remain a significant source of perioperative morbidity.[1,2]

Proper positioning requires the cooperation of anesthesia providers, surgeons, and nurses to ensure patient well-being and safety while permitting surgical exposure. During surgery, patients should be placed in a position that they would tolerate when awake whenever possible. Jewelry and hair ornaments are removed. Peripheral joint extremities are padded, and the normal lumbar spine curvature is supported. The head should remain in a midline position without substantial extension or flexion. No pressure should be placed on the eyes. Surgeons wish to have optimal exposure for the procedure and patients may remain in the same position for long periods of time; therefore, prevention of positioning-related complications often requires compromise and judgment. The duration of more extreme positions, when necessary, should be limited as much as possible. The need for tilting of the operating room table during surgery should be anticipated before draping, and the patient secured accordingly. Use of safety straps and prevention of a patient falling off the operating room table to the floor are fundamental.

CARDIOVASCULAR CONCERNS

Complex arterial, venous, and cardiac physiologic responses can blunt the effects of positional changes upon arterial blood pressure and maintain perfusion to vital organs. Central, regional, and local mechanisms are involved. This activity is particularly important for humans who maintain an upright posture because of the vertical distance from the heart to the brain and its need for constant perfusion.

Normally, as a human being reclines from an erect to a supine position, venous return to the heart increases as pooled blood from the lower extremities redistributes toward the heart. Preload, stroke volume, and cardiac output are augmented. The resultant increase in arterial blood pressure activates afferent baroreceptors from the aorta (via the vagus nerve) and within the walls of the carotid sinuses (via the glossopharyngeal nerve) to decrease sympathetic outflow and increase parasympathetic impulses to the sinoatrial node and myocardium. The result is a compensatory decrease in heart rate, stroke volume, and cardiac output. Mechanoreceptors from the atria and ventricle are also activated to decrease sympathetic outflow to muscle and splanchnic vascular beds. Lastly, atrial reflexes are activated to regulate renal sympathetic nerve activity, plasma renin, atrial natriuretic peptide, and arginine vasopressin levels.[3] As a result, systemic arterial blood pressure is maintained within a narrow range during postural changes in the nonanesthetized setting.

General anesthesia, muscle relaxation, positive pressure ventilation, and neuraxial blockade interfere with venous return to the heart, arterial tone, and autoregulatory mechanisms, rendering patients under anesthesia especially vulnerable to relatively uncompensated circulatory effects of changes in position. The use of spinal or epidural anesthesia causes a significant sympathectomy across all affected dermatomes, independent of the presence of general anesthesia, reducing preload and potentially blunting cardiac responses if the sympathetic output to the heart is affected. Positive pressure ventilation increases mean intrathoracic pressure, diminishing the venous pressure gradient from peripheral capillaries to the right atrium. Because relatively small pressure gradients are active in the venous circulation, this may significantly affect cardiac filling and, consequently, cardiac output. Positive end-expiratory pressure (PEEP) further increases mean intrathoracic pressure, as do conditions associated with low lung compliance such as airways disease, obesity, ascites, and light anesthesia. Venous return and cardiac output may be further compromised.[4]

For these reasons, arterial blood pressure is often particularly labile immediately following the initiation of anesthesia and during patient positioning. The anesthesia provider needs to anticipate, monitor, and treat these effects and to assess the safety of positional changes for each patient. Frequent arterial blood pressure measurements should be made following induction of anesthesia or initiation of neuraxial blockade. Intravenous fluid administration may need to be increased, the level of anesthesia adjusted, or vasopressors given, during this hemodynamic transition. Temporary use of head-down positions may be helpful. At times, a delay in repositioning of the patient for surgery may be necessary until arterial blood pressure reaches an acceptable level of homeostasis. Interruptions in monitoring to facilitate positioning or

turning of the operating room table must be minimized during this dynamic period. Patient positioning is always secondary to patient safety.

PULMONARY CONCERNS

Anesthetized human beings who are breathing spontaneously have a reduced tidal volume and functional residual capacity and an increased closing volume when compared with the nonanesthetized state. Positive pressure ventilation with muscle relaxation may ameliorate ventilation-perfusion mismatches under general anesthesia by maintaining adequate minute ventilation and limiting atelectasis. However, the diaphragm assumes an abnormal shape due to the loss of muscle tone and is displaced less in the dependent portions of the lung.[5] This decreases ventilation-perfusion matching and consequently arterial Po_2. Patients undergoing neuraxial anesthesia lose abdominal and thoracic muscle function in affected dermatomes. However, diaphragmatic function is retained if general anesthesia and muscle relaxation are not concurrently administered. In addition to these effects of anesthesia, patient position has distinct effects on pulmonary function. In particular, any position that limits movement of the diaphragm, chest wall, or abdomen may increase atelectasis and intrapulmonary shunt.

Spontaneous ventilation results from relatively small negative intrathoracic pressure shifts during inspiration due to diaphragmatic displacement and chest wall expansion. This pressure decrease also promotes venous return to the thorax by reducing the pressure in the great veins and right atrium compared to the periphery. Normal distribution of ventilation is determined by the excursion of the diaphragm, movement of the chest wall, and compliance of the lung. When a human being shifts from standing to supine position, functional residual capacity decreases due to cephalad displacement of the diaphragm. The relative contribution to ventilation of the chest wall compared to the diaphragm decreases from 30% to only 10%. With spontaneous ventilation in either position, diaphragmatic movement is greatest adjacent to the most dependent portions of the lung, helping to bring new ventilation to the zones of the lung that are preferentially perfused. The preferential perfusion of the dependent portions is dominated by gravity, but other factors such as pulmonary vascular length may also be important. Perfusion appears to follow a central-to-peripheral spectrum in each lobe that is maintained with changes in cardiac output.[6–8]

The prone position has been utilized to improve respiratory function in patients with adult respiratory distress syndrome (ARDS).[9] In anesthetized patients, the prone position has advantages over the supine position with regard to lung volumes and oxygenation without adverse effects upon respiratory mechanics.[10,11] This benefit has also been demonstrated in obese[12] and pediatric patients.[13] When patients are prone, weight should be distributed to the thoracic cage and bony pelvis, allowing the abdomen to move with respiration.

SPECIFIC POSITIONS

Supine

The most common position for surgery is the *supine*, or *dorsal decubitus*, position (Fig. 19-1A). Because the entire body is close to the level of the heart, hemodynamic reserve is best maintained. However, because compensatory mechanisms are blunted by anesthesia, even a few degrees of head-down (Trendelenburg) position or head-up (reverse Trendelenburg) position are sufficient to cause significant cardiovascular changes.

ASSOCIATED ARM POSITION

In a supine patient, one or both arms may be abducted out to the side or adducted (tucked) alongside the body. It is recommended that upper extremity abduction be limited to less than 90 degrees to minimize the likelihood of brachial plexus injury by caudad pressure in the axilla

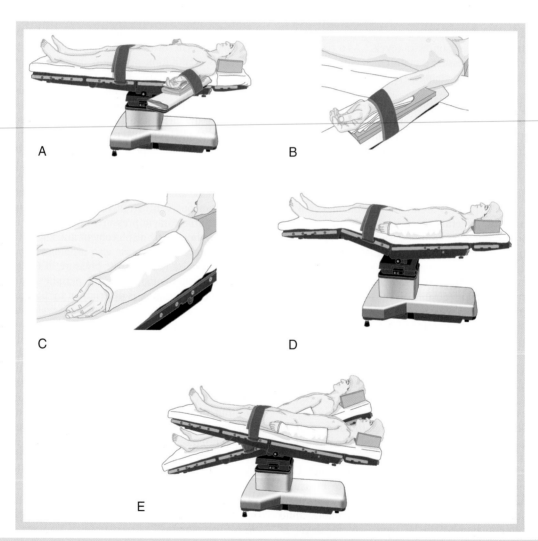

Figure 19-1 A, Supine. Note the asymmetry of the base of the table, placing the patient's center of gravity over the base if positioned in the usual direction. **B,** Arm position on the arm board. Abduction of the arm should be limited to less than 90 degrees whenever possible. The arm is supinated, and the elbow is padded. **C,** Arm tucked at patient's side. Arm in neutral position with palm to hip. The elbow is padded, and one needs to ensure that the arm is supported. **D,** Lawn-chair position. Flexion of the hips and knees decreases tension on the back. **E,** Trendelenburg position (head tilted down) and reverse Trendelenburg position (head tilted up). Shoulder braces should be avoided to prevent brachial plexus compression injuries.

from the head of the humerus. The hand and forearm are either supinated or kept in a neutral position with the palm toward the body to reduce external pressure on the ulnar nerve (Fig. 19-1B).[14-16] When the arms are adducted, they are usually held alongside the body with a "draw sheet" that passes under the body and over the arm and is then tucked directly under the torso (not the mattress) to ensure that the arm remains properly placed next to the body. Alternatively, when access to the chest or abdomen is not necessary, curved arm cradles may be used. In all cases the arms are placed in a neutral position.[14] The elbows, as well as any protruding objects such as intravenous fluid lines and stopcocks, are padded (Fig. 19-1C).

VARIATIONS OF THE SUPINE POSITION

Several variations of the supine position are frequently used. The *lawn-chair position* (Fig. 19-1D), in which the hips and knees are slightly flexed, reduces stress on the back, hips, and knees and is better tolerated by patients who are awake or undergoing monitored anesthesia care. In addition, because the legs are slightly above the heart, venous drainage from the lower extremity is facilitated. Also, the xiphoid to pubic distance is decreased, reducing the tension on the ventral abdominal musculature and easing closure of laparotomy incisions. Proper positioning of the patient's hips on the operating room table requires manipulation of the table. Typically the back of the bed is raised, the legs below the knees are lowered to an equivalent angle, and a slight Trendelenburg tilt is used to level the hips with the shoulders, if desired. This position reduces venous pooling in the legs and permits an arm board or table to be parallel with the floor if desired for upper extremity surgery.

The *frog-leg position*, in which the hips and knees are flexed and the hips are externally rotated with the soles of the feet facing each other, allows access to the perineum, medial thighs, genitalia, and rectum. Care must be taken to minimize stress and postoperative pain in the hips and prevent dislocation by supporting the knees appropriately.

Tilting a supine patient head down, the *Trendelenburg position* (Fig. 19-1E), is often used to increase venous return during hypotension, to improve exposure during abdominal and laparoscopic surgery, and during central line placement to prevent air emboli and facilitate cannulation. It is linked by name to a 19th century German surgeon, Friedrich Trendelenburg, who described its use for abdominal surgery. Nonsliding mattresses are recommended to prevent the patient from sliding cephalad. Shoulder braces are not recommended because of considerable risk of compression injury to the brachial plexus.

The Trendelenburg position has significant cardiovascular and respiratory consequences. The head-down position increases central venous, intracranial, and intraocular pressures. Prolonged head-down position can also lead to swelling of the face, conjunctiva, larynx, and tongue with an increased potential for postoperative upper airway obstruction. The cephalad movement of abdominal viscera against the diaphragm also decreases functional residual capacity and pulmonary compliance. In spontaneously ventilating patients the work of breathing increases. In mechanically ventilated patients, airway pressures must be higher to ensure adequate ventilation. The stomach also lies above the glottis. Therefore, endotracheal intubation is often preferred to protect the airway from pulmonary aspiration of gastric contents and to reduce atelectasis. Because of the risk of edema to the trachea and mucosa surrounding the airway during surgeries in which patients have been in the Trendelenburg position for prolonged periods of time, an air leak should be verified around the endotracheal tube or the larynx visualized prior to extubation.

The *reverse Trendelenburg* position (Fig. 19-1E), supine with the head tilted upward, is often employed to facilitate upper abdominal surgery by shifting the abdominal contents caudad. This is increasingly popular due to the growing number of laparoscopic surgeries. Again, patients must be prevented from slipping on the table, and more frequent monitoring of arterial blood pressure may be prudent to detect hypotension due to decreased venous return. In addition, the position of the head above the heart reduces perfusion pressure to the brain and should be taken into consideration when determining optimal blood pressure.

In all positions in which the head is at a different level than the heart, the effect of the hydrostatic gradient upon cerebral arterial and venous pressures should be carefully considered in terms of cerebral perfusion pressure. Careful documentation of any potential arterial pressure gradients is especially prudent.

COMPLICATIONS

Pressure alopecia due to ischemic hair follicles is related to prolonged immobilization of the head with its full weight falling on a limited area, usually the occiput. Lumps such as those due to monitoring cable connectors, should not be placed under head padding, as they may create focal areas of pressure. Hypothermia and hypotension during surgery may increase the incidence of this complication. Consequently, it is prudent to cushion the head well, and during prolonged surgery, periodic rotation of the head to redistribute the weight may be considered.

Backache may occur in the supine position as the normal lumbar lordotic curvature, particularly the tone of the paraspinous musculature is lost during general anesthesia with muscle relaxation or a neuraxial block. Consequently, patients with extensive kyphosis, scoliosis, or a previous history of back pain may require extra padding of the spine or slight flexion at the hip and knee. Lastly, tissues overlying all bony prominences, such as the heels and sacrum, must be padded to prevent soft tissue ischemia due to pressure, especially during prolonged surgery.[17]

III

Peripheral nerve injury, discussed in a later section, is a complex phenomenon with a multifactorial etiology. The American Society of Anesthesiologists (ASA) released an updated practice advisory in 2010 to help prevent perioperative neuropathies.[14] Ulnar neuropathy is the most common lesion. Although there is no direct evidence that positioning or padding alone can prevent perioperative ulnar neuropathies, the committee has recommended to limit arm abduction in the supine patient to less than 90 degrees at the shoulder with the hand and forearm either supinated or kept in a neutral position. Regardless of the position of the upper extremities, maintaining the head in a relatively midline position can help minimize the risk of stretch injury to the brachial plexus.[18]

With obese patients, caution is advised when placing them in reverse axis on the operating room table. The *base of the operating room table is asymmetrical*, with the torso usually over the foot of the table. However, patients are often positioned with the torso over the open side of the table to improve surgical access or to permit use of equipment such as C-arm x-ray devices. This places the heaviest portion of the body, and therefore the patient's center of gravity, opposite the weighted foot of the table, with substantial leverage. The operating room table can tilt and tip over if sufficient weight is placed away from the base, particularly if extensions are used or the bed is tilted in the Trendelenburg position. Operating room table weight limits should be strictly observed; they differ substantially with regard to normal and reverse positioning.

Lithotomy

The classic *lithotomy position* (Fig. 19-2A to C) is frequently used during gynecologic, rectal, and urologic surgeries. The hips are flexed 80 to 100 degrees from

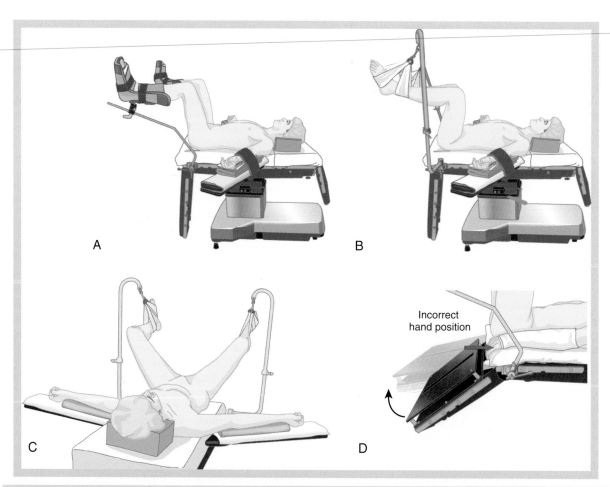

Figure 19-2 A, Lithotomy position. Hips are flexed 80 to 100 degrees with the lower leg parallel to the body. Arms are on armrests away from the hinge point of the foot section. **B,** Lithotomy position with "candy cane" supports. **C,** Lithotomy position with correct position of "candy cane" stirrups away from lateral fibular head. **D,** Improper position of arms in lithotomy position with fingers at risk for compression when the lower section of the bed is raised.

the trunk and the legs are abducted 30 to 45 degrees from the midline. The knees are flexed until the lower legs are parallel to the torso, and the legs are held by supports or stirrups, usually "candy cane," knee crutch, or calf support style. The foot section of the operating room table is lowered. If the arms are on the operating table alongside the patient, the hands and fingers may lie near the open edge of the lowered section of the table. When raising the foot of the table at the end of surgery, strict attention to the position of the hand must be paid to avoid a potentially disastrous crush injury to the fingers (Fig. 19-2D). For this reason, positioning the arms on armrests far from the table hinge point is recommended at all times when patients are in lithotomy position.

Initiation of the lithotomy position requires coordinated positioning of the lower extremities by two assistants to avoid torsion of the lumbar spine. Both legs should be raised together, flexing the hips and knees simultaneously. The lower extremities should be padded to prevent compression against the stirrups. Following the surgery, the patient must also be returned to the supine position in a coordinated manner. As mentioned, the hands should be positioned to prevent entrapment in any moving or articulating sections of the operating room table. The legs should be removed from the holders simultaneously, knees brought together in the midline, and the legs slowly straightened and lowered onto the operating room table.

The lithotomy position may also cause significant physiologic changes. When the legs are elevated, preload increases, causing a transient increase in cardiac output and, to a lesser extent, cerebral venous and intracranial pressure in otherwise healthy patients. In addition, the lithotomy position causes the abdominal viscera to displace the diaphragm cephalad, reducing lung compliance and potentially resulting in a decreased tidal volume. If the patient is obese or a large abdominal mass is present (tumor, gravid uterus), abdominal pressure may increase significantly enough to obstruct venous return to the heart. Lastly, the normal lordotic curvature of the lumbar spine is lost in the lithotomy position, potentially aggravating any previous lower back pain.[19]

In a retrospective review of 198,461 patients undergoing surgery in the lithotomy position from 1957 to 1991, injury to the common peroneal nerve was the most common lower extremity motor neuropathy, representing 78% of nerve injuries. A potential cause of the injury was the compression of the nerve between the lateral head of the fibula and the bar holding the legs. When the "candy cane" stirrups are used, special attention must be paid to avoid compression (Fig. 19-2C). The injury was more common with patients who had low body mass index, recent cigarette smoking, or prolonged duration of surgery.[20] In a prospective review of 991 patients undergoing surgery in the lithotomy position from 1997 to 1998, there were no motor neuropathies in the lower extremity

although paresthesias in the distribution of the obturator, lateral femoral cutaneous, sciatic, and peroneal nerves were found.[21]

Lower extremity compartment syndrome is a rare complication associated with the lithotomy position. It occurs when perfusion to an extremity is inadequate, resulting in ischemia, edema, and extensive rhabdomyolysis from increased tissue pressure within a fascial compartment. In a large retrospective review of 572,498 surgeries, the incidence of compartment syndromes was higher in the lithotomy (1 in 8720) and lateral decubitus (1 in 9711) positions as compared to the supine (1 in 92,441) position. Long surgical procedure time was the only distinguishing characteristic of the surgeries in which patients developed lower extremity compartment syndromes.[22] Compartment pressures increase over time in the lithotomy position. Therefore, it is recommended to periodically lower the legs to the level of the body if surgery extends beyond several hours.[23-25]

Lateral Decubitus

The lateral decubitus position (Fig. 19-3A) is most frequently used for surgery involving the thorax, retroperitoneal structures, or hip. The patient rests upon the nonoperative side and is balanced with anterior and posterior support such as bedding rolls or a deflatable beanbag, as well as a somewhat flexed dependent leg. The arms are usually positioned in front of the patient. The dependent arm rests upon a padded arm board perpendicular to the torso. The nondependent arm is often supported over folded bedding or suspended with an armrest or foam cradle (Fig. 19-3B). If possible, the arm should not be abducted more than 90 degrees. For some high thoracotomies, the nondependent arm may need to be elevated above the shoulder plane for exposure, but vigilance is warranted to prevent neurovascular compromise.

The act of positioning a patient in the lateral decubitus position requires the cooperation of the entire operating room staff to prevent potential injuries. The patient's head must be kept in a neutral position to prevent excessive lateral rotation of the neck and stretch injuries to the brachial plexus. This positioning may require additional head support (Fig. 19-3B). The dependent ear should be checked to avoid folding and undue pressure. The eyes should be securely taped before repositioning if the patient is asleep. The dependent eye must be checked frequently for external compression.

To avoid compression injury to the dependent brachial plexus or vascular compression, an "axillary roll" (generally a liter bag of intravenous fluid) is frequently placed just caudal to the dependent axilla (Fig. 19-3C). This "roll" should never be placed in the axilla. Its purpose is to ensure that the weight of the thorax is borne by the chest wall caudad to the axilla and avoid compression of the axillary contents. Many practitioners do not

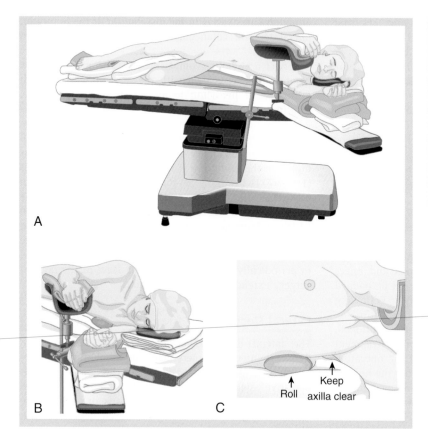

Figure 19-3 **A,** Lateral decubitus position. Note flexion of the lower leg, padding between the legs, and proper support of both arms. **B,** Lateral decubitus position showing placement of arms and head. Note additional padding under headrest to ensure alignment of head with spine. Headrest should be kept away from the dependent eye. **C,** Use of axillary roll in lateral decubitus position. The roll, in this case a bag of intravenous fluid, is placed well away from the axilla to prevent compression of the axillary artery and brachial plexus.

A

B   C

Roll   Keep
        axilla clear

use a roll if the deflatable beanbag is used to cradle the torso; however, the beanbag must not compress the axilla. Regardless of positioning technique, the arterial pulse should be monitored in the dependent arm for early detection of compression to axillary neurovascular structures. Vascular compression and venous engorgement in the dependent arm may alter the pulse oximetry reading; a low saturation reading may reflect compromised circulation. Hypotension measured in the dependent arm may be due to axillary arterial compression; therefore, the ability to measure arterial blood pressure in both arms is helpful. When a kidney rest is used, it must be properly placed under the dependent iliac crest to prevent inadvertent compression of the inferior vena cava. Lastly, a pillow or other padding is generally placed between the knees with the dependent leg flexed to minimize excessive pressure on bony prominences and stretch of low extremity nerves.

The lateral decubitus position can compromise pulmonary function.[26] In a patient who is mechanically ventilated, the combination of the lateral weight of the mediastinum and disproportionate cephalad pressure of abdominal contents on the dependent diaphragm decreases compliance of the dependent lung and favors ventilation of the nondependent lung. At the same time,

pulmonary blood flow to the underventilated, dependent lung increases because of the effect of gravity. Consequently, ventilation-perfusion matching worsens, potentially affecting alveolar ventilation and gas exchange.

The lateral decubitus position is preferred during thoracic surgery and one-lung ventilation. The minute ventilation of the dependent lung is usually increased when the nondependent lung is collapsed. The increase in minute ventilation combined with decreased compliance due to positioning may further exacerbate the airway pressure required to achieve adequate ventilation. Head-down tilt in the lateral position worsens pulmonary function yet further, increasing shunt fraction.[27]

Patients may be flexed while in the lateral position to spread the ribs during thoracotomies or to improve exposure of the retroperitoneum for renal surgeries. The point of flexion, and the kidney rest if raised, should lie under the iliac crest rather than the flank or ribcage to minimize compression of the dependent lung. This position is often accompanied by a component of reverse Trendelenburg positioning, creating the potential for venous pooling in the lower body. For these reasons, use of the flexed, lateral position is discouraged when not actively needed for surgical exposure.

Prone

The *prone* or *ventral decubitus position* (Fig. 19-4A) is used primarily for surgical access to the posterior fossa of the skull, the posterior spine, the buttocks and perirectal area, and the lower extremities. As with the supine position, if the legs are in the same plane with the torso,

hemodynamic reserve is relatively maintained, but if there is any significant lowering of the legs or tilt of the entire table, venous return may be decreased or augmented. Pulmonary function may be superior to the supine or lateral decubitus positions if there is no significant abdominal pressure and the patient is properly positioned.[28,29] The legs should be padded and flexed slightly at the

Figure 19-4 A, Prone position with Wilson frame. Arms are abducted less than 90 degrees whenever possible. Pressure points are padded, and chest and abdomen are supported away from the bed to minimize abdominal pressure and preserve pulmonary compliance. Foam head pillow has cutouts for eyes and nose and a slot to permit the endotracheal tube to exit. Eyes must be checked frequently. **B,** Mirror system for prone position. Bony structures of the head and face are supported, and monitoring of eyes and airway is facilitated with a plastic mirror. **C,** Prone position with horseshoe adapter. Head height is adjusted to position neck in a neutral position. **D,** Prone position, face seen from below. Horseshoe adapter permits superior access to airway and visualization of eyes. Width may be adjusted to ensure proper support by facial bones.

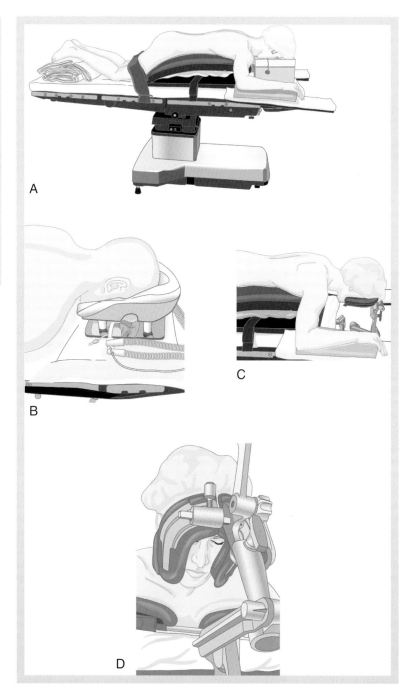

knees and hips. The head may be supported face-down with its weight borne by the bony structures or turned to the side.

Both arms may be positioned to the patient's sides, and tucked in the neutral position as described for the supine patient, or placed next to the patient's head on arm boards—sometimes called the prone "superman" position. Extra padding under the elbow will be needed to prevent compression of the ulnar nerve. Again, the arms should not be abducted greater than 90 degrees to prevent excessive stretching of the brachial plexus, especially in patients with the head turned. Finally, elastic stockings and active compression devices will be needed for the lower extremities to minimize pooling of the blood, especially if there is any flexion of the body.

When general anesthesia is planned, the trachea is first intubated while the patient is still on the stretcher, and all intravascular access is obtained as needed. The endotracheal tube is well secured to prevent dislodgment and loosening of tape due to drainage of saliva when prone. With the coordination of the entire operating room staff, the patient is then turned prone onto the operating room table, keeping the neck in line with the spine during the move. The anesthesia provider is primarily responsible for coordinating the move and for the repositioning of the head. An exception might be cases in which rigid pin fixation is used and the surgeon holds the pin frame. Blood pressure cuffs should be disconnected and arterial and venous lines on the side that rotates furthest to avoid dislodgment, although some prefer to disconnect all lines and monitors before moving. Pulse oximetry can usually be maintained if applied to the "inside" arm, and complete monitoring should be reinstituted as rapidly as possible. Endotracheal tube position and adequate ventilation are reassessed immediately following the move.

Head position is critical. The patient's head may be turned to the side once prone if neck mobility is adequate. However, as in the lateral decubitus position, the dependent eye must be checked frequently for external compression. In addition, in patients with cervical arthritis or cerebrovascular disease, lateral rotation of the neck may compromise carotid or vertebral arterial blood flow or jugular venous drainage. In most cases, the head is kept in a neutral position using a surgical pillow, horseshoe headrest, or Mayfield head pins. A number of commercially available pillows are specially designed for the prone position. Most, including disposable foam versions, support the forehead, malar regions, and the chin with a cutout for the eyes, nose, and mouth. Regardless of whether the pillow or head device is used, the anesthesia provider should consider using a wire-reinforced endotracheal tube when positioning a patient prone to avoid kinking of the tube if it exits the mouth at a right angle to the head-holder. In addition, the face is not always visible, making eye checks more difficult. Mirror systems

are available to facilitate confirmation that the eyes are not impinged, although direct visualization or tactile confirmation of at least the initial appearance is prudent. (Fig. 19-4B). The horseshoe headrest supports only the forehead and malar regions and allows excellent access to the airway; however, it is more rigid and therefore potentially dangerous if the head moves (Fig. 19-4C and D). Mayfield rigid pins support the head without any direct pressure on the face, allow access to the airway, and hold the head firmly in one position that can be finely adjusted for optimal neurosurgical exposure (Fig. 19-5A). Rigid pin fixation is rarely used outside cranial or cervical spine surgeries. When properly applied, the pins will cause significant periosteal stimulation. Patient movement must be prevented when the head is held in rigid pins; skidding out of pins can result in scalp lacerations or cervical spine injury. Because horseshoe and pin headrests attach to adjustable articulating supports, any slippage or failure of this bracketing device may lead to complications if the head suddenly drops. Regardless of the technique employed to support the head, the eyes and the airway must be checked periodically to ensure that the weight is borne only by the bony structures of the face and that there is no pressure on the eyes. Verification of proper position is performed frequently and noted in the anesthetic record. The face should be rechecked if any patient motion occurs during surgery, or if the table is significantly repositioned. The prone position is a risk factor for perioperative visual loss, which is discussed in a separate section later in this chapter.

Because the abdominal wall is easily displaced, external pressure on the abdomen may elevate intra-abdominal pressure in the prone position. This compromises respiration and transmits elevated venous pressures to the abdominal and spine vessels including the epidural veins. During spinal surgery, relatively low venous pressure is desirable to minimize bleeding and facilitate surgical exposure. External pressure on the abdomen may push the diaphragm cephalad, decreasing functional residual capacity and pulmonary compliance and increasing peak airway pressure. Abdominal pressure may also impede venous return through compression of the inferior vena cava. For these reasons, careful attention must be paid to the ability of the abdomen to hang relatively free and to move with respiration. The thorax is generally supported by firm rolls or bolsters placed along each side from the clavicle to the iliac crest. Multiple commercial rolls and bolsters are available including the Wilson frame (Fig. 19-4A), Jackson table, Relton frame, and the Mouradian/Simmons modification of the Relton frame. All devices and special operating room tables for the prone position serve to minimize abdominal compression and maintain normal pulmonary compliance. To prevent tissue injury, pendulous structures (e.g., male genitalia and female breasts) should be clear

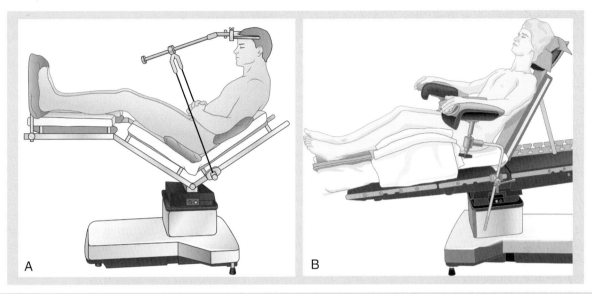

Figure 19-5 **A,** Sitting position with Mayfield head pins. The patient is typically semirecumbent rather than sitting as the legs are kept as high as possible to promote venous return. Arms must be supported to prevent shoulder traction. Note that the head holder support is preferably attached to the back section rather than the thigh section of the table so that the patient's back may be adjusted or lowered emergently without first detaching the head holder. **B,** Sitting position adapted for shoulder surgery. Note the absence of pressure over the ulnar area of the elbow.

of compression; the breasts should be placed medial to the bolsters. The lower portion of each roll or bolster must be placed under its respective iliac crest to prevent pressure injury to the genitalia and the femoral vasculature.[30] The prone position presents special risks for morbidly obese patients whose respiration is already compromised and who may be difficult to reposition quickly. At times, alternate positioning options should be discussed with the surgeon to ensure patient safety.

Sitting

The *sitting position* (Fig. 19-5B), although infrequently used due to the perception of risk from venous and paradoxical air embolism, offers advantages to the surgeon in approaching the posterior cervical spine and the posterior fossa. The main advantages of the sitting position over the prone position for neurosurgical and cervical spine surgeries are excellent surgical exposure, decreased blood in the operative field, and, possibly, reduced perioperative blood loss.[31] The main advantages to the anesthesia provider are superior access to the airway, reduced facial swelling, and improved ventilation, particularly in obese patients. A variation of the sitting position, the "beach chair" position, is increasingly used for shoulder surgeries including arthroscopic procedures. Its attraction to the surgeon is superior access to the shoulder from both the anterior and posterior aspect, and potential for great mobility of the arm at the shoulder joint.

The head may be fixed in pins for neurosurgery, or taped in place with adequate support for other surgeries. Because gravity is pulling the arms caudad, they must be supported to the point of slight elevation of the shoulders to avoid traction on the shoulder muscles and potential stretching of upper extremity neurovascular structures. The knees are usually slightly flexed for balance and to reduce stretching of the sciatic nerve, and the feet are supported and padded.[32]

The hemodynamic effects of placing a supine patient in the sitting position are dramatic. Due to the pooling of blood into the lower body under general anesthesia (see previous discussion), patients are particularly prone to hypotensive episodes. Incremental positioning and the use of intravenous fluids, vasopressors, and appropriate adjustments of anesthetic depth can reduce the degree and duration of hypotension. Elastic stockings and active leg compression devices can help maintain venous return.

Head and neck position has been associated with complications during surgery to the posterior spine or skull in the sitting position. Excessive cervical flexion has a number of adverse consequences. It can impede both arterial and venous blood flow causing hypoperfusion or venous congestion of the brain. It may impede normal respiratory excursion. Excessive flexion can also obstruct the endotracheal tube and place significant pressure on the tongue, leading to macroglossia. In general, maintaining at least two fingers' distance between the mandible and the sternum is recommended for a normal-sized adult,

III

and patients should not be positioned at the extreme of their range of motion.[33] Extra caution with neck flexion is advised if transesophageal echocardiography (TEE) is used for air embolism monitoring, as the esophageal probe lies between the flexed spine and the airway and endotracheal tube, adding potential for compression of laryngeal structures and the tongue.

Due to the elevation of the surgical field above the heart and the inability of the dural venous sinuses to collapse because of their bony attachments, the risk of venous air embolism is a constant concern. Arrhythmia, desaturation, pulmonary hypertension, circulatory compromise, or cardiac arrest may occur if sufficient quantities are entrained. If the foramen ovale is patent, even small amounts of venous air may result in a stroke or myocardial infarction due to paradoxical embolism. TEE has demonstrated some degree of venous air in a large majority of patients studied during neurosurgery in the sitting position, up to 100%.[34,35] Because of the risk of paradoxical embolus, screening contrast echocardiography to investigate the patency of the interatrial septum is often performed prior to sitting position intracranial or cervical spine surgery. However, septal patency may not always be detected. Adequate hydration and early detection of entrained air with the use of TEE or precordial Doppler ultrasound may decrease the incidence and severity of venous air embolism.[34]

PERIPHERAL NERVE INJURY

Peripheral nerve injury remains a serious perioperative complication and a significant source of professional liability despite its infrequent incidence of approximately 0.11% of 81,000 anesthetic procedures reviewed from 1987 to 1993[36] and 0.03% of 380,000 anesthetic procedures performed from 1997 to 2007.[37] Injuries occur when peripheral nerves are subjected to compression, stretch, ischemia, metabolic derangement, and direct trauma/laceration during surgery.[38] Because sensation is blocked by unconsciousness or regional anesthesia, early warning symptoms of pain with normal spontaneous repositioning are absent. In 1984 the ASA developed a Closed Claims Project to evaluate adverse anesthetic outcomes from the closed claims files of 35 U.S. liability insurance companies. Since the initial report in 1990, the incidence of nerve injury has remained essentially constant, representing 18% of all claims during 1990 to 1994, second only to death (22%).[1,3] Among the total 670 claims filed, ulnar neuropathy remained the most frequent site of injury (28%), followed by the brachial plexus (20%), lumbosacral nerve root (16%), and spinal cord (13%) (Table 19-1). However, the distribution of nerve injuries has changed significantly over time. Ulnar neuropathy decreased from 37% in 1980 to 1984 to 17% in the 1990s, and spinal cord

Table 19-1 Nerve Injury Claims in the American Society of Anesthesiologists Closed Claims Project Database

Nerve	Distribution of Claims for Nerve Injury			
	Number of Claims in Current Database (N = 4183)	Percentage of Total (N = 670)	Number of Claims since 1990 Report	Percentage of Total since 1990 (N = 445)
Ulnar	190	28	113	25
Brachial plexus	137	20	83	19
Lumbosacral nerve root	105	16	67	15
Spinal cord	84	13	73	16
Sciatic*	34	5	23	5
Median	28	4	19	4
Radial	18	3	13	3
Femoral	15	2	9	2
Other single nerves	43	6	35	8
Multiple nerves	16	2	10	2
Total	**670**	**100**	**445**	**100**

*Includes peroneal nerve.
From Cheney FW, Domino KB, Caplan RA, Posner KL. Nerve injury associated with anesthesia: A closed claims analysis. Anesthesiology 1999; 90(4):1062-1069.

Table 19-2 Most Common Nerve Injuries in American Society of Anesthesiologists Closed Claims Project Database after 1990[1,2]

Nerve Injury	Recommendations for Prevention
Ulnar nerve (25%)	▪ Avoid excessive pressure on the postcondylar groove of the humerus. ▪ Keep the hand and forearm either supinated or in a neutral position.
Brachial plexus (19%)	▪ Avoid the use of shoulder braces in patients in the Trendelenburg position (use nonsliding mattresses). ▪ Avoid excessive lateral rotation of the head either in the supine or prone position. ▪ Limit abduction of the arm to less than 90 degrees in the supine position. ▪ Avoid the placement of high "axillary" roll in the decubitus position—keep the roll out of the axilla. ▪ Use ultrasound imaging to find the internal jugular vein for central line placement.
Spinal cord (16%) and lumbosacral nerve root (15%)	▪ Be aware that the fraction of spinal cord injuries is increasing, probably in relation to use of epidural catheters for pain management. ▪ Follow current guidelines for regional anesthesia in anticoagulated patients.[70]
Sciatic and peroneal (5%) nerves	▪ Minimize time of surgery in the lithotomy position. ▪ Use two assistants to coordinate the simultaneous movement of both legs to and from the lithotomy position. ▪ Avoid excessive flexion of the hips, extension of the knees, or torsion of the lumbar spine. ▪ Avoid excessive pressure on peroneal nerve at the fibular head.
Median (4%) and radial (3%) nerves	▪ Be aware that 25% of injuries to the median and radial nerves were associated with axillary block, and 25% of injuries were associated with traumatic insertion or infiltration of an intravenous line.

injury increased from 8% in 1980 to 1984 to 27% in the 1990s. Spinal cord injury and lumbosacral nerve root neuropathy were predominantly associated with regional anesthesia. Epidural hematoma and chemical injury represented 29% of the known mechanisms of injury among the claims filed. The injuries were probably related to the use of neuraxial block in patients who are receiving anticoagulation drugs and the increased usage of blocks for chronic pain management (Table 19-2).[1,39,40]

With the exception of spinal cord injury, the mechanism of nerve injury remains largely unknown. Most injuries, particularly injuries to nerves of the upper extremity such as the ulnar nerve and brachial plexus, occurred in the presence of adequate positioning and padding. Because of the significant morbidity rate associated with peripheral nerve injury, in 2000 the ASA published a practice advisory for the prevention of peripheral neuropathies.[14] However, the advisory was not based on scientific evidence but the consensus of a consultant expert group. Only 6 out of 509 positioning studies reviewed "...exhibited sufficiently acceptable methods and analyses that provided a clear indication of the relationships between interventions and outcomes of interest"[14] (See Table 19-3).

Because of the paucity of clear data on the causes and therefore the prevention of peripheral injuries, individual practices vary with regard to specific padding and positional details. Prolonged duration is a risk factor. Good sense would avoid positions that permit stretching of the nerves and pressure to anatomic locations known to carry nerves prone to injury, such as the ulnar cubital tunnel and the peroneal nerve coursing over the fibular head. Whenever possible, the patient's position should appear as natural as possible. Padding and support should distribute weight over as wide an area as possible. Currently, no padding material has been shown to be superior. The presence of anesthesia and muscle relaxation increases the danger of malposition-induced injury.

In a retrospective study of 1000 consecutive spine surgeries that used somatosensory evoked potential (SSEP) monitoring, five arm positions were compared with regard to SSEP changes in the upper extremities. A modification of arm position reversed 92% of upper extremity SSEP changes. The incidence of position-related upper extremity SSEP changes was significantly higher in the prone "superman" (7%) and lateral decubitus (7.5%) positions compared with the supine arms out, supine arms tucked, and prone arms tucked positions (1.8% to 3.2%). Reversible SSEP changes were not associated with postoperative deficits.[41]

Ulnar Nerve

The etiology of perioperative ulnar neuropathy is complex and incompletely understood. The ulnar nerve lies in a superficial position at the elbow. Although the incidence is low, the morbidity associated with ulnar neuropathy can be severe. In a prospective study among

Table 19-3 An Updated Report by the American Society of Anesthesiologists Task Force on Prevention of Perioperative Peripheral Neuropathies[14]

I. Preoperative History and Physical Assessment

- When judged appropriate, it is helpful to ascertain that patients can comfortably tolerate the anticipated operative position.
- Body habitus, preexisting neurologic symptoms, diabetes mellitus, peripheral vascular disease, alcohol dependency, arthritis, and gender (e.g., male gender and its association with ulnar neuropathy) are important elements of a preoperative history.

II. Positioning Strategies for the Upper Extremities

Arm abduction in supine patients should be limited to 90°. Patients who are positioned prone may comfortably tolerate arm abduction greater than 90°.

- *Supine Patient with Arm on an Armboard:* The upper extremity should be positioned to decrease pressure on the postcondylar groove of the humerus (ulnar groove). Either supination or the neutral forearm positions facilitates this action.
- *Supine Patient with Arms Tucked at Side:* The forearm should be in a neutral position. Flexion of the elbow may increase the risk of ulnar neuropathy, but there is no consensus on an acceptable degree of flexion during the perioperative period. Prolonged pressure on the radial nerve in the spiral groove of the humerus should be avoided. Extension of the elbow beyond the range that is comfortable during the preoperative assessment may stretch the median nerve. Periodic perioperative assessments may ensure maintenance of the desired position.

III. Specific Positioning Strategies for the Lower Extremities

- *Stretching of the Hamstring Muscle Group:* Positions that stretch the hamstring muscle group beyond the range that is comfortable during the preoperative assessment may stretch the sciatic nerve.
- *Limiting Hip Flexion:* Since the sciatic nerve or its branches cross both the hip and the knee joints, extension and flexion of these joints, respectively, should be considered when determining the degree of hip flexion. Neither extension nor flexion of the hip increases the risk of femoral neuropathy. Prolonged pressure on the peroneal nerve at the fibular head should be avoided.

IV. Protective Padding

- *Padded Armboards:* Padded armboards may decrease the risk of upper extremity neuropathy.
- *Chest Rolls:* The use of chest rolls in the laterally positioned patient may decrease the risk of upper extremity neuropathy.
- *Padding at the Elbow:* Padding at the elbow may decrease the risk of upper extremity neuropathy.
- *Padding to Protect the Peroneal (Fibular) Nerve:* The use of specific padding to prevent pressure of a hard surface against the peroneal nerve at the fibular head may decrease the risk of peroneal neuropathy.
- *Complications from the Use of Padding:* The inappropriate use of padding (*e.g.*, padding too tight) may increase the risk of perioperative neuropathy.

V. Equipment:
The use of properly functioning automated blood pressure cuffs on the arm (i.e., placed above the antecubital fossa) does not change the risk of upper extremity neuropathy. The use of shoulder braces in a steep head-down position may increase the risk of perioperative neuropathies.

VI. Postoperative Assessment:
A simple postoperative assessment of extremity nerve function may lead to early recognition of peripheral neuropathies.

VII. Documentation:
Documentation of specific perioperative positioning actions may be useful for continuous improvement processes, and may result in improvements by helping practitioners focus attention on relevant aspects of patient positioning, and providing information on positioning strategies that eventually leads to improvements in patient care.

American Society of Anesthesiologists Task Force on Prevention of Perioperative Peripheral Neuropathies: Practice advisory for the prevention of perioperative peripheral neuropathies: An updated report by the American Society of Anesthesiologists Task Force on Prevention of Perioperative Peripheral Neuropathies, Anesthesiology, in Press, 2011.

1502 patients undergoing noncardiac surgery, 7 patients developed perioperative ulnar neuropathy, of which 3 patients had residual symptoms after 2 years.[42] The neuropathy, if permanent, results in the inability to abduct or oppose the fifth finger, diminished sensation in the fourth and fifth fingers, and eventual atrophy of the intrinsic muscle of the hands creating a "claw-like" hand.

Previously, the injury was thought to be associated with hyperflexion of the elbow and compression by the operating room table of the nerve at the condylar groove and the cubital tunnel against the posterior aspect of the medial epicondyle of the humerus. Current consensus is that the etiology of ulnar nerve palsy is multifactorial and not always preventable. In a large retrospective review of perioperative ulnar neuropathy lasting longer than 3 months, the onset of symptoms occurred more than 24 hours postoperatively in 57% of patients, 70% were male, and 9% experienced bilateral symptoms. Very thin or obese patients were at increased risk, as were those with prolonged postoperative bed rest. There was no association with intraoperative patient position or anesthetic technique.[43] The Closed Claims Project also demonstrated that perioperative ulnar neuropathy occurred predominately in males, an older population, and with a delayed onset (median of 3 days).[1] In addition, although most ulnar damage claims were associated with general anesthesia, payment was also made for claims where the patient had been awake or sedated during regional anesthesia involving the lower extremity. Interestingly, in a prospective study of medical patients who did not undergo surgical procedures, 2 of 986 patients developed ulnar neuropathy.[44] The large predominance of ulnar injury in males may possibly be explained by anatomic differences. Males have a more developed and thickened flexor retinaculum with less protective adipose tissue and a larger (1.5×) tubercle of the coronoid process that can predispose to nerve compression in the cubital tunnel.[45,46] Other risk factors including diabetes mellitus, vitamin deficiency, alcoholism, cigarette smoking, and cancer, will need further studies to be substantiated. In the ASA Closed Claims Project, only 9% of ulnar injury claims had an explicit mechanism of injury, and in 27% of claims, the padding of the elbows were explicitly stated.[1] Postoperative ulnar nerve palsy can occur without any apparent cause, even when padding and positioning of the patient's arm were done carefully and documented in the anesthetic record.[16]

Brachial Plexus

The brachial plexus is susceptible to injury from stretching or compression due to its long superficial course in the axilla between two points of fixation, the vertebra and the axillary fascia, in association with the mobile clavicle and humerus. The patient often complains of sensory deficit in the distribution of the ulnar nerve. Injury is most commonly associated with arm abduction greater than 90 degrees, lateral rotation of the head, asymmetrical retraction of the sternum for internal mammary artery dissection during cardiac surgery, and direct trauma. To avoid brachial plexus injury, patients should ideally be positioned with the head midline, arms kept at the sides, the elbow mildly flexed, and the forearm supinated.

In cardiac surgery patients requiring median sternotomy brachial plexus injury has been specifically associated with the C8-T1 nerve roots. In a prospective study in which the incidence of injury was 4.9%, the authors found that 73% of the injuries occurred on the same side as the internal jugular vein cannulation.[47] Among noncardiac surgery patients, the incidence is reported to be 0.02%.[48] Interestingly, in the ASA Closed Claims Project, 16% of brachial plexus injury occurred during a regional block, particularly the axillary block.[1]

Brachial plexus injury can occur with direct compression, particularly with the use of shoulder braces in patients undergoing surgery in the Trendelenburg position. The nerves are vulnerable to compression as they pass between the clavicle and the first rib. Medial placement of the braces can compress the proximal roots, and lateral placement of the braces can stretch the plexus by displacing the shoulders. The patient with injury often complains of painless motor deficit in the distribution of the radial and median nerves. In the ASA Closed Claims Project, 10% of brachial plexus injuries were directly attributed to patient positioning. Of those, half involved the use of shoulder braces in patients in the Trendelenburg position.[1] Consequently, nonsliding mattresses should be used in place of shoulder braces.

Other Upper Extremity Nerves

Although quite rare, the radial nerve can be injured from direct pressure as it traverses the spiral groove of the humerus in the lower third of the arm. The injury often manifests as a wrist drop with an inability to abduct the thumb or extend the metacarpophalangeal joints. Isolated median nerve injury most often occurs during the insertion of an intravenous needle into the antecubital fossa in an anesthetized patient where the nerve is adjacent to the medial cubital and basilic veins. Patients with this injury are unable to oppose the first and fifth digits and have decreased sensation over the palmar surface of the lateral ½. Surprisingly, in an evaluation of the ASA Closed Claims Project database from 1970 to 2001, Liau found that peripheral intravenous and arterial line insertion accounted for 2.1% of all claims filed, particularly among patients undergoing cardiac surgery where the arms are tucked and the lines are not visible for inspection.[49] Nerve injury accounted for 17% of intravenous line complications second only to skin slough or necrosis (28%) and swelling, inflammation, and infection (17%).

Lower Extremity Nerves

Injuries to the sciatic and common peroneal nerves occur most often in the lithotomy position. Because of its fixation between the sciatic notch and the neck of the fibula, the sciatic nerve can be stretched with external rotation of the leg. Hyperflexion of the hips or extension of the knees can also aggravate nerve stretch in this position. The common peroneal nerve, a branch of the sciatic, can be damaged from the compression of the nerve between the head of the fibula and the frame of the leg support. Most often, patients who suffer injury will complain of a foot drop and the inability to extend the toes in a dorsal direction or evert the foot.

In a prospective study of 991 patients undergoing surgery under general anesthesia in the lithotomy position, the incidence of lower extremity neuropathies was 1.5%, with injuries to the sciatic and peroneal nerves representing 40% of the cases. Interestingly, symptoms were predominantly paresthesia with onset within 4 hours of surgery and resolution generally within 6 months. No motor deficits were noted, but in a previous retrospective study, the same authors found the incidence of severe motor disability in patients undergoing surgery in the lithotomy position to be 1 in 3608.[20,21]

Injury to the femoral or obturator nerves generally occurs during lower abdominal surgical procedures with excessive retraction. The obturator nerve can also be injured during a difficult forceps delivery or by excessive flexion of the thigh to the groin. A femoral neuropathy will present with decreased flexion of the hip, decreased extension of the knee, or a loss of sensation over the superior aspect of the thigh and medial/anteromedial side of the leg. An obturator neuropathy will present with inability to adduct the leg and decreased sensation over the medial thigh.

PERIOPERATIVE EYE INJURY AND VISUAL LOSS

Although quite rare, with an incidence of 0.056% in one retrospective review,[50] perioperative eye injuries are a source of significant morbidity and liability. In the ASA Closed Claims Project Database, eye complications accounted for 3% of all claims and were associated with greater monetary settlements as compared to nonocular injuries.[1]

Corneal abrasion continues to be the most common type of perioperative eye injury and is associated with direct trauma to the cornea from facemasks, surgical drapes, or other foreign objects. Corneal abrasion can also be associated with decreased basal tear production or swelling of the dependent eye in patients in the prone position. Patients complain of pain associated with a foreign body sensation in the eye upon awakening from surgery. This can also occur from a dried section of cornea. Symptoms are generally transient, and treatment comprises supportive care and antibiotic ointment to prevent bacterial infection. In a prospective study of 671 patients undergoing nonocular surgery, 4.2% of patients reported a new onset of blurred vision lasting at least 3 days after surgery. For most patients, the symptoms resolved within 2 months without complication. However, 1% required visits to eye-care providers.[51] Precautionary measures to reduce the incidence of corneal abrasion include early and careful taping of the eyelids following induction of anesthesia, care regarding dangling objects when leaning over patients, and close observation as patients awaken. Before they are completely awake, patients often try to rub their eye or nose with pulse oximeter probes, arm boards, and intravenous lines attached, inadvertently endangering their eyes.

Postoperative visual loss is a devastating complication that has been associated with specific surgeries and patient risk factors. Risk varies with type of surgery. The incidence varies from a range of 1/60,965 to 1/125,234 for patients undergoing noncardiac, nonocular surgeries[50,52] to 0.06% to 0.113% for patients undergoing cardiac surgery with cardiopulmonary bypass,[53,54] and

0.09% for patients undergoing spine surgery in the prone position.[55] Ischemic optic neuropathy (ION) and to a lesser extent central retinal arterial occlusion from direct retinal pressure are the conditions most cited as potential causes. Perioperative factors associated with an increased risk of ION include prolonged hypotension, long duration of surgery especially in the prone position, large blood loss, large crystalloid use, anemia or hemodilution, and increased intraocular or venous pressure from the prone position.[56,57] Intraocular pressure increases in the dependent eye in the lateral decubitus position as well.[58] Patient risk factors associated with ION include hypertension, diabetes, atherosclerosis, morbid obesity, and tobacco use. However, with the exception of obvious external compression of the eyes, the cause of perioperative visual loss appears to be multifactorial in nature with no consistent underlying mechanism.

In 1999, the ASA Committee on Professional Liability established the ASA Postoperative Visual Loss (POVL) Registry to better understand the complication. By 2005, 131 cases were reported to the registry; 73% of these reported cases involved patients undergoing spine surgeries and 9% involved cardiac surgery.[59-61] Of 93 patients with postoperative visual loss following prone spine surgery, Lee and associates reported that 89% were diagnosed with ION, predominantly posterior, and 11% with central retinal artery occlusion (CRAO). In patients who were diagnosed with ION, 66% had documented bilateral involvement, of which 42% had eventual improvement in vision although often clinically insignificant. Compared to CRAO, patients with ION had significantly higher anesthetic duration (9.8 ± 3.1 vs. 6.5 ± 2.2 hours), estimated blood loss (median 2 vs. 0.75 L), and crystalloid infusion (9.7 ± 4.7 vs. 4.6 ± 1.7 L). Patients with ION were also relatively healthy (64% ASA I and II) and 72% were male.[61] In 2006, the ASA issued a practice advisory for perioperative visual loss associated with spine surgery. Unfortunately, no definite recommendations were made concerning the issue of induced hypotension, use of vasopressors, or transfusion threshold due to the multifactorial nature and the low incidence of the injury. Despite a lack of direct evidence, several suggestions were made for high-risk patients undergoing complex spine surgery:[62]

1. Discuss the possibility of staging the spine surgery in consultation with the surgeon.
2. Avoid excessive increase in intraocular pressure from head position below the body as well as external compression of the abdomen or chest. Keep the head neutral.
3. Use colloids along with crystalloids to maintain intravascular volume. Consider placement of a central venous line for monitoring preload.
4. For patients who are anticipated preoperatively to undergo prolonged procedures, to have substantial blood loss, or both, consider informing the patients of a small, unpredictable risk of perioperative visual loss.

5. Additional recommendations include careful attention to factors related to oxygen delivery including oxygen tension, maintenance of adequate intravascular volume and cardiac output, and frequent eye checks, which may help prevent central retinal artery occlusion, although the required frequency has not been established.[63]

Until the causative factors of this devastating type of injury are better defined, it is likely that debate regarding patient management strategies will continue. With regard to patient positioning, the anesthesiologist should be aware that intraocular pressures are elevated in the dependent eye in the lateral position and both eyes in the prone position in the absence of any external pressure. It is sensible to document eye checks frequently, and to limit time in the prone position whenever possible. Fortunately, in a retrospective review of 5.6 million patients in the Nationwide Inpatient Sample, the largest United States all-payer hospital inpatient care database, the rate of POVL decreased from 1996 to 2005,[64] perhaps due to an increase in awareness of the complication.

EVALUATION AND TREATMENT OF PERIOPERATIVE NEUROPATHIES

When a nerve injury becomes apparent postoperatively, it is essential to perform and document a directed physical examination to correlate the extent of sensory or motor deficits with the preoperative examination as well as any intraoperative events. It is prudent to seek neurologic consultation to help define the neurogenic basis, localize the site of the lesion, and determine the severity of injury for guiding prognostication.[65,66] With proper diagnosis and management, most injuries resolve, but months to years may be required.[38]

For motor neuropathy, an electromyogram (EMG) can be performed to determine the exact location of the injury. An EMG examination involves recording the electrical activity of muscle from a needle electrode inserted within it. If present, abnormalities may point to the affected component within the motor unit, which consists of the anterior horn cell, its axon and neuromuscular junctions, and the muscle fibers that it innervates. From a medicolegal standpoint, the presence of abnormal spontaneous activity in the acute setting may suggest the nerve injury was present preoperatively. In addition, depending on the pattern of abnormalities, an EMG study may distinguish between radiculopathies, plexopathies, and neuropathies.

Nerve conduction studies, which assess both motor and sensory nerves, may be more useful to evaluate potential peripheral nerve injuries such as ulnar neuropathy. Nerve conduction studies may reveal a subclinical polyneuropathy that made the individual nerves more susceptible to injury and also may help distinguish between axon loss

and demyelination, which has significant implications regarding expected clinical course and overall prognosis.

Most sensory neuropathies are generally transient and require only reassurance to the patient with follow-up, whereas most motor neuropathies include demyelination of peripheral fibers of a nerve trunk (neurapraxia) and generally take 4 to 6 weeks for recovery. Injury to the axon within an intact nerve sheath (axonotmesis) or complete nerve disruption (neurotmesis) can cause severe pain and disability. When reversible, recovery often takes 3 to 12 months. Interim physical therapy is recommended to prevent contractures and muscle atrophy.[65,66]

If a new sensory or motor deficit is found postoperatively, electrophysiologic evaluation by a neurologist within the first week may provide useful information concerning the characteristic and temporal pattern of the injury. However, another examination after 4 weeks when enough time has elapsed for the electrophysiologic changes to evolve will provide more definitive information about the site, nature, and severity of the nerve injury. Regardless, electrophysiologic testing must be interpreted within the clinical content for which it was obtained. No single test can define the etiology of injury.

ANESTHESIA OUTSIDE THE OPERATING ROOM

Anesthesia care providers are increasingly involved with procedures performed in remote locations such as for gastrointestinal endoscopy, cardiac catheterization, interventional radiology, neuroradiology, magnetic resonance imaging/computed tomography, and office-based procedures.[67] Anesthesia care is sometimes requested specifically because the patient is not expected to tolerate the position required for the procedure due to co-morbidities such as congestive heart failure, pulmonary disease, or morbid obesity. Additionally, positions that are generally safe for patients who are awake may pose serious risks to those under anesthesia.

Vigilance is particularly important outside the operating room to maintain patient safety because of the less familiar environment, relative lack of positioning equipment, and variability in staff and nursing training with regard to patient positioning. For example, many locations do not routinely have safety straps or arm supports available. Diagnostic tables are much less versatile than operating room tables and usually lack the ability to initiate the Trendelenburg position to rapidly augment venous return and cardiac output. Also, in some settings, such as magnetic resonance imaging, radiation therapy, and computed tomography, the anesthesia provider is not continuously in direct proximity to the patient.

Currently, the number of claims in the ASA Closed Claims Project database for injury during anesthesia care in remote locations is very small (87 vs. 3287 claims for

III

operating room procedures). Compared to operating room claims, remote location claims typically involved an older and sicker patient population undergoing monitored anesthesia care. More than a third of claims involved emergent procedures; 21% of all claims did not require any anesthesia (emergent endotracheal intubation or resuscitation). Not surprisingly, 54% of all claims were associated with death (vs. 29% for operating room claims) with a more frequent incidence of respiratory events, suggesting oversedation and inadequate oxygenation/ventilation. Remote location claims were also more often judged as being preventable with better monitoring (32% vs. 8% for operating room claims).[68,69] In such an environment, where practice patterns have often evolved in the context of nonanesthetized patients, the anesthesia provider will be primarily responsible for verifying the safety of each patient's position and for implementing guidelines for patients under anesthesia.

CONCLUSION

The positioning of patients under anesthesia care is a major responsibility requiring great attention to detail and constant vigilance. Rapid positioning and optimal surgical exposure are virtues that may be appreciated instantly; however, the potential for lasting harm to patients from improper positioning and physiologic compromise must guide our actions. Each position has significant physiologic effects on ventilation and circulation. In addition, despite increased awareness, position-related complications including peripheral nerve injuries continue to remain a significant source of patient morbidity. The entire operative team, including anesthesia providers, must work together when positioning each patient to ensure the patient's comfort and safety in addition to the desired surgical exposure. Ideally, the final position should appear natural: a position that the patient would comfortably tolerate if awake and not sedated for the anticipated duration of the procedure.

QUESTIONS OF THE DAY

1. What is the impact of the Trendelenburg position on cardiac, pulmonary, and upper airway physiology and anatomy?

2. What are the potential adverse effects of excessive abdominal pressure in a patient undergoing surgery in the prone position? How can this be prevented?

3. What are the risk factors for postoperative ulnar nerve palsy? Which ones are preventable?

4. What are the most common causes of postoperative visual loss in a patient undergoing spine surgery in the prone position?

REFERENCES

1. Cheney FW, Domino KB, Caplan RA, et al: Nerve injury associated with anesthesia: A closed claims analysis, *Anesthesiology* 90(4):1062–1069, 1999.

2. Cheney FW: The American Society of Anesthesiologists Closed Claims Project: What have we learned, how has it affected practice, and how will it affect practice in the future? *Anesthesiology* 91(2):552–556, 1999.

3. O'Brien TJ, Ebert TJ: Physiologic changes associated with the supine position. In Martin JT, Warner MA, editors: *Positioning in Anesthesia and Surgery*, ed 3, Philadelphia, 1997, WB Saunders.

4. Luecke T, Pelosi P: Clinical review: Positive end-expiratory pressure and cardiac output, *Crit Care* 9:607–621, 2005.

5. Froese AB: Gravity, the belly, and the diaphragm: You can't ignore physics, *Anesthesiology* 104:193–196, 2006.

6. Hakim TS, Lisbona R, Dean GW: Gravity-independent inequality in pulmonary blood flow in humans, *J Appl Physiol* 63:1114–1121, 1987.

7. Burrowes KS, Tawhai MH: Computational predictions of pulmonary blood flow gradients: Gravity versus structure, *Respir Physiol Neurobiol* 154:515–523, 2006.

8. Galvin I, Drummond GB, Nirmalan M: Distribution of blood flow and ventilation in the lung: Gravity is not the only factor, *Br J Anaesth* 98:420–428, 2007.

9. Girard TD, Bernard GR: Mechanical ventilation in ARDS: A state-of-the-art review, *Chest* 131:921–929, 2007.

10. Pelosi P, Croci M, Calappi E, et al: The prone positioning during general anesthesia minimally affects respiratory mechanics while improving functional residual capacity and increasing oxygen tension, *Anesth Analg* 80:955–960, 1995.

11. Soro M, Garcia-Perez ML, Belda FJ, et al: Effects of prone position on alveolar dead space and gas exchange during general anaesthesia in surgery of long duration, *Eur J Anaesthesiol* 24:431–437, 2007.

12. Pelosi P, Croci M, Calappi E, et al: Prone positioning improves pulmonary function in obese patients during general anesthesia, *Anesth Analg* 83:578–583, 1996.

13. von Ungern-Sternberg BS, Hammer J, Frei FJ, et al: Prone equals prone? Impact of positioning techniques on respiratory function in anesthetized and paralyzed healthy children, *Intensive Care Med* 33:1771–1777, 2007.

14. American Society of Anesthesiologists Task Force on Prevention of Perioperative Peripheral Neuropathies: Practice advisory for the prevention of perioperative peripheral neuropathies: An updated report by the American Society of Anesthesiologists Task Force on Prevention of Perioperative Peripheral Neuropathies, *Anesthesiology,* in Press, 2011.

15. Prielipp RC, Morell RC, Walker FO, et al: Ulnar nerve pressure: influence of arm position and relationship to somatosensory evoked potentials, *Anesthesiology* 91:345–354, 1999.

16. Stewart JD, Shantz SH: Perioperative ulnar neuropathies: A medicolegal review, *Can J Neurol Sci* 30:15–19, 2003.

17. Warner M: Supine positions. In Martin JT, Warner MA, editors: *Positioning in Anesthesia and Surgery*, ed 3, Philadelphia, 1997, WB Saunders.

18. Coppieters MW, Van de Velde M, Stappaerts KH: Positioning in anesthesiology: Toward a better

understanding of stretch-induced perioperative neuropathies, *Anesthesiology* 97:75–81, 2002.

19. Martin JT: Lithotomy. In Martin JT, Warner MA, editors: *Positioning in Anesthesia and Surgery*, ed 3, Philadelphia, 1997, WB Saunders.

20. Warner MA, Martin JT, Schroeder DR, et al: Lower-extremity motor neuropathy associated with surgery performed on patients in a lithotomy position, *Anesthesiology* 81:6–12, 1994.

21. Warner MA, Warner DO, Harper CM, et al: Lower extremity neuropathies associated with lithotomy positions, *Anesthesiology* 93:938–942, 2000.

22. Warner ME, LaMaster LM, Thoeming AK, et al: Compartment syndrome in surgical patients, *Anesthesiology* 94:705–708, 2001.

23. Chase J, Harford F, Pinzur MS, et al: Intraoperative lower extremity compartment pressures in lithotomy-positioned patients, *Dis Colon Rectum* 43:678–680, 2000.

24. Wassenaar EB, van den Brand JG, van der Werken C: Compartment syndrome of the lower leg after surgery in the modified lithotomy position: Report of seven cases, *Dis Colon Rectum* 49:1449–1453, 2006.

25. Turnbull D, Farid A, Hutchinson S, et al: Calf compartment pressures in the Lloyd-Davies position: A cause for concern? *Anaesthesia* 57:905–908, 2002.

26. Dunn PF: Physiology of the lateral decubitus position and one-lung ventilation, *Int Anesthesiol Clin* 38:25–53, 2000.

27. Choi YS, Bang SO, Shim JK, et al: Effects of head-down tilt on intrapulmonary shunt fraction and oxygenation during one-lung ventilation in the lateral decubitus position, *J Thorac Cardiovasc Surg* 134:613–618, 2007.

28. Douglas WW, Rehder K, Beynen FM, et al: Improved oxygenation in patients with acute respiratory failure: The prone position, *Am Rev Respir Dis* 115:559–566, 1977.

29. Lumb AB, Nunn JF: Respiratory function and ribcage contribution to ventilation in body positions commonly used during anesthesia, *Anesth Analg* 73:422–426, 1991.

30. Martin JT: The ventral decubitus (prone) positions. In Martin JT, Warner MA, editors: *Positioning in Anesthesia and Surgery*, ed 3, Philadelphia, 1997, WB Saunders.

31. Black S, Ockert DB, Oliver WC Jr, et al: Outcome following posterior fossa craniectomy in patients in the sitting or horizontal positions, *Anesthesiology* 69:49–56, 1988.

32. Newberg Milde L: The head-elevated position. In Martin JT, Warner MA, editors: *Positioning in Anesthesia and Surgery*, ed 3, Philadelphia, 1997, WB Saunders.

33. Warner M: Positioning the head and neck. In Martin JT, Warner MA, editors: *Positioning in Anesthesia and Surgery*, ed 3, Philadelphia, 1997, WB Saunders.

34. Mammoto T, Hayashi Y, Ohnishi Y, et al: Incidence of venous and paradoxical air embolism in neurosurgical patients in the sitting position: Detection by transesophageal echocardiography, *Acta Anaesthesiol Scand* 42:643–647, 1998.

35. Papadopoulos G, Kuhly P, Brock M, et al: Venous and paradoxical air embolism in the sitting position. A prospective study with transoesophageal echocardiography, *Acta Neurochir (Wien)* 126:140–143, 1994.

36. Blitt C, Kaufer-Bratt C, Ashby J, et al: QA program reveals safety issues, promotes development of guidelines, *Anesth Patient Safety Found Newsl* 9:17, 1994.

37. Welch MB, Brummett CM, Welch TD, et al: Perioperative peripheral nerve injuries: A retrospective study of 380,680 cases during a 10-year period at a single institution, *Anesthesiology* 111:490–497, 2009.

38. Winfree CJ, Kline DG: Intraoperative positioning nerve injuries, *Surg Neurol* 63:5–18, 2005.

39. Lee LA, Posner KL, Domino KB, et al: Injuries associated with regional anesthesia in the 1980s and 1990s: A closed claims analysis, *Anesthesiology* 101:143–152, 2004.

40. Fitzgibbon DR, Posner KL, Domino KB, et al: Chronic pain management: American Society of Anesthesiologists Closed Claims Project, *Anesthesiology* 100:98–105, 2004.

41. Kamel IR, Drum ET, Koch SA, et al: The use of somatosensory evoked potentials to determine the relationship between patient positioning and impending upper extremity nerve injury during spine surgery: A retrospective analysis, *Anesth Analg* 102:1538–1542, 2006.

42. Warner MA, Warner DO, Matsumoto JY, et al: Ulnar neuropathy in surgical patients, *Anesthesiology* 90:54–59, 1999.

43. Warner MA, Warner ME, Martin JT: Ulnar neuropathy. Incidence, outcome, and risk factors in sedated or anesthetized patients, *Anesthesiology* 81:1332–1340, 1994.

44. Warner MA, Warner DO, Harper CM, et al: Ulnar neuropathy in medical patients, *Anesthesiology* 92:613–615, 2000.

45. Contreras MG, Warner MA, Charboneau WJ, et al: Anatomy of the ulnar nerve at the elbow: Potential relationship of acute ulnar neuropathy to gender differences, *Clin Anat* 11:372–378, 1998.

46. Morell RC, Prielipp RC, Harwood TN, et al: Men are more susceptible than women to direct pressure on unmyelinated ulnar nerve fibers, *Anesth Analg* 97:1183–1188, 2003.

47. Hanson MR, Breuer AC, Furlan AJ, et al: Mechanism and frequency of brachial plexus injury in open-heart surgery: A prospective analysis, *Ann Thorac Surg* 36:675–679, 1983.

48. Cooper DE, Jenkins RS, Bready L, et al: The prevention of injuries of the brachial plexus secondary to malposition of the patient during surgery, *Clin Orthop Relat Res* 33–41, 1988.

49. Liau D: Injuries and liability related to peripheral catheters: A closed claim analysis, *ASA Newsl* 70:11–13, 2006.

50. Roth S, Thisted RA, Erickson JP, et al: Eye injuries after nonocular surgery. A study of 60,965 anesthetics from 1988 to 1992, *Anesthesiology* 85:1020–1027, 1996.

51. Warner ME, Fronapfel PJ, Hebl JR, et al: Perioperative visual changes, *Anesthesiology* 96:855–859, 2002.

52. Warner ME, Warner MA, Garrity JA, et al: The frequency of perioperative vision loss, *Anesth Analg* 93:1417–1421, 2001.

53. Kalyani SD, Miller NR, Dong LM, et al: Incidence of and risk factors for perioperative optic neuropathy after cardiac surgery, *Ann Thorac Surg* 78:34–37, 2004.

54. Nuttall GA, Garrity JA, Dearani JA, et al: Risk factors for ischemic optic neuropathy after cardiopulmonary bypass: A matched case/control study, *Anesth Analg* 93:1410–1416, 2001.

55. Roth S, Barach P: Postoperative visual loss: Still no answers—yet, *Anesthesiology* 95:575–577, 2001.

56. Hunt K, Bajekal R, Calder I, et al: Changes in intraocular pressure in anesthetized prone patients, *J Neurosurg Anesthesiol* 16:287–290, 2004.

57. Cheng MA, Todorov A, Tempelhoff R, et al: The effect of prone positioning on intraocular pressure in anesthetized patients, *Anesthesiology* 95:1351–1355, 2001.

58. Hwang JW, Jeon YT, Kim JH, et al: The effect of the lateral decubitus position on the intraocular pressure in anesthetized patients undergoing lung surgery, *Acta Anaesthesiol Scand* 50:988–992, 2006.

59. Lee L: ASA Postoperative Visual Loss Registry: Preliminary analysis of factors associated with spine operations, *ASA Newsl* 67:7–8, 2003.

III

60. Ho VT, Newman NJ, Song S, et al: Ischemic optic neuropathy following spine surgery, *J Neurosurg Anesthesiol* 17:38–44, 2005.

61. Lee LA, Roth S, Posner KL, et al: The American Society of Anesthesiologists Postoperative Visual Loss Registry: Analysis of 93 spine surgery cases with postoperative visual loss, *Anesthesiology* 105:652–659, 2006.

62. American Society of Anesthesiologists Task Force on Perioperative Blindness: Practice advisory for perioperative visual loss associated with spine surgery, *Anesthesiology* 104:1319–1328, 2006.

63. Weiskopf RB, Feiner J, Lieberman J, et al: Visual loss after spinal surgery, *Anesthesiology* 106:1250–1251, 2007.

64. Shen Y, Drum M, Roth S: The prevalence of perioperative visual loss in the United States: A 10-year study from 1996 to 2005 of spinal, orthopedic, cardiac, and general surgery, *Anesth Analg* 109:1534–1545, 2009.

65. Aminoff MJ: Electrophysiologic testing for the diagnosis of peripheral nerve injuries, *Anesthesiology* 100:1298–1303, 2004.

66. Dylewsky W, McAlpine FS: Peripheral nervous system. In Martin JT, Warner MA, editors: *Positioning in Anesthesia and Surgery*, ed 3, Philadelphia, 1997, WB Saunders.

67. Lalwani K: Demographics and trends in nonoperating-room anesthesia, *Curr Opin Anaesthesiol* 19:430–435, 2006.

68. Robbertze R, Posner KL, Domino KB: Closed claims review of anesthesia for procedures outside the operating room, *Curr Opin Anaesthesiol* 19:436–442, 2006.

69. Metzner J, Posner KL, Domino KB: The risk and safety of anesthesia at remote locations: The US closed claims analysis, *Curr Opin Anaesthesiol* 22:502–508, 2009.

70. Horlocker TT, Wedel DJ, Benzon H, et al: Regional anesthesia in the anticoagulated patient: Defining the risks (the second ASRA Consensus Conference on Neuraxial Anesthesia and Anticoagulation), *Reg Anesth Pain Med* 28:172–197, 2003.

20 ANESTHETIC MONITORING

Anil de Silva

Monitoring of anesthetized patients is designed to collect data that reflect the patient's ongoing physiologic conditions and any responses that may result from therapeutic interventions. Monitoring allows the anesthesiologist to react to adverse physiologic changes or trends before they result in irreversible damage. The vigilance of the anesthesiologist is enhanced by the use of monitoring equipment and provides objective data to the anesthesiologist's own subjective observations.

The American Society of Anesthesiologists (ASA) has adopted basic anesthetic monitoring standards (see Appendix B). These standards mandate the use of pulse oximetry, capnography, an oxygen analyzer, disconnect alarms, body temperature measurements, and a visual display of an electrocardiogram (ECG) during the intraoperative period in all patients undergoing anesthesia. Systemic blood pressure and heart rate must be evaluated every 5 minutes. The use of a peripheral nerve stimulator to monitor the effect of neuromuscular blocking drugs (see Chapter 12) may become a standard-required monitor. The choice of intraoperative monitoring may be expanded beyond the ASA basic standards depending on the patient's medical condition and the complexity of the intraoperative procedure. The anesthesia provider's medical judgment will determine whether the potential risk of using any monitor (especially invasive monitors) is outweighed by the potential benefits provided (Fig. 20-1)[1] (Table 20-1).

ELECTROCARDIOGRAPHY

The ECG displays cardiac rhythm and rate and can also detect cardiac ischemia. The standard bipolar limb leads I, II, and III, and the augmented unipolar leads aVR, aVL, and aVF provide the clinician with important, though limited, views of the myocardium. Because the electrical vector of lead II parallels the atrial and ventricular depolarization waves, one can normally obtain large P waves and QRS complexes when using this limb lead. However, monitoring of cardiac ischemia is significantly enhanced by use of the precordial leads V_1 through V_6.

Normal Electrocardiogram

A normal ECG is composed of a P wave, PR interval, QRS complex, ST segment, and T wave, perhaps followed by a U wave (Fig. 20-2). The P wave is created by a wave of depolarization generated by the sinoatrial node, which is normally situated in the right atrium. The impulse travels through the atrioventricular node through the bundle of His down the Purkinje fibers to the ventricle. The QRS complex ensues when the ventricle contracts in response to the electrical stimulation. A T wave follows the QRS complex with the commencement of repolarization.

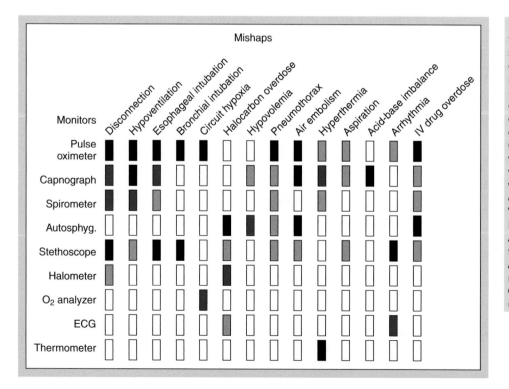

Figure 20-1 Estimate of the relative value of several monitors for detection of a variety of potential intraoperative mishaps. Most mishaps can be detected to some degree with the pulse oximeter or capnograph (or both). Dark red, high value; black, moderate value; light red, low value; white, no value. ECG, electrocardiogram. (From Whitcher C, Ream AK, Parsons D, et al. Anesthetic mishaps and the cost of monitoring: A proposed standard for monitoring equipment. J Clin Monit 1988;4:5-15, used with permission.)

Table 20-1 Measured and Calculated Hemodynamic Variables

Variable	Normal Value	Range
Systolic blood pressure (mm Hg)	120/80	90-140/70-90
Mean arterial pressure (mm Hg)	93	77-97
Heart rate (beats/min)	72	60-80
Mean right atrial pressure (mm Hg)	5	0-10
Right ventricular pressure (mm Hg)	25/5	15-30/0-10
Pulmonary artery pressure (mm Hg)	23/10	15-30/5-15
Mean pulmonary artery pressure (mm Hg)	15	10-20
Pulmonary artery occlusion pressure (mm Hg)	10	5-15
Mean left atrial pressure (mm Hg)	8	4-12
Cardiac output (L/min)	5	4-6
Stroke volume (mL/beat)	70	60-90
Systemic vascular resistance (dynes/sec/cm^5)	1200	900-1500
Pulmonary vascular resistance (dynes/sec/cm^5)	100	50-150

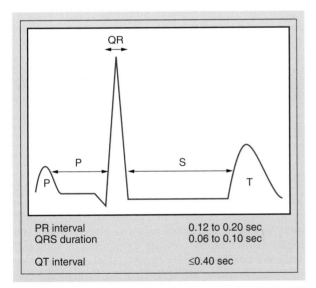

PR interval	0.12 to 0.20 sec
QRS duration	0.06 to 0.10 sec
QT interval	≤0.40 sec

Figure 20-2 A normal electrocardiogram is composed of a P wave, PR interval, QRS complex, ST segment, and T wave.

Evidence of Myocardial Ischemia

The ECG displays ischemia by means of changes in the rate of repolarization of ischemic myocardial tissue. Thus the ST segment and T wave portions of the ECG signal are primarily affected. Generally the T wave is affected initially, followed by ST segment changes as the ischemia worsens. Myocardial necrosis is displayed by the production of Q waves.

Use of lead V_5 alone results in the ECG detection of 75% of ischemic episodes in men aged 50 to 60. The addition of lead V_4 increases the sensitivity of the ECG to 90%. The combination of leads II, V_4, and V_5 results in detection of up to 96% of ischemic episodes.[2]

ARTERIAL BLOOD PRESSURE CUFF MONITORING

The most common techniques of arterial blood pressure measurement involve variations of the Riva-Rocci method. The Riva-Rocci method involves the placement of an inflatable cuff around a limb. The cuff is inflated until the pulse distal to the cuff disappears. Deflation then is begun until the pulse reappears—this point reflects the systolic pressure of the patient (Table 20-2).

Korotkoff Method

A stethoscope placed over the artery distal to the occluding cuff will detect a sound when the systolic pressure exceeds the cuff pressure (Korotkoff technique). Systolic blood pressure is consistent with the first sound heard

Table 20-2 Recommendations for the Use of Noninvasive Blood Pressure Devices

- Do not wrap the cuff tightly.
- Do not apply the cuff across a joint, bony prominence, or superficial nerve (ulnar nerve, peroneal nerve).
- Select the maximum cycle time consistent with safe monitoring.
- Inspect the cuff site periodically during prolonged cuff application.
- Record cuff location and cycle time.
- Keep alarms enabled.

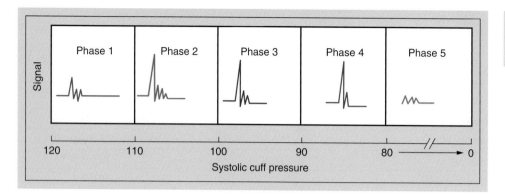

Figure 20-3 Phases of Korotkoff sounds during deflation of the blood pressure cuff.

(phase 1) during deflation of the blood pressure cuff (Fig. 20-3). As the cuff is deflated the sound changes in quality (phases 2 and 3). Phase 4 occurs with sudden onset of a muffled sound, followed by phase 5, which is the absence of any sound. Diastolic blood pressure is considered to be the pressure observed at phase 4 or 5. The American Heart Association recommends using phase 5 as the diastolic pressure except in cases in which the sound may not dependably disappear.

The size of the blood pressure cuff influences the measurement of blood pressure. A cuff that is too small will result in a reading that is inappropriately high; a larger cuff than indicated may show a lower than accurate decreased blood pressure reading. The cuff is appropriately sized when its width is 40% the circumference of the arm.[3] Variations in arterial blood pressure may also result with changes in posture. The diastolic blood pressure is routinely somewhat higher in the sitting patient (also see Chapter 19).

Oscillometric Method

The oscillometric method as described by von Recklinghausen in 1931[4] may also be used to determine arterial blood pressure. The cuff is inflated until oscillations on the blood pressure gauge are no longer seen. This point is considered the systolic pressure. The cuff is then further deflated until the point of maximum oscillations occurs—this peak is thought to correlate with the mean blood pressure. Diastolic blood pressure cannot be measured using this technique.

DINAMAP Method

The DINAMAP (device for indirect noninvasive automatic mean arterial pressure) is an automated blood pressure measurement device, and it uses the oscillometric technique. The oscillometric variation is compared at each reduction in cuff pressure. Automated blood pressure measurements generally correlate well with the systolic and mean blood pressures as measured with intra-arterial catheters. However, the diastolic pressure is usually about 10 mm Hg higher with automated devices than with direct arterial measurements.

Finometer

The Finometer utilizes the principle of the "unloaded arterial wall." A cuff is placed on a finger and inflated till the transmural pressure across the digital arteries is equal to zero. The magnitude of the plethysmograph is maximized at this point because arterial wall compliance is greatest. Blood pressure is measured by the photoplethysmographic detection of changes in light intensity transmitted through the finger. The Finometer is quite accurate when compared to direct arterial blood pressure measurements. The difference is generally between 2 and 4 mm Hg.[5]

Direct Arterial Pressure Monitoring

Continuous blood pressure monitoring is accomplished by placement of a catheter in a peripheral (usually radial) artery, which is connected to a transducer system and display. Direct blood pressure monitoring is indicated (1) during cardiopulmonary bypass, (2) when wide swings in blood pressure are expected, (3) when rigorous control of blood pressure is necessary, and (4) when there is a need for multiple analyses of arterial blood gas measurements.

CANNULATION SITE

The most frequently chosen site for arterial cannulation is the radial artery, which is close to the skin surface and is relatively easily palpable compared to some deeper arterial sites. Other acceptable sites for arterial pressure monitoring are the brachial, axillary, dorsalis pedis, and femoral arteries (Table 20-3).

Complications resulting from arterial cannulation include distal ischemia, infection, and hemorrhage. The rate of distal ischemia after radial artery catheterization is less than 0.1%.[6]

Table 20-3 Sites for Monitoring Systemic Blood Pressure with an Indwelling Catheter

Arterial Cannulation Site	Clinical Consideration(s)
Radial artery	Most commonly selected site
Ulnar artery	Principal source of blood flow to the hand
Brachial artery	Near the median nerve
Femoral artery	Accessible in low-flow states Risk for local and retroperitoneal hematoma
Dorsalis pedis artery	Higher systolic blood pressure displayed

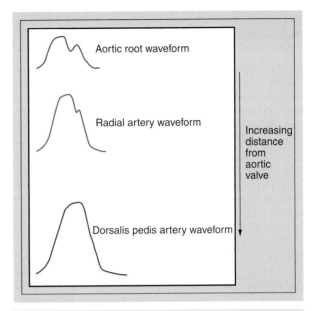

Figure 20-4 The shape of the arterial pulse wave changes as the waveform progresses distally from the central aorta.

The placement site of the catheter in various arterial systems determines the shape of the systemic blood pressure wave (Table 20-4). As the pressure wave is measured at sequentially further distances from the heart, the high-frequency components such as the dicrotic notch begin to disappear. There is more resonance such that the systolic peak is higher and the diastolic trough is lower as the blood pressure wave travels away from the heart (Fig. 20-4). Mean arterial pressure remains approximately the same at all measurement sites.

TECHNIQUE OF MEASUREMENT

The transducer is the hardware essential for direct blood pressure monitoring. All pressure transducers use a diaphragm with low compliance characteristics, which will bend and cause a volume change in response to an applied pressure. The most commonly used types of transducers are the Wheatstone bridge and the unbonded strain gauge. The transducer must be zeroed at whatever level is most appropriate for the patient. Although there may be certain inaccuracies, many clinicians will place the transducer at a level corresponding to the center of the heart. Zeroing exposes the transducer system to the ambient atmospheric pressure. Once the transducer system is closed off from the atmospheric pressure all subsequent pressure changes will be considered to be changes in physiologic pressure.[7] For every 15 cm in height that the transducer is moved up or down there is a corresponding change of 10 mm Hg in the blood pressure reading.

Table 20-4 Central Venous Pressure Catheter Placement Sites

Site	Advantage(s)	Disadvantage(s)
Right internal jugular vein	Good landmarks Predictable anatomy Accessible from the head of the operating room table	Carotid artery puncture Trauma to the brachial plexus
Left internal jugular vein	Same as for right internal jugular vein	Same as for right internal jugular vein Thoracic duct damage
Subclavian vein	Good landmarks Remains patent despite hypovolemia Patient comfort when awake	Pneumothorax
External jugular vein	Superficial location	Often difficult to thread the catheter into the central circulation
Antecubital vein	Safety	Often difficult to thread the catheter into the central circulation

CENTRAL VENOUS PRESSURE MONITORING

Central venous pressure (CVP) monitoring is used to monitor right ventricular filling when it is the clinically critical structure or to measure left ventricular filling when there is a correlation between left and right ventricles. A normal CVP reading ranges between 2 and approximately 7 mm Hg. The filling pressure is used as an indicator of cardiac volume with the understanding that adequate volumes will generate optimal cardiac contractility. When the ventricle is underfilled, large volume changes will generate little increase in the CVP, but small volume changes will generate large increases in CVP in an overfilled ventricle.

The CVP waveform consists of three positive waveforms called a, c, and v and two negative slopes called the x and y depressions (Fig. 20-5). The a wave represents the right atrial pressure increase during the phase of atrial contraction. The c wave is caused by the bulging of the closed tricuspid valve into the right atrium during the beginning of ventricular systole. The x descent occurs during ventricular systole and corresponds to atrial relaxation. The v wave then occurs, representing filling of the atrium while the tricuspid valve is closed. The y descent occurs when the tricuspid valve opens and the atrium starts to empty.[8]

Clinical Uses

The CVP waveform is used diagnostically in many different clinical situations. It is typically used to help in the assessment of a patient's intravascular volume status (see Table 20-4). The CVP may also be profitably used to monitor atrial dysrhythmias, right-sided cardiac valvular defects, tamponade, and ischemia.[8] In particular, in the case of atrial fibrillation the a wave will vanish and be replaced by a more discernible c wave. Tricuspid regurgitation can be diagnosed by noticing a prominent c-v wave as a regurgitant quantity of blood traverses the tricuspid valve in a retrograde fashion, thus elevating both c and v waves. Tamponade will exhibit an elevated CVP waveform and loss of the y descent. In the case of atrioventricular dissociation the contraction of the atrium against a closed tricuspid valve will elicit a particularly enlarged a wave called a "cannon" wave.

PULMONARY ARTERY CATHETER MEASUREMENTS

The PA (pulmonary artery) catheter is 110 cm long with a balloon at the tip with a capacity of 1.5 mL. The PA catheter may be used to measure cardiac output, mixed venous oxygen tension, pulmonary arterial and right atrial pressures, and, indirectly, LVEDP (left ventricular end-diastolic pressure) (Table 20-5). Complications from the placement of PA catheters are infrequent (<0.5% of insertions) but include dysrhythmias, catheter knotting, cardiac valve injury, and pulmonary artery rupture.[9] The waveform displayed from the distal end of a PA catheter from its venous insertion site reflects the position of the distal catheter tip in the vascular system (Fig. 20-6).

Pulmonary Artery Occlusive Pressure

Wedge pressure or pulmonary artery occlusive pressure (PAOP) is frequently used as a measure of LVEDP (Table 20-6). To measure the occlusive pressure, the distal balloon is inflated, thus isolating the distal lumen; theoretically, blood flow ceases between the tip of the catheter and left atrium. During diastole, when the mitral valve is open, the pressure between the left atrium and left

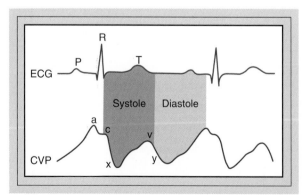

Figure 20-5 Central venous pressure (CVP) waveforms in relation to electrical events on the electrocardiogram (ECG). (From Mark JB. Central venous pressure monitoring: Clinical insights beyond the numbers. J Cardiothoracic Vasc Anesth 1991;5:164.)

Table 20-5 Possible Clinical Indications for Insertion of a Pulmonary Artery Catheter

Poor left ventricular function (ejection fraction <0.4; cardiac index <2 L/min/m^2)
Assessment of intravascular fluid volume
Evaluation of the response to fluid administration or administration of drugs (vasopressors, vasodilators, inotropes)
Valvular heart disease
Recent myocardial infarction
Adult respiratory distress syndrome
Massive trauma (shock, hemorrhage)
Major vascular surgery (cross-clamping of the aorta, large fluid shifts)

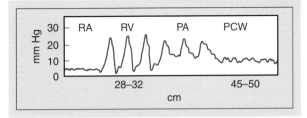

Figure 20-6 Schematic depiction of pressure waveforms as a pulmonary artery catheter passes through the right atrium (RA), right ventricle (RV), and pulmonary artery (PA). Note the narrowing of pulse pressure ("diastolic step-up") as the catheter enters the PA. Loss of a pulsatile trace as the catheter is advanced through the PA reflects pulmonary capillary wedge (PCW) pressure, which is also designated pulmonary artery occlusive pressure. Insertion of the pulmonary artery catheter through the right internal jugular vein should result in an RV tracing after the catheter has been advanced 28 to 32 cm and a PCW tracing at 45 to 50 cm.

ventricle should equalize, thus allowing the tip of the catheter to register the LVEDP.

Normal occlusive pressure is about 8 to 12 mm Hg, but a larger cardiac output can often be obtained by increasing the pressure to 14 to 18 mm Hg. An occlusive pressure more than 18 mm Hg can cause dyspnea, while one more than 20 mm Hg can cause the onset of fluid movement into alveoli. A pressure more than 30 mm Hg indicates frank pulmonary edema.

Measurement of Cardiac Output

Cardiac output is measured by utilizing a modification of the Stewart-Hamilton equation that takes into account temperature changes between the injectate and PA blood, which is proportional to pulmonary blood flow (cardiac output). The possibilities for inaccuracies in cardiac output determination are multiple. An error of 0.5 mL out of a 10-mL injectate volume can alter the output by 5%. A 1° C increase in the temperature of the injectate can cause an error of 3% in the cardiac output. In addition, a decrement in the volume of the injectate will increase the calculated cardiac output.[10]

Measurement of Mixed Venous Oxygen Partial Pressure

The PA catheter is often used to measure the mixed venous oxygen tension. This value is a global representation of total body oxygen supply and demand. Normal Pvo_2 is about 40 mm Hg with a saturation of 75%. A reduction in Pvo_2 may be attributed to a reduction in O_2 delivery (secondary to a reduction in O_2 content per deciliter or a reduction in cardiac output), or an increase in O_2 consumption (secondary to an increased metabolic state).

ECHOCARDIOGRAPHY

Conventionally, hemodynamic monitoring of the cardiovascular system has been accomplished by use of intravascular catheters. However the advent of echocardiography has revolutionized the field (Table 20-7).[11] The use of transesophageal echocardiography (TEE) allows for the rapid and accurate determination of left ventricular ejection fraction, myocardial ischemia, and left ventricular preload. It also allows the anesthesiologist to inspect the integrity of the interior myocardial structures such as the septal tissues and valves. In the hands of an expert clinician, a TEE can also indicate issues with systemic vascular resistance and pulmonary arterial pressures, aortic dissections, and other less common anomalies.

The use of TEE allows the clinician to rapidly diagnose the etiologic basis of hypotension by estimating left

Table 20-7 Clinical Information Derived from Intraoperative Transesophageal Echocardiography

Regional (segmental) wall motion abnormalities (myocardial ischemia)
Stroke volume (ejection fraction)
Cardiac valve function (aortic, mitral)
Intracardiac air
Effects of anesthesia and surgery on cardiac function
Adequacy of intravascular fluid volume

Table 20-6 Use of the Pulmonary Artery Catheter to Evaluate Hemodynamic Disorders

Disorder	Central Venous Pressure	Pulmonary Artery Occlusive Pressure (PAOP)	Pulmonary Artery End-Diastolic Pressure (PAEDP)
Hypovolemia	Decreased	Decreased	PAEDP = PAOP
Left ventricular failure	Increased	Increased	PAEDP = PAOP
Right ventricular failure	Increased	No change	PAEDP = PAOP
Pulmonary embolism	Increased	No change	PAEDP > PAOP
Cardiac tamponade	Increased	Increased	PAEDP = PAOP

ventricular end-diastolic area and ejection fraction. For example, a decreased LV end-diastolic area coupled with an increased ejection fraction most likely indicates hypovolemia, whereas an increased end-diastolic area and a decreased ejection fraction may indicate cardiac failure.[12]

An incidence of about 0.1% of oral and pharyngeal injuries occur with the introduction of the TEE probe into the esophagus. Esophageal rupture has been reported. Bronchial and arterial compression can occur especially in the infant.

Technology

Echocardiography uses ultrasound waves emitted by a piezoelectric crystal to penetrate tissue. This high-frequency sound is inaudible. The sound energy strikes various tissue planes and is subsequently reflected back to the crystal. The energy striking the crystal is analyzed with regard to attenuation, time delay, and frequency change and the results are displayed in a format that gives the clinician information as to velocity, distance, and density.

M-MODE ECHOCARDIOGRAPHY

M-mode echocardiography offers a unidimensional view of the myocardium. It represents the tissue densities and velocities encountered by a thin beam of ultrasound energy that is directed at the heart. M-mode echocardiography is best used in determining velocities.

B-MODE ECHOCARDIOGRAPHY

Two-dimensional (B-mode) echocardiography displays a two-dimensional image of the myocardium. The ultrasound energy is swept through the heart in a planar fashion, thus giving one a cross-sectional view of the heart. The cross section is updated every few milliseconds and so it is possible to view changes in myocardial performance immediately.

Velocity

Velocity is monitored in echocardiography by using the principle of the Doppler shift in sound wave frequencies. When the emitted ultrasound strikes a moving red blood cell the shift in the frequency of the reflected sound energy represents the velocity of the red blood cell.

PULSED-WAVE DOPPLER

Pulsed-wave Doppler uses one crystal for both the emission and the reception of the ultrasound energy (Fig. 20-7). The crystal emits ultrasound for a specified period of time and then waits for the reflected energy to return. The number of ultrasound emissions per minute is defined as the *pulse repetition frequency*. Because the crystal will not emit another sound until the reflected sound energy returns,

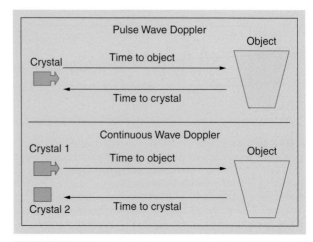

Figure 20-7 Timing differences between Doppler modalities.

the velocities it can measure using this technique are necessarily slow. The advantage, however, is that the location of the tissue with the velocity being measured is known. The maximal Doppler shift measurable is limited to one half the pulse repetition frequency, which is known as the Nyquist limit. Velocities which give a Doppler shift higher than the Nyquist limit are inaccurate. This phenomenon is known as *aliasing*. The pulsed-wave Doppler signal scans the myocardium in a planar fashion and a wedge-shaped cross section of the myocardium is displayed. As the TEE probe is moved up and down the esophagus, different cross sections of the myocardium may be examined.

CONTINUOUS-WAVE DOPPLER

Continuous-wave Doppler differs from pulsed-wave Doppler by virtue of its use of two crystals: one for ultrasound emission, and one for the detection of the returning energy. The continuous production of sound energy allows one to measure very high Doppler shifts and thus obtain information on higher velocities. However, the ability to locate the tissue reflecting the energy is lost: instead, an average of the velocities along the path of the ultrasound beam is acquired.[12]

Color Doppler Imaging

Color Doppler imaging is a technology based on pulse-wave Doppler. However, color Doppler overlays a color grid on the traditional gray-scale cross-sectional view seen for pulsed-wave Doppler. Blood flowing toward the transducer head is seen as a shade of red and flow away from the transducer is seen as blue. The velocity of the flow is characterized by deeper shades of blue and red. With the interposition of color on the image, the clinician is able to better correlate blood flow with the structural elements of the heart.

PULSE OXIMETRY

Pulse oximetry is based upon an application of the Beers-Lambert law, which relates concentration of solute to intensity of light transmitted through the solution. The solute in question is hemoglobin. The typical pulse oximeter illuminates the tissue sample with two wavelengths of light: 660-nm red light (which is well absorbed by oxyhemoglobin), and 940-nm infrared light (which is well absorbed by deoxyhemoglobin) (Fig. 20-8). An increased absorbance of red light transmitted through tissue during cardiac systole is related to arterial hemoglobin saturation. The pulse oximeter determines the amount of absorbance that will be attributed to the pulsatile arterialized blood and then divides it by the nonpulsatile baseline absorbance, which is attributed to capillary and venous blood. The amount of increased absorbance seen in the pulsatile component is a measure of the arterial oxygen saturation.[13]

Measurement Errors

Most pulse oximeters are two-wavelength devices, which only measure light absorbance from oxyhemoglobin and deoxyhemoglobin. Thus, any other substance that also absorbs light at the same wavelengths will lead to measurement errors (Table 20-8).

METHEMOGLOBIN

Methemoglobin absorbs light almost equally well in both the red and infrared wavelengths. Thus, a large quantity of methemoglobin will force the ratio between pulse-added absorbance and baseline absorbance toward unity, which conforms to an arterial saturation of 85%.

CARBOXYHEMOGLOBIN

Carboxyhemoglobin absorbs red light, but not infrared light; in this case the pulse oximeter reported oxygen saturation will vary widely.

Table 20-8 Factors That Influence the Accuracy of Pulse Oximetry

Low blood flow conditions
Patient movement
Ambient light
Dysfunctional hemoglobin (carboxyhemoglobin, methemoglobin)
Methylene blue
Altered relationship between $Paco_2$ and Sao_2 (shift in the oxyhemoglobin dissociation curve)

INTRAVASCULAR DYES

Intravascular dyes will also cause errors in pulse oximeter measurements of oxygen saturation. Methylene blue forces the arterial oxygen saturation to drop to about 65%. Other dyes, including indigo carmine and indocyanine green, will cause spurious drops in measured saturation as well.

A recent development is continuous, non-invasive monitoring of blood hemoglobin concentrations via the pulse oximeter device (also see Chapter 24).

EVOKED POTENTIALS (Also See Chapter 30)

Evoked potentials (visual, auditory, somatosensory, motor) are the electrical signals produced by the nervous system in response to various stimuli. Certain changes in the potentials can indicate neuronal pathway dysfunction. Evoked potentials are generally described in terms of latency, amplitude, and site of the stimulus. The potentials are displayed as a plot of voltage changes versus time (Fig. 20-9). Latency describes the time between the stimulus and the subsequently generated potential. Amplitude is a measure of the peak of the displayed waveform from its baseline.[14]

Figure 20-8 Light emission and absorbance in the pulse oximeter.

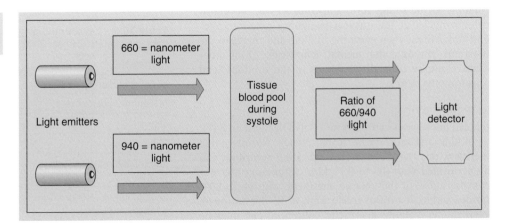

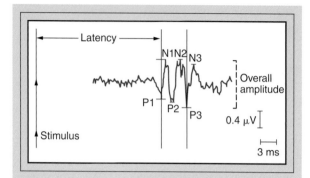

Figure 20-9 A typical somatosensory evoked potential consisting of three positive peaks (P1, P2, and P3) and three negative peaks (N1, N2, N3). More than a 50% decrease in the amplitude of the positive peaks or loss of one or more of the negative peaks, or both, may indicate the effects of volatile anesthetics or interference with the transmission of sensory nerve signals. (From Loghnan BA, Hall GM. Spinal cord monitoring 1989. Br J Anaesth 1989;63:587-594, used with permission.)

Somatosensory Evoked Potentials

Somatosensory evoked potentials (SSEPs) are generally monitored by placing surface or subcutaneous stimulating electrodes near the median or ulnar nerves of the arm or the posterior tibial nerves of the legs. The recording electrodes are often placed on the scalp or close to the spinal cord. Lower limb SSEPs generally monitor the integrity of the dorsal columns of the spinal cord. Thus, they are often used during surgery on the spinal cord or vertebral column. The vascular supply of the dorsal columns is obtained from the posterior spinal arteries; thus, SSEP serves to warn against posterior spinal cord ischemia.

TECHNOLOGY

A square wave signal with a time interval between 0.2 and 2 msec is applied to the nerve. The electrical signal then enters the dorsal root ganglia, traverses the posterior columns of the spinal cord, and continues to the dorsal column nuclei at the cervical medullary junction. Second-order fibers then cross the midline and travel to the thalamus through the medial lemniscus. Third-order fibers continue from the thalamus to the frontoparietal sensorimotor cortex.

INTERPRETATION

Inhaled anesthetics cause a dose-related decrease in SSEP amplitude and an increase in its latency. Nitrous oxide increases this tendency. In general, SSEP recording can be performed with 0.5 to 0.75 MAC (minimum alveolar concentration) of the volatile anesthetic with up to 60% nitrous oxide. If nitrous oxide were to be discontinued, even higher volatile anesthetic concentrations may be

used. Barbiturates have a variable effect on SSEP, depending on the dosage. Higher barbiturate plasma levels do cause a decrease in amplitude and an increase in latency. Benzodiazepines administered as preanesthetic medication appear to cause only a slight change in SSEP. Opioids, such as fentanyl, may also interfere with SSEP, whereas muscle relaxants do not affect SSEP.

CLINICAL USES

SSEP monitoring is essential when operating in the region of major peripheral nerves, plexuses, or spinal cord. Although serious neurologic injury may result when an SSEP shows a prolonged increase in latency and a decrease in amplitude, the extent of the change required remains unclear.[15]

Motor Evoked Potentials

Motor pathways located within the corticospinal tracts are not monitored by SSEPs, and monitoring of motor evoked potentials has not been widely practiced. The stimulating electrode must be placed on the scalp or perhaps lower down the motor pathway, and the recording electrode is placed on the contracting muscle. Motor evoked potentials are generally difficult to obtain and are prone to inaccuracy. Their sensitivity to anesthetics and muscle relaxants (in contrast to SSEPs) increase the difficulty of clinical interpretation.

CAPNOGRAPHY

The carbon dioxide waveform is helpful in (1) determining that the patient is in fact being ventilated, (2) as an estimate of $Paco_2$, and (3) as an evaluation of dead space (Table 20-9). The carbon dioxide waveform itself is characterized by four phases: (1) an inspiratory baseline, (2) an expiratory upstroke, (3) an expiratory plateau, and (4) an inspiratory downstroke (Fig. 20-10). A sustained carbon dioxide waveform (>30 mm Hg) confirms that

Table 20-9 Causes of Changes in the Exhaled Concentration of Carbon Dioxide

Increase	Decrease
Hypoventilation	Hyperventilation
Malignant hyperthermia	Hypothermia
Sepsis	Low cardiac output
Rebreathing	Pulmonary embolism
Administration of bicarbonate	Accidental disconnection or tracheal extubation
Insufflation of carbon dioxide during laparoscopy	Cardiac arrest

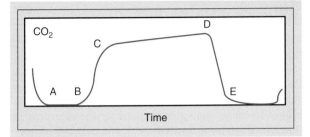

Figure 20-10 The capnogram is divided into four distinct phases. Phase A-B represents the exhalation of anatomic dead space, which is normally devoid of carbon dioxide. Phase B-C is present on the capnogram as a sharp upstroke that is determined by the evenness of ventilation and alveolar emptying. A slow rate of rise in this phase may reflect chronic obstructive pulmonary disease or acute airway obstruction, including bronchospasm. Phase C-D reflects the exhalation of alveolar gas, with point D being designated the end-tidal carbon dioxide concentration. Phase D-E reflects the beginning of inspiration and entrainment of gases lacking carbon dioxide. Normally, unless rebreathing of carbon dioxide occurs, the baseline approaches zero.

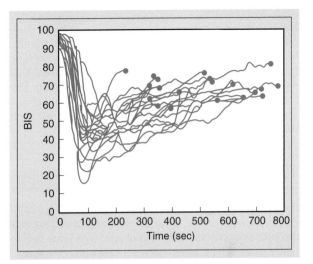

Figure 20-11 Plot of the bispectral index (BIS) against time from induction of anesthesia to recovery of consciousness after the administration of propofol. (From Flaishon RI, Windsor A, Sigl J, et al. Recovery of consciousness after thiopental or propofol: Bispectral index and the isolated forearm technique. Anesthesiology 1997;86;613-619, used with permission.)

III

an endotracheal tube is placed in the trachea, although a tube placed in the pharynx can occasionally exhibit a carbon dioxide waveform. However, a tube placed in the esophagus should be distinguishable from a tracheal intubation because any carbon dioxide present in the stomach will quickly vanish (usually within three "tidal volumes") and the waveform will become essentially a flat line. Healthy, conscious people exhale gas from alveoli that are all essentially well perfused and ventilated; therefore, dead space ranges from 2% to 3% and the differential between arterial and end-tidal carbon dioxide is about 0.6 mm Hg.[16]

BRAIN ELECTRICAL ACTIVITY MONITORING

Most of the devices designed to monitor brain electrical activity for the purpose of assessing anesthetic effect record electroencephalographic (EEG) activity from electrodes placed on the patient's forehead. Systems may be subdivided into those that process spontaneous EEG and electromyographic (EMG) activity (bispectral index [BIS], entropy, Narcotrend, Patient State Analyzer) and those that acquire evoked responses to auditory stimuli (auditory evoked potentials).

Bispectral Index Monitoring (Also See Chapter 46)

The bispectral index (BIS) monitor attempts to measure the effects of anesthesia on a patient's level of consciousness by algorithmically processing the patient's EEG and

converting it to a single number, which probably represents the patient's state of awareness (Fig. 20-11).[17] A BIS number lower than 60 is thought to represent a state at which the patient is unable to respond to verbal commands. A BIS number higher than 70 is believed to correspond to a higher likelihood of awareness. A BIS number of 100 represents the awake state. BIS numbers between 45 and 60 are, in general, considered to be optimal for a relatively healthy patient undergoing a routine general anesthetic and surgery.

CLINICAL USES

The problem of awareness during surgery may be more frequent than most anesthesia providers realize. Awareness with recall during anesthesia may occur in up to 1 in 500 cases. In obstetric, cardiac, and trauma patients, the incidence may approach 1%.[18,19] Therefore, if the BIS monitor is effective in reducing the incidence of awareness, the monitor would likely be very useful. So far, this conclusion is not clear.

The BIS monitor allows clinicians to employ reduced amounts of anesthetic for light sedation cases and may enable anesthesia providers to modify their anesthetics to allow for a faster wake-up. However, if the BIS monitor is used primarily to decrease the amount of anesthetic administered for reasons of cost and efficiency, it is possible that an even more frequent incidence of recall might result.[20] Conversely, a recent study on the use of the BIS monitor showed no decrease in the incidence of awareness with the use of volatile anesthetics.[21]

DISADVANTAGES

The BIS monitor is subject to artifact. For example, how can a patient with head trauma and a low BIS number be evaluated for adequate sedation? Factors such as hypothermia and electromyographic contamination of the EEG signal can also degrade the utility of the BIS. Physiologic conditions that may result in central nervous system effects (such as hepatic failure) may also affect the BIS number.

TEMPERATURE MONITORING

Changes in body temperature are frequent intraoperative events during surgical procedures. The exposed state of the patient causes the skin to cool and even more importantly, the administered general anesthetics cause a decline in thermoregulatory functioning. Most general anesthetics have vasodilatory properties, which cause a flow of thermal energy from core areas of the body to more peripheral areas. In general, core temperatures decline by approximately 1° C to 1.5° C in the first hour after anesthetic induction. After the initial hour, body heat continues to decrease secondary to factors such as initial body thermal content, environmental temperature, and the size of the surgical incision. Core heat loss continues from redistributive effects, but peripheral heat loss persists via pathways of radiation, conduction, convection, and evaporation.[22]

Hypothermia

Hypothermia cannot be considered a benign condition. Mild hypothermia can delay recovery from anesthesia. Shivering can increase oxygen utilization, systemic blood pressure, and heart rate and can result in myocardial ischemia in elderly or physiologically weakened patients. More profound hypothermia may be directly related to myocardial dysrhythmias. Coagulation times and wound healing are also impaired.[23]

Body Temperature Monitoring Sites

The body temperature monitoring site must be chosen for the accuracy with which it registers the central thermal content. The best core temperature monitors are the PA catheter, which measures blood temperature within the pulmonary artery, and the tympanic membrane monitor, which measures the temperature of the carotid artery. Bladder fluid temperature is close to core temperature, whereas rectal temperature is a relatively poor substitute. Many anesthesiologists employ an esophageal temperature monitor, but it may be better used to indicate the trend of heat gain or loss. Axillary and skin temperature monitors are highly prone to artifact.

INHALED ANESTHETIC MONITORING

Monitoring the inhaled and exhaled concentrations of inhaled anesthetics is essential for confirming the identification and determining the delivered levels of these drugs. Errors in the amount and choice of inhaled anesthetics can result in clinically significant morbidity. Several different technologies are used for the identification and examination of inhaled anesthetic concentrations.

Monochromatic Infrared Spectrometry

In monochromatic infrared spectrometry, an infrared beam with a wavelength of 3.3 μm is passed through a representative gas sample. Because the absorption spectrum of halogenated agents is very similar at this wavelength of light, it is critically important to program the correct agent into the monitor.

Polychromatic Infrared Spectrometer

The polychromatic infrared spectrometer emits infrared light with a wavelength of 7 to 13 μm. The absorption spectrum of inhalational agents is relatively different at this wavelength. As a result, this monitor can automatically identify the inhaled anesthetic drug, as well as describe the concentration of gas being delivered. Should the anesthesiologist switch from one to another inhaled anesthetic, this monitor can measure the concentrations of both drugs simultaneously.[24]

Mass Spectrometry

Mass spectrometers ionize the gas sample and then allow the ionized particles to fall on a magnetized plate. Because of the differing atomic weights of the ionized particles it is possible to identify the type of particles and concentration of anesthetic drug. This technology uses a central machine, which draws gases from multiple operating rooms simultaneously. The system analyzes the gas from each room sequentially thus providing near but not completely constant gas monitoring. This type of centralized monitoring is quite expensive and is infrequently used in today's operating rooms.

Raman Scattering Spectrometry

The Raman scattering spectrometer emits an intense beam of light into a sample of gas. Collision of a photon and gas molecule causes the photon to change its energy characteristics and emerge at a substantially different wavelength typical for the particular gas. The change in frequency allows the Raman monitor to identify the type and concentration of the specific inhaled anesthetic gas or vapor.

QUESTIONS OF THE DAY

1. Which ECG leads are most useful for intraoperative monitoring in the adult?
2. What is the oscillometric method of blood pressure monitoring?
3. What are the clinically important differences between the use of pulsed-wave Doppler versus continuous-wave Doppler in echocardiography?
4. What is the rationale for monitoring somatosensory evoked potentials (SSEPs) during spine surgery?
5. Which body temperature monitoring sites are the most accurate? Which are the least accurate?

REFERENCES

1. Whitcher C, Ream AK, Parsons D, et al: Anesthetic mishaps and the cost of monitoring: A proposed standard for monitoring equipment, *J Clin Monit* 4:5–15, 1988.
2. Slogoff S, Keats AS: Does perioperative myocardial ischemia lead to postoperative myocardial infarction? *Anesthesiology* 73:1074–1081, 1985.
3. Pickering TG: Principles and techniques of blood pressure measurement, *Cardiol Clin* 20: 207–223, 2002.
4. von Recklinghausen H: Neue Wege der Blutdruckmessung, *Wschr Klin Med* 113:4, 1930.
5. Penaz J: Photo-electric measurement of blood pressure, volume and flow in the finger, *Dig 10th Int Conf Med Biol Eng* 104:1973.
6. Slogoff S, Keats AS, Arlund C: On the safety of radial arery cannulation, *Anesthesiology* 59:42–47, 1983.
7. Courtois M, Fattal P, Kovacs S, et al: Anatomically and physiologically based reference level for measurement of intracardiac pressures, *Circulation* 92:1994–2000, 1995.
8. Mark JB: Central venous pressure monitoring: Clinical insights beyond the numbers, *J Cardiothorac Vasc Anesth* 5:163–173, 1991.
9. Roizen M, Berger D, Gabel R, et al: Practice guidelines for pulmonary artery catheterization, *Anesthesiology* 99:988–1014, 2003.
10. Sharkey S: Beyond the wedge: Clinical physiology and the Swan-Ganz catheter, *Am J Med* 83:111–122, 1987.
11. Sutton DC, Cahalan MK: Pro: TEE is a routine monitor, *J Cardiothorac Vasc Anesth* 7:357–360, 1993.
12. Cahalan M: *Intraoperative Transesophageal Echocardiography. An Interactive Text and Atlas*, New York, 1997, Churchill Livingstone.
13. Severinghaus JW, Kehheher JF: Recent developments in pulse oximetry, *Anesthesiology* 76:1018–1038, 1992.
14. Loghnan BA, Hall GM: Spinal cord monitoring 1989, *Br J Anaesth* 63:587–594, 1989.
15. Kumar AB, Makhija NA: Evoked potential monitoring in anaesthesia and analgesia, *Anaesthesia* 55:225–241, 2001.
16. Gravenstein JS, Paulus DA, Hayes JJ: *Capnography in Clinical Practice*, Boston, 1989, Butterworths.
17. Flaishon RI, Windsor A, Sigl J, et al: Recovery of consciousness after thiopental or propofol: Bispectral index and the isolated forearm technique, *Anesthesiology* 86: 613–619, 1997.
18. Ghoneim NM: Learning and consciousness during general anesthesia, *Anesthesiology* 76:279–305, 1992.
19. Myles PS, Leslie K, McNeil J, et al: A randomised controlled trial of BIS monitoring to prevent awareness during anesthesia: The B-Aware Trial, *Lancet* 363:1757–1763, 2004.
20. O'Connor MF, Daves SM, Tung A, et al: BIS monitoring to prevent awareness during general anesthesia, *Anesthesiology* 94:520–522, 2000.
21. Avidan MS, Zhang L, Burnside BA, et al: Anesthesia awareness and the bispectral index, *N Engl J Med* 358:1097–1108, 2008.
22. Sessler D: Perioperative heat balance, *Anesthesiology* 92:578–600, 2000.
23. Cereda Maurizio MG: Intraoperative temperature monitoring, *Int Anesthesiol Clin* 42:41–54, 2004.
24. Walder B, Lauber R, Zbinden AM: Accuracy and cross-sensitivity of 10 different anesthetic gas monitors, *J Clin Monit* 9:364–373, 1993.

III

B STANDARDS FOR BASIC ANESTHETIC MONITORING†

These standards apply to all anesthesia care, although in emergency circumstances, appropriate life support measures take precedence. These standards may be exceeded at any time based on the judgment of the responsible anesthesia provider. They are intended to encourage quality patient care, but observing them cannot guarantee any specific patient outcome. They are subject to revision from time to time, as warranted by the evolution of technology and practice. They apply to all general anesthetics, regional anesthetics, and monitored anesthesia care. This set of standards addresses only the issue of basic anesthetic monitoring, which is one component of anesthesia care. In certain rare or unusual circumstances, (1) some of these methods of monitoring may be clinically impractical, and (2) appropriate use of the described monitoring methods may fail to detect untoward clinical developments. Brief interruptions in continual† monitoring may be unavoidable. These standards are not intended for application to the care of the obstetrical patient in labor or in the conduct of pain management.

STANDARD I

Qualified anesthesia personnel shall be present in the room throughout the conduct of all general anesthetics, regional anesthetics, and monitored anesthesia care.

Objective

Because of rapid changes in patient status during anesthesia, qualified anesthesia personnel shall be continuously present to monitor the patient and provide anesthesia care. In the event of a direct known hazard (e.g., radiation) to the anesthesia personnel, which might require intermittent remote observation of the patient, some provision for monitoring the patient must be made. In the event that an emergency requires the temporary absence of the person primarily responsible for the anesthetic, the best judgment of the anesthesia provider will be exercised in comparing the emergency with the anesthetized patient's condition and in the selection of the person left responsible for the anesthetic during the temporary absence.

STANDARD II

During all anesthetics, the patient's oxygenation, ventilation, circulation, and temperature shall be continually evaluated.

OXYGENATION

Objective

To ensure adequate oxygen concentration in the inspired gas and blood during all anesthetics.

Methods

1. Inspired gas: During every administration of general anesthesia using an anesthesia machine, the concentration of oxygen in the patient breathing system shall be measured by an oxygen analyzer with a low-oxygen concentration limit alarm in use.*
2. Blood oxygenation: During all anesthetics, a quantitative method of assessing oxygenation such as pulse

---

†Note that "continual" is defined as "repeated regularly and frequently in steady rapid succession," whereas "continuous" means "prolonged without any interruption at any time."

*Under extenuating circumstances, the responsible anesthesiologist may waive the requirements marked with an asterisk (*); it is recommended that when this is done, it should be so stated (including the reasons) in a note in the patient's medical record.

oximetry shall be employed.* When a pulse oximeter is utilized, the variable-pitch pulse tone and the low threshold alarm shall be audible to the anesthesia provider or the anesthesia care team personnel.* Adequate illumination and exposure of the patient are necessary to assess color.*

VENTILATION

Objective

To ensure adequate ventilation of the patient during all anesthetics.

Methods

1. Every patient receiving general anesthesia shall have the adequacy of ventilation continually evaluated. Qualitative clinical signs such as chest excursion, observation of the reservoir breathing bag, and auscultation of breath sounds are useful. Continual monitoring for the presence of expired carbon dioxide shall be performed unless invalidated by the nature of the patient, procedure, or equipment. Quantitative monitoring of the volume of expired gas is strongly encouraged.*

2. When an endotracheal tube or laryngeal mask is inserted, its correct positioning must be verified by clinical assessment and by identification of carbon dioxide in the expired gas. Continual end-tidal carbon dioxide analysis, in use from the time of endotracheal tube/laryngeal mask placement until extubation/removal or initiation of transfer to a postoperative care location, shall be performed using a quantitative method such as capnography, capnometry, or mass spectroscopy.* When capnography or capnometry is utilized, the end-tidal CO_2 alarm shall be audible to the anesthesia providers or the anesthesia care team personnel.*

3. When ventilation is controlled by a mechanical ventilator, there shall be in continuous use a device that is capable of detecting disconnection of components of the breathing system. The device must give an audible signal when its alarm threshold is exceeded.

4. During regional anesthesia (with no sedation) or local anesthesia (with no sedation), the adequacy of ventilation shall be evaluated by continual observation of qualitative clinical signs. During moderate or deep sedation, the adequacy of ventilation shall be evaluated by continual observation of qualitative clinical signs and monitoring for the presence of exhaled carbon dioxide unless precluded or invalidated by the nature of the patient, procedure, or equipment.

CIRCULATION

Objective

To ensure adequacy of the patient's circulatory function during all anesthetics.

Methods

1. Every patient receiving anesthesia shall have the electrocardiogram continuously displayed from the beginning of anesthesia until preparing to leave the anesthetizing location.*

2. Every patient receiving anesthesia shall have arterial blood pressure and heart rate determined and evaluated at least every 5 minutes.*

3. Every patient receiving general anesthesia shall have, in addition to the above, circulatory function continually evaluated by at least one of the following: palpation of a pulse, auscultation of heart sounds, monitoring of a tracing of intra-arterial pressure, ultrasound peripheral pulse monitoring, or pulse plethysmography or oximetry.

BODY TEMPERATURE

Objective

To aid in maintenance of appropriate body temperature during all anesthetics.

Methods

Every patient receiving anesthesia shall have temperature monitored when clinically significant changes in body temperature are intended, anticipated, or suspected.

---

*Under extenuating circumstances, the responsible anesthesiologist may waive the requirements marked with an asterisk (*); it is recommended that when this is done, it should be so stated (including the reasons) in a note in the patient's medical record.

---

†Standards for Basic Anesthetic Monitoring is reprinted with permission of the American Society of Anesthesiologists, 520 N. Northwest Highway, Park Ridge, IL 60068-2573.
These standards were approved by the ASA House of Delegates on October 21, 1986, and last amended on October 20, 2010 with an effective date of July 1, 2011.

21 ACID-BASE BALANCE AND BLOOD GAS ANALYSIS

Linda L. Liu

The concentrations of hydrogen and bicarbonate ions in plasma must be precisely regulated to optimize enzyme activity, oxygen transport, and rates of chemical reactions within cells. Each day approximately 15,000 mmol of carbon dioxide (which can generate carbonic acid as it combines with water) and 50 to 100 mEq of nonvolatile acid (mostly sulfuric acid) are produced and must be eliminated safely. The body is able to maintain this intricate acid-base balance by utilizing buffers, pulmonary excretion of carbon dioxide, and renal elimination of acid. This chapter will define concepts important for understanding acids and bases, discuss clinical measurements of blood gases and their interpretation, and present a diagnostic approach to common acid-base disturbances.

DEFINITIONS

Acids and Bases

An acid was defined by Bronsted as a molecule that can act as a proton (H^+) donor, and a base is a molecule that can act as a proton acceptor. In physiologic solutions, a strong acid is a substance that readily and irreversibly gives up an H^+, and a strong base avidly binds H^+. In contrast, biologic molecules are either weak acids or bases, which reversibly donate H^+, or reversibly bind H^+.

Acidemia and Acidosis

A blood pH less than 7.35 is called acidemia and a pH greater than 7.45 is called alkalemia, regardless of the mechanism. The underlying process that lowers the pH is called an acidosis, and the process that raises the pH is known as an alkalosis. A patient can have a mixed disorder with both an acidosis and an alkalosis concurrently, but can only be either acidemic or alkalemic. The last two terms are mutually exclusive.

Base Excess

Base excess (BE) is usually defined as the amount of strong acid (hydrochloric acid for base excess greater than zero) or strong base (sodium hydroxide for base excess less than zero) required to return 1 L of whole blood exposed in vitro to a P_{CO_2} of 40 mm Hg to a pH of 7.4.[1] Instead of an actual titration, the blood gas machine calculates the base excess with algorithms utilizing plasma pH, blood P_{CO_2}, and hemoglobin concentration. The number is supposed to refer to the nonrespiratory or metabolic component of an acid-base disturbance. A BE less than zero (negative) suggests the presence of a metabolic acidosis, and a value greater than zero (positive) suggests the presence of a metabolic alkalosis. In vitro, the number has been accurate, but in the living organism, because ions do cross beyond vascular and cellular boundaries, a primary acute change in Pa_{CO_2} sometimes can cause the BE to move in the opposite direction, despite an unchanged metabolic acid-base status.[2] Anesthesia providers often use the base excess as a surrogate measure for lactic acidosis to help determine adequacy of volume resuscitation.

REGULATION OF THE HYDROGEN ION CONCENTRATION

At 37° C, the normal hydrogen ion concentration in arterial blood and extracellular fluid is 35 to 45 nmol/L, which is equivalent to an arterial pH of 7.45 to 7.35, respectively. The normal plasma bicarbonate ion concentration is 24 ± 2 mEq/L. The intracellular hydrogen ion concentration is approximately 160 nmol/L, which is equivalent to a pH of 6.8.

Physiologic changes to acid-base disturbances are corrected by three systems—buffers, ventilation, and renal response. The buffer systems provide an immediate chemical response. The ventilatory response occurs in minutes whenever possible, and lastly, the renal response can provide nearly complete restoration of the pH, but it can take days.

Buffer Systems

A buffer is defined as a substance within a solution that can prevent extreme changes in pH. A buffer system is composed of a base molecule and its weak conjugate acid. The base molecules of the buffer system bind excess hydrogen ions, and the weak acid protonates excess base molecules. The *dissociation ionization constant* (pKa) indicates the strength of an acid and is derived from the classic Henderson-Hasselbalch equation (Fig. 21-1). The pKa is the pH at which an acid is 50% protonated and 50% deprotonated. The smaller the pKa value, the stronger the acid. The most important buffer systems in blood, in order of importance, are the (1) bicarbonate buffer

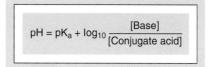

$$pH = pK_a + \log_{10} \frac{[Base]}{[Conjugate\ acid]}$$

Figure 21-1 Henderson-Hasselbalch equation. [Base], concentration of base; [Conjugate acid], concentration of conjugate acid.

system (H_2CO_3/HCO_3^-), (2) hemoglobin buffer system (HbH/Hb), (3) other protein buffer systems (PrH/Pr$^-$), (4) phosphate buffer system ($H_2PO_4^-/HPO_4^{2-}$), and (5) ammonia buffer system (NH_3/NH_4^+).

BICARBONATE BUFFER SYSTEM

Carbon dioxide, generated through aerobic metabolism, slowly combines with water to form carbonic acid, which spontaneously and rapidly deprotonates to form bicarbonate (Fig. 21-2). In this system, the base molecule is bicarbonate, and its weak conjugate acid is carbonic acid. Less than 1% of the dissolved carbon dioxide undergoes this reaction because it is so slow. However, the enzyme carbonic anhydrase, present in the endothelium, erythrocytes, and kidneys, catalyzes this reaction to greatly accelerate the formation of carbonic acid and make this the most important buffering system in the human body when combined with renal control of bicarbonate and pulmonary control of carbon dioxide.

HEMOGLOBIN BUFFER SYSTEM

The hemoglobin protein is the second most important buffering system because of multiple histidine residues. Histidine is an effective buffer from pH 5.7 to 7.7 (pKa 6.8) because it contains multiple protonatable sites on the imidazole side chains. Buffering by hemoglobin depends on the bicarbonate system in order to get the carbon dioxide intracellularly. Carbon dioxide freely diffuses into erythrocytes, where carbonic anhydrase resides. There, it combines with water to form carbonic acid, which rapidly deprotonates. The protons generated are bound up by hemoglobin. The bicarbonate anions are exchanged electroneutrally back into plasma with extracellular chloride (chloride or Hamburger shift) (Fig. 21-3). At the lungs, the reverse process occurs.

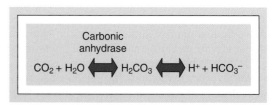

$$CO_2 + H_2O \xrightleftharpoons[\text{Carbonic anhydrase}]{} H_2CO_3 \xrightleftharpoons{} H^+ + HCO_3^-$$

Figure 21-2 Hydration of carbon dioxide results in carbonic acid, which dissociates into bicarbonate and hydrogen ions.

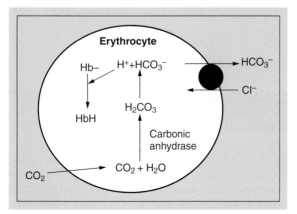

Figure 21-3 Hemoglobin buffering system: Carbon dioxide freely diffuses into erythrocytes, where it combines with water to form carbonic acid, which rapidly deprotonates. The protons generated are bound up by hemoglobin. The bicarbonate anions are exchanged back into plasma with chloride.

Chloride ions move out of the red blood cells as bicarbonate enters for conversion back to carbon dioxide. The carbon dioxide is released back into plasma and is eliminated by the lungs. This process allows a large fraction of extrapulmonary carbon dioxide to be transported back to the lungs as plasma bicarbonate.

Oxygenated and deoxygenated hemoglobin have different affinities for hydrogen ions and carbon dioxide. Deoxyhemoglobin takes up more hydrogen ions, which shifts the carbon dioxide/bicarbonate equilibrium to produce more bicarbonate and facilitates removal of carbon dioxide from peripheral tissues for release into the lungs. Oxyhemoglobin favors the release of hydrogen ions and shifts the equilibrium to more carbon dioxide formation. At physiologic pH, a small amount of carbon dioxide is also carried as carbaminohemoglobin. Deoxyhemoglobin has a greater affinity (3.5 times) for carbon dioxide, so venous blood carries more carbon dioxide than arterial blood. These two mechanisms combine to account for the difference in carbon dioxide content of arterial versus venous plasma (25.6 mmol/L vs. 27.7 mmol/L, respectively) (Haldane effect).

Ventilatory Response

Central chemoreceptors lie on the anterolateral surface of the medulla and respond to changes in cerebrospinal fluid pH. Carbon dioxide diffuses across the blood-brain barrier to elevate cerebrospinal fluid (CSF) hydrogen ion concentration, which activates the chemoreceptors and increases alveolar ventilation. The relationship between $Paco_2$ and minute ventilation is almost linear except at very high arterial $Paco_2$, when carbon dioxide narcosis develops, and at very low arterial $Paco_2$, when the apneic threshold is reached. There is a very wide variation in individual $Paco_2$/ventilation response curves, but minute ventilation generally increases 1 to 4 L/min for every 1 mm Hg increase in $Paco_2$. Under anesthesia, spontaneous ventilation will cease when the $Paco_2$ decreases to less than below the apneic threshold, whereas in the awake patient, cortical influences prevent apnea, so the apneic threshold is not ordinarily observed.

Peripheral chemoreceptors are at the bifurcation of the common carotid arteries and surrounding the aortic arch. The carotid bodies are the principal peripheral chemoreceptors, and are sensitive to changes in Pao_2, $Paco_2$, pH, and arterial perfusion pressure. They communicate with the central respiratory centers via the glossopharyngeal nerves. Unlike the central chemoreceptors, which are more sensitive to hydrogen ions, the carotid bodies are most sensitive to Pao_2. Bilateral carotid endarterectomies abolish the peripheral chemoreceptor response, and patients have almost no hypoxic ventilatory drive.

The stimulus from central and peripheral chemoreceptors to either increase or decrease alveolar ventilation diminishes as the pH approaches 7.4 such that complete correction or overcorrection is not possible. The pulmonary response to metabolic alkalosis is usually less than the response to metabolic acidosis. The reason is because progressive hypoventilation results in hypoxemia when breathing room air. Hypoxia activates oxygen-sensitive chemoreceptors and limits the compensatory decrease in minute ventilation. Because of this, the $Paco_2$ usually does not rise above 55 mm Hg in response to metabolic alkalosis for patients not receiving oxygen supplementation.

Renal Response

Renal effects are slower in onset and may not be maximal for up to 5 days. The response occurs via three mechanisms: (1) reabsorption of the filtered HCO_3^-, (2) excretion of titratable acids, and (3) production of ammonia (Fig. 21-4).[3] Carbon dioxide combines with water in the renal tubular cell. With the help of carbonic anhydrase, the bicarbonate produced enters the bloodstream while the hydrogen ion is exchanged with sodium and is released into the renal tubule. There, H^+ combines with filtered bicarbonate and dissociates into carbon dioxide and water with help from carbonic anhydrase located in the luminal brush border, and the carbon dioxide diffuses back into the renal tubular cell. The proximal tubule reabsorbs 80% to 90% of the bicarbonate, while the distal tubule takes care of the remaining 10% to 20%. Once the bicarbonate is reclaimed, further hydrogen ions can combine with HPO_4^{2-} to form HPO_4^-, which is eliminated in the urine. The last important urinary buffer is ammonia. Ammonia is formed from deamination of glutamine. The ammonia passively crosses the cell membrane to enter the tubular fluid. In the tubular fluid, it combines with hydrogen ion to form NH_4^+, which is trapped within the tubule and excreted in the urine. All of these steps

Figure 21-4 Three mechanisms of renal compensation during acidosis to sequester hydrogen ions and reabsorb bicarbonate: (1) reabsorption of the filtered HCO_3^-, (2) excretion of titratable acids, and (3) production of ammonia.

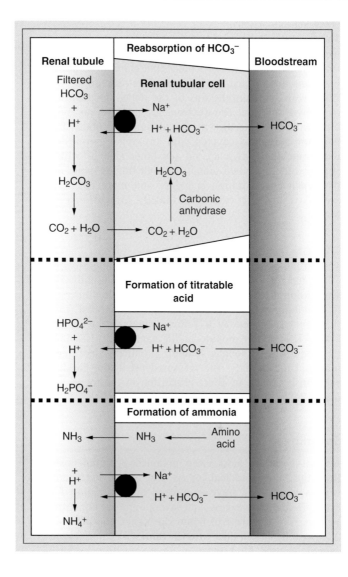

allow for generation and return of bicarbonate into the bloodstream. The large amount of bicarbonate filtered by the kidneys allows for rapid excretion if necessary for compensation during alkalosis. The kidneys are highly effective in protecting the body against alkalosis except in association with sodium deficiency or mineralocorticoid excess.

MEASUREMENT OF ARTERIAL BLOOD GASES

The ability to measure arterial and venous blood gases has revolutionized patient care during anesthesia and in the intensive care unit. Although pulse oximetry and capnography can be monitored continuously

intraoperatively, analysis of arterial blood gases have increased our diagnostic ability and the accuracy of our measurements.

Blood Gas and pH Electrodes

pH ELECTRODE

The pH electrode is a silver/silver chloride electrode encased in a special pH-sensitive glass that contains a buffer solution with a known pH. The electrode is placed in a blood sample and measures changes in voltage. The potential difference generated across the glass and a reference electrode is proportional to the difference in hydrogen ion concentration. Both electrodes must be kept at $37°$ C and calibrated with buffer solutions of known pH.

OXYGEN ELECTRODE

The O_2 electrode is known as the Clark or polarographic electrode.[4] It has a silver/silver chloride reference electrode that is immersed in a potassium chloride solution. Electrons are formed by the oxidation reaction of the silver with the chloride ions of the potassium chloride electrolyte solution. The electrons are then free to combine with O_2 molecules at the platinum cathode. The platinum surface is covered with an oxygen-permeable membrane (polyethylene), on the other side of which is placed the unknown sample. Current flow is increased if oxygen concentration is higher and more electrons are taken up. The current is directly proportional to the Po_2.

CARBON DIOXIDE ELECTRODE

The carbon dioxide sensor was first described by Stow in 1957, and then modified by Bradley and Severinghaus.[5] The carbon dioxide electrode is a pH electrode immersed in a sodium bicarbonate solution and is separated from the blood specimen by a Teflon semipermeable membrane. The carbon dioxide in the sample diffuses into the sodium bicarbonate solution producing hydrogen ions and bicarbonate. The measured pH in the bathing solution is altered in direct proportion to the logarithm of the Pco_2.

Sampling

Arterial blood is most often obtained percutaneously from the radial, brachial, or femoral artery. Peripheral venous blood may serve as a good approximation for Pco_2, pH, and base excess, and save an arterial puncture. Venous Pco_2 is only 4 to 6 mm Hg higher and pH only 0.03 to 0.04 lower than arterial values.[6] Venous blood cannot be used for estimation of oxygenation because venous Po_2 (Pvo_2) is significantly lower than Pao_2. Also, depending on the site of the venous blood draw, differences in tissue metabolic activity may alter Pvo_2.

A heparinized, bubble-free, fresh blood sample is required for blood gas analysis. Heparin is acidic, and excessive amounts of this anticoagulant in the sampling syringe could falsely lower the measured pH. Air bubbles should be removed because equilibration of oxygen and carbon dioxide in the blood with the corresponding partial pressures in the air bubble could influence the measured results. A delay in analysis can lead to oxygen consumption and carbon dioxide generation by the metabolically active white blood cells. Usually this error is small and can be reduced by placing the sample on ice. In some leukemia patients with a markedly elevated white blood cell count, this error can be large and lead to a falsely low Po_2 even though the patient's oxygenation is acceptable. This phenomenon is often referred to as leukocyte larceny.[7]

Temperature Correction

Decreases in temperature decrease the partial pressure of a gas in solution, even though the total gas content does not change. Both Pco_2 and Po_2 decrease during hypothermia, but serum bicarbonate is unchanged. This leads to an increase in pH if the blood could be measured at the patient's temperature. A blood gas with a pH of 7.4 and Pco_2 of 40 mm Hg at 37° C will have a pH of 7.58 and a Pco_2 of 23 mm Hg at 25° C.[8] Unfortunately, all blood gas samples are measured at 37° C, which raises the issue of how to best manage the arterial blood gas (ABG) measurement in hypothermic patients. This has led to two schools of thought: alpha stat and pH stat.

ALPHA STAT

Alpha refers to the protonation state of the imidazole side chain of histidine. The pKa of histidine changes with temperature so that its protonation state is relatively constant regardless of temperature. The term *alpha stat* developed because as the patient's pH was allowed to drift with temperature, the protonation state of the histidine residues remained "static." This concept arose from the observation that "cold-blooded" poikilothermic animals functioned well over a wide range of body temperatures, yet they relied on a similar complement of enzymes as "warm-blooded" homeothermic animals. During cardiopulmonary bypass, an anesthesia provider using alpha stat would manage the patient based on an ABG measured at 37° C and strive to keep that pH at 7.4, while the patient's true pH would be higher.

pH STAT

pH stat is different from alpha stat in that it requires keeping a patient's pH static at 7.4 based on the core temperature (similar to that of a hibernating, homeothermic animal). During cardiopulmonary bypass, an anesthesia provider using pH stat would manage the patient based on an ABG that is corrected for the patient's temperature. With hypothermia, this usually means adding carbon dioxide so that the patient's temperature-correct blood gas has a pH of 7.4. The lower pH and higher Pco_2 maintained during pH stat may improve cerebrovascular perfusion during hypothermia; however, there is still debate about which method provides better outcomes.[9]

Oxygenation

The same physical properties exist for oxygen and hypothermia as for carbon dioxide. Decreases in temperature decrease the partial pressure of a gas in solution, so temperature correction of Po_2 remains relatively important for assessing oxygenation at the extremes of temperature. To be exact, the change in Po_2 with respect to temperature depends on the degree that hemoglobin is saturated with oxygen, but as a guideline, the Po_2 is decreased approximately 6% for every 1° C that the patient's body temperature is below 37° C. P_{O_2} is increased approximately 6% for every 1° C that the body temperature exceeds 37° C.[10]

DIFFERENTIAL DIAGNOSIS OF ACID-BASE DISTURBANCES

Acid-base disturbances are categorized as respiratory or metabolic acidosis (pHa lower than 7.35) or alkalosis (pHa higher than 7.45). These disorders are further stratified into acute versus chronic based on their duration, which is gauged clinically by the patient's compensatory responses. It must be kept in mind that a patient may have a mixed acid-base disorder. The approach to managing acid-base disorders should first involve searching for the causes, rather than an immediate attempt to normalize the pH. Sometimes the treatment may be more detrimental than the original acid-base problem.

Adverse Responses to Acidemia and Alkalemia

Adverse responses can be associated with severe acidemia or alkalemia. Consequences of severe acidosis can occur regardless of whether the acidosis is of respiratory, metabolic, or mixed origin. Acidemia usually leads to decreased myocardial contractility and release of catecholamines. With mild acidosis, the release of catecholamines mitigates the myocardial depression. Permissve hypercapnia, which is used as a protective lung ventilation strategy for acute respiratory distress syndrome (ARDS) patients, has been quite well tolerated. No significant impact on systemic vascular resistance, pulmonary vascular resistance, cardiac output, or systemic oxygen delivery has been seen.[11] With severe acidemia (pH < 7.2), myocardial responsiveness to catecholamines decreases, so myocardial depression and hypotension predominates (Fig. 21-5). Respiratory acidosis may produce more rapid and profound myocardial dysfunction than metabolic acidosis because of the rapid entry of carbon dioxide into the cardiac cell. In the brain, this rapid increase in carbon dioxide can lead to confusion, loss of consciousness, and seizures. This is probably due to an abrupt decrease of intracellular pH, because chronic increases in carbon dioxide as high as 150 mm Hg are typically well tolerated.

Severe alkalemia (pH > 7.6) can lead to decreased cerebral and coronary blood flow due to arteriolar vasoconstriction. The consequences of severe alkalosis are also more prominent with respiratory than with metabolic causes because of the rapid movement of carbon dioxide across cell membranes.[12] Acute hyperventilation can produce confusion, myoclonus, asterixis, depressed consciousness, and seizures.

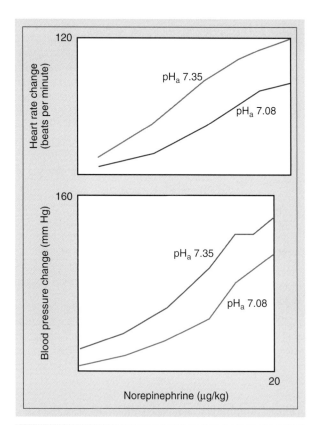

Figure 21-5 Diminished hemodynamic response to intravenously administered norepinephrine in a canine model of lactic acidosis. (From Ford GD, Cline WH, Fleming WW. Am J Physiol 1968;215:1123-1129, used with permission.)

Respiratory Acidosis

Respiratory acidosis occurs when alveolar minute ventilation is inadequate relative to carbon dioxide production (Table 21-1). This can occur with a normal or elevated minute ventilation if carbon dioxide production is increased from sepsis or overfeeding or if there is decreased carbon dioxide elimination from ARDS or obstructive lung disease. Decreased carbon dioxide elimination from a low minute ventilation can occur with volatile or intravenous anesthetics, neuromuscular blocking agents, or neuromuscular disease. The last cause of respiratory acidosis is from increased rebreathing or absorption, found with exhausted soda lime, an incompetent one-way valve, or laparoscopic surgery.

COMPENSATORY RESPONSES AND TREATMENT

Over the course of hours to days the kidneys compensate for the respiratory acidosis by increased hydrogen ion secretion and bicarbonate reabsorption. After a few days, the P_{CO_2} will remain elevated, but the pH will be near normal, which is the hallmark of a chronic respiratory

Table 21-1 Causes of Respiratory Acidosis
Increased production
Malignant hyperthermia
Hyperthyroidism
Sepsis
Overfeeding
Decreased elimination
Intrinsic pulmonary disease (pneumonia, ARDS, fibrosis, edema)
Upper airway obstruction (laryngospasm, foreign body, OSA)
Lower airway obstruction (asthma, COPD)
Chest wall restriction (obesity, scoliosis, burns)
CNS depression (anesthetics, opioids, CNS lesions)
Decreased skeletal muscle strength (residual effects of neuromuscular blocking drugs, myopathy, neuropathy)
Increased rebreathing or absorption
Exhausted soda lime
Incompetent one-way valve
Laparoscopic surgery

ARDS, acute respiratory distress syndrome; CNS, central nervous system; COPD, chronic obstructive pulmonary disease, OSA, obstructive sleep apnea.

Table 21-2 Causes of Respiratory Alkalosis
Increased minute ventilation
Hypoxia (high altitude, low F_{IO_2}, severe anemia)
Iatrogenic (mechanical ventilation)
Anxiety and pain
CNS disease (tumor, infection, trauma)
Fever, sepsis
Drugs (salicylates, progesterone, doxapram)
Liver disease
Pregnancy
Restrictive lung disease
Pulmonary embolism
Decreased production
Hypothermia
Skeletal muscle paralysis

CNS, central nervous system.

acidosis. Respiratory acidosis with a pH less than 7.2 indicates the need for tracheal intubation or increased ventilatory support. In patients with chronic respiratory acidosis, the key is to avoid overventilation. The alkalosis from overventilation and relative hypocapnia can result in central nervous system (CNS) irritability and cardiac ischemia. Also, the kidneys will now start to lose bicarbonate. The increased bicarbonate has allowed the patient to maintain a normal pH with a relatively lower alveolar minute ventilation. Losing the bicarbonate will increase their work of breathing when ventilatory support is decreased, making it difficult to wean from the ventilator.

Respiratory Alkalosis

Respiratory alkalosis occurs when alveolar minute ventilation is increased relative to carbon dioxide production. In a few cases, it can be due to decreased production from hypothermia, or skeletal muscle paralysis can also cause respiratory alkalosis. More often, it is due to increased alveolar minute ventilation from a variety of causes (iatrogenic, CNS disease, liver disease, drugs, or pain) (Table 21-2). $Paco_2$ is diminished relative to bicarbonate levels, resulting in a pH greater than 7.45. The decreased $Paco_2$ and increased pH trigger the peripheral and central chemoreceptors to decrease the stimulus to breathe. During prolonged respiratory alkalosis, active transport of bicarbonate ions out of CSF causes the central chemoreceptors to reset to a lower $Paco_2$ level.

COMPENSATORY RESPONSES AND TREATMENT
Respiratory alkalosis is compensated for by decreased reabsorption of bicarbonate ions from the renal tubules and increased urinary excretion of bicarbonate. Treatment of respiratory alkalosis is directed at correcting the underlying disorder. Mild alkalemia usually does not require treatment. In rare cases, severe acute respiratory alkalosis (pH > 7.6) may require sedation. During general anesthesia, acute respiratory alkalosis is easily remedied by decreasing total minute ventilation.

Metabolic Acidosis

Metabolic acidosis is present when accumulation of any acid in the body other than carbon dioxide results in a pH lower than 7.35 (Table 21-3). An increase in ventilatory elimination of carbon dioxide starts in minutes after

Table 21-3 Causes of Metabolic Acidosis
Anion Gap Acidosis
M methanol, ethylene glycol
U uremia
L lactic acidosis = CHF, sepsis, cyanide toxicity
E ethanol
P paraldehyde
A aspirin, INH
K ketones = starvation, diabetic
Nongap Acidosis
Administration of 0.9% NaCl
GI losses—diarrhea, ileostomy, neobladder, pancreatic fistula
Renal losses—RTA
Drugs—acetazolamide

CHF, congestive heart failure; GI, gastrointestinal; INH, isoniazid; RTA, renal tubular acidosis.

the development of metabolic acidosis to provide a near normal pH. Some patients, however, may not be able to sustain the increased minute ventilation, and require tracheal intubation and mechanical ventilation.

ANION GAP

The best way to categorize the differential diagnosis for a metabolic acidosis is to divide these causes into those that cause and do not cause an anion gap. The anion gap is the difference between measured cations (sodium) and measured anions (chloride and bicarbonate) and represents the concentration of anions in serum that are unaccounted for in this equation (Fig. 21-6). A normal anion gap value is 8 to 12 mEq/L and is mostly composed of anionic serum albumin.[13] A patient with a low serum albumin concentration would likely have a lower anion gap value (each 1.0 g/dL decrease or increase in serum albumin below or above 4.4 g/dL lowers or raises the actual concentration of unmeasured anions by approximately 2.3 to 2.5 mEq/L). An increase in the anion gap occurs when the anion replacing bicarbonate is not one that is routinely measured. The most common unmeasured anions are lactic acid and keto acids. Metabolic acidosis with a normal anion gap occurs when chloride replaces the lost bicarbonate such as with a bicarbonate-wasting process in the kidneys (renal tubular acidosis) or gastrointestinal tract (diarrhea). Aggressive fluid resuscitation with normal saline (>30 mL/kg/hour) will induce a nongap metabolic acidosis secondary to excessive chloride administration, which impairs bicarbonate reabsorption in the kidneys.[14]

STRONG ION DIFFERENCE

A second way to look at categorizing metabolic acidoses is by the strong ion difference (SID) introduced by Peter Stewart in the 1980s.[15] His major tenet is that although serum bicarbonate and base excess can be used to determine the extent of a clinical acid-base disorder, they do not help determine the mechanism of the abnormality. Instead, he proposed that the independent variables responsible for changes in acid-base balance are the strong ion difference (the difference between the completely dissociated cations and anions in plasma) (Fig. 21-7), the plasma concentration of nonvolatile weak acids (ATot), and the arterial carbon dioxide tension (Pa_{CO_2}). The strong ion approach distinguishes six primary acid-base disturbances (strong ion, nonvolatile buffer, or respiratory acidosis and alkalosis) instead of the four primary acid-base disturbances (respiratory or metabolic acidosis and alkalosis) differentiated by the traditional Henderson-Hasselbalch equation. Under normal conditions, the SID is approximately 40 mEq/L. Processes that increase the strong ion difference increase blood pH, whereas processes that reduce it decrease pH. For instance, in the case of massive volume resuscitation with normal saline, the major ions are Na^+ and Cl^-, which gives the fluid an SID of 0. Because infusions of saline would lower the normal SID of 40, this leads to a strong ion acidosis. With the Stewart approach, administering a solution with a high SID, such as sodium bicarbonate or THAM, should treat the resultant strong ion acidosis

The major practical difference between the two theories (Stewart vs. Henderson-Hasselbalch) is the inclusion of the serum albumin concentration in the Stewart approach, which provides some increase in accuracy in certain clinical settings. If changes in serum albumin concentration are accounted for in measurement of the anion gap, the more complex Stewart approach does not appear to offer a clinically significant advantage over the traditional approach to acid-base disturbances.[16]

COMPENSATORY RESPONSES AND TREATMENT

The compensatory responses for a metabolic acidosis include increased alveolar ventilation from carotid body stimulation and renal tubule secretion of hydrogen ions into urine. Chronic metabolic acidosis, as seen with chronic renal failure, is commonly associated with loss of bone mass because buffers present in bone are used to neutralize the nonvolatile acids.

Treatment of metabolic acidosis is based on whether an anion gap is present or not. Intravenous administration of sodium bicarbonate is often given for a nongap metabolic acidosis because the problem is bicarbonate loss. Management of an anion gap metabolic acidosis is guided by diagnosis and treatment of the underlying

$$\text{Anion gap} = [Na^+] - ([Cl^-] + [HCO_3^-])$$

Figure 21-6 Calculation of the anion gap: the difference between the cations and the anions equals the concentration of unmeasured anions in serum.

Figure 21-7 Calculation of the strong ion difference: the difference between the completely dissociated cations and anions in plasma.

$$
\begin{aligned}
SID &= [\text{strong cations}] - [\text{strong anions}] \\
&= [Na^+] + [K^+] + [Ca^{2+}] + [Mg^{2+}] - ([Cl^-] + [SO_4^{2-}] + [\text{organic acids}^-]) \\
&\approx [Na^+] + [K^+] - [Cl^-]
\end{aligned}
$$

cause in order to remove the nonvolatile acids in the circulation. Tissue hypoxia leading to lactic acidosis should be corrected if possible with oxygen, fluid resuscitation, and circulatory support. Diabetic ketoacidosis requires intravenous fluid and insulin therapy. Minute ventilation can be increased in a patient who is mechanically ventilated to compensate until more definitive treatment takes effect. Bicarbonate therapy is more controversial, but may be considered in the setting of extreme metabolic acidosis as a temporizing measure, particularly when a patient is deteriorating. Sodium bicarbonate administration generates carbon dioxide, which unless eliminated by ventilation, can worsen any intracellular and extracellular acidosis.[17] A common approach is to administer a small dose of sodium bicarbonate, and then repeat the pH measurement and monitor hemodynamics to determine the impact of treatment. Newer alkalinizing agents that do not generate carbon dioxide have been developed but have not yet been shown to reduce mortality rate in patients with severe metabolic acidosis. Such agents include Carbicarb, which is equimolar sodium carbonate and sodium bicarbonate, and THAM, which is tris(hydroxymethyl)aminomethane. Alkalinizing agents, because of their osmotic properties, introduce the risk of causing hypervolemia and hypertonicity.

Metabolic Alkalosis

Metabolic alkalosis is present when the pH is higher than 7.45 due to gain of bicarbonate ions or loss of hydrogen ions. The loss of hydrogen ions is usually from the stomach or the kidney. The stimulus for bicarbonate reabsorption or gain is usually from hypovolemia, hypokalemia, or hyperaldosteronism (Table 21-4). In hypovolemia, because of insufficient chloride ions, bicarbonate is reabsorbed with sodium. With the adoption of low tidal volumes (4 to 6 mL/kg) and permissive hypercapnia for ventilatory management of ARDS patients, a compensatory metabolic alkalosis is often a common finding for the critically ill patient.

Table 21-4 Causes of Metabolic Alkalosis
Chloride Responsive
Renal loss—diuretic therapy
GI loss—vomiting, NG suction
Alkali administration—citrate in blood products, acetate in TPN, bicarbonate
Chloride Resistant
Hyperaldosteronism
Refeeding syndrome
Profound hypokalemia

GI, gastrointestinal; NG, nasogastric; TPN, total parenteral nutrition.

COMPENSATORY RESPONSES AND TREATMENT

Compensatory responses for metabolic alkalosis include increased reabsorption of hydrogen ions by renal tubule cells, decreased secretion of hydrogen ions by renal tubule cells, and alveolar hypoventilation. The efficiency of the renal compensatory mechanism is dependent on the presence of cations (sodium, potassium) and chloride. Lack of these ions impairs the ability of the kidneys to excrete excess bicarbonate and results in incomplete renal compensation. Respiratory compensation for pure metabolic alkalosis, in contrast to metabolic acidosis, is never more than 75% complete. As a result, the pH remains increased in patients with primary metabolic alkalosis. Treatment of metabolic alkalosis should be aimed at reducing the acid loss by stopping gastric drainage or fluid repletion with saline and potassium chloride, which allows the kidneys to excrete excess bicarbonate ions. Occasionally, a trial of acetazolamide may be useful in causing a bicarbonaturia. Life-threatening metabolic alkalosis is rarely encountered.

Diagnosis

The diagnosis of an acid-base disorder should occur in a structured fashion. Figure 21-8 shows a stepwise algorithm for blood gas interpretation. Step 1, which determines oxygenation, will be discussed later in this chapter. Step 2 is to determine whether the patient is acidemic (pH < 7.35) or alkalemic (pH > 7.45). Step 3 looks at whether the etiology is from a primary metabolic or respiratory process. Metabolic processes involve a change in bicarbonate concentration from 24 mEq/L, and respiratory processes involve a change in Pco_2 from 40 mm Hg. If the primary process is respiratory in origin, then step 4 is to assess whether the abnormality is chronic or acute (Table 21-5). If a metabolic alkalosis is present, then the next step is to skip to step 7 and determine whether appropriate respiratory compensation is present (Table 21-6). If the measured Pco_2 is more than expected, a concurrent respiratory acidosis is present. If the measured Pco_2 is less than expected, then a concurrent respiratory alkalosis is present. If a metabolic acidosis is present, then an anion gap should be calculated (step 5). If there is a gap, then a $\triangle$gap should be determined. The $\triangle$gap is the excess anion gap (anion gap minus 12) added back to the serum bicarbonate level. If the number is less than 22 mEq/L, then a concurrent nongap metabolic acidosis is present. If the number is more than 26 mEq/L, then a concurrent metabolic alkalosis is present. The last step, step 7, is to determine whether an appropriate respiratory compensation is present for the metabolic acidosis. If measured Pco_2 is greater than calculated from Winter's formula, then the compensation is not adequate and a respiratory acidosis is also present (see Table 21-6). If the measured Pco_2 is less than calculated, then a respiratory alkalosis is present. See sample calculations in Figure 21-9.

Figure 21-8 Seven steps for acid-base diagnosis. Δgap = anion gap − 12 + [HCO₃⁻]. If Δgap is less than 22 mEq/L, then concurrent nongap metabolic acidosis exists. If Δgap is greater than 26 mEq/L, then concurrent metabolic alkalosis exists.

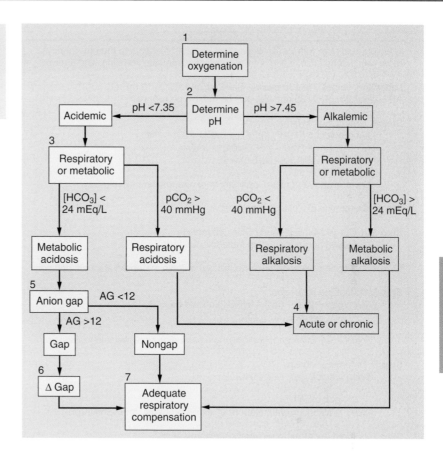

Table 21-5 Determining Whether Respiratory Process Is Acute or Chronic
Acute Process
pH Δ 0.08 for every 10 mm Hg Δ in Pco₂ from 40 mm Hg
Chronic Process
pH Δ 0.03 for every 10 mm Hg Δ in Pco₂ from 40 mm Hg

Table 21-6 Determining Appropriate Compensation in Acid-Base Disorders
Metabolic Acidosis
Winter's formula:
$\quad$ Pco₂ = (1.5 × HCO₃⁻) + 8
If measured Pco₂ > calculated Pco₂, then concurrent respiratory acidosis is present.
If measured Pco₂ < calculated Pco₂, then concurrent respiratory alkalosis is present.
Metabolic Alkalosis
Pco₂ = (0.7 × HCO₃⁻) + 21
If measured Pco₂ > calculated Pco₂, then concurrent respiratory acidosis is present.
If measured Pco₂ < calculated Pco₂, then concurrent respiratory alkalosis is present.

OTHER INFORMATION PROVIDED BY BLOOD GASES AND pH

Aside from acid-base problems, additional measurements and information available from a blood gas include the patient's ability to ventilate and oxygenate and cardiac output estimates.

Ventilation

Paco₂ reflects the adequacy of ventilation for removing carbon dioxide from blood. A measured Paco₂ above 45 mm Hg suggests that a patient is hypoventilating relative to carbon dioxide production, whereas a Paco₂ below 35 mm Hg suggests that a patient is hyperventilating. Increased dead space ventilation markedly decreases the efficiency of ventilation. The Vᴅ/Vᴛ ratio is the fraction of each tidal volume that is involved in dead space ventilation. This value is usually less than 0.3 due to anatomic dead space. When minute ventilation is held constant during anesthesia, the gradient between Paco₂ and end-tidal CO₂ (ETco₂) will increase if dead space is increased (pulmonary embolus or reduced cardiac output).

A 23-year-old man with insulin dependent diabetes presents to the emergency room with somnolence, influenza like symptoms, nausea, vomiting, and anorexia.

Laboratory values: Na 130 mEq/L, Cl 80 mEq/L, HCO_3 10 mEq/L
ABG: pH 7.20, pCO_2 35 mm Hg, pO_2 68 mm Hg on room air

Step 1: Determine oxygenation:

$$\text{A-a gradient} = [(P_B\text{-}P_{H_2O})FIO_2 - PaCO_2/RQ] - PaO_2$$
$$= (150 - PaCO_2/0.8) - PaO_2$$
$$= (150 - 35/0.8) - 68$$
$$= 38$$

There is an A-a gradient, possibly from pneumonia or aspiration.

Step 2: Determine pH: pH <7.4, so acidosis

Step 3: $[HCO_3]$ <24 mEq/L and pCO_2 <40 mm Hg
Primary abnormality is from metabolic acidosis.

Step 4: Not applicable here since we are going down metabolic acidosis pathway.

Step 5: Determine anion gap
$$\text{Anion gap} = [Na] - ([Cl] + [HCO_3]) \text{ should be} <12$$
$$= 130 - (80 + 10)$$
$$= 40 \text{ mEq/L}$$
There is an anion gap, probably from starvation or diabetic ketoacidosis.

Step 6: Determine Δ gap
$$\Delta \text{ gap} = \text{anion gap} - 12 + [HCO_3]$$
$$= 40 - 12 + 10$$
$$= 38 \text{ mEq/L}$$
There is a concurrent metabolic alkalosis probably from vomiting.

Step 7: Is there appropriate respiratory compensation?
$$\text{Winter's formula} = 1.5 [HCO_3] + 8 = \text{expected } pCO_2$$
$$= 1.5 (10) + 8$$
$$= 23 \text{ mm Hg}$$
There is also a respiratory acidosis probably from somnolence.

Figure 21-9 Example for calculating acid-base abnormalities.

Oxygenation

Oxygenation is assessed by measurement of Pa_{O_2}. Arterial hypoxemia may be caused by (1) a low P_{O_2} in the inhaled gases (altitude, accidental occurrence during anesthesia), (2) hypoventilation, or (3) venous admixture with or without decreased mixed venous oxygen content. Acute hypoxia causes activation of the sympathetic nervous system with endogenous catecholamine release, which augments blood pressure and cardiac output despite the vasodilating effects of hypoxemia.[18] The increased cardiac output will increase oxygen delivery from the lungs to peripheral tissues.

ALVEOLAR GAS EQUATION

To judge the efficiency of gas exchange, the alveolar oxygen tension much be calculated first. The alveolar gas equation estimates the partial pressure of alveolar oxygen by accounting for barometric pressure, water vapor pressure, and the inspired oxygen concentration (Fig. 21-10). Atmospheric oxygen is a constant 21% of barometric pressure; however, barometric pressure diminishes with altitude such that the decrease in inspired oxygen can become significant. Hypoventilation leads to increased P_{CO_2}, which encroaches on the space available in the alveolus for oxygen and dilutes the oxygen concentration. The alveolar gas equation estimates this decrease in alveolar oxygen concentration by subtracting an amount equal to the carbon dioxide divided by the respiratory quotient.

ALVEOLAR-ARTERIAL GRADIENT

Calculation of the alveolar-arterial (A-a) gradient provides an estimate of venous admixture as the cause of hypoxia (see Fig. 21-10). Venous admixture refers to deoxygenated venous blood mixing with oxygenated arterial blood through shunting. The A-a gradient formula calculates the difference in oxygen partial pressure between alveolar (Pa_{O_2}) and arterial (Pa_{O_2}) blood. Normally, the A-a gradient is less than 15 mm Hg while breathing room air due to shunting via the thebesian and bronchial veins. Age increases the A-a gradient due to progressive increase in closing capacity relative to functional residual capacity

Figure 21-10 The alveolar gas equation, calculation of alveolar-arterial (A-a) gradient, and estimation of percentage of shunt.

Alveolar gas equation: $P_{A}O_2 = (P_b\text{-}P_{H_2O})FIO_2 - PaCO_2/RQ$

$P_{A}O_2$ = alveolar partial pressure oxygen (mm Hg)
P_b = barometric pressure (760 mm Hg at sea level)
P_{H_2O} = partial pressure of water vapor (47 mm Hg at 37° C)
FIO_2 = fraction inspired oxygen concentration
RQ = respiratory quotient (0.8 for normal diet)

A-a gradient = $P_{A}O_2 - PaO_2$

For patient with PaO_2 of 363 mm Hg and $PaCO_2$ of 40 mm Hg breathing FIO_2 1.0

$$P_{A}O_2 = (760 - 47)(1.0) - 40/0.8$$
$$= (713) - 50$$
$$= 663 \text{ mm Hg}$$

A-a gradient = 663 − 363
= 300 mm Hg

% shunt = 1% for every 20 mm Hg of A-a gradient
= 300/20
= 15%

(FRC). Increased inspired FIO_2 can lead to a larger gradient (up to 60 mm Hg while breathing FIO_2 1.0). Vasodilating drugs (nitroglycerin, nitroprusside, inhaled anesthetics), which inhibit hypoxic pulmonary vasoconstriction and increase $\dot{V}/\dot{Q}$ mismatch, can also increase the A-a gradient.

Larger A-a gradients suggest the presence of pathologic shunting, such as right-to-left intrapulmonary shunts (atelectasis, pneumonia, endobronchial intubation) or intracardiac shunts (congenital heart disease). The A-a gradient provides an assessment of the patient's shunt fraction and is more sensitive than pulse oximetry. A patient may have an SaO_2 of 100% but have a PaO_2 of only 90 mm Hg while breathing 100% oxygen. Significant shunting secondary to a pulmonary or cardiac process has occurred despite the reassuring pulse oximeter reading. In patients with large shunts (>50%), administration of 100% oxygen will be unable to raise PaO_2.

To estimate the amount of shunt present, when PaO_2 is higher than 150 mm Hg, the shunt fraction is approximately 1% of cardiac output for every 20 mm Hg difference in the A-a gradient. Below a PaO_2 of 150 mm Hg or when cardiac output is increased relative to metabolism, this guideline will underestimate the actual amount of venous admixture.

P/F RATIO

The PaO_2/FIO_2 (P/F) ratio is a simple alternative to the A-a gradient to communicate the degree of hypoxia. Standards have been created to define the P/F ratio for acute lung injury (ALI) versus ARDS in order to recruit more homogeneous research subjects. Patients with ALI need to have a P/F ratio below 300, while ARDS patients should have a P/F ratio below 200. A ratio under 200 suggests a shunt fraction greater than 20%.

Cardiac Output Estimates

Normal mixed venous PO_2 ($P\bar{v}O_2$) is 40 mm Hg and is a balance between oxygen delivery and tissue oxygen consumption. A true $P\bar{v}O_2$ should reflect blood from the superior and inferior vena cava and the heart. It is usually obtained from the distal port of an unwedged pulmonary artery (PA) catheter. Owing to the complexity and risks of placing a PA catheter, many clinicians simply follow the trend from a central line placed in the superior vena cava. If tissue oxygen consumption is unchanged, changes in $P\bar{v}O_2$ reflect direct changes in cardiac output. The $P\bar{v}O_2$ will decrease when there is inadequate cardiac output because the peripheral tissues have to increase oxygen extraction for aerobic metabolism. The $P\bar{v}O_2$ will increase when there is high cardiac output (sepsis), peripheral shunting (AV fistulas), or impaired oxygen extraction (cyanide toxicity).

FICK EQUATION

If PaO_2, $P\bar{v}O_2$, and hemoglobin are measured, the cardiac output can then be calculated by using the Fick equation (Fig. 21-11), which states that the delivery of oxygen in the veins must equal the delivery of oxygen in the arteries minus what is consumed (VO_2). The delivery of oxygen is cardiac output multiplied by the amount of oxygen carried in the blood. The total amount of oxygen in the blood is the amount bound to hemoglobin and the amount dissolved in solution. Because the vast majority of the oxygen content in blood is bound to hemoglobin,

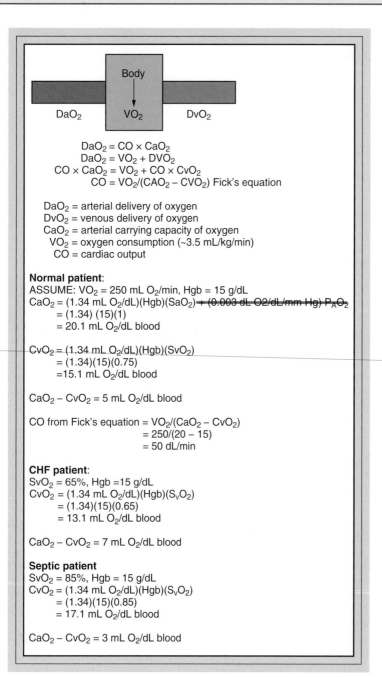

Figure 21-11 Calculation of cardiac output via Fick's equation, arterial and mixed venous oxygen content, and arteriovenous difference in normal, septic, and heart failure patients.

$DaO_2 = CO \times CaO_2$
$DaO_2 = VO_2 + DVO_2$
$CO \times CaO_2 = VO_2 + CO \times CvO_2$
$CO = VO_2/(CAO_2 - CVO_2)$ Fick's equation

DaO_2 = arterial delivery of oxygen
DvO_2 = venous delivery of oxygen
CaO_2 = arterial carrying capacity of oxygen
VO_2 = oxygen consumption (~3.5 mL/kg/min)
CO = cardiac output

Normal patient:
ASSUME: VO_2 = 250 mL O_2/min, Hgb = 15 g/dL
$CaO_2 = (1.34$ mL O_2/dL$)($Hgb$)($SaO_2$) ~~+ (0.003 dL O2/dL/mm Hg) P_AO_2~~
    $= (1.34)(15)(1)$
    $= 20.1$ mL O_2/dL blood

~~$CvO_2 = (1.34$ mL O_2/dL$)($Hgb$)($SvO_2$)~~
    $= (1.34)(15)(0.75)$
    $= 15.1$ mL O_2/dL blood

$CaO_2 - CvO_2 = 5$ mL O_2/dL blood

CO from Fick's equation $= VO_2/(CaO_2 - CvO_2)$
                $= 250/(20 - 15)$
                $= 50$ dL/min

CHF patient:
SvO_2 = 65%, Hgb =15 g/dL
$CvO_2 = (1.34$ mL O_2/dL$)($Hgb$)($S_vO_2$)
    $= (1.34)(15)(0.65)$
    $= 13.1$ mL O_2/dL blood

$CaO_2 - CvO_2 = 7$ mL O_2/dL blood

Septic patient:
SvO_2 = 85%, Hgb = 15 g/dL
$CvO_2 = (1.34$ mL O_2/dL$)($Hgb$)($S_vO_2$)
    $= (1.34)(15)(0.85)$
    $= 17.1$ mL O_2/dL blood

$CaO_2 - CvO_2 = 3$ mL O_2/dL blood

the amount dissolved can often be left out of the equation in order to simplify calculations. The amount dissolved becomes important in situations such as severe anemia, when the amount carried by hemoglobin is low.

ARTERIOVENOUS DIFFERENCE

The difference between the arterial and mixed venous oxygen content (arteriovenous difference) is a good estimate of the adequacy of oxygen delivery (see Fig. 21-11).

The normal arteriovenous difference is 4 to 6 mL/dL of blood. When tissue oxygen consumption is constant, a decreased cardiac output (congestive heart failure) leads to higher oxygen extraction, which increases the arteriovenous difference. An increased cardiac output (sepsis) or lower extraction (cyanide poisoning) leads to a lower arteriovenous difference.

When the delivery of oxygen is first reduced, oxygen consumption remains normal because of the body's ability to increase extraction. With further reductions in oxygen delivery, a critical point is reached when oxygen consumption becomes proportional to delivery. When oxygen consumption becomes supply dependent, cellular hypoxia occurs, which leads to progressive lactic acidosis and eventual death if uncorrected (Fig. 21-12).

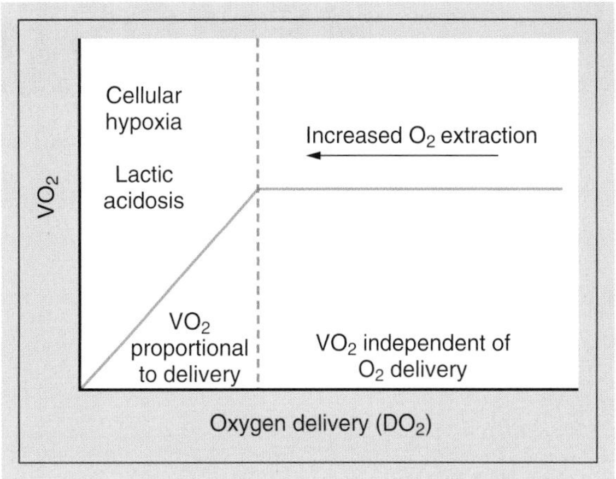

QUESTIONS OF THE DAY

1. What are the two most important physiologic buffer systems in blood? How do they work? In a patient with metabolic alkalosis, what mechanism serves to limit the respiratory compensation?
2. What is the compensatory renal response in a patient with respiratory acidosis? What is the expected time course?
3. What is the strong ion difference (SID)? How does management of acid-base disturbances using the SID differ from the traditional approach?

ACKNOWLEDGMENT

The editors and publisher would like to thank Dr. Joseph F. Cotten for contributing a chapter on this topic to the prior edition of this work. It has served as the foundation for the current chapter.

Figure 21-12 Relationship of oxygen consumption (VO_2) to oxygen delivery (DO_2): when oxygen consumption becomes supply dependent, cellular hypoxia occurs, which leads to progressive lactic acidosis and eventually death.

III

REFERENCES

1. Adrogue HJ, Gennari FJ, Galla JH, et al: Assessing acid-base disorders, *Kidney Int* 76:1239–1247, 2009.
2. Morgan TJ: The Stewart approach—One clinician's perspective, *Clin Biochem Rev* 30:41–54, 2009.
3. McNamara J, Worthley LIG: Acid-base balance: Part 1, physiology, *Crit Care Resusc* 3:181–187, 2001.
4. Clark LC: Monitor and control of blood and tissue O_2 tensions, *Trans Am Soc Artif Intern Organs* 2:41–48, 1956.
5. Severinghaus JW, Bradley AF: Electrodes for blood pO_2 and pCO_2 determination, *J Appl Physiol* 13:515–520, 1958.
6. Williamson DC, Munson ES: Correlation of peripheral venous and arterial blood gas values during general anesthesia, *Anesth Analg* 61:950–952, 1982.
7. Fox MJ, Brody JS, Weintraub LR: Leukocyte larceny: A cause of spurious hypoxemia, *Am J Med* 67:742–746, 1979.

8. Ashwood ER, Kost G, Kenny M: Temperature correction of blood-gas and pH measurements, *Clin Chem* 29:1877–1885, 1983.
9. Piccioni MA, Leirner AA, Auler JO: Comparison of pH-stat versus alpha-stat during hypothermic cardiopulmonary bypass in the prevention and control of acidosis in cardiac surgery, *Artif Organs* 28:347–352, 2004.
10. Ashwood ER, Kost G, Kenny M: Temperature correction of blood-gas and pH measurements, *Clin Chem* 29:1877–1885, 1983.
11. McIntyre RC, Haenel JB, Moore FA, et al: Cardiopulmonary effects of permissive hypercapnia in the management of adult respiratory distress syndrome, *J Trauma* 37:433–438, 1994.
12. Adrogue HJ, Madias NE: Management of life-threatening acid-base disorders, *N Engl J Med* 338:26–34, 1998 107–111.
13. Fidkowski C, Helstrom J: Diagnosing metabolic acidosis in the critically ill:

Bridging the anion gap, Stewart, and base excess methods, *Can J Anaesth* 56:247–256, 2009.
14. Scheingraber S, Rehm M, Schmisch C, et al: Rapid saline infusion produces hyperchloremic acidosis in patients undergoing gynecologic surgery, *Anesthesiology* 90:1265–1270, 1999.
15. Stewart PA: Modern quantitative acid-base chemistry, *Can J Physiol Pharmacol* 61:1444–1461, 1983.
16. Dubin A, Menises MM, Masvicius FD, et al: Comparison of three different methods of evaluation of metabolic acid-base disorders, *Crit Care Med* 35:1254–1270, 2007.
17. Hindman BJ: Sodium bicarbonate in the treatment of subtypes of acute lactic acidosis: Physiologic considerations, *Anesthesiology* 72:1064–1076, 1990.
18. Rose CE, Althous JA, Kaiser DL, et al: Acute hypoxemia and hypercapnia: Increase in plasma catecholamines in conscious dogs, *Am J Physiol* 245: H924–H929, 1983.

22 HEMOSTASIS

Greg Stratmann

Blood coagulation and inflammation are two lifesaving responses to invasion of the vasculature. Although this chapter discusses only coagulation, it is important to recognize that the two processes evolved together and are intimately tied to one another in health and disease. Physiologic coagulation results in hemostasis whereas pathologic coagulation causes thrombosis. Interdependent, often competing physiologic systems in blood and in tissue both maintain intravascular fluidity and isolate, plug, and resolve endovascular interruptions. Trauma, surgery, and hereditary or spontaneous disease may favor one system over others, which can cause either hemorrhage or thrombosis. New therapeutic drugs and perioperative practices have been introduced to prevent or restore hemostatic imbalance to normal, halt hemorrhage, and inhibit thrombosis.

COAGULATION

Mechanisms of Coagulation

Hemostasis requires a rapid response to injury including vascular smooth muscle contraction, platelet activation, and blood coagulation. The coagulation process has traditionally been viewed as a cascading system of sequentially activated enzymes culminating in the generation of cross-linked fibrin. Two separate systems of coagulation were proposed—an intravascular (intrinsic) and an extravascular (extrinsic) system. Activation of either system culminates in a common pathway leading to the generation of thrombin, which converts fibrinogen to fibrin. We have learned that this view of coagulation is not entirely accurate. For example, it appears that the intrinsic pathway is not important in physiologic coagulation despite some of its downstream constituents that are shared by the extrinsic pathway being critical to coagulation. This is based on the observation that with the exception of factor XI, absence of most upstream factors of the intrinsic system causes thrombosis, not bleeding. Even absence of factor XI usually only causes minor bleeding and only in some patients. This illustrates that the separation into the two pathways was an artificial construct of questionable clinical relevance. Coagulation is now understood to be a cell-based process occurring on the surface of tissue factor–bearing (subendothelial) cells and platelets that involves elements of both systems (Fig. 22-1).

Events at the Site of Vascular Injury

At the site of vascular injury, platelets adhere to collagen or von Willebrand factor (vWF) forming an initial platelet plug. At the same time, tissue factor on the surface of perivascular subendothelial cells is exposed to circulating blood. Tissue factor binds with circulating factor VII and forms an active catalytic tissue factor–factor VIIa

complex. This tissue factor–factor VIIa complex rapidly cleaves amino acid sequences from factors IX and X and thereby converts each factor from the inactive to the active form (factor IXa and factor Xa). Factor Xa remains localized and activates factor V to form a factor Xa–factor Va complex (prothrombinase complex) on tissue factor–bearing cells. The prothrombinase complex catalyzes the conversion of small amounts of prothrombin to thrombin. This initial small amount of thrombin is not sufficient to convert fibrinogen to fibrin but serves as a priming mechanism for a second round of the clotting process, which occurs on activated platelets. Thrombin rapidly catalyzes the activation of additional factors, such as factors X, IX, and XI. It also separates factor VIII from vWF and activates it to form factor VIIIa. Importantly, thrombin activates platelets at the site of injury. In contrast to factor Xa, factor IXa does not remain localized to tissue factor–bearing cells. Being the only activated clotting factor that can travel some distance without being immediately inactivated by natural inhibitors of the coagulation system, it binds to the surface of activated platelets where it contributes to the full size thrombin burst.

Role of Activated Platelets

Activated platelets degranulate and release, among others, large amounts of calcium and factors V and VIII that are necessary of efficient coagulation. Factor IXa complexes with factor VIIIa on the surface of activated platelets to form the "tenase" complex. Tenase complexes recruit and activate more factor X from plasma, which is part of the prothrombinase complex. Platelet membrane-bound prothrombinase complexes convert large amounts of plasmatic prothrombin to thrombin. Sufficient thrombin is now formed to generate fibrin from fibrinogen and activate factor XIII to cross-link fibrin monomers. The cross-linked fibrin meshwork shrinks and traps activated platelets and red blood cells to form a strong blood clot.

Physiologic Control of Coagulation

A potent system of checks and balances limiting clot formation is activated as soon as coagulation is initiated. Coagulation is terminated mainly by the action of inhibitor proteins and anticoagulant proteases. The three major categories of regulatory molecules are (1) serine protease inhibitors (serpins), (2) heparins, and (3) anticoagulant proteases.

Serpins are described as (1) antithrombin (once called antithrombin III), (2) heparin cofactor II, (3) α_2-macroglobulins, and (4) tissue factor pathway inhibitor. Antithrombin inhibits thrombin and factors VIIa, IXa, Xa, and XIa. Endogenous heparin found on the endothelial cell surface speeds the action of antithrombin 1000-fold, and this serves to protect normal endothelium from spontaneous

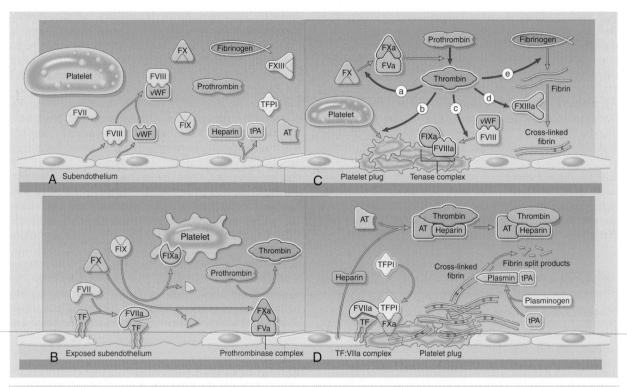

Figure 22-1 A, Normal endothelium. Procoagulants (factors [F] VII, VIII, IX, X, XIII, prothrombin), fibrinogen, and platelets circulate in their inactive forms. Anticoagulants (tissue factor pathway inhibitor [TFPI], heparin, and tissue plasminogen activator [tPA]) actively prevent endothelial spontaneous thrombus formation. **B,** Vascular injury, initial phase. Subendothelial tissue factor (TF) exposed to circulating FVII forms a TF:VII complex. TF:VII activates FIX and FX. FIXa binds to platelets. FXa activates FV to form prothrombinase complex, which converts localized, small amounts of prothrombin to thrombin. **C,** Vascular injury, role of thrombin. Thrombin (a) activates FX and FV to form prothrombinase complexes that generate the secondary thrombin burst, (b) activates platelets, (c) separates FVIII from von Willebrand factor (vWF) and activates FVIII, (d) converts fibrinogen to fibrin, (e) activates factor XI, and (f) activates FXIII, the stabilizer of cross-linked fibrin. Stable clot is formed. **D,** Control of coagulation and fibrin clot dissolution. Antithrombin (AT) binds heparin and potently inhibits thrombin activity. TFPI binds to FXa to inhibit the TF:VIIa complex. Plasminogen is activated to plasmin by tPA and cleaves fibrin into soluble fibrin split products.

thrombus formation and localizes the coagulation process to activated endothelium. α_2-Macroglobulins trap, inactivate, and rapidly clear circulating activated coagulation factors, thereby contributing to systemic control of generalized activation states such as disseminated intravascular coagulation (DIC). Tissue factor pathway inhibitor is a kunin protein that regulates the tissue factor–factor VIIa complex and becomes more potent after binding factor Xa. Thrombomodulin is a membrane protein receptor that binds thrombin and alters the thrombin molecule. Altered thrombin activates protein C. Activated protein C inactivates factor Va and factor VIIIa. Protein S accelerates the action of protein C.

Fibrin Clot Dissolution (Fibrinolysis)

Normally, plasmin circulates in the blood in the inactive plasminogen form, and normal endothelium secretes plasminogen activator inhibitor type 1 to inhibit the activation of plasminogen. When endothelium is activated by injury, tissue plasminogen activator is secreted and plasminogen is activated to plasmin. The plasmin formed is now able to degrade fibrin to soluble products (D-dimers, fibrin degradation products), and these products inhibit thrombin activity. Because tissue plasminogen activator also binds to plasmin's substrate (fibrin), conversion of plasminogen to plasmin remains localized to areas of thrombus. Circulating plasmin, in comparison, is inhibited by a much more powerful (100 times) second inhibitor, α_2-antiplasmin. Generally, surgery and massive trauma induce a hypercoagulable state with elevation of acute-phase reactants that also retard the normal process of fibrinolysis.

Rarely, uncontrolled systemic fibrinolysis is activated in the setting of surgery, cardiopulmonary bypass, or massive trauma by unknown mechanisms. Plasmin activity becomes systemic and degrades both local fibrin and circulating fibrinogen. Systemic antifibrinolytics such as ε-aminocaproic acid and tranexamic acid have been useful in the setting of systemic fibrinolysis.

COMMON LABORATORY TESTS OF HEMOSTASIS (Table 22-1)

Given that any available coagulation test assesses only a very limited aspect of the poorly understood, impeccably timed interplay of cellular and molecular elements leading to hemostasis, it is no surprise that they are not useful in predicting surgical bleeding.[2] The usefulness of routine coagulation tests is mostly to guide heparin and warfarin (Coumadin) therapy.

Tests of Platelet Function

PLATELET COUNT
Platelet levels are quantified by optical or impedance measurements on automated instruments as part of the complete blood count. Even minimal platelet activation, as with a difficult blood draw, can cause platelet clumping and result in artifactually decreased counts on automated analyzers. Most clinical laboratories examine stained blood films for clumping if the platelet count is less than 100,000 cells/μL.

BLEEDING TIME
To calculate the bleeding time, a standardized incision 9 mm long and 1 mm deep is made on the volar surface of the forearm, with backpressure maintained by inflating a blood pressure cuff on the upper part of the arm to 40 mm Hg of pressure. Excess blood is blotted away every 30 seconds with filter paper without disturbing the wound edge. Although this test is the single best predictor of functional platelet disorders, the test must be performed in a standardized controlled setting, is difficult to control, and is often not readily available.

The bleeding time is prolonged with platelet counts less than 100,000 cells/μL with poor predictive values for perioperative bleeding. Scarring at the test site may result.

PLATELET FUNCTION ANALYSIS
The presence of dysfunctional platelet adhesion is assessed with this assay, provided that the hematocrit is greater than 35% and the platelet count is normal. Anticoagulated whole blood is exposed to high-shear flow conditions, and membrane-bound collagen coated with either adenosine diphosphate (ADP) or epinephrine initiates the release of platelet granules and membrane adhesion. The time to instrument aperture occlusion as a result of platelet thrombus formation is measured. Common causes of platelet dysfunction such as uremia, antiplatelet medications, von Willebrand's disease, other hereditary platelet disorders, and post–cardiopulmonary bypass platelet dysfunction can be detected but not distinguished with this test.

PLATELET AGGREGATION STUDIES
Platelet aggregation studies are not performed intraoperatively and are infrequently performed perioperatively. Preoperative evaluation of patients with potential platelet disorders may include measurement of the response of platelets to aggregating agents (collagen, ADP, epinephrine, and ristocetin). Platelet aggregometers measure increasing plasma clarity as platelets aggregate and decrease light scatter. Low ADP concentrations induce a biphasic aggregation pattern. Samples from individuals with Glanzmann's thrombasthenia do not aggregate with ADP, epinephrine, or collagen. Patients with von Willebrand's disease and Bernard-Soulier syndrome have a normal response to epinephrine, collagen, and ADP but do not respond to ristocetin. Aspirin ingestion, uremia, liver disease, and myeloproliferative syndromes can also be differentiated with this test.

Table 22-1 Common Laboratory Tests of Hemostasis and Normal Ranges

Platelet Tests	Coagulation Tests	Fibrinolysis Tests
Platelet count: 140,000-450,000 cells/μL	Prothrombin time: 11.5-14.5 sec*	Thrombin time: 22.1-31.2 sec
Bleeding time: <11 min	Partial thromboplastin time: 24.5-35.2 sec*	Fibrinogen-fibrin degradation products: >5 μg/dL
Platelet function analysis	Thrombin time: 22.1-31.2 sec*	Fibrin D-dimer assay: <250 μg/mL
Collagen/epinephrine: 94-193 sec	Fibrinogen: 175-433 mg/dL	
Collagen/adenosine diphosphate: 71-118 sec	Activated coagulation time: 70-180 sec	
Platelet aggregation (response to aggregating agents: collagen, adenosine diphosphate, epinephrine, and ristocetin)		

*The normal range varies with reagent lots.

Tests of Coagulation

PROTHROMBIN TIME

Citrated plasma is recalcified, and tissue thromboplastin is added to activate factor X in the presence of factor VII. The time until clot formation is measured in seconds. Low levels of factors VII, X, and V, prothrombin, and fibrinogen prolong the PT. Factor VII deficiency is the only cause of a prolonged prothrombin time (PT) with a normal partial thromboplastin time (PTT). The international normalized ratio (INR) standardizes reagent differences between PT results across laboratories and is useful in monitoring oral anticoagulant treatment.

PARTIAL THROMBOPLASTIN TIME

Citrated plasma is recalcified, and phospholipids are added to initiate coagulation. Plasma activators such as kaolin, celite, ellagic acid, or silica speed the reaction by providing the surface for contact activation of factor XII. The time to clot formation is measured in seconds. Low levels of factors VIII, IX, XI, and XII prolong the PTT. Adequate amounts of factor X, factor V, prothrombin, and fibrinogen must also be present. Factor VII is not required for a normal PTT. This test is useful to monitor heparin therapy.

THROMBIN TIME

Citrated plasma is recalcified, and thrombin is added. The time until clot formation is measured in seconds. This test measures thrombin-fibrinogen interaction and is prolonged with low levels of fibrinogen (<100 mg/dL), in the presence of abnormal fibrinogen, and in the presence of circulating anticoagulants such as heparin. The PT and PTT will both be prolonged in all conditions in which the thrombin time is prolonged.

FIBRINOGEN LEVELS

Several types of tests are available to quantify fibrinogen in milligrams per deciliter. Classic methods add thrombin to recalcified plasma to convert all fibrinogen to fibrin and measure the amount of clot protein or the time until clot formation. The amount of fibrinogen is extrapolated. Immunologic methods are useful when dysfibrinogenemia is suspected.

ACTIVATED CLOTTING TIME

The activated clotting time (ACT) measures the amount of time in seconds required for whole blood to clot in a test tube. Finely divided clay (celite or kaolin) shortens the time until clotting and reduces test variability. The ACT is used to monitor heparin therapy in the operating room. Heparin therapy can also be monitored in central laboratories with the PTT.

THROMBOELASTOGRAPHY

Causes of abnormal coagulation are determined by using viscoelastic measures of the time until blood clot formation, consolidation, and lysis in this system. Measures include (1) the time until initial clot formation (r value), which is dependent on the clotting factor concentration and sensitive to anticoagulant medication; (2) the time until clot formation (α-angle), which is dependent on fibrinogen and platelets; (3) the absolute clot strength (maximum amplitude [MA]), for which sufficient platelets and normal platelet aggregation are needed; and (4) the degree of clot lysis (the amplitude 60 minutes after MA or A60), with abnormal A60 being indicative of hyperfibrinolysis or antifibrinolytic therapy. Like other tests operating in low shear stress environments, thromboelastography models venous rather than arterial coagulation. Thromboelastography assesses platelet aggregation but not platelet adhesion, nor the effects of aspirin, uremia, or von Willebrand's disease.

Tests of Fibrinolysis

The plasmin released during fibrinolysis cleaves fibrin and fibrinogen. Decreased amounts of fibrinogen and increased amounts of fibrin degradation products can be found in plasma and can in turn prolong the thrombin time.

FIBRINOPEPTIDES AND FIBRIN MONOMER LEVELS

Thrombin releases two peptides (fibrinopeptides A and B) from fibrinogen to generate a fibrin monomer. Fibrin monomers polymerize and cross-link in the presence of factor XIII. Elevated levels of fibrinopeptide or fibrin monomer suggest intravascular coagulation.

FIBRIN DEGRADATION PRODUCTS

Normally, plasmin degrades fibrin, but excessive plasmin activity also cleaves fibrinogen. Fibrin degradation products cannot clot and interfere with clotting of the remaining fibrinogen. High concentrations of fibrin degradation products also inhibit platelet plug formation. Elevated levels suggest conditions of intravascular fibrin deposition with resultant secondary fibrinolysis, such as DIC.

D-DIMER LEVELS

This monoclonal antibody test measures blood levels of D-dimer fragments that are released when plasmin cleaves cross-linked fibrin. Elevated D-dimer levels are present with fibrinolytic states and in more than 90% of patients with thrombotic or thromboembolic disorders. D-dimer levels are not elevated in primary fibrinolysis because the fibrin is not cross-linked.

DISORDERS ASSOCIATED WITH ALTERED HEMOSTASIS DURING SURGERY

Disorders Favoring Bleeding

Hereditary and acquired coagulation factor and platelet disorders, some systemic diseases, and certain environmental conditions can cause excessive bleeding in the

Table 22-2 Diseases Associated with Altered Hemostasis during Surgery

Increased Incidence of Bleeding	Increased Incidence of Thrombosis	Initiators of Disseminated Intravascular Coagulation
Hereditary coagulation factor deficiency Factors I, II, VII, IX, X, XI, XII	Blood stasis Vascular damage	Crush injury Acute hemolytic transfusion reaction
Hereditary platelet disorders von Willebrand's disease Bernard-Soulier syndrome Glanzmann's thrombasthenia Storage pool disease	Hereditary hypercoagulable states Procoagulant mutations Antithrombin deficiency Protein C deficiency Protein S deficiency	Abruptio placentae Cardiopulmonary bypass Intravascular emboli (fat, air) Sepsis Liver disease
Spontaneous coagulation factor disorders	Anticoagulant mutations	Arterial hypoxemia
Liver disease	Factor V Leiden	Acidosis
Drugs: warfarin	Homocystinemia	Acute pancreatitis
Coagulation factor inhibitors	Mutant factor II or VIII	Immune complex disease
Spontaneous platelet disorders	Factor XII deficiency (rare)	Allergic reactions
Renal disease	Dysfibrinogenemia	Transplant rejection
HELLP syndrome	Increased platelet turnover	Cancer (pancreas, prostate)
Acute immune thrombocytopenia	Prosthetic heart valves	
Drugs	Valvular heart disease	
Heparin, aspirin, nonsteroidal anti-inflammatory drugs, digitalis, thiazide diuretics, abciximab, ethyl alcohol	Spontaneous hypercoagulable states	
Elevated plasma proteins	Antiphospholipid antibody	
Multiple myeloma	Lupus anticoagulant	
Dysproteinurias	Anticardiolipin antibody	
Myeloproliferative disorders		
Hypothermia		

HELLP, *h*emolysis, increased *l*iver function tests, *l*ow *p*latelet count.

operating room. In general, levels of coagulation factors of less than 20% to 30% of normal or platelet counts of less than 50,000 cells/μL are associated with uncontrolled intraoperative bleeding. Severe congenital coagulation factor deficiencies lead to impaired conversion of fibrinogen to fibrin. These diseases typically manifest in early childhood as subcutaneous, intramuscular, and intra-articular hemorrhage after minor trauma. Congenital platelet disorders are associated with mucosal bleeding, epistaxis, prolonged bleeding after dental procedures, and menorrhagia in women (Table 22-2).

Hereditary Coagulation Factor and Platelet Disorders

Hemophilia A (factor VIII deficiency), hemophilia B (Christmas disease or factor IX deficiency), and von Willebrand's disease account for the majority of perioperative bleeding secondary to hereditary diseases (Table 22-3). Of the three diseases, von Willebrand's disease is the most common, with a prevalence as high as 1% to 2% in some populations. The prevalence of hemophilia A is estimated to be 1 per 10,000 persons, with hemophilia B being less frequent (1 per 100,000 persons). Factor XII deficiency is associated with clotting rather than bleeding. Factor VIII and IX deficiencies are inherited on the X chromosome. Factor XI deficiency can be associated with bleeding. The other factor deficiencies are autosomal recessive inherited diseases.

TREATMENT

Deficiencies in both factor VIII and factor IX are treated with specific factor concentrate (recombinant, intermediate purity, or ultrahigh purity) replacement. Mild forms of factor VIII deficiency can be treated with cryoprecipitate and adjuvant therapy as needed. Perioperatively, coagulant

Table 22-3 Coagulation Factor Synthesis and Disorders Associated with Coagulation Factor Deficiencies

Coagulation factors synthesized in the liver	Fibrinogen (factor I); factors II, VII, IX, X; protein C; protein S
Coagulation factors synthesized in endothelial cells	Factor VIII, von Willebrand factor
Coagulation factor with the shortest half-life	Factor VII (3-6 hours)
Vitamin K-dependent factors	Factors II, VII, IX, X
Most common inherited bleeding disorder	von Willebrand's disease
Level of circulating coagulant factor below which bleeding occurs	Plasma levels ≤ 30%
Hemophilia A	Factor VIII deficiency
Hemophilia B (Christmas disease)	Factor IX deficiency

Von Willebrand's Disease

Von Willebrand's disease is the most common cause of unsuspected hereditary bleeding in the operating room. Arterial hemostasis is initiated by platelet adhesion to damaged vessel wall, mediated by vWF or collagen. Synthesized in vascular endothelial cells and megakaryocytes, vWF is stored in platelets and secreted into plasma and the subendothelial matrix, where it mediates platelet adhesion to damaged vessel wall. Furthermore vWF is important in platelet aggregation and protection of factor VIII from inactivation and clearance. When quantitative or qualitative deficits of vWF exist, platelet adhesion, platelet aggregation, and factor VIII levels are insufficient, causing the clinical features of both defective platelet plug formation and defective fibrin formation.

PHENOTYPES

Three phenotypes of von Willebrand's disease are recognized (Table 22-4). Types 1 and 2 are transmitted predominantly as autosomal dominant traits, and type 3, the least frequent and most severe form, is transmitted as an autosomal recessive trait. Type 1 accounts for 60% to 80% of cases and is a mild to moderate quantitative deficiency of vWF, with factor VIII levels being decreased to 5% to 30% of normal. Type 2 accounts for 20% to 30% of cases and is a qualitative vWF deficiency with several subtypes. Type 3 accounts for 1% to 5% of cases and is characterized by very low to undetectable levels of vWF and very low levels of factor VIII. The symptoms of type 3 von

activity is maintained by replacement therapy at 50% to 100% of normal levels until wound healing is complete. Adjuvant therapy consists of the intravenous infusion of desmopressin (DDAVP) and antifibrinolytics. DDAVP (0.3 µg/kg IV) induces the release of stored vWF and factor VIII into plasma. Antifibrinolytics (tranexamic acid, 10 to 15 mg/kg IV every 8 to 12 hours, or ε-aminocaproic acid, 50 to 60 mg/kg IV every 4 to 6 hours) retard clot resolution.

Table 22-4 Classification of von Willebrand's Disease

Type	Characteristic	Frequency	Inheritance	Diagnosis	Treatment
1	Not enough vWF	70-80%	AD	vWF:Ag, vWF:RCo, FVIII	1. DDAVP 2. FVIII/vWF concentrate
2	Qualitative defect of vWF	15-20%	AD		
A	↓ binding of vWF to platelets, ↓ large multimers	Common		vWF:RCo << vWF:Ag (↓ large multimers)	
B	↑ binding of vWF to platelets, ↓ large multimers			RIPA (much less ristocetin required for aggregation)	FVIII/vWF concentrate (DDAVP contraindicated)
M	↓ vWF function despite normal large multimers	Rare		↓ vWF:RCo compared with vWF:Ag	1. FVIII/vWF concentrate 2. DDAVP
N	↓ binding of VWF to FVIII	Rare			1. FVIII/vWF concentrate? 2. DDAVP?
3	Absent vWF	Very rare	AR	vWF:Ag	1. FVIII/vWF concentrate/ rFVIII 2. Platelet concentrate

AD, autosomal dominant; AR, autosomal recessive; FVIII, coagulation factor VIII; rFVIIa, recombinant factor VIIa; RIPA, ristocetin-induced platelet aggregation; vWF, von Willebrand factor; vWF:Ag, von Willebrand factor antigen; vWF:RCo, von Willebrand factor ristocetin cofactor activity; ↓, decreased; ↑, increased; <<, much lower than; ?, uncertain.

Willebrand's disease are similar to those of moderately severe factor VIII deficiency. An abnormal bleeding time (normal in factor VIII deficiency), electrophoresis of von Willebrand antigens, ristocetin cofactor, or platelet function analysis distinguishes between the two diseases.

TREATMENT

Episodes of spontaneous or perioperative bleeding associated with von Willebrand's disease can be treated with DDAVP (with the exception of type 2B), cryoprecipitate (7 to 10 mL/kg IV), or intermediate-purity factor VIII concentrates (Humate-P and Profilate), which contain large amount of vWF. Recombinant or ultrahigh purity factor VIII concentrates is not used because it does not contain vWF. DDAVP is contraindicated for the treatment of type 2B von Willebrand's disease because of transient thrombocytopenia after its administration. It is also not recommended in patients with unstable coronary artery disease because the ultralarge vWF multimers released by DDAVP can aggregate platelets at sites of high fluid shear stress and increase the risk for myocardial infarction.

Spontaneous Coagulation Factor Disorders

Vitamin K deficiency, liver disease, antibody to coagulation factors, and some therapeutic drugs cause acquired coagulation disorders.

VITAMIN K DEFICIENCY

Vitamin K is fat soluble with limited tissue storage. A dietary source or bacterial synthesis of vitamin K in the intestine is needed to make functional factors II, VII, IX, and X, protein C, and protein S. Fasting patients or patients with diseases involving impaired intestinal absorption (obstructive jaundice, sprue, or regional ileitis) are vulnerable to vitamin K deficiency when intestinal bacterial flora is compromised by antibiotic therapy.

LIVER DISEASE

With the exception of factor VIII, plasma clotting factors are synthesized in the liver. Therefore, liver disease that is severe enough to cause decreased synthetic function will lead to decreased factor levels and an increased risk for uncontrolled bleeding. PT is often used as a surrogate test of hepatic synthetic capability. Fibrinolysis is also increased in liver disease as a result of impaired clearance of plasminogen activators and impaired synthesis of fibrinolysis inhibitors. Thrombocytopenia is caused by decreased hepatic production of thrombopoetic factors and splenic platelet sequestration among other pathophysiologic states.[3]

ACQUIRED COAGULATION DEFECTS

Antibodies to coagulation factors develop in some patients with autoimmune disease and occasional hemophiliac patients treated with factor replacement therapy. These antibodies usually act as inhibitors neutralizing factor activity. Clinically, patients will have severe bleeding after minor injury. Less commonly, antibody may bind to factor without neutralizing factor activity but create a deficiency by rapidly clearing antigen-antibody complexes. Factor VIII inhibitors may be present in patients with rheumatoid arthritis or ulcerative colitis and in older persons with no known cause. Patients with factor VIII inhibitors have a prolonged PTT and a normal PT, thrombin time, and bleeding time. Acquired inhibitors to factors VIII, IX, or XI can be associated with significant intraoperative bleeding.

Spontaneous Platelet Disorders

Bleeding as a result of platelet disorders is characterized by a prolonged bleeding time (>11 minutes). Poor platelet function may be due to thrombocytopenia (<100,000 cells/μL) or to qualitative platelet disorders. Both these conditions result in a prolonged bleeding time and abnormal findings on platelet function analysis (see Table 22-1).

THROMBOCYTOPENIA

Thrombocytopenia is caused by either insufficient platelet production or peripheral platelet destruction/sequestration (Table 22-5). Heparin-induced thrombocytopenia occurs in 5% of treated patients and is the most common cause of drug-induced thrombocytopenia and thrombosis. Thrombocytopenia during pregnancy is associated with a spectrum of disorders, including gestational thrombocytopenia, preeclampsia, and pregnancy-associated hypertensive disorders, of which the HELLP syndrome (hemolysis, increased liver function test results, low platelet count) is the most severe form. Normally, a third of peripheral platelets

Table 22-5 Causes of Peripheral Platelet Destruction

Idiopathic antiplatelet antibody formation
Viral infection
Human immunodeficiency virus
Cytomegalovirus
Hepatitis B
Malignancy
Chronic lymphocytic leukemia
Lymphoma
Colon cancer
Collagen vascular disease
Drugs
Heparin
Quinine
Quinidine
Digitoxin
Thiazide
Multiple blood transfusions

sequester in the spleen, with a portion of these platelets released into circulation at times of vascular stress. Splenic sequestration of platelets increases with splenomegaly, and these platelets are not available for release.

QUALITATIVE PLATELET DISORDERS

Despite adequate numbers, poor platelet function increases bleeding risk, prolongs the bleeding time, and variably affects measures of platelet aggregation. Drugs such as alcohol, aspirin, and nonsteroidal anti-inflammatory drugs (NSAIDs) commonly impair platelet function. Impaired platelet granule release is seen in severe uremia. Treatment with transfused platelets is not effective because both the patient's native platelets and the transfused platelets function abnormally. High levels of circulating fibrin-fibrinogen split products inhibit platelet aggregation and thereby lead to impaired hemostatic plug formation. Increased fibrin-fibrinogen split products are present in hepatic failure as a result of decreased clearance of these fibrin split products, in DIC, and with conditions of therapeutically induced fibrinolysis such as treatment with streptokinase or urokinase. High levels of abnormal serum proteins (multiple myeloma, dysproteinemias, or transfused dextran solutions) also inhibit normal platelet function.

Intraoperative Conditions Facilitating Bleeding

Hypothermia, acidosis, and anemia contribute to intraoperative bleeding (see Table 22-2). Hypothermia with temperatures of 34° C or less is associated with poor platelet function and decreased procoagulant activity. The formation and strength of hemostatic plugs are impaired in the presence of low plasma viscosity. Plasma viscosity decreases with increasing anemia. Aggressive intravenous fluid resuscitation can dilute plasma coagulation factors and platelet numbers below amounts needed for effective hemostasis.

DISORDERS FAVORING THROMBOSIS

Hereditary Hypercoagulable States

Inherited deficiency of antithrombin, protein C, or protein S and qualitative abnormalities in factor V (factor V Leiden) or prothrombin (prothrombin 20210) and MTHFR mutation with elevated homocysteine are the commonly recognized conditions leading to intraoperative deep vein thrombosis and pulmonary embolism (see Table 22-2). Individuals with factor V Leiden are resistant to activated protein C and may constitute as many as 4% to 8% of the normal population. Hyperhomocysteinemia (tetramethylhydrofolate reductase deficiency) treated with folate is also associated with hypercoagulability. Hereditary conditions should be suspected in patients with a positive family history, recurrent thromboembolic disease, or

thromboemboli at a young age without predisposing factors or at an unusual site. Optimally, laboratory tests to aid in diagnosis should be performed after resolution of the episode and in the absence of anticoagulation.

Antiphospholipid Syndrome

A heterogeneous and relatively new disease, antiphospholipid syndrome manifests in a variety of arterial and venous macrovascular and microvascular thromboses.[4] The lupus anticoagulant is an example of an antiphospholipid antibody that is present in 5% to 10% of patients with systemic lupus erythematosus. It is also found in patients with other immunologic disorders and after treatment with certain drugs (chlorpromazine, procainamide, quinidine). Laboratory findings consist of a prolonged PTT, normal to slightly prolonged PT, and normal thrombin time, suggesting that a bleeding disorder should be present, when in fact the problem is abnormal clotting or sludging of blood.

Spontaneous Hypercoagulable States

A diverse group of conditions are associated with perioperative thrombosis. Venous thrombosis is associated with venous stasis, hypercoagulable states, and vascular damage. Surgery imposes all three of these predisposing conditions. Venous blood flow is impaired in pregnancy and with abdominal tumors, varicose veins, or conditions involving vascular damage such as vasculitis. Common hypercoagulable states include inflammatory conditions such as sepsis, coronary artery disease, diabetes mellitus, malignancy, nephritic syndrome, prolonged bed rest, and postoperative status. Patients with artificial heart valves, atrial fibrillation, and certain types of valvular heart disease have an increased risk for the development of arterial thrombosis.

Disseminated Intravascular Coagulation: Systemic Bleeding and Thrombosis

DIC is an acquired disorder characterized by uncontrolled intravascular activation of coagulation and fibrinolysis with bleeding and thrombosis. Generalized intravascular thrombin generation and fibrin deposition in small blood vessels lead to the formation of microvascular thrombi. Tissue hypoxia and multiorgan failure follow. Normal regulatory control of thrombin and plasmin is impaired, thereby allowing these proteolytic enzymes to activate and consume circulating coagulation factors, fibrinogen, and platelets.

DIAGNOSIS

DIC should not be thought of as a disease but rather as a syndrome with variable severity and chronicity that is initiated by multiple different stimuli (see Table 22-2).

No single laboratory test definitively identifies DIC. The combination of a decreased platelet count, decreased fibrinogen, prolonged PT and PTT, and elevated fibrin degradation products or D-dimers is present in DIC. Once elevated, D-dimers remain increased for days, thus making serial test measurements more sensitive and specific than single measurements. Both fibrin degradation products and D-dimers are elevated with trauma or recent surgery and with liver and kidney disease. Coagulation test results in patients with severe liver disease may be similar to those in patients with DIC, although D-dimer levels may not be as high and platelet counts may not be as low. Factor VIII activity is helpful in discriminating between these conditions because factor VIII is consumed in DIC and factor VIII levels are normal in liver disease.

TREATMENT

Definitive treatment consists of removing the inciting stimulus when possible. Patients with active bleeding should be supported with platelet, plasma, cryoprecipitate, and red blood cell transfusion as needed. There is no evidence that transfusion of these products worsens DIC. Heparin treatment has little role unless thrombosis is profound.

ANTICOAGULANTS, THROMBOLYTICS, AND ANTIPLATELET DRUGS

Anticoagulants (coumarin derivatives, heparin, low-molecular-weight heparin [LMWH], fondaparinux, direct thrombin inhibitors), antiplatelet drugs (aspirin, ADP receptor antagonists [clopidogrel and ticlopidine], glycoprotein IIb/IIIa [GPIIb/IIIa] antagonists [abciximab, eptifibatide, tirofiban], dipyridamole), and thrombolytics are used for the prevention and treatment of stroke, myocardial infarction, and deep vein thrombosis/pulmonary embolism in many patients undergoing surgery. Perioperative use of these drugs has an impact on the risk-benefit ratio of spinal, epidural, and regional anesthetic techniques. Intraoperative anticoagulation of varying degrees is required during certain operations and procedures, with the anesthesiologist administering, monitoring, and at times reversing the anticoagulant effect.

Coumarin Derivatives

Vitamin K antagonists such as warfarin (Coumadin) inhibit vitamin K epoxide reductase, an intracellular enzyme that recycles vitamin K. Oral warfarin reaches effective plasma concentrations in 90 minutes, with the full anticoagulant effect developing over a period of several days. Several factor half-lives are required to deplete normal factor to the 20% to 30% level needed for effective anticoagulation. Initiation of the anticoagulant and

antithrombotic effects of warfarin depends on the plasma factor VII concentration because factor VII has the shortest half-life (3 to 6 hours). Heparinization during the initial phase of warfarin therapy serves two purposes. Insufficient antithrombotic activity during the time required to lower plasma prothrombin levels and the initial warfarin-induced hypercoagulable state caused by early reductions in the anticoagulant proteins C and S are avoided.

MONITORING

Warfarin effect is monitored in the laboratory by using the PT (INR standardized). Because pharmacokinetic and pharmacodynamic factors vary widely from patient to patient, frequent PT determination is necessary. Warfarin has a very narrow therapeutic window between bleeding and prevention/treatment of thrombosis, and drugs, foods, and alcohol can profoundly alter the pharmacokinetic profile of warfarin. Warfarin is contraindicated in pregnancy because fetal exposure can lead to embryopathy.

Heparin

Heparin is the most commonly used anticoagulant drug in the operating room. It is a highly negatively charged sugar that is extracted from mast cells, pig intestinal mucosa, or bovine lung. Saccharide units of very different size are stripped from the proteoglycan skeleton, which accounts for the large variation in size of unfractionated heparin (5000 to 30,000 kd). Advantages of unfractionated heparin over LMWH or pentasaccharide drugs are its immediate onset, efficacy against thrombin, short half-time of 30 to 60 minutes, and reversibility with protamine, a highly positively charged protein isolated from salmon. The need for close monitoring of heparin therapy reflects its unpredictable pharmacokinetics caused by heparin binding to plasma proteins, macrophages, endothelial cells, and proteins released from activated platelets and endothelial cells.

CLINICAL USES

Heparin is the anticoagulant of choice for cardiac surgery, vascular surgery, and percutaneous interventional procedures such as neuroangiography or ablation of cardiac arrhythmogenic pathways. Full-dose heparin for cardiac surgery is administered as an intravenous bolus of 300 to 400 U/kg. An ACT greater than 400 seconds is usually considered safe for initiation of cardiopulmonary bypass. Protamine at approximately 1 mg to 100 units of heparin is commonly used to reverse the activity of heparin at the conclusion of cardiopulmonary bypass. Most vascular and percutaneous interventional procedures require lower levels of anticoagulation, and intravenous doses of 3000 to 5000 units of heparin are administered to achieve an ACT of twice baseline or less. Protamine reversal of anticoagulation is not usually required. Bolus heparin can cause a moderate decrease in systemic vascular resistance and systemic blood pressure, for unclear reasons.

HEPARIN RESISTANCE

Heparin resistance is present when the usual heparin doses do not result in adequate prolongation of the PTT or ACT. Insufficient antithrombin or excessive heparin-binding proteins (factor VIII, fibrinogen, and other acute-phase proteins) are thought to be the cause. If insufficient anticoagulation persists after the administration of additional heparin, fresh frozen plasma may be used in an attempt to increase antithrombin plasma concentrations.

COMPLICATIONS

The major complications of heparin therapy include heparin-induced thrombocytopenia (HIT) types 1 and 2 and osteopenia (Table 22-6). HIT type 1 is not mediated by immunoglobulin G (IgG), is self-limited, and does not require intervention. HIT type 2 is the most feared non-hemorrhagic complication of heparin treatment and is usually due to antiplatelet factor 4 antibodies causing platelet aggregation. The diagnosis of HIT type 2 is recognized by a decrease in the platelet count to less than 100,000 cells/μL or less than 50% of baseline 5 to 10 days after the initiation of heparin therapy and recovery of the platelet count after discontinuation of heparin. HIT type 2 has a mortality rate of 20% to 30%. Heparin (including heparin flushes or heparin-coated central venous catheters) should be avoided once the diagnosis is suspected and alternative anticoagulants used. Heparin-platelet factor 4 antibody testing confirms the diagnosis.

Low-Molecular-Weight Heparin

LMWH is produced by cleaving heparin into shorter fragments. The pentasaccharide unit binds to and activates antithrombin, but the shorter saccharide units make LMWH ineffective in inhibiting thrombin directly. Instead, the LMWH/antithrombin complex binds to and inactivates factor Xa and indirectly inhibits thrombin production.

LMWH has a delayed onset of 20 to 60 minutes and a longer half-time than heparin and can be administered subcutaneously either once or twice daily. The predictable anticoagulant effect obviates the need for regular monitoring, thus making it a better choice for outpatient therapy, except in some clinical situations (obese patients, patients with renal disease, or neonates) in which anti-factor Xa levels are monitored. Most LMWH preparations are eliminated by the kidneys. LMWH derivatives are not associated with osteopenia and have a much lower risk of heparin-induced thrombocytopenia. Disadvantages of LMWH include less reliable reversal with protamine and increased risk of bleeding during long-term use compared to unfractionated heparin.

Pentasaccharide (Fondaparinux)

Pentasaccharide (fondaparinux) contains only the pentasaccharide unit necessary for binding and activation of antithrombin. Like LMWH the length of the saccharide chain is insufficient for antithrombin to effectively bind and inhibit thrombin. Therefore, antithrombin-mediated anti-Xa activity confers the therapeutic efficacy of pentasaccharide. Its longer half-life as compared with LMWH allows once-daily subcutaneous administration. Like LMWH, therapy does not require laboratory monitoring. Pentasaccharides do not cause HIT. The risk of bleeding during long-term therapy with pentasaccharide exceeds that of LMWH.

Direct Thrombin Inhibitors

Direct thrombin inhibitors are the most important alternative to heparin available. When used perioperatively, direct thrombin inhibitors all share a high risk of bleeding due to inability to reverse the pharmacologic effects. Argatroban and hirudin are licensed for use in patients with heparin-induced thrombocytopenia. Bivalirudin is used for anticoagulation during percutaneous coronary intervention and as an adjunct to thrombolytics in patients with acute myocardial infarction. All three have been used for intraoperative anticoagulation, including

Table 22-6 Heparin-Induced Thrombocytopenia (HIT)	
HIT Type 1	**HIT Type 2**
Not immunoglobulin G-mediated	Immunoglobulin G-mediated
Self-limited	Progressive (mortality rate of 20% to 30%)
Onset 1 to 2 days after the start of heparin	Onset 5 to 10 days after the start of heparin
Platelet count usually >100,000 cells/μL	Platelet count often <100 cells/mL
Incidence: 20% to 25% of heparin-treated patients	Incidence: 1% to 3% of heparin-treated patients
No treatment necessary	Stop heparin therapy and use an alternative anticoagulant Measure platelet factor 4 antibodies Perform serotonin release assay

surgery involving cardiopulmonary bypass. The relatively long half-life of hirudin (2.8 hours) makes this drug a poor choice for intraoperative use. Bivalirudin, with a half-life of 30 minutes, is a more attractive choice. Argatroban, with a half-life of 45 minutes, is an alternative direct thrombin inhibitor in patients with renal insufficiency because argatroban is hepatically eliminated. Argatroban anticoagulation is monitored with either the ACT or PTT. Neither the ACT nor the PTT is reliable for monitoring either bivalirudin or hirudin therapy. Bleeding remains a major concern with the use of direct thrombin inhibitors, including the drugs with a short half-life. To avoid using direct thrombin inhibitors in patients with confirmed antibody-positive HIT type 2, surgeons can delay surgery for 3 months (to allow spontaneous disappearance of antibodies) or use plasmapheresis (for rapid antibody clearance).

Thrombolytics

Thrombolytics are classified as native tissue plasminogen activators, streptokinase and urokinase, or as exogenous tissue plasminogen activator formulations, alteplase and tenecteplase. Native tissue plasminogen activators are potent activators of plasmin and act by cleaving a single bond from plasminogen to form plasmin. Exogenous tissue plasminogen activator formulations are more fibrin-selective, with less selectivity for circulating plasminogen. Tissue plasminogen activators are both thrombolytics and anticoagulants because fibrinolysis generates increased amounts of circulating fibrin degradation products, which inhibit platelet aggregation by binding to platelet surfaces without participating in the process of coagulation. Surgery or puncture of noncompressible vessels is contraindicated within a 10-day period after the use of thrombolytic drugs.

Antiplatelet Drugs

Percutaneous coronary interventions with bare metal or drug-eluting stents have become increasingly popular. Owing to the thrombogenicity of the stents, these procedures require prolonged and combined antiplatelet therapy with obvious implications for the perioperative period. Antiplatelet drugs include cyclooxygenase (COX) inhibitors, thienopyridine derivatives, and platelet GPIIb/IIIa antagonists.

CYCLOOXYGENASE INHIBITORS

COX inhibitors include (1) nonselective inhibitors (aspirin and NSAIDs) and (2) selective agents inhibiting only COX-2. Aspirin irreversibly inhibits COX-1-mediated platelet granule release over the platelet's lifetime. NSAIDs (naproxen, piroxicam, and ibuprofen) reversibly inhibit platelet COX and prevent thromboxane A_2 synthesis. Platelet function normalizes 3 days after discontinuing the use of NSAIDs. Platelet function is not affected by COX-2-specific inhibitors because platelets do not express COX-2.

THIENOPYRIDINE DERIVATIVES

The thienopyridine derivatives ticlopidine and clopidogrel interfere with platelet function by interfering with fibrinogen binding to platelets and thus inhibiting ADP-induced primary and secondary platelet aggregation. Platelet functions normalize 7 days after discontinuing clopidogrel and 14 to 21 days after discontinuing ticlopidine.

GPIIb/IIIa ANTAGONISTS

Available GPIIb/IIIa platelet receptor antagonists include abciximab, eptifibatide, and tirofiban. These drugs are potent inhibitors of platelet aggregation because binding of fibrinogen and vWF to platelet GPIIb/IIIa receptors is blocked. Platelet aggregation normalizes 8 hours after discontinuing eptifibatide and tirofiban and 24 to 48 hours after discontinuing abciximab.

AN APPROACH TO PATIENTS WHO ARE ANTICOAGULATED

Patients who are chronically anticoagulated present a particular challenge in the perioperative setting. Therapeutic levels of warfarin can result in excessive bleeding, and reversing the action of warfarin is associated with perioperative thromboembolism. The risk for a thrombotic complication after stopping warfarin therapy depends on the surgical procedure, the original indication for warfarin therapy, and the degree of the rebound hypercoagulable state associated with warfarin cessation. A multidisciplinary discussion probably ought to take place a few weeks prior to elective surgery.

Cardiothoracic and major abdominal surgeries have the highest risk for venous thrombosis after warfarin reversal. Figure 22-2 shows the relationship between indications for warfarin therapy and risk of perioperative thrombosis as well as the therapeutic consequences for the anesthesiologist.

High Risk for Thrombosis

PREOPERATIVE HEPARINIZATION

In patients with a high perioperative thrombotic risk, preoperative therapeutic heparinization, either with intravenous unfractionated heparin or with LMWH, is indicated as a bridge between discontinuation of oral anticoagulation therapy and surgery. Intravenous heparin should be discontinued 6 hours before the surgical procedure, and the last dose of LMWH should be given 12 hours before the procedure. Heparin should not be restarted until 12 hours after the surgical procedure, even in high-risk patients, because the risk for severe hemorrhage is significant. Preoperative heparinization is avoided in patients with a high likelihood of perioperative bleeding, such as elderly patients or those with known risk factors

III

(thrombocytopenia, concurrent aspirin or NSAID therapy, recent history of bleeding in the gastrointestinal, genitourinary, or central nervous system) (see Fig. 22-2).

POSTOPERATIVE HEPARINIZATION

When restarted postoperatively, intravenous heparin is initiated at the maintenance dose, with a loading dose omitted, and is discontinued when the warfarin-induced INR is greater than 2.0 for more than 24 hours. In high-risk patients a more careful approach is to continue heparin for a full 5 days. Therapeutic doses of LMWH and fondaparinux are at least as effective as full-dose unfractionated heparin and allow subcutaneous administration without laboratory monitoring. This is an advantage in patients who can be discharged within 5 days of surgery because it allows reinitiation of warfarin therapy to be accomplished as an outpatient (see Fig. 22-2).

Intermediate or Low Risk for Thrombosis

Patients at intermediate or low risk for perioperative thrombosis require only postoperative pharmacologic therapy. In patients at low risk, prophylactic subcutaneous unfractionated heparin, LMWH, or fondaparinux is probably all that is required to supplement physical means of deep vein thrombosis prophylaxis (pneumatic compression devices, early ambulation) while anticoagulation is reestablished. It is unclear whether prophylactic or therapeutic dosing of these drugs is more appropriate for patients at intermediate risk (see Fig. 22-2).

Restoration of Vitamin K Activity

In emergency circumstances, vitamin K activity can be restored by the transfusion of fresh frozen plasma (10 to 15 mL/kg IV). Prothrombin complex concentrate (25 to 50 IU/kg), a highly thrombogenic factor IX concentrate that contains variable concentrations of vitamin K–dependent coagulation factors, is also effective. The risk-benefit ratio of treatment with prothrombin complex, however, must be considered when the risk for perioperative thrombosis is high. Although vitamin K–dependent coagulation factors are quickly restored with these products, the factor half-life is only 4 to 6 hours, thus necessitating the concomitant oral administration of vitamin K (1 mg). Intravenous administration of vitamin K carries a higher risk of anaphylaxis. Larger doses of vitamin K should be avoided because of postoperative warfarin resistance.

AN APPROACH TO PATIENTS RECEIVING ANTIPLATELET THERAPY

Percutaneous coronary interventions are commonly performed these days and require antiplatelet therapy for 4 weeks to 12 months, depending on whether a bare metal stent or a drug-eluting stent has been inserted.[5] Drug-eluting stents effectively retard intimal hyperplasia but also delay formation of an antithrombotic intimal layer, rendering patients with these stents at risk for perioperative heart attacks if antiplatelet drugs are

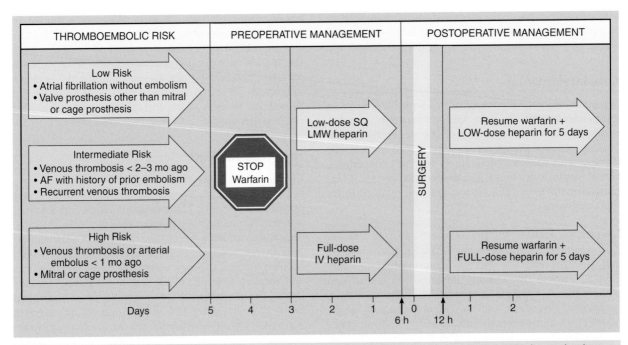

Figure 22-2 Perioperative management of an anticoagulated patient. AF, atrial fibrillation; IV, intravenous; LWM, low molecular weight; SQ, subcutaneous.

Figure 22-3 Perioperative management of a patient on antiplatelet medication. The table within the figure shows the result of the risk assessment of perioperative bleeding versus clotting and the flow diagram is an example of the perioperative management of a patient on aspirin and clopidogrel whose perioperative thrombotic and bleeding risks were considered high. D/C, Discontinue; GpIIb/IIIa, glycoprotein IIb/IIIa antagonist; ICU, intensive care unit; PFA, platelet function analysis; TEG, thromboelastogram; UFH, unfractionated heparin; ?, uncertain.

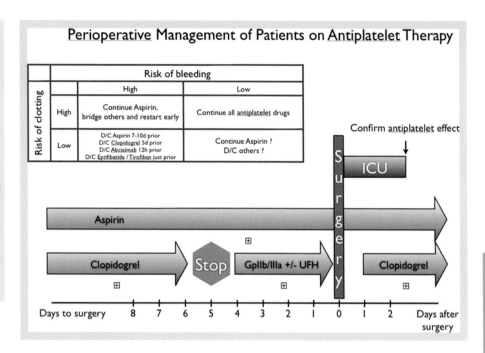

discontinued. If the antiplatelet drugs are continued, the risk of bleeding increases, depending on the surgical procedure. Elective surgery should be delayed until antiplatelet therapy is no longer recommended. For procedures that cannot be delayed, negotiating the balance between risk of bleeding and risk of thrombosis requires a multidisciplinary approach including, but not limited to, cardiology, surgery, anesthesia, and intensive care.[6] A possible approach based on an assessment of this balance is suggested in Figure 22-3. If the risk of bleeding and the risk of thrombosis are both high, this theoretical and unproven approach might include bridging therapy: a switch of a long-acting antiplatelet drug to a short-acting antiplatelet agent possibly in combination with unfractionated heparin. This requires hospitalization, which, given the nature of the surgery is a likely scenario to begin with. After surgery the antiplatelet agents should be restarted as soon as safely possible, ideally in an intensive care unit. Transitioning to the ward requires, among others, confirmation of antiplatelet efficacy and hemostasis. Confirmation of antiplatelet efficacy is achieved by platelet aggregometry or modified thromboelastography.[7]

NEURAXIAL INTERVENTIONS IN PATIENTS BEING TREATED WITH ANTICOAGULANT DRUGS

The introduction of potent antithrombotic drugs to prevent and treat perioperative thrombosis has raised awareness about the risks of bleeding and neurologic injury with neuraxial interventions. Developing definitive recommendations that improve patient safety is complicated by the low incidence of untoward outcomes, including epidural hematoma leading to paralysis. Current consensus conference recommendations on neuraxial anesthesia and anticoagulation by the American Society of Regional Anesthesia are periodically updated as additional information becomes available (Table 22-7).[8]

AN INTRAOPERATIVE APPROACH TO UNCONTROLLED BLEEDING

Laboratory tests (platelet count, PT, PTT, fibrinogen) are indicated to aid in diagnosis and to determine appropriate replacement therapy in the presence of uncontrolled intraoperative bleeding without apparent surgical cause. Estimates of circulating levels of either coagulation factors or platelets based on the estimated blood loss during surgery are often inaccurate but necessary under circumstances in which laboratory testing is not available. In the absence of coagulation test results, fresh frozen plasma is often transfused after blood loss equivalent to one blood volume, and platelets are transfused after blood loss equivalent to two blood volumes.

Coagulation Factor Deficiency

Blood loss caused by a low level of one or more coagulation factors (PT or PTT prolonged to 1.5 times the normal range) is replaced with fresh frozen plasma (10 to 15 mL/kg IV). Platelet counts lower than 50,000 to 80,000 cells/μL

Table 22-7 American Association of Regional Anesthesia Guidelines for Neuraxial Anesthesia in Anticoagulated Patients

Medication	Event	Recommendation(s)*
Antiplatelet Medications	Neuraxial interventions	
Nonsteroidal anti-inflammatory drugs		No contraindication
Aspirin		No contraindication
Ticlopidine		Discontinue 14 days preoperatively
Clopidogrel		Discontinue 7 days preoperatively
GPIIb/IIIa inhibitors		
Abciximab		Discontinue 7 days preoperatively
Eptifibatide		Discontinue 4 to 8 hours preoperatively
Tirofiban		Discontinue 14 days preoperatively
Dipyridamole		Discontinue
Other Agents		
Unfractionated heparin		
Subcutaneous	Neuraxial interventions	No contraindication; measure platelet count if >4 days of heparin treatment
	After intervention	If >4 days of heparin treatment, measure platelet count before removing catheter
Intravenous	Vascular surgery and neuraxial interventions	Avoid in presence of other coagulopathies Delay heparin for 1 hour after catheter placement No restrictions before procedure with dosing every 12 hours; delay if difficult catheter placement is anticipated
	After intervention	Catheter removal 2 to 4 hours after heparin dosing and normal PTT or ACT No mandatory delay if traumatic, but wait 1 hour after catheter removal to administer repeat heparin dose
	Cardiac surgery with full heparinization and neuraxial interventions	No data
Warfarin	Neuraxial interventions	Stop warfarin 4 to 5 days preoperatively Document normal INR before intervention
	After intervention	Remove catheter when INR <1.5
Low-molecular-weight heparin	Neuraxial interventions	Delay 10 to 12 hours after dose Delay 24 hours after traumatic (bloody) tap or with twice-daily dosing
	After intervention	Once-daily dosing: remove catheter 10 to12 hour after last dose and start next dose 2 hours later Twice-daily dosing: remove catheter 2 hours before first dose
Thrombolytics	Neuraxial interventions After intervention	No safety data; avoid for first 10 days if possible Remove catheter when fibrinogen normalizes Frequent neurologic checks (minimize degree of sensory and motor blockade)

*Antiplatelet medications combined with unfractionated heparin, low-molecular-weight heparin, oral anticoagulants, and thrombolytics increase the frequency of bleeding.
ACT, activated clotting time; GPIIb/IIIa, glycoprotein IIb/IIIa; INR, international normalized ratio; PTT, partial thromboplastin time.
Adapted from Horlocker TT, Wedel DJ, Benzon H, et al. Regional anesthesia in the anticoagulated patient: Defining the risks (The Second ASRA Consensus Conference on Neuraxial Anesthesia and Anticoagulation). Reg Anesth Pain Med 2003;28:172-197.

are increased by administering concentrated platelets. One platelet pheresis unit contains a minimum of 6×10^6 cells/μL and generally raises the platelet count by 30,000 to 60,000 cells/μL in a 70-kg patient. Cryoprecipitate (1 concentrate per 10-kg body weight) can be used to augment fibrinogen levels less than 125 mg/dL. Each fresh frozen plasma and platelet pheresis unit has approximately twice the amount of fibrinogen contained in 1 cryoprecipitate concentrate. Cryoprecipitate contains high concentrations of factor VIII and vWF.

Recombinant Factor Concentrates

Although designed and licensed for the treatment of bleeding in hemophilia patients with inhibitors to factor concentrates, prothrombin complex concentrate and recombinant factor VIIa have been found to be useful but expensive treatments of uncontrolled intraoperative bleeding that is unresponsive to replacement of blood components. Prothrombin complex concentrate contains variable concentrations of coagulation factors and may be associated with a high thrombotic risk. Factor VIIa, at doses of 30 to 90 µg/kg, may be effective as rapid rescue treatment of uncontrolled bleeding that is unresponsive to conventional replacement therapy in trauma and surgery. Redosing may be needed after 2 hours if bleeding recurs.

Other Hemostatic Drugs

Other hemostatic drugs useful perioperatively include DDAVP and the antifibrinolytics ε-aminocaproic acid and tranexamic acid. DDAVP (0.3 µg/kg IV) releases vWF from endothelial cells, with maximum effect occurring within 30 to 60 minutes. DDAVP has proved useful for the prevention of bleeding in some forms of von Willebrand's disease and in mild forms of factor VIII deficiency and for bleeding associated with uremia.

QUESTIONS OF THE DAY

1. Abnormally low levels of what coagulation factors lead to a prolonged prothrombin time (PT)?
2. Which coagulation factors are deficient in patients with hemophilia A and hemophilia B? What is the appropriate perioperative management?
3. What laboratory tests can be used to confirm the diagnosis of von Willebrand's disease?
4. What constellation of laboratory abnormalities is consistent with disseminated intravascular coagulation (DIC)?
5. How should the perioperative anticoagulation regimen be managed for a patient receiving chronic anticoagulation with warfarin? Assume the procedure carries a high risk of thrombosis (e.g., total hip replacement).

ACKNOWLEDGEMENT

The editors and publisher would like to thank Drs. Elizabeth Donnegan and Tin-Na Kan for contributing to the chapter on this topic in the prior edition. It has served as the foundation for the chapter.

REFERENCES

1. Roberts HR, Hoffman M, Monroe DM: A cell-based model of thrombin generation, *Semin Thromb Hemost* 32(Suppl 1):32–38, 2006.
2. Watson HG, Greaves M: Can we predict bleeding? *Semin Thromb Hemost* 34:97–103, 2008.
3. Wada H, Usui M, Sakuragawa N: Hemostatic abnormalities and liver diseases, *Semin Thromb Hemost* 34:772–778, 2008.
4. Edwards CJ, Hughes GR: Hughes syndrome (the antiphospholipid syndrome): 25 years old, *Mod Rheumatol* 18:119–124, 2008.
5. O'Riordan JM, Margey RJ, Blake G, et al: Antiplatelet agents in the perioperative period, *Arch Surg* 144:69–76, 2009.
6. Howard-Alpe GM, de Bono J, Hudsmith L, et al: Coronary artery stents and non-cardiac surgery, *Br J Anaesth* 98:560–574, 2007.
7. Agarwal S, Coakley M, Reddy K, et al: Quantifying the effect of antiplatelet therapy: A comparison of the platelet function analyzer (PFA-100) and modified thromboelastography (mTEG) with light transmission platelet aggregometry, *Anesthesiology* 105:676–683, 2006.
8. Horlocker TT, Wedel DJ, Benzon H, et al: Regional anesthesia in the anticoagulated patient: Defining the risks (the second ASRA Consensus Conference on Neuraxial Anesthesia and Anticoagulation), *Reg Anesth Pain Med* 28:172–197, 2003.

III

FLUID MANAGEMENT

Alan David Kaye

The goal of perioperative fluid management is to provide the appropriate amount of parenteral fluid to maintain intravascular volume and cardiac preload, oxygen-carrying capacity, coagulation status, acid-base homeostasis, and electrolyte balance. In addition to surgical considerations (blood loss, evaporative loss, third spacing), certain conditions and changes that occur during the perioperative period can make the management of fluid balance a challenge, including preoperative fluid volume status, preexisting disease states, and the effect of anesthetic drugs on normal physiologic functions. All these factors must be considered when devising a rational approach to fluid management for patients during the perioperative period.

OVERVIEW OF FLUID AND ELECTROLYTE PHYSIOLOGY

Water is the major component of all fluid compartments within the body.[1] Total body water represents approximately 60% of body weight in an average adult. In a 70-kg man, total body water is about 600 mL/kg, or 40 L. The relative percentage of water varies significantly with age, gender, and adiposity. Total body water can be divided into two basic components, intracellular and extracellular. The compartments are separated by water-permeable cell membranes. In the adult, the intracellular fluid volume represents two thirds of total body water, and extracellular fluid volume represents one third. The major components of the extracellular compartment are the blood volume (60 to 65 mL/kg) and the interstitial fluid volume (120 to 165 mL/kg). The plasma volume, representing the noncellular component of blood, is a fraction of the blood volume based on the hematocrit. Typical plasma volume in the adult is 30 to 35 mL/kg. The blood volume is distributed as 15% in the arterial system and 85% in the venous system. Plasma is continuously seeking equilibrium with the interstitial fluid. A major difference between plasma and interstitial fluid

Table 23-1 Daily Loss of Water

Source of Loss	Amount of Loss (mL)	
	Normal Activity and Temperature	*Normal Activity and High Temperature*
Urine	1400	1200
Sweat	100	1400
Feces	100	100
Insensible losses	700	600
Total	**2300**	**3300**

Adapted from Rhoades RA, Tanner GA. Medical Physiology. Boston, Little, Brown, 1995.

Table 23-2 Normal Electrolyte Composition in Body Compartments

Electrolyte	Plasma (mEq/L)	Intracellular Fluid (mEq/L)	Extracellular Fluid (mEq/L)
Sodium	142	10	140
Potassium	4	150	4.5
Magnesium	2	40	2
Calcium	5	1	5
Chloride	103	103	117
Bicarbonate	25	7	28

Adapted from Rhoades RA, Tanner GA. Medical Physiology. Boston, Little, Brown, 1995.

is the much higher concentration of proteins in plasma, resulting in a plasma oncotic pressure 20 mm Hg greater than the interstitial oncotic pressure. This gradient helps maintain the intravascular volume. The sources of daily water loss are listed in Table 23-1. Electrolyte balance is also influenced by parenteral fluid administration. The normal composition of electrolytes in body compartments is listed in Table 23-2. Some patients present for surgery with electrolyte abnormalities related to loss of specific gastrointestinal fluids (Table 23-3). Maintenance

requirements for the adult include daily intake of 1.5 to 2.5 L of water, 50 to 100 mEq sodium and 40 to 80 mEq potassium via entereral or parenteral routes.[2]

PERIOPERATIVE FLUID BALANCE

Physiologic changes in the perioperative period lead to shifts in fluid balance (Table 23-4). The traditional view is that preoperative fasting (NPO) produces an "NPO deficit" equal to the maintenance fluid requirement multiplied by the duration of fasting from fluid intake. However, the insensible and urinary losses during this time may not lead to an actual decrease in the blood volume.[3] In addition, although a patient may have fasted for many hours, the recommended duration of preoperative fasting from clear liquids is only 2 hours. Surgical trauma and inflammation probably create extracellular fluid sequestration into a "third space" not in equilibrium with the interstitial or plasma compartments. In a 2008 review, Chappell and associates question the existence of a third space, and instead consider the fluid shift to occur from the vascular to the interstitial space.[4] Patients undergoing major surgical procedures require intravenous fluid replacement beyond simple blood loss, and the anesthesia provider plays a vital role in assessing and administering appropriate fluid therapy.

FLUID REPLACEMENT SOLUTIONS

There are many crystalloid and colloid solutions that are appropriate for typical adult surgical and obstetric patients (Table 23-5). Because the goals of fluid administration include providing adequate oxygen-carrying capacity and coagulation factors, some patients may require blood product transfusions, which are addressed in Chapter 24.

Crystalloids

Crystalloids are solutions that contain water and electrolytes. They are grouped as balanced, isotonic, hypertonic,

Table 23-3 Volume and Composition of Gastrointestinal Fluids

Fluid Source	24-Hour Volume (mL)	Na$^+$ (mEq/L)	K$^+$ (mEq/L)	Cl$^-$ (mEq/L)	HCO$_3^-$ (mEq/L)
Saliva	500–2000	2–10	20–30	8–18	30
Stomach	1000–2000	60–100	10–20	100–130	0
Pancreas	300–800	135–145	5–10	70–90	95–120
Bile	300–600	135–145	5–10	90–130	30–40
Jejunum	2000–4000	120–140	5–10	90–140	30–40
Ileum	1000–2000	80–150	2–8	45–140	30
Colon	—	60	30	40	—

Table 23-4 Perioperative Shifts in Fluid Balance

Event	Potential Impact	Magnitude
Preoperative fasting	Continued insensible and urinary losses causing hypovolemia	Depends on duration of fasting; may not lead to decreased blood volume
Vasodilation from general or regional anesthetic	Venodilation causing decreased preload	Depends on individual patient and anesthetic drugs administered
Insensible losses from intraoperative surgical exposure	Hypovolemia	Depends on type and duration of exposure
Fluid shift from surgical trauma and inflammation	Can lead to third space fluid accumulation and/or increased interstitial fluid volume	Depends on trauma of surgery and volume of fluid administered
Blood loss	Reduced blood volume, decreased interstitial volume	Depends on amount of blood loss

Table 23-5 Composition of Replacement Fluids

Fluid	Na^+ (mEq/L)	K^+ (mEq/L) (g/L)	Glucose (g/L)	Osm	pH	Other
5% Albumin	145 ± 15	<2.5	0	330	7.4	COP = 32-35 mm Hg
Plasmanate	145 ± 15	<2.0			7.4	COP = 20 mm Hg
10% Dextran 40	0	0	0	255	4.0	
HES 450/0.7	154	0	0	310	5.9	
0.9% NaCl	154	0	0	308	6.0	
Lactated Ringer's	130	4	0	273	6.5	Lactate = 28 mEq/L
5% Dextrose	0	0	50	252	4.5	
D_5LR	130	4	50	525	5.0	
$D_5$0.45% NaCl	77	0	50	406	4.0	
Normosol-R	140	5	0	294	6.6	Mg = 3, acetate = 27, gluconate = 23 mEq/L

COP, colloid oncotic pressure; D_5LR, 5% dextrose in lactated Ringer's solution; $D_5$0.45% NaCl, 5% dextrose in 0.45% NaCl; Osm, osmolarity.

and hypotonic salt solutions. Crystalloid solutions distribute freely within the intravascular and interstitial compartments; therefore, approximately one third of intravenously administered crystalloid remains intravascular.

BALANCED SALT SOLUTIONS
Balanced salt solutions have an electrolyte composition similar to that of extracellular fluid (ECF) (e.g., lactated Ringer's solution, Plasma-Lyte, Normosol). With respect to sodium, they are hypotonic. A buffer is included (e.g., lactate in lactated Ringer's), which is metabolized in vivo to generate bicarbonate. Compared with 0.9% NaCl, these solutions provide small quantities of other electrolytes.

NORMAL SALINE
Normal saline (0.9% NaCl) is slightly hypertonic and contains more chloride than ECF. When used in large volumes, mild hyperchloremic (non-anion gap) metabolic acidosis) results, though the clinical significance may be

limited. Normal saline contains no buffer or other electrolytes. In fact, normal saline is preferred to lactated Ringer's solution (which contains a hypotonic concentration of sodium) when brain injury, hypochloremic metabolic alkalosis, or hyponatremia occurs. Many patients with hyperkalemia, including patients with renal failure, routinely receive normal saline because it contains no potassium. Because it is nearly isotonic, normal saline is an ideal solution for dilution of packed red blood cells (PRBC). Plasma-Lyte is also acceptable for dilution of PRBC, but lactated Ringer's should not be used because of its calcium content.

HYPERTONIC SALT SOLUTIONS
Hypertonic salt solutions are less commonly used, and their sodium concentrations range from 250 to 1200 mEq/L. The greater the sodium concentration, the lower the total volume required for satisfactory resuscitation. This difference reflects the movement due to osmotic

forces of water from the intracellular space into the extracellular space. The reduced volume of water injected may reduce edema formation. This effect could be important in patients predisposed to tissue edema (e.g., prolonged bowel surgery, burns, brain injuries). However, the intravascular half-life of hypertonic solutions is no longer than that for isotonic solutions of an equivalent sodium load. In most studies, sustained plasma volume expansion was achieved only when colloid was present in the resuscitation solution. Moreover, the osmolality of these solutions can cause hemolysis at the point of injection.[5]

FIVE PERCENT DEXTROSE

Five percent dextrose functions as free water, because the dextrose is metabolized. It is iso-osmotic and does not cause the hemolysis that would occur if pure water were injected intravenously. It may be used to correct hypernatremia but is most often used in the prevention of hypoglycemia in diabetic patients who have had insulin administered, or in patients receiving high concentrations of dextrose via total parenteral nutrition immediately prior to surgery.

Colloids

Colloid solutions are composed of large-molecular weight substances that remain in the intravascular space longer than crystalloids. Typically, the initial volume of distribution is equivalent to the plasma volume. For example, the half-life of albumin in the circulation is normally 16 hours, although it can be as short as 2 to 3 hours in pathophysiologic conditions.[6] The synthetic colloids, processed albumin, and protein fractions have minimal or no risks of infection. They are more expensive than crystalloids, but are less expensive and have fewer risks than blood products.

FIVE PERCENT ALBUMIN

Five percent albumin or plasma protein fractions (e.g., Plasmanate) have a colloid osmotic pressure of about 20 mm Hg (i.e., near-normal colloid osmotic pressure). Preparation methods remove viruses and bacteria. Albumin has minimal effects on coagulation.[7]

DEXTRAN

The dextran solutions are water-soluble glucose polymers synthesized from sucrose by certain bacteria. The mean molecular weight of dextran 40 is about 40,000 daltons (40 kDa), and the mean molecular mass of dextran 70 is about 70,000 daltons (70 kDa). A colloid solution of 6% dextran 70 is administered for the same indications as 5% albumin. Dextran 40 is used in vascular surgery to prevent thrombosis but is rarely used as a volume expander. Both dextran solutions are ultimately degraded enzymatically to glucose. Side effects include anaphylactic or anaphylactoid reactions in about 1 in every 3300 administrations, increased bleeding time caused by decreased platelet adhesiveness (at doses of 20 mL/kg/24 hours), rouleaux formation (i.e., interfering with cross-matching of blood), and rare cases of noncardiogenic pulmonary edema thought to be a direct toxic effect on pulmonary capillaries after intravascular absorption.[8,9]

HYDROXYETHYL STARCH

Hydroxyethyl starches (HES) are synthetic colloid solutions that are modifications of natural polysaccharides.[10,11] Like the dextrans, they are characterized by their concentration and average molecular weight. Six percent solutions are isotonic. The average molecular weight can be low (<70 kDa), medium (130 to 270 kDa), or high (>450 kDa). Two other characteristics of HES are important: the molar substitution and C_2 to C_6 ratio. The molar substitution refers to the number of hydroxyethyl residues per 10 glucose subunits. HES preparations with 7 hydroxyethyl residues per 10 glucose subunits (a ratio of 0.7) are called hetastarches. Generally, the higher the molecular weight and molar substitution, the more prolonged the volume effect, but with more potential side effects. The C_2 to C_6 ratio describes the pattern of hydroxyethyl substitution on specific carbon atoms of the HES glucose subunits. HES preparations with higher C_2 to C_6 ratios are more resistant to breakdown by amylase, and have prolonged duration of action without increasing side effects. HES preparations are described by their concentration, average molecular weight, and molar substitution. For example, the first HES product available in the United States, Hespan, is 6% HES 450/0.7. Two other preparations available in the United States include Hextend (6% HES 670/0.7) and Voluven (6% HES 130/0.4). Duration of HES volume expansion ranges from 2 to 5 hours depending on preparation.

The incidence of side effects varies with different HES preparations but includes coagulation disturbances, renal toxicity, and tissue storage. HES interferes with von Willebrand factor, factor VIII, and platelet function. The higher molecular weight HES solutions may have more deleterious hemostatic effects than lower molecular weight solutions. The solvent may also have an impact, as Hespan (dissolved in saline) causes more thromboelastographic changes than Hextend (dissolved in balanced salt solution).[12] The effects of HES on renal function are controversial, with most reports of renal toxicity occurring with the older, high-molecular-weight HES preparations.[11] The primary manifestation of HES tissue storage is pruritus, which can occur in up to 22% of patients.[10]

Crystalloids versus Colloids

Much controversy exists about the role of crystalloids and colloids in fluid therapy, leading to a prolonged "crystalloid versus colloid" debate. Proponents of colloid fluid point out that resuscitation with crystalloid solution dilutes the plasma proteins, with a subsequent reduction of plasma oncotic pressure resulting in fluid filtration from the intravascular to the interstitial compartment, favoring the development of gastrointestinal tract edema. Administration of colloid after acute blood loss (1 mL of colloid solution for each milliliter of blood loss) may lead to more rapid improvement of filling pressures, arterial blood pressure, and heart rate.[13]

Proponents of crystalloid solutions have argued that albumin molecules normally enter the pulmonary interstitial compartment freely and then are cleared through the lymphatic system returning to the systemic circulation. Additional albumin should merely increase the albumin pool cleared by the lymphatics. Isotonic crystalloid solutions are effective plasma volume expanders for resuscitation without the addition of a variety of colloid fluids. The additional cost and potential risks of colloids compared with crystalloids is another argument against colloid administration. There have been many crystalloid versus colloid clinical studies over the years. The largest randomized trial of saline versus albumin fluid resuscitation involved nearly 7000 patients in an intensive care population, and showed no difference in any major outcome.[14] However, a subgroup of patients with traumatic brain injury had increased mortality rate in the albumin resuscitation group.[15] Though the biologic mechanism was not clear, it may be prudent to minimize use of albumin and other colloids in this patient population. Finally, there is also controversy regarding which colloid is superior, a so-called "colloid versus colloid" debate.

PERIOPERATIVE FLUID STRATEGIES

The traditional approach to perioperative fluid management reflects concepts developed over 40 years ago. These guidelines are intended to facilitate initiating therapy, and represent a starting point for patients without other major co-morbidities of vital organs. The choice of fluid and rate of administration must be adjusted to achieve physiologic goals, using careful observation of the patient's response as the basis for ongoing modification.

Routine Maintenance Fluids

Routine maintenance fluids are described for a 25-kg and 90-kg postoperative patient (Table 23-6). These examples are based on the 4-2-1 rule (see Table 23-4), which provides a close approximation of water requirements.

Routine Intraoperative Fluids

Key aspects of the traditional approach include replacement of preoperative deficits, maintenance fluids, third space fluids, insensible loss, and blood loss (Table 23-7). The total fluid requirement is composed of compensatory intravascular volume expansion (CVE), deficit replacement, maintenance fluids, restoration of losses (e.g., blood loss), and substitution for fluid redistribution (i.e., third space fluids):

$$\text{Rate of fluid} = \text{CVE} + \text{Deficit} + \text{Maintenance administration} + \text{Loss} + \text{Third space}$$

COMPENSATORY INTRAVASCULAR VOLUME EXPANSION

Intravascular volume must usually be supplemented to compensate for the venodilation and cardiac depression caused by anesthesia. Increasing cardiac preload by infusing fluid intravascularly to take advantage of the Starling mechanism often returns stroke volume to an

Table 23-6 Calculations of Maintenance Fluid Requirements by the 4-2-1 Rule

Example 1: 25-kg patient, maintenance fluid: 65 mL/hour			
Body Weight (kg)	Fluid Rate (mL/kg)	Weight Category (kg)	Fluid (mL/hr)
0-10	4	10	40
11-20	2	10	20
21+	1	5	5
Total	—	25	65
Example 1: 90-kg patient, maintenance fluid: 130 mL/hour			
Body Weight (kg)	Fluid Rate (mL/kg)	Weight Category (kg)	Fluid (mL/hr)
0-10	4	10	40
11-20	2	10	20
21+	1	70	70
Total	—	90	130

Table 23-7 Fluid Calculations for a Hypothetical Intra-abdominal Surgery with Crystalloid Replacement

Time	Fluid Replacement Component (mL)						
	Compensatory	Deficit	Maintenance	Blood Loss*	Third Space	This Hour[†]	Cumulative[‡]
Preinduction	350	220	110	0	0	680	680
I-S[‖]	—	220	110	0	0	330	1010
First hour[¶]		220	110	300	350	980	1990
Second hour[¶]		220	110	300	350	980	2970
Third hour[¶]		220	110	150	350	830	3800
Fourth hour[¶]		0	110	0	200	310	4110

Key assumptions:
- Patient weight = 70 kg, starting hemoglobin 15 g/dL
- Compensatory volume expansion 5 mL/kg
- Maintenance fluids (by 4-2-1 rule) = 110 mL/hour
- Preoperative deficit = maintenance fluid rate × 10 hours NPO
- Crystalloid fluid replacement for 250 mL blood loss = EBL × 3 = 750 mL
- Third space fluid loss = 5 mg/kg/hour for first 3 hours, 3 mg/kg/hour for last hour of surgery
- Patient was hemodynamically stable throughout case, with satisfactory urine output

*Reflects fluid replacement for blood loss.
[†]Total fluid administered during the hour.
[‡]Grand total since beginning the case.
[‖]Induction until intra-abdominal surgical entry (assumed to be 1 hour).
[¶]Operative time.
EBL, estimated blood loss; I-S, induction until intra-abdominal surgical entry (assumed to be 1 hour); NPO, nil per os (fasted).

acceptable range. Postoperatively, venodilation and myocardial depression rapidly subside when administration of the anesthetic is stopped. Patients with impaired cardiac or renal responses may then become acutely hypervolemic. CVE with 5 to 7 mL/kg of balanced salt solution should occur before or simultaneous with the onset of anesthesia.

FLUID DEFICITS
The fluid deficit equals the maintenance fluid requirement multiplied by the hours since last intake ("NPO deficit") plus unreplaced preoperative external and interstitial/third space losses (e.g., vomiting, diarrhea). When hypovolemia is present, sufficient fluid should be infused to restore mean arterial pressure, heart rate, and filling pressures to near-normal values before induction. If sufficient time is available, restoration of normal urine flow rate is also desirable. The fluid infusion rate for normal patients should then be set to deliver three to four times the maintenance rate until the calculated deficit has been corrected.

The maintenance fluid meets ongoing basal needs for water and electrolytes. The onset of surgical stimulation elicits changes in catecholamines, cortisol, and growth hormone. These tend to reduce insulin secretion or impede its glucose-lowering effect, leading to hyperglycemia. If dextrose-containing solutions are infused at the usual 5% concentration at the rates often required during surgery, severe hyperglycemia will result. Thus, the fluid used for volume maintenance should not contain dextrose.

External losses (e.g., blood, ascites) should be replaced to maintain normal blood volume and normal composition of the ECF volume. Blood loss can be replaced initially with 3 mL of balanced salt solution or 0.9% NaCl for each milliliter of blood loss.

The electrolyte composition of gastrointestinal tract losses is site dependent (see Table 23-3). Most gastrointestinal losses removed at the time of surgery entered the bowel lumen preoperatively and should be considered to be part of the deficit. Evaporation from exposed viscera is entirely water, but the electrolyte is left behind, leading to a need for free water.

Surgical trauma and inflammation can result in extracellular fluid sequestration into a "third space" or the interstitial space. Traditional approaches include replacement with crystalloid at a rate proportional to surgical incision and exposure (e.g., 4 to 6 mL/kg/hour for bowel resection).

Liberal versus Restrictive Fluid Management

The routine intraoperative fluid management strategy described here has been criticized. For example, in pulmonary surgery, the risk of postpneumonectomy pulmonary edema is clearly associated with the amount of administered fluid. As a result, "fluid-conservative" or "dry" fluid strategies are now commonly employed for patients undergoing lung surgery.[16] In addition, "low central venous pressure (CVP)" approaches are used to reduce venous bleeding during liver resection.

Excessive perioperative fluid administration may also lead to edema of the gastrointestinal tract, contributing to ileus. In fact, perioperative fluid restriction can lead to improved outcomes after major elective gastrointestinal surgery.[17] There are several approaches to fluid restriction described, including the following:

- Replacement of blood loss on a "mL per mL" basis with colloid
- No replacement of interstitial/third space loss or urine output during surgery
- No fluid loading prior to epidural analgesia used during general anesthesia
- Administration of colloid bolus for signs of hypovolemia
- Postoperative restriction of fluids with administration of diuretics for weight gain above a certain threshold, e.g., 1 kg

A fluid regimen according to a more restricted approach is represented in Table 23-8. Unfortunately, definitions of "liberal" and "restrictive" fluid regimens are not standardized, and the importance of fluid management depends on the stress of the surgical procedure. For example, liberal fluid administration may be appropriate in a patient undergoing outpatient surgery (risk of postoperative nausea and vomiting may be reduced), but more judicious fluid management may be warranted in a patient undergoing major abdominal or pulmonary surgery.[4]

Monitoring Adequacy of Fluid Replacement

Whether a liberal or restrictive intravenous fluid replacement strategy is used, the anesthesia provider must be prepared to adjust the composition and rate of the fluids administered. Evaluation of intravascular volume status can be challenging, especially if invasive monitors are not being used. Anesthetic drugs can cause hypotension and mask traditional signs of hypovolemia such as tachycardia. Decreased intraoperative urine output does not necessarily indicate hypovolemia. If the surgical blood loss is negligible, serial hemoglobin levels can be followed to assess volume status. With an arterial line in place, analysis of respiratory changes during positive pressure ventilation (e.g., systolic pressure variation) may be useful to predict fluid responsiveness.[18] Finally, use of monitors such as central venous pressure, pulmonary artery pressure, cardiac output, or transesophageal echocardiography may be used to assess volume status and guide perioperative fluid therapy.

In summary, management of fluid therapy may influence intraoperative and postoperative morbidity and mortality rates. Providing sufficient intravascular fluid volume is essential for adequate perfusion of vital organs. Although quantitative considerations are of primary concern, oxygen-carrying capacity, coagulation, and electrolyte and acid-base balance are also of critical importance. Definitive answers regarding the amount of fluid to administer, and the best solution (crystalloid versus colloid) for resuscitation and maintenance do not exist at

Table 23-8 Fluid Calculations for a Hypothetical Intra-abdominal Surgery with "Restricted" Fluid Regimen

Time	Fluid Replacement Component (mL)					
	Deficit	Maintenance	Blood Loss*	Third Space	This Hour[†]	Cumulative[‡]
Preinduction	500	110	0	0	610	610
I-S[‖]	0	110	0	0	110	720
First hour[¶]	0	110	100	0	210	930
Second hour[¶]	0	110	100	0	210	1240
Third hour[¶]	0	110	50	0	160	1400
Fourth hour[¶]	0	110	0	0	110	1510 (includes 250 mL colloid)

Key assumptions:
- Patient weight = 70 kg, starting hemoglobin 15 g/dL
- Maintenance fluids (by 4-2-1 rule) = 110 mL/hour
- Preoperative deficit = 500 mL crystalloid replacement
- Colloid fluid replacement for 250 mL blood loss = EBL = 250 mL
- Third space fluid loss = not replaced
- Patient was hemodynamically stable throughout case, with satisfactory urine output

*Reflects fluid replacement for blood loss.
[†]Total fluid administered during the hour.
[‡]Grand total since beginning the case.
[‖]Induction until intra-abdominal surgical entry (assumed to be 1 hour).
[¶]Operative time.
EBL, estimated blood loss; I-S, induction until intra-abdominal surgical entry (assumed to be 1 hour).

present; sound clinical judgment remains the cornerstone of providing optimal fluid management.

QUESTIONS OF THE DAY

1. What is the normal distribution of total body water in the adult? What is the normal ratio of plasma to interstitial water content?
2. How does intravenous 5% dextrose distribute within the total body water?
3. What are the risks of intravenous dextran administration?
4. What are the most important properties of hydroxyethyl starches with respect to their duration of action and side effects?

5. What are the practical differences between "restrictive" and "liberal" fluid management strategies? What patient populations are most likely to benefit from a restrictive fluid strategy?

ACKNOWLEDGMENT

The editors and publisher would like to thank Dr. Alicia G. Kalamas for contributing a chapter on this topic to the prior edition of this work. It has served as the foundation for the current chapter.

REFERENCES

1. Rhoades RA, Tanner GA: *Medical Physiology*, Boston, 1995, Little, Brown, pp 448–449.
2. Powell-Tuck J, Gosling P, Lobo DN, et al: *British Consensus Guidelines on Intravenous Fluid Therapy for Adult Surgical Patients (GIFTASUP)*, 2008. Retrieved February 28, 2010 from http://www.ics.ac.uk/intensive_care_professional/standards_and_guidelines/british_consensus_guidelines_on_intravenous_fluid_therapy_for_adult_surgical_patients__giftasup__2008.
3. Jacob M, Chappell D, Conzen P, et al: Blood volume is normal after preoperative overnight fasting, *Acta Anaesthesiol Scand* 52:522–529, 2008.
4. Chappell D, Jacob M, Hofmann-Kiefer K, et al: A rational approach to perioperative fluid management, *Anesthesiology* 109:723–740, 2008.
5. Rocha e Silva M, Velasco IT, Portirio MF: Hypertonic saline resuscitation: Saturated salt-dextran solutions are equally effective, but induce hemolysis in dogs, *Crit Care Med* 18:203, 1990.
6. Tuullis JL: Albumin. Background and uses, *JAMA* 237:355, 1977.

7. Boldt J: Use of albumin: An update, *Br J Anaesth* 104:276–284, 2010.
8. Ibister JP, Fisher MM: Adverse effects of plasma volume expanders, *Anaesth Intensive Care* 8:145, 1980.
9. Mangar D, Gerson JI, Constantine RM, et al: Pulmonary edema and coagulopathy due to Hyskon (32% dextran-70) administration, *Anesth Analg* 68:686–687, 1989.
10. Bailey AG, McNaull PP, Jooste E, et al: Perioperative crystalloid and colloid fluid management in children: Where are we and how did we get here? *Anesth Analg* 10:375–390, 2010.
11. Westphal M, James MF, Kozek-Langenecker S, et al: Hydroxyethyl starches: Different products—different effects, *Anesthesiology* 111:187–202, 2009.
12. Martin G, Bennett-Guerrero E, Wakeling H, et al: A prospective, randomized comparison of thromboelastographic coagulation profile in patients receiving lactated Ringer's solution, 6% hetastarch in a balanced-saline vehicle, or 6% hetastarch in saline during major surgery, *J Cardiothorac Vasc Anesth* 16:441–446, 2002.

13. McIlroy DR, Kharasch ED: Acute intravascular volume expansion with rapidly administered crystalloid or colloid in the setting of moderate hypovolemia, *Anesth Analg* 96:1572–1577, 2003.
14. SAFE Study Investigators: Finfer S, Bellomo R, Boyce N, et al: A comparison of albumin and saline for fluid resuscitation in the intensive care unit, *N Engl J Med* 350:2247–2256, 2004.
15. SAFE Study Investigators: Myburgh J, Cooper DJ, Finfer S, et al: Saline or albumin for fluid resuscitation in patients with traumatic brain injury, *N Engl J Med* 357:874–884, 2007.
16. Holte K, Sharrock NE, Kehlet H: Pathophysiology and clinical implications of perioperative fluid excess, *Br J Anaesth* 89:622–632, 2002.
17. Joshi GP: Intraoperative fluid restriction improves outcome after major elective gastrointestinal surgery, *Anesth Analg* 101:601–605, 2005.
18. Magder S: Clinical usefulness of respiratory variations in arterial pressure, *Am J Respir Crit Care Med* 169:151–155, 2004.

III

24 BLOOD THERAPY

Ronald D. Miller

Allogeneic blood transfusions are given for inadequate oxygen-carrying capacity/delivery and correction of coagulation deficits. Blood transfusion can secondarily provide additional intravascular fluid volume. "Practice Guidelines for Perioperative Blood Transfusions and Adjuvant Therapies" provides information and recommendations regarding blood therapy from the American Society of Anesthesiologists.[1]

BLOOD THERAPY PROCEDURES

Determination of the blood types of the recipient and donor is the first step in selecting blood for transfusion therapy. Routine typing of blood is performed to identify the antigens (A, B, Rh) on the membranes of erythrocytes (Table 24-1). Naturally occurring antibodies (anti-B, anti-A) are formed whenever erythrocyte membranes lack A or B antigens (or both). These antibodies are capable of causing rapid intravascular destruction of erythrocytes that contain the corresponding antigens.

Cross-Match

The major cross-match occurs when the donor's erythrocytes are incubated with the recipient's plasma. Incubation of the donor's plasma with the recipient's erythrocytes constitutes a minor cross-match. Agglutination occurs if either the major or minor cross-match is incompatible. The major cross-match also checks for immunoglobulin G antibodies (Kell, Kidd). Type-specific blood means that only the ABO-Rh type has been determined. The chance of a significant hemolytic reaction related to the transfusion of type-specific blood is about 1 in 1000.

Emergency Transfusion

In an emergency situation that requires transfusion before compatibility testing is completed, the most desirable

Table 24-1 Blood Groups: Typing and Cross-Matching

Blood Group	Antigen on Erythrocyte	Plasma Antibodies	Incidence (%) White	Incidence (%) African American
A	A	Anti-B	40	27
B	B	Anti-A	11	20
AB	AB	None	4	4
O	None	Anti-A, anti-B	45	40
Rh	Rh		42	17

approach is to transfuse type-specific, partially cross-matched blood. The donor erythrocytes are mixed with recipient plasma, centrifuged, and observed for macroscopic agglutination. If the time required to complete this examination (should require < 5 minutes) is not acceptable, the second option is to administer type-specific, non–cross-matched blood. The least attractive option is to administer O-negative packed red blood cells. O-negative whole blood is not selected because it may contain high titers of anti-A and anti-B hemolytic antibodies. Even if the patient's blood type becomes known and available, after 2 units of type O-negative packed red blood cells have been transfused, subsequent transfusions should continue with O-negative blood.

Type and Screen

Blood that has been typed and screened has been typed for A, B, and Rh antigens and screened for common antibodies. This approach is used when the scheduled surgical procedure is unlikely to require transfusion of blood (hysterectomy, cholecystectomy) but is one in which blood should be available. Blood typing and screening permit more cost-efficient use of stored blood because the blood is available to more than one patient. The chance of a significant hemolytic reaction related to the use of typed and screened blood is approximately 1 in 10,000 units transfused.

Blood Storage

Blood can be stored in a variety of solutions that contain phosphate, dextrose, and possibly adenine at temperatures of $1°$ C to $6°$ C. Storage time (70% viability of transfused erythrocytes 24 hours after transfusion) is 21 to 35 days, depending on the storage medium. Adenine increases erythrocyte survival by allowing the cells to resynthesize the adenosine triphosphate needed to fuel metabolic reactions. Changes that occur in blood during storage reflect the length of storage and the type of preservative used. For many years, fresher blood (<5 days of storage) has been recommended for critically ill patients in an effort to improve the delivery of oxygen (2,3-diphosphoglycerate [2,3-DPG] concentrations better maintained). More recently, administration of younger blood (i.e., stored < 14 days) has been associated with better outcomes (e.g., decreased mortality rate and fewer postoperative complications, especially with major surgery.[2] The extent to which the clinician must consider the duration of storage as a criterion for selection of a blood product for transfusion is being evaluated by studies funded by the National Institutes of Health.

DECISION TO TRANSFUSE

The decision to transfuse should be based on a combination of (1) monitoring for blood loss, (2) monitoring for inadequate perfusion and oxygenation of vital organs, and (3) monitoring for transfusion indicators, especially the hemoglobin concentration.

Monitoring for Blood Loss

Visual estimation is the simplest technique for quantifying intraoperative blood loss. The estimate is based on blood on sponges and drapes and in suction devices.

Monitoring for Inadequate Perfusion and Oxygenation of Vital Organs

Standard monitors, including those measuring arterial blood pressure, heart rate, urine output, electrocardiogram, and oxygen saturation, are commonly used. Analysis of arterial blood gases, mixed venous oxygen saturation, and echocardiography may be useful in selected patients. Tachycardia is an insensitive and nonspecific indicator of hypovolemia, especially in patients receiving a volatile anesthetic. Maintenance of adequate systemic blood pressure and central venous pressure (6 to 12 mm Hg) suggests adequate intravascular blood volume. Urinary output usually declines during moderate to severe hypovolemia and the resulting tissue hypoperfusion. Arterial pH may decrease only when tissue hypoperfusion becomes severe.

Monitoring for Transfusion Indicators (Especially Hemoglobin Concentration)

The decision to transfuse is based on the risk that anemia poses to an individual patient and the patient's ability to compensate for decreased oxygen-carrying capacity, as well as the inherent risks associated with transfusion. In the past 20 years, a "restrictive" blood policy has been encouraged, that is, "give blood only when absolutely necessary." This "restrictive" approach was based on an appropriate fear of transmitting hepatitis or HIV. However,

Table 24-2 Estimated Risk of Infection Transmitted by Blood Transfusion

Hepatitis B	1 in 220,000
Hepatitis C	1 in 1.6 million
HIV	1 in 1.8 million
HTLV-I	1 in 640,000
West Nile virus	1 in >1 million

HIV, human immunodeficiency virus; HTLV-I, human T-cell lymphotropic virus type I.

transmission of such diseases is now rare (Table 24-2). Blood transfusons, given in response to proper indications, do not increase patient mortality rate.[3,4] Lastly, preoperative anemia should be treated (e.g., with recombinant human erythropoietin and iron); this action decreases not only the need for intraoperative blood transfusions but the overall morbidity and mortality rates.[5] Healthy patients with hemoglobin values more than 10 g/dL rarely require transfusion, whereas those with hemoglobin values less than 6 g/dL almost always require transfusion, especially when anemia or surgical bleeding (or both) is acute and continuing. Determination of whether intermediate hemoglobin concentrations (6 to 10 g/dL) justify or require transfusion should be based on the patient's risk for complications of inadequate oxygenation. For example, certain clinical situations (coronary artery disease, chronic lung disease, surgery associated with large blood loss) may warrant transfusion of blood at a higher hemoglobin value than in otherwise healthy patients. A hemoglobin concentration of 8 g/dL may be an appropriate threshold for transfusion in surgical patients with no risk factors for ischemia, whereas a transfusion threshold of 10 g/dL may be justified in patients who are considered to be at risk (emphysema, coronary artery disease). Controlled studies to determine the hemoglobin concentration at which blood transfusion improves outcome in a surgical patient with acute blood loss are few.

Transfusion of packed red blood cells in patients with hemoglobin concentrations higher than 10 to 12 g/dL does not substantially increase oxygen delivery. Further decreases in the hemoglobin concentration can sometimes be offset by increases in cardiac output. The exact hemoglobin value at which cardiac output increases varies among individuals and is influenced by age, whether the anemia is acute or chronic, and sometimes anesthesia. For example, the cardiovascular response to anemia is decreased in the elderly and by general anesthesia. The focus on hemoglobin has existed for many years and still continues.[6] Furthermore, a new noninvasive spectrophotometric monitor (Masimo SpHb) attached to a finger will allow continuous monitoring of hemoglobin levels.

Whether this monitor presently can be used for transfusion decisions without a laboratory co-oximeter determination is not clear.[7] For sure, this new monitor will provide more opportunity for defining the relationship between hemoglobin levels and transfusion requirements.

BLOOD COMPONENTS

Packed Red Blood Cells

Packed red blood cells (250- to 300-mL volume with a hematocrit of 70% to 80%) are used for treatment of the anemia usually associated with surgical blood loss. The major goal is to increase the oxygen-carrying capacity of blood. Although packed red blood cells can increase intravascular fluid volume, nonblood products, such as crystalloids and colloids, can also achieve that end point. A single unit of packed red blood cells will increase adult hemoglobin concentrations about 1 g/dL. Administration of packed red blood cells can be facilitated by reconstituting them in crystalloid solutions, such as 50 to 100 mL of saline. The use of hypotonic glucose solutions may theoretically cause hemolysis, whereas the calcium present in lactated Ringer's solution may cause clotting if mixed with packed red blood cells.

COMPLICATIONS

Complications associated with packed red blood cells are similar to those of whole blood. An exception would be the chance for development of citrate intoxication, which would be less with packed red blood cells than with whole blood because less citrate is infused. Removal of plasma decreases the concentration of factors I (fibrinogen), V, and VIII as compared with whole blood.

DECISION TO ADMINISTER PACKED RED BLOOD CELLS

The decision to administer packed red blood cells should be based on measured blood loss and inadequate oxygen-carrying capacity.

Acute Blood Loss

Acute blood loss in the range of 1500 to 2000 mL (approximately 30% of an adult patient's blood volume) may exceed the ability of crystalloids to replace blood volume without jeopardizing the oxygen-carrying capacity of the blood. Hypotension and tachycardia are likely, but these compensatory responses may be blunted by anesthesia or other drugs (β-adrenergic blocking drugs). Compensatory vasoconstriction may conceal the signs of acute blood loss until at least 10% of the blood volume is lost, and healthy patients may lose up to 20% of their blood volume before signs of hypovolemia occur. To ensure an adequate oxygen content in blood, packed red blood cells should be administered when blood loss is sufficiently large. Whole blood, when available, is gradually being used more frequently, and this practice decreases the incidence of hypofibrinogenemia and perhaps coagulopathies associated with administration of packed red blood cells.[1] In the Vietnam conflict, fresh whole blood (typed and cross-matched, but not cooled) was quite effective especially with massive transfusion-associated coagulopathies.[8] Almost 40 years later in Iraq, military physicians use fresh whole blood from prescreened "walking donors" which also can treat or prevent thrombocytopenia. In fact, warm fresh whole blood may be more efficacious than stored component therapy when treating critically ill patients requiring massive blood transfusions.[9] Also, whole blood may be preferable to packed red blood cells when replacing blood losses that exceed 30% of the blood volume. Alternatively, specific ratios of red blood cell transfusions with fresh frozen plasma and platelets are being recommended.[10] For example, 1.5 red blood cells with 1.0 units of fresh frozen plasma has been proposed. Then 1.0 platelets for 6 units of red blood cells has been recommended in patients with large blood losses and trauma.[10]

With acute blood loss, interstitial fluid and extravascular protein are transferred to the intravascular space, which tends to maintain plasma volume. For this reason, when crystalloid solutions are used to replace blood loss, they should be given in amounts equal to about three times the amount of blood loss, not only to replenish intravascular fluid volume but also to replenish the fluid lost from interstitial spaces. Albumin and hetastarch are examples of solutions that are useful for acute expansion of the intravascular fluid volume. In contrast to crystalloid solutions, albumin and hetastarch are more likely to remain in the intravascular space for prolonged periods (about 12 hours). These solutions avoid complications associated with blood-containing products but do not improve the oxygen-carrying capacity of the blood and, in large volumes (>20 mL/kg), may cause coagulation defects.

Platelets

Administration of platelets allows specific treatment of thrombocytopenia without the infusion of unnecessary blood components. Platelets are derived from volunteer donors (cytapheresis and plateletpheresis). Pooled platelet concentrates are derived from whole blood donation and can be called "random-donor platelets." During surgery, platelet transfusions are probably not required unless the platelet count is less than 50,000 cells/mm[3] as determined by laboratory analysis or in predetermined ratios with red blood cells as described previously.

COMPLICATIONS

The risks associated with platelet concentrate infusions are (1) sensitization reactions because of human leukocyte antigens on the cell membranes of platelets and (2) transmission of infectious diseases, which is rare.

Table 24-3 Transfusion-Related Fatalities in the United States, 2005-2009

Cause of Fatalities	Number of Fatalities	
	2005-2009	2009 Alone
Transfusion-related acute lung injury	127	13
Hemolytic transfusion reaction (non-ABO)	42	8
Microbial infections	33	5
Hemolytic transfusion reaction	26	4
Anaphylaxis	7	1

Data from the U.S. Food and Drug Administration (2009).

One of the leading causes of transfusion-related fatalities in the United States is bacterial contamination, which is most likely to occur in platelet concentrates (Table 24-3). Platelet-related sepsis can be fatal and occurs as frequently as 1 in 5000 transfusions; it is probably underrecognized because of the many other confounding variables present in critically ill patients. When donor platelets are cultured before infusion, the incidence of sepsis may be significantly reduced but sepsis is still possible. The fact that platelets are stored at 20° C to 24° C instead of 4° C probably accounts for the greater risk of bacterial growth than with other blood products. As a result, any patient in whom a fever develops within 6 hours of receiving platelet concentrates should be considered to possibly be manifesting platelet-induced sepsis, and empirical antibiotic therapy should be instituted.

Fresh Frozen Plasma

Fresh frozen plasma (FFP) is the fluid portion obtained from a single unit of whole blood that is frozen within 6 hours of collection. All coagulation factors, except platelets, are present in FFP, which explains the use of this component for the treatment of hemorrhage from presumed coagulation factor deficiencies. FFP transfusions during surgery are probably not necessary unless the prothrombin time (PT) or partial thromboplastin time (PTT), or both, are at least 1.5 times longer than normal. More recently, FFP is given in specific ratios with red blood cells in trauma patients. Other indications for FFP are urgent reversal of warfarin and management of heparin resistance. FFP's role as a cause of transfusion-related acute lung injury (TRALI) will be discussed later.

Cryoprecipitate

Cryoprecipitate is the fraction of plasma that precipitates when FFP is thawed. This component is useful for treating hemophilia A (contains high concentrations of factor

VIII in a small volume) that is unresponsive to desmopressin. Cryoprecipitate can also be used to treat hypofibrinogenemia (as induced by packed red blood cells) because it contains more fibrinogen than FFP.

COMPLICATIONS OF BLOOD THERAPY

Blood transfusions are extremely valuable in clinical medicine and have become increasingly safer mainly because of more effective donor screening and pretransfusion blood testing (see Table 24-2). Complications of blood therapy, like an adverse effect of any therapy, must be considered when evaluating the risk-to-benefit ratio for treatment of individual patients with blood products. The risk of having a fatal outcome from blood transfusion is remote but possible. The leading causes of a fatal outcome from blood transfusion are transfusion-related acute lung injury (TRALI), hemolytic transfusion reaction, and bacterial contamination (see Table 24-3).

Anesthesiologists are among the most likely physicians to administer blood products to patients; therefore, it is imperative that complications of this therapy be fully appreciated. Transmission of infectious diseases, hepatitis, and human immunodeficiency virus (HIV) and hemolytic transfusion reactions have probably been the most feared complications of transfusion therapy, but they are now not the most common. Because of these fears there have been concerns that transfusions are sometimes underused.[11]

Transmission of Infectious Diseases

The incidence of infection from blood transfusions has markedly decreased. For example, in 1980, the frequency of hepatitis was as high as 10%. Improved donor blood testing has dramatically decreased the risk of transmission of hepatitis C and HIV to less than 1 in 1 million transfusions (see Table 24-2). Although many factors account for the marked decreased incidence of transmission of infectious agents by blood transfusion, the most important one is improved testing of donor blood. Currently, hepatitis C, HIV, and West Nile virus (WNV) are tested by nucleic acid technology. In 2002, more than 30 cases of transfusion-transmitted WNV occurred. By 2003, nearly universal screening of donor blood by nucleic acid technology has reduced the incidence to that of HIV. Chagas' disease has become an increasing transfusion problem in the Southwest United States. Development and use of screening tests should markedly decrease the problem.

Other less commonly transmitted infectious agents include hepatitis B, human T-cell lymphotropic virus, cytomegalovirus, malaria, and possibly variant Creutzfeldt-Jakob disease.

Transfusion-Related Acute Lung Injury

TRALI is the leading cause of transfusion-related deaths (see Table 24-3). TRALI is acute lung injury that occurs within 6 hours after transfusion of a blood product, especially packed red blood cells or FFP. Exclusion of female blood donors and fresher blood (i.e., storage <14 days) decrease the risk of TRALI.[12] It is characterized by dyspnea and arterial hypoxemia secondary to noncardiogenic pulmonary edema. The diagnosis of TRALI is confirmed when pulmonary edema occurs in the absence of left atrial hypertension and the pulmonary edema fluid has a high protein content. Immediate actions to take when TRALI is suspected include (1) stopping the transfusion, (2) supporting the patient's vital signs, (3) determining the protein concentration of the pulmonary edema fluid via the endotracheal tube, (4) obtaining a complete blood count and chest radiograph, and (5) notifying the blood bank of possible TRALI so that other associated units can be quarantined.

Because the diagnosis is sometimes difficult to make, follow-up paperwork is especially important, including sending a blood specimen and bags of units of blood given to the blood bank. All copies of transfusion forms and anesthetic records will be required by the blood bank.

Transfusion-Related Immunomodulation

Blood transfusion suppresses cell-mediated immunity, which when combined with similar effects produced by surgical trauma, may place patients at risk for postoperative infection. The association with long-term prognosis in cancer surgery is unclear, but there is a suggestion of a correlation between tumor recurrence and blood transfusions.[13,14] Conversely, patients who receive blood transfusions may have more extensive disease and a poorer prognosis independent of the administration of blood. As such, the role of blood transfusions in postoperative infections and cancer is difficult to ascertain. Packed red blood cells, which contain less plasma than whole blood does, may produce less immunosuppression, thus suggesting that plasma contains an undefined immunosuppressive factor.

Removing most of the white blood cells from blood and platelets (leukoreduction) is becoming increasingly common. This practice reduces the incidence of nonhemolytic febrile transfusion reactions and the transmission of leukocyte-associated viruses. Other possible benefits (reduction of cancer recurrence and postoperative infections) are more speculative.

Metabolic Abnormalities

Metabolic abnormalities that accompany the storage of whole blood include accumulation of hydrogen ions and potassium and decreased 2,3-DPG concentrations. The citrate present in the blood preservative may produce changes in the recipient.

HYDROGEN IONS

The addition of most preservatives promptly increases the hydrogen ion content of stored whole blood. Continued metabolic function of erythrocytes results in additional production of hydrogen ions with the pH of stored blood being as low as 7.0. Despite these changes, metabolic acidosis is not a consistent occurrence in recipients of blood products, even with rapid infusion of large volumes of stored blood. Therefore, intravenous administration of sodium bicarbonate to patients receiving transfusions of whole blood should be determined by measurement of pH and not be based on arbitrary regimens.

POTASSIUM

The potassium content of stored blood increases progressively with the duration of storage, but even massive transfusions rarely increase plasma potassium concentrations. Failure of plasma potassium concentrations to increase most likely reflects the small amount of potassium actually present in 1 unit of stored blood. For example, because 1 unit of whole blood contains only 300 mL of plasma, a measured potassium concentration of 21 mEq/L would represent the administration of less than 7 mEq of potassium to the patient.

DECREASED 2,3-DIPHOSPHOGLYCERATE

Storage of blood is associated with a progressive decrease in concentrations of 2,3-DPG in erythrocytes, which results in increased affinity of hemoglobin for oxygen (decreased P_{50} values). Conceivably, this increased affinity could make less oxygen available for tissues and jeopardize tissue oxygen delivery. There is speculation that fresh blood (with more oxygen available for tissues) should be used for critically ill patients. Despite these observations, the clinical significance of the 2,3-DPG oxygen affinity changes remains unconfirmed.

CITRATE

Citrate metabolism to bicarbonate may contribute to metabolic alkalosis, whereas binding of calcium by citrate could result in hypocalcemia. Indeed, metabolic alkalosis rather than metabolic acidosis can follow massive blood transfusions. Hypocalcemia as a result of citrate binding of calcium is rare because of mobilization of calcium stores from bone and the ability of the liver to rapidly metabolize citrate to bicarbonate. Therefore, arbitrary administration of calcium in the absence of objective evidence of hypocalcemia (prolonged QT intervals on the electrocardiogram, measured decrease in plasma ionized calcium concentrations) is not indicated. Supplemental calcium may be needed when (1) the rate of blood infusion is more rapid than 50 mL/min, (2) hypothermia or liver disease interferes with the metabolism of citrate, or (3) the patient is a neonate. Patients undergoing liver transplantation are the most likely to experience citrate intoxication, and these patients may require calcium administration during a massive transfusion of stored blood.

Hypothermia

Administration of blood stored at less than 6° C can result in a decrease in the patient's body temperature. Passage of blood through specially designed warmers greatly decreases the likelihood of transfusion-related hypothermia. Unrecognized malfunction of these warmers, causing them to overheat, may result in hemolysis of the blood being transfused.

Coagulation

The conclusion that excessive microvascular bleeding is occurring should be the combined judgment of both the surgical and anesthesia teams. Laboratory tests are only a supplement to clinically determined excessive microvascular bleeding. Blood loss should be determined by checking suction canisters, surgical sponges, and drains. A decision needs to be made regarding whether the blood loss is from inadequate surgical control of vascular bleeding or a coagulopathy. A platelet count, PT or international normalized ratio (INR), PTT, and fibrinogen level can confirm both the presence and type of coagulopathy. Platelet concentrates may be administered if the platelet count is less than 50,000 cells/mm.[3,8] A qualitative platelet defect (antiplatelet drugs, cardiopulmonary bypass) may require platelet concentrates to be given, even with a normal platelet count. Administration of FFP should be considered when the PT is greater than 1.5 times normal or the INR is more than 2.0 and if laboratory tests are unavailable, more than one blood volume (about 70 mL/kg) has been given, and excessive microvascular bleeding is present. The dose of FFP (10 to 15 mL/kg) should achieve at least 30% of most plasma factor concentrations. As indicated previously, specific ratios of FFP and platelets with administration of red blood cells seem to decrease coagulation problems in patients with trauma and massive blood loss.

Cryoprecipitate should be considered if fibrinogen levels are less than 100 mg/dL. Also, a highly purified, lyophilized virus-inactivated fibrinogen concentrate from human plasma (Riastap, CSL Behring, Kankakee, Ill.) can be used to treat hypofibrinogenemia and is effective in some broader based coagulopathies.[15] Low blood fibrinogen levels are increasingly associated with coagulopathies and massive blood transfusions. Accordingly, fibrinogen administration via Riastap or cryoprecipitate is increasingly recognized as being important in treating patients with significant blood loss.[16] In addition, desmopressin or a topical hemostatic (fibrin glue) may be used for excessive bleeding. Recombinant

III

activated factor VII may be considered as a "rescue" drug when standard therapy has failed to successfully treat a coagulopathy (microvascular bleeding).[17] It apparently enhances thrombin generation on already activated platelets. It also has the risk of inducing thromboembolic complications.[17]

Transfusion Reactions

Although transfusion reactions are traditionally categorized as febrile, allergic, and hemolytic, anesthesia, especially general anesthesia, may mask the signs and symptoms of all types of transfusion reactions.[18] The possibility of a transfusion reaction during anesthesia should be suspected in the presence of hyperthermia, increased peak airway pressure, or an acute change in urine output or color.

In considering the occurrence of transfusion reactions, it is important to periodically check for signs and symptoms of bacterial contamination, TRALI, and hemolytic transfusion reactions, including urticaria, hypotension, tachycardia, increased peak airway pressure, hyperthermia, decreased urine output, hemoglobinuria, and microvascular bleeding.[1] Before instituting therapy for transfusion reactions, stop the blood transfusion and order appropriate diagnostic testing.[1]

FEBRILE REACTIONS

Febrile reactions are the most common adverse nonhemolytic response to the transfusion of blood, and they accompany 0.5% to 1% of transfusions. The most likely explanation for febrile reactions is an interaction between recipient antibodies and antigens present on the leukocytes or platelets of the donor. The patient's temperature rarely increases above 38° C, and the condition is treated by slowing the infusion and administering antipyretics. Severe febrile reactions accompanied by chills and shivering may require discontinuation of the blood transfusion.

ALLERGIC REACTIONS

Allergic reactions to properly typed and cross-matched blood are manifested as increases in body temperature, pruritus, and urticaria. Treatment often includes intravenous administration of antihistamines and, in severe cases, discontinuation of the blood transfusion. Examination of plasma and urine for free hemoglobin is useful to rule out hemolytic reactions.

HEMOLYTIC REACTIONS

Hemolytic reactions occur when the wrong blood type is administered to a patient. The common factor in the production of intravascular hemolysis and the development of spontaneous hemorrhage is activation of the complement system. With the exception of hypotension, the immediate signs (lumbar and substernal pain, fever, chills, dyspnea, skin flushing) of hemolytic reactions are masked by general anesthesia. Even hypotension may be attributed to other causes in an anesthetized patient. The appearance of free hemoglobin in plasma or urine is presumptive evidence of a hemolytic reaction. Acute renal failure reflects precipitation of stromal and lipid contents (not free hemoglobin) of hemolyzed erythrocytes in distal renal tubules. Disseminated intravascular coagulation causing a coagulopathy is initiated by material released from hemolyzed erythrocytes.

Treatment

Treatment of acute hemolytic reactions is immediate discontinuation of the incompatible blood transfusion and maintenance of urine output by infusion of crystalloid solutions and administration of mannitol or furosemide. The use of sodium bicarbonate to alkalinize the urine and improve the solubility of hemoglobin degradation products in the renal tubules is of unproven value, as is the administration of corticosteroids.

AUTOLOGOUS BLOOD TRANSFUSIONS

Types of autologous blood transfusion are (1) predeposited (preoperative) autologous donation (PAD), (2) intraoperative and postoperative blood salvage, and (3) normovolemic hemodilution. Two primary reasons for the use of autologous blood are to decrease or eliminate complications from allogeneic blood transfusions and to conserve blood resources. In the 1980s, both patient and physician fear escalated because of a legitimate concern regarding infectious diseases, especially hepatitis C and HIV. Although there is still an inherent belief that PAD blood is safer, the markedly reduced rate of infectious disease transmission from allogeneic blood makes that view difficult to prove. Furthermore, PAD blood is more expensive and not very effective in reducing allogeneic blood transfusion. Therefore, PAD is not generally a cost-effective alternative to allogeneic blood.

Predeposited Autologous Donation

Patients scheduled for elective surgery that may require transfusion of blood may choose to predonate (predeposit) blood for possible transfusion in the perioperative period. Patient-donors must have a hemoglobin concentration of at least 11 g/dL. Most patients can donate 10.5 mL/kg of blood approximately every 5 to 7 days (maximum, 2 to 3 units), with the last unit collected 72 hours or more before surgery to permit restoration of plasma volume. Oral iron supplementation is recommended when blood is withdrawn within a few days preceding surgery. Treatment with recombinant erythropoietin is very expensive, but it increases the amount of blood that patients can predeposit by as much as 25%.

Intraoperative and Postoperative Blood Salvage

Intraoperative blood salvage for reinfusion into the patient decreases the amount of allogeneic blood needed. Typically, semiautomated systems are used in which the red blood cells are collected and washed and then delivered to a reservoir for future administration either intraoperatively or postoperatively. The presence of infection or malignant disease at the operative site is considered a contraindication to blood salvage. Complications of intraoperative salvage include dilutional coagulopathy, reinfusion of excessive anticoagulant (heparin), hemolysis, air embolism, and disseminated intravascular coagulation. A documented quality assurance program, as recommended by the American Association of Blood Banks, is required for those who use intraoperative salvage techniques.

Normovolemic Hemodilution

Normovolemic hemodilution consists of withdrawing a portion of the patient's blood volume early in the intraoperative period and concurrent infusion of crystalloids or colloids to maintain intravascular volume. The end point is a hematocrit of 27% to 33%, depending on the patient's cardiovascular and respiratory status. By initially hemodiluting the patient, fewer red blood cells will be lost per millimeter of blood loss during surgery. At the conclusion of surgery, the patient's blood, with its enhanced oxygen-carrying capacity by virtue of a higher hematocrit and its greater clotting ability by virtue of platelets and other coagulation factors, is reinfused. Whether the use of this technique actually decreases allogeneic blood administration is questionable. The survival of recovered red blood cells appears to be similar to that of transfused allogeneic cells.

CONCLUSIONS AND FUTURE DIRECTIONS

Transfusion of blood products has become increasingly safer, especially because of the dramatically decreased incidence of infectious disease transmission (see Table 24-2). If given in accordance with proper indications, patient mortality rate is not increased because of receiving blood transfusions per se.[3,4] As indicated previously, increasingly, emphasis is being placed on defining "ratios" of blood products that should be given (e.g., 1:1 packed red blood cells with fresh frozen plasma or platelets).[19,20] Alternatively, perhaps in the future whole blood will be given more often. Other possibilities include hemoglobin-based oxygen carriers (HBOC) (synthetic blood). For over 20 years with all of their advantages (e.g., no typing and cross-matching), we hoped that one or more of these products would partially replace human blood transfusions. However, a Food and Drug Administration and National Institutes of Health conference in 2008 indicated that HBOC products will not be available soon.[21] Also, the ultimate impact that the length of time blood has been stored will have on transfusion practice overall is not clear.[2] Lastly, consistent with the practice of medicine overall, well-designed protocols will increasingly be the basis upon which transfusion practice is based.[22]

QUESTIONS OF THE DAY

1. A patient requires packed red blood cell transfusion. How is a cross-match performed? What are the risks of hemolytic transfusion reaction if type-specific, non-cross-matched red blood cells are administered instead?
2. What are the risks associated with transfusion of platelet concentrates?
3. What is the risk of transmission of hepatitis C and human immunodeficiency virus (HIV) with blood transfusion in the United States?
4. What conditions predispose a patient to citrate toxicity from blood product transfusions?
5. What are the manifestations of hemolytic transfusion reaction in a patient receiving general anesthesia? What is the appropriate initial management?

REFERENCES

1. American Society of Anesthesiologists Task Force: Practice guidelines for perioperative blood transfusions and adjuvant therapies, *Anesthesiology* 105:198–208, 2006.
2. Adamson JW: New blood, old blood, or no blood? *N Engl J Med* 358:1295–1296, 2008.
3. Vincent JL, Sakr Y, Sprung C, et al: Are blood transfuions associated with greater mortality rates? *Anesthesiology* 108:31–39, 2008.

4. Weightman WM, Gibbs NM, Sheminant MR, et al: Moderate exposure to allogeneic blood products is not associated with reduced long-term survival after surgery for coronary artery disease, *Anesthesiology* 111:327–333, 2009.
5. Beattie WS, Karkouti K, Wijeysundera DN, et al: Risk associated with preoperative anemia in noncardiac surgery, *Anesthesiology* 110:574–581, 2009.

6. Weiskppf RB: Emergency transfusion for acute severe anemia: A caluated risk, *Anesth Analg* 111:1088–1092, 2010.
7. Miller RD, Ward TA, Shiboski S, et al: A comparison of three methods of hemoglobin monitoring in patients undergoing spine surgery, *Anesth Analg* 112: April, 2011.
8. Miller RD: Massive blood transfusions: The impact of Vietnam military data on modern civilian transfusion

III

medicine, *Anesthesiology* 110:1412–1416, 2009.

9. Spinella PC: Warm fresh whole blood transfusion for severe hemorrhage: U.S. military and potential civilian applications, *Crit Care Med* 36: S340–S345, 2008.

10. Inaba K, Lustenberger T, Talving P, et al: The impact of platelet transfusions in massively transfused trauma patients, *J Am Coll Surg* 211:573–579, 2010.

11. Sexena S, Wehrli G, Makarewicz K, et al: Monitoring for underutilization of RBC components and platelets, *Transfusion* 41:587–595, 2001.

12. Benson AB, Moss M: Trauma and acute respiratory distress syndrome, *Anesthesiology* 110:216–217, 2009.

13. Spahn DR, Moch H, Hofmann A, et al: Patient blood management, *Anesthesiology* 109:951–953, 2008.

14. Arad S, Glasner A, Abiri N, et al: Blood transfusion promotes cancer progression, *Anesthesiology* 109:989–1987, 2008.

15. Rahe-Meyer N, Pichlmaier M, Haverich A, et al: Bleeding managnement with fibrinogen concentrate targeting a high-normal plasma fibringogen level: A pilot study, *Br J Anaesth* 102:785–792, 2009.

16. Stinger HK, Spinella PC, Perkins JG, et al: The ratio of fibrinogen to red cells transfused affects survival in casualties receiving massive transfuions at an army combat support hospital, *J Trauma* 64:S79–S85, 2008.

17. Aledort LM: Off-label use of recombinant activated Factor VII–safe or not safe? *N Eng J Med* 363:1853–1854, 2010.

18. Kopko PM, Holland PV: Mechanisms of severe transfusion reaction, *Transfus Clin Biol* 8:278–281, 2001.

19. Holcomb JB, Wade CE, Michalek JE, et al: Increased plasma and platelet to red blood cell ratios improves outcome in 466 massively transfused civilian trauma patients, *Ann Surg* 248:447–458, 2008.

20. Perkins JG, Andrew PC, Blackbourne LH, et al: An evaluation of the impact of apheresis platelets used in the setting of massively transfused trauma patients, *J Trauma* 66:S77–S84, 2009.

21. Silverman TA, Weiskoph RB, planning committee: Hemoglobin-based oxygen carriers, *Anesthesiology* 111:946–963, 2009.

22. Cotton BA, Dossett LA, Au BK, et al: Room for (performance) improvement: Provider-related factors associated with poor outcomes in massive transfusions, *J Trauma* 67:1004–1012, 2009.

SPECIAL ANESTHETIC CONSIDERATIONS

25 CARDIOVASCULAR DISEASE

Art Wallace

Cardiovascular disease is the leading cause of death in the United States, Canada, Europe, and Japan.[1] Many of the risk factors identified to predict perioperative death are cardiac. Coronary artery disease, peripheral vascular disease, and risk for coronary artery disease increase operative risk.[2,3] Recent myocardial infarction, the presence of congestive heart failure, and aortic stenosis are the most common major risk factors. Management of anesthesia for patients with cardiovascular disease requires an understanding of the pathophysiology of the disease process; appropriate preoperative testing; application of perioperative risk reduction strategies; careful selection of anesthetic, analgesic, neuromuscular, and autonomic blocking drugs; and use of monitors to match the needs created by this disease.

CORONARY ARTERY DISEASE

Coronary artery disease (ischemic heart disease), often asymptomatic, is a common accompaniment of aging in the American population. Of the adult patients who undergo surgery annually in the United States, about 40% will either have, or be at risk for, coronary artery disease.[1] Patients who undergo anesthesia for noncardiac surgery have increased rates of morbidity and mortality when coronary artery disease is present. History, physical examination with specific attention to cardiac and respiratory disease and risks, and evaluation of exercise tolerance, cardiac symptoms, and electrocardiogram (ECG) are important components of the routine preoperative cardiac evaluation (also see Chapter 13).[4] The most common symptoms of cardiac disease are shortness of breath with exercise in men and fatigue in women. The presence of angina, angina at rest, orthopnea, paroxysmal nocturnal dyspnea, and dizziness or fainting should also be evaluated.

More specialized procedures, such as ambulatory ECG monitoring (Holter monitoring), exercise stress testing, transthoracic or transesophageal echocardiography, radionuclide ventriculography (determination of ejection fraction), dipyridamole-thallium scintigraphy (mimics the coronary vasodilator response but not the heart rate response associated with exercise), cardiac catheterization, and angiography, are performed on selected patients. Invasive preoperative testing does not add appreciably to the information provided by routine history and physical examination and electrocardiographic data for predicting adverse outcomes.[1] For example, echocardiographic determination of ejection fraction does not improve upon the ability to predict the presence of a preoperative myocardial infarction beyond that of a careful preoperative clinical evaluation. Thallium scintigraphy, which evaluates adequacy of coronary blood flow, does not predict patients at risk for perioperative cardiac events.[5,6] Ultimately, the history and physical examination with specific attention to signs and symptoms of

new onset of angina, change in anginal pattern, unstable angina, recent myocardial infarction, congestive heart failure, or aortic stenosis, and presence of appropriate medical therapy should determine whether patients are in the best medical condition possible before elective cardiac or noncardiac surgery.

Patient History

Important aspects of the history taken from patients with coronary artery disease before noncardiac surgery include cardiac reserve, characteristics of angina pectoris, the presence of a prior myocardial infarction, and the medical, interventional cardiology, and cardiac surgical therapy for those conditions. Potential interactions of medications used in the treatment of coronary artery disease with drugs used to produce anesthesia must also be considered. Coexisting noncardiac diseases include hypertension, peripheral vascular disease, chronic obstructive pulmonary disease from cigarette smoking, renal dysfunction associated with chronic hypertension, and diabetes mellitus. A thorough evaluation needs to recognize that patients can remain asymptomatic despite 50% to 70% stenosis of a major coronary artery.

CARDIAC RESERVE

Limited exercise tolerance in the absence of significant pulmonary disease is the most striking evidence of decreased cardiac reserve. Inability to lie flat, awakening from sleep with angina or shortness of breath, or angina at rest or with minimal exertion are evidence of significant cardiac disease. If a patient can climb two to three flights of stairs without symptoms, cardiac reserve is probably adequate.

ANGINA PECTORIS

Angina pectoris is stable when no change has occurred for at least 60 days in precipitating factors, frequency, and duration. Chest pain or shortness of breath produced with less than normal activity or at rest, or lasting for increasingly longer periods, is characteristic of unstable angina pectoris and may signal an impending myocardial infarction. Dyspnea following the onset of angina pectoris probably indicates acute left ventricular dysfunction due to myocardial ischemia. Angina pectoris due to spasm of the coronary arteries (variant or Prinzmetal's angina) differs from classic angina pectoris in that it may occur at rest and then be absent during vigorous exertion. Silent myocardial ischemia does not evoke angina pectoris (asymptomatic) and usually occurs at a slower heart rate and lower systemic arterial blood pressure than those present during exercise-induced myocardial ischemia. About 70% of ischemic episodes are not associated with angina pectoris and as many as 15% of acute myocardial infarctions are silent. Women and diabetics have a more frequent incidence of painless myocardial ischemia and infarctions. The most common symptom in men is shortness of breath with exertion and in women it is fatigue.

The heart rate or systolic blood pressure at which angina pectoris or evidence of myocardial ischemia is indicated on the ECG is useful preoperative information. An increased heart rate is more likely than hypertension to produce signs of myocardial ischemia (Fig. 25-1). Tachycardia increases myocardial oxygen requirements while at the same time decreases the duration of diastole, thereby decreasing coronary blood flow and the delivery of oxygen to the left ventricle. Conversely, hypertension, while increasing oxygen consumption, simultaneously increases coronary perfusion despite the presence of atherosclerotic coronary arteries.

PRIOR MYOCARDIAL INFARCTION

The incidence of myocardial reinfarction in the perioperative period is related to the time elapsed since the previous myocardial infarction (Table 25-1).[7-10] The incidence of perioperative myocardial reinfarction does not stabilize at 5% to 6% until 6 months after the prior myocardial infarction. Thus, elective surgery, especially thoracic, upper abdominal, or other major procedures are delayed for a period of 2 to 6 months after a myocardial infarction. Even after 6 months, the 5% to 6% incidence of myocardial reinfarction is about 50 times more frequent than the 0.13% incidence of perioperative myocardial infarction in patients undergoing similar operations but in the absence

Time Elapsed Since Previous Myocardial Infarction	Reported Incidence			
	Tarhan et al[7]	Steen et al[8]	Rao et al[9]	Shah et al[10]
0-3 months	37%	27%	5.7%	4.3%
4 to 6 months	16%	11%	2.3%	0
>6 months	5%	6%		5.7%

Table 25-1 Incidence of Perioperative Myocardial Infarction

of a prior myocardial infarction. Most perioperative myocardial reinfarctions occur in the first 48 to 72 hours postoperatively. However, if ischemia is initiated by the stress of surgery, the risk of myocardial infarction is increased for several months after surgery.[2,11]

Several factors influence the incidence of myocardial infarction in the perioperative period. For example, the incidence of myocardial reinfarction is increased in patients undergoing intrathoracic or intra-abdominal operations lasting longer than 3 hours. Factors that do not predispose to a myocardial reinfarction include the (1) site of the previous myocardial infarction, (2) history of prior aortocoronary bypass graft surgery, (3) site of the operative procedure if the duration of the surgery is shorter than 3 hours, and (4) techniques used to produce anesthesia. Giving β-adrenergic blocking drugs 7 to 30 days prior to surgery and continued for 30 days postoperatively reduces the risk of cardiac morbidity (myocardial infarction or cardiac death) by 90% (also see Chapter 7).[12,13] Giving β-adrenergic blocking drugs just prior to surgery and continuing for 7 days reduces the mortality risk by 50%.[14,15] Perioperative clonidine administration reduces the 30-day and 2-year mortality risks.[16] Statin therapy with fluvastatin for 30 days before and after surgery, in addition to β-blockade, reduces risk of myocardial infarction and death by an additional 50%.[17] Intensive hemodynamic monitoring using an intra-arterial catheter and prompt pharmacologic intervention or fluid infusion to treat physiologic hemodynamic alterations from the normal range may decrease the risk of perioperative cardiac morbidity in high-risk patients (see Table 25-1).[9]

CURRENT MEDICATIONS

Drugs most likely taken by patients with coronary artery disease are β-adrenergic antagonists, nitrates, calcium channel blockers, angiotensin-converting enzyme inhibitors, drugs that decrease blood lipids, diuretics, antihypertensives, and platelet inhibitors. Potential adverse interactions of these drugs with anesthetics is an important preoperative consideration (see Chapters 7 to 9 and 22). All patients with known coronary artery disease, known peripheral vascular disease, or with two risk factors for

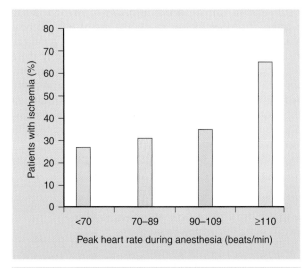

Figure 25-1 The incidence of myocardial ischemia increases with heart rates with the greatest effect at heart rates above 110 beats/min. (From Slogoff S, Keats AS. Does chronic treatment with calcium entry blocking drugs reduce perioperative myocardial ischemia? Anesthesiology 1988;68:676-680, used with permission.)

IV

coronary artery disease (e.g., being elderly, hypertension, diabetes, significant smoking history, or hyperlipidemia) should receive a perioperative β-adrenergic blocking drug unless there is a specific contraindication.[12-15] Even though chronic obstructive pulmonary disease (COPD) is not a contraindication to perioperative β-adrenergic blockade,[14,15] reactive asthma is. In patients who cannot tolerate β-blockers, the α_2-agonist clonidine may be used.[16] Patients with coronary artery disease or vascular disease should receive a statin unless there is a specific contraindication.[17] Despite the potential for adverse drug interactions, cardiac medications being taken preoperatively should be continued without interruption through the perioperative period. Discontinuation of β-adrenergic blockers,[18] calcium channel blockers, nitrates, statins, or angiotensin-converting enzyme inhibitors in the perioperative period increases perioperative morbidity and mortality rates and should be avoided.

Electrocardiogram (Also See Chapter 20)

The preoperative ECG should be examined for evidence of (1) myocardial ischemia, (2) prior myocardial infarction, (3) cardiac hypertrophy, (4) abnormal cardiac rhythm or conduction disturbances, and (5) electrolyte abnormalities. The exercise ECG simulates sympathetic nervous system stimulation as may accompany perioperative events such as direct laryngoscopy, tracheal intubation, and surgical incision. The resting ECG in the absence of angina pectoris may be normal despite extensive coronary artery disease. Nevertheless, an ECG demonstrating ST-segment depression more than 1 mm, particularly during angina pectoris, confirms the presence of myocardial ischemia. Furthermore, the ECG lead demonstrating changes of myocardial ischemia can help determine the specific diseased coronary artery (Table 25-2). Of particular importance is that a prior myocardial infarction, especially if subendocardial, may not be accompanied by persistent changes on the ECG. The preoperative presence of ventricular premature beats may signal their likely occurrence intraoperatively. A PR interval on the ECG longer than 200 milliseconds may be

related to digitalis therapy. Conversely, the block of conduction of cardiac impulses below the atrioventricular node (right bundle branch block, left bundle branch block, or intraventricular conduction delay) most likely reflects pathologic changes rather than drug effect.

Risk Stratification versus Risk Reduction

One of the standard approaches to the perioperative care of patients with cardiac disease is risk stratification. Risk stratification consists of a preoperative history and physical examination followed by some series of tests thought to predict perioperative cardiac morbidity and mortality risk. These tests may include persantine thallium, echocardiography, Holter monitoring, dobutamine stress echocardiography, and angiography, and may lead to angioplasty with or without an intracoronary stent or coronary artery bypass surgery. As indicated previously, preoperative risk stratification with invasive testing adds little to a careful history and physical examination followed by prophylactic medical therapy.[5,6,12-16] Furthermore, the risk of angiography and an intracoronary stent or coronary artery bypass graft (CABG) surgery prior to a surgical procedure does not reduce total risk.[19,20] The combined risk of two procedures exceeds that of the original operation.[19,21,22] Despite the lack of proven benefit of prophylactic invasive testing combined with either CABG or coronary angioplasty with stenting over medical therapy, the American College of Cardiology (ACC) and American Heart Association (AHA) have developed a protocol entitled ACC/AHA Guideline Perioperative Cardiovascular Evaluation for Noncardiac Surgery.[23-26] (See Figure 25-2). The use of this protocol is difficult to apply in practice with conflicting guidance on indications for testing with physicians ordering more tests than suggested by the guidelines.[27] Furthermore, the ACC/AHA guidelines have not been shown to actually reduce perioperative risk. Perioperative risk reduction therapy with β-adrenergic blockers, clonidine, statins, and aspirin may be superior to risk stratification with invasive testing, angioplasty, and CABG.[12-17,19-21]

Table 25-2 Area of Myocardial Ischemia as Reflected by the Electrocardiogram

Electrocardiogram Leads	Coronary Artery Responsible for Myocardial Ischemia	Area of Myocardium That May Be Involved
II, III, aVF	Right coronary artery	Right atrium Sinus node Atrioventricular node Right ventricle
V_3-V_5	Left anterior descending coronary artery	Anterolateral aspects of the left ventricle
I, aVL	Circumflex coronary artery	Lateral aspects of the left ventricle

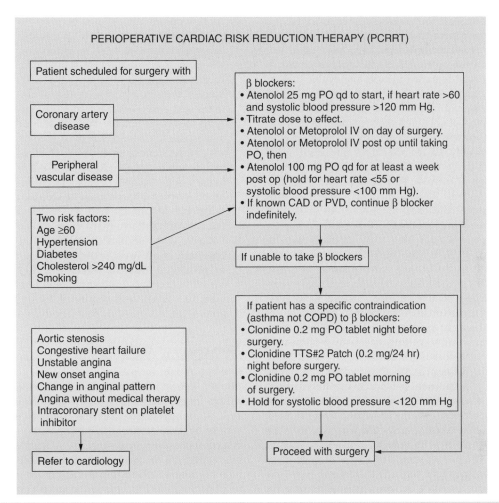

PERIOPERATIVE CARDIAC RISK REDUCTION THERAPY (PCRRT)

Patient scheduled for surgery with

Coronary artery disease

Peripheral vascular disease

Two risk factors:
Age ≥60
Hypertension
Diabetes
Cholesterol >240 mg/dL
Smoking

Aortic stenosis
Congestive heart failure
Unstable angina
New onset angina
Change in anginal pattern
Angina without medical therapy
Intracoronary stent on platelet
  inhibitor

Refer to cardiology

β blockers:
• Atenolol 25 mg PO qd to start, if heart rate >60 and systolic blood pressure >120 mm Hg.
• Titrate dose to effect.
• Atenolol or Metoprolol IV on day of surgery.
• Atenolol or Metoprolol IV post op until taking PO, then
• Atenolol 100 mg PO qd for at least a week post op (hold for heart rate <55 or systolic blood pressure <100 mm Hg).
• If known CAD or PVD, continue β blocker indefinitely.

If unable to take β blockers

If patient has a specific contraindication (asthma not COPD) to β blockers:
• Clonidine 0.2 mg PO tablet night before surgery.
• Clonidine TTS#2 Patch (0.2 mg/24 hr) night before surgery.
• Clonidine 0.2 mg PO tablet morning of surgery.
• Hold for systolic blood pressure <120 mm Hg

Proceed with surgery

Figure 25-2 Perioperative cardiac risk reduction therapy with beta-blockers and clonidine protocol. All patients with known coronary artery disease, vascular disease, or two risk factors for coronary artery disease should be placed on prophylactic anti-ischemic agent therapy with a long-acting β-blocker unless there is a specific contraindication. If there is a contraindication to β-blockade, then prophylactic therapy with clonidine is an alternative.[12-16] COPD, chronic obstructive pulmonary disease; PVD, peripheral vascular disease. (From American College of Cardiology (ACC) and American Heart Association (AHA): ACC/AHA Guideline Perioperative Cardiovascular Evaluation for Noncardiac Surgery. Anesth Analg 1994;5:1052-1064, used with permission.)

IV

PERIOPERATIVE CARDIAC RISK REDUCTION THERAPY
Recommendations for the administration of prophylactic medical therapy to stable patients with known coronary artery disease or at risk for such disease have been established (see Fig. 25-2). The protocol is as follows:

1. All patients who have either coronary artery disease (CAD), peripheral vascular disease (PVD), or two risk factors for coronary artery disease (age ≥ 60 years, cigarette smoking, diabetes, hypertension, cholesterol ≥ 240 mg/dL) should receive perioperative β-adrenergic blockade unless they have a specific intolerance to β-blockers. Patients with renal failure or renal insufficiency may also benefit from therapy.

2. If a patient has an absolute contraindication to perioperative β-blockers, clonidine may be used as an alternative. Clonidine should be administered as follows:
   a. Clonidine 0.2 mg PO on the night before surgery as well as a clonidine TTS#2 (0.2 mg/24 hours) patch. Withhold the tablet for systolic blood pressure less than 120 mm Hg.
   b. Clonidine 0.2 mg PO on morning of surgery.
   c. Leave the patch on for a week.

3. β-Adrenergic blocking drugs should be given as soon as the patient is identified as having CAD, PVD, or risk factors. If the surgeon identifies the patient as having risk, the surgeon should initiate the medication to the

patient. Likewise, if the anesthesia preoperative clinic identifies the patient, β-blockers should be started. If the patient is not identified until the morning of surgery, intravenous atenolol or metoprolol should be used. If the drug is started prior to the day of surgery, atenolol 25 mg PO daily is an appropriate starting dose.

4. β-Blockade should be continued until at least 30 days postoperatively, if not indefinitely, in patients with coronary artery disease or peripheral vascular disease. In patients with only risk factors, 7 days may be sufficient.

5. The optimal time to start β-blockade is at the time of identification of the risk. This process should be multitiered to avoid missing patients. The following approach should be used to provide the maximum benefit at the minimum cost.

   a. The surgeon should give a β-blocker if patients have CAD, PVD, or two risk factors. Atenolol 25 mg PO daily is an appropriate starting dose.

   b. If a medical or cardiology consult is requested by surgery, the most common advice is: start a β-blocker.

   c. The anesthesia preoperative clinic checks to see if the patients at risk are receiving a β-blocker. If the patient is not getting adequate β-adrenergic blockade, the dose is increased.

   d. On the day of surgery, treatment with or increasing the dose of intravenous β-blockers should be considered. Intravenous metoprolol in 5-mg boluses is used. The standard dose is 10 mg IV (withhold for heart rate less than 50 beats/min or systolic blood pressure less than 100 mm Hg). Intraoperative doses are used as needed. The patient should receive additional doses in the postanesthetic care unit as needed.

   e. The patient receives the drug postoperatively for 30 days. If the patient is NPO, the patient receives intravenous metoprolol (5 to 10 mg q6 hours) unless systolic blood pressure is less than 100 mm Hg or heart rate less than 50 beats/min. If the patient is taking oral medications, the patient receives atenolol 100 mg PO daily if the heart rate is more rapid than 65 beats/min and the systolic blood pressure is more than 100 mm Hg. If the heart rate is between 55 and 65 beats/min, the dose is 50 mg. There is a "hold order" for heart rate less than 50 beats/min or systolic blood pressure less than 100 mm Hg.

   f. The patient receives the drug for at least 30 days postoperatively.

   g. Many patients should receive the drug for life (patients with known CAD, known PVD, and hypertension).

6. Preoperative testing and revascularization[22] should be used only as needed for specific indications not prophylaxis.[28] If a patient is identified with new onset angina, unstable angina, a change in the anginal pattern, or congestive failure, then further risk stratification is appropriate. If the patient is stable with known CAD, PVD, or two risk factors for CAD, the patient should receive a β-adrenergic blocker.[12-16]

7. Additional attention should be given to patients with congestive heart failure (CHF), aortic stenosis, intracoronary stents on platelet inhibitors, or renal failure. All patients who have CHF should be evaluated by a cardiologist for the initiation of β-blocker therapy. Beta blocker therapy reduces the risk of death from CHF. Many patients with CHF are profoundly improved by β-blockade, but the dose must be titrated slowly and is usually supervised by a cardiologist. Patients with aortic stenosis should be evaluated by cardiology, and β-adrenergic blockade initiated with a cardiologist's supervision. Patients with intracoronary stents on platelet inhibitors should be seen by a cardiologist. *Warning*: Discontinuation of platelet inhibitors in patients with intracoronary stents can be lethal.[20]

8. Patients with an indication for statin therapy and especially those with known coronary artery disease or peripheral vascular disease should be considered for statin therapy.[17] Therapy should be started 30 days prior to surgery and continued for at least 30 days after surgery,[17] possibly indefinitely.

Management of Anesthesia

Anesthesia care for patients with known coronary artery disease, known peripheral vascular disease, or two risk factors for coronary artery disease (age older than or equal to 60 years, hypertension, diabetes, significant smoking history, or hyperlipidemia) should begin as soon as the patient is identified as needing surgery.[12-16] All patients with new-onset angina, a change in anginal pattern, unstable angina, angina without medical therapy, aortic stenosis, congestive heart failure, or an intracoronary stent on a platelet inhibitor should be referred to cardiology. Patients with recently placed intracoronary stents on platelet inhibitors have a high risk of intracoronary thrombosis and death when the platelet inhibitors are discontinued for perioperative care.[20,29,30] Patients with bare metal stents may require 3 or more months of antiplatelet therapy.[29] Patients with drug-eluting intracoronary stents may require platelet inhibitors for a year or more.[30] Patients with stable coronary disease on medical therapy with no evidence of congestive heart failure or aortic stenosis should be started on an oral β-blocker (atenolol 25 mg/day PO) and a statin drug.[17] Patients with congestive heart failure should have β-blockers initiated by cardiology over a prolonged period. The dose of β-blockers should be increased as tolerated. β-Blockers should be avoided in patients with a history of high-grade atrioventricular (AV) block without a pacemaker, reactive asthma, or an intolerance for β-blockers. Diabetes is an indication for perioperative β-blockade. For maximal effect, β-blockers should be started as soon as the patient is identified as needing surgery (optimally 7 to 30 days before surgery).[12] If a patient is identified the day of surgery, intravenous atenolol or metoprolol can be started in the preoperative area (atenolol or metoprolol 10 mg IV if heart rate is more rapid than 55 beats/min or systolic blood pressure is higher than 100 mm Hg) and continued postoperatively.[15] Perioperative β-blockers should be continued for at least 7 days postoperatively.[15] In patients with more frequent risks (those with known coronary artery disease or peripheral vascular disease) β-blockers should be continued at least 30 days if not indefinitely.[12,13] In patients with cardiac risk (coronary disease, peripheral vascular disease, or two risk factors for coronary disease) who cannot tolerate β-blockade, the α_2-agonist clonidine reduces the risk of 30-day and 2-year mortality.[16] Clonidine (#2TTS = 0.2 mg/day patch plus a 0.2-mg tablet) is started the night before surgery. A second tablet of clonidine 0.2 mg PO is given on the morning of surgery. The patch takes 24 hours to achieve adequate blood levels, so the tablet plus patch makes an infusion and bolus of drug. The patch is discontinued after 7 days and autotapers the drug. Esmolol boluses during surgery do not constitute perioperative β-blockade and are not adequate to reduce perioperative cardiac risk.[16] Appropriate dosing of β-blockers is appropriate to avoid hypotension, bradycardia, and possible sequelae.[31]

The intraoperative anesthetic management as well as postoperative pain management of patients with coronary artery disease includes modulation of sympathetic nervous system responses and rigorous control of hemodynamic variables.[1] Management of anesthesia should be based on a preoperative evaluation of left ventricular function and should sustain a favorable balance between myocardial oxygen requirements and myocardial oxygen delivery to prevent myocardial ischemia (Tables 25-3 and 25-4). Persistent tachycardia, systolic hypertension, arterial hypoxemia, or diastolic hypotension can adversely influence this delicate balance.

Persistent and excessive changes in heart rate and systemic blood pressure should be minimized (Fig. 25-1).[32] Maintaining heart rate and systemic blood pressure within 20% of the awake values is commonly recommended.

Table 25-3 Evaluation of Left Ventricular Function

Assessment Feature	Good Function	Impaired Function
Previous myocardial infarction	No	Yes
Evidence of congestive heart failure	No	Yes
Ejection fraction	>0.55	<0.4
Left ventricular end-diastolic pressure	<12 mm Hg	>18 mm Hg
Cardiac index	>2.5 L/min/m²	<2 L/min/m²
Areas of ventricular dyskinesia	No	Yes

Table 25-4 Determinants of Myocardial Oxygen Requirements and Delivery

Myocardial Oxygen Requirements
Heart rate
Systolic blood pressure
Myocardial contractility
Ventricular volume

Myocardial Oxygen Delivery
Coronary blood flow
Oxygen content of arterial blood

Monitoring with an intra-arterial catheter facilitates the ability to maintain stable systemic blood pressures. Nevertheless, about one half of all new perioperative ischemic episodes are not preceded by, or associated with, significant changes in heart rate or systemic blood pressure.[33] A single 1-minute episode of myocardial ischemia detected by 1-mm ST-segment elevation or depression increases the risk of cardiac events tenfold and the risk for death twofold.[3,34] Tachycardia for 5 minutes above 120 beats/min in the postoperative period can increase the risk of death tenfold. The only clinically proven method to reduce the risk of perioperative myocardial ischemia and associated death is perioperative β-blockade[12–15] (atenolol or metoprolol) or α_2-agonist therapy with clonidine.[16]

MONITORING (Also See Chapter 20)

Anticipation of problems and avoidance of potential disasters is a key component in successful anesthetic management in patients with cardiovascular disease. Prophylactic therapy and more extensive monitoring reduce risk. Continuous intra-arterial pressure monitoring can reduce the risk of hemodynamic events by early identification of problems. Continuous ECG monitoring rapidly identifies arrhythmias, tachycardia, and myocardial ischemia. Monitoring should be continuous if possible. Rapid changes in hemodynamics can quickly lead to cardiac arrest; monitoring can quickly identify those changes and permits prompt therapy prior to further complications. When operations are completed, monitoring should be continued into the recovery room or intensive care unit (ICU). When patients are transferred from the operating room table to the gurney or ICU bed, or are turned from supine to prone or back to supine, monitoring should be as continuous as possible. Unconscious patients with cardiac disease may have rapid hemodynamic collapse with transfers from the operating room table to the gurney or ICU bed or when turned over and should be monitored during transfers. If arterial blood pressure, ECG, and saturation are monitored, the problem can be quickly identified and corrected prior to serious sequelae. Intravascular volume, vasoconstrictors, β-agonists, β-blockers, anticholinergics, and vasodilator

IV

drugs should be immediately available. Loss of a pulse oximeter signal or desaturation can imply hypoxia or inadequate arterial blood pressure or cardiac output and should signal an immediate search for a cause and corrective action. The pulse oximeter is a monitor both of oxygen saturation and perfusion. If the pulse oximeter loses a signal, adequacy of perfusion should be assessed. Loss of the pulse oximeter signal may be the first warning of impending hemodynamic collapse. Continuous monitoring and prophylactic therapy can reduce the risk in patients with cardiovascular disease.

The intensity of monitoring in the perioperative period is influenced by the complexity of the operative procedure and the severity of the coronary artery disease. The five-lead ECG serves as a noninvasive monitor of the balance between myocardial oxygen requirements and myocardial oxygen delivery in unconscious patients (see Chapter 20). When this balance is unfavorably altered, myocardial ischemia occurs, as evidenced on the ECG by at least a 1-mm downsloping of the ST segment from baseline. A precordial V_5 lead is a useful selection for detecting ST-segment changes characteristic of ischemia of the left ventricle during anesthesia. Intra-arterial pressure monitoring can speed the identification and treatment of hemodynamic changes. Monitoring should be continuous if possible. Ventricular wall motion abnormalities observed by transesophageal echocardiography may be the most sensitive indicator of myocardial ischemia, but this monitor is expensive, invasive, and requires additional training before use. Intraoperative monitoring of pulmonary artery pressures or use of transesophageal echocardiography should be reserved for selected high-risk patients (cardiac surgery, recent myocardial infarction, current congestive heart failure, unstable angina).[1] Continuous cardiac output monitoring may improve intravascular fluid management.[35]

INDUCTION OF ANESTHESIA

Preoperative anxiety can lead to preoperative myocardial ischemia.[36] Myocardial ischemia predisposes to subsequent myocardial ischemia. Preoperative β-blocker therapy or clonidine reduces the incidence of myocardial ischemia.[36,37] Patients should receive their routine medications except for oral hypoglycemic drugs. Preoperative sedative medication is intended to produce sedation and reduce anxiety, which if unopposed, could lead to secretion of catecholamines and an increase in myocardial oxygen requirements because of an increase in heart rate and systemic blood pressure. Oral administration of benzodiazepines (diazepam PO) is an effective pharmacologic approach frequently selected to allay anxiety. Supplemental oxygen may be needed if narcotics are combined with benzodiazepines for sedation.

Induction of anesthesia is acceptably accomplished with the intravenous administration of rapidly acting drugs. Preinduction placement of an intra-arterial catheter to monitor blood pressure allows rapid pharmacologic manipulations and a very stable induction of anesthesia. An infusion of phenylephrine (0.2 to 0.4 μg/kg/min) started prophylactically stabilizes arterial blood pressure and can eliminate most hemodynamic changes with induction. Etomidate is a popular anesthetic to induce anesthesia because of its limited inhibition of the sympathetic nervous system and limited hemodynamic effects[38] (also see Chapter 9). The lack of inhibition of autonomic reflexes by etomidate may lead to hypertension with laryngoscopy and endotracheal intubation. Propofol is popular secondary to its antiemetic effects and rapid recovery, but the dose should be reduced to avoid hypotension with induction. Fentanyl and midazolam in combination with an infusion of phenylephrine and a nondepolarizing muscle relaxant cause minimal changes in arterial blood pressure or heart rate.

Ketamine is not often used to induce anesthesia for patients with coronary disease because of the associated increase in heart rate and systemic blood pressure, which may increase myocardial oxygen requirements. When giving desflurane, the inspired concentration should be slowly increased because of sympathetic stimulation and associated tachycardia, pulmonary hypertension, myocardial ischemia, and bronchospasm.[39] Tracheal intubation is facilitated by the administration of succinylcholine or a nondepolarizing neuromuscular blocking drug (also see Chapter 12).

Myocardial ischemia may accompany the tachycardia and hypertension that results from the stimulation of direct laryngoscopy as necessary for tracheal intubation. Adequate anesthesia and a brief duration of direct laryngoscopy is important in minimizing the magnitude of these circulatory changes. When the duration of direct laryngoscopy is not likely to be brief, or when hypertension coexists, the addition of other drugs to minimize the pressor response produced by tracheal intubation should be considered. For example, laryngotracheal lidocaine (2 mg/kg) administered just before placing the tube in the trachea produces rapid topical anesthesia of the tracheal mucosa and minimizes the magnitude and duration of the systemic blood pressure increase. Alternatively, lidocaine (1.5 mg/kg IV), administered just before initiating direct laryngoscopy, is efficacious.

Opioids (fentanyl, sufentanil, alfentanil, or remifentanil) before initiating direct laryngoscopy reduce the stimulation produced by tracheal intubation. β-Adrenergic blockers are effective in attenuating heart rate increases associated with tracheal intubation. Tachycardia should be avoided in all patients with coronary disease, vascular disease, or risk factors for coronary disease.

MAINTENANCE OF ANESTHESIA

The choice of anesthesia is often based on left ventricular function (see Table 25-3). For example, patients with coronary artery disease but normal left ventricular function may develop tachycardia and hypertension in response to intense stimulation. Controlled myocardial depression produced by a volatile anesthetic with or without nitrous oxide may be appropriate if the primary goal is to prevent increased myocardial oxygen requirements. Equally acceptable for the maintenance of anesthesia is the use of a nitrous oxide–opioid technique with the addition of a volatile anesthetic as necessary to treat acute increases in systemic blood pressure as produced by a change in the level of surgical stimulation. When hypertension is treated with a volatile anesthetic (isoflurane, desflurane, sevoflurane), the drug-induced decrease in systemic vascular resistance is more responsible for decreases in systemic blood pressure than is drug-induced myocardial depression. The ability to rapidly increase the alveolar concentration of sevoflurane makes this drug uniquely efficacious for treating sudden increases in systemic blood pressure. Abrupt and large increases in the delivered concentrations of desflurane, may be accompanied by stimulation of the sympathetic nervous system and transient increases in systemic blood pressure, heart rate, pulmonary hypertension, and myocardial ischemia (see Chapter 8).[39]

Volatile anesthetics are vasodilators. Under unusual clinical circumstances, potent coronary vasodilators could divert blood flow from ischemic areas of myocardium (blood vessels already fully dilated) to nonischemic areas of myocardium supplied by vessels capable of vasodilation. Regional myocardial ischemia associated with drug-induced vasodilation is known as coronary artery steal. There are reports that the incidence of myocardial ischemia is either unchanged or increased in patients with coronary artery disease and anesthetized with isoflurane compared with those receiving a different volatile anesthetic or an opioid-based anesthetic.[40–42] Volatile anesthetics to varying degrees (halothane, isoflurane, sevoflurane, and desflurane) induce ischemic preconditioning and may protect the myocardium from subsequent ischemia.[43,44] All facts considered, volatile anesthetics may be either beneficial in patients with coronary artery disease because they decrease myocardial oxygen requirements and induce ischemic preconditioning, or detrimental because they decrease systemic blood pressure and coronary perfusion pressure or produce coronary artery steal (isoflurane) or tachycardia (desflurane).[45] A large clinical trial in patients undergoing cardiac surgery failed to demonstrate a difference between halothane, enflurane, isoflurane, and narcotic-based anesthetics.[46] Avoiding tachycardia with the use of long-acting (metoprolol or atenolol) β-blockers is more important than anesthetic choice.[12–16,18,46] Intraoperative bolus doses of short-acting β-blockers (esmolol) have not been shown to be effective in reducing perioperative cardiac risk. Prophylactic perioperative administration of long-acting β-blockers (metoprolol or atenolol) is needed to reduce perioperative risk.[16]

Patients with impaired left ventricular function, as associated with a prior myocardial infarction, may not tolerate direct myocardial depression produced by volatile anesthetics. In these patients, the use of short-acting opioids with nitrous oxide may be a more acceptable selection. Nitrous oxide, when administered to patients who have received opioids for anesthesia, may produce undesirable decreases in systemic blood pressure and cardiac output. High-dose fentanyl (50 to 100 µg/kg IV) or equivalent doses of sufentanil or alfentanil as the primary anesthetic with benzodiazepines added to ensure amnesia may be useful for patients who cannot tolerate the myocardial depression from even low concentrations of anesthetics. Yet, this technique is not clearly better than moderate dose narcotics with an inhaled volatile or intravenous anesthetic.[46]

A regional anesthetic is an excellent technique in patients with coronary artery disease (also see Chapters 17 and 18). Regional anesthesia for peripheral surgery (orthopedic, podiatric, peripheral vascular) and lower abdominal surgery (gynecologic and urologic) is a very safe technique for patients with cardiac risk. However, flow through critically narrowed coronary arteries is pressure-dependent. Therefore, decreases in systemic blood pressure associated with a regional anesthetic that are more than 20% of the preblock value probably should be treated with an intravenous infusion of crystalloid solutions or a vasoconstrictor such as phenylephrine. Phenylephrine improves coronary perfusion pressure but at the expense of increasing afterload and myocardial oxygen requirements. Nevertheless, the increase in coronary perfusion pressure is likely to more than offset any increase in myocardial oxygen requirements. Perioperative β-blockers or clonidine should be used in patients with cardiac risk undergoing surgery using regional anesthesia.

NEUROMUSCULAR BLOCKING DRUGS (Also See Chapter 12)

The choice of nondepolarizing neuromuscular blocking drug during maintenance of anesthesia for patients with coronary artery disease may be influenced by the circulatory effects of these drugs. Vecuronium, rocuronium, and cisatracurium do not evoke histamine release and associated decreases in systemic blood pressure, even with the rapid intravenous administration of large doses. Likewise, the systemic blood pressure lowering effects of atracurium and mivacurium, are usually modest, especially if the drug is injected over 30 to 45 seconds to minimize the likelihood of drug-induced histamine release. None of these neuromuscular blocking drugs will adversely alter myocardial oxygen requirements. Pancuronium increases heart rate and systemic blood pressure, but these changes are usually less than 15% above predrug values, making this drug a possible choice for administration to patients with coronary artery disease. Furthermore, circulatory

IV

changes produced by pancuronium can be used to offset negative inotropic or chronotropic effects of drugs being used for anesthesia. In contrast to pancuronium, the other nondepolarizing neuromuscular blocking drugs would not be expected to offset decreases in systemic blood pressure or heart rate as associated with the administration of large doses of opioids. Use of pancuronium has decreased with the increased use of more selective neuromuscular blocking drugs (vecuronium, rocuronium, and cisatracurium).

Nondepolarizing neuromuscular blockade in patients with coronary artery disease can be safely antagonized with anticholinesterase drugs combined with an anticholinergic drug. Glycopyrrolate has more titratable chronotropic effects than atropine. Tachycardia after reversal of nondepolarizing muscle relaxants can still occur. One of the common causes of postoperative myocardial ischemia and infarction is tachycardia after emergence, which may be the result of the combination of emergence, surgical pain, and reversal of nondepolarizing muscle relaxants. The addition of long-acting intravenous β-blockers should be used to avoid tachycardia, which may lead to myocardial ischemia in this period. The use of sugammadex should eliminate these cardiovascular problems with reversal of neuromuscular blockade.

TREATMENT OF MYOCARDIAL ISCHEMIA

The appearance of signs of myocardial ischemia on the ECG supports the aggressive treatment of adverse changes in heart rate or systemic blood pressure. Only 5% of perioperative myocardial ischemia found on Holter ECG is identified by clinicians. Prophylactic therapy with long-acting β-blockers or clonidine is essential to reduce perioperative risk.[12-16] Tachycardia is treated with the administration of atenolol, metoprolol, propranolol, or esmolol. Excessive increases in systemic blood pressure respond to narcotics, increases in inhaled agents, β-blockers, or continuous intravenous infusion of nitroprusside. Nitroglycerin is a more appropriate choice than nitroprusside when myocardial ischemia is associated with a normal systemic blood pressure. Hypotension should be treated with a phenylephrine infusion to rapidly restore pressure-dependent perfusion through atherosclerotic coronary arteries. In addition to drugs, the intravenous infusion of fluids to restore systemic blood pressure helps myocardial oxygen requirements. A disadvantage of this approach is the time necessary for intravenous fluid treatment to be effective.

The use of pulmonary artery catheters, in selected patients, may be helpful for monitoring responses to intravenous fluid replacement and the therapeutic effects of drugs on left ventricular function. Right atrial (central venous) pressure may not reliably reflect left-sided heart filling pressure in the presence of left ventricular dysfunction due to coronary artery disease if the ejection fraction is less than 50%. In healthy patients who have a reduced need for monitoring, right atrial pressure is more likely to correlate with pulmonary artery occlusion pressure in patients with coronary artery disease when the ejection fraction is larger than 0.5 and when there is no evidence of left ventricular dysfunction.[47,48] Abrupt increases in the pulmonary artery pressure may also reflect acute myocardial ischemia; however, when compared with transesophageal echocardiography monitoring (TEE), monitoring with a pulmonary artery catheter is not a highly sensitive approach for detecting myocardial ischemia. TEE also provides an assessment of regional wall motion, global ventricular function, valvular function, intravascular fluid volume, and associated ventricular filling. TEE is more expensive than pulmonary artery catheterization but the information is more accurate and useful than pulmonary artery catheter data.

Decreases in body temperature that occur intraoperatively may predispose to shivering on awakening, leading to abrupt increases in myocardial oxygen requirements. Attempts to minimize decreases in body temperature and provision of supplemental oxygen are of obvious importance. Postoperative pain relief is important as pain-induced activation of the sympathetic nervous system can increase myocardial oxygen requirements.

Postoperative Care (Also See Chapter 39)

Postoperative care of the patient with coronary artery disease is based on provision of perioperative anti-ischemic agents (β-blockers or clonidine, statins), analgesia, and if needed, sedation to blunt excessive sympathetic nervous system activity and facilitate rigorous control of hemodynamic variables. Intensive and continuous postoperative monitoring is useful for detecting myocardial ischemia, which is often asymptomatic. In addition to detecting it, the occurrence of myocardial ischemia should be prevented. Episodes of myocardial ischemia lead to increased risk and increasingly frequent episodes.[2,37,49] Reducing the incidence of episodes of myocardial ischemia with β-blockers or clonidine reduces 30-day and 2-year mortality rates.[36,37] All patients with known coronary artery disease, known peripheral vascular disease, or two risk factors for coronary artery disease (including the elderly, hypertension, diabetes, significant smoking history, or hyperlipidemia) should receive a perioperative β-blocker unless there is a specific contraindication.[12-15] They should receive β-blockers as soon as they are identified as being at risk for cardiac complications.[12,13] Patients with lower risk should take the drug for at least 7 days postoperatively.[14,15] Patients with known coronary disease or vascular disease should take the drug for at least 30 days, if not permanently.[12,13] Chronic obstructive pulmonary disease (COPD) is not a contraindication to perioperative β-blockade, but reactive asthma is. Diabetes is not a contraindication for perioperative β-blockade; it is an indication. In patients who cannot tolerate β-blockers, the α_2-agonist clonidine may be used.[16] All medications have a therapeutic index and β-blockers are no exception. The dose of perioperative β-blockers should follow standard manufacturer guidelines to avoid hypotension, bradycardia, morbidity, and death.[31]

The major determinant of pulmonary complications (atelectasis, pneumonia) after cardiac surgery is poor cardiac function. Early mobilization and pain control are likely to minimize the incidence of clinically significant pulmonary complications.

VALVULAR HEART DISEASE (Also See Chapter 26)

The most frequently encountered forms of valvular heart disease produce pressure overload (mitral stenosis, aortic stenosis) or volume overload (mitral regurgitation, aortic regurgitation).[50] The net effect of valvular heart disease is interference with forward flow of blood from the heart into the systemic circulation. Transesophageal echocardiography has revolutionized the evaluation and intraoperative management of valvular heart disease (Table 25-5). Selection of anesthetic drugs and neuromuscular blocking drugs for patients with valvular heart disease is often based on the likely effects of drug-induced changes in cardiac rhythm, heart rate, systemic blood pressure, systemic vascular resistance, and pulmonary vascular resistance relative to maintenance of cardiac output in these patients. Although no specific general anesthetic is superior, when cardiac reserve is minimal, an anesthetic combination of opioids, an amnestic benzodiazepine, and an inhaled anesthetic is common. Dexmedetomidine infusions may be extremely useful in combination with other drugs. Patients with valvular heart disease should receive appropriate antibiotics in the perioperative period for protection against infective endocarditis. Monitoring intra-arterial pressure is helpful in patients with clinically significant valvular heart disease.

Mitral Stenosis

Mitral stenosis is characterized by mechanical obstruction of left ventricular diastolic filling secondary to a progressive decrease in the orifice of the mitral valve.

Table 25-5 Diagnosis: Echocardiography and Valvular Heart Disease

- Determine significance of cardiac murmurs (most often aortic stenosis).
- Identify hemodynamic abnormalities associated with physical findings (most often mitral regurgitation).
- Determine transvalvular pressure gradient.
- Determine cardiac valve regurgitation.
- Evaluate prosthetic valve function.

The obstruction produces an increase in left atrial and pulmonary venous pressure. Increased pulmonary vascular resistance is likely when the left atrial pressure is chronically higher than 25 mm Hg. Distention of the left atrium predisposes to atrial fibrillation, which can result in stasis of blood, the formation of thrombi, and systemic emboli. Chronic anticoagulation or antiplatelet therapy (or both) of patients with atrial fibrillation can reduce the risk of systemic embolic events. Mitral stenosis is commonly due to the fusion of the mitral valve leaflets during the healing process of acute rheumatic carditis. Symptoms of mitral stenosis do not usually develop until about 20 years after the initial episode of rheumatic fever. A sudden increase in the demand for cardiac output as produced by pregnancy or sepsis, however, may unmask previously asymptomatic mitral stenosis.

Patients with mitral stenosis who are being chronically treated with digitalis for the control of heart rate should continue to take this drug throughout the perioperative period. Adequate digitalis effect for heart rate control is generally reflected by a ventricular rate less than 80 beats/min. Because diuretic therapy is common in these patients, the serum potassium concentration should be measured preoperatively. Other common antiarrhythmic drugs such as β-blockers should also be continued. The discontinuation of anticoagulant or antiplatelet therapy should be discussed with the surgeon and cardiologist. Patients should be switched from warfarin (Coumadin) therapy to heparin therapy prior to surgery depending on the type of case. Also, patients with mitral stenosis can be more susceptible than normal individuals to the ventilatory depressant effects of sedative drugs used for preoperative medication. If patients are given sedative drugs, supplemental oxygen may increase the margin of safety. Most medications that patients are taking, except anticoagulants, antiplatelet agents, and oral hypoglycemic agents, should be continued throughout the preoperative period. Patients with diabetes may benefit from an intravenous insulin infusion with frequent glucose monitoring.[51]

MANAGEMENT OF ANESTHESIA
Preinduction of anesthesia placement of intra-arterial pressure monitoring can speed the identification and treatment of hemodynamic changes in patients with clinically significant valvular disease. Induction of anesthesia in the presence of mitral stenosis can be achieved with intravenous drugs, with the possible exception of ketamine, which may be avoided because of its propensity to increase the heart rate. Tracheal intubation is facilitated by the administration of a neuromuscular blocking drug. Neuromuscular blocking drugs with minimal effect on heart rate are commonly chosen. Drugs used for maintenance of anesthesia should cause minimal changes in heart rate and in systemic and pulmonary vascular resistance. Furthermore, these drugs should not

greatly decrease myocardial contractility. No one anesthetic has been proved to be superior. These goals can be achieved with combinations of an opioid and low concentrations of a volatile anesthetic or intravenous anesthetics such as propofol or dexmedetomidine. Although nitrous oxide can increase pulmonary vascular resistance, this increase is not sufficiently great to justify avoiding this drug in all patients with mitral stenosis.[52] The effect of nitrous oxide on pulmonary vascular resistance, however, seems to be accentuated when coexisting pulmonary hypertension is severe. Avoiding the use of nitrous oxide allows higher inspired oxygen concentrations and may reduce pulmonary vasoconstriction. Rapid increases in the concentration of desflurane may cause tachycardia, bronchospasm, and pulmonary hypertension and should be avoided. Control of arterial blood pressure with a prophylactic intravenous infusion of the vasoconstrictors phenylephrine can reduce hemodynamic changes with induction of anesthesia.

Nondepolarizing neuromuscular blocking drugs with minimal circulatory effects are useful in patients with mitral stenosis. Pancuronium is less appropriate because of its ability to increase the speed of transmission of cardiac impulses through the atrioventricular node, which could lead to excessive increases in heart rate. Such increases may be problematic in the presence of atrial fibrillation because the ventricular response to atrial impulses is determined by the degree of atrioventricular conduction. The adverse effects of drug-induced tachycardia in response to drug-assisted antagonism of nondepolarizing neuromuscular blocking drugs should be avoided (Table 25-6). Sugammadex, which can replace neostigmine, does not cause cardiovascular changes. If cases are prolonged and neuromuscular blockade is not required for the conduct of the case, allowing the nondepolarizing neuromuscular blockade to be eliminated through metabolism may reduce the risk of tachycardia with drug-assisted antagonism. Intraoperative intravenous fluid therapy must be carefully titrated because these patients are susceptible to intravascular volume overload and to the development of left ventricular failure and pulmonary edema. Likewise, the head-down position may not be well tolerated because the pulmonary blood volume is already increased.

Monitoring intra-arterial pressure and possibly right atrial pressure is a helpful guide to the adequacy of intravascular fluid replacement. An increase in right atrial pressure could also reflect pulmonary vasoconstriction, suggesting the need to check for causes, which may include nitrous oxide, desflurane, acidosis, hypoxia, increased mitral regurgitation, or light anesthesia.

Postoperatively, patients with mitral stenosis are at high risk for developing pulmonary edema and right-sided heart failure. Mechanical support of ventilation of the lungs may be necessary, particularly after major thoracic or abdominal surgery. The shift from positive-pressure ventilation to spontaneous ventilation with weaning and extubation may lead to increased venous return and increased central venous pressures with worsening of heart failure.

Mitral Regurgitation

Mitral regurgitation is characterized by left atrial volume overload and decreased left ventricular forward stroke volume due to the backflow of part of each stroke volume through the incompetent mitral valve back into the left atrium. This regurgitant flow is responsible for the characteristic V waves seen on the recording of the pulmonary artery occlusion pressure.[53] Mitral regurgitation secondary to rheumatic fever usually has a component of mitral stenosis. Dilated cardiomyopathy, which may be from ischemia, multiple myocardial infarctions, viral or parasitic infections, or other causes, may cause mitral regurgitation. Isolated mitral regurgitation may be acute, reflecting papillary muscle dysfunction after a myocardial infarction or rupture of chordae tendineae secondary to infective endocarditis.

MANAGEMENT OF ANESTHESIA

Management of anesthesia in patients with mitral regurgitation should avoid decreases in the forward left ventricular stroke volume. Conversely, cardiac output can be improved by mild increases in heart rate and mild decreases in systemic vascular resistance (Table 25-7). Preinduction placement of intra-arterial pressure monitoring can speed the identification and treatment of hemodynamic changes in patients with clinically significant valvular disease.

Table 25-6 Anesthetic Considerations in the Patients with Mitral Stenosis

- Avoid sinus tachycardia or rapid ventricular response rate during atrial fibrillation.
- Avoid marked increases in central blood volume associated with overtransfusion or head-down position.
- Avoid drug-induced decreases in systemic vascular resistance.
- Avoid events such as arterial hypoxemia or hypoventilation that may exacerbate pulmonary hypertension and evoke right ventricular failure.

Table 25-7 Anesthetic Considerations in Patients with Mitral Regurgitation

- Avoid sudden decreases in heart rate.
- Avoid sudden decreases in systemic vascular resistance.
- Minimize drug-induced myocardial depression.
- Monitor the magnitude of the V wave as a reflection of mitral regurgitant flow.

A general anesthetic is the usual choice for patients with mitral regurgitation. Although decreases in systemic vascular resistance are theoretically beneficial, the rapid onset and uncontrolled nature of this response with a spinal anesthetic may detract from the use of this technique. Local or regional anesthesia may be used safely for surgery on peripheral body sites. Additional monitoring with continuous intra-arterial pressure monitoring can improve the identification of hypotension and improve the margin of safety. Continuous spinal anesthetics may allow a slow titration of the regional block and can be a good choice of anesthetic. Maintenance of general anesthesia can be provided with volatile anesthetic, with or without nitrous oxide, or a continuous infusion of intravenous anesthetic. The concentration of volatile anesthetic can be adjusted to attenuate undesirable increases in systemic blood pressure and systemic vascular resistance that can accompany surgical stimulation. Avoiding the use of nitrous oxide allows higher inspired oxygen concentrations and may reduce pulmonary vasoconstriction. Rapid increases in the concentration of desflurane may cause tachycardia, bronchospasm, and pulmonary hypertension and should be avoided. Control of blood pressure with a prophylactic intravenous infusion of the vasoconstrictor phenylephrine can reduce hemodynamic changes with induction. Nondepolarizing neuromuscular blocking drugs that lack significant circulatory effects are useful. Intravascular fluid volume must be maintained by prompt replacement of blood loss to ensure adequate venous return and ejection of an optimal forward left ventricular stroke volume.

Aortic Stenosis

Aortic stenosis is characterized by increased left ventricular systolic pressure to maintain the forward stroke volume through a narrowed aortic valve. The magnitude of the pressure gradient across the valve serves as an estimate of the severity of valvular stenosis. Hemodynamically significant aortic stenosis is associated with pressure gradients less than 50 mm Hg or valve areas less than 1.2 cm^2. A peak systolic gradient exceeding 50 mm Hg in the presence of normal cardiac output or an effective aortic orifice less than about 0.75 cm^2 in an average-sized adult (i.e., 0.4 cm^2/m^2 of body surface area or less than approximately one fourth of the normal orifice) is generally considered to represent critical aortic stenosis. The combination of symptoms (angina, congestive failure, or fainting), signs (serious left ventricular dysfunction and progressive cardiomegaly), and a reduced valve area also may make the diagnosis of critical aortic stenosis requiring surgical replacement. Increased intraventricular pressures are accompanied by compensatory increases in the thickness of the left ventricular wall. Angina pectoris occurs often in these patients in the absence of coronary artery disease, reflecting an increased myocardial oxygen demand because of the increased amounts of ventricular muscle associated with myocardial hypertrophy in combination with higher intraventricular pressures. There is a decrease in oxygen delivery secondary to the aortic valve pressure gradient in combination with an increase in oxygen requirements from the increase in left ventricular pressure and stroke work.

Isolated nonrheumatic aortic stenosis usually results from progressive calcification and stenosis of a congenitally abnormal (usually bicuspid) valve. Aortic stenosis due to rheumatic fever almost always occurs in association with mitral valve disease. Likewise, aortic stenosis is usually accompanied by some degree of aortic regurgitation. Regardless of the etiology of aortic stenosis, the natural history of the disease includes a long latent period, often 30 years or more, before symptoms occur. Because aortic stenosis may be asymptomatic, it is important to listen for this cardiac murmur (systolic murmur in the second right intercostal space that may radiate to the right carotid) in patients scheduled for surgery. The incidence of sudden death is increased in patients with aortic stenosis.

MANAGEMENT OF ANESTHESIA

Goals during management of anesthesia in patients with aortic stenosis are maintenance of normal sinus rhythm and avoidance of extreme and prolonged alterations in heart rate, systemic vascular resistance, and intravascular fluid volume (Table 25-8). Preservation of normal sinus rhythm is critical because the left ventricle is dependent on properly timed atrial contractions to ensure optimal left ventricular filling and stroke volume. Marked increases in heart rate (higher than 100 beats/min) decrease the time for left ventricular filling and ejection, and decrease coronary blood flow while increasing myocardial oxygen consumption. Coronary blood flow to the left ventricle occurs during diastolic and changes in heart rate primarily effect diastolic time. Bradycardia (lower than 50 beats/min) can lead to acute overdistention of the left ventricle. Tachycardia may lead to myocardial ischemia and ventricular dysfunction. In view of the

IV

Table 25-8 Anesthetic Considerations in Patients with Aortic Stenosis

Intra-arterial pressure monitoring
Rapid availability or prophylactic administration of intravenous vasoconstrictors (phenylephrine)
Maintenance of normal sinus rhythm
Avoidance of extreme bradycardia or tachycardia
Avoidance of sudden decreases in systemic vascular resistance
Optimization of intravascular fluid volume

obstruction to left ventricular ejection, decreases in systemic vascular resistance may be associated with large decreases in systemic blood pressure and coronary blood flow and myocardial ischemia. Intra-arterial pressure monitoring is essential and can speed identification and treatment of hemodynamic changes. Prophylactic infusions of vasoconstrictors, such as phenylephrine, may reduce hemodynamic changes.

A general anesthetic may be preferred to a regional anesthetic because sympathetic nervous system blockade can lead to undesirable decreases in systemic vascular resistance. If surgery is peripheral, a regional anesthetic with careful intra-arterial pressure monitoring can be equally successful. Maintenance of general anesthesia can be achieved with both intravenous and inhaled anesthetics. A potential disadvantage of volatile inhaled anesthetics is depression of sinus node automaticity, which may lead to junctional rhythm and decreased left ventricular filling due to loss of properly timed atrial contractions. Techniques with peripheral vasodilation should be used carefully. A prophylactic intravenous infusion of phenylephrine can be started prior to induction to reduce hemodynamic changes. The most important technique for the management of patients with aortic stenosis is intra-arterial pressure monitoring with careful avoidance of hypotension.

Intravascular fluid volume must be maintained by prompt replacement of blood loss and liberal administration of intravenous fluids. If a pulmonary artery catheter is placed, it should be remembered that the occlusion pressure may overestimate the left ventricular end-diastolic volume because of the decreased compliance of the left ventricle that accompanies chronic aortic stenosis. A cardiac defibrillator should be promptly available when anesthesia is administered to patients with aortic stenosis since external cardiac compressions are unlikely to generate an adequate stroke volume across a stenosed aortic valve.

Aortic Regurgitation

Aortic regurgitation is characterized by decreased forward left ventricular stroke volume due to regurgitation of part of the ejected stroke volume from the aorta back into the left ventricle through an incompetent aortic valve. A gradual onset of aortic regurgitation results in marked left ventricular hypertrophy and eventually dilation. Increased myocardial oxygen requirements secondary to left ventricular hypertrophy, plus a characteristic decrease in aortic diastolic pressure that decreases coronary blood flow, can manifest as angina pectoris in the absence of coronary artery disease. Coronary blood flow to the left ventricle occurs during diastole. In severe or acute aortic regurgitation with low diastolic pressures and elevated end-diastolic ventricular pressures, coronary blood flow can be severely compromised. The combination of a low diastolic pressure from aortic regurgitation with the increase in left ventricular diastolic pressure substantially decreases the coronary perfusion pressure gradient. Acute aortic regurgitation is most often due to infective endocarditis, trauma, or dissection of a thoracic aortic aneurysm. Chronic aortic regurgitation is usually due to prior rheumatic fever. In contrast to aortic stenosis, the occurrence of sudden death in patients with aortic regurgitation is rare.

MANAGEMENT OF ANESTHESIA

Management of anesthesia for noncardiac surgery in patients with aortic regurgitation is as described for patients with mitral regurgitation (see Table 25-7). Preinduction intra-arterial pressure monitoring can speed the identification and treatment of hemodynamic changes and should be used for patients with significant aortic regurgitation. Anesthetics with minimal effects on systemic vascular resistance or cardiac function should be selected.

Mitral Valve Prolapse

Mitral valve prolapse (click-murmur syndrome, Barlow syndrome) is characterized by an abnormality of the mitral valve support structure that permits prolapse of the valve into the left atrium during contraction of the left ventricle.[54] Previous estimates that mitral valve prolapse was present in 5% to 15% of individuals are most likely erroneously high.[55] Transesophageal or transthoracic echocardiography can confirm the diagnosis of mitral valve prolapse, particularly in the absence of the characteristic systolic murmur. The incidence of mitral valve prolapse in patients probably increases with musculoskeletal abnormalities, including Marfan syndrome, pectus excavatum, and kyphoscoliosis.

Despite the prevalence of mitral valve prolapse, most patients are asymptomatic, emphasizing the usually benign course of this abnormality. Nevertheless, serious complications may accompany mitral valve prolapse (Table 25-9). For example, mitral valve prolapse is probably the most common cause of pure mitral regurgitation, which may progress to the need for surgical intervention. Infective endocarditis is a potential complication, and transient ischemic attacks in patients younger than 45 years of age are often associated with mitral

Table 25-9 Complications Associated with Mitral Valve Prolapse

Mitral regurgitation
Infective endocarditis
Transient ischemic events
Cardiac dysrhythmias
Sudden death (extremely rare)

valve prolapse. Sudden death is an extremely rare complication of mitral valve prolapse, which may be due to a ventricular cardiac dysrhythmia.

MANAGEMENT OF ANESTHESIA

Management of anesthesia for patients with mitral valve prolapse should avoid events that can increase cardiac emptying, which can accentuate prolapse of the mitral valve into the left atrium.[56] Perioperative events that can increase cardiac emptying include (1) sympathetic nervous system stimulation, (2) decreased systemic vascular resistance, and (3) performance of surgery with patients in the head-up or sitting position. Adequate intravascular fluid volume is of prime importance in the preoperative period. Although intravenous anesthetics can be used to induce anesthesia, a sudden prolonged decrease in systemic vascular resistance must be avoided. Also, intra-arterial pressure monitoring can facilitate recognition and treatment of hemodynamic changes during induction of anesthesia. Prophylactic infusions of phenylephrine can reduce systemic vasodilation with induction of anesthesia. Ketamine and pancuronium are not recommended because of their ability to increase cardiac contractility and heart rate. Yet, these drugs are probably given to patients with undiagnosed and asymptomatic mitral valve prolapse without problems.

Addition of a narcotic to the anesthetic can minimize sympathetic nervous system activation due to noxious intraoperative stimulation. Volatile anesthetics should be titrated to avoid excessive decreases in systemic vascular resistance. Regional anesthetic can be used so long as undesirable decreases in systemic vascular resistance are avoided, which dictates appropriate monitoring. Prompt replacement of blood loss and generous administration of intravenous fluids will contribute to maintenance of an optimal intravascular fluid volume and decrease the potential adverse effects of positive-pressure ventilation. Lidocaine, amiodarone, metoprolol, and esmolol should be available to treat cardiac dysrhythmias. If a vasoconstriction is needed to treat hypotension, an α-agonist, such as phenylephrine, should probably be used.

DISTURBANCES OF CARDIAC CONDUCTION AND RHYTHM (Also See Chapter 20)

The ECG is a valuable tool for diagnosing disturbances of cardiac conduction and rhythm. Ambulatory ECG monitoring (Holter monitoring) is useful in documenting the occurrence of life-threatening cardiac dysrhythmias and assessing the efficacy of antidysrhythmic drug therapy. The incidence of intraoperative cardiac dysrhythmias depends on the definition (benign versus life-threatening), patient characteristics, and the type of surgery (frequent incidence during cardiothoracic surgery).[56] The following questions should be asked when interpreting the ECG:

1. What is the heart rate?
2. Are P waves present, and what is their relationship to the QRS complexes?
3. What is the duration of the PR interval (normal 120 to 200 msec)?
4. What is the duration of the QRS complex (normal 50 to 120 msec)?
5. Is the ventricular rhythm regular?
6. Are there early cardiac beats or abnormal pauses after a preceding QRS complex?
7. Is there evidence of prior myocardial infarction or ventricular hypertrophy?
8. Is there evidence of myocardial ischemia?
9. Is there a conduction disturbance such as left bundle branch block, right bundle branch block, or intraventricular conduction delay?

Heart Block

Disturbances of conduction of cardiac impulses can be classified according to the site of the conduction block relative to the atrioventricular node (Table 25-10). Heart block occurring above the atrioventricular node is usually benign and transient. Heart block occurring below the atrioventricular node tends to be progressive and permanent.

A theoretical concern in patients with bifascicular heart block is that perioperative events, such as alterations in systemic blood pressure, arterial oxygenation, or electrolyte concentrations, might compromise conduction in the one remaining intact fascicle, leading to the acute onset intraoperatively of third-degree atrioventricular heart block. However, surgery performed during a general or regional anesthetic has not been shown to

Table 25-10 Classification of Heart Block
First-degree atrioventricular heart block
Second-degree atrioventricular heart block
Mobitz type I (Wenckebach)
Mobitz type II
Unifascicular heart block
Left anterior hemiblock
Left posterior hemiblock
Right bundle branch block
Left bundle branch block
Bifascicular heart block
Right bundle branch block plus anterior hemiblock
Right bundle branch block plus posterior hemiblock
Third-degree (trifascicular, complete) atrioventricular heart block

IV

predispose to the development of third-degree atrioventricular heart block in patients with coexisting bifascicular block. Therefore, placement of a prophylactic artificial cardiac pacemaker is not required before anesthesia and surgery, but it should be available.

Third-degree atrioventricular heart block is treated by placement of an artificial cardiac pacemaker. An artificial cardiac pacemaker can be inserted intravenously (endocardial lead) or by the subcostal approach (epicardial or myocardial lead). An alternative to emergency transvenous artificial cardiac pacemaker placement is noninvasive transcutaneous or temporary esophageal cardiac pacing. A continuous intravenous infusion of isoproterenol acting as a pharmacologic cardiac pacemaker may be necessary to maintain an adequate heart rate until artificial electrical cardiac pacing can be established.

Sick Sinus Syndrome

Sick sinus syndrome is characterized by inappropriate sinus bradycardia associated with degenerative changes in the sinoatrial node. Frequently, bradycardia due to this syndrome is complicated by episodes of supraventricular tachycardia. Artificial cardiac pacemakers may be indicated when therapeutic plasma concentrations of drugs necessary to control tachycardia result in bradycardia. The increased incidence of pulmonary embolism in these patients may be a reason to initiate anticoagulation.

Ventricular Premature Beats

Ventricular premature beats (VPCs) are recognized on the ECG by (1) premature occurrence, (2) the absence of a P wave preceding the QRS complex, (3) a wide and often bizarre QRS complex, (4) an inverted T wave, and (5) a compensatory pause that follows the premature beat. The primary goal with VPCs should be to identify any underlying cause (myocardial ischemia, arterial hypoxemia, hypercarbia, hypertension, hypokalemia, mechanical irritation of the ventricles) if possible and correct it. Ventricular premature beats can be treated with lidocaine (1 to 2 mg/kg IV) when they (1) are frequent (more than 6 premature beats/min), (2) are multifocal, (3) occur in salvos of 3 or more, or (4) take place during the ascending limb of the T wave (R on T phenomenon) that corresponds to the relative refractory period of the ventricle.

Ventricular Tachycardia

Ventricular tachycardia is defined as the appearance of at least three consecutive wide QRS complexes (longer than 120 msec) on the ECG occurring at an effective heart rate more rapid than 120 beats/min. Ventricular tachycardia not associated with hypotension is initially treated with the intravenous administration of amiodarone, lidocaine, or procainamide. Torsade-de-point responds to magnesium. Symptomatic ventricular tachycardia is best treated with external electrical cardioversion. The presence of ventricular tachycardia should elicit an immediate search for a cause such as myocardial ischemia, hypoxia, electrolyte abnormalities, or myocardial stimulation by the surgeons.

Pre-Excitation Syndromes

Pre-excitation syndromes are characterized by activation of a portion of the ventricles by cardiac impulses that travel from the atria via accessory (anomalous) conduction pathways. These pathways bypass the atrioventricular node such that activation of the ventricles occurs earlier than it would if impulses reached the ventricles by normal pathways.

WOLFF-PARKINSON-WHITE SYNDROME

The Wolff-Parkinson-White syndrome is the most common pre-excitation syndrome, with an incidence of approximately 0.3% of the general population. The lack of physiologic delay in transmission of cardiac impulses along the Kent fibers results in the characteristic short PR interval (less than 120 msec) on the ECG. The wide QRS complex and delta wave on the ECG reflect the composite of cardiac impulses conducted by normal and accessory pathways. Paroxysmal atrial tachycardia is the most frequent cardiac dysrhythmia. More patients with Wolff-Parkinson-White syndrome are frequently treated by catheter ablation of accessory pathways as identified by electrophysiologic mapping. Supraventricular tachycardias such as atrial fibrillation or atrial flutter with one-to-one conduction may lead to hemodynamic collapse in patients with Wolff-Parkinson-White syndrome.

MANAGEMENT OF ANESTHESIA

The goal during management of anesthesia in the presence of a pre-excitation syndrome is to avoid events (anxiety) or drugs (anticholinergics, ketamine, pancuronium) that might increase sympathetic nervous system activity and predispose to tachydysrhythmias.[56] All cardiac antidysrhythmic drugs should be continued throughout the perioperative period. Anesthesia can be induced with intravenous anesthetic, with the possible exception of ketamine. Tracheal intubation should be performed only after a sufficient concentration or dose of anesthetic has been given to reliably blunt sympathetic nervous system stimulation evoked by instrumentation of the upper airway. Intravenous β-adrenergic blockers (atenolol, metoprolol, propranolol, or esmolol) can be used to avoid tachycardia during induction of anesthesia. Neuromuscular blocking drugs with minimal effects on heart rate should be used.

The onset of paroxysmal atrial tachycardia or fibrillation in the perioperative period can be treated with the intravenous administration of drugs that abruptly prolong the refractory period of the atrioventricular node (adenosine) or lengthen the refractory period of accessory pathways (procainamide). β-Adrenergic blockers may be used to control heart rate. Digitalis and verapamil may decrease the refractory period of accessory pathways responsible for atrial fibrillation, resulting in an increase in ventricular response rate during this dysrhythmia and should be avoided. Electrical cardioversion is indicated when tachydysrhythmias are life-threatening.

Prolonged QT Interval Syndrome

A prolonged QT interval (longer than 440 msec on the ECG) syndrome is associated with ventricular dysrhythmias, syncope, and sudden death. Treatment probably should include β-adrenergic antagonists or left stellate ganglion block. The effectiveness of a left stellate ganglion block supports the hypothesis that this syndrome results from a congenital imbalance of autonomic innervation to the heart produced by decreases in right cardiac sympathetic nerve activity. Management of anesthesia includes avoidance of events or drugs that are likely to activate the sympathetic nervous system and availability of β-antagonists (metoprolol, atenolol, propranolol, or esmolol) or electrical cardioversion to treat life-threatening ventricular dysrhythmias.[56] Inhaled and intravenous anesthetics can prolong the QT interval on the ECG in normal patients. Fortunately, these anesthetics do not produce additional prolonged QT interval in those patients with this syndrome in a predictable manner.[57] Many medications have the potential to prolong the QT interval (droperidol)[58,59] and should be avoided if possible, in patients with prolonged QT syndrome.

ARTIFICIAL CARDIAC PACEMAKERS

Preoperative evaluation of the patient with an artificial cardiac pacemaker in place includes determination of the reason for placing the pacemaker, assessment of its present function, as well as the brand, model, magnet mode, and availability of a programmer for this specific device and a person who knows how to operate the programmer.[60] Many implanted electrical devices can be used. A device under the skin may not be a pacemaker. Implanted devices include deep brain stimulators, automatic implantable cardiac defibrillators, intravenous pumps, spinal stimulators for chronic pain, bladder stimulators for neurogenic bladder, gastric stimulators for the treatment of obesity, intravenous ports, and vagal stimulators for sleep.

Special considerations are necessary for devices where the patient's life depends on the device. If a device is a cardiac pacemaker placed for third-degree heart block, appropriate experts regarding the continuous operation of that device and monitoring of its operation need to be immediately available. If a pacemaker implanted for third-degree heart block is to be disconnected to change the stimulator, transvenous pacing may be needed. If the device is an automatic defibrillator, it will need to be inactivated during electrical-surgical cautery to avoid the device erroneously detecting ventricular dysrhythmias and defibrillating, which would waste battery life and possibly cause R on T phenomena (see electrocardiogram) and ventricular fibrillation. The device should be reactivated after the surgical procedure and interrogated for proper function. The magnet mode of many implanted devices is now programmable. The magnet mode cannot automatically be assumed to be "safe." The specific magnet mode for a patient's device should be identified as some magnet modes change with device state or are programmable. Magnet mode for many pacemakers is asynchronous at 99 beats/min. If the patient has a spontaneous heart rate of 60 to 80 beats/min, the asynchronous mode at 99 beats/min would be safe. However, in some devices, the magnet mode shifts to asynchronous at 50 beats/min at the end of battery life. Asynchronous pacing at 50 beats/min may lead to R on T phenomena if the patient has a spontaneous heart rate above 50 beats/min. The specific magnet mode should be identified and used only when needed given the circumstances of the case.

Intraoperative monitoring of patients with artificial cardiac pacemakers includes the ECG and possible intra-arterial pressure monitoring so as to detect the appearance of asystole promptly. Atropine, isoproterenol, and an external pacemaker should be available if the artificial cardiac pacemaker ceases to function. If electrocautery interferes with the ECG, monitoring intra-arterial pressure, or arterial oxygenation, auscultation through an esophageal stethoscope or a palpable pulse confirms continued cardiac activity. Monitoring systemic blood pressure with an intra-arterial catheter provides immediate evidence of loss of pacemaker function and should be considered in patients with third-degree heart block. Inhibition of pulse generator activity by electromagnetic interference most commonly from electrosurgical cautery, which is interpreted as spontaneous cardiac activity by the artificial cardiac pacemaker, is most likely when the ground plate for electrocautery is placed too near the pulse generator or unipolar cautery is used. For this reason, the ground plate should be placed as far as possible from the pulse generator. Bipolar electrocautery may also reduce interference between electrosurgical cautery and the pacemaker. If surface pads are placed for external pacing or defibrillation, they should be placed away from the implanted device to reduce current passing down the pacing lead and hyperpolarizing a small segment of myocardium, which could interfere with pacemaker capture after defibrillation. Automatic implantable cardioversion devices sense ventricular fibrillation or ventricular tachycardia. They provide a cardioversion shock through implanted cardiac leads. Electrocautery signals can be misinterpreted as ventricular dysrhythmias, thus triggering unnecessary shocks and decreasing battery life. These devices should be reprogrammed to the standby mode prior to elective surgery and returned postoperatively to full function with interrogation of proper operation.

Selection of drugs or techniques for anesthesia is not influenced by the presence of artificial cardiac pacemakers as there is no evidence that the threshold and subsequent response of these devices is altered by drugs administered in the perioperative period. However, patients with artificial cardiac pacemakers or implanted cardioversion devices have a frequent incidence of coexisting cardiac disease and should be monitored carefully and anesthetized with care. Patients with defibrillators frequently have poor ventricular function. Insertion of a pulmonary artery catheter will not disturb epicardial electrodes but might dislodge recently placed (within 2 weeks) transvenous endocardial electrodes.[61] Pulmonary artery catheters are not necessary for cases with minimal fluid shifts.

ESSENTIAL HYPERTENSION

Essential hypertension is arbitrarily defined as sustained increases in systemic blood pressure (systolic blood pressure higher than 160 mm Hg or a diastolic blood pressure higher than 90 mm Hg) independent of any known cause. Treatment of essential hypertension with appropriate drug therapy decreases the incidence of stroke and congestive heart failure. Hypertension is a risk factor for coronary artery disease, and the longer the patient has hypertension the higher the risk of end organ damage. Patients with two risk factors (hypertension, smoking, diabetes, elevated cholesterol, or the elderly) for coronary artery disease should be treated as if they have coronary artery disease.

Management of anesthesia for patients with essential hypertension includes preoperative evaluation of drug therapy and extent of the disease plus a consideration of the implications of exaggerated systemic blood pressure responses elicited by painful intraoperative stimulation.[62]

Preoperative Evaluation (Also See Chapter 13)

Preoperative evaluation of patients with essential hypertension begins with a determination of the adequacy of systemic blood pressure control and a review of the pharmacology of the antihypertensive drugs being used for therapy (see Chapter 7). Antihypertensive drugs should be continued throughout the perioperative period. Evidence of major organ dysfunction (congestive heart failure, coronary artery disease, cerebral ischemia, renal dysfunction) must be sought. Patients with essential hypertension have an increased risk of coronary artery disease. Evidence of

peripheral vascular disease should be recognized, as all patients with peripheral vascular disease have coronary artery disease. About 50% of patients with evidence of peripheral vascular disease will have more than 50% stenosis of one or more coronary arteries even in the absence of angina pectoris and the presence of a normal resting ECG. Additional monitoring, including intra-arterial catheter monitoring, is justified for significant operations. Patients with increased pulse pressure have increased perioperative and long-term complications.[63] Essential hypertension is associated with a shift to the right of the curve for the autoregulation of cerebral blood flow, emphasizing that these patients are more vulnerable to cerebral ischemia should perfusion pressures decrease. Detection of renal dysfunction due to chronic hypertension may influence the selection of drugs, particularly if elimination from the plasma depends on renal clearance or metabolites of the drugs are known potential nephrotoxins (fluoride from metabolism of sevoflurane).

Hypertension should be treated preoperatively because the incidence of hypotension and evidence of myocardial ischemia on the ECG during the maintenance of anesthesia is increased in patients who remain hypertensive before the induction of anesthesia.[62] Perioperative therapy with β-adrenergic blockers for at least 7 days and continued for 30 days postoperatively reduces the risk of cardiac morbidity and death 90% for patients at risk.[12–15] Perioperative therapy with clonidine started the night before surgery and continued for 4 days reduces the 30-day and 2-year mortality rates.[16] Administration of intravenous β-blockers just prior to surgery and continued for 7 days reduces the risk of death 50%.[14,15] Prophylactic cardiac risk reduction therapy with β-blockers or clonidine of patients with coronary artery disease, peripheral vascular disease, or two risk factors (age greater than or equal to 60, hypertension, cholesterol higher than 240 mg/dL, diabetes, or smoking) reduces risk of perioperative death.[12–16] Appropriate dosing of β-adrenergic blockers is important to avoid sequelae.[31]

Despite therapy, systemic blood pressure increases during the intraoperative period are more likely to occur in patients with a history of essential hypertension regardless of the degree of pharmacologic control of systemic blood pressure established preoperatively. Furthermore, the incidence of postoperative cardiac complications is not increased when hypertensive patients undergo elective operations as long as the preoperative diastolic blood pressure is not more than 110 mm Hg and heart rate is controlled. Pretreatment with a β-blocker or the α_2-agonist, such as clonidine, may be useful in blunting exaggerated sympathetic nervous system responses and reduces perioperative mortality rate.[14–16]

Induction of Anesthesia

Induction of anesthesia with intravenous drugs is acceptable, remembering that an exaggerated decrease in systemic blood pressure may occur, particularly if hypertension is present preoperatively. Sodium thiopental, propofol, midazolam, synthetic opioids (fentanyl, sufentanil, alfentanil, remifentanil), and etomidate all have been used to induce anesthesia. Any anesthetic is acceptable if used with appropriate dosing and careful monitoring. Etomidate or combinations of midazolam and fentanyl are frequently used because of their limited hemodynamic effects. Ketamine is rarely selected for induction of anesthesia in patients with essential hypertension because it can increase systemic blood pressure and cause tachycardia, which may lead to myocardial ischemia. Placement of an intra-arterial pressure monitor prior to induction of anesthesia and prophylactic infusions of the vasoconstrictor phenylephrine can reduce hemodynamic perturbations with induction of anesthesia. Hemodynamic changes with induction most likely reflect unmasking of decreased intravascular fluid volume due to chronic hypertension combined with a stiffening of the arterial vasculature.

Hypertension can occur during direct laryngoscopy for tracheal intubation in patients with essential hypertension but may be attenuated with administration of opioids and β-adrenergic blockers. Tachycardia may lead to episodes of myocardial ischemia. A single 1-minute episode of myocardial ischemia increases the risk of perioperative cardiac morbidity tenfold and death twofold. The risk of myocardial ischemia can be reduced by prophylactic therapy with β-blockers or clonidine.[14–16]

Maximal attenuation of sympathetic nervous system responses should be attempted during direct laryngoscopy by administering anesthetics, intravenous opioids, and β-blockers before attempting tracheal intubation. Careful attention to the airway is critical in all anesthetics, and the risks are even more intense in patients with cardiac disease. If the patient has a recognized difficult airway precluding direct laryngoscopy, heart rate control is of prime importance, including possibly selecting alternative approaches such as fiberoptic intubation. Hypoxia, tachycardia, hypotension, hypertension, and myocardial ischemia must be avoided. Yet, an excessive concentration or dose of anesthetic drugs can produce hypotension, which is as undesirable as hypertension. An important concept for limiting pressor responses elicited by tracheal intubation is to limit the duration of direct laryngoscopy to less than 15 seconds if possible. In addition, the administration of laryngotracheal lidocaine immediately before placement of the tube in the trachea will minimize any additional pressor response.

Maintenance of Anesthesia

The goal during maintenance of anesthesia is to adjust the concentrations of anesthetics so tachycardia and wide fluctuations in systemic blood pressure can be avoided (Table 25-11). No anesthetic technique has been shown to be superior. Combinations of volatile anesthetics with

Table 25-11 Management of Anesthesia for Patients with Essential Hypertension

Preoperative Evaluation
- Determine the adequacy of systemic blood pressure control.
- Review the pharmacology of antihypertensive drugs.
- Evaluate associated organ dysfunction (cardiac, central nervous system, renal).
- Consider the administration of prophylactic anti-ischemic therapy (perioperative β-blockade or clonidine).
- Choose appropriate monitors and consider intra-arterial pressure monitoring.

Induction of Anesthesia and Tracheal Intubation
- Anticipate exaggerated systemic blood pressure changes.
- Consider initiation of prophylactic infusion of phenylephrine to reduce hemodynamic perturbation with induction.
- Minimize the pressor response during tracheal intubation by limiting the duration of direct laryngoscopy to <15 seconds.

Maintenance of Anesthesia
- Use a volatile anesthetic and vasoconstrictors to control systemic arterial blood pressure.
- Monitor the electrocardiogram for evidence of myocardial ischemia (avoidance is better than detection).
- Anticipate excessive increases in systemic blood pressure with emergence.

Postoperative Management
- Ensure effective pain control.
- Patient's blood pressure will return to preoperative level or greater after emergence from anesthesia, be ready to treat as needed.
- Continue perioperative anti-ischemic therapy for at least a week in low-risk patients, 30 days in those at higher risk, and permanently in patients with known coronary artery disease or vascular disease.

IV

or without nitrous oxide and a narcotic are commonly used. Changes in the concentration of volatile anesthetics allow rapid adjustments in the depth of anesthesia in response to increases or decreases in arterial blood pressure. Changes in surgical stimulation may lead to changes in blood pressure and heart rate. Additional doses of narcotics, β-blockers, and changes in the dose of volatile anesthetic can be used to control hemodynamics. Heart rate control is the most critical element for preventing cardiac morbidity and death. Heart rates above 120 beats/min increase mortality rate. Volatile anesthetics are useful for attenuating activity of the sympathetic nervous system, which is responsible for these pressor responses. The ability to rapidly increase the alveolar concentration of sevoflurane (because of its low blood solubilities) makes this volatile anesthetic uniquely efficacious for treating sudden increases in systemic blood pressure (see the discussion under "Coronary Artery Disease," at "Maintenance of Anesthesia"). Rapid changes in desflurane concentration may lead to tachycardia, hypertension, pulmonary hypertension, and myocardial ischemia and should be avoided. A positive feedback situation can occur with desflurane anesthetics whereby a surgical stimulus can raise blood pressure, the anesthetist raises the desflurane concentration, which stimulates the sympathetic system causing the blood pressure to increase, which causes the anesthetist to further increase the desflurane concentration, which further raises the blood pressure.

Both intravenous and inhaled anesthetics can be used. For example, a nitrous oxide–opioid technique is acceptable for the maintenance of anesthesia, but the addition of a volatile anesthetic is often necessary to prevent hypertension, particularly during periods of maximal surgical stimulation. Total intravenous anesthesia (combinations of dexmedetomidine, propofol, narcotics, and benzodiazepines) can also be used. Continuous intravenous infusions of phenylephrine, nitroprusside, nitroglycerine, carvedilol, or esmolol can be used to maintain normotension during the intraoperative period. Hypotension that occurs during maintenance of anesthesia is often treated by decreasing the concentrations of volatile anesthetic while infusing fluids intravenously to increase intravascular fluid volume. Sympathomimetics, such as ephedrine, or vasoconstrictors such as phenylephrine may be necessary to restore perfusion pressures until the underlying cause of the hypotension can be corrected.

The choice of intraoperative monitors for patients with coexisting essential hypertension is influenced by the complexity of the surgery. The ECG is monitored with the goal of recognizing changes suggestive of myocardial ischemia. Invasive monitoring with an intra-arterial pressure monitor is commonly used. Pulmonary artery catheters may be considered if major surgery is planned and there is evidence preoperatively of left ventricular dysfunction, although there is no evidence that demonstrates improved outcomes with pulmonary artery catheter monitoring. Monitoring with transesophageal echocardiography is an alternative to placement of a pulmonary artery catheter.

A regional anesthetic is an excellent choice in patients with multiple medical conditions scheduled for peripheral surgery. Whatever the choice of anesthetic, β-adrenergic blockers, α_2-agonist clonidine, and sedatives can be used to reduce sympathetic nervous system stimulation. Patients with cardiac disease who are scheduled for elective surgery can have episodes of myocardial ischemia in the days prior to surgery. The night before surgery is stressful and prophylactic β-blockade or clonidine can reduce the risk of sympathetic stimulation resulting in tachycardia and subsequent myocardial ischemia. There is the erroneous belief that minor surgery causes minor stress. Patients scheduled for ophthalmic surgery, a minor outpatient procedure, commonly have sympathetic stimulation resulting in preoperative hypertension. Prophylactic therapy with β-blockers or clonidine can reduce the preoperative hypertensive episodes and myocardial ischemia. Appropriate dosing of all medications is essential and inappropriate dosing may lead to hypotension, bradycardia, and increased morbidity and mortality rates.[31] All medications have a therapeutic index. Withholding antihypertensive medications may lead to withdrawal phenomena and increase the morbidity and mortality rates.

Postoperative Management

Hypertension in the early postoperative period is a frequent occurrence in patients with a preoperative diagnosis of essential hypertension. Prophylactic or therapeutic administration of β-blockers or clonidine can reduce these episodes of hypertension and reduce risk of perioperative ischemia and death. If hypertension persists despite β-blockers and adequate analgesia, it may be necessary to pharmacologically decrease systemic blood pressure utilizing a continuous intravenous infusion of nitroprusside, nitroglycerin, or intermittent injections of hydralazine (5 to 20 mg IV) or labetalol (0.1 to 0.5 mg/kg IV). Tachycardia in the postoperative period must be actively avoided as it increases morbidity and mortality rates. A heart rate of 120 beats/min raises the risk of postoperative death. Clearly the arterial blood pressure needs to be controlled during the entire perioperative period. The patient needs preoperative, intraoperative, and postoperative hemodynamic and autonomic control to prevent associated cardiac morbidity and death. Anesthesia care for patients with cardiac disease truly needs to be perioperative for optimal outcomes. If a patient needs a medication to control blood pressure and heart rate while at home, he will likely need it during surgery and postoperative care. Withdrawal of antihypertensive and anti-ischemic medications in the perioperative period increases cardiac risk.[23,25,26]

CONGESTIVE HEART FAILURE

Elective surgery should not be performed on patients with congestive heart failure unless optimally treated. The preoperative presence of congestive heart failure is associated with significant postoperative morbidity or mortality rates. Cardiology consultation is frequently helpful in patients with congestive failure as consideration of surgical or interventional revascularization and improvement of medical therapy can improve cardiac function. Preoperative initiation of β-blockers and vasodilator therapy with angiotensin-converting enzyme inhibitors can improve ventricular function and reduce operative risk. These drugs should be started by physicians with expertise in treating congestive failure and the doses increased slowly as tolerated over 3 to 6 months as the heart function recovers.

Management of Anesthesia

When surgery cannot be delayed, however, the drugs and techniques chosen to provide anesthesia must be selected with the goal of minimizing detrimental effects on cardiac output. Optimal cardiac output can be obtained when the impedance of the vasculature (preload and afterload) match the impedance of the heart and can be achieved by careful preload and afterload management.

Etomidate may be useful for the induction of anesthesia in the presence of congestive heart failure because of its limited effect on the sympathetic nervous system. Small concentrations of volatile anesthetics can maintain anesthesia, but cardiac depression should be avoided if possible. In the presence of severe congestive heart failure, the use of opioids in large doses as the primary anesthetic in combination with amnestic benzodiazepines (midazolam) may be justified, although no evidence supports this approach over the use of a primary volatile anesthetic combined with narcotics.[46] Positive-pressure ventilation of the lungs may be beneficial by decreasing pulmonary congestion, improving arterial oxygenation, and eliminating the work of breathing. The resumption of negative intrathoracic pressures with spontaneous ventilation following extubation can lead to increased filling pressures and worsening heart failure. Invasive monitoring of intra-arterial blood pressure is helpful. Use of pulmonary arterial catheters can be helpful in hemodynamic management but no evidence exists that they reduce operative risk or improve outcome. Maintenance of blood pressure with vasoconstrictors (phenylephrine) should precede increasing myocardial contractility with continuous intravenous infusions of inotropic drugs such as epinephrine, dopamine, and dobutamine. The use of β-adrenergic agonists in patients with congestive heart failure may decrease chance of survival and should only be used when necessary.

Regional anesthesia should be considered for patients with congestive heart failure requiring peripheral or minor surgery. Anesthetics with minimal hemodynamic effects are optimal. If the surgery precludes such a choice, general anesthesia with careful hemodynamic control with intra-arterial pressure monitoring, infusions of vasoconstrictors, and possibly inotropic drugs, with the careful avoidance of tachycardia, should be used.

HYPERTROPHIC CARDIOMYOPATHY

Hypertrophic cardiomyopathy (idiopathic hypertrophic subaortic stenosis) is characterized by obstruction to left ventricular outflow produced by asymmetrical hypertrophy of the intraventricular septal muscle.[64] Associated left ventricular hypertrophy in an attempt to overcome the obstruction may be so massive that the volume of the left ventricular chamber is decreased. Despite these adverse changes, the stroke volume remains normal or increased owing to the hypercontractile state of the myocardium. This disease is often hereditary, and the genetic defect seems to be an increased density of calcium channels manifesting as myocardial hypertrophy.

Management of Anesthesia

The goal during management of anesthesia for patients with hypertrophic cardiomyopathy is to decrease the pressure gradient across the left ventricular outflow obstruction (Table 25-12). Decreases in myocardial contractility and increases in preload (ventricular volume) and afterload will decrease the magnitude of left ventricular outflow obstruction. Volatile anesthetics are useful for maintenance of anesthesia, providing mild depression of myocardial contractility. Theoretically, isoflurane, desflurane, and sevoflurane would be less ideal choices than halothane because these drugs decrease systemic vascular resistance more than does halothane. Rapid increases in desflurane may cause sympathetic stimulation with tachycardia, hypertension, bronchospasm, and pulmonary hypertension and should be avoided. Primary opioid anesthetics may not be optimal as they do not produce myocardial depression and can decrease systemic vascular resistance. High potency opioids stimulate the vagus nerve, lower heart rate, and can decrease sympathetic stimulation improving hemodynamics. Combinations of volatile agents (sevoflurane or isoflurane) with an opioid are commonly selected.

Table 25-12 Events that Decrease Left Ventricular Outflow Obstruction in the Presence of Hypertrophic Cardiomyopathy

Decreased Myocardial Contractility
β-Adrenergic blockade (atenolol, metoprolol, propranolol, esmolol)
Volatile anesthetic (sevoflurane or isoflurane)

Increased Preload
Increased intravascular fluid volume
Bradycardia (fentanyl or sufentanil)

Increased Afterload
α-Adrenergic stimulation (phenylephrine infusions)

Intraoperative hypotension is generally treated with intravenous fluids or an α-agonist such as phenylephrine. Drugs with β-agonist activity are not likely to be used to treat hypotension because any increase in cardiac contractility or heart rate could increase left ventricular outflow obstruction. When hypertension occurs, an increased delivered concentration of isoflurane or sevoflurane can be used. Vasodilators, such as nitroprusside or nitroglycerin, should be used with caution because decreases in systemic vascular resistance can increase left ventricular outflow obstruction.

PULMONARY HYPERTENSION AND COR PULMONALE

Cor pulmonale is the designation for right ventricular hypertrophy and eventual cardiac dysfunction that occurs secondary to chronic pulmonary hypertension. Elective operations in patients with cor pulmonale should not be performed until any reversible component of the coexisting pulmonary vascular disease has been treated.

Management of Anesthesia

Goals during management of anesthesia in patients with cor pulmonale are to avoid events or drugs that could increase pulmonary vascular resistance. Volatile anesthetics are useful for relaxing vascular smooth muscle and attenuating airway responsiveness to stimuli produced by a tracheal tube. Pulmonary vasodilation with prostaglandins (epoprostenol, treprostinil, iloprost, beraprost), endothelin receptor antagonists (bosentan, sitaxsentan, ambrisentan), inhaled nitric oxide, inhaled milrinone, type 5 phosphodiesterase inhibitors (sildenafil, vardenafil), or soluble guanylate cyclase activators (cinaciguat, riociguat) have been tried with variable success. Patients with pulmonary hypertension have significant increased risk and should be treated with extreme care. Nitrous oxide may increase pulmonary vascular resistance and should probably be avoided.[52] Another disadvantage of nitrous oxide is the associated decrease in the inspired concentration of oxygen necessitated by the administration of this drug.

Intra-arterial pressure monitoring is very helpful for hemodynamic management. Monitoring of pulmonary arterial or right atrial pressure (or both) may be helpful to detect any adverse effect on pulmonary vasculature. TEE monitoring can be very helpful in blood volume management. In severe cor pulmonale, inotropic support with β-agonists can improve cardiac function. Therapy should be chosen based on the hemodynamic problem (volume, systemic vascular resistance, chronotropy, inotropy, and pulmonary hypertension). β-Agonists must be used carefully to avoid myocardial ischemia. In severe right ventricular failure, combinations of β-agonists and phosphodiesterase inhibitors (amrinone or milrinone) can provide synergistic improvements in ventricular function and vasodilation, thus improving cardiac output.

CARDIAC TAMPONADE

Cardiac tamponade is characterized by (1) decreases in diastolic filling of the ventricles, (2) decreases in stroke volume, and (3) decreases in systemic blood pressure due to increased intrapericardial pressure from accumulation of fluid in the pericardial space (Table 25-13). Decreased stroke volume from inadequate ventricular filling results in activation of the sympathetic nervous system (tachycardia, vasoconstriction) in attempts to maintain the cardiac output. Cardiac output and systemic blood pressure are maintained only as long as the pressure in the central veins exceeds the right ventricular end-diastolic pressure. Institution of general anesthesia and positive-pressure ventilation of the lungs in the presence of cardiac tamponade can lead to profound hypotension or death, reflecting anesthetic-induced peripheral vasodilation, direct myocardial depression, and decreased venous return. When percutaneous pericardiocentesis cannot be performed using local anesthesia, the induction and maintenance of general anesthesia are extremely dangerous but may be achieved while carefully maintaining spontaneous respiration. Potential adverse effects of increased intrathoracic pressure from controlled respiration on venous return must be taken seriously. If possible, positive-pressure ventilation of the lungs should be avoided until drainage of the pericardial space is imminent. With this in mind, tracheal intubation with topical anesthesia has been suggested.

Table 25-13	Manifestations of Cardiac Tamponade
Primary diastolic dysfunction from increased pericardial pressure
Hypotension
Tachycardia
Increased systemic vascular resistance
Low cardiac output
Equalization of left and right diastolic filling pressures
Exaggeration of blood pressure variation with respiration
Fixed and reduced stroke volume (cardiac output and systemic blood pressure dependent on heart rate)
Failure to respond to volume and multiple inotropes with cardiogenic shock

Management of Anesthesia

Prior to the induction of general anesthesia in patients with significant cardiac tamponade, the patient should be positioned on the operating room table. Intra-arterial monitoring is helpful if time permits. The chest and abdomen should be prepped and draped for surgery. The surgeons should be scrubbed, gowned, gloved, and at the operating room table ready for incision prior to anesthetic induction. It is optimal if anesthetic induction, intubation, incision, and drainage of the pericardial tamponade can occur in extremely rapid succession (less than 60 seconds). Although continuous intravenous infusions of catecholamines (epinephrine, norepinephrine, dopamine, dobutamine, or isoproterenol) and vasoconstrictors may be necessary to maintain cardiac output and blood pressure, the primary therapy is pericardial drainage. A common sign of cardiac tamponade is hemodynamic collapse and cardiogenic shock unresponsive to fluids and inotropes. Systolic ventricular function is not the problem; diastolic dysfunction from increased pericardial pressure is the primary problem. Once the pericardium is drained, venous return can enter the heart and hemodynamics will rapidly normalize.

ANEURYSMS OF THE AORTA

Aneurysms of the aorta most often involve the abdominal aorta but may involve any part including thoracic or abdominal. Most patients are hypertensive, and many have associated atherosclerosis. A dissecting aneurysm denotes a tear in the intima of the aorta that allows blood to enter and penetrate between the walls of the vessel, producing a false lumen. Ultimately, the dissection may reenter the lumen through another tear in the intima or rupture through the adventitia.

Elective repair of an abdominal aneurysm is often recommended when the estimated diameter of the aneurysm is more than 5 cm. The incidence of spontaneous rupture increases dramatically when the size of the aneurysm exceeds this diameter. Extension of the abdominal aneurysm to include the renal arteries occurs in about 5% of patients.

Management of Anesthesia

All surgery patients with vascular disease should be considered for prophylactic β-blocker and statin therapy. Perioperative administration of β-blockers reduces perioperative mortality rate 50% to 90%. β-Blockers should be started as soon as patients are identified as needing surgery. Starting β-blockers 7 to 30 days preoperatively and continuing for at least 30 days postoperatively is most effective, with a 90% reduction in mortality rate.[12,13]

Starting β-blockers on the day of surgery and continuing for 7 days reduces mortality rate 50%.[15] Clonidine reduces 30-day and 2-year mortality rates[16] and may be used in patients with specific contraindications (reactive asthma or atrioventricular block or allergy) to β-blockade. Perioperative statin use reduces risk of mortality an additional 50% over the benefits of β-blockers and should be started 30 days preoperatively and continued at least 30 days postoperatively, if not indefinitely.[17]

The surgical approach certainly influences the anesthetic. Endovascular aneurysm repair is less invasive and may require only regional anesthesia, although in prolonged cases general anesthesia is preferred. Open procedures for aortic aneurysm surgery are major procedures and require general anesthesia. All patients undergoing anesthesia for resection of an abdominal aortic aneurysm should have monitoring of intra-arterial pressures. The use of pulmonary arterial pressure monitoring is controversial.[47,48] Patients with coexisting coronary artery disease are likely to develop increases in the pulmonary artery occlusion pressure and evidence of myocardial ischemia during cross-clamping of the abdominal aorta. Transesophageal echocardiography may be useful in evaluating the adequacy of intravascular volume replacement and in the recognition of cardiac wall motion abnormalities associated with myocardial ischemia, although no data support its use as a risk reduction strategy. Intraoperatively, myocardial ischemia is treated by decreasing heart rate with β-blockers and maintaining systemic blood pressure and filling pressures to acceptable levels by pharmacologic interventions, which may include continuous intravenous infusion of phenylephrine (for hypotension), nitroprusside, or nitroglycerine (for hypertension). Preoperative hydration with a balanced salt solution and prompt intraoperative replacement of blood loss as guided by data obtained from the pulmonary artery catheter, echocardiography, or continuous cardiac output devices are considered useful for maintaining intravascular fluid volume and thus renal function. Diuresis is often facilitated by intraoperative administration of a diuretic (mannitol, furosemide, or both) with or without dopamine. Despite these interventions, glomerular filtration rate and renal blood flow are not predictably improved.[65]

Hypotension can accompany unclamping of the abdominal aorta, presumably reflecting sudden increases in vascular resistance and venous compliance with reperfusion. Systemic blood pressure decreases can be minimized by infusing intravenous fluids to maintain the pulmonary artery occlusion pressure between 10 and 20 mm Hg before removal of the aortic cross-clamp. Gradual removal of the aortic cross-clamp minimizes decreases in systemic blood pressure by allowing time for return of pooled venous blood to the circulation. The exact cause of hypotension and vasodilation following removal of the aorta is unclear.

IV

CARDIOPULMONARY BYPASS
(Also See Chapter 26)

Cardiopulmonary bypass (extracorporeal circulation) support is used to stabilize the myocardium reducing motion during coronary artery bypass surgery and allow ascending aortic and intraventricular procedures (valve repair or replacement). Cardiopulmonary bypass is characterized by gravity drainage of blood from the vena cava into a reservoir, followed by its pumping through a heat exchanger, oxygenator, and filter, followed by its return to the arterial system, usually the ascending aorta, by means of a centrifugal or roller pump (Fig. 25-3).[66] In the presence of a competent aortic valve, the heart is excluded from the patient's circulation by either a single venous cannula inserted into the right atrium (see Fig. 25-3) and advanced into the inferior vena cava, or by dual catheters placed into the superior and inferior

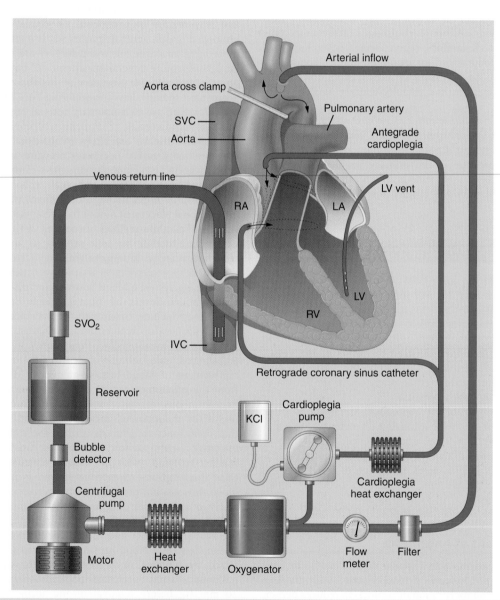

Figure 25-3 Schematic diagram of a cardiopulmonary bypass circuit. Blood from cannulas placed through the right atrium and into the inferior vena cava drains by gravity into a reservoir and then is pumped by a centrifugal pump through a heat exchanger, oxygenator, and filter prior to return to the ascending aorta. Blood mixed with cardioplegia solution is pumped alternatively into the proximal ascending aorta or into the coronary sinus. Venting can be from a cannula placed through the right superior pulmonary vein into the left ventricle, or from the ascending aorta antegrade cardioplegia cannula, or the pulmonary artery.

venae cavae so that all returning blood enters the large cannulas in these vessels. If the aortic valve is not competent, venting of the left ventricle may be necessary (1) through a drain placed from the right superior pulmonary vein into the left ventricle, (2) by aspirating from the antegrade cardioplegia line placed in the proximal ascending aorta, or (3) via a pulmonary venous drain. Otherwise, retrograde blood flow through the incompetent aortic valve could cause distention of the left ventricle and damage ventricular function. Venting of blood returning via the thebesian or bronchial veins may also be necessary. An aortic cross-clamp is placed between the antegrade cardioplegia catheter and the arterial inflow catheter to separate the heart from the circulation and allow cardioplegic arrest. The ventricle should not be overdistended in any situation in which it is not pumping. If the aortic cross-clamp is removed and ventricular contraction has not returned, the ventricle may become overdistended in situations with aortic valve insufficiency. When the heart is isolated from the circulation, total cardiopulmonary bypass is present, and ventilation of the lungs is no longer necessary to maintain oxygenation. However, in any situation in which there is a pulsatile pulmonary pressure detected by pulmonary arterial catheter measurement, there is partial pulmonary bypass, and the lungs should be ventilated to avoid pumping desaturated blood systemically. Gravity-dependent venous drainage to the cardiopulmonary bypass machine can be improved by raising the level of the operating table or placing a small negative pressure on the cardiotomy reservoir.

The use of extracorporeal circulatory support is dangerous and requires special precautions. Prior to going on cardiopulmonary bypass it is important to review a checklist of required items. Checklists are effective in improving anesthetic care. The checklist prior to going on cardiopulmonary bypass follows the acronym HADDSUE, pronounced HAD TO SUE, making it easy to remember (Table 25-14).

Components of the Cardiopulmonary Bypass Circuit

The bypass pump produces nonpulsatile flow into the patient's aorta by either a centrifugal or roller pump. The centrifugal pump has three disks rotating at 3000 to 4000 rpm that use blood viscosity to pump blood. Centrifugal pumps are superior to roller pumps because they are less traumatic to blood cells, do not pump air bubbles secondary to air being less dense than blood, and are afterload-dependent, avoiding the risk of line rupture with clamping of the arterial inflow circuit. Roller pumps compress the fluid-filled tubing between the roller and curved metal back plate and are able to pump air and can have tube rupture with arterial inflow clamping. The necessary cardiac index delivered by the bypass pump is determined by the patient's body temperature and oxygen consumption. For normothermia or mild hypothermia, a cardiac index of 2 to 4 $L/min/m^2$ is satisfactory, although flows of about half these levels have been used successfully. Low flows have the advantage of less blood trauma and less noncoronary collateral blood flow, which might result in better myocardial protection. Blood is oxygenated by a membrane or bubble oxygenator. Membrane oxygenators use a blood-membrane-gas interface rather than a blood-gas interface and produce less trauma to the blood compared with bubble oxygenators. Because membrane oxygenators cause less

Table 25-14	Protocol to Initiate Cardiopulmonary Bypass: HADDSUE
Heparin	Was heparin administered? If the surgeon is placing sutures in the aorta for aortic cannulation, ask about heparin. Do not allow a surgeon to initiate cardiopulmonary bypass without heparin administration or alternative profound anticoagulant, the results will immediately be fatal.
ACT	Did the heparin increase the ACT to 450 seconds or greater? Were antifibrinolytics given?
Drugs	Were additional nondepolarizing muscle relaxants and/or anesthetics administered to prevent inspiration during venous cannula placement, which could result in gas emboli?
Drips	Did you discuss any infusions with the perfusionist that may interfere with hemodynamic management during bypass? Blood pressure on cardiopulmonary bypass depends on flow and resistance. Drugs that affect resistance will affect blood pressure. Drugs that affect venous capacity will reduce venous return to the reservoir and force a reduction in pump flow.
Swan	Pull back the pulmonary arterial catheter 5 cm to avoid pulmonary arterial injury or pulmonary infarction during bypass.
Urine	Measure the total urine output so that the urine produced during bypass can be tabulated. Urine output can be quite variable during bypass depending on the extracorporeal circulatory prime, volume administered, intrinsic hormonal response to cardiopulmonary bypass, and renal function.
Emboli	Check the aortic cannula visually to detect any emboli.

ACT, activated clotting time.

trauma to blood components than bubble oxygenators, membrane-based oxygenator systems are the norm. Bubble oxygenators consisted of an oxygenator column, a defoaming section to remove air bubbles, and an arterial reservoir. They are not commonly used today. With either form of oxygenator Pa_{O_2} is maintained by adjusting the concentration of oxygen into the oxygenator. Air-oxygen mixing may be used to avoid hyperoxia. Carbon dioxide levels are controlled between 35 and 45 mm Hg by controlling the sweep (the total free gas flow through the oxygenator). In the past carbon dioxide was added to maintain Pa_{CO_2} and pH at levels considered normal for 37° C. Carbon dioxide is no longer added to cardiopulmonary bypass circuits to maintain blood gases. Bypass circuits are flushed with carbon dioxide prior to priming to speed priming and reduce gas emboli in the circuit. Carbon dioxide is also continuously flushed into the pericardial cavity to replace air during bypass in an effort to reduce the significance of gas emboli during bypass. Carbon dioxide is more easily absorbed than the nitrogen in air reducing the duration that gas emboli take be resorbed.

Heat exchangers are incorporated into bypass circuits to control the patient's body temperature by heating or cooling blood as it circulates. Hot or cold water entering the unit at one end with blood entering at the other provides an efficient countercurrent flow system. Metabolic requirements are decreased about 8% for every degree Celsius decrease in body temperature below 37° C. The optimal temperature management for cardiopulmonary bypass is not entirely clear. Eighteen degrees (18° C) is used prior to circulatory arrest and 28° C is common during aortic cross-clamping with rewarming to 37° C prior to weaning from bypass. Newer protocols maintain temperature between 31° C and 33° C. Normothermic (37° C) bypass is associated with an increase in cerebrovascular accidents.[67]

Blood from the pericardial cavity and the opened heart, as during a valve replacement, is returned to a cardiotomy reservoir, where it is filtered, defoamed, and pumped to the oxygenator for recirculation. The cardiotomy suction may be a major cause of hemolysis and emboli during cardiopulmonary bypass. Filters are incorporated in the cardiotomy reservoir and the arterial circuit to act as traps for particulate debris (blood clot, latex, talc, fat, Silastic, polyethylene, etc.) that could act as systemic emboli.

The tubing used for the cardiopulmonary bypass system is flushed with carbon dioxide, then filled (primed) with crystalloid. Additives to the circuit may include albumin, hetastarch, blood, bicarbonate, heparin, and antibiotics. The goal is a predetermined solution that is calculated to produce a specific hematocrit with institution of total cardiopulmonary bypass. Because whole body hypothermia (18° C to 28° C) may be utilized, the pump prime often contains little or no blood, such that the hematocrit of blood during cardiopulmonary bypass is 20% to 30%. Hemodilution is important for decreasing

viscosity during hypothermia. It is mandatory that all air be cleared from the arterial side of the circuit before institution of cardiopulmonary bypass. Indeed, pumping of air into the patient by the cardiopulmonary bypass machine is an ever-present hazard. Carbon dioxide flushing prior to priming and continuous flushing of the pericardium reduce gas emboli risk. Patients who suffer gas emboli can be treated with hyperbaric oxygen with improvements in neurologic function even 24 hours after embolization.[68] Early treatment may have better results.

Heparin-induced anticoagulation of the patient is mandatory before placement of the venous and aortic cannulas used for cardiopulmonary bypass. The usual initial dose of heparin administered intravenously is 300 to 400 units/kg. The adequacy of anticoagulation is subsequently confirmed by determination of the activated coagulation time, which is typically maintained at greater than 450 seconds during cardiopulmonary bypass (when baseline normal is 90 to 120 seconds).[66]

Monitoring During Cardiopulmonary Bypass

Institution of cardiopulmonary bypass is often associated with decreases in mean arterial pressure, presumably reflecting the dramatic decreases in viscosity that result from infusion of prime solutions and activation of systemic inflammatory response. In addition, peripheral vasodilation may accompany decreased oxygen delivery that occurs in the early period of hemodilution. Administration of an α-agonist, such as phenylephrine, to increase perfusion pressures to higher than 40 mm Hg in the early period after institution of cardiopulmonary bypass may be recommended on the assumption that perfusion pressure is important for maintenance of cerebral blood flow. The correct blood pressure during bypass is debatable. Lower pressures may reduce cerebral blood flow and reduce emboli load to the brain. Higher pressures may improve cerebral blood flow and reduce watershed infarction but higher pressures come from higher flows and more emboli per unit time. Pressures less than 40 mm Hg are avoided if possible in adults. Pressures higher than 60 mm Hg are used during rewarming. Pressures up to 80 to 90 mm Hg may be used in patients with cerebral vascular disease. Evidence to support these recommendations is limited.

After the initial decrease, mean arterial pressure during cardiopulmonary bypass often begins to increase spontaneously, perhaps reflecting activation of the renin-angiotensin system or sympathetic nervous system. Mean arterial pressures higher than 100 mm Hg can lead to impairment of tissue perfusion as well as the risk of intracranial hemorrhage. Furthermore, noncoronary collateral blood flow is likely to be increased as mean arterial pressure increases, resulting in perfusion of the heart with blood at higher temperatures than desired for optimal cellular protection. Hypertension is often treated by decreasing systemic vascular resistance with volatile agents administered through the oxygenator or the continuous intravenous administration of nitroprusside. Nitroglycerine has reduced effect on cardiopulmonary bypass because its action is predominantly venodilation and arterial pressures during bypass are primarily dependent on systemic vascular resistance.

An increasing central venous pressure with or without facial edema (eyelids and scleras) may reflect improper placement of the vena cava cannula resulting in obstruction to venous drainage. For example, insertion of a cannula too far into the superior vena cava can obstruct the right innominate vein, leading to an increase of cerebral venous pressure with associated cerebral edema. Placement of a cannula too far into the inferior vena cava results in abdominal distention. Confirmatory evidence of misplacement of a vena cava cannula is inadequate venous return from the patient to the cardiopulmonary bypass machine. Prompt withdrawal of the vena cava cannula to a more proximal position should immediately improve venous drainage.

A pulmonary artery catheter detects increases in pulmonary artery pressures caused by malfunction of the left ventricular vent and the associated inadequate decompression of the left ventricle. Persistent left ventricular distention can result in damage to the contractile elements of the myocardium.

Blood gases and pH are monitored frequently during cardiopulmonary bypass. A mixed venous P_{O_2} lower than 30 mm Hg associated with metabolic acidosis suggests inadequate tissue perfusion. Temperature correction of Pa_{CO_2} and pH is probably not necessary (see Chapter 17). Urine output may serve as a guide to the adequacy of renal perfusion, with an output of 1 mL/kg/hour being a common expectation.

During total cardiopulmonary bypass, the lungs are left quiescent with or without moderate continuous positive airway pressure. The best composition of gases in the lungs during this period is unsettled. Continued ventilation of the lungs with oxygen may be appropriate when there is some pulmonary blood flow, as evidenced by a pulsatile pulmonary artery trace. If there is a pulsatile pulmonary arterial pressure or systemic arterial pressure, the lungs should be ventilated because there is only partial cardiopulmonary bypass.

Esophageal, rectal, bladder, and blood temperatures are monitored routinely. Rapid rewarming caused by a high blood-to-body temperature gradient is avoided to avoid gas emboli. Drug-induced vasodilation as produced by a volatile anesthetic or nitroprusside may speed the rewarming process, as reflected by a more rapid approach of the rectal (core) to esophageal (blood) temperature, but should be used carefully. Measurement of urinary bladder temperature may be a superior alternative to monitoring rectal temperature, as bladder temperature may reflect core temperatures better than rectal.

Myocardial Preservation

The goal of myocardial preservation is to decrease myocardial damage introduced by the period of ischemia associated with cardiopulmonary bypass. This goal is achieved by decreasing myocardial oxygen consumption by infusing cardioplegia solutions containing potassium into the aortic root, which in the presence of a distally cross-clamped aorta and competent aortic valve ensures diversion of the solution into the coronary arteries. Alternatively, the cardioplegia solution may be administered in retrograde fashion through a cannula placed into the coronary sinus. Monitoring of coronary sinus pressures during retrograde administration is used to assess catheter placement. If the pressure at the distal tip of the coronary sinus catheter during cardioplegia administration at 200 mL/min is equal to central venous pressure, the catheter is not in the coronary sinus but is most likely in the right atrium. If the pressure is very high (>100 mm Hg) the coronary sinus catheter is up against a vascular wall. If the pressure in the coronary sinus catheter is 40 to 60 mm Hg during a 200 mL/min infusion, the catheter is correctly positioned. Positioning of the coronary sinus catheter should be checked with transesophageal echocardiography and manual feel by the surgeon. If the catheter is in too deep, cardioplegia to the right ventricle will be compromised, resulting in poor right ventricular protection. An additional route for infusion of cardioplegia solutions is directly into newly placed bypass grafts.

Potassium in the cardioplegia solution blocks the initial phase of myocardial depolarization, resulting in cessation of electrical and mechanical activity. The cold solution produces selective hypothermia of the cardiac muscle. At 30° C, the normally contracting heart muscle consumes oxygen at a rate of 8 to 10 mL/100 g/min. Oxygen consumption in the fibrillating ventricle at 22° C is 2 mL/100 g/min. The electromechanically quiet heart at 22° C consumes oxygen at a rate of 0.3 mL/100 g/min. The effectiveness of cold cardioplegia is monitored by measuring heart temperature with a temperature probe placed into the left ventricular muscle plus the absence of any visible electrical activity on the ECG. Cold cardioplegia infusions are supplemented by total-body hypothermia and localized epicardial surface cooling using ice or cold irrigation solutions placed in the pericardial space. Cardioplegia solutions may also contain many additives, including blood, insulin, glucose, aspartate, glutamate, calcium, magnesium, nitroglycerine, superoxide dismutase, at the discretion of the surgeon. None of these additives are definitively better than cold blood cardioplegia with a short cross-clamp time. Adequate myocardial preservation is suggested by good myocardial contractility without the need for inotropic drugs at the conclusion of cardiopulmonary bypass.

A side effect of cardioplegia solutions is an increased incidence of atrioventricular heart block due to intramyocardial hyperkalemia. This heart block usually

IV

resolves in 1 to 2 hours and can be treated temporarily by use of an artificial cardiac pacemaker. Intramyocardial hyperkalemia also produces decreased myocardial contractility. Systemic hyperkalemia can occur when coronary sinus blood containing cardioplegia solution is returned to the oxygenator for subsequent circulation. Decreased renal function during cardiopulmonary bypass will also contribute to hyperkalemia. If hyperkalemia persists at the conclusion of cardiopulmonary bypass, regular insulin (10 to 20 units IV) can be given in combination with glucose (25 to 50 mg IV) in an attempt to shift potassium into the cells. Alternatively, furosemide can be used. The perfusionist can also add crystalloid solutions to the bypass circuit and then use a hemoconcentrator to ultrafiltrate the blood and thereby eliminate potassium.

Management of Anesthesia

Drugs selected for maintenance of anesthesia in patients undergoing cardiopulmonary bypass are influenced by the patient's cardiac disease. Patients with diabetes or those who develop glucose intolerance during surgery should have infusions of insulin with a target of glucose between 120 and 150 mg/dL. Avoidance of hypoglycemia is essential to avoid neurologic injury. Hyperglycemia may lead to increased risk of infections and neurologic sequelae. Infusions of dexmedetomidine are associated with reduced risk of delirium.[69] Institution of cardiopulmonary bypass may produce a sudden dilution of circulating drug concentrations. For this reason, supplemental anesthetics, such as benzodiazepines or opioids, may be needed. An additional dose of nondepolarizing muscle relaxant should be administered just prior to placement of the venous cannula to avoid inspiratory efforts entraining air. Anesthetic depth can also be increased by volatile anesthetics from vaporizers incorporated into the cardiopulmonary bypass circuit. The effect of hemodilution on drug concentrations is likely to be offset by a decreased need for drugs during hypothermia. Anesthetic requirements seem to be minimal following rewarming to a normal body temperature at the conclusion of cardiopulmonary bypass. Therefore, additional anesthesia is not routinely required during rewarming or the early period after the conclusion of cardiopulmonary bypass. However, additional anesthetic will be needed to maintain tracheal intubation for transfer and postoperative ventilation in the intensive care unit. An intravenous anesthetic (propofol or dexmedetomidine) with minimal hemodynamic effects can be given in the procedure and continued into the ICU. Dexmedetomidine-induced sedation may reduce the risk of postoperative delirium after cardiac surgery.[69]

Discontinuation of Cardiopulmonary Bypass

Optimal anesthetic care can be achieved with checklists. The checklist for weaning from cardiopulmonary bypass consists of the mnemonic WRMVP (Table 25-15), as in

Table 25-15 Checklist for Weaning from Cardiopulmonary Bypass: WRMVP	
Warm	Body temperature (37° C) is likely to decrease rapidly after cardiopulmonary bypass if patient is not adequately rewarmed, with resultant metabolic acidosis and poor myocardial contractility.
Rhythm	Confirm that the patient has a stable cardiac rhythm.
Monitors	Confirm that the monitors are turned on; pulse oximeter is essential for arterial oxygen saturation and cardiac output.
Ventilator	Confirm that it is turned on.
Perfusion	Confirm heart beating, presence of vasodilation.

Wide Receiver Most Valuable Player (a wide receiver is a football position for our non–United States readers):

1. Warm: Is the patient at 37° C?
2. Rhythm: Does the patient have a stable cardiac rhythm?
3. Monitors: Are the monitors turned back on? How about the pulse oximeter? The pulse oximeter is essential postoperatively both as a monitor of arterial oxygen saturation and cardiac output. If the pulse oximeter is not working, it may be that perfusion is inadequate. The pulse oximeter is an excellent low cardiac output alarm.
4. Ventilator: Is the ventilator back on? It is easy to forget this and rapid desaturation after bypass detected from the pulse oximeter should be quickly identified.
5. Perfusion: Is the heart beating? Is the vasculature appropriate for the cardiac function? Very few hearts following cardiopulmonary bypass are adequate to maintain blood pressure in the face of profound systemic vasodilation. The systemic vascular resistance should be normal (not profoundly vasodilated or constricted).

Cardiopulmonary bypass is discontinued when the patient is hemodynamically stable and normothermia has been reestablished. In the absence of adequate rewarming before discontinuation of cardiopulmonary bypass, body temperature is likely to decrease rapidly in the postcardiopulmonary bypass period, resulting in metabolic acidosis and poor myocardial contractility. When the left side of the heart has been opened, as during valve replacement surgery, it is mandatory to remove all air from the cardiac chambers and pulmonary veins before permitting the heart to eject blood into the aorta. Otherwise, systemic air emboli can occur with disastrous cardiac and central nervous system effects. The presence of air can be checked with transesophageal echocardiography. Unrecognized air in the coronary arteries may be a cause of sudden onset of poor myocardial contractility after discontinuation of cardiopulmonary bypass. Air embolization with neurologic defects can be treated with hyperbaric oxygen even 24 hours after surgery with improvements in neurologic outcome.[68] Measurement of cardiac filling pressures, determination of thermodilution cardiac outputs, and calculation of systemic and pulmonary vascular resistance are helpful for guiding intravenous fluid replacement and the appropriate selection of drugs in the early postcardiopulmonary bypass period (Table 25-16). Alternatively, transesophageal echocardiography can be used to estimate the adequacy of intravascular fluid volume and myocardial contractility. Transesophageal echocardiography is also useful for evaluating cardiac valve function and intracardiac blood flow patterns, particularly following surgical repair or replacement.

The most common hemodynamic abnormality after cardiopulmonary bypass is low systemic vascular resistance (SVR). It is very difficult to wean from cardiopulmonary bypass with a systemic vascular resistance that is low. SVR can be calculated from the following:

$$\text{Mean arterial pressure (mm Hg)} - \text{central venous pressure (mm Hg)} / \text{pump flow (L/min)} \times 80$$

Systemic vascular resistance should be between 1200 and 1400 prior to weaning from bypass. The units of SVR are dynes · seconds/centimeters5 (dyn·s/cm5). Systemic vascular resistance can be normalized with a vasoconstrictor prior to weaning from cardiopulmonary bypass. The goal should be to match the vascular input impedance to the cardiac output impedance to optimize energy transfer. It is much easier to adjust the vasculature to match the heart, than force the heart to tolerate a dilated vasculature. On occasion, an inotropic drug, such as epinephrine, norepinephrine, dopamine, or dobutamine, is needed. In cases of severe ventricular dysfunction, a combination of drugs (epinephrine or norepinephrine and amrinone or milrinone) with an intra-aortic balloon pump or left ventricular assist device is necessary to maintain optimal cardiac output. The use of combinations of β-agonists and phosphodiesterase inhibitors produce synergistic increases in cardiac function. The vasoconstriction of epinephrine or norepinephrine is counterbalanced by the vasodilation of the phosphodiesterase inhibitor. Careful measurement of systemic vascular resistance and supplementation with a vasoconstrictor such as phenylephrine is frequently needed to maintain a normal systemic vascular resistance. If β-agonists are needed, frequent attention must be given to measurement and control of potassium, glucose, calcium, pH, and the presence of arrhythmias. Gas emboli to the coronaries may suddenly and profoundly reduce ventricular function. Posterior papillary muscle dysfunction at the conclusion of cardiopulmonary bypass may result in mitral regurgitation as evidenced by the presence of prominent V waves on the pulmonary artery occlusion pressure tracing. This dysfunction may reflect less than optimal cardioplegic protection of the posterior myocardium, which is most vulnerable to warming effects from blood in the adjacent descending aorta, as well as perfusion with warm blood representing noncoronary collateral circulation. Acute mitral regurgitation can also occur with volume overload from excessive fluid administration; it can be managed simply by the use of the reverse Trendelenburg position to reduce venous return to the heart.

A mechanical complement to inotropic support of cardiac output is the intra-aortic balloon pump. The intra-aortic balloon pump (a 25-cm long balloon mounted on a 90-cm stiff plastic catheter) is typically inserted percutaneously through the femoral artery and advanced so that the tip is just distal to the left subclavian artery. The balloon is timed to inflate during diastole to augment diastolic blood pressure and increase the gradient for coronary perfusion improving coronary

IV

Table 25-16 Diagnosis and Treatment of Cardiovascular Dysfunction after Cardiopulmonary Bypass

Systemic Blood Pressure	Atrial Pressure	Cardiac Output	Diagnosis	Therapy
Decreased	Decreased	Decreased	Hypovolemia	Administer volume
Decreased	Decreased	Increased	Vasodilation Low blood viscosity	Vasoconstrictor Erythrocyte transfusion
Decreased	Increased	Decreased	Left ventricular dysfunction	Inotrope Inodilator Vasodilator Mechanical assistance
Increased	Increased	Decreased	Vasoconstriction Left ventricular dysfunction	Vasodilator Inotrope
Increased	Decreased	Increased	Hyperdynamic	Volatile anesthetic β-Antagonist

blood flow. The balloon deflates immediately before systole, thus decreasing afterload and lowering oxygen requirements. Coronary blood flow is increased, with little or no increase in cardiac work, which may result in improvements in cardiac output. Aortic insufficiency may be worsened by intra-aortic balloon inflation. Rapid heart rates and cardiac dysrhythmias interfere with proper balloon timing and optimal augmentation of cardiac output. Temporary ventricular assist can also be provided by catheters with impellers that rely on the Archimedes screw technology. The impeller device comes in two sizes capable of 2.5 or 5.0 L/min flow.

When an adequate systemic blood pressure and cardiac output have been maintained for several minutes, the vena caval cannula is removed and protamine administration is begun to reverse heparin anticoagulation. Protamine administration is dangerous and frequently is associated with hypotension from release of histamine. Occasionally there is severe pulmonary hypertension or even anaphylaxis from protamine administration. Protamine should be administered after a test dose slowly to avoid catastrophic hemodynamic collapse. Administration of the vasoconstrictor phenylephrine can be used to maintain blood pressure. In cases of hemodynamic collapse even epinephrine boluses will be inadequate, and return to cardiopulmonary bypass after emergency reheparinization can be life-saving. NPH insulin is made with protamine. Diabetics who use NPH insulin may be at increased risk for protamine reactions. Protamine allergic reactions may be reduced with a combination of histamine blockade (H$_1$ [diphenhydramine] and H$_2$ blocker [cimetidine]) and a steroid (hydrocortisone). The aortic cannula is removed after protamine administration is safely concluded. Pharmacologic measures to decrease bleeding include administration of antifibrinolytics (aminocaproic acid, tranexamic acid, and formerly aprotinin) and desmopressin (improves platelet function in patients with von Willibrand's disease). Blood loss throughout the procedure as well as the blood in the bypass tubing can be salvaged, washed, and retransfused using "cell saver" devices.

Administration of nitrous oxide after cardiopulmonary bypass is not recommended because this gas could unmask the presence of air in the heart or coronary arteries. For this reason, anesthesia is most often supplemented, when necessary, by the intravenous administration of propofol, dexmedetomidine, opioids, benzodiazepines, or alternatively with low inhaled concentrations of volatile anesthetics. Intravenous anesthetics such as propofol infusions,[70] dexmedetomidine infusions,[69] or opioids and benzodiazepines are continued after bypass and continued into the ICU to provide sedation prior to extubation. Dexmedetomidine sedation may reduce postoperative delirium after cardiac surgery.[69] The time to tracheal extubation is shortening after cardiopulmonary bypass but some period of time of postoperative intubation is common after leaving the operating room. Once the Pao$_2$ with an Fio$_2$ of 0.40 is above 80 mm Hg, the bleeding is controlled, the patient is awake, and neuromuscular function has recovered, extubation can be considered. There is no benefit from prolonged postoperative ventilation in cardiac surgery. The blood and fluid that remain in the cardiopulmonary bypass circuit are washed and collected into sterile plastic bags as packed cells for possible reinfusion to the patient. High resistance to blood flow in the arm induced by vasoconstriction may result in a falsely low systemic blood pressure reading from the radial artery in the early period after cardiopulmonary bypass. If there is a question of inadequate arterial blood pressure, direct pressure measurement from the ascending aorta can be instantly obtained. Placement of a femoral arterial catheter is needed if there is a gradient between central and radial pressure. Any gradient between central aortic and radial artery blood pressure usually disappears within 60 minutes.

The large financial cost of cardiac surgery is due in part to the duration of intensive care required for these patients. Improvements in anesthetic, surgical, and perfusion techniques serve to decrease the need for prolonged care of these patients in an ICU. The concept known as "fast track" as applied to cardiac surgical patients includes early postoperative awakening and tracheal extubation.[71]

Off-Pump Coronary Artery Bypass Graft Surgery

In an effort to minimize postoperative morbidity, coronary artery bypass graft (CABG) surgery may be accomplished in selected patients without institution of cardiopulmonary bypass and in the presence of a spontaneously beating heart and normothermia. Cardiopulmonary bypass using extracorporeal circulatory support was developed because it is difficult to safely produce a high-quality anastomosis between a vessel and a coronary artery while the heart is beating. Off-pump CABG was developed to reduce the sequelae of extracorporeal circulatory support, which may include stroke, global encephalopathy, renal failure, pulmonary injury, and death. Off-pump CABG surgery is limited by several considerations including the quality of the distal anastomosis and long-term graft patency is of primary concern. There are several problems with off-pump CABG or "beating heart" surgery. The first is motion of the coronary artery making suture placement for the anastomosis difficult. Anticoagulation with heparin is achieved and the activated clotting time (ACT) is measured. There is some debate on the appropriate ACT levels of an off-pump CABG with some surgeons using standard doses appropriate for cardiopulmonary bypass (300 to 400 units/kg ACT > 450 seconds) and others using lower dose heparin (200 unit/kg). Antifibrinolytics (aprotinin, aminocaproic acid, or transexemic acid) are not used if the patient is not going on extracorporeal circulatory support. The ability to immediately go on extracorporeal circulatory support must be available during the conduct of off-pump CABG should the patient have circulatory collapse or cardiac arrest. Blood flow in the target coronary artery is usually stopped by placement of a proximal and distal latex suture, which is lifted up, consequently arresting flow. Alternatively, a silicon stent can be placed in the target coronary artery during production of the anastomosis to maintain coronary flow. The silicon stent is removed just prior to tightening the suture. Stopping the coronary blood flow in the target coronary artery may cause myocardial ischemia, ventricular arrhythmias, ventricular dysfunction, heart block, hemodynamic collapse, and cardiac arrest. When flow is resumed in the coronary artery reperfusion arrhythmias may occur. Prophylactic antiarrhythmic therapy should be administered prior to off-pump CABG. Magnesium (2 g IV slowly) combined with lidocaine (100 mg bolus followed by 2 mg/min) infusion works well. Intravenous amiodarone should be used in patients who demonstrate a tendency toward ventricular tachycardia or fibrillation.

The technology for the off-pump CABG was developed in the 1990s and initially stabilized the heart with a retractor that simply pushed on the myocardium while it was lifted into the retractor with stay sutures. This system was difficult to use because ventricular diastolic filling was compromised by external pressure on the heart. The development of a retractor that used a vacuum foot (Octopus) to stabilize the heart eliminated the external pressure on the myocardium and improved ventricular diastolic function during the distal anastomosis. Coronary grafts to the inferior and lateral circulation were difficult to perform because retraction of the heart reduced diastolic filling and caused hemodynamic collapse. The use of suction retractors (Starfish and Urchin) for lateral and anterior displacement of the heart during production of the lateral and inferior anastomosis in combination with steep Trendelenburg positioning greatly stabilized hemodynamics. Careful cooperation between the cardiac surgeon and cardiac anesthesiologist is essential for off-pump CABG. Surgical positioning must be performed in conjunction with anesthesia. The surgeon must not open the coronary artery for a distal anastomosis without ensuring that the patient will hemodynamically tolerate the 10- to 15-minute anastomosis. Communication between the cardiac surgeon and cardiac anesthesiologist is especially critical during this process. Some surgeons use a 5-minute period of ischemic preconditioning prior to a 5-minute recovery period followed by the anastomosis. The 5-minute preconditioning period can be used to optimize hemodynamics and test to see if the patient will tolerate the anastomosis. Ischemic preconditioning may reduce ischemic injury at the cost of a longer operative time.

Anastomosis of the left internal mammary artery (LIMA) to the left anterior descending (LAD) coronary artery was the first off-pump bypass and is technically simplest and most important for reducing myocardial ischemia. The LIMA to LAD anastomosis is usually conducted first, which improves coronary blood flow to the LAD circulation. Saphenous vein grafts (SVG) are then placed to the obtuse marginal (OM) branches off the circumflex artery and finally to the posterior descending artery (PDA), which usually branches from the right coronary artery. Placement of the lateral wall grafts to the obtuse marginal branches requires shifting the heart to the right, which may be better tolerated by opening the right pleural space and placing lifting-stay sutures into the inferior pericardium. Steep Trendelenburg with right tilt will improve hemodynamics. Intravascular administration of colloid and vasoconstriction with phenylephrine should be used to maintain arterial blood pressure. The ECG amplitude may diminish dramatically making ST segments difficult to observe secondary to myocardial positioning. Transesophageal echocardiography of the ventricle may be impossible secondary to lifting of the ventricle off the esophagus. Anastomosis to the posterior descending coronary artery can be produced with steep Trendelenburg, volume loading, and vasoconstriction with phenylephrine. Low cardiac outputs can be tolerated for the brief period of the distal anastomosis. Completion of the proximal aortic anastomosis for the saphenous vein grafts requires placement of a side biter clamp on the ascending aorta. Devices that staple the proximal anastomosis are available and may reduce the use of side biter clamps with less aortic trauma. Arterial blood pressure can be decreased to assist placement of this clamp with increasing inspired concentrations of volatile anesthetics or cardiac manipulation to reduce venous return. Once the distal and proximal anastomoses are complete any air in the saphenous vein graft must be removed to avoid coronary gas emboli. Removal of the aortic side biter should only be done once any remaining air is removed from the saphenous vein grafts to avoid systemic gas emboli. Heparin anticoagulation should then be carefully reversed with protamine. Protamine reactions, which include hypotension, pulmonary hypertension, and anaphylaxis, are more difficult to treat in off-pump CABG because rapid return to extracorporeal circulatory support will require full reheparinization, bypass circuit priming, followed by proximal aortic cannula and right atrial venous cannula placement. If hypotension occurs following protamine administration, rapid treatment with the vasoconstrictor phenylephrine is frequently needed. Severe reactions to protamine may be treated with intravenous epinephrine, diphenhydramine, H_2 blockade, steroids, intravascular fluid administration, and if necessary reheparinization, and initiation of extracorporeal circulatory support. The use of off-pump CABG is becoming less

IV

frequent after the publication of the ROOBY trial which showed a reduction in graft patency and poorer outcomes in the off-pump group.[72]

MANAGEMENT OF ANESTHESIA

Anesthesia for off-pump CABG is very similar to anesthesia for on-pump CABG with a few notable exceptions. Patients for off-pump CABG have similar medical conditions, medical therapies, and requirements for care as those receiving on-pump CABG. All preoperative medications with the exception of oral hypoglycemic agents should be continued in the perioperative period. Patients with diabetes should be managed with intravenous insulin infusions and frequent blood glucose determinations. Coumadin (warfarin) should be stopped at least 7 days prior to an operation. Platelet inhibitors, with the exception of aspirin, should be discontinued preoperatively depending on clearance. Preoperative heparin infusions can be continued into the operating room and discontinued after full heparinization. Preoperative sedation with a benzodiazepine (diazepam 10 mg PO) and nasal cannula oxygen is effective at reducing sympathetic stimulation. Induction of anesthesia should have the goal to maintain arterial blood pressure within 10% to 20% of baseline. Baseline measurements of heart rate, blood pressure, pulmonary artery pressures, central venous pressures, and cardiac output can be obtained using intra-arterial and pulmonary arterial catheters allowing preinduction optimization of hemodynamics. If severe pulmonary hypertension or low cardiac output is identified, a discussion of the case with the cardiac surgeon is warranted. An infusion of the vasoconstrictor phenylephrine may be started prior to induction of anesthesia and then titrated to maintain blood pressure. Any intravenous anesthetic can be used to induce anesthesia, but benzodiazepines (midazolam) and narcotics (fentanyl) are common. Sufentanil decreases heart rate more than fentanyl, which may or may not be advantageous. Dexmedetomidine can be used to supplement other agents and may reduce stress response and postoperative delirium.[69] Etomidate, propofol, and thiopental are also effective for induction of anesthesia, but doses should be reduced in patients at risk for hypotension. Once anesthetic induction is complete, a muscle relaxant can be given. Bradycardia (heart rates between 45 and 60 beats/min) is helpful during conduct of the distal anastomosis, so use of pancuronium may be avoided. If reflux is a concern, a modified rapid sequence induction with cricoid pressure is warranted. If the patient is thought to have a difficult airway, the standard difficult airway protocols should be used with special attention to avoid tachycardia and sympathetic stimulation. Intubation of cardiac surgery patients should follow the standard protocols for airway management, the only difference being that the tolerance for tachycardia, hypotension, or hypertension is greatly reduced and myocardial ischemia, ventricular arrhythmias, and hemodynamic collapse are the possible rapid sequelae of complications. Maintenance of anesthesia is usually with a volatile agent (isoflurane or sevoflurane) in combination with an opioid (fentanyl or sufentanil). Nitrous oxide should be avoided secondary to reduction in F_{IO_2}, potential for pulmonary vasoconstriction, and potential to increase the volume of gas emboli. Maintenance infusions of propofol, dexmedetomidine, or remifentanil are also commonly used. If remifentanil is chosen, inadvertent discontinuation of the infusion should be avoided because the metabolism is rapid. Cardiac depression may be more with remifentanil than fentanyl or sufentanil, making its use more difficult in patients with limited cardiac reserve. Prophylactic antiarrhythmic therapy (lidocaine and magnesium or amiodarone) is appropriate to avoid arrhythmias from manual manipulation of the heart, from ischemia during the distal anastomosis, and upon reperfusion after completion of the anastomosis. Anticoagulation is achieved with heparin and monitored with ACT (activated clotting time) or heparin assay. Hemodynamic stability during the distal anastomosis is achieved with careful surgical manipulation and retraction of the heart, table positioning, infusions of vasoconstrictors, and volume. Inotropic stimulation with β-agonists has the potential to raise the heart rate, making completion of the distal anastomosis more difficult and lowering the threshold for ventricular arrhythmias. If β-agonists are needed to support cardiac output during conduct of the distal anastomosis, use of extracorporeal circulatory support should be considered. Heparin anticoagulation is reversed with protamine after completion of the proximal and distal anastomosis and is confirmed by measurement of an ACT near baseline (120 to 140 seconds). The period and requirements for postoperative ventilation and sedation may be reduced in off-pump CABG and extubation should be performed once hemodynamics are stable, bleeding is controlled, oxygen requirements are reduced ($F_{IO_2} = 0.40$ with P_{O_2} more than 80 mm Hg), neuromuscular blockade has been reversed, and the patient is awake and breathing spontaneously with the help of continuous positive-pressure ventilation. Postoperative β-blockade may reduce the incidence of atrial fibrillation and myocardial ischemia and should be started as soon as hemodynamics will tolerate. Aspirin therapy should be resumed once bleeding is controlled. Discontinuation of anti-ischemic and vasodilator agents (β-blockers, calcium channel blockers, nitrates, and angiotensin inhibitors) should be avoided because withdrawal phenomena may lead to increased morbidity and mortality rates.

Cardiac surgery is continually advancing with hybrid operations, off-pump CABG, minimal access, surgical ventricular restoration, left ventricular assist devices, artificial hearts, and robotic mitral and coronary artery bypass surgery. Vigilance, cooperation, team work, and a very clear understanding of the surgical plans and hemodynamic consequences of procedures are essential to reduce the morbidity and mortality rates of these operations.

QUESTIONS OF THE DAY

1. What factors influence the risk of perioperative myocardial infarction?

2. Which patients are most likely to benefit from perioperative β-blockade?

3. What are the hemodynamic goals for management of patients with aortic stenosis who are undergoing anesthesia?

4. What is the "magnet mode" of a programmable cardiac pacemaker? Why should the specific magnet mode be known during the perioperative period?

5. What factors reduce left ventricular outflow obstruction in a patient with hypertrophic cardiomyopathy?

6. What are the clinical manifestations of cardiac tamponade? What are the most important aspects of anesthesia management for a patient with cardiac tamponade who requires a pericardial window?

REFERENCES

1. Mangano DT, Goldman L: Preoperative assessment of patients with known or suspected coronary disease, *N Engl J Med* 333:1750–1756, 1995.

2. Mangano DT, Browner WS, Hollenberg M, et al: Long-term cardiac prognosis following noncardiac surgery. The Study of Perioperative Ischemia Research Group, *JAMA* 268:233–239, 1992.

3. Mangano DT, Browner WS, Hollenberg M, et al: Association of perioperative myocardial ischemia with cardiac morbidity and mortality in men undergoing noncardiac surgery. The Study of Perioperative Ischemia Research Group, *N Engl J Med* 323:1781–1788, 1990.

4. Fleisher LA, Barash PG: Preoperative cardiac evaluation for noncardiac surgery: A functional approach, *Anesth Analg* 74:586–598, 1992.

5. Mangano DT, London MJ, Tubau JF, et al: Dipyridamole thallium-201 scintigraphy as a preoperative screening test. A reexamination of its predictive potential. Study of Perioperative Ischemia Research Group, *Circulation* 84:493–502, 1991.

6. Baron JF, Mundler O, Bertrand M, et al: Dipyridamole-thallium scintigraphy and gated radionuclide angiography to assess cardiac risk before abdominal aortic surgery, *N Engl J Med* 330:663–669, 1994.

7. Tarhan S, Moffitt EA, Taylor WF, et al: Myocardial infarction after general anesthesia, *Anesth Analg* 56:455–461, 1977.

8. Steen PA, Tinker JH, Tarhan S: Myocardial reinfarction after anesthesia and surgery, *JAMA* 239:2566–2570, 1978.

9. Rao TL, Jacobs KH, El-Etr AA: Reinfarction following anesthesia in patients with myocardial infarction, *Anesthesiology* 59:499–505, 1983.

10. Shah KB, Kleinman BS, Sami H, et al: Reevaluation of perioperative myocardial infarction in patients with prior myocardial infarction undergoing noncardiac operations, *Anesth Analg* 71:231–235, 1990.

11. Mangano DT, Layug EL, Wallace A, et al: Effect of atenolol on mortality and cardiovascular morbidity after noncardiac surgery. Multicenter Study of Perioperative Ischemia Research Group [published erratum appears in *N Engl J Med* 1997; 336: 1039], *N Engl J Med* 335:1713–1720, 1996.

12. Poldermans D, Boersma E, Bax JJ, et al: The effect of bisoprolol on perioperative mortality and myocardial infarction in high-risk patients undergoing vascular surgery. Dutch Echocardiographic Cardiac Risk Evaluation Applying Stress Echocardiography Study Group, *N Engl J Med* 341:1789–1794, 1999.

13. Poldermans D, Boersma E, Bax JJ, et al: Bisoprolol reduces cardiac death and myocardial infarction in high-risk patients as long as 2 years after successful major vascular surgery, *Eur Heart J* 22:1353–1358, 2001.

14. Wallace A, Layug B, Tateo I, et al: Prophylactic atenolol reduces postoperative myocardial ischemia. McSPI Research Group, *Anesthesiology* 88:7–17, 1998.

15. Mangano DT, Layug EL, Wallace A: Effect of atenolol on mortality and cardiovascular morbidity after noncardiac surgery. Multicenter Study of Perioperative Ischemia Research Group, *N Engl J Med* 335:1713–1720, 1996.

16. Wallace AW, Galindez D, Salahieh A, et al: Effect of clonidine on cardiovascular morbidity and mortality after noncardiac surgery, *Anesthesiology* 101:284–293, 2004.

17. Schouten O, Boersma E, Hoeks SE, et al: Fluvastatin and perioperative events in patients undergoing vascular surgery, *N Engl J Med* 361:980–989, 2009.

18. Slogoff S, Keats AS, Ott E: Preoperative propranolol therapy and aortocoronary bypass operation, *JAMA* 240:1487–1490, 1978.

19. McFalls EO, Ward HB, Moritz TE: Coronary-artery revascularization before elective major vascular surgery, *N Engl J Med* 351:2795–2804, 2004.

20. Kaluza GL, Joseph J, Lee JR, et al: Catastrophic outcomes of noncardiac surgery soon after coronary stenting, *J Am Coll Cardiol* 35:1288–1294, 2000.

21. Hueb W, Soares PR, Gersh BJ: The medicine, angioplasty, or surgery study (MASS-II): A randomized, controlled clinical trial of three therapeutic strategies for multivessel coronary artery disease: One-year results, *J Am Coll Cardiol* 43:1743–1751, 2004.

22. Shelton RJ, Velavan P, Nikitin NP, et al: Clinical trials update from the American Heart Association meeting: ACORN-CSD, primary care trial of chronic disease management, PEACE, CREATE, SHIELD, A-HeFT, GEMINI, vitamin E meta-analysis, ESCAPE, CARP, and SCD-HeFT cost-effectiveness study. Disparate opinions regarding indications for coronary artery revascularization before elective vascular surgery. Myocardial revascularization before carotid endarterectomy. How to avoid cardiac ischemic events associated with aortic surgery, *Eur J Heart Fail* 7:127–135, 2005.

23. Eagle KA, Berger PB, Calkins H, et al: ACC/AHA Guideline Update for Perioperative Cardiovascular Evaluation for Noncardiac Surgery—Executive Summary. A report of the American College of Cardiology/American Heart Association Task Force on Practice Guidelines (Committee to Update the 1996 Guidelines on Perioperative Cardiovascular Evaluation for Noncardiac Surgery). *Anesth Analg* 94:1052–1064, 2002.

24. Eagle KA, Berger PB, Calkins H, et al: ACC/AHA guideline update for perioperative cardiovascular evaluation for noncardiac surgery—Executive summary: A report of the American College of Cardiology/American Heart Association Task Force on Practice Guidelines (Committee to Update the 1996 Guidelines on Perioperative Cardiovascular Evaluation for Noncardiac Surgery). *J Am Coll Cardiol* 39:542–553, 2002.

25. Fleischmann KE, Beckman JA, Buller CE, et al: 2009 ACCF/AHA

IV

Focused Update on Perioperative Beta Blockade. A Report of the American College of Cardiology Foundation/ American Heart Association Task Force on Practice Guidelines, *Circulation* 120:2123–2151, 2009.

26. Fleisher LA, Beckman JA, Brown KA, et al: ACC/AHA 2006 guideline update on perioperative cardiovascular evaluation for noncardiac surgery: Focused update on perioperative beta-blocker therapy: A report of the American College of Cardiology/American Heart Association Task Force on Practice Guidelines (Writing Committee to Update the 2002 Guidelines on Perioperative Cardiovascular Evaluation for Noncardiac Surgery): Developed in collaboration with the American Society of Echocardiography, American Society of Nuclear Cardiology, Heart Rhythm Society, Society of Cardiovascular Anesthesiologists, Society for Cardiovascular Angiography and Interventions, and Society for Vascular Medicine and Biology, *Circulation* 113:2662–2674, 2006.

27. Gordon AJ, Macpherson DS: Guideline chaos: Conflicting recommendations for preoperative cardiac assessment, *Am J Cardiol* 91:1299–1303, 2003.

28. Krupski WC, Nehler MR: How to avoid cardiac ischemic events associated with aortic surgery, *Semin Vasc Surg* 14:235–244, 2001.

29. Nuttall GA, Brown MJ, Stombaugh JW, et al: Time and cardiac risk of surgery after bare-metal stent percutaneous coronary intervention, *Anesthesiology* 109:588–595, 2008.

30. Rabbitts JA, Nuttall GA, Brown MJ, et al: Cardiac risk of noncardiac surgery after percutaneous coronary intervention with drug-eluting stents, *Anesthesiology* 109:596–604, 2008.

31. Devereaux PJ, Yang H, Yusuf S, et al: Effects of extended-release metoprolol succinate in patients undergoing non-cardiac surgery (POISE trial): A randomised controlled trial, *Lancet* 371:1839–1847, 2008.

32. Slogoff S, Keats AS: Does chronic treatment with calcium entry blocking drugs reduce perioperative myocardial ischemia? *Anesthesiology* 68:676–680, 1988.

33. Slogoff S, Keats AS: Further observations on perioperative myocardial ischemia, *Anesthesiology* 65:539–542, 1986.

34. Mangano DT, Browner WS, Hollenberg M, et al: Long-term cardiac prognosis following noncardiac surgery. The Study of Perioperative Ischemia Research Group, *JAMA* 268:233–239, 1992.

35. Wakeling HG, McFall MR, Jenkins CS, et al: Intraoperative oesophageal Doppler guided fluid management shortens postoperative hospital stay after major bowel surgery, *Br J Anaesth* 95:634–642, 2005.

36. Wallace AW, Galindez D, Salahieh A, et al: Effect of clonidine on cardiovascular morbidity and mortality after noncardiac surgery, *Anesthesiology* 101:284–293, 2004.

37. Wallace A, Layug B, Tateo I, et al: Prophylactic atenolol reduces postoperative myocardial ischemia. McSPI Research Group, *Anesthesiology* 88:7–17, 1998.

38. Ebert TJ, Muzi M, Berens R, et al: Sympathetic responses to induction of anesthesia in humans with propofol or etomidate, *Anesthesiology* 76:725–733, 1992.

39. Helman JD, Leung JM, Bellows WH, et al: The risk of myocardial ischemia in patients receiving desflurane versus sufentanil anesthesia for coronary artery bypass graft surgery. The SPI Research Group, *Anesthesiology* 77:47–62, 1992.

40. Slogoff S, Keats AS, Dear WE, et al: Steal-prone coronary anatomy and myocardial ischemia associated with four primary anesthetic agents in humans, *Anesth Analg* 72:22–27, 1991.

41. Diana P, Tullock WC, Gorcsan J, et al: A comparison between isoflurane and enflurane in coronary artery bypass patients, *Anesth Analg* 77:221–226, 1993.

42. Leung JM, Goehner P, O'Kelly BF, et al: Isoflurane anesthesia and myocardial ischemia: Comparative risk versus sufentanil anesthesia in patients undergoing coronary artery bypass graft surgery. The SPI (Study of Perioperative Ischemia) Research Group, *Anesthesiology* 74:838–847, 1991.

43. Hanley PJ, Ray J, Brandt U, et al: Halothane, isoflurane and sevoflurane inhibit NADH:ubiquinone oxidoreductase (complex I) of cardiac mitochondria, *J Physiol* 544:687–693, 2002.

44. Cason BA, Gamperl AK, Slocum RE, et al: Anesthetic-induced preconditioning: Previous administration of isoflurane decreases myocardial infarct size in rabbits, *Anesthesiology* 87:1182–1190, 1997.

45. Helman JD, Leung JM, Bellows WH, et al: The risk of myocardial ischemia in patients receiving desflurane versus sufentanil anesthesia for coronary artery bypass graft surgery. The SPI Research Group [see comments], *Anesthesiology* 77:47–62, 1992.

46. Slogoff S, Keats AS: Randomized trial of primary anesthetic agents on outcome of coronary artery bypass operations, *Anesthesiology* 70:179–188, 1989.

47. Practice guidelines for pulmonary artery catheterization. A report by the American Society of Anesthesiologists Task Force on Pulmonary Artery Catheterization, *Anesthesiology* 78:380–394, 1993.

48. Practice guidelines for pulmonary artery catheterization. An updated report by the American Society of Anesthesiologists Task Force on Pulmonary Artery Catheterization, *Anesthesiology* 99:988–1014, 2003.

49. Mangano DT: Dynamic predictors of perioperative risk. Study of Perioperative Ischemia (SPI) Research Group, *J Card Surg* 5:231–236, 1990.

50. Carabello BA, Crawford FA Jr: Valvular heart disease, *N Engl J Med* 337:32–41, 1997.

51. van den Berghe G, Wouters P, Weekers F, et al: Intensive insulin therapy in the critically ill patients, *N Engl J Med* 345:1359–1367, 2001.

52. Hilgenberg JC, McCammon RL, Stoelting RK: Pulmonary and systemic vascular responses to nitrous oxide in patients with mitral stenosis and pulmonary hypertension, *Anesth Analg* 59:323–326, 1980.

53. Greenberg BH, Rahimtoola SH: Vasodilator therapy for valvular heart disease, *JAMA* 246:269–272, 1981.

54. Hanson EW, Neerhut RK, Lynch C 3rd: Mitral valve prolapse, *Anesthesiology* 85:178–195, 1996.

55. Freed LA, Levy D, Levine RA, et al: Prevalence and clinical outcome of mitral-valve prolapse, *N Engl J Med* 341:1–7, 1999.

56. Atlee JL: Perioperative cardiac dysrhythmias: Diagnosis and management, *Anesthesiology* 86:1397–1424, 1997.

57. Gallagher JD, Weindling SN, Anderson G, et al: Effects of sevoflurane on QT interval in a patient with congenital long QT syndrome, *Anesthesiology* 89:1569–1573, 1998.

58. Michalets EL, Smith LK, Van Tassel ED: Torsade de pointes resulting from the addition of droperidol to an existing cytochrome P450 drug interaction, *Ann Pharmacother* 32:761–765, 1998.

59. Guy JM, Andre-Fouet X, Porte J, et al: [Torsades de pointes and prolongation of the duration of QT interval after injection of droperidol], *Ann Cardiol Angeiol (Paris)* 40:541–545, 1991.

60. Kusumoto FM, Goldschlager N: Cardiac pacing, *N Engl J Med* 334:89–97, 1996.

61. Zaidan JR: Pacemakers, *Anesthesiology* 60:319–334, 1984.

62. Dagnino J, Prys-Roberts C: Studies of anaesthesia in relation to hypertension. VI: Cardiovascular responses to extradural blockade of treated and untreated hypertensive patients, *Br J Anaesth* 56:1065–1073, 1984.

63. Nikolov NM, Fontes ML, White WD, et al: Pulse pressure and long-term survival after coronary artery bypass graft surgery, *Anesth Analg* 110:335–340, 2010.

64. Spirito P, Seidman CE, McKenna WJ, et al: The management of hypertrophic cardiomyopathy, *N Engl J Med* 336:775–785, 1997.

65. Pass LJ, Eberhart RC, Brown JC, et al: The effect of mannitol and dopamine on the renal response to thoracic aortic cross-clamping, *J Thorac Cardiovasc Surg* 95:608–612, 1988.

66. Despotis GJ, Gravlee G, Filos K, et al: Anticoagulation monitoring during cardiac surgery: A review of current and emerging techniques, *Anesthesiology* 91:1122–1151, 1999.

67. Martin TD, Craver JM, Gott JP, et al: Prospective, randomized trial of retrograde warm blood cardioplegia: Myocardial benefit and neurologic threat, *Ann Thorac Surg* 57:298–302, 1994, discussion 302–304.

68. Gibson AJ, Davis FM: Hyperbaric oxygen therapy in the treatment of postcardiac surgical strokes—A case series and review of the literature, *Anaesth Intens Care* 38:175–184, 2010.

69. Maldonado JR, Wysong A, van der Starre PJ, et al: Dexmedetomidine and the reduction of postoperative delirium after cardiac surgery, *Psychosomatics* 50:206–217, 2009.

70. Wahr JA, Plunkett JJ, Ramsay JG, et al: Cardiovascular responses during sedation after coronary revascularization. Incidence of myocardial ischemia and hemodynamic episodes with propofol versus midazolam. Institutions of the McSPI Research Group, *Anesthesiology* 84:1350–1360, 1996.

71. Engelman RM, Rousou JA, Flack JE 3rd, et al: Fast-track recovery of the coronary bypass patient, *Ann Thorac Surg* 58:1742–1746, 1994.

72. Shroyer AL, Grover FL, Hattler B, et al: On-pump versus off-pump coronary-artery bypass surgery, *N Engl J Med* 361:1827–1837, 2009.

IV

26 CONGENITAL HEART DISEASE

Jin J. Huang, James E. Baker, and Isobel A. Russell

Categorization of the many types of congenital heart disease (CHD) may be based on distinctive anatomic or physiologic features of the defects (Table 26-1). Sometimes complete comprehension of the anatomic complexities in a patient with CHD may be difficult because of a wide range of anatomic lesions. Fortunately many lesions share similar pathophysiologic conditions despite their anatomic variations. When these conditions are understood, then successful management of a patient with complex CHD can be achieved.

FUNDAMENTAL PATHOPHYSIOLOGY IN CONGENITAL HEART DISEASE

Normally, pulmonary blood flow (Qp) and systemic blood flow (Qs) do not mix, and the entire cardiac output flows sequentially from one circulation to the other. All of the systemic venous return is directed to the pulmonary circulation and, likewise, all of the pulmonary venous return is directed to the systemic arterial circulation. Shunting occurs when a portion of the venous return of one circulation is redirected back to the arterial outflow of the same circulation.[1] This redirected flow occurs when there is an abnormal communication or a defect between two otherwise separate structures. The direction of the shunt flow is dictated by the relative pressures of the communicating structures, while the amount of shunting usually is limited by the size of the defect. Small defects tend to be *restrictive* with limited flow and large defects tend to be *nonrestrictive* with unimpaired flow [1]

Left-to-Right Shunts

A left-to-right (L → R) shunt occurs when part of the pulmonary venous return is redirected toward the pulmonary arterial system.[1] This may occur at any of numerous locations, including the pulmonary veins (anomalous pulmonary venous return), the atrial septum (atrial septal

Table 26-1	Categorization of Congenital Heart Disease
Acyanotic versus cyanotic—VSD versus TOF
Simple versus complex—ASD versus HLHS
Left-to-right shunt versus right-to-left shunt versus mixing lesions—ASD versus TOF versus HLHS

ASD, atrial septal defect; HLHS, hypoplastic left heart syndrome; TOF, tetralogy of Fallot; VSD, ventricular septal defect.

defect), the ventricular septum (ventricular septal defect), and at the great vessels (patent ductus arteriosus). The portion of the pulmonary blood flow that is redirected toward the pulmonary artery is *recirculated* pulmonary blood flow, and that which is appropriately directed toward the systemic circulation (Qs) is *effective* pulmonary blood flow (Qep). Their sum is the total pulmonary blood flow (Qp) (Fig. 26-1). The physiologic effect of a left-to-right shunt is that Qp is greater than Qs (Qp > Qs), which can result in hypotension and pulmonary edema. Prolonged hypotension can lead to circulatory shock with multiple organ failure and lactic acidosis, and the long-term effects of pulmonary overflow may be an increase of pulmonary vascular resistance and abnormal cardiac chamber dilation.

Right-to-Left Shunts

A right-to-left (R → L) shunt occurs when a portion of the systemic venous return is redirected to the systemic arterial outflow without first circulating through the lungs. The hallmark of lesions producing a right-to-left shunt is arterial oxygen desaturation. Because the pulmonary venous return mixes with recirculated systemic venous blood, the resulting arterial oxygen saturation will be decreased. The degree of desaturation depends upon the magnitude of right-to-left shunting as well as the degree of desaturation of the systemic venous return.[2]

Mixing Lesions

Whereas a shunt connotes a communication between pulmonary and systemic venous circulations with *partial* mixing, many forms of CHD result in a *complete* blending of the two. Mixing lesions therefore are conditions in which oxygen content is equilibrated between the two circulations, yielding identical or nearly identical oxygen saturation at both the pulmonary and systemic arterial level.[2]

As with right-to-left shunts, one of the chief characteristics of mixing lesions is systemic arterial oxygen desaturation, the final value of which depends on the volume flow

IV

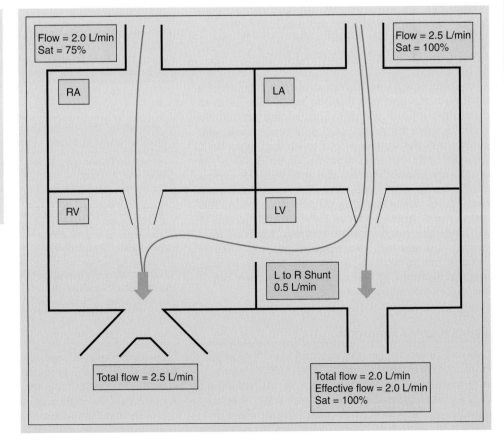

Figure 26-1 Schematic diagram of a ventricular septal defect. A left-to-right shunt occurs at a septal defect with 0.5 L/min flow. Thus, total pulmonary flow is 2.5 L/min, of which the 2 L/min is the effective pulmonary flow; 2 L/min is also the systemic flow (Qs < Qp). LA, left atrium; LV, left ventricle; RA, right atrium; RV, right ventricle; Qs, systemic flow; Qp, pulmonary flow

Flow = 2.0 L/min
Sat = 75%

Flow = 2.5 L/min
Sat = 100%

RA

LA

RV

LV

L to R Shunt
0.5 L/min

Total flow = 2.5 L/min

Total flow = 2.0 L/min
Effective flow = 2.0 L/min
Sat = 100%

of the two contributing circulations as well as the difference in the individual oxygen saturation. A decrease in pulmonary venous saturation from apnea or atelectasis will decrease the saturation of the final mixed circulation. A decrease in the systemic venous saturation will also cause the final systemic arterial saturation to decrease. A decrease in systemic venous saturation may result from either an increase of systemic oxygen consumption (e.g., fever) or a decrease in systemic oxygen delivery (e.g., low cardiac output, anemia).

THE SIGNIFICANCE OF Qp:Qs RATIO IN MIXING LESIONS

The ideal Qp:Qs ratio is 1 because equal blood flows tend to maximize the *effective* component of each circulation and minimize the wasteful *recirculated* component. Any preferential flow toward the aorta will increase systemic blood flow, but at the expense of greater desaturation, and therefore less oxygen delivery. Any preferential flow toward the pulmonary artery will increase pulmonary blood flow, resulting in greater oxygen saturation of the mixed blood, but at the expense of systemic cardiac output, and therefore less oxygen delivery.

Qp:Qs ratio is determined by the relative resistance to flow of the two circulations: pulmonary vascular resistance (PVR) and systemic vascular resistance (SVR). If PVR exceeds SVR, Qs will exceed Qp. Likewise, if SVR exceeds PVR, Qp will exceed Qs. SVR and PVR are both affected by many factors listed in Table 26-2.[3]

THE SIGNIFICANCE OF THE PATENT DUCTUS ARTERIOSUS

Mixing lesions with one functional ventricle often require a patent ductus arteriosus (PDA) to supply blood flow to the underdeveloped side. Shunting through the PDA in systole is either left to right (e.g., pulmonary atresia with intact ventricular septum) or right to left (e.g., hypoplastic left-sided heart syndrome), depending on which side of the heart is hypoplastic. Shunting during diastole, however, is usually left to right through the PDA because the aorta has a higher resting tone than the pulmonary artery. This means that a large amount of blood can be diverted to the lungs and away from the coronary arteries during diastole. Consequently the myocardium may become ischemic and infarcted due to coronary ischemia. Maneuvers that decrease PVR will cause more pulmonary runoff and exacerbate coronary ischemia.

Eisenmenger's Syndrome

CHD may subject the lungs to abnormal blood flow or pulmonary artery pressure (Table 26-3). Over time, the pulmonary vasculature may undergo a process of remodeling with a gradual increase in PVR that may result in pulmonary hypertension, even if the underlying hemodynamic problem is corrected.[3] When pulmonary hypertension becomes irreversible and pulmonary pressure becomes supersystemic, blood is preferentially directed toward the systemic circulation and the direction of the shunt is R → L even if the original shunting pattern was L → R. This condition is called Eisenmenger's syndrome and often is a contraindication for surgical correction of the shunt.

Table 26-2 Impact of Anesthetic Management on Peripheral and Systemic Vascular Resistance

Events That Increase Systemic Vascular Resistance
Light anesthesia
Sympathetic nervous system activation
Administration of α-agonists
Physical manipulations (e.g., compression of the femoral arteries by flexing the hips of infants and small children)

Events That Decrease Systemic Vascular Resistance
Deep anesthesia
Administration of vasodilating drugs—nitrates, intravenous and inhaled anesthetics

Events That Increase Pulmonary Vascular Resistance
Alveolar hypoxemia (e.g., from low inspired oxygen concentrations)
Hypercapnia
Acidosis
High lung volumes or pressures—tend to collapse pulmonary capillaries
Low lung volumes with atelectasis—tend to collapse larger pulmonary blood vessels
Light anesthesia
Sympathetic nervous system stimulation
Hypothermia

Events That Decrease Pulmonary Vascular Resistance
Hyperventilation
Hypocarbia
Alkalosis
Oxygenation
Inhaled nitric oxide
Warmth
Bronchodilators (e.g., albuterol)

Table 26-3 Defects Resulting in Increased Pulmonary Blood Flow and Pulmonary Artery Pressure over Time

Increased Pulmonary Blood Flow
Atrial septal defect
Anomalous pulmonary venous return

Increased Pulmonary Artery Pressure
Ventricular septal defect
Atrioventricular canal defect
Aortopulmonary window
Truncus arteriosus
Transposition of the great arteries
Double-inlet left ventricle
Patent ductus arteriosus

PERIOPERATIVE MANAGEMENT

Surgery for CHD should be planned with the cooperative input of a multidisciplinary team that includes surgeons, cardiologists, critical care specialists, and anesthesiologists. Aspects of the patient's condition that can be improved before surgery should be identified. For the anesthesiologist, the physiology of the cardiac lesion and the subsequent effects of the planned surgical palliative or corrective procedure should be understood.

History and Physical Examination

A review of the patient's history should include attention to details that are of importance to pediatric anesthetic care in general, such as pertinent pregnancy details, prematurity, and postnatal course. Patients with CHD frequently have associated syndromes (trisomy 21, DiGeorge syndrome) or evidence of chronic illness (renal dysfunction, pulmonary edema, imbalances in electrolyte and glucose metabolism). Preoperative medications and laboratory studies (complete blood count, electrolytes, coagulation studies, indices of renal and hepatic function) should be known and understood.

The anesthesiologist should review the available diagnostic studies such as the echocardiograms (Fig. 26-2) and cardiac catheterization studies (Fig. 26-3). Magnetic resonance imaging (MRI) can also provide invaluable

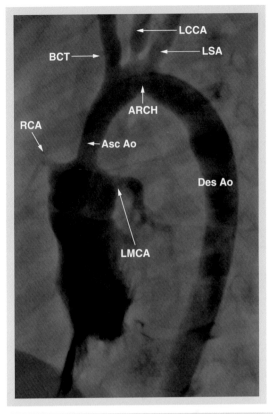

Figure 26-3 Angiogram of the aorta during systole showing narrowing of the ascending aorta. This is an example of supravalvular aortic stenosis. The left main coronary artery is dilated and the orifice of the left common carotid artery is stenosed. Asc Ao, ascending aorta; Des Ao, descending aorta; BCT, brachiocephalic trunk; LCCA, left common carotid artery; LSA, left subclavian artery; LMCA, left main coronary artery; RCA, right coronary artery.

anatomic details (Fig. 26-4). Electrocardiograms and chest radiographs are part of the routine preoperative evaluation. Medical or surgical interventions that have been instituted previously and any interim change or deterioration in the patient's status should be evaluated. Previous sternotomy is a risk factor for increased operative blood loss and cardiac trauma during dissection as a result of adhesions to the sternum and chest wall. Many hospitalized neonates require continuous infusions of inotropic drugs or other medications such as prostaglandin E_1 to maintain stability while awaiting surgery.

Physical examination should include an assessment of airway problems (trisomy 21), signs of congestive heart failure (tachypnea, wheezing, dilated neck veins), cyanosis, nutritional status, and any other coexisting conditions. Outpatients who have been scheduled for elective surgery should be evaluated the day of surgery for new onset of signs or symptoms of an intercurrent illness such as an upper respiratory tract infection. Inpatients should

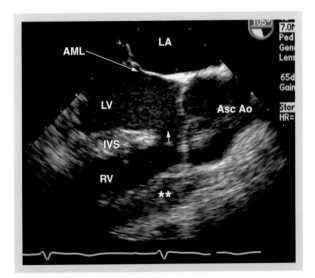

Figure 26-2 Transesophageal echocardiogram of an adult with unrepaired tetralogy of Fallot. Note that the aorta is straddling over both ventricles, and a ventricular defect (*block arrow*) is seen immediately below the aortic valve. Right ventricle is hypertrophied (**). AML, anterior mitral leaflet; Asc Ao, ascending aorta; IVS, interventricular septum; LA, left atrium; LV, left ventricle; RV, right ventricle.

IV

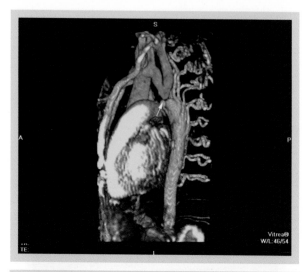

Figure 26-4 Three-dimensional magnetic resonance image of a coarctation of aorta (*block arrow*). Note the numerous collateral arteries to the descending aorta.

be evaluated for their hospital course along with any new developing problems such as an elevated white blood cell count, which could indicate the presence of some type of inflammatory process.

Preparation for Surgery

All patients should follow the standard American Society of Anesthesiologists (ASA) guidelines for fasting instructions. Outpatients taking cardiac medications should generally be advised to continue therapy up to and including the day of surgery, although preference may vary among anesthesiologists regarding diuretics and angiotensin-converting enzyme inhibitors. Antiplatelet medications, such as aspirin and clopidogrel (Plavix), are usually not given several days before surgery.

OPERATING ROOM SETUP

Preparation of the operating room should include readiness of age-appropriate airway equipment, intravenous equipment (Buretrol infusion sets and fluid warmers), and invasive monitors (catheters and transducers). All intravenous administration sets should be meticulously de-aired to prevent paradoxical arterial embolization of intravenous air bubbles. Any warming blankets or surface cooling equipment should be made available, and adjustment of the operating room temperature should precede entry of the patient (27° C for small or premature infants and 24° C for older children). Hemodynamic medications should be prepared in weight-appropriate dilutions before surgery. Preparation may include readiness of specialized equipment such as transesophageal echocardiography or nitric oxide delivery systems.

Induction of Anesthesia

Induction of anesthesia for patients with CHD may involve the use of inhaled or intravenous anesthetics (Tables 26-4 and 26-5). The goal is to execute a smooth anesthetic induction to avoid increased anxiety, crying, coughing, or breath-holding. These events may aggravate unfavorable physiologic effects such as increased right-to-left shunting and dynamic right ventricular outflow tract obstruction in susceptible patients.

INHALATION INDUCTION OF ANESTHESIA

Awake infants and children without intravenous access are frequently amenable to an inhaled induction of anesthesia. This strategy is typically reserved for those with minimal or

Table 26-4 Anesthetics Used for Induction of Anesthesia in Congenital Heart Disease

Sevoflurane	1.5%-3.5% (ET) Decrease SVR, contractility Decrease dose if N_2O used; may cause myocardial depression
Halothane	0.8%-2.0% (ET) Decreases contractility, HR More pronounced myocardial depression with decreased CO, dysrhythmia, and ventricular irritability
Fentanyl	20-50 µg/kg Non-significant effect on contractility, SVR May cause loss of sympathetic tone, bradycardia May cause chest wall rigidity with rapid administration or large doses
Sufentanil	5-10 µg/kg Similar to fentanyl
Ketamine (IV)	1-2 mg/kg Increases HR, increase or no change in SVR, PVR Actually a myocardial depressant with sympathetic stimulant properties; may decrease contractility in patients with depleted SNS May cause bronchorrhea (prevented with atropine, 20 µg/kg)
Ketamine (IM)	3-5 mg/kg
Etomidate (IV)	0.2-0.3 mg/kg Preserves HR, SVR, PVR, contractility May inhibit endogenous corticosteroid production; burning pain at the injection site

BP, blood pressure; CHF, congestive heart failure; CO, cardiac output; ET, end-tidal; HR, heart rate; IM, intramuscular; IV, intravenous; PVR, pulmonary vascular resistance; SVR, systemic vascular resistance; SNS, sympathetic nervous system.

Table 26-5 Common Congenital Cardiac Lesions: Summary of Anesthetic Goals and Induction Strategies

General Goals and Principles

- Avoid air entrapment in intravenous and pressure tubing; meticulous clearing techniques.
- Avoid dehydration; careful orders regarding NPO status (following ASA guidelines).
- Avoid myocardial depression.
- Maintain sinus rhythm whenever possible.
- Well-sedated, cooperative patient is ideal.
- Premedication is indicated for patients older than 1 year (oral midazolam, 0.5 - 1 mg/kg).
- Close monitoring after sedation.

Lesions Characterized by Excessive Pulmonary Blood Flow

Atrial Septal Defects

- Avoid further decreases in pulmonary vascular resistance (hyperventilation, high F_{O_2}).
- Consider early tracheal extubation.

Ventricular Septal Defects

- Avoid decreases in pulmonary vascular resistance.
- Avoid excessive myocardial depression, particularly in patients with congestive heart failure—inhaled induction may be rapid.

Atrioventricular Septal Defects

- Avoid decreases in pulmonary vascular resistance before cardiopulmonary bypass.
- Prepare to treat pulmonary hypertension (100% oxygen, hyperventilation, alkalinization, deep sedation).
- Have nitric oxide available and ready.
- Inotropic support frequently is required.

Truncus Arteriosus

- Neonates are critically ill and require close management of systemic and pulmonary vascular resistance to balance systemic and pulmonary blood flow.
- Addition of carbon dioxide or nitrogen may be needed to decrease F_{O_2} to 17%.

Hypoplastic Left Heart Syndrome

Surgical correction occurs in three stages:

Stage I: Norwood procedure
- Ascending aorta and arch reconstruction.
- PDA ligation.
- Construction of a reliable pulmonary blood flow source using a BT shunt or Sano shunt.
- Anesthetic management includes pre-bypass PGE_1 infusion, maintenance of nearly equal pulmonary and systemic blood flow for adequate systemic perfusion, precautions against air embolism, maintenance of anesthesia with intravenous drugs, and postbypass maintenance of a high hematocrit and probably a need for inotropic support.

Stage II: Glenn procedure
- Creation of a direct connection between the superior vena cava and pulmonary artery.
- Anesthetic management includes maintenance of a high hematocrit, elevation of the head of the bed to facilitate venous drainage, avoidance of central lines to reduce the risk for pulmonary artery thrombus and recognition that positive-pressure ventilation of the patient's lungs may decrease pulmonary blood flow and cardiac output.
- Mild hypoventilation may increase oxygen saturation.

Stage III: Fontan procedure
- Rerouting of blood flow from the inferior vena cava into the pulmonary circulation, usually accomplished using an extracardiac conduit.
- Preload to the heart is completely passive. Management of a patient status post Fontan procedure should focus on maintaining reasonable preload, i.e., passive flow from systemic veins to the pulmonary artery and eventually to the common atrium.
- Poor prognostic factors are high pulmonary vascular resistance, tricuspid regurgitation, and decreased ventricular function.

Continued

Table 26-5 Common Congenital Cardiac Lesions: Summary of Anesthetic Goals and Induction Strategies—cont'd

Lesions with Inadequate Pulmonary Blood Flow

Transposition of the Great Arteries (TGA)
- PGE_1 infusion is maintained before cardiopulmonary bypass.
- Patient may need Rashkind's procedure (atrial septectomy) if patent ductus does not provide adequate mixing for survival.
- Manipulation of pulmonary vascular resistance before cardiopulmonary bypass.
- Opioid-based anesthetic.

Tetralogy of Fallot (see Fig. 26-2)
- Adequate preoperative hydration is essential.
- Manipulations are indicated to decrease pulmonary vascular resistance and improve pulmonary blood flow.
- Hypercyanotic episodes are treated by intravenous fluid administration, sedation, and pharmacologically induced increases in systemic vascular resistance (phenylephrine).
- Avoid increases in heart rate, which may worsen infundibular pulmonary stenosis.
- Rate of induction of anesthesia with a volatile anesthetic may be slowed because of a right-to-left shunt.

Tricuspid Atresia or Pulmonary Atresia with Intact Ventricular Septum
- Usually the right ventricle is diminutive or hypoplastic.
- Surgical approach involves an aortopulmonary shunt and subsequent Glenn and Fontan procedures.

Total Anomalous Pulmonary Venous Return
- Severe cyanosis is treated with high FIo_2.
- Avoid systemic acidosis and high hematocrit.

Obstructive Lesions

Coarctation of the Aorta (see Fig. 26-4)
- Arterial monitoring in the right arm.
- Use cuffed endotracheal tube to provide adequate ventilation to patients requiring the thoracotomy position.
- Avoid acidosis.

Aortic Stenosis
- Avoid tachycardia, dysrhythmias, hypotension.
- Decrease myocardial oxygen demand.
- Maintain preload and afterload.

Subvalvular Aortic Stenosis
- Avoid tachycardia, dysrhythmias, hypotension.
- Decrease myocardial oxygen demand.
- Maintain preload and afterload.

Supravalvular Aortic Stenosis (see Fig. 26-3)
- Associated with William's syndrome.
- Patient may have concomitant pulmonary artery stenosis.
- Avoid tachycardia, dysrhythmias, hypotension.
- Coronary abnormalities common.
- Avoid acute afterload reduction.

ASA, American Society of Anesthesiologists; FIo_2, inspired oxygen concentration; NPO, nil per os ("nothing by mouth"); PGE_1, prostaglandin E_1.

well-controlled congestive heart failure because a dose-dependent reduction in myocardial contractility occurs with volatile anesthetics. Sevoflurane is the preferred volatile anesthetic because of its lack of pungency and airway irritant effect and the absence of cardiac sensitization to catecholamines.[4] Nitrous oxide may hasten the induction of anesthesia and decrease the necessary concentration of sevoflurane. Concerns regarding the propensity of nitrous oxide to increase PVR have not been substantiated in patients with CHD. Yet, the use of nitrous oxide decreases FIo_2, which may impair protection against increased PVR. When used during induction of anesthesia, nitrous oxide is often discontinued thereafter because of its property of expanding intravascular air bubbles.

Placement of a pulse oximetry probe is minimally distressing to an anxious, awake child and provides ample monitoring for the initial stages of an inhaled induction of anesthesia. Other noninvasive monitors may be placed in a timely fashion once a light plane of anesthesia has been achieved. Intravenous access is secured when anesthetic depth is adequate, at which time additional intravenous anesthetics, neuromuscular blocking drugs, and possibly anticholinergics may be given before laryngoscopy and tracheal intubation.

INTRAVENOUS INDUCTION OF ANESTHESIA

Patients with poorly controlled congestive heart failure, moderately impaired ventricular function, significant right-to-left shunting, or complete mixing lesions may benefit from the increased stability afforded by intravenous induction of anesthesia. Frequently, these patients come to the operating room from a critical care setting with intravenous access. Traditionally, intravenous opioids have been used in this setting because they produce little or no myocardial depression and also lack vasodilating properties in both the pulmonary and systemic vascular beds.[5] Other intravenous drugs that are used in patients with CHD include benzodiazepines, etomidate, and ketamine. Propofol can cause hypotension or increased right-to-left shunting in most of these patients. Ketamine preserves or augments sympathetic nervous system tone and, in so doing, maintains a high degree of circulatory stability. Concern regarding ketamine's propensity to increase PVR has not been substantiated in patients with CHD.[6] Ketamine may be administered intramuscularly to achieve stable induction of anesthesia and allow subsequent vascular cannulation to proceed in an anesthetized patient. Obviously, an unintentional injection of air should be avoided during the administration of all intravenous drugs because the presence of circulatory mixing or shunting in patients with CHD poses a real risk for paradoxical embolization.

AIRWAY MANAGEMENT

The size of the endotracheal tube should be individualized to age and size of the patient. Tracheal intubation is usually facilitated by the administration of a neuromuscular blocking drug (also see Chapter 12). The selection of the drug should depend on the patient (age, type of lesion, renal function) and the characteristics of the drug (duration of action, hemodynamic properties, and mode of elimination). Pancuronium has a long half-life and may be desirable in some patients for its vagolytic effect in offsetting bradycardia. Both vecuronium and rocuronium have an intermediate duration of action but rocuronium has a faster onset of action than vecuronium. Succinylcholine is also fast acting, has a very short half-life, but

may cause bradycardia, ventricular arrhythmias, and asystole in some children without pretreatment with atropine.

The approach to ventilatory management hinges upon how the circulatory system will be affected by changes in PVR in relationship to the SVR. The ventilation strategy should have minimal impact on blood flow across shunts or on tenuously balanced pulmonary-to-systemic flow ratios. The cardiac lesion must be understood in order to predict the effect of increasing or decreasing PVR. This understanding will help govern such parameters as fraction of inspired oxygen (F_{IO_2}), minute ventilation, use of positive end-expiratory pressure, and peak inspiratory airway pressure.

MONITORING (Also See Chapter 34)

Invasive monitoring is usually established after induction of anesthesia in most patients. Patients undergoing cardiac surgery generally require arterial line placement, as well as some form of central venous access. When selecting the site for arterial line placement, the underlying cardiac lesion should be considered. For example, in a patient who has a Blalock-Taussig shunt (diversion of the subclavian artery to the ipsilateral pulmonary artery), the arterial line should be placed contralaterally. Similarly, patients with coarctation of the aorta may have unreliable pressure measurement in the left upper extremity either because of the location of the coarctation or because of aortic cross-clamp placement at or near the left subclavian artery during surgery. The internal jugular vein is a common choice for central pressure monitoring and infusion of medications intraoperatively. Also, right atrial catheters can be placed intraoperatively by the surgeon before separation from bypass. Transesophageal echocardiography (TEE) has become an invaluable monitoring tool in the operating room to further delineate the anatomy not clearly demonstrated by preoperative transthoracic echocardiography (TTE), to rule out additional defects, and to assess the quality of the repair.

BLOOD PRODUCTS (Also See Chapter 24)

Many operations for CHD will require blood product administration, and the likelihood increases with smaller infants, lower preoperative hematocrit levels, repeat sternotomy incisions, and long cardiopulmonary bypass (CPB) times. Judgment and experience dictate how much and what type of blood products should be made available at the start of surgery, and many centers use standardized blood ordering schedules based on the surgical procedure and the child's age or weight. Generally, small infants are allocated the freshest blood (less than 5 days of storage) available because older blood may become significantly hyperkalemic and develop leftward shifting of the oxygen-hemoglobin dissociation curve. Blood should be administered with the use of appropriate filters and warming devices because small infants are particularly susceptible to intraoperative hypothermia

IV

and even to bradydysrhythmias from boluses of hypothermic blood products. Having blood products available in the operating room before the skin incision is appropriate in cases of repeat sternotomy inasmuch as these patients may be at risk for severe bleeding from unintentional injury to major cardiac structures.

ANTIFIBRINOLYTIC DRUGS

Antifibrinolytic drugs reduce blood loss and transfusion requirements during surgery for CHD. Aminocaproic acid and tranexamic acid are examples of commonly used drugs. Aprotinin may be more efficacious, but is rarely used because of being associated with increased morbidity and mortality rates.[7]

Maintenance of Anesthesia

Before CPB, anesthesia is maintained with a combination of intravenous opioids, volatile anesthetics (doses <1 minimum alveolar concentration [MAC]), and neuromuscular blocking drugs. Use of a small concentration of a volatile anesthetic minimizes the myocardial depressant effects of the drug while also decreasing the total dose of opioids that would otherwise be necessary to ensure adequate anesthetic depth. It is not unusual to administer large doses of opioids (fentanyl, 50 to 100 μg/kg IV, or sufentanil, 10 to 20 μg/kg IV) may be given over the course of an operation.[5] These opioids may be administered in divided doses (fentanyl, 0.5 to 10 μg/kg, or sufentanil, 1 to 2 μg/kg) according to judgment of anesthetic depth or in anticipation of noxious surgical stimuli. Alternatively, opioids may be delivered as a continuous intravenous infusion. Patients who are critically ill or have complex cardiac anomalies may benefit from high-dose opioid techniques so that the hypotensive and myocardial depressant effects of the volatile anesthetics may be avoided or minimized. In contrast, patients with good cardiac reserve who are undergoing procedures for simple defects (atrial septal defect, ventricular septal defect, patent ductus arteriosus, coarctation of the aorta) may benefit from limited opioid use (fentanyl <20 μg/kg) and more reliance on volatile anesthetics so that postoperative tracheal extubation is not delayed.[5] Nitrous oxide is commonly omitted from anesthesia because of concern for expansion of unintentional intravascular air emboli.

MONITORING CHANGES IN SHUNT RATIOS

The potential for significant changes in the circulatory system after anesthetic induction warrant early and possibly repeated measurement of arterial blood gases to allow early correction or refinement of pulmonary ventilation variables, as well as acid-base disorders, before the development of important circulatory derangements. In patients with shunts or mixing lesions, pulse oximetry also provides a continuous monitor of changes in the balance between pulmonary and systemic blood flow or changes in shunt direction or magnitude.

ANTICOAGULATION

Anticoagulation with unfractionated heparin (3 to 4 mg/kg) delivered intravenously is achieved before cannulation for CPB. The subsequent anticoagulation effect is assessed by measuring the activated clotting time (ACT). Target ACT values may vary with institutional preference, but 480 seconds is typical. Additional heparin is administered if target values are not initially obtained. Heparin concentration assays may also be used instead of or as a supplement to the ACT.

Cardiopulmonary Bypass

Most procedures for repair of congenital cardiac defects require use of CPB. As with adults, CPB for infants and children entails diversion of systemic venous return to the CPB machine and return of blood to the arterial system. Venous blood is drained passively (by gravity) through two venous cannulas, one for each vena cava. The cannulas converge through a Y-connector to a cardiotomy reservoir, which allows rapid administration of blood products, crystalloid and colloid solutions, medications, and blood suctioned from the field by the surgeon ("pump suction"). The cardiotomy reservoir also provides a temporary buffer in the event that venous return is temporarily interrupted. Blood is next conducted to a pump mechanism, which is generally a centrifugal pump. This pump is adjustable and permits delivery of a specified rate of blood flow to the patient. Generally, flow rates are adjusted to maintain an age-appropriate mean arterial pressure. Blood is then channeled through a membrane oxygenator, which equilibrates the blood with a supply of fresh gas; in this way, oxygen is added and carbon dioxide is removed. The perfusionist controls oxygenation and ventilation by adjusting the blend (FIO_2) and flow rate (sweep) of the fresh gas. Modern oxygenator circuits also allow rapid adjustment of blood temperature by running cooled or warmed water through a coil in contact with the blood path. Blood is then conducted back to the patient through tubing connected to a cannula positioned in the ascending aorta. An arterial filter is generally used downstream from the oxygenator to prevent microembolization of debris to the arterial tree.[8]

A still and bloodless heart is achieved by complete diversion of venous return to the CPB machine, subsequent aortic cross-clamping, and immediate administration of a cardioplegia solution. Because the act of aortic cross-clamping renders the heart ischemic, the cardioplegia solution has a dual purpose of providing both mechanical quiescence and myocardial protection. As with adults, these effects are achieved through the use of a cold (4° C) hyperkalemic crystalloid solution. Hypothermia and electromechanical arrest each contribute to minimizing myocardial oxygen requirements and lengthening the tolerable period of myocardial ischemia.

CALCULATION OF PHYSIOLOGIC VARIABLES

The perfusionist and the anesthesiologist should consider the patient's size in order to calculate the necessary flow rate to maintain metabolic function. Equally important is the patient's estimated blood volume because it determines the degree of hemodilution that will be realized when the patient's blood mixes with the obligatory "priming volume" of fluid that occupies the CPB machine's tubing, oxygenator, and cardiotomy reservoir at the onset of CPB. Whereas adult patients frequently have acceptable degrees of anemia as a result of this hemodilution, infants and small children require smaller, shorter tubing and lower-volume cardiotomy reservoirs to minimize this effect. Most infants require some blood product to be mixed with the circuit prime to preserve adequate oxygen-carrying capacity while on CPB. The amount of blood product required is a function of the patient's starting hematocrit, estimated blood volume, circuit prime volume, and the lowest acceptable limit of anemia (institutional and physician preferences vary but are commonly in the range of a hematocrit of 20% to 30%).

BODY TEMPERATURE DURING CARDIOPULMONARY BYPASS

Institutional, surgeon, or anesthesiologist preference also provides the perfusionist with a target patient temperature to be achieved while on CPB. Mild (30° C to 35.5° C) to moderate (25° C to 30° C) systemic hypothermia reduces metabolic oxygen requirements (7% per degree Celsius) and provides protective effects on both cerebral and myocardial tissue.[8] Hypothermia is usually achieved by active cooling of CPB blood with a heat exchange device incorporated in the membrane oxygenator. Active rewarming is initiated toward the end of CPB. Deleterious effects of post-CPB hypothermia may include myocardial ischemia, cardiac dysrhythmias, elevated PVR, coagulation failure, or renal dysfunction.

DEEP HYPOTHERMIC CIRCULATORY ARREST

Deep hypothermic circulatory arrest is used in situations in which adequate surgical repair is precluded by CPB cannula placement or by the requirement to repair the aorta at or near the arch.[9-11] Sufficiently cooled, patients may safely undergo periods of complete circulatory arrest to permit surgical repair in a bloodless field unencumbered by CPB cannulas. Cardiac cannulation and active cooling by CPB are required to lower core temperature to approximately 18° C. After surgical repair, CPB is reestablished, and the patient is rewarmed and reperfused.

TERMINATION OF CARDIOPULMONARY BYPASS

Successful termination of CPB requires close communication between the anesthesiologist, the cardiac surgeon, and the perfusionist. Rewarming is effected via the CPB machine and is initiated at the request of the surgeon at an appropriate point during the surgical procedure. Pulmonary ventilation is commenced when the surgeon no longer requires the lungs to be collapsed in the surgical field.

CARDIAC RHYTHM

Ventricular fibrillation can occur after removal of the aortic cross-clamp and reperfusion of the coronary arteries, especially when the hypothermia has not been fully corrected. It may revert spontaneously to a sinus rhythm but often requires electrical defibrillation. Acid-base or electrolyte disorders (hyperkalemia) may contribute to disturbances in cardiac rhythm. Relative bradycardia or atrioventricular node conduction failure can be corrected by means of temporary cardiac pacing. Many patients with good cardiac reserve who have endured relatively short periods (<1.5 hours) of aortic cross-clamping and the attendant myocardial ischemia may be able to separate from CPB without inotropic assistance. Many others will require infusion of inotropic drugs to achieve adequate cardiac output and systemic blood pressure. In particular, those with preexisting myocardial dysfunction, congestive heart failure, or hemodynamic instability are likely to require pharmacologic assistance for successful separation from CPB (Table 26-6).

VENTILATION AND PULMONARY VASCULAR RESISTANCE

The approach to PVR and ventilation of the patient's lungs must be carefully considered before separation from CPB. Patients with simple defects that have been repaired are no longer at risk for shunting and unbalanced Qp/Qs ratios. For this reason, such patients are typically ventilated with 100% FIO_2 at the time of separation from CPB, with minute ventilation targeted to avoid respiratory acidosis. Patients with long-standing excessive pulmonary blood flow may have underlying pulmonary hypertension and may be at risk for pulmonary hypertensive crisis at the time of separation from CPB. These patients may benefit from maneuvers that minimize PVR (see Table 26-2).

PRESENCE OF A RESIDUAL MIXING LESION

Difficulty arises when a palliative procedure has left the patient with a mixing lesion. This situation is exemplified by surgical treatment of hypoplastic left-sided heart syndrome (Norwood procedure) that results in a single ventricle supplying blood flow to both the pulmonary and systemic circulation (see Table 26-5). In such circumstances which circulation will be likely to receive most of the cardiac output must be anticipated and adjusted so that PVR and SVR tend to yield a balanced circulation. Pulse oximetry is an invaluable tool in this particular situation because a patient with a complete mixing lesion will tend to have systemic oxygen saturation near 80% when the systemic and pulmonary circulations are balanced. Systemic saturation greater than 85% to 90% indicates excessive pulmonary blood flow (possibly with resultant systemic hypoperfusion or hypotension), whereas saturation lower than 75% indicates inadequate pulmonary blood flow. The best possible milieu in the setting of the underlying defect must be provided in order to promote satisfactory cardiac output, adequate oxygenation, and a balanced circulation.

IV

Table 26-6 Common Vasoactive Drugs

Drug	Dose Range	Comments
Dopamine	3-20 µg/kg/min	Lower maximum effect than with epinephrine and norepinephrine Tachycardia
Epinephrine	0.02-0.1 µg/kg/min	Drug of choice when maximum inotropic effect is required Strong effect at the medium- to high-dose range Tachycardia
Norepinephrine	0.02-0.1 µg/kg/min	Strong alpha, beta effects, with activity at lower doses than with epinephrine
Milrinone	0.25-1 µg/kg/min	Can lower both PVR and SVR No tachycardia May need α-agonist to prevent hypotension Loading dose typically is 25-50 µg/kg
Dobutamine	1-20 µg/kg/min	Lower maximum effect than with epinephrine and norepinephrine May decrease SVR or BP because of peripheral β_2-vasodilation

BP, blood pressure; PVR, pulmonary vascular resistance; SVR, systemic vascular resistance

DIFFICULTY IN SEPARATION OF THE PATIENT FROM CARDIOPULMONARY BYPASS

Difficulty in separation from CPB may reflect multiple physiologic derangements but most often is due to inadequate pulmonary blood flow or inadequate systemic blood flow (Table 26-7). After separation from CPB, systemic arterial blood pressure, systemic oxygenation, and acid-base status must be closely monitored. Data derived from a central venous or pulmonary artery catheter may be helpful in diagnosing hemodynamic problems. Transesophageal echocardiography is useful in evaluating the surgical repair of CHD and cardiac function in the period after separation from CPB. In the event that pharmacologic support of cardiac contractility, vascular tone, and management of ventilation fails to achieve circulatory stability, patients may require resumption of CPB support. In some cases, a period of "rest" on CPB allows resolution of cross-clamp–related ischemic ventricular dysfunction, whereas in other situations, revision of the surgical repair may be indicated. If the patient cannot be separated from CPB despite surgical revision and maximal inotropic support, then extracorporeal life support may be instituted and continued until adequate cardiac and pulmonary function is regained.

REVERSAL OF HEPARIN

Reversal of heparin is achieved with protamine (approximately 1 mg/kg of active heparin) by means of slow infusion (over at least a 10-minute period) after concluding that a return to CPB will not be necessary. Like adults, pediatric patients are susceptible to important complications of protamine administration, including anaphylactic, anaphylactoid, hypotensive, or severe pulmonary hypertensive reactions.

COAGULOPATHY

Although return of the ACT to baseline indicates successful reversal of heparin, a residual increase of the ACT may indicate coagulation factor or platelet deficiency. Hypothermia and hypocalcemia may contribute to in vivo coagulopathy but will not be reflected in the ACT or other laboratory tests of coagulation. Early measurement of the platelet count, prothrombin time, and partial thromboplastin time will facilitate appropriate blood product therapy in the event that hemostasis is not achieved with protamine. Often, however, the degree of clinical coagulopathy necessitates empirical administration of platelets, fresh frozen plasma, or other factor preparations before the results of such investigations become available.

BLOOD COMPONENT AND INTRAVASCULAR VOLUME THERAPY (Also See Chapter 24)

Blood component and intravascular volume therapy must be administered very carefully to infants because their total intravascular volume is small in comparison to adults. Unless critically hypovolemic, blood product or volume therapy should proceed in aliquots of approximately 5 mL/kg to prevent excessive intravascular volume

Table 26-7 Causes of Difficulty in Separation from Cardiopulmonary Bypass

Inadequate pulmonary blood flow (associated with arterial hypoxemia)

Inadequate systemic blood flow (associated with hypotension and metabolic acidosis

Valvular dysfunction

Dynamic outflow obstruction (decreases in cardiac output related to hyperdynamic or hypovolemic states)

Decreased systemic vascular resistance (associated with long cardiopulmonary bypass times)

Cardiac rhythm disturbances

Hypovolemia

and possible ventricular dysfunction. Citrated blood products may cause important degrees of hypocalcemia, and calcium replacement may thus be necessary. Dilutional anemia can occur when administering platelet or plasma preparations. Fluid-warming devices prevent the delivery of cold fluid boluses to cardiac conduction tissue, as well as the development of systemic hypothermia.

ACTIVATED RECOMBINANT FACTOR VII

Recombinant activated factor VII (rFVIIa) is approved by the Food and Drug Administration (FDA) for use in the prevention and treatment of bleeding in patients with hemophilia A or B with inhibitors to factor VIII or IX, factor VII deficiency, or Glanzmann's thrombasthenia.[12] Its role in pediatric cardiac surgery has not been delineated, although its use is growing. Generally rFVIIa is recommended when conventional hemostatic therapy has failed to stop the bleeding after separation from bypass.[13] The dose is typically 90 to 120 µg/kg every 2 hours for excessive bleeding.

POSTOPERATIVE CARE (Also See Chapter 34)

Children undergoing surgery for CHD are managed in an intensive care setting, where continuous invasive monitoring is possible along with one-to-one nursing care. Mechanical ventilation of the patient's lungs is continued for variable intervals, depending on the type of surgery performed and the overall status of the patient. Sedation is maintained throughout the period of ongoing tracheal intubation. Critical care management entails the continuation of hemodynamic drug infusions and possibly electrical pacing of cardiac rhythm. Early postoperative management frequently involves correction of various electrolyte, glucose, and hematologic parameters. Mediastinal bleeding is assessed frequently. A high index of suspicion is always maintained for the possible requirement for revision of the surgical repair, and bedside echocardiography is frequently undertaken in the intensive care unit to clarify hemodynamic problems.

QUESTIONS OF THE DAY

1. What is a "mixing lesion"? What characteristics are similar to a right-to-left shunt?
2. What is Eisenmenger's syndrome? What congenital heart lesions are associated with its development?
3. In a patient receiving general anesthesia, what steps can be taken to reduce pulmonary vascular resistance?
4. What is the appropriate management for a hypercyanotic episode in a patient with tetralogy of Fallot?

ACKNOWLEDGMENT

The editors and publisher would like to thank Dr. James E. Baker for contributing a chapter on this topic to the prior edition of this work. It has served as the foundation of the current chapter.

IV

REFERENCES

1. Walker SG: Anesthesia for left-to-right shunt lesions. In Andropoulos DB, Stayer SA, Russell IA, editors: *Anesthesia for Congenital Heart Disease*, ed 2, West Sussex, 2010, Wiley-Blackwell, pp 373–397.
2. Mossad EB, Joglar J: Preoperative evaluation and preparation. In Andropoulous DB, Stayer SA, Russell IA, Mossad EB, editors: *Anesthesia for Congenital Heart Disease*, ed 2, West Sussex, 2010, Wiley-Blackwell, pp 223–243.
3. Fischer LG, Van Aken H, Burkle H: Management of pulmonary hypertension: Physiological and pharmacological considerations for anesthesiologists, *Anesth Analg* 96:1603–1616, 2003.
4. Russell IA, Miller Hance WC, Gregory G, et al: The safety and efficacy of sevoflurane anesthesia in infants and children with congenital heart disease, *Anesth Analg* 92(5):1152–1158, 2001.
5. Duncan HP, Cloote A, Weir PM, et al: Reducing stress responses in the pre-bypass phase of open heart surgery in infants and young children: A comparison of different fentanyl doses, *Br J Anaesth* 84:556–564, 2000.
6. Williams GD, Philip BM, Chu LF, et al: Ketamine does not increase pulmonary vascular resistance in children with pulmonary hypertension undergoing sevoflurane anesthesia and spontaneous ventilation, *Anesth Analg* 105:1578–1584, 2007.
7. Fergusson DA, Hebert PC, Mazer CD, et al: A Comparison of aprotinin and lysine analogues in high-risk cardiac surgery, *N Engl J Med* 358:2319–2331, 2008.
8. Vinas M: Extracorporeal circulation. In Kambam J, editor: *Cardiac Anesthesia for Infants and Children*, St Louis, 1994, Mosby-Year Book, pp 20–32.
9. Jonas RA: Deep hypothermic circulatory arrest: Current status and indications, *Semin Thorac Cardiovasc Surg Pediatr Card Surg Annu* 5:76–88, 2002.
10. Wypij D, Newburger JW, Rappaport LA, et al: The effect of duration of deep hypothermic circulatory arrest in infant heart surgery on late neurodevelopment: The Boston Circulatory Arrest Trial, *J Thorac Cardiovasc Surg* 126:1397–1403, 2003.
11. Hickey PR: Neurologic sequelae associated with deep hypothermic circulatory arrest, *Ann Thorac Surg* 65:S65–S69, 1998 discussion S69–S70, S74–S76.
12. Warren O, Mandal K, Hadjianastassiou V, et al: Recombinant activated factor VII in cardiac surgery: A systemic review, *Ann Thorac Surg* 83:707–714, 2007.
13. Warren OJ, Rogers PL, Watret AL, et al: Defining the role of recombinant activated factor VII in pediatric cardiac surgery: Where should we go from here? *Pediatr Crit Care Med* 10:572–582, 2009.

CHRONIC PULMONARY DISEASE

Luca M. Bigatello and Venkatesh Srinivasa

Chronic pulmonary disease (CPD) is an independent predictor of morbidity in patients undergoing thoracic and upper abdominal surgery.[1] In addition, CPD is present in nearly all patients undergoing lung resection surgery. Anesthesia for lung resection surgery presents unique challenges to the anesthesia provider both because of the increased operative risk due to CPD and because of the technical difficulty of providing adequate ventilation while surgery is being performed on the lung. Asthma and chronic obstructive pulmonary disease (COPD) constitute the two main forms of CPD.

ASTHMA

Asthma affects as many as 300 million people worldwide, and it is the most common chronic disease in children[2] (also see Chapter 34). Asthma is a disease defined by the presence of chronic inflammatory changes in the airways, airway hyperresponsiveness, and reversible expiratory airflow obstruction. Airway hyperresponsiveness may result in the development of bronchoconstriction in response to stimuli (allergens, exercise, and mechanical airway stimulation) that have little or no effect on normal airways. Airway hyperresponsiveness elicited during bronchoprovocation with methacholine and subsequent bronchodilation with albuterol help diagnose asthma.

Clinical Presentation

The classic symptoms associated with asthma are cough, shortness of breath, and wheezing. The intensity of these symptoms is variable, ranging from cough with or without sputum production to chest pain and tightness. Some asthmatic patients may experience symptoms exclusively with exertion ("exercise-induced asthma"), and this diagnosis is a consideration in the pediatric and young adult population. High-pitched, musical wheezes are characteristic of asthma, although they are not specific. The presence or absence of wheezing by physical examination is a poor predictor of the severity of airflow obstruction, which needs to be confirmed and quantified by spirometry. Pulmonary function studies demonstrate evidence of airflow obstruction, either by curvilinearity in the expiratory loop of the flow-volume curve for those with mild obstruction or by decreased forced expiratory volume in 1 second (FEV_1) in addition to curvilinearity (Fig. 27-1). Elimination of obstruction after the administration of a bronchodilator drug suggests a diagnosis of asthma. An increase in FEV_1 % predicted of more than 12% and an increase in FEV_1 of more than 0.2 L suggest acute bronchodilator responsiveness and variability in airflow obstruction. Patients with COPD do not demonstrate reversibility of airflow obstruction to the same degree as do those with asthma, a characteristic that can help distinguish these two causes of airflow obstruction.

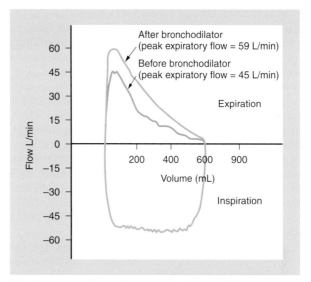

Figure 27-1 Flow-volume loop showing a response to bronchodilator administration. The expiratory segment of the loop (*top*) is concave due to expiratory flow limitation. Administration of an inhaled bronchodilator partially normalizes the shape of the curve. From MacIntyre NM, Branson RD. Mechanical Ventilation. Philadelphia, WB Saunders, 2001, p 17.

Treatment of Asthma and Bronchospasm

Pharmacologic therapy is based on the use of bronchodilator and anti-inflammatory drugs. Short-acting, inhaled β_2-adrenergic agonists and anticholinergics are potent bronchodilators that are used to treat acute symptoms for all stages of severity. Albuterol is the prototype short-acting β_2-agonist that produces rapid (in minutes) and dose-dependent bronchodilation. Its total dose during severe bronchospasm is limited by side effects—essentially tachycardia. Levo-albuterol causes less tachycardia, but it is not used routinely because of its increased cost. Ipratropium bromide is the prototype short-acting anticholinergic, which produces fairly rapid (within 10 to15 minutes) bronchodilation. Given its longer duration of action, ipratropium is used at longer intervals than albuterol, usually every 4 to 6 hours. Tachycardia is the most common side effect.

Long-acting β_2-adrenergic agonists (e.g., salmeterol and formoterol) and anticholinergics (e.g., thiotropium) are useful in the treatment of moderately persistent asthma (defined as the occurrence of daytime as well as nocturnal symptoms more than once weekly), but have little indication in the treatment of acute bronchospasm. These longer acting drugs can be replaced by the correspondent short-acting molecules in perioperative patients with respiratory complications.

IV

A very small dose of intravenous epinephrine (0.25 to 1 µg/min) is a potent bronchodilator that can be used as a second-line intervention, with appropriate monitoring and experienced supervision. Tachyarrhythmias are the most common complication, but they are of short duration as are the beneficial effects of epinephrine.

Leukotriene receptor antagonists and synthesis inhibitors (e.g., montelukast, zafirlukast, and zileuton) in adults, and cromolyn sodium in children, are effective maintenance drugs for chronic asthma. These drugs can be continued in the perioperative period, but have no indication in the treatment of acute bronchospasm. Methylxanthines, such as theophylline and aminophylline, are weak bronchodilators with significant proarrhythmic effects, and probably should not be used to treat an acute asthma attack nor of acute perioperative bronchospasm.

Corticosteroids (beclometasone, fluticasone) are extremely effective bronchodilators. Inhaled corticosteroids are effective in the chronic treatment of asthma, and intravenous corticosteroids can be part of the treatment of acute bronchospasm, recognizing that their onset of action is slow and early use enhances effectiveness.

All volatile anesthetics are potent bronchodilators[3] and have been used as a second-line treatment of *status asthmaticus*. They act through cathecholamine-independent mechanisms, and can be additive to ongoing therapy; their use, though, is based on anecdotal observation, and no guidelines on dosage and duration of therapy are available.

Anesthetic Considerations

An accurate preoperative evaluation of asthmatic patients includes knowing the pattern of use of bronchodilators, the frequency of emergency room visits, and the occurrence of hospitalization and tracheal intubation. Any signs of recent deterioration, such as increasing use of bronchodilators, worsening dyspnea, or a new respiratory infection, should prompt further evaluation with the specific question as to whether the current therapeutic regimen is adequate. Optimal treatment should be continued throughout the perioperative period.[4]

Patients with mild and well-controlled asthma can be safely anesthetized with any technique, as long as airway irritation is minimized. For example, general anesthesia through a laryngeal mask airway (LMA) is less stimulating to the airway than through an endotracheal tube.[5] If general anesthesia is chosen, additional inhaled bronchodilator therapy immediately prior to induction of anesthesia is effective in blunting the onset of bronchospasm. Regional anesthesia, when applicable, should always be considered in the severely asthmatic patient (see Chapter 18).

The goal during induction and maintenance of general anesthesia in patients with asthma is to depress airway reflexes and avoid bronchoconstriction in response to mechanical stimulation of the airway. A sufficient depth of anesthesia should be established before tracheal intubation. Propofol has a bronchodilator effect,[6] in contrast to thiopental (bronchospasm) or ketamine (increased secretions), which have essentially no indication in asthmatic patients. An inhaled induction of anesthesia with isoflurane or sevoflurane is a valid alternative, although the advent of propofol has decreased the use of this technique, particularly in adults. Desflurane is a volatile anesthetic which is not recommended because it increases secretions and irritation of the proximal airway.[7] Although intravenous lidocaine is often recommended to blunt airway reflexes during induction of anesthesia, its effectiveness has not been reliably documented.[8] All opiates blunt airway reflexes and can be helpful during the induction of general anesthesia. Muscle relaxants, often recommended during severe acute bronchospasm, do not affect smooth musculature, and their alleged utility is likely related to the facilitation of mechanical ventilation that occurs with relaxation of the skeletal musculature of the chest wall. Both opiates (morphine) and some muscle relaxants may cause bronchospasm through the release of histamine; safe choices include fentanyl, rocuronium and cisatracurium.

Intraoperatively, the need for a slow respiratory rate with sufficient time for exhalation limits the degree of expiratory flow obstruction. As this breathing pattern may result in hypercapnia, end-tidal CO_2 and possibly $PaCO_2$ are monitored, as the end-tidal to $PaCO_2$ difference may be significantly altered in asthma and COPD owing to increased dead space ventilation.

Upon emergence, extubation of the trachea can be considered during deep anesthesia, and ventilation continued by mask. This maneuver (deep extubation) is effective if performed in the appropriate patients (not in those at increased risk for aspiration of gastric content) and with the necessary airway management skills. Alternatively, tracheas can be extubated in traditional ways, paying close attention to avoid airway irritation as described earlier.

Intraoperative Bronchospasm

Airway instrumentation can cause severe reflex bronchoconstriction and bronchospasm in asthmatic patients with hyperactive airways. Acute bronchospasm usually presents with wheezing, increased peak inspiratory pressure or decreased tidal volume (depending on the mode of ventilation), and a typically slower phase III upslope of the capnogram.[9] However, occasionally severe bronchospasm can cause complete airway obstruction with no breath sounds heard and ventilation nearly impossible. While considering mechanical causes of obstruction such as a kinked endotracheal tube or a mucous plug (fiberoptic bronchoscopy may be useful for this purpose), anesthesia should be augmented with an intravenous anesthetic such as propofol. As ventilation becomes possible, inhaled anesthetics (see earlier) and inhaled bronchodilators become effective. Concomitant attention to the hemodynamics is due, as the massive alveolar hyperinflation as well as the increasing depth of anesthesia may result in severe hypotension. Severe intraoperative bronchospasm is a dreaded complication of anesthesia practice that has led to intraoperative deaths. Its immediate recognition and prompt summoning of help from other clinicians are of paramount importance.

CHRONIC OBSTRUCTIVE PULMONARY DISEASE

COPD is a progressive disease of the lungs due primarily to the toxic effects of cigarette smoking. COPD affects more than 200 million people, of which approximately 15 million are in the United States. Deaths from COPD are projected to increase significantly over the next decade if interventions to reduce risks (smoking) are not implemented.[10] In a highly simplified way, COPD is characterized by the progressive destruction of lung parenchyma, inflammation, and predisposition to infections. From a mechanical standpoint, the hallmark of COPD is the loss of elastic recoil of the lungs and the increase in airway resistance, which lead to expiratory flow limitation, lung hyperinflation, and the increased work of breathing. From the standpoint of gas exchange, a mismatch between ventilation and perfusion leads to hypoxemia, which is responsible for polycythemia, pulmonary hypertension, and eventually the need for supplemental oxygen. In addition, the mismatch of ventilation and perfusion, lung hyperinflation, and poor ventilatory mechanics lead to dead space ventilation, increased ventilatory burden, and eventually a decrease in alveolar ventilation and chronic hypercarbia. The chronic inflammation, blunting of the ciliary function, and unfavorable respiratory mechanics lead to recurrent episodes of lung infection, clinically known as COPD exacerbations.[11]

Clinical Presentation

COPD consists of two entities—emphysema and chronic bronchitis. Emphysema is characterized by loss of elastic recoil of the lungs, which results in alveolar hyperinflation and collapse of the airways during exhalation. Chronic bronchitis is characterized by the presence of cough and sputum production that recur for extended periods of time. In most COPD patients, these two entities overlap, and from a clinical standpoint the two conditions can be considered together as COPD (Table 27-1).

Treatment

COPD is a preventable and somewhat treatable disease. Smoking cessation is universally helpful because it reduces the carboxyhemoglobin blood level immediately and airway inflammation over a period of time. In addition to smoking cessation, pharmacologic therapy improves symptoms and may slow the progression of the disease. Pharmacologic treatment is aimed at improving airflow obstruction through the use of inhaled bronchodilators and anti-inflammatory drugs that have been described under the Asthma section. Methylxanthines are still occasionally used in the treatment of COPD, although their effectiveness is erratic and their side effects substantial. In chronically hypoxemic patients, oxygen inhalation at home improves dyspnea.

Acute Exacerbation of COPD

Acute exacerbations of COPD are characterized by acute worsening of dyspnea, increased sputum volume, and sputum purulence.[12] Acute exacerbations are common in the course of COPD and have an average mortality rate of 3% to 4% when requiring hospitalization and of 10% to 25% when requiring treatment in the intensive care unit (ICU). After an acute exacerbation, patients experience at least a temporary worsening in dyspnea and quality of life, and are expected to be readmitted to the hospital at least once over the next 6 months.[12] Treatment of an acute

IV

Table 27-1 NAEPP Guidelines for a Stepwise Approach in Asthma Management

Severity (before Treatment)	Symptoms and Spirometry	Medications to Maintain Control
Severe persistent	Continual daytime, frequent nighttime $FEV_1 \leq 60\%$ of predicted	High-dose inhaled corticosteroids PLUS long-acting inhaled β-agonist
Moderate persistent	Daily daytime, >1 night/week FEV_1 60%-80%	Low- to medium-dose inhaled corticosteroids plus long-acting inhaled β-agonist
Mild persistent	>2 days/week daytime, >2 nights/month $FEV_1 \geq$ 80%	Low-dose inhaled corticosteroids
Mild intermittent	≤2 days/week daytime, ≤2 nights/month $FEV_1 \geq$ 80%	No daily medication required

FEV_1, forced expiratory volume in 1 second.
Modified from National Asthma Education and Prevention Program. National Heart, Lung, and Blood Institute, 2002.

exacerbation is multifactorial, including bronchodilators, antibiotics, and a "steroid taper" starting at 60 mg of prednisone per day. If mechanical ventilatory support is considered, noninvasive positive pressure ventilation has become the first choice of treatment because it decreases the chance of tracheal intubation and the onset of pneumonia, and possibly improves survival.[13] The suspicion of an ongoing acute exacerbation in a patient with COPD scheduled to undergo elective surgery must be considered carefully, as it would place the patient at higher risk for perioperative respiratory complications.

Preoperative Evaluation (Also see Chapter 13)

Except for the case of lung resection surgery (see later discussion) the preoperative evaluation of COPD patients is largely based on clinical assessment. Most COPD patients with mild to moderate symptoms (e.g., GOLD stages 0 to III, see Table 27-1) should be able to proceed with their planned surgery without additional workup. However, patients with a more intense level of compromise (GOLD stages II to IV, see Table 27-1) and patients with acute exacerbations require additional consideration, possibly involving the evaluation by a pneumonologist. This evaluation focuses on the assessment of their functional status and the uncovering of untreated bronchospasm, worsening dyspnea, hypoxemia, and signs of a new respiratory infection. In these cases, therapy must be optimal, and surgery may have to be postponed.

Management of Anesthesia

The presence of COPD implies similar considerations as described for asthma, except that airway hyperresponsiveness is on the average less severe in COPD than in asthma. Airway manipulation is more forgiving in COPD, and the choice of regional over general anesthesia may be less frequently recommended than with asthma. Nonetheless, using an LMA results in a lesser increase of airway resistance than endotracheal intubation and should be considered. Placement of an epidural catheter to optimize perioperative analgesia is sensible for COPD patients undergoing thoracic and upper abdominal surgery. A balanced technique of an inhaled anesthetic and opioid is a common choice for anesthesia. Much debate has existed around the use of nitrous oxide (N_2O), although its use is both not strictly necessary and generally safe. One important cue when using N_2O is its ability to diffuse in closed spaces, thus potentially leading to the enlargement of an emphysematous bulla or a pneumothorax.

Intraoperative Ventilation

Similar considerations to those described for asthma apply to the delivery of mechanical ventilation to patients with COPD. A breathing pattern of normal tidal volume and a slow respiratory rate will minimize the development of air trapping. Mild hypercapnia secondary to hypoventilation is generally well tolerated in stable patients, but higher $PaCO_2$ levels will increase pulmonary artery pressure, which may be poorly tolerated in patients with a compromised right ventricular function. Bronchodilation and pulmonary toilet through blind suctioning or fiberoptic bronchoscopy are measures that can temporarily aid airflow and allow safe extubation of the trachea. Although most patients should have no reason to remain tracheally intubated at the end of the procedure, postoperative mechanical ventilation may be necessary in selected patients because of either the magnitude of the operation or the severity of their COPD. Prolongation of mechanical ventilation for the time necessary to optimize respiratory mechanics, the patient's wakefulness, and muscular strength should not be considered an ominous sign. Despite the frequent recommendation by consultant physicians to avoid postoperative endotracheal intubation of patients with severe COPD, there is really no physiologic reason as to why these patients cannot be safely extubated once the perioperative changes in respiratory function subside (within a few hours to a few days), unless the surgery itself reduces respiratory function permanently (e.g., lung resections, see later discussion) or a new cardiorespiratory event has occurred.

PULMONARY HYPERTENSION

Pulmonary hypertension is defined as an increase in mean pulmonary artery pressure (PAP) above 25 mm Hg at rest or 30 mm Hg with exercise. Most cases of pulmonary hypertension are secondary to cardiac or pulmonary disease. In a minority of cases, the etiology is unknown and the pulmonary hypertension is considered primary.[14] Pulmonary hypertension is relatively rare compared to asthma and COPD, but can be associated with significant perioperative morbidity.

Pathophysiology

In chronic pulmonary hypertension of various etiology, the increase in the afterload to the right side of the heart causes the right ventricle to progressively dilate, hypertrophy, and eventually lose in systolic function, which decrease the stroke volume and filling of the left ventricle. In addition, dilatation of the right ventricle causes bulging of the interventricular septum into the left ventricular cavity, further compromising its filling. The ultimate result is a decrease in cardiac output, reduced coronary perfusion, and the clinical signs of right ventricular failure, including peripheral edema, hepatomegaly, jugular veins distention, and eventually hypoxemia and dyspnea.[15]

Preoperative Evaluation (Also See Chapter 13)

Preoperative evaluation of patients with known pulmonary hypertension is aimed at identifying the severity of the disease and the adequacy of physiologic compensation. The gold standard for evaluating the degree of pulmonary hypertension, right-sided heart catheterization, also determines cardiac output and provides the opportunity to evaluate the response to vasodilators. In patients with previously diagnosed pulmonary hypertension, systolic pulmonary artery pressure can be estimated noninvasively by the echocardiogram. The echocardiogram also offers important information as to the status of the right ventricular function and left ventricular filling. In patients with moderate to severe pulmonary hypertension with signs of right ventricular failure, an expert cardiologic evaluation should advise whether treatment has been optimized preoperatively.

Management of Anesthesia

Intraoperative considerations for patients with pulmonary hypertension include maintaining adequate preload, minimizing tachycardia and dysrhythmias that may decrease cardiac output, and avoiding hypoxemia and hypercapnia, which can both cause acute increases in PAP. Monitoring with arterial and pulmonary artery lines should be considered in severe symptomatic patients who need to undergo major surgery. Acute increases in PAP may result in opening of the *foramen ovale* with consequent right-to-left shunt and severe hypoxemia. Under such circumstances, the shunt should be reversed first by correcting the underlying stimuli if possible (hypoxemia, hypercarbia, light anesthesia) and decreasing intrathoracic pressure, for example, by lowering the level of positive end-expiratory pressure (PEEP) whether applied or intrinsic (auto-PEEP). In addition, pharmacologic treatment is based on the use of vasodilators such as inhaled nitric oxide,[16] intravenous and inhaled prostacyclin (epoprostenol and iloprost),[17] calcium channel blockers, and phosphodiesterase inhibitors such as milrinone.

Postoperative Management

Morbidity and death in the postoperative period are significant concerns, with possible causes including pulmonary vasospasm, increases in pulmonary artery pressure, pulmonary thromboembolism, cardiac dysrhythmias, and heightened sympathetic nervous system tone. Large-volume intravascular fluid shifts, arterial hypoxemia, and hypovolemia should be avoided.

OBSTRUCTIVE SLEEP APNEA

Patients with obstructive sleep apnea (OSA) are at increased risk for postoperative complications. OSA is affecting 24% of men and 9% of women in the general population of the United States. Obesity is the most significant risk factor for the development of OSA and is an independent risk factor for the development of perioperative complications during weight loss surgery.[18] Patients with OSA have a high Mallampati score, have a low functional residual capacity, and may have an increased risk of oxygen desaturation during induction of anesthesia.[19] Co-morbid medical illnesses such as systemic hypertension, pulmonary hypertension, cardiovascular disease, and congestive heart failure are also more prevalent in patients with OSA than in the general population, a fact that contributes to their postoperative morbidity. Treatment of OSA by noninvasive ventilation results in better control of systemic hypertension.

Management of Anesthesia

Evaluation of the oral cavity in patients with OSA may not reveal the true nature of their pharyngeal space. Fat is deposited in the lateral pharyngeal walls and correlates with the severity of OSA. Neck circumference reflects pharyngeal fat deposition and correlates more strongly with the incidence and severity of OSA than general obesity does.

Relaxation of the upper airway musculature in response to benzodiazepines may significantly reduce the pharyngeal space and result in longer periods of hypopnea, arterial hypoxemia, and hypercapnia in patients with OSA than in the general population. Any medications that depress the central nervous system can cause airway obstruction because airway patency and skeletal muscle tone, maintained in the awake state, may be lost at the onset of sleep. In addition, opioid analgesics may decrease the central respiratory drive and thus further add to the possible complications of sedation.

Being prepared for difficult airway management is important and a plan should be charted before initiating direct laryngoscopy for tracheal intubation. Administration of oxygen is necessary before induction of anesthesia in obese patients with OSA because of their reduced functional residual capacity and risk for arterial hypoxemia. Tracheal extubation should be performed only when the patient is breathing spontaneously with adequate tidal volumes, oxygenation, and ventilation.

Postoperative Management (Also See Chapter 39)

Respiratory depression and apnea in the postoperative period can occur in patients with OSA, especially in the setting of opioid administration for pain control. In patients with OSA who hypoventilate (obesity-hypoventilation syndrome), documentation of preoperative analysis of arterial blood gases is necessary to establish the baseline set point for ventilation, an important factor when considering respiratory drive after extubation of the trachea.

IV

Relative hyperventilation intraoperatively to maintain a normal $PaCO_2$ in subjects who chronically hypoventilate may result in prolonged apnea when attempting tracheal extubation.

ANESTHESIA FOR LUNG RESECTION

The major challenges in anesthesia for thoracic surgery are establishing adequate separation of the lungs, maintaining gas exchange, and ensuring circulatory stability during one-lung ventilation. One-lung ventilation involves lung separation and deliberate ventilation of the dependent lung by isolating its bronchus from that of the nondependent lung (the operative site) with specially designed endotracheal tubes. In addition, thoracic surgery often involves thoracotomy incisions, which are associated with severe pain and potentially deleterious changes in cardiopulmonary physiology after surgery. Some of these physiologic changes can be minimized by thoracic epidural analgesia for effective postoperative pain management (see Chapter 40).

Preoperative Evaluation and Preparation

Patients undergoing thoracic surgery are at high risk for postoperative pulmonary complications, due to the predictable presence of CPD, the impact of a thoracotomy incision, and the possible removal of functional lung parenchyma. Risk factors associated with increased perioperative morbidity and mortality rates include the extent of lung resection (pneumonectomy > lobectomy > wedge resection), age older than 70 years, and inexperience of the operating surgeon.[20]

In patients with anatomically resectable lung cancer, pulmonary function testing, lung perfusion scanning, and exercise testing to measure maximum oxygen consumption may predict postoperative pulmonary function and outcome (Fig. 27-2). The preoperative physiologic assessment should include spirometry to measure the FEV_1. Depending on the number of segments of the lung that will be resected (Fig. 27-3), an estimate of the postoperative FEV_1 is obtained. A predicted postoperative FEV_1 (ppo FEV_1) = preoperative FEV_1% × (1 - % functional lung tissue removed/100) of less than 40% is associated with poor outcomes. In addition to spirometry, the diffusing capacity of the lung for carbon monoxide (DL_{CO}) should be measured in patients with diffuse parenchymal lung disease (by radiologic studies) or in patients with dyspnea out of proportion to their preoperative FEV_1. Similar to FEV_1, a DL_{CO} less than 40% predicted is associated with an increased risk for perioperative complications, including death, from a standard lung cancer resection.[21]

If postoperative FEV_1 or DL_{CO} is less than 40% as predicted by lung scan, an exercise study should be obtained. A significant decrease in oxygen consumption (<10 mL/kg/min) as measured by exercise testing predicts a postoperative mortality rate of 25% to 50% and should prompt discussion of alternatives to surgical resection.[21]

Smoking Cessation

Smoking increases airway irritability and secretions, decreases mucociliary transport, and increases the incidence of postoperative pulmonary complications. Cessation of smoking for 12 to 24 hours before surgery decreases the level of carboxyhemoglobin, and shifts the oxyhemoglobin dissociation curve to the right, thus increasing the oxygen available to tissues. In contrast to these short-term effects, improvement in mucociliary transport and small airway function and decreases in sputum production require prolonged abstinence (8 to 12 weeks) from smoking. The incidence of postoperative pulmonary complications decreases with abstinence from cigarette smoking for more than 8 weeks in patients undergoing coronary artery bypass surgery, and more than 4 weeks in patients undergoing pulmonary surgery.[22] Surgery can be a "teachable moment for smoking cessation."[23] Estimates derived from national surgical utilization data show that approximately 8% of people who quit smoking in the United States annually do so at the time of undergoing a surgical procedure. Major surgery doubled the likelihood of quitting.[23]

Management of Anesthesia

Anesthesia for thoracic surgery aims to provide adequate surgical conditions (one-lung ventilation), maintain stable hemodynamics and gas exchange, and provide rapid recovery after the surgery. A practical approach is to induce general anesthesia with intravenous propofol and maintain it with a volatile anesthetic supplemented with intravenous opioids, and fully control ventilation. Volatile anesthetics depress airway reflexes and do not seem to significantly inhibit regional hypoxic pulmonary vasoconstriction, thus aiding in maintaining an adequate PaO_2.[24] If N_2O is administered, the inhaled concentration is often limited to 50% until the adequacy of oxygenation can be confirmed by pulse oximetry or measurement of PaO_2. Nitrous oxide may exacerbate preexisting pulmonary hypertension and is therefore not appropriate for patients with increased PAP. In addition, N_2O is contraindicated in situations in which it has the potential to expand within a closed airspace, such as during closure of a thoracotomy after pneumonectomy when there is no thoracostomy drain. Nondepolarizing neuromuscular blocking drugs are needed to facilitate endotracheal intubation and mechanical ventilation. Ketamine or etomidate may be useful for induction of anesthesia in patients with hemodynamic instability.

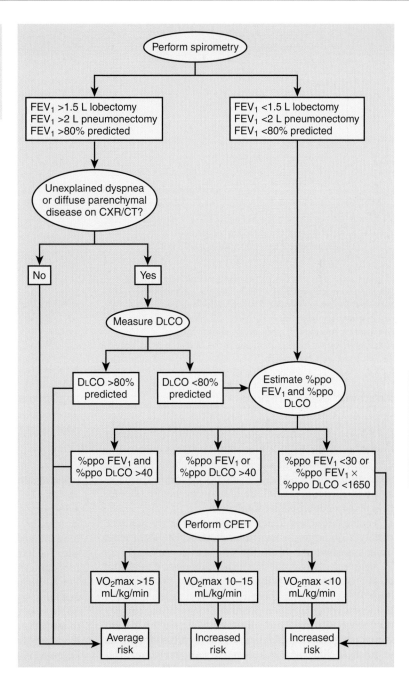

Figure 27-2 Preoperative physiologic assessment of surgical risk before lung resection. From Beckles MA, Spiro SG, Colice GL, Rudd RM. The physiologic evaluation of patients with lung cancer being considered for resectional surgery. Chest 2003;123:105S–114S.

For effective postoperative pain control (also see Chapter 40), a thoracic epidural catheter can be inserted preoperatively with the patient sedated but conscious. Intra-arterial and central venous catheters probably should be inserted for all patients undergoing lobectomy or pneumonectomy to facilitate monitoring hemodynamics and analysis of arterial blood gases. To avoid risk of acute lung injury,[25] intravenous fluids should be given in limited amounts in patients undergoing lung resection, in particular pneumonectomy.

Isolation of the Lungs

Delivering ventilation selectively to one lung is perhaps the most important anesthetic procedure in patients undergoing thoracic surgery. Separation of the lungs permits intraoperative one-lung ventilation, which greatly facilitates the surgical procedure. Double-lumen (endobronchial) tubes (DLTs) and bronchial blockers (BBs) with single-lumen endotracheal tubes enable anatomic isolation of the lungs and facilitate lung separation.

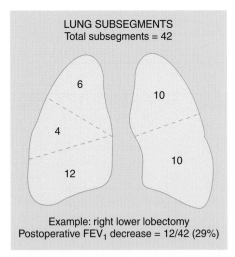

LUNG SUBSEGMENTS
Total subsegments = 42

6

10

4

10

12

Example: right lower lobectomy
Postoperative FEV₁ decrease = 12/42 (29%)

Figure 27-3 The number of segments of the lung that it is planned to resect are used to calculate the postoperative FEV_1 (see text). From Slinger PD, Johnston MR. Preoperative assessment for lung cancer surgery. In Slinger PD (ed). Progress in Thoracic Anesthesia, a Society of Cardiovascular Anesthesiologists Monograph. Lippincott, Williams & Wilkins, 2004, used with permission.

Anatomic Considerations

The tracheobronchial anatomy should first be assessed by reviewing preoperative radiologic studies. In addition, bronchoscopy is helpful immediately before surgery for detecting abnormal anatomy that may complicate lung separation. For example, a markedly distorted carina or a proximal endobronchial tumor may necessitate fiberoptic-guided endobronchial intubation.

Tracheobronchial dimensions in general are approximately 20% larger in men than women. The right main bronchus diverges from the trachea at an angle of 25 degrees, whereas the left main bronchus diverges at 45 degrees. The right main bronchus is shorter but wider (Fig. 27-4). Although there is variation in tracheal and bronchial width in the population, a significant correlation between tracheal and bronchial width occurs in individual patients (bronchial diameter is predicted to be 0.68 of tracheal diameter). Based on these dimensional relationships, a left-sided DLT is preferred because uniform ventilation to all lobes will most likely be achieved. Measurement of tracheal width from a posteroanterior chest roentgenogram can help select the size of a left-sided DLT.[26]

Left-Sided Double-Lumen Tube

Placement of a left-sided DLT is the most reliable and widely used approach for endobronchial intubation in one-lung ventilation (Fig. 27-5). Several manufacturers produce clear polyvinyl chloride tubes with high-volume,

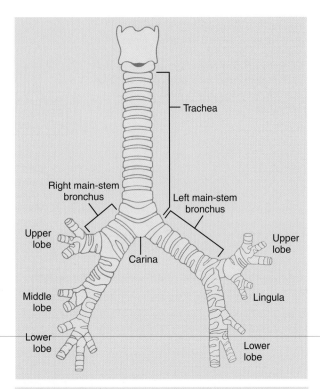

Trachea

Right main-stem bronchus

Left main-stem bronchus

Upper lobe

Carina

Upper lobe

Middle lobe

Lingula

Lower lobe

Lower lobe

Figure 27-4 Tracheobronchial anatomy. Right main stem bronchus: length, 1.8 ± 0.8 cm; width, 1.6 ± 0.2 cm. Left main stem bronchus: length, 4.8 ± 0.8 cm; width, 1.3 ± 0.2 cm.

low-pressure tracheal and bronchial cuffs. In general, a 35- or 37-French tube can be used for most women and a 39-French tube for most men. Endobronchial intubation is usually accomplished by direct laryngoscopy after induction of general anesthesia and neuromuscular blockade. The left-sided DLT tube is held so that the distal curve faces anteriorly while the proximal lumen is to the right. The bronchial cuff is inserted through the vocal cords, and the stylet is removed. Next, the tube is rotated 90 degrees to the left, thus directing the bronchial lumen to the left main stem bronchus. The tube is advanced until moderate resistance to further passage is encountered. Force should never be used during advancement of the tube; resistance usually indicates impingement within the airway, both proximally and in main stem bronchus. An estimate of the appropriate depth of placement of the DLT can be based on the patient's height. The average depth of insertion referenced to the corner of the mouth is 29 cm for patients 170 cm tall, and for each 10-cm increase or decrease in height, the average depth of placement correspondingly changes by 1 cm. Correct DLT position must be confirmed by fiberoptic bronchoscopy (Fig. 27-6). Dependence on physical examination to confirm proper position of a left-sided DLT is not reliable, with fiberoptic assessment showing malpositioning in

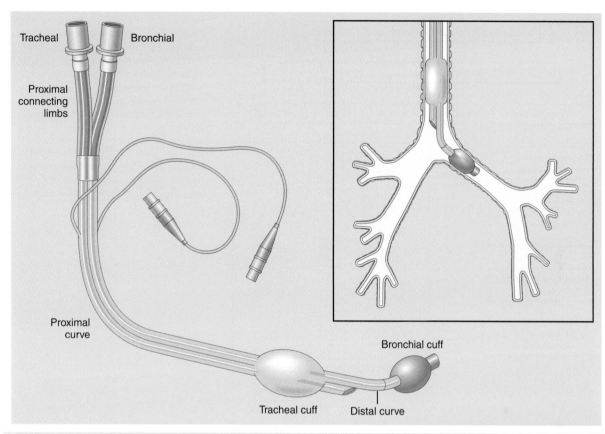

Figure 27-5 Left-sided double-lumen endobronchial tube.

20% to 48% of placements considered to be appropriate on the basis of auscultation.[27] If clamping of the left main stem bronchus is necessary intraoperatively, the DLT is withdrawn under fiberoptic guidance to just above the carina, and ventilation of the right lung is then continued through the bronchial lumen. This approach may be used effectively for lung separation during left pneumonectomy.

Fiberoptic Visualization of a Left-Sided Double-Lumen Tube

A 3.6-mm fiberoptic bronchoscope (pediatric broncho-scope) is initially passed through the tracheal lumen. Correct position of the DLT is confirmed by visualization of the carina, a nonobstructed view of the right main stem bronchus, and a view of the tube entering the left main stem, with the blue bronchial cuff below the carina (Fig. 27-7A). In addition, the line encircling the bronchial lumen tube should be visualized. This line is 4 cm from the distal lumen, and it should ideally be positioned at or slightly above the carina. Fiberoptic visualization through the bronchial lumen will reveal the bronchial carina and the left lower and upper lobes (Fig. 27-7B).

Malposition of a left-sided DLT may occur during initial placement, after surgical positioning, or during surgery. A malpositioned tube is usually detected by clinical signs and changes in lung mechanics. Two algorithms that define three types of malpositioned left-sided DLTs are shown in Figure 27-8A and B.

Right-Sided Double-Lumen Tube

The short and variable distance of the right upper lobe ori-fice from the carina makes the use of a right-sided DLT prob-lematic for most procedures requiring lung separation. A small change in the position of the tube may result in inadequate lung separation, collapse of the right upper lobe, or both. Nevertheless, in some situations (e.g., obstruction by tumor, disruption after trauma, or distortion secondary to a thoracic aortic aneurysm) it is best to avoid intubation of the left main stem bronchus. Right-sided DLTs are designed to incorporate a separate opening in the bronchial lumen to allow ventilation of the right upper lobe (Fig. 27-9). Confirmation of correct right-sided DLT position by physical examination alone results in a 90% chance of malposition, with most being too deep. Proper positioning of a right-sided DLT must include fiberoptic guidance.[28]

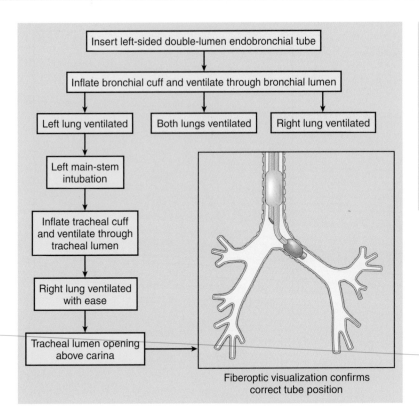

Insert left-sided double-lumen endobronchial tube

↓

Inflate bronchial cuff and ventilate through bronchial lumen

Left lung ventilated

Both lungs ventilated

Right lung ventilated

↓

Left main-stem intubation

↓

Inflate tracheal cuff and ventilate through tracheal lumen

↓

Right lung ventilated with ease

↓

Tracheal lumen opening above carina

Fiberoptic visualization confirms correct tube position

Figure 27-6 Algorithm for determining the position for a left-sided double-lumen tube: a series of cuff inflations and hand-bag breaths is performed. The sequence starts by inflating the bronchial cuff slowly, with 1 to 3 mL of air. Initial ventilation through the bronchial lumen should produce left-lung ventilation. A malpositioned tube could result in either the right lung only or both lungs being ventilated. Next, the tracheal cuff is inflated. Ventilation through the tracheal lumen should produce only right-lung ventilation, indicating that the tracheal lumen is above the carina.

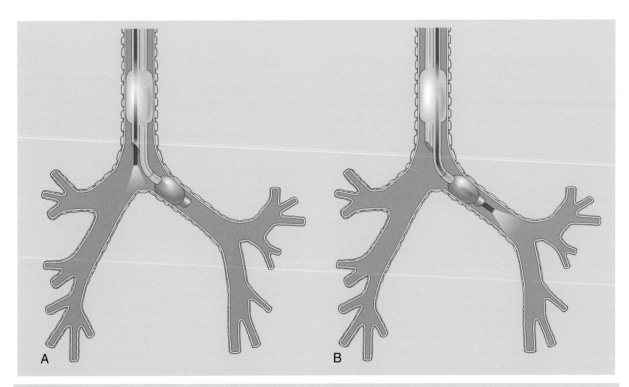

A B

Figure 27-7 Fiberoptic visualization confirming correct position of a left-sided double-lumen tube.

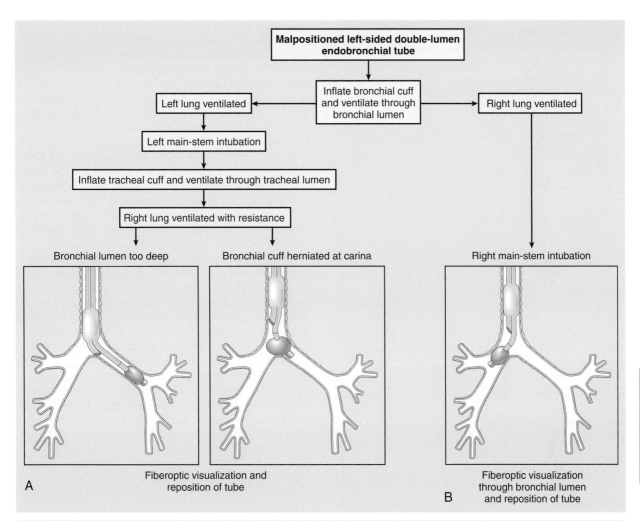

Figure 27-8 Malpositioned left-sided double-lumen tube (DLT). **A,** Ventilation through the bronchial lumen results in left-lung ventilation, but ventilation through the tracheal lumen has an abnormally elevated resistance. Fiberoptic visualization through the tracheal lumen identifies either a bronchial lumen that is too deep in the left main stem bronchus (*left panel*) or a bronchial cuff that has herniated over the carina (*right panel*). Repositioning is accomplished with fiberoptic guidance. **B,** The left-sided DLT is accidentally inserted into the right main stem bronchus. Ventilation through the bronchial lumen results in right-lung ventilation. Correction is accomplished by advancing the fiberscope through the bronchial lumen and identifying the bronchus intermedius. With both cuffs deflated, the DLT and fiberscope are withdrawn simultaneously until the carina comes into view. Next, the fiberscope is advanced into the left main bronchus till 1 cm above the bronchial carina. The tube is advanced until the rim of the bronchial lumen comes into view. The fiberscope is then inserted into the tracheal lumen, confirming correct tube position.

Bronchial Blockers

Lung separation can also be achieved with a single-lumen endotracheal tube and fiberoptically guided placement of a BB.[29] The BB technique can be useful if postoperative ventilation will be required because it eliminates the need to exchange the DLT for a single-lumen tube. Using a BB is especially helpful when managing a difficult airway. For example, in patients requiring an awake, fiberoptic intubation where DLT placement may be impossible, use of a BB may be the only practical approach to lung separation. Several BB systems are available; we will briefly describe three of the most common.

The Univent BB tube has two compartments: a main lumen for conventional air passage, and a small lumen embedded in the anterior wall of the endotracheal tube that permits passage of the movable BB (Fig. 27-10). The BB is a relatively stiff catheter that has an internal channel measuring 2 mm through which oxygen may be insufflated. After tracheal intubation with the BB retracted, initial positioning

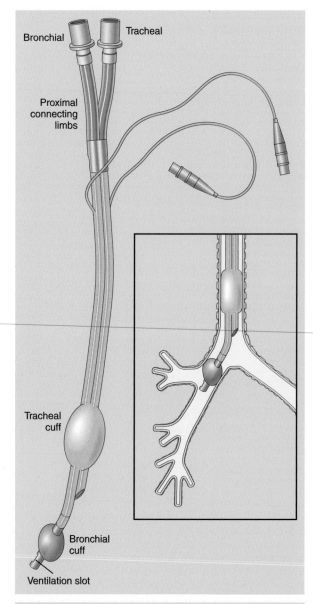

Bronchial

Tracheal

Proximal
connecting
limbs

Tracheal
cuff

Bronchial
cuff

Ventilation slot

Figure 27-9 Right-sided double-lumen endobronchial tube.

The Arndt endobronchial blocker consists of a 9-French, double-lumen, wire-guided endobronchial catheter and a multiairway adapter that allows independent passage of the BB and fiberscope (Fig 27-12).[29] The BB and a pediatric fiberscope are placed through a conventional endotracheal tube (8.0 mm internal diameter). The BB is coupled to the bronchoscope through the guide loop (protruding at the distal end of the catheter), and the bronchoscope is advanced into the desired main stem bronchus. The BB is advanced while steadying the bronchoscope until the guide loop is seen to exit at the end of it. The bronchoscope is then retracted, and endobronchial placement of the BB is confirmed. After final positioning of the patient, endobronchial blockade is visualized by inflating the 3-cm-long elliptical cuff with approximately 6 mL of air, and the guide loop is removed.

The Cohen tip deflecting endobronchial blocker is introduced into a single-lumen endotracheal tube previously inserted. To establish single-lung ventilation, the flexible tip of the bronchial blocker is directed into the desired bronchus (left or right) by using the control wheel on the proximal end of the blocker. The whole maneuver is done under bronchoscopic guidance.[30]

Arndt and Cohen BBs are relatively new. Although experience with these BBs is still limited, they provide equivalent surgical exposure to left-sided DLTs during left-sided open or video-assisted thoracoscopic surgery. However, BBs required longer time to position and more frequent intraoperative manipulation (Fig. 27-13).[31]

GAS EXCHANGE DURING ONE-LUNG VENTILATION

The intrapulmonary distribution of blood flow is regulated by gravity, lung volume, and regional vascular resistance. As a result, in the lateral decubitus position, the dependent lung receives a greater proportion of the cardiac output (about 60%). During thoracotomy and mechanical ventilation, the proportion of tidal ventilation to the operated (nondependent) lung increases once the chest is opened because lung and chest wall compliance increase. In contrast, the dependent hemithorax has lower compliance and low ventilation per unit lung volume because of the weight of the nondependent hemithorax, the mediastinum, and the abdominal contents, which is no longer offset by the subatmospheric pressure in the nondependent hemithorax. These factors promote atelectasis in the dependent lung. Thus, the nondependent lung is well ventilated but poorly perfused (high ventilation-to-perfusion [$\dot{V}/\dot{Q}$] ratio), and the dependent lung is well perfused but poorly ventilated (low $\dot{V}/\dot{Q}$ ratio). These $\dot{V}/\dot{Q}$ imbalances lead to altered pulmonary gas exchange.

Once the nondependent lung is isolated and no longer ventilated (one-lung ventilation), an iatrogenic

is accomplished by the tube rotation method. Rotating the tube to the right or left positions the BB so that it may be advanced into the corresponding main stem bronchus. Fiberoptic visualization should be used to confirm appropriate main stem intubation and to guide the depth of insertion. For right-sided placement, the BB should be positioned so that inflation of the cuff will cause partial herniation into the right upper lobe (Fig. 27-11A). For left-sided placement, the BB should be inserted deep into the main stem bronchus to minimize dislodgment into the trachea with surgical manipulation (Fig. 27-11B).

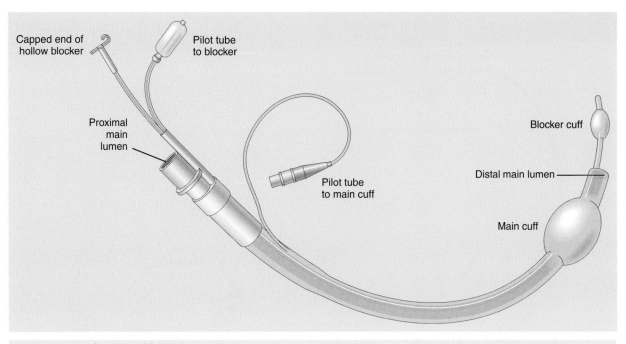

Figure 27-10 Univent bronchial blocker system.

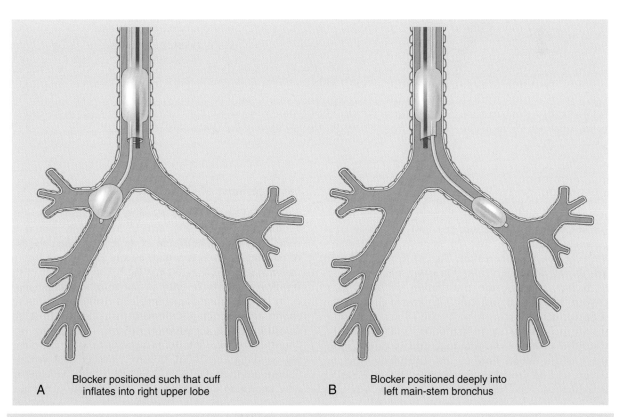

A   Blocker positioned such that cuff inflates into right upper lobe

B   Blocker positioned deeply into left main-stem bronchus

Figure 27-11 Positioning of the Univent bronchial blocker (see text).

IV

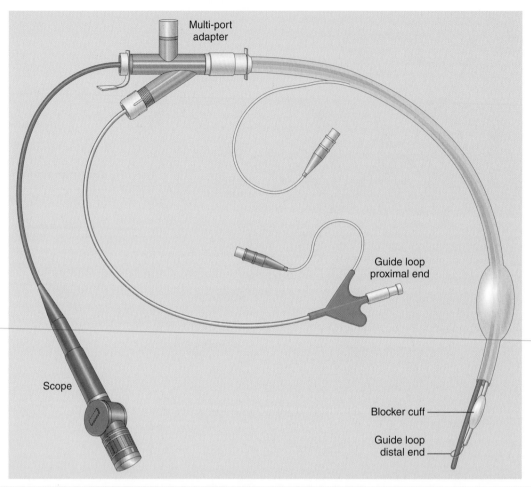

Figure 27-12 Arndt bronchial blocker. The Arndt endobronchial blocker and a pediatric bronchoscope are connected through a multiport airway adapter. The blocker is coupled to the bronchoscope through the guide loop at the distal end of the blocker. The bronchoscope and blocker are then advanced together into the main bronchus of the lung to be blocked.

right-to-left intrapulmonary shunt is introduced, due to the continued perfusion of both lungs. After the initiation of one-lung ventilation, the PaO$_2$ decreases progressively during the first 20 minutes, and remains relatively constant thereafter. The wide variability in PaO$_2$ during one-lung ventilation is the result of multiple factors affecting the distribution of blood flow between the lungs. Blood flow is decreased through the collapsed, nondependent lung by the effects of gravity, hypoxic pulmonary vasoconstriction, and potentially, by surgical compression. Although gravity directs more than half the blood flow to the dependent lung, an increase in PAP from the underlying COPD (see earlier discussion) and the new formation of atelectasis may limit blood flow diversion from the collapsed, nondependent lung.

Management of One-Lung Ventilation

An FiO$_2$ of nearly 1.0 is recommended during one-lung ventilation; nevertheless, arterial hypoxemia cannot be completely prevented (Table 27-2). In approximately 25% of patients, PaO$_2$ is less than 80 mm Hg, and in 10% of patients, it is less than 60 mm Hg.[32] The use of air in the inspired gas mixture prior to one-lung ventilation may delay lung deflation during one-lung ventilation due to the slower reabsorption of nitrogen than oxygen from the alveoli that have not passively deflated.[33] Ventilating with large tidal volumes (8 to 10 mL/kg) used to be the norm during one-lung ventilation. However, smaller tidal volumes (lung-protective ventilation, 5 to 7 mL/kg tidal volume) are now known to be beneficial in patients with acute lung injury/acute respiratory distress syndrome.[34] Ventilation with small tidal volumes improves postoperative respiratory

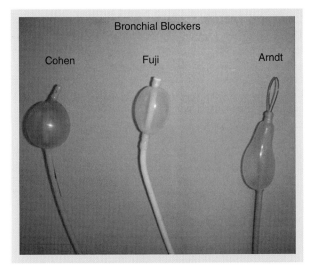

Bronchial Blockers

Cohen   Fuji   Arndt

Figure 27-13 The three types of bronchial blockers. The 9 French Cohen tip-deflecting endobronchial blocker (Cook Critical Care, Bloomington, IN) allows the establishment of single-lung ventilation by directing its flexible tip left or right into the desired bronchus using a control wheel device on the proximal end of the blocker, in combination with fiberoptic bronchoscope guidance. The wire-guided endobronchial blocker (Arndt blocker, Cook Critical Care) contains a wire loop in the inner lumen; when used as a snare with a fiberoptic bronchoscope, it allows directed placement. The snare is then removed and a 1.4-mm lumen may be used as a suction channel or for oxygen insufflation. The 9 French Fuji Uni-blocker, (Fuji Corp., Tokyo, Japan) has a fixed distal curve, which allows it to be rotated for manipulation into position with fiberoptic guidance. It is also available in a 5 Fr size. Unlike its predecessor, the Univent, the Uni-blocker is used with a standard endotracheal tube. From Narayanaswamy M, McRae K, Slinger P, et al. Choosing a lung isolation device for thoracic surgery: A randomized trial of three bronchial blockers versus double-lumen tubes. Anesth Analg 2009;108:1097-1101.

Table 27-2 Approach to Management of One-Lung Ventilation

- Deliver an FiO_2 close to 1.0.
- Adjust respiratory frequency to maintain a minute ventilation close to the level of two-lung ventilation, allowing for slight increases in $PaCO_2$.
- Follow continuous pulse oximetry, and measure arterial blood gas tensions after 15-20 minutes of one-lung ventilation and thereafter as indicated.
- Response to hypoxemia (in sequence):
  - Reconfirm proper position of the double-lumen tube by fiberoptic bronchoscopy.
  - Apply a sustained inflation to the dependent lung, and titrate 5-10 cm H_2O PEEP to the dependent lung.
  - Partially reinflate the nondependent lung and insufflate oxygen with CPAP of 5-10 cm H_2O.
  - Ask the surgeon to transiently occlude the pulmonary artery feeding the nondependent lung.
  - If hypoxemia is still uncorrected, resume two-lung ventilation.

CPAP, continuous positive airway pressure; PEEP, positive end-expiratory pressure.

IV

outcomes in patients undergoing lung resection for cancer, as evidenced by significantly reduced incidences of acute lung injury and atelectasis along with reduced utilization of intensive care unit resources (also see Chapter 41).[35]

Patients who are at particular risk of developing hypoxemia during one-lung ventilation include those with a low PaO_2 prior to lung isolation, those with a high percentage of ventilation or perfusion to the operative lung on preoperative scan, and, somewhat counterintuitively, those with preserved spirometric indices.[36] The latter phenomenon is likely due to the fact that lungs with normal expiratory recoil (i.e., normal FEV_1, no COPD or asthma) will collapse fully upon opening the respective lumen of the tracheal tube to air. In contrast, lungs with COPD or asthma have lost much of their elastic recoil and will tend to remain somewhat inflated for longer periods of time, thus allowing the residual alveolar oxygen to be absorbed. If hypoxemia develops during one-lung ventilation (see Table 27-2), proper positioning of the DLT should first be confirmed with the fiberoptic scope because dislodgment of the tube is not uncommon after positioning of the patient for surgery and again after surgical manipulation. The most effective approach to improve oxygenation is the application of 5 to 10 cm H_2O continuous positive airway pressure (CPAP) to the nondependent lung.[37] This level of CPAP results in minimal lung inflation and generally does not interfere with surgery. A slow inflation of 2 L/min of oxygen into the nonventilated lung for 2 seconds and repeated every 10 seconds for 5 minutes or until the saturation rises to 98%, has been shown to improve oxygenation during one-lung ventilation.[38] However, CPAP to the nondependent lung may interfere with the surgical dissection, and attempts to recruit lung parenchyma in the dependent lung may be tried first. Because atelectasis in the dependent lung can occur, a sustained lung inflation of 30 to 40 cm H_2O for 15 to 30 seconds may increase PaO_2.[39] Application of PEEP following manual recruitment generally prolongs its effect. Hemodynamic effects from the application of sustained inflations or PEEP can be significant as the increased intrathoracic pressure can significantly impede venous return and decrease cardiac output and arterial blood pressure.

CONCLUSION OF SURGERY

Reexpansion of the lungs is an important maneuver at the conclusion of thoracic surgery to prevent persistent atelectasis. Furthermore, chest tubes are placed to drain fluid and air and to promote continued expansion of the lung. Chest tubes should be set to continuous suction and must not be allowed to kink because sudden increases in intrathoracic pressure, as with coughing, may increase the air leak and cause tension pneumothorax if air cannot escape. Placement of chest tubes is not necessary after pneumonectomy. Instead, intrapleural pressure on the operated side is adjusted by aspirating air to slightly below atmospheric pressure. Excessive negative pressure can cause hypotension by shifting the mediastinum and compromising cardiac output.

Patients should be tracheally extubated at the conclusion of the surgery, to minimize the complications associated with mechanical ventilation (barotrauma, ventilator-associated pneumonia). If mechanical ventilation of the lungs must be continued into the postoperative period, it will be necessary to replace the DLT with a single-lumen tube.

POSTOPERATIVE PULMONARY COMPLICATIONS

Postoperative pulmonary complications after thoracic surgery include atelectasis, hypoxemia, and hypoventilation, sometimes requiring the institution of mechanical ventilation and leading to the development of pneumonia and acute lung injury.[40] The severity of these complications may be related to intraoperative problems (surgical trauma, aspiration of infected secretions around the endotracheal tube), the severity of preexisting lung disease, or postoperative inability to mobilize secretions and effectively expand the operative lung. A most effective way to prevent this sequence of events seems to be to promote early mobilization, which reestablishes physiologic lung volumes and gas exchange. Early mobilization is probably superior to traditional chest physical therapy and incentive spirometry. In patients who are developing severe impairment of gas exchange, application of noninvasive positive-pressure ventilation for limited periods of time may avoid tracheal intubation and prolonged mechanical ventilation.[41]

Pain Management (Also See Chapter 40)

Thoracic epidural analgesia provides effective postoperative pain relief, improved pulmonary function, and prompt mobility. Thoracic epidural analgesia was associated with lower mortality rate (OR [odds ratio] = 0.4; CI [confidence interval] 0.2 to 0.8) and fewer respiratory complications (OR = 0.6; CI 0.3 to 0.9).[42]

MEDIASTINOSCOPY

Mediastinoscopy is often performed before thoracotomy to establish the diagnosis or resectability of lung carcinoma. Although generally a low-morbidity procedure, vigilance needs to be paid because of the occasional occurrence of hemorrhage and pneumothorax. Given the small surgical incision, and limited access to the operative field, bleeding can be difficult to control and can rapidly become serious. Hence, central venous access is prudent.

QUESTIONS OF THE DAY

1. What are the potential manifestations of acute bronchospasm in the patient receiving general anesthesia? What is the initial management?
2. What are the goals of preoperative assessment in a patient with known pulmonary hypertension?
3. What are the physiologic benefits of smoking cessation after 24 hours of abstinence and 12 weeks of abstinence?
4. What are the three major malpositions of a left-sided double-lumen endotracheal tube?
5. Which patients are at greatest risk of developing hypoxemia during one-lung ventilation?

ACKNOWLEDGMENT

The editors and publisher would like to thank Drs. Anh Innes, Jeanine Wiener-Kronish, and Jeffrey Katz for contributing a chapter on this topic to the prior edition of this work. It has served as the foundation for the current chapter.

REFERENCES

1. Smetana GW: A 68 year-old man with COPD contemplating colon surgery, *JAMA* 297:2121–2130, 2007.
2. The Global Initiative for Asthma: http://www.ginasthma.com/.
3. Rooke GA, Choi JH, Bishop MJ: The effect of isoflurane, halothane, sevoflurane and thiopental/nitrous oxide on respiratory system resistance after tracheal intubation, *Anesthesiology* 86:1294–1299, 1997.
4. Burburan SM, Xisto DG, Rocco PR: Anaesthetic management in asthma, *Minerva Anestesiol* 73:357–365, 2007.
5. Tanaka A, Isono S, Ishikawa T, et al: Laryngeal resistance before and after minor surgery, *Anesthesiology* 99:252–258, 2003.
6. Eames WO, Rooke GA, Wu RS, et al: Comparison of the effects of etomidate, propofol, and thiopental on

respiratory resistance after tracheal intubation, *Anesthesiology* 84:1306–1311, 1996.

7. Goff MJ, Arain SR, Ficke DJ, et al: Absence of bronchodilation during desflurane anesthesia: A comparison to sevoflurane and thiopental, *Anesthesiology* 93:404–408, 2000.

8. Maslow AD, Regan MM, Israel E, et al: Inhaled albuterol, but not intravenous lidocaine, protects against intubation-induced bronchoconstriction in asthma, *Anesthesiology* 93:1198–1204, 2000.

9. Hess D, Crimi E: Respiratory monitoring. In Bigatello LM, editor: *Critical Care Handbook of the Massachusetts General Hospital*, Philadelphia, 2010, Lippincott Williams & Wilkins.

10. The Global Initiative for Chronic Obstructive Lung Disease: http://www.goldcopd.com/.

11. Sutherland ER, Cherniack RM: Management of chronic obstructive pulmonary disease, *N Engl J Med* 350:2689–2697, 2004.

12. Celli BR, Barnes PJ: Exacerbations of chronic obstructive pulmonary disease, *Eur Respir J* 29:1224–1238, 2007.

13. Mehta S, Hill NS: Noninvasive ventilation, *Am J Respir Crit Care Med* 163:540–577, 2001.

14. World Symposium on Primary Pulmonary Hypertension: Evian. France, 1998, World Health Organization.

15. Blaise G, Langleben D, Hubert B: Pulmonary arterial hypertension. Pathophysiology and anesthetic approach, *Anesthesiology* 99:1415–1432, 2003.

16. Bigatello LM, Hess D, Dennehy KC, et al: Sildenafil can increase the response to inhaled nitric oxide, *Anesthesiology* 92:1827–1829, 2000.

17. Fiser SM, Cope JT, Kron IL, et al: Aerosolized prostacyclin (epoprostenol) as an alternative to inhaled nitric oxide for patients with reperfusion injury after lung transplantation, *J Thorac Cardiovasc Surg* 121:981–982, 2001.

18. Vetter ML, Vinnard CL, Wadden TA, et al: Perioperative safety and bariatric surgery, *N Engl J Med* 361:445–454, 2009.

19. Isono S: Obstructive sleep apnea of obese adults: Pathophysiology and perioperative airway management, *Anesthesiology* 110:908–921, 2009.

20. Beckles MA, Spiro SG, Colice GL, et al: The physiologic evaluation of patients with lung cancer being considered for resectional surgery, *Chest* 123:105S–114S, 2003.

21. Colice GL, Shafazand S, Griffin JP, et al: Physiologic evaluation of the patient with lung cancer being considered for resectional surgery: ACCP evidenced-based clinical practice guidelines, 2nd ed, *Chest* 132:161S–177S, 2007.

22. Warner MA, Divertie MB, Tinker JH: Preoperative cessation of smoking and pulmonary complications in coronary artery bypass patients, *Anesthesiology* 60:380–383, 1984.

23. Shi YU, Warner DO: Surgery as a teachable moment for smoking cessation, *Anesthesiology* 112:102–107, 2010.

24. Benumof JL, Augustine SD, Gibbons JA: Halothane and isoflurane only slightly impair arterial oxygenation during one-lung ventilation in patients undergoing thoracotomy, *Anesthesiology* 67:910–915, 1987.

25. Bigatello LM, Allain R, Gaissert HA: Acute lung injury after pulmonary resection, *Minerva Anestesiol* 70:159–166, 2004.

26. Brodsky JB, Macario A, Mark JB: Tracheal diameter predicts double-lumen tube size: A method for selecting left double-lumen tubes, *Anesth Analg* 82:861–864, 1996.

27. Alliaume B, Coddens J, Deloof T: Reliability of auscultation in positioning of double-lumen endobronchial tubes, *Can J Anaesth* 39:687–690, 1992.

28. Campos JH, Massa FC: Is there a better right-sided tube for one-lung ventilation? A comparison of the right-sided double-lumen tube with the single-lumen tube with right-sided enclosed bronchial blocker, *Anesth Analg* 86:696–700, 1998.

29. Campos JH: An update on bronchial blockers during lung separation techniques in adults, *Anesth Analg* 97:1266–1274, 2003.

30. Cohen E: The Cohen flexitip endobronchial blocker: An alternative to a double-lumen tube, *Anesth Analg* 101:1877–1879, 2005.

31. Narayanaswamy M, McRae K, Slinger P, et al: Choosing a lung isolation device for thoracic surgery: A randomized trial of three bronchial

blockers versus double-lumen tubes, *Anesth Analg* 108:1097–1101, 2009.

32. Katz JA, Laverne RG, Fairley HB, et al: Pulmonary oxygen exchange during endobronchial anesthesia: Effect of tidal volume and PEEP, *Anesthesiology* 56:164–171, 1982.

33. Ko R, McRae K, Darling G, et al: The use of air in the inspired gas mixture during two-lung ventilation delays lung collapse during one-lung ventilation, *Anesth Analg* 108:1092–1096, 2009.

34. The Acute Respiratory Distress Syndrome Network: Ventilation with lower tidal volumes as compared with traditional tidal volumes for acute lung injury and the acute respiratory distress syndrome, *N Eng J Med* 342:1301–1308, 2000.

35. Licker M, Diaper J, Villiger Y, et al: Impact of intraoperative lung-protective interventions in patients undergoing lung cancer surgery, *Crit Care* 13:R41, 2009.

36. Slinger PD, Johnston MR: Preoperative assessment for lung cancer surgery. In Slinger PD, editor: *Progress in Thoracic Anesthesia, a Society of Cardiovascular Anesthesiologists Monograph. Philadelphia*, Williams & Wilkins, 2004, Lippincott.

37. Capan LM, Turndorf H, Patel C, et al: Optimization of arterial oxygenation during one-lung anesthesia, *Anesth Analg* 59:847–851, 1980.

38. Russell WJ: Intermittent positive airway pressure to manage hypoxia during one-lung anaesthesia, *Anaesth Intensive Care* 37:432–434, 2009.

39. Tusman G, Bohm SH, Sipmann FS, et al: Lung recruitment improves the efficiency of ventilation and gas exchange during one-lung ventilation anesthesia, *Anesth Analg* 98:1604–1609, 2004.

40. Weissman C: Pulmonary function after cardiac and thoracic surgery, *Anesth Analg* 88:1272–1279, 1999.

41. Auriant I, Jallot A, Hervé P, et al: Noninvasive ventilation reduces mortality in acute respiratory failure following lung resection, *Am J Respir Crit Care Med* 164:1231–1235, 2001.

42. Licker MJ, Widikker I, Robert J, et al: Operative mortality and respiratory complications after lung resection for cancer: Impact of chronic obstructive pulmonary disease and time trends, *Ann Thorac Surg* 81:1830–1837, 2006.

28 RENAL, LIVER, AND BILIARY TRACT DISEASE

Vinod Malhotra and Anup Pamnani

RENAL DISEASE

Normal renal function is important for the excretion of anesthetics and medications, maintaining fluid and acid–base balance, and regulating hemoglobin levels. Multiple preoperative risk factors have been identified that predict renal dysfunction in the postoperative period (Table 28-1).[1] Recently, the term acute kidney injury (AKI) has been coined to reflect a more physiologic way of thinking about acute reductions in kidney function. Such terminology reflects an increased understanding of the clinical significance of minor declines in kidney function.[2,3]

Renal Blood Flow

Although the kidneys represent only 0.5% of total body weight, their blood flow is equivalent to about 20% of cardiac output. Approximately two thirds of renal blood flow is distributed to the renal cortex. Renal blood flow and the glomerular filtration rate (GFR) remain relatively constant at renal arterial pressures in the range of 80 to 180 mm Hg (Fig. 28-1). This ability to maintain renal blood flow at a constant rate despite changes in perfusion pressure is known as autoregulation. It is achieved by adjustment of afferent arteriolar tone, which alters the resistance to blood flow. Autoregulation protects the glomerular capillaries from high systemic blood pressure during acute hypertensive episodes and maintains GFR and renal tubule function during modest decreases in systemic blood pressure. When mean arterial blood pressure is outside the autoregulatory range, renal blood flow becomes pressure dependent. Autoregulation is reset by chronic hypertension and maybe abolished in the diabetic kidney.

Renal blood flow is also strongly influenced by the activity of the sympathetic nervous system and by release of renin and other hormones. Sympathetic nervous system stimulation can produce renal vasoconstriction and a marked decrease in renal blood flow even if systemic

Table 28-1 Predictors of Postoperative Acute Kidney Injury

Advanced Age
Emergent surgery
Liver disease
High-risk surgery
Body mass index
Peripheral vascular occlusive disease
Chronic obstructive pulmonary disease

blood pressure is within the autoregulatory range. Any decrease in renal blood flow will initiate the release of renin, which can further decrease renal blood flow.

Glomerular Filtration Rate

Glomerular filtration rate reflects glomerular function and is a measure of the ability of the glomerular membrane to allow filtration. About 90% of the fluid filtered at the glomeruli is reabsorbed from renal tubules into peritubular capillaries and thus returned to the circulation (Fig. 28-2). Normal GFR is 125 mL/min and is heavily dependent on glomerular filtration pressure (GFP). GFP, in turn, is a function of renal artery pressure, afferent and efferent arteriolar tone, and glomerular oncotic pressure. Hydrostatic pressure within the glomerular capillaries is about 50 mm Hg. This pressure acts to force water and other low-molecular-weight substances such as electrolytes through the glomerular capillaries into Bowman's space. Plasma oncotic pressure is about 25 mm Hg at the afferent arteriole and with filtration increases

to about 35 mm Hg at the efferent arteriole. Despite a relatively low net filtration pressure, the glomerular capillaries are able to filter plasma at a rate equivalent to about 125 mL/min. GFR is reduced by significantly decreased mean arterial pressure or renal blood flow. Afferent arteriolar constriction decreases GFR by decreasing glomerular flow. Conversely, afferent arteriolar dilation and mild efferent vasoconstriction increase GFP and GFR.

Humoral Mediators of Renal Function

RENIN-ANGIOTENSIN-ALDOSTERONE SYSTEM
Renin is a proteolytic enzyme secreted by the juxtaglomerular apparatus of the kidneys in response to (1) sympathetic nervous system stimulation, (2) decreased renal perfusion pressure, and (3) decreases in the delivery of sodium to the distal convoluted renal tubules. Renin acts on angiotensinogen (a circulating globulin in plasma) to form angiotensin I. Angiotensin I is converted in the lungs by angiotensin-converting enzyme to angiotensin II. Angiotensin II, a potent vasoconstrictor, is an important stimulus for the release of aldosterone from the adrenal cortex. It selectively increases efferent renal arteriolar tone at low levels and causes afferent arteriolar constriction at higher levels.

PROSTAGLANDINS
Prostaglandins are produced in the renal medulla via the enzymes phospholipase A_2 and cyclooxygenase and released in response to sympathetic nervous system stimulation, hypotension, and increased levels of angiotensin II. During periods of hemodynamic instability, prostaglandins act to modulate the effects of arginine vasopressin (AVP),

IV

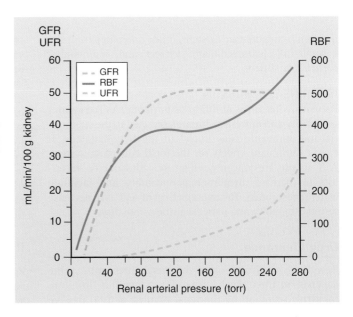

Figure 28-1 Autoregulation of renal blood flow (RBF) and the glomerular filtration rate (GFR). The relationships between RBF, GFR, and urine flow rate (UFR) and mean renal arterial pressure in dogs are shown as renal arterial pressure is varied from 20 to 280 mm Hg. Autoregulation of RBF and GFR is observed between about 80 mm Hg and 180 mm Hg. (Redrawn from Hemmings HC. Anesthetics, adjuvants and drugs and the kidney. In Malhotra V [ed]. Anesthesia for Renal and Genitourinary Surgery. New York, McGraw-Hill, 1996, p 18.)

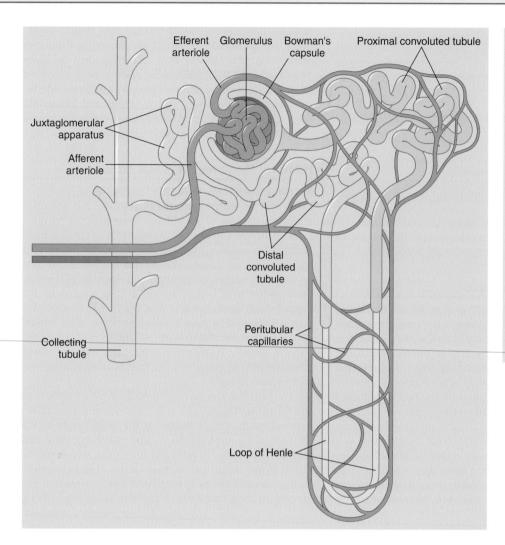

Efferent arteriole • Glomerulus • Bowman's capsule • Proximal convoluted tubule • Juxtaglomerular apparatus • Afferent arteriole • Distal convoluted tubule • Peritubular capillaries • Collecting tubule • Loop of Henle

Figure 28-2 Anatomy of a nephron. The glomerulus is formed by the invaginated and blind end of the nephron known as Bowman's capsule. Hydrostatic pressure in these capillaries causes water and low-molecular-weight substances to filter through the glomerulus. Glomerular filtrate travels along the renal tubule (proximal convoluted tubule, loop of Henle, distal convoluted tubule), during which most of its water and various amounts of solutes are reabsorbed from the renal tubular lumen into peritubular capillaries. The remaining glomerular filtrate becomes urine.

the renin-angiotensin system, and norepinephrine by vasodilating juxtamedullary vessels and maintaining cortical blood flow.

ARGININE VASOPRESSIN

Previously known as antidiuretic hormone, AVP regulates osmolality and diuresis. Although secreted in the supraoptic and paraventricular nuclei in the hypothalamus, it exerts significant effects on the renal collecting system. AVP actions are concentrated on collecting duct V_2 receptors to increase membrane permeability and facilitate water reabsorption. The overall effect of AVP is to decrease serum osmolality and increase urine osmolality.

Drug Clearance

Excretion of drugs or their metabolites into urine depends on three mechanisms: (1) glomerular filtration, (2) active secretion by the renal tubules, and (3) passive reabsorption by the tubules. The glomerular filtration of small molecules characteristic of anesthetic drugs depends on the GFR and the fractional plasma protein binding. Drugs that are highly protein bound will be inefficiently filtered at the glomerulus. Un-ionized acidic and basic compounds undergo passive reabsorption by backdiffusion in the proximal and distal renal tubules. Ionized forms of these weak acids and bases, on the other hand, are trapped within renal tubules, accounting for increased renal elimination by either alkalinization or acidification of urine. Conjugation of drugs in the liver to water-soluble metabolites is another mechanism by which renal excretion of substances is achieved.

Renal Function Tests

Renal function can be evaluated preoperatively by using several laboratory tests (Table 28-2). These tests are not sensitive measurements, and significant renal disease

Table 28-2 Tests Used for Evaluation of Renal Function

Test	Normal Value	Factors That Influence Interpretation
Test of Glomerular Filtration		
Blood urea nitrogen	8-20 mg/dL	Dehydration Variable protein intake Gastrointestinal bleeding Catabolism
Serum creatinine	0.5-1.2 mg/dL	Age Skeletal muscle mass Catabolism
Creatinine clearance	120 mL/min	Accurate urine volume measurement
Tests of Tubular Function		
Urine specific gravity Urine osmolality Urine sodium	1.003-1.030 350-500 mOsm 20-40 mEq	All are affected by dehydration, solutes, filtrates, proteins, diuretics, dehydration, drugs, and extremes of age.

(more than a 50% decrease in renal function) can exist while laboratory values remain normal. Furthermore, the normal values established in healthy individuals may not be adjusted for age or applicable during anesthesia. Trends are more useful for evaluating renal function than a single laboratory measurement.[4]

SERUM CREATININE

Serum creatinine concentration, which reflects the balance between creatinine production by muscle and its renal excretion, is often used as a marker of GFR. In contrast to blood urea nitrogen (BUN) concentration, serum creatinine level is not influenced by protein metabolism or the rate of fluid flow through renal tubules. It is, however, influenced by skeletal muscle mass. Furthermore, increases in serum creatinine are not typically noted until GFR has declined by at least 50%. Thus, increased creatinine level may serve as a late marker of renal injury. For example, elderly patients, with known decreases in GFR, frequently display normal serum creatinine concentrations due to decreased creatinine production as a consequence of the decrease in skeletal muscle mass. Indeed, mild increases in the serum creatinine concentration in elderly patients may suggest significant renal disease. Likewise, in patients with chronic renal failure, serum creatinine concentrations may not accurately reflect the GFR because of (1) decreased creatinine production, (2) the presence of decreased skeletal muscle mass, or (3) nonrenal (gastrointestinal tract) excretion of creatinine. GFR can be estimated from serum creatinine by a variety of methods including the following formula:

$$\text{GFR} = (140 - \text{age}) \times \text{weight (in kg)/serum creatinine} \times 72$$

BLOOD UREA NITROGEN

BUN concentrations, which are normally 10 to 20 mg/dL, vary with changes in GFR. The relationship between serum creatinine and BUN levels is particularly useful in diagnosing the etiology of renal failure. Like serum creatinine, elevations in BUN level are frequently a late sign of renal injury and are affected by dietary intake, coexisting illnesses, and intravascular fluid volume. For example, high-protein diets or gastrointestinal bleeding can increase the production of urea and thereby result in increased BUN concentrations (azotemia) despite a normal GFR. Other causes of increased BUN concentrations in the presence of normal GFR are increased catabolism during febrile illnesses and dehydration. Conversely, BUN concentrations can remain normal in the presence of low-protein diets despite decreases in GFR.

Increased BUN concentrations relative to serum creatinine in the presence of dehydration most likely reflect increased urea absorption due to decreased urinary flow through the renal tubules, which results in a BUN-to-creatinine ratio greater than 20. Although BUN concentration is susceptible to multiple extraneous influences, values more than 50 mg/dL inevitably reflect a decreased GFR.

CREATININE CLEARANCE

Creatinine clearance (normal, 110 to 150 mL/min) is a measurement of the ability of the glomeruli to excrete creatinine into urine for a given serum creatinine concentration. Because clearance does not depend on corrections for age or the presence of a steady state, it is a more reliable measurement of GFR than the serum BUN and creatinine values. The principal disadvantage of this test, however, is the need for timed (2 hours may be as

IV

acceptable as 24 hours) urine collections. Creatinine clearance (CrCl) and by proxy GFR can be calculated from the formula

$$GFR = CrCl = Ucr \times V/Pcr$$

where Ucr is urine creatinine, Pcr is plasma creatinine drawn at midpoint of the timed collection, and V is urinary flow rate.

PROTEINURIA

Small amounts of protein are normally filtered through glomerular capillaries and then reabsorbed in the proximal convoluted tubules. Proteinuria (excretion of more than 150 mg of protein per day) is most likely due to abnormally high filtration rather than impaired reabsorption by the renal tubules. Intermittent proteinuria occasionally occurs in healthy individuals when standing and disappears when supine. Other nonrenal causes of proteinuria include exercise, fever, and congestive heart failure.

URINE INDICES

Measurement of urine osmolality and urinary sodium, and calculation of the fractional excretion of sodium can help differentiate between prerenal and renal tubular causes of azotemia.

OTHER LABORATORY MEASUREMENTS

Measurement of serum calcium, uric acid, and creatinine kinase concentrations and serum osmolality may be useful in the differential diagnosis of acute renal failure secondary to conditions such as rhabdomyolysis, nephrotoxic drugs, or malignancy.

Pharmacology of Diuretics

THIAZIDE DIURETICS

Thiazide diuretics (hydrochlorothiazide, chlorthalidone) are generally administered for the treatment of essential hypertension and for mobilization of the edema fluid that is associated with renal, hepatic, or cardiac dysfunction. Diuresis occurs as a result of the inhibition of reabsorption of sodium and chloride ions from the early distal renal tubules. Side effects associated with diuretic-induced hypokalemia may include (1) skeletal muscle weakness,

(2) increased risk for digitalis toxicity, and (3) enhancement of nondepolarizing neuromuscular blocking drugs (Table 28-3).[5,6]

LOOP DIURETICS

Loop diuretics (ethacrynic acid, furosemide, bumetanide) inhibit the reabsorption of sodium and chloride and augment the secretion of potassium, primarily in the loop of Henle. Intravenous administration of these drugs produces a diuretic response within minutes. Chronic administration of loop diuretics may result in hypochloremic, hypokalemic metabolic alkalosis and, in rare instances, deafness.

OSMOTIC DIURETICS

The most frequently administered osmotic diuretic is the six-carbon sugar mannitol. Mannitol produces diuresis because it is filtered by the glomeruli and not reabsorbed within the renal tubules. This leads to increased osmolarity of the renal tubule fluid and associated excretion of water.

Mannitol increases fluid movement from intracellular spaces into extracellular spaces such that intravascular fluid volume expands acutely. This redistribution of fluid from intracellular to extracellular compartments decreases brain size and intracranial pressure. Mannitol may further diminish intracranial pressure by decreasing the rate of cerebrospinal fluid formation.

ALDOSTERONE ANTAGONISTS

Spironolactone blocks the renal tubular effects of aldosterone and offsets the loss of potassium that is associated with the administration of thiazide diuretics. Fluid overload secondary to cirrhosis of the liver is often treated with spironolactone. The most serious toxic effect of spironolactone is hyperkalemia. Serum potassium concentration should be followed closely in patients taking spironolactone.

DOPAMINE AND FENOLDOPAM

Dopamine dilates renal arterioles, via its agonist action at the DA1 receptor, leading to increased renal blood flow and GFR. Treatment with low-dose dopamine (0.5 to 3 µg/kg/min) may augment urine output but studies display little benefit in altering the course of renal failure with

Table 28-3 Side Effects of Diuretics

Diuretic Class	Hypokalemic, Hypochloremic Metabolic Alkalosis	Hyperkalemia	Hyperglycemia
Thiazide diuretics	Yes	No	Yes
Loop diuretics	Yes	No	Minimal
Osmotic diuretics	No	No	No
Aldosterone antagonists	No	Yes	No

this therapy. In addition, dose-dependent side effects of dopamine include tachydysrhythmias, pulmonary shunting, and tissue ischemia (gastrointestinal tract, digits).[7-9]

Fenoldopam, a dopamine analog, also possesses DA1 agonist activity but lacks the adrenergic activity of dopamine. It also increases renal blood flow and GFR and may have beneficial effects in the treatment of acute kidney injury. However, its role in the treatment of renal failure is unclear at this time. It is presently approved for short-term parenteral treatment of severe hypertension.[7,10]

Pathophysiology of End-Stage Renal Disease

End-stage renal disease (ESRD) causes profound physiologic changes that affect several organs (Tables 28-4 and 28-5).

CARDIOVASCULAR DISEASE

Cardiovascular disease is the predominant cause of death in patients with ESRD. Acute myocardial infarction, cardiac arrest of unknown etiology, cardiac dysrhythmias, and cardiomyopathy account for more than 50% of deaths in patients maintained on dialysis. Hypertension deserves particular mention as it is very commonly encountered in the patient with ESRD. Systemic hypertension in these patients can be severe and refractory to antihypertensive therapy. Hypervolemia and excess activation of the renin-angiotensin-aldosterone system are the most common etiologies. .

Additionally, the accumulation of uremic toxins and metabolic acids may contribute to poor myocardial performance. The presence of ESRD with significantly depressed cardiac function does not necessarily contraindicate renal transplantation because cardiac ventricular function often improves after transplantation.

Uremia causes changes in lipid metabolism that lead to increased concentrations of serum triglycerides and reduced levels of protective high-density lipoproteins. Thus, ESRD accelerates the progression of atherosclerosis. Pericardial disease and cardiac dysrhythmias can also be encountered in patients with ESRD. Pericardial effusions are resolved when patients are adequately dialyzed.[11]

METABOLIC DISEASE

A large number of patients with ESRD manifest diabetes mellitus. Kidney failure as a result of diabetes develops in nearly 30% to 40% of patients with ESRD, and these patients account for 30% of those on the waiting list for kidney transplantation. In fact, nephropathy develops in nearly 60% of insulin-dependent diabetic patients. Patients with ESRD and diabetes have a higher cardiovascular risk than do patients with renal failure alone.[11]

Once patients are unable to excrete their dietary fluid and electrolyte loads, abnormalities in plasma electrolyte concentrations (sodium, potassium, calcium, magnesium, and phosphate) can develop. The most life-threatening electrolyte abnormality is hyperkalemia.

ANEMIA AND ABNORMAL COAGULATION

Patients with renal failure generally display a normochromic, normocytic anemia because of decreased erythropoiesis and retained toxins that are secondary to renal failure. Treatment with recombinant erythropoietin can frequently raise hemoglobin levels, which reduces symptoms of fatigue and improves both cerebral and cardiac function. Occasionally, recombinant erythropoietin therapy may exacerbate preexisting essential hypertension. Renal failure patients may also display uremia-induced defects in platelet function.

Management of Anesthesia in Patients with End-Stage Renal Disease

General anesthesia with the trachea intubated provides acceptable hemodynamics, excellent skeletal muscle relaxation, and a predictable depth of anesthesia in patients with ESRD who are undergoing major operations. Patients with advanced stages of co-morbid conditions may require more extensive monitoring, such as continuous monitoring of systemic blood pressure and perhaps central venous pressure. Large swings in arterial blood pressure may occur with hypotension being more likely than hypertension during maintenance of anesthesia

Table 28-4 Changes Characteristic of Chronic Renal Disease
Anemia
Depressed ejection fraction
Decreased platelet adhesiveness
Hyperkalemia
Unpredictable intravascular fluid volume
Metabolic acidosis
Systemic hypertension
Pericardial effusion
Decreased sympathetic nervous system activity

Table 28-5 Stages of Chronic Renal Failure	
Stage	Glomerular Filtration (mL/min/1.73 m^2)
1	>90
2	60-89
3	30-59
4	15-29
5	<15

IV

particularly if the patient has recently been hemodialyzed in preparation for the procedure. Those with the most severe co-morbid conditions, such as symptomatic coronary artery disease or a history of congestive heart failure, may benefit from monitoring with a pulmonary artery catheter or transesophageal echocardiography. The status of hemodialysis shunts or fistulas should be monitored (presence of a thrill) during positioning and intraoperatively to confirm continued patency. Peripheral lines and blood pressure monitoring cuffs should not be placed in proximity to such implanted vascular access devices.

Patients with uremia and other co-morbid conditions (diabetes mellitus) are at an increased risk for aspiration of gastric contents during induction of anesthesia. The use of a rapid sequence induction of anesthesia technique may be indicated in such patients. Succinylcholine is not contraindicated in patients with ESRD. The increase in serum potassium concentration after a large dose of succinylcholine is approximately 0.6 mEq/L for patients both with and without ESRD. This increase can be tolerated without imposing a significant cardiac risk, even in the presence of an initial serum potassium concentration higher than 5 mEq/L.

Several strategies have been successfully used to achieve adequate heart rate and arterial blood pressure control during induction of anesthesia. Moderate to large doses of opioids such as fentanyl can blunt the response to laryngoscopy. However, systemic blood pressure is frequently more difficult to maintain after induction of anesthesia, and hypotension may require treatment with vasoconstrictors. The short-acting β-adrenergic blocker esmolol may be used to blunt the hemodynamic response to tracheal intubation and is ideally suited for patients with an adequate ejection fraction.

Drugs or their metabolites that depend on renal elimination (pancuronium, morphine, meperidine) should be used cautiously or avoided. Atracurium and cisatracurium may be particularly useful as they are metabolized by spontaneous Hoffman degradation and plasma cholinesterase, which makes their duration of action independent of liver or kidney function. Similarly, fentanyl, sufentanil, alfentanil, and remifentanil are alternatives to morphine which is transformed to long-acting renally excreted metabolites (e.g., morphine-6-glucuronide).

Choices of inhaled anesthetics include desflurane, isoflurane, and sevoflurane. The metabolism of sevoflurane to inorganic fluoride has been implicated in experimental studies of renal toxicity, although no controlled human studies are available to indicate either safety concerns or danger when using sevoflurane in the setting of ESRD.

Differential Diagnosis of Perioperative Oliguria

PRERENAL OLIGURIA

Prerenal oliguria is characterized by the excretion of concentrated urine that contains minimal amounts of sodium (Table 28-6). Excretion of highly concentrated and sodium-poor urine confirms that renal tubular function is intact and reflects an attempt by the kidneys to conserve sodium and restore intravascular fluid volume in response to decreased renal blood flow. The decreased renal blood flow most likely reflects an acute decrease in intravascular fluid volume or decreased cardiac output. Other causes of decreased renal blood flow are sepsis, liver failure, and congestive heart failure.[11]

The initial management of patients with perioperative oliguria is influenced by their risk for the development of acute renal failure. A brisk diuresis in response to a fluid challenge suggests that an acute decrease in intravascular fluid volume is the cause of the prerenal oliguria. When intravascular fluid replacement does not result in increased urine output, intrinsic renal disease or hemodynamic causes should be considered. Prompt recognition and treatment of prerenal oliguria is critical as prolonged severe ischemia can lead to necrosis of renal tubules and convert reversible injury to irreversible intrarenal disease.

Administration of diuretics to maintain or stimulate urine flow in the perioperative period is controversial. Some believe that prevention of renal tubule urine stasis with diuretics can prevent prerenal oliguria from progressing to acute tubular necrosis. Nevertheless, urine

Table 28-6 Oliguria versus Acute Tubular Necrosis: Preoperative Differential Diagnosis

Diagnostic Feature	Prerenal Oliguria	Acute Tubular Necrosis
Fractional excretion of sodium	<1%	>3%
Urine specific gravity	>1.015	1.01-1.015
Urine sodium (mEq/L)	<40	>40
Urine osmolality (mOsm/L)	>400	<400
Causes	Decreased renal blood flow (hypotension, hypovolemia, decreased cardiac output)	Renal ischemia Nephrotoxins Free hemoglobin or myoglobin

output that is enhanced by the administration of a diuretic does not necessarily predict postoperative renal function. There is no evidence that drug-induced diuresis (dopamine, furosemide, mannitol) in the presence of low cardiac output or hypovolemia (or both) protects renal function. Likewise, there is no evidence that the incidence of acute renal failure is decreased when low-dose dopamine is administered to high-risk patients (abdominal aortic cross-clamping, cardiopulmonary bypass).

INTRINSIC RENAL DISEASE

Acute tubular necrosis, glomerulonephritis, and acute interstitial nephritis are intrinsic renal causes of oliguria. In contrast to oliguria secondary to hypovolemia, the urine of patients with acute tubular necrosis is poorly concentrated and contains excessive amounts of sodium (see Table 28-6). Intrinsic renal disease is the most severe of the different forms of oliguria and is typically the hardest to reverse.

POSTRENAL OLIGURIA

An obstruction that is distal to the renal collecting system usually involves a mechanical problem such as a blood clot in the ureter, bladder, or urethra. Surgical ligation, renal calculi, and edema are other postrenal causes of low urine output. Another common postrenal cause is bladder catheter obstruction. Postrenal oliguria is frequently reversible once the source of the obstruction is removed.

LIVER DISEASE

The liver is responsible for the production of essential plasma proteins, the metabolism and detoxification of drugs and deleterious xenobiotics, the absorption of critical nutrients, and carbohydrate metabolism. Impaired liver function affects nearly every organ system in the body.

Hepatic Blood Flow

The liver is unique in that it receives a dual afferent blood supply that is equal to about 25% of cardiac output (Fig. 28-3). Approximately 70% of hepatic blood flow is supplied by the portal vein with the remainder supplied by the hepatic artery. Under normal conditions, each blood vessel contributes roughly 50% to the liver's oxygen supply. Portal vein flow is not regulated and is susceptible to systemic hypotension and decreases in cardiac output.

INTRINSIC REGULATION OF HEPATIC BLOOD FLOW

Reduction in portal flow (up to a 50% reduction) is compensated by modulating hepatic artery tone to maintain perfusion to the liver. This is primarily mediated via

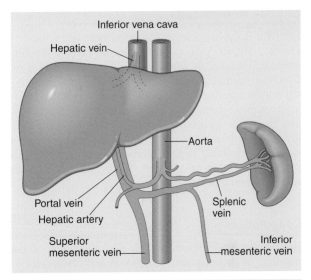

Figure 28-3 Schematic depiction of the dual afferent blood supply to the liver provided by the portal vein and hepatic artery. About 70% of hepatic blood flow is via the portal vein, with the remainder via the hepatic artery. Total hepatic blood flow is directly proportional to perfusion pressure across the liver and inversely related to splanchnic vascular resistance. Cirrhosis of the liver increases resistance to blood flow through the portal vein and decreases hepatic blood flow.

the hepatic arterial buffer response, which reciprocally varies hepatic arterial blood flow to changes in portal flow mediated by adenosine. The response is stimulated by low pH and O_2 content and increased P_{CO_2}. Volatile anesthetics and cirrhosis of the liver attenuate this reciprocal relationship and render the liver vulnerable to ischemia.

Extrinsic Determinants of Hepatic Blood Flow

Hepatic perfusion pressure (mean arterial or portal vein pressure minus hepatic vein pressure) and splanchnic vascular resistance determine hepatic blood flow. The splanchnic vessels receive vasomotor innervation from the sympathetic nervous system. Splanchnic nerve stimulation (pain, arterial hypoxemia, surgical stress) increases splanchnic vascular resistance and decreases hepatic blood flow. Surgical stimulation and the proximity of the operative site to the liver are important determinants of the magnitude of the decrease in hepatic blood flow seen during general anesthesia. β-Adrenergic receptor blockers such as propranolol are associated with decreases in hepatic blood flow. Positive-pressure ventilation of the lungs, congestive heart failure, and fluid overload cause increased central venous pressure, resulting in increased hepatic venous pressure, which effectively decreases hepatic perfusion pressure and blood flow.

Glucose Homeostasis

The liver is the main organ for the storage and release of glucose. Hepatocytes extract glucose via an insulin-mediated mechanism, where it can be stored as glycogen. Glucagon-mediated catabolism of glycogen (glycogenolysis) releases glucose back into the systemic circulation for maintenance of euglycemia. Surgical stress, starvation, and sympathetic nervous system activation stimulates glycogen depolymerization to glucose. When glycogen stores are depleted hepatic gluconeogenesis from substrates such as lactate, glycerol, and certain amino acids restores blood glucose levels.

Coagulation

Hepatocytes are responsible for the synthesis of the majority of procoagulant proteins as well as regulators such as proteins C and S and antithrombin III. An important exception to this is factor VIII, which is partially produced in endothelial cells. Vitamin K, which is absorbed by bile secretion into the gastrointestinal tract, plays an important role in catalysis of some of the procoagulant proteins to produce factors II, VII, IX, and X. Laboratory studies such as prothrombin time (international normalized ratio [INR]), partial thromboplastin time, and fibrinogen levels can be used to evaluate impaired coagulation and hepatic function. Impaired laboratory studies reflect significant hepatic dysfunction because most coagulation factors maintain function at up to 20% to 30% of their normal levels.

Drug Metabolism

Hepatic drug metabolism is characterized by the conversion of lipid-soluble drugs to more water-soluble forms to facilitate renal excretion, transformation to pharmacologically less active substances, and excretion in bile. Three major pathways are utilized to accomplish these goals. Phase 1 metabolism involves an increase in polarity of drugs via cytochrome P and mixed function oxidases. Phase 2 metabolism involves conjugation of metabolites to water-soluble substrates, and phase 3 elimination relies on energy-dependent excretion of drugs into bile. Chronic liver disease may interfere with the metabolism of drugs because of the decreased number of enzyme-containing hepatocytes or the decreased hepatic blood flow that typically accompanies cirrhosis of the liver. Prolonged elimination half-times for morphine, alfentanil, diazepam, lidocaine, pancuronium, and vecuronium have been demonstrated in patients with cirrhosis of the liver. Likewise, chronic drug therapy can inhibit hepatic enzymes and inhibit metabolism of anesthetic drugs leading to higher circulating blood levels. Conversely, enzyme induction, particularly of cytochrome P isoforms, can also occur as a response to chronic therapy with drugs like phenytoin, INH, and rifampin or as a result of alcohol abuse. Such induction of hepatic enzymes can increase metabolism of administered anesthetic and therapeutic drugs, thereby reducing plasma levels.

Heme Metabolism

While fetal erythrocyte production occurs exclusively in the liver, hepatic hematopoiesis accounts for only 20% of adult heme synthesis with the remainder produced in the bone marrow. Heme synthesis occurs from glycine and succinyl CoA through a reaction catalyzed by ALA synthetase. ALA synthetase is the rate-limiting step in the heme synthesis pathway and is regulated by feedback inhibition by its end product heme. Porphyrias are rare genetic diseases characterized by interruption of feedback inhibition of ALA synthetase

Heme degradation, primarily by the reticuloendothelial system, results in formation of bilirubin as an end product. Formed bilirubin is then bound to plasma albumin for transport to the liver, where it is extracted and conjugated for secretion into canalicular bile. The majority of bilirubin excretion occurs in the gut, although a small portion is recirculated to the liver via the enterohepatic circulation. This accounts for the small amount of bilirubin conjugates present in blood. Conjugated bilirubin is water soluble and about 10% is excreted in the urine.

Cholesterol and Lipid Metabolism

The liver stores dietary fat as triglycerides, cholesterol, and phospholipids and releases free fatty acids via triglyceride hydrolysis. In addition, it synthesizes free fatty acids from glucose, lipids, and protein. The liver also plays an important role in regulation of cholesterol uptake, metabolism, and transport. Bile salts, the end product of cholesterol synthesis, serve as regulators of lipid metabolism. Elimination of cholesterol is achieved by biliary secretion and by excretion of bile acids.

Protein Metabolism

The liver plays a vital role in protein metabolism. Numerous biologically active proteins including albumin, cytokines, hormones, and coagulation factors are manufactured in the liver. In addition, nonessential amino acid synthesis can also occur in hepatocytes when necessary. Protein degradation is another important function of the liver. The urea (Krebs) cycle is utilized by hepatocytes to convert the end products of amino acid degradation, such as ammonia and other nitrogenous waste products, to urea which is readily excreted by the kidney. Severe hepatic dysfunction, such as that which occurs in end-stage liver disease, leads to accumulation of ammonia in the serum resulting in hepatic encephalopathy.

Pathophysiology of End-Stage Liver Disease

HYPERDYNAMIC CIRCULATION

Severe parenchymal disease that has advanced to the point of cirrhosis usually results in a hyperdynamic circulation. Hemodynamic measurements generally reveal normal to low systemic blood pressure, increased cardiac output, and decreased systemic vascular resistance. Decreased systemic vascular resistance is a result of vasodilation and abnormal anatomic and physiologic shunting. Physiologic shunting is the passage of blood from the arterial to the venous side of the circulation without effectively traversing a capillary bed blood. Abnormal blood vessels, such as those seen in the skin as spider angiomas, represent an anatomic shunt.[12]

PORTAL HYPERTENSION

High resistance to blood flow through the liver, a hallmark of end-stage liver disease, causes an accumulation of blood in the vascular beds that are immediately upstream of the liver. Vessels draining the esophagus, stomach, spleen, and intestines dilate and hypertrophy, which leads to the development of splenomegaly and esophageal, gastric, and intra-abdominal varices. Symptoms of portal hypertension include anorexia, nausea, ascites, esophageal varices, spider nevi, and hepatic encephalopathy. It is central to the pathogenesis of a variety of complications associated with end-stage liver disease including massive hemorrhage, increased susceptibility to infection, renal failure, and mental status changes.

PULMONARY COMPLICATIONS

End-stage liver disease can be associated with the hepatopulmonary syndrome and portopulmonary hypertension. Hepatopulmonary syndrome develops as a result of intrapulmonary arteriovenous communications that are not ventilated, impairment of hypoxic pulmonary vasoconstriction, atelectasis, and restrictive pulmonary disease secondary to ascites and pleural effusion. Arterial hypoxemia, secondary to the hepatopulmonary syndrome, may improve somewhat with supplemental oxygen in the early stages of the disease but oxygen may not be effective with disease progression.

Portopulmonary hypertension is an increase in intrapulmonary vascular pressure in patients with portal hypertension. The cause is not well established. This syndrome occurs in less than 5% of patients, including the liver transplant population. Nevertheless, these patients are at increased risk for acute right-sided heart failure if physiologic conditions that increase pulmonary vascular resistance (acidosis, arterial hypoxemia, hypercapnia) occur during anesthesia. Hepatic hydrothorax, pleural effusions occurring in the absence of cardiopulmonary disease, can also occur in up to 10% of cirrhotic patients.

HEPATIC ENCEPHALOPATHY

Altered mental state is a frequent complication of both acute and chronic liver failure with a clinically variable presentation ranging from minor changes in brain function to deep coma. The etiology of this complex neuropsychiatric syndrome is multifactorial. Serum concentration of a number of chemicals, which are normally filtered by the healthy liver and are present in higher concentrations with hepatic dysfunction, are believed to play an important role. Ammonia is heavily implicated as a precipitating factor of episodes of hepatic encephalopathy (HE). Other etiologic factors include disruption of the blood-brain barrier, increased central nervous system inhibitory neurotransmission, and altered cerebral energy metabolism. The reversibility of symptoms of HE with administration of flumazenil support an important role for the GABA (γ-aminobutyric acid) receptor activation in HE pathogenesis. It is also important to rule out other causes of altered mental status in the patient with liver disease, such as intracranial bleeding or masses, hypoglycemia, or a postictal state. As effective treatments for many of the putative etiologic factors in HE do not yet exist, current treatment still revolves around reducing the production and absorption of the ammonia. Typically, neomycin (to reduce ammonia production by urease-producing bacteria) or the administration of lactulose (to reduce ammonia absorption) are employed.[13]

IMPAIRED DRUG BINDING

When liver disease is so severe that albumin production is decreased, fewer sites are available for drug binding. This limited availability can increase levels of the unbound, pharmacologically active fraction of drugs such as thiopental and alfentanil. Increased drug sensitivity as a result of decreased protein binding is most likely to be manifested when plasma albumin concentrations are lower than 2.5 g/dL.

ASCITES

Ascites is a common complication of cirrhosis affecting up to 50% of cirrhotic patients. The development of ascites is associated with significant morbidity and heralds the end stages of cirrhosis. Complications associated with ascites include marked abdominal distention (leading to atelectasis and restrictive pulmonary disease), spontaneous bacterial peritonitis, and circulatory instability due to compression of the inferior vena cava and right atrium. Although the exact mechanism of ascites is unclear, excess sodium retention by the kidney, decreased oncotic pressure due to hypoalbuminemia, and portal hypertension appear to play a central role. Initial therapy includes fluid restriction, reduction of sodium intake, and administration of diuretics. In severe cases, abdominal paracentesis can be effective at transiently reducing abdominal distention and restoring hemodynamic stability.[14,15]

RENAL DYSFUNCTION AND HEPATORENAL SYNDROME

Renal dysfunction can develop in a significant portion of patients with cirrhosis. A variety of etiologic factors

IV

including diuretic therapy, reduced intravascular volume secondary to ascites or gastrointestinal hemorrhage, nephrotoxic drugs, and sepsis can provoke acute renal failure and ultimately acute tubular necrosis in cirrhotic patients.

In the absence of obvious factors precipitating renal failure, the hepatorenal syndrome (HRS) can be diagnosed. HRS is characterized by intense renal vasoconstriction as an end-stage response to decreased effective arterial blood volume. Type 1 HRS, typically presenting as rapidly progressing prerenal failure, is associated with a poor prognosis in the absence of therapeutic intervention. Conversely, type 2 HRS presents with a milder degree of renal dysfunction. Treatment with octreotide, glucagons, and midodrine have shown some promise at reversing type 1 HRS.[16]

Effects of Anesthesia and Surgery on the Liver

IMPACT OF ANESTHETICS ON HEPATIC BLOOD FLOW

Inhaled anesthetics and regional anesthesia both typically decrease hepatic blood flow 20% to 30% in the absence of surgical stimulation. These changes reflect drug- or technique-induced effects on hepatic perfusion pressure or splanchnic vascular resistance, or both. For example, the various degrees of reduction in hepatic blood flow that are associated with volatile anesthetics, as well as regional anesthesia (T5 sensory level), are most likely due to decreased hepatic perfusion pressure. There is some experimental evidence that autoregulation (increased hepatic artery blood flow offsetting decreases in portal vein blood flow) of hepatic blood flow is best maintained with isoflurane. However, hepatic blood flow during the administration of desflurane and sevoflurane is maintained by a similar mechanism.

VOLATILE ANESTHETIC–INDUCED HEPATIC DYSFUNCTION

A rare, but life-threatening form of hepatic dysfunction may reflect an immune-mediated hepatotoxicity caused by halothane. Two patterns of hepatic injury have been associated with use of halothane. A mild form occurs in up to 20% of patients and is associated with minimal sequelae, and a rare fulminant form is associated with a fatality rate of 50% to 70%. Risk factors for development of this condition include prior exposure to halothane, age above 40, obesity, and female gender. Isoflurane and desflurane are also capable of causing hepatic dysfunction, but the incidence of hepatitis after exposure to these volatile anesthetics is extremely rare, mainly because of the decreased magnitude of metabolism in comparison to halothane. Given its rare incidence and the disappearance of halothane in modern clinical practice in North America, volatile anesthetic–induced hepatic dysfunction remains a diagnosis of exclusion in the patient presenting with hepatitis in the perioperative period.[17,18]

Management of Anesthesia in Patients with End-Stage Liver Disease

PREOPERATIVE EVALUATION OF LIVER DISEASE

Liver function tests (Table 28-7) are used to detect the presence of liver disease preoperatively and to establish the diagnosis when postoperative liver dysfunction occurs. The Child-Pugh System and Model for End-Stage Liver Disease (MELD) score are two methods of evaluating severity of liver dysfunction (Table 28-8). Patients with Child-Pugh class C liver dysfunction or MELD score greater than 14 have an increased risk for perioperative morbidity and death. Morbidity and mortality rates after elective operations are higher in patients with preexisting cirrhosis of the liver than in patients undergoing similar operations but in the absence of liver disease.[15,19,20]

Unfortunately, liver function tests are rarely specific. Postoperative liver dysfunction is greater in the presence of coexisting liver disease. Furthermore, the large reserve of the liver means that considerable hepatic damage can be present before liver function test results become altered. Indeed, cirrhosis of the liver may cause little alteration in liver function. It may take an additional stress, such as anesthesia and surgery, to reveal the underlying liver disease. Inadequate hepatocyte function during anesthesia and surgery will be manifested as metabolic acidosis intraoperatively.

INTRAOPERATIVE MANAGEMENT

Most major operations in patients with significant liver diseases involve the use of general anesthesia. Regional techniques can be considered in selected patients with acceptable coagulation. The magnitude of the operation determines the extent of invasive monitoring that is required. Major operations during which blood loss is

Table 28-7 Liver Function Tests with Normal Values	
Test	**Normal Values***
Albumin	3.5-5.5 g/dL
Bilirubin	0.3-1.1 mg/dL
Unconjugated bilirubin (indirect reacting)	0.2-0.7 mg/dL
Conjugated bilirubin (direct reacting)	0.1-0.4 mg/dL
Aspartate aminotransferase (i.e., SGOT)	10-40 U/mL
Alanine aminotransferase (i.e., SGPT)	5-35 U/mL
Alkaline phosphatase	10-30 U/mL
Prothrombin time	12-14 sec

*Normal values for each individual laboratory should be considered in interpreting liver function test results.
SGOT, serum glutamic-oxaloacetic [acid] transaminase; SGPT, serum glumate-pyruvate transaminase.

Table 28-8 Child-Pugh Classification System and MELD Score Formula for Liver Disease

Finding	Child-Turcotte-Pugh Score		
	A	**B**	**C**
Serum bilirubin (mg/dL)	<2.0	2.0-3.0	>3.0
Serum albumin (g/dL)	>3.5	2.8-3.5	<2.8
Prothrombin time (seconds prolonged)	1-4 sec	4-6 sec	>6 sec
Ascites	None	Slight	Moderate
Encephalopathy	None	Minimal	Advanced
MELD (Model for End-Stage Liver Disease) Score Formula			

MELD score = (0.957 × $\log_e$ [serum creatinine (mg/dL)] + 0.378 × $\log_e$ [total serum bilirubin (mg/dL)] + 1.120 × $\log_e$ [INR]) × 10
Minimum for all values is 1.
Maximum value for creatinine is 4.

likely require continuous means of monitoring systemic blood pressure (arterial line) and filling pressure (central venous line). Those patients with significant other co-morbidities (including cardiac diseases) undergoing procedures involving large anticipated blood loss may require placement of a pulmonary artery catheter. Correction of a severe coagulopathy before vascular line placement may be considered, whereas the use of ultrasound may facilitate central venous cannulation. Communication with the blood bank before surgery is crucial to ensure adequate availability of red blood cells, platelets, and clotting factors, including fresh frozen plasma and cryoprecipitate. In patients with esophageal varices there exists a risk of bleeding from insertion of a trans-esophageal echocardiography (TEE) probe.

Induction and Maintenance of Anesthesia

Most patients have well-preserved cardiac function and no significant systemic or pulmonary hypertension. Induction of anesthesia can be achieved with an intravenous anesthetic such as propofol, thiopental, or etomidate, along with opioids and short- or intermediate-acting neuromuscular blocking drugs. Intravenous anesthetics have minimal impact on hepatic blood flow provided arterial blood pressure is adequately maintained. Thus, arterial blood pressure should be preserved and sympathetic stimulation avoided, which also has an adverse effect on hepatic blood flow. A rapid-sequence or modified rapid-sequence induction of anesthesia is warranted if patients have significant ascites or delayed gastric emptying. Hypotension after induction of anesthesia occurs commonly as a result of the low systemic vascular resistance and relative hypovolemia. This can usually be treated with small doses of vasoconstrictors such as phenylephrine. With the exception of halothane, all volatile anesthetics are suitable for patients with severe liver disease. No optimal anesthetic technique has been established for the maintenance of anesthesia.

Coagulopathy

Coagulopathy and surgical blood loss are treated by the administration of red blood cells, fresh frozen plasma, platelets, and cryoprecipitate. Pharmacologic treatment of hepatic-associated coagulopathy may include ε-aminocaproic acid, tranexamic acid, conjugated estrogen, and activated recombinant factor VII. Thromboelastography may be helpful in identifying the cause of coagulopathy and can guide administration of coagulation products.

Postoperative Jaundice

Halothane or other volatile anesthetics are often implicated as the cause of postoperative jaundice, but there are many other and probably more likely causes (Table 28-9). A surgical cause of postoperative jaundice is likely if the operation involved the liver or biliary tract. Similarly, multiple blood transfusions and resorption of surgical hematoma can lead to jaundice in the perioperative period. Drugs, including antibiotics, and other metabolic or infectious causes must also be considered in the differential diagnosis of postoperative jaundice.

Management of Anesthesia in Intoxicated Patients

Acutely intoxicated patients require less anesthesia because there is an additive depressant effect between alcohol and anesthetics. Lowered minimum alveolar

IV

Table 28-9   Classification and Causes of Postoperative Liver Dysfunction

Diagnostic Feature	Prehepatic	Intrahepatic	Posthepatic
Bilirubin	Increased (unconjugated fraction)	Increased (conjugated fraction)	Increased (conjugated fraction)
Aminotransferase enzymes	No change	Markedly increased	Normal to slightly increased
Alkaline phosphatase	No change	No change to slightly increased	Markedly increased
Prothrombin time	No change	Prolonged	No change to prolonged
Albumin	No change	Decreased	No change to decreased
Causes	Hemolysis Hematoma reabsorption Bilirubin overload from whole blood	Viruses Drugs Sepsis Arterial hypoxemia Congestive heart failure Cirrhosis	Stones Cancer Sepsis

concentration (MAC) levels in the acutely intoxicated patient may also reduce the amount of volatile anesthetic needed to maintain anesthesia. Intoxicated patients are more vulnerable to regurgitation of gastric contents and aspiration pneumonia because alcohol slows gastric emptying and decreases the tone of the lower esophageal sphincter.

Alcohol Withdrawal Syndrome

Initial symptoms of alcohol withdrawal, including agitation, tachycardia, and signs of increased sympathetic stimulation, may be subtle and mistaken for other common perioperative complications such as pain and delirium. A history of chronic alcohol use, however, should always prompt consideration of this entity in the differential diagnosis, and prophylactic benzodiazepine treatment can be promptly initiated. Manifestations of severe alcohol withdrawal syndrome (delirium tremens) usually appear 48 to 72 hours after cessation of drinking. This syndrome represents a medical emergency. Such patients may manifest tremulousness and hallucinations. There is significantly increased activity of the sympathetic nervous system with subsequent catecholamine release, leading to diaphoresis, hyperpyrexia, cardiac dysrhythmias, and hemodynamic instability. In some patients, grand mal seizures may be the first indication of alcohol withdrawal syndrome. When seizures occur, hypoglycemia and other possible causes, including brain injury, should also be ruled out.

TREATMENT

Treatment of delirium tremens must be aggressive and consists of benzodiazepine administration at regular intervals. A β-antagonist (propranolol or esmolol) should be used to control the heart rate. If mental status declines significantly, airway protection may be achieved by endotracheal intubation. Correction of fluid, electrolyte (magnesium, potassium), and metabolic (thiamine) derangements is important. Despite aggressive treatment, mortality rate from delirium tremens is about 10%. Death is often due to hemodynamic instability, cardiac dysrhythmias, or seizures.[21]

DISEASES OF THE BILIARY TRACT

Gallstones are reported to be present in 10% of men and 20% of women between 55 and 65 years of age. These patients usually have normal liver function test results, except for increased serum bilirubin or alkaline phosphatase concentrations due to choledocholithiasis (common bile duct stone) or chronic cholangitis. Gilbert's syndrome, a benign disorder causing elevation in unconjugated bilirubin, is one of the most common causes of jaundice and may occasionally be mistaken for postoperative hepatobiliary dysfunction. Conversely, Dubin-Johnson and Rotor's syndromes are congenital disorders leading to elevated conjugated bilirubin levels that can be exacerbated by surgery.

Management of Anesthesia

Anesthesia for cholecystectomy or exploration of the common bile duct, or both, is influenced by the effect of the drugs used for anesthesia on intraluminal pressure in the biliary tract. Specifically, opioids can produce spasm of the choledochoduodenal sphincter, which increases common bile duct pressure. Such spasm may impair the passage of contrast medium into the duodenum and erroneously suggest the need for sphincteroplasty or the presence of common bile duct stones. However, opioids have been used in many instances without adverse effect, which emphasizes the fact that not all patients respond to opioids with choledochoduodenal sphincter spasm. Treatment of biliary spasm includes naloxone, glucagons, and nitroglycerin.

LAPAROSCOPIC CHOLECYSTECTOMY

Anesthetic considerations for laparoscopic cholecystectomy are similar to those for other laparoscopic procedures.[22] For example, insufflation of the abdominal cavity (pneumoperitoneum) with carbon dioxide introduced through a needle placed via a supraumbilical incision results in increased intra-abdominal pressure that may interfere with ventilation of the lungs and venous return. During laparoscopic cholecystectomy, placement of the patient in the reverse Trendelenburg position favors movement of the abdominal contents away from the operative site and may facilitate mechanical ventilation of the lungs. This position, however, may further interfere with venous return. Generous fluid replacement during laparoscopic cholecystectomy may facilitate recovery from this surgery.

Monitoring end-tidal carbon dioxide concentrations during laparoscopic abdominal surgical procedures is useful because of the unpredictability of systemic absorption of the carbon dioxide used to create the pneumoperitoneum. Intraoperative decompression of the stomach with a nasogastric or orogastric tube may decrease the risk for visceral puncture at the time of needle insertion and may subsequently improve laparoscopic visualization. Administration of nitrous oxide during laparoscopic cholecystectomy is not usually recommended because of the remote possibility that it could expand bowel gas volume, causing interference with surgical working conditions.[23] Loss of hemostasis or injury to the hepatic artery or liver may require prompt intervention via a conventional laparotomy incision.

QUESTIONS OF THE DAY

1. How is creatinine clearance (CrCl) measured? How accurate are the estimates of CrCl based on single measurements of serum creatinine or blood urea nitrogen (BUN)?
2. What is the most common cause of death in patients with end-stage renal disease (ESRD)?
3. What are the potential causes of perioperative oliguria? How can these causes be distinguished clinically?
4. What are the major pathways of hepatic drug metabolism?
5. What is the classic hemodynamic profile (e.g., blood pressure, cardiac output, systemic vascular resistance) of a patient with end-stage liver disease (ESLD)?
6. What are the criteria used to determine the Child-Pugh and the Model for End-Stage Liver Disease (MELD) scores? What do these scores predict?

ACKNOWLEDGMENTS

The editors and publisher would like to thank Drs. C.S. Yost and Claus U. Niemann for contributing a chapter on this topic to the prior edition of this work. It has served as the foundation for the current chapter.

IV

REFERENCES

1. Kheterpal S, Tremper KK, Englesbe MJ, et al: Predictors of postoperative acute renal failure after noncardiac surgery in patients with previously normal renal function, *Anesthesiology* 107:892–902, 2007.
2. Mehta R, Kellum JA, Shah SV, et al: Acute Kidney Injury Network: Report of an initiative to improve outcomes in acute kidney injury, *Crit Care* 11:2634–2653, 2007.
3. Hoste E, Clermont G, Kersten A, et al: RIFLE criteria for acute kidney injury are associated with hospital mortality in critically ill patients: A cohort analysis, *Crit Care* 10:R73, 2006.
4. Singri N, Ahya SN, Levin ML, et al: Acute renal failure, *JAMA* 289:747–751, 2003.
5. Wang DJ, Gottlieb SS: Diuretics: Still the mainstay of treatment, *Crit Care Med* 36(1 Suppl):S89–S94, 2008.
6. Brater DC: Diuretic therapy, *N Engl J Med* 339:387–402, 1998.
7. Sear JW: Kidney dysfunction in the postoperative period, *Br J Anaesth* 95:20–32, 2005.
8. ANZICS Clinical Trials Group: Low-dose dopamine in patients with early renal dysfunction: A placebo-controlled randomized trial, *Lancet* 356:2139–2143, 2000.
9. Friedrich JO, Adhikari N, Herridge MS, et al: Meta-analysis: Low dose dopamine increases urine output but does not prevent renal dysfunction or death, *Ann Intern Med* 142:510–524, 2005.
10. Landoni G, Biondi-Zoccai GG, Tumlin JA, et al: Beneficial impact of fenoldopam in critically ill patients with or at risk for acute renal failure: A meta-analysis of randomized clinical trials, *Am J Kidney Dis* 49:56–68, 2007.
11. Sladen RN: Anesthetic considerations for the patient with renal failure, *Anesthesiol Clin North Am* 18:863–882, 2000.
12. Moller S, Henriksen JH: Cardiovascular complications of cirrhosis, *Gut* 57:268–278, 2008.
13. Sundaram V, Shaikh OS: Hepatic encephalopathy: Pathophysiology and emerging therapies, *Med Clin North Am* 93:819–836, 2009.
14. Gines P, Cardenas A, Arroyo V, et al: Management of cirrhosis and ascites, *N Engl J Med* 350:1646–1654, 2004.
15. Schuppan D, Afdhal NH: Liver cirrhosis, *Lancet* 371:838–851, 2008.
16. Gines P, Schrier RW: Renal failure in cirrhosis, *N Engl J Med* 361:1279–1290, 2009.
17. Njoku D, Laster MJ, Gong DH, et al: Biotransformation of halothane, enflurane, isoflurane, and desflurane to trifluoroacetylated liver proteins: Association between protein acylation and hepatic injury, *Anesth Analg* 84:173–178, 1997.
18. Elliott RH, Strunin L: Hepatotoxicity of volatile anaesthetics, *Br J Anaesth* 70:339–348, 1993.

19. Muilenburg DJ, Singh A, Torzilli G, et al: Surgery in the patient with liver disease, *Anesthesiol Clin* 27:721–737, 2009.

20. Ziser A, Plevak DJ, Wiesner RH, et al: Morbidity and mortality in cirrhotic patients undergoing anesthesia and surgery, *Anesthesiology* 90:42–53, 1999.

21. Kosten TR, O'Connor PG: Management of drug and alcohol withdrawal, *N Engl J Med* 348:1786–1795, 2003.

22. Gerges FJ, Kanazi GE, Jabbour-Khoury SI: Anesthesia for laparoscopy: A review, *J Clin Anesth* 18:67–78, 2006.

23. Taylor E, Feinstein R, White PF, et al: Anesthesia for laparoscopic cholecystectomy. Is nitrous oxide contraindicated? *Anesthesiology* 76:541–543, 1992.

NUTRITIONAL AND GASTROINTESTINAL DISEASE

Steven A. Hyman and William R. Furman

NUTRITIONAL DISORDERS

Morbid Obesity

Approximately 1.7 billion people worldwide[1] are considered overweight, which is defined as a body mass index (BMI, weight in kg/height in m^2) more than 25 to 30. The Centers for Disease Control report that approximately 33% of U.S. adults older than 20 years of age are overweight and 34% are obese (BMI 30 to 40).[2,3] A desirable BMI is 18 to 25.[4] Morbid obesity is defined by a BMI of 40 or more. Superobesity (BMI $\geq$ 50) and super-superobesity (BMI $\geq$ 60) are an increasingly frequent health care challenge. The prevalence of obesity has doubled since 1980.

The morbidity associated with obesity can affect virtually any part of the body and may account for 2.5 million deaths per year. Pulmonary manifestations of obesity include a small residual volume (with rapidly decreasing oxygen saturations during apnea), restrictive lung disease, and obstructive sleep apnea. Hypertension, stroke, and right-sided heart failure are associated with morbid obesity, as are colon and breast cancer. Increased intra-abdominal pressure may predispose to hiatal hernias and gastroesophageal reflux. Skeletal diseases are also common, including back pain and osteoarthritis, particularly affecting the knees. Endocrine abnormalities may lead to reproductive hormonal imbalances and impaired fertility, and these patients may also be at increased risk for depression and other psychological illnesses.

The combination of many of the complications of obesity is now called the "metabolic syndrome." The metabolic syndrome has six components: abdominal obesity, atherogenic dyslipidemia, hypertension, insulin resistance (glucose intolerance), a proinflammatory state, and a prothrombotic state. The metabolic syndrome is diagnosed by the presence of three of the five following factors: abdominal obesity, increased triglycerides, low high-density lipids, hypertension, and increased fasting blood glucose levels. The diagnosis and treatment are important because obesity alone predicts approximately 25% of all new-onset cardiovascular disease.[5]

The pathophysiology of morbid obesity is multifactorial and involves genetic, environmental, metabolic, and psychosocial factors. Caloric consumption is important, but the urge to eat (or overeat) can be modulated by hormones[6] or inflammation.[7] Treatment must be multifaceted; weight loss is not as easy as simply not eating because fasting releases several orexigenic (appetite-stimulating) hormones.

PERIOPERATIVE CONSIDERATIONS

In the 1970s, fasted, obese patients were thought to have larger, more acidic gastric fluid volumes than nonobese patients and therefore would be at increased risk for pulmonary aspiration of gastric contents.[8] Actually just the opposite may be true. Nondiabetic obese patients may have a smaller volume at higher pH than do lean nondiabetic patients.[9]

Obesity may increase the risk of a difficult laryngeal intubation,[10-13] especially in males and patients with a higher Mallampati airway evaluation score.[14,15] Surprisingly, the time to tracheal intubation and the decreasing levels of SpO_2 (oxygen saturation as measured by pulse oximetry) levels are the same in obese patients as in lean ones.[10]

The care of obese patients present several logistical issues because of their size and shape. These issues include intravenous access, arterial blood pressure monitoring, positioning, endotracheal intubation and emergency techniques. Because of the amount of subcutaneous fat, peripheral intravenous line placement may be difficult. As a result, central venous catheterization may be required for access, independent of the nature of the surgical procedure. Arterial blood pressure monitoring may be made difficult by the conical shape of the upper arm. Most blood pressure cuffs are designed for a more cylindrical profile and may not remain in position or function correctly on a cone-shaped arm. Practical options in this situation include utilizing the forearm or inserting an arterial catheter for blood pressure monitoring.

An obese patient may be wider than the horizontal surface of the operating table, and the table must be able to support the patient's weight and be able to move into positions required by the surgeon. At times, extreme positions of tilt are needed, which demands that the patient be well secured and that potential pressure points be addressed.

Induction of anesthesia may be complicated by a rapid decrease in oxygen saturation owing to a smaller functional residual capacity. Reverse Trendelenburg position (head up) can be helpful in reducing atelectasis in dependent areas of the lung and may also move chest and breast tissue caudally, allowing easier access to the mouth for endotracheal intubation. No anesthetic drug has a distinct advantage in the obese patient, but emergence can be slow because elimination of some anesthetics from adipose tissues takes more time in patients with a smaller lean body mass.

BARIATRIC SURGERY

Surgical treatment of obesity was first described in 1954 with the creation of the jejunoileal bypass (JIB). The JIB was a malabsorptive operation that was used to treat everything from hyperlipidemia and atherosclerosis[16] to obesity.[17] The JIB was abandoned by the 1980s because of unacceptable complications, including uveitis, kidney dysfunction, intestinal bacterial overgrowth, and liver damage.

Subsequent operations were directed toward restriction of the intestinal tract with the goal of achieving weight loss through decreased intake. Examples of commonly performed restrictive operations are the gastric bypass, gastric sleeve, and adjustable gastric band. In 2006, there were approximately 177,000 bariatric operations performed, representing treatment of less than 1% of eligible patients in the United States. Each procedure has its own set of advantages, and the overall surgical risk is infrequent (0.17%, approximately the same as gallbladder surgery).

Most people who undergo bariatric procedures are morbidly obese (BMI $\geq$ 40), but surgical weight loss is more effective than conventional therapy if BMI is at 30 or higher. Patients generally have improvements in quality of life and reduced co-morbidities.[4,18] Bariatric surgery improves hypertension, diabetes, and obstructive sleep apnea.[19-22]

Appetite and insulin-regulating hormonal function may be changed by bariatric surgery, thus promoting weight loss. Ghrelin, an orexigenic hormone secreted by the gastric fundus and proximal small intestine, is increased in the face of nonsurgical weight loss, but ghrelin levels are either unchanged or decreased after bariatric procedures. Several other intestinal hormones that regulate appetite and glucose metabolism are affected more favorably by bariatric surgery than by fasting. These hormones include glucagon-like peptide-1, glucose-dependent insulinotropic peptide, and peptide YY, which are all secreted by the gastrointestinal tract in response to food.

Malnutrition

Malnutrition occurs when caloric requirements exceed intake. Decreased intake, impaired absorption, or increased metabolic rate may cause profound malnutrition in a very short time. Malnutrition may be present when there is weight loss of 10% to 20% over a short time, when weight is less than 90% of ideal body weight, or when BMI is less than 18.5. Healthy patients may quickly become malnourished after an accident or acute illness.

Critically ill patients develop malnutrition if they are not fed. Feeding may take place enterally, through an enteric feeding tube, or parenterally, through an intravenous catheter. The preferred method of nutritional replacement usually is enteral nutrition. Enteral feeding maintains the absorptive villi of the gastrointestinal tract and reduces pathologic bacterial transfer across the gastrointestinal mucosa and into the blood stream. Patient outcomes improve in terms of decreased infectious complications and fewer ventilator and intensive care unit days. Long-term feeding usually requires a gastrostomy or jejunostomy tube. Postpyloric placement is frequently preferred because it prevents regurgitation and possible aspiration of gastric contents. However, gastric feeding tubes have infrequent aspiration rates as well.[23] In patients who have pancreatitis, jejunal placement helps avoid stimulation of pancreatic enzyme secretions.

Intravenous feeding (total parenteral nutrition, or TPN) is required when the gastrointestinal tract is not functional. Peripheral parenteral nutrition may be used for brief periods, but long-term alimentation requires a central venous access device. TPN lacks the beneficial effects of enteral feeding on the gut and carries risks of catheter sepsis, thrombosis, hyperglycemia, iatrogenic hypoglycemia (from insulin added to the feeding solution in response to hyperglycemia), and fatty liver.

PERIOPERATIVE CONSIDERATIONS

Acute nutritional replacement in a malnourished patient may cause a refeeding syndrome, characterized by complications of increased ATP (adenosine triphosphate) production and metabolic rate. ATP production may cause a significant decrease in plasma phosphate, leading to respiratory and cardiac failure. An increased metabolic rate may cause a significant increase in CO_2 production, leading to respiratory acidosis. The refeeding syndrome can be avoided by slowly increasing the nutritional intake toward caloric goals.

In the perioperative setting malnourished patients may have muscular (including respiratory) weakness and may be immunocompromised. For severely malnourished patients, TPN or enteral feeding should be considered for 7 to 10 days prior to an elective surgical procedure as it takes several days to achieve goal feeding levels.

An important clinical issue commonly arises for enterally fed critically ill patients (such as burn and trauma patients) who require surgical treatment. A decision must be made regarding how long to fast such a patient prior to induction of anesthesia. The risk of pulmonary aspiration must be weighed against the benefit of continuing to keep the nutritional intake at the patient's goal level. In essence, nutrition should be continued as much as possible. A short fast (45 minutes) from nutritional administration should be done when the feeding tube is placed beyond the ligament of Treitz.[24] When TPN is in use, insulin is typically part of the infusion, and therefore, blood glucose monitoring should be done for procedures greater than 2 hours in duration.

GASTROINTESTINAL DISEASE

Inflammatory Bowel Disease

Inflammatory bowel disease (IBD) affects an estimated 1.5 million Americans and results from an aberrant response by the bowel mucosal immune system to normal luminal flora.[25,26] IBD is divided into two categories: ulcerative colitis (UC) and Crohn's disease (CD). UC is restricted to the large intestine and manifests itself as inflammation and loss of colonic mucosa. CD can affect any part of the digestive tract and may cause transmural inflammation leading to abscesses or granulomatous disease. Although they are distinct entities, distinction between the two diseases may be difficult when CD manifests itself by only affecting the colon.

The trigger for the activation of the immune system in IBD is multifactorial. There is evidence of a genetic basis for susceptibility to the disease and an increased risk in close family members. Caucasian patients are more likely to develop IBD than other patients. Jewish patients have a more frequent risk for CD. In addition, several environmental factors including smoking, appendectomy, antibiotics, oral contraceptives, and nonsteroidal anti-inflammatory drugs (NSAIDs) are associated with increased risk. Diagnosis may be suspected based on symptoms of chronic abdominal pain, fever, and diarrhea and is confirmed by endoscopy and biopsy.

Although the primary mode of therapy is nonoperative, 60% to 70% of patients with IBD require surgical treatment at some point. Reasons include complications of the disease (fistulas, strictures, or toxic megacolon), complications of surgery (small bowel obstruction due to postoperative scarring), cancer prevention (colectomy in the case of UC), plus other reasons unrelated to the intestinal disease.

PERIOPERATIVE CONSIDERATIONS

CD and UC are chronic diseases that are typically managed by using up to six different classes of medications: antidiarrheal, anti-inflammatory, immunosuppressant, antibiotic, anti-TNF (tumor necrosis factor), and other investigational drugs. Patients who are taking steroids should continue to do so prior to surgery and may require supplementation in anticipation of adrenal insufficiency.

Specific anesthetics are neither preferred nor contraindicated for patients with IBD, but certain of their medications may have anesthetic implications. In general, potential interactions between anesthetic and antineoplastic drugs are not clear.[27] Cyclosporine increases the minimum alveolar concentration (MAC) of volatile

IV

anesthetics[28] and possibly barbiturates or fentanyl.[29] Azathioprine has phosphodiesterase effects and may partially antagonize nondepolarizing neuromuscular blockade.[30,31] Cyclosporine and infliximab may enhance the nondepolarizing neuromuscular blocking drugs,[32,33] as may aminoglycoside antibiotics. The clinical consequences of these interactions is minimal.

Gastroesophageal Reflux Disease

Gastroesophageal reflux disease (GERD) is defined as the retrograde movement of gastric contents through the lower esophageal sphincter (LES) into the esophagus.[34] Retrograde movement of gastric contents past both the LES and the upper esophageal sphincter into the pharynx can lead to pulmonary aspiration of gastric acid and particulate matter.

GERD is an extremely common syndrome. In the general population, 20% of people have heartburn (the most reliable symptom) at least once per week and 4% to 10% have heartburn daily. Besides heartburn, the most common symptoms are noncardiac chest pain, dysphagia, pharyngitis, cough, asthma, hoarseness, laryngitis, sinusitis, and dental erosions.

Reflux occurs when the LES is incompetent or when LES pressure (LESP) is less than intra-abdominal (or intra-gastric) pressure. GERD can occur as a result of esophageal dysmotility or a hiatal hernia. In a patient with a hiatal hernia, the LES may be displaced cephalad into the thoracic cavity so that it loses the diaphragmatic contribution to LES function. The diaphragm can also obstruct the esophagus. GERD is associated with other conditions, including pregnancy, obesity, obstructive sleep apnea, gastric hypersecretion, gastric outlet obstruction, gastric neuropathy, and increased intra-abdominal pressure. The risk of pulmonary aspiration of gastric contents during induction of anesthesia in patients with GERD, or the above mentioned predisposing factors is not well established. In contrast, increased intra-abdominal (gastric) pressure and pregnancy are important risk factors. Significant GERD occurs with at least 30% to 50% of pregnant women. The mechanism is primarily a progesterone-mediated relaxation of LES tone, but there also may be contributions from delayed gastric emptying, and decreased bowel transit.[35]

Initial management of GERD usually consists of a combination of lifestyle management and drug therapy using medications that are moderately effective and have limited side effects. Lifestyle management includes elevating the head of the bed, eating food high in proteins and red pepper, and avoiding smoking, coffee, and foods and drugs known to relax the LES. Symptoms may be relieved by antacids and mucoprotective drugs, but if not, further medical management includes prokinetic drugs and drugs that reduce gastric acid secretion.

Prokinetics minimize contact time of gastric contents with the esophagus by blocking dopamine or serotonin (5-HT) receptors. Metoclopramide (a 5-HT receptor antagonist) can produce choreoathetosis and other extrapyramidal side effects. Histamine (H_2) receptor blockers decrease gastric acid secretion by gastric parietal cells; however, they may increase the production of gastrin and decrease LES pressure.[36] In some patients, particularly the elderly, H_2 receptor blocking drugs may cause adverse central nervous system side effects including confusion, agitation, and psychosis.[37] Proton pump inhibitors (PPIs) are the most potent therapy for severe erosive esophagitis. Omeprazole may inhibit the metabolism and elimination of warfarin, digoxin, phenytoin, and benzodiazepines.

PERIOPERATIVE CONSIDERATIONS

The customary approach to induction of general anesthesia in the patient at risk for pulmonary aspiration of gastric acid is the rapid sequence induction (RSI) using cricoid pressure (CP) to obstruct any potential flow of gastric contents into the pharynx and trachea (also see Chapter 14). The putative benefits of the RSI and CP remain controversial.[38] CP can be ineffective, especially if not properly applied, and can have undesired side effects including potentially increasing the risk of regurgitation and of failed tracheal intubation.[39] Furthermore, improperly performed CP sometimes might not properly align the cricoid and esophagus with the solid cervical spine underneath.[40] However, the significance of this failure of alignment is by no means a settled issue. One view is that if the cricoid and esophagus are displaced laterally, they may be over muscle and might not occlude the upper esophagus.[41] However the exact opposite view, that lateral displacement does not impair barrier function, has also been articulated.[40,42]

CP is not a benign procedure and can be associated with several complications (Table 29-1). Also, complications are more likely in the elderly, children, pregnant women, patients with cervical injury, and patients with difficult airways, and when there is difficulty palpating the cricoid cartilage.

Surgical management of symptomatic reflux disease may be treated with an antireflux operation—most commonly the Nissen fundoplication in adults. This operation is typically performed laparoscopically. The Nissen fundoplication consists of reducing the herniated stomach, repairing the diaphragmatic defect, and performing a gastric wrap to prevent the stomach and LES from retracting into the thorax. Important postoperative events include discomfort from carbon dioxide gas accumulation under the diaphragm and postoperative nausea and vomiting. Subcutaneous air may also appear in the neck and chest. This is benign and self-limited because CO_2 gas is rapidly reabsorbed by the body. Likewise, pneumoperitoneum and pneumomediastinum are common, occurring in up to 86% of patients due to dissection of the phrenoesophageal

Table 29-1 Categories of Patients at Risk from Inappropriately Applied Cricoid Pressure

Patient Group at Risk	Reason
Elderly	Esophageal rupture, laryngeal obstruction
Children	Laryngeal obstruction
Parturient	May require more pressure
Laryngeal trauma	May require surgical repair after cricoid pressure
Cervical spine trauma	May displace an unstable cervical spine
Difficult airway	May worsen visualization

Adapted from Brimacombe JR, Berry AM. Cricoid pressure. Can J Anaesth 1997;44:414-425.

ligament.[43] Pneumothorax, in contrast, is not a normal consequence of laparoscopic surgery. Nausea and vomiting are more serious complications in the setting of esophageal surgery, as esophageal rupture could be the result.

ENDOCRINE DISORDERS

Diabetes Mellitus

Diabetes mellitus is characterized by increased blood glucose levels due to a relative lack of endogenous insulin. It affects 15 to 20 million Americans (7% to 8% of the population) and complicates most organ systems.[44] Previously, diabetes was classified in terms of insulin requirement (insulin-dependent versus non–insulin-dependent) but this system has proved less satisfactory because nearly all diabetics develop a need for insulin at some point. The current classification is type 1 (T1DM) or type 2 (T2DM) diabetes.[45] T1DM is typically characterized by the absence of insulin production from the pancreas, whereas T2DM involves a relative lack of insulin plus resistance to endogenous insulin.

Blood glucose control is required in both types, but T1DM always requires insulin to prevent hyperglycemia, ketoacidosis, and other complications. Type 2 diabetics may require insulin, but often only require oral hypoglycemic agents, weight loss, or dietary management. Type 1 diabetes is commonly heralded at an early age by a dramatic episode of ketoacidosis. The onset of T2DM usually is more insidious. Type 2 diabetics constitute the majority and, unlike type 1 diabetics, are often overweight. Dietary control and weight loss are important in T2DM, but the cornerstone of management of both types is pharmacologic.

Insulin is categorized as rapid, intermediate, or long acting. In the outpatient setting it is usually given by subcutaneous injection. For tight control, especially for type 1 diabetics, rapid-acting insulin may be administered by a continuous infusion pump that is worn by the patient. Although insulin may be used in T2DM as one of several treatment options, it is essential in T1DM for normoglycemia and to prevent ketoacidosis because these patients always have an insulin requirement.

Oral drugs influence diabetes by several mechanisms. Glyburide and repaglinide increase pancreatic insulin production; metformin reduces glucose load by decreasing hepatic production; acarbose reduces intestinal absorption; and, rosiglitazone increases glucose uptake by fat and muscle.

During hyperglycemia, glucose can permanently combine with hemoglobin in erythrocytes and form hemoglobin A_{1c} (glycohemoglobin). Because erythrocytes normally have a 120-day lifespan, Hb A_{1c} levels give an indication of how well the diabetes is being controlled over time. Normal Hb A_{1c} levels are less than 6%, and risk of complications of diabetes increases with increasing Hb A_{1c} levels.

Complications are common in long-standing diabetes and result largely from microangiopathy and macroangiopathy. Diabetes is a well-recognized risk factor for large and small vessel coronary artery disease, and was originally advanced as an indication for perioperative β-adrenergic blockade.[46,47] Diabetes in young and-middle-aged adults is the leading cause of renal failure requiring hemodialysis. Retinopathy occurs in 80% to 90% of those who require insulin for at least 20 years. Autonomic neuropathy occurs in 20% to 40% of patients with long-standing diabetes, particularly those with peripheral sensory neuropathy, renal failure, or systemic hypertension. Cardiac autonomic neuropathy may mask angina pectoris and obscure the presence of coronary artery disease. Gastroparesis, which may cause delayed gastric emptying, is a sign of autonomic neuropathy affecting the vagus nerves.

PERIOPERATIVE CONSIDERATIONS

A patient with well-controlled diabetes may not require special treatment before and during surgery, although reducing the morning dose of insulin by 30% to 50% in order to prevent hypoglycemia due to fasting is common. Sulfonylurea drugs may be continued until the evening before surgery; however, these drugs may also produce hypoglycemia in the absence of morning caloric intake.

Recommendations regarding biguanides such as metformin have changed in recent years. The first biguanide introduced, phenformin, was associated with lactic acidosis and was eventually replaced in clinical use by metformin. In the 1990s, a common recommendation was made for metformin to be discontinued 48 hours preoperatively to avoid risk of fatal lactic acidosis. This recommendation was based on case reports[48,49] and was questioned in a recent metaanalysis.[50]

IV

Preoperative measurement of blood glucose is usually performed prior to anesthesia; however, the desired intra-operative glucose level is not clear. Perioperative concerns related to increased glucose levels include the risk of diabetic ketoacidosis, the risk of severe dehydration and coma related to the hyperosmolar hyperglycemic nonketotic state, the adverse effect of hyperglycemia on neurologic outcome after cerebral ischemia,[51,52] and the impact of hyperglycemia on the risk of surgical wound infection. The optimal level of glucose control in the perioperative and critical care setting remains controversial. Attempts to maintain glucose levels less than 108 mg/dL in critically ill patients may result in more frequent cardiovascular mortality rates compared to those patients in whom the level was controlled in the 140 to180 mg/dL range.[53,54]

Hyperthyroidism and Thyroid Storm

Hyperthyroidism, or thyrotoxicosis, is characterized by increasing circulating levels of unbound thyroid hormones triiodothyronine (T_3) and tetraiodothyronine (thyroxine, or T_4). The most common cause is Graves' disease, an autoimmune condition in which thyrotropin receptor antibodies continuously mimic the effect of thyroid-stimulating hormone (TSH). However, it may also be caused by the following:

- Struma ovarii, which is the presence of thyroid tissue in an ovarian teratoma
- Human chorionic gonadotropin (hCG)–secreting hydatidiform mole[55]
- Pregnancy, because hCG has weak TSH activity[56]
- The administration of iodinated contrast dye to a susceptible patient
- Amiodarone (which can lead to both hypo- and hyperthyroidism)

The principal signs and symptoms of hyperthyroidism are cardiac, neurologic, and constitutional.[57] Thyroid hormone increases cardiac sensitivity to catecholamines, resulting in hypertension and tachyarrhythmias. Other signs of severe hyperthyroidism include high-output congestive heart failure or angina,[58] even in the absence of coronary plaques. Tremor, hyperreflexia, and irritability are common neurologic manifestations. Periodic paralysis, characterized by hypokalemia and proximal muscle weakness, may also occur. Fever and heat intolerance are common. Gastrointestinal symptoms include nausea, vomiting, and diarrhea as well as hepatic dysfunction and jaundice. Diagnosis is confirmed by demonstrating increased thyroid hormone levels in blood.[59]

Thyroid storm is characterized by worsening of the signs and symptoms of thyrotoxicosis, including severe cardiac dysfunction, hyperglycemia, hypercalcemia, hyperbilirubinemia, altered mental status, seizures, and coma. It may be triggered in a thyrotoxic patient by any of several stresses:

- Infection
- Stroke
- Trauma, especially to the thyroid gland[60]
- Surgery
- Diabetic ketoacidosis
- Drugs: pseudoephedrine, aspirin, excess iodine intake, contrast dye, amiodarone
- Incorrect antithyroid drug discontinuation

The distinction between thyrotoxicosis and thyroid storm is one of degree, with thyroid storm being the most severe form of the disorder. All hyperthyroid patients are at risk to develop thyroid storm, which is a life-threatening emergent clinical syndrome that has a ~30% mortality rate in spite of treatment. For this reason, the general rule regarding surgery in the setting of thyrotoxicosis or thyroid storm is to undertake only that which cannot be delayed until control of thyroid hormone secretion and effect has been accomplished, either with medical management or through ablation of the thyroid using radioiodine.

PERIOPERATIVE CONSIDERATIONS

The initial medical treatment for hyperthyroidism is to reduce thyroid hormone synthesis. This is accomplished by administration of a thioamide such as propylthiouracil (PTU) or methimazole (MMI). PTU and MMI inhibit thyroid peroxidase (TPO), the enzyme that catalyzes the incorporation of iodide into thyroglobulin to produce T_3 and T_4. At least an hour after giving the thioamide, large doses of stable iodide may be given. This step takes advantage of a paradoxical effect, called the Wolff-Chaikoff effect.[57] Rather than catalyze additional incorporation of iodide into thyroglobulin, as might be expected, large amounts of iodide suppress gene transcription of TPO, further reducing the gland's capacity to produce and release hormone. This benefit is temporary, lasting about a week.

In addition, especially in cases of thyroid storm, β-adrenergic blockade is used to reduce adrenergic symptoms. Propranolol is the β-blocker traditionally selected because it also inhibits peripheral conversion of T_4 to the more potent hormone T_3; however, other β-adrenergic blockers such as atenolol, metoprolol, and esmolol have been used and are not contraindicated. Corticosteroids are recommended to treat the relative adrenal insufficiency that results from accelerated metabolism in the context of thyroid storm. Cortisol levels tend to be in the normal range in these patients, but they ought to be higher to be appropriate to the level of stress. Plasmapheresis has been utilized as an adjunct method to reduce circulating thyroid hormone levels by removing T_3 and T_4 from the blood stream.[61]

The goal of anesthesia is to avoid an increase in heart rate or sympathetic activation. Conversely, anesthetics and techniques that reduce or blunt sympathetic activity are usually favored. If correct, ketamine would not be ideal to induce anesthesia or provide analgesia. Rather, fentanyl and its congeners would be favored for analgesia. Isoflurane, sevoflurane, and desflurane would all be useful for maintenance of general anesthesia, with the warning that high inspiratory concentrations of desflurane might not be advantageous. Regional anesthesia, when practical, might also be efficacious in avoiding sympathetic activation. Intraoperative thyroid storm may be difficult to distinguish from malignant hyperthermia. Dantrolene is beneficial in either situation and should be considered if there is suspicion of either condition.[62]

Hypothyroidism

Hypothyroidism is characterized by decreased circulating levels of unbound thyroid hormones triiodothyronine (T_3) and tetraiodothyronine (thyroxine, or T_4). Hypothyroidism may be congenital (cretinism) or acquired. The most common acquired cause in adults is Hashimoto's thyroiditis, a chronic autoimmune disease characterized by progressive destruction of the thyroid gland. Medical or surgical treatment of hyperthyroidism may lead to iatrogenic hypothyroidism. Hypothyroidism after radioactive iodine treatment of hyperthyroidism occurs in at least 50% of patients within 10 years after treatment. Secondary hypothyroidism may occur as a consequence of hypothalamic or pituitary disease or after surgery on these structures. The absence of dietary iodine causes hypothyroidism and an enlarged gland ("endemic goiter").

The onset of hypothyroidism usually is insidious and the symptoms are often nonspecific. Adults may have easy fatigability, lethargy, weakness, and weight gain. The skin is usually dry and the hair brittle. In severe cases, myxedema develops and is characterized by a reduced cardiac output, attenuated deep tendon reflexes, and nonpitting pretibial edema. Untreated, hypothyroidism may progress to include electrolyte disturbance, hypoventilation, hypothermia, and coma. Laboratory diagnosis is confirmed by measuring low T_3 and T_4 levels in blood. Primary hypothyroidism is diagnosed by low T_3 and T_4 levels but an elevated TSH. In secondary hypothyroidism, all thyroid-related hormones are reduced. Subclinical hypothyroidism, manifested as an increased plasma TSH concentration, is present in about 5% of the American population, with a prevalence of more than 13% in otherwise healthy elderly patients, especially women.[63]

Hypothyroidism is treated with oral administration of synthetic levothyroxine, 75 to 150 mg/day. Thyroid replacement is initiated slowly because acute cardiac ischemia can develop in patients with coronary artery disease from the sudden increase in myocardial oxygen demand as the metabolism and cardiac output increase. Although intravenous thyroid replacement therapy is available, its use is limited to severe presentations such as myxedema coma.

PERIOPERATIVE CONSIDERATIONS
Asymptomatic mild to moderate hypothyroidism does not increase the risk of perioperative morbidity.[64] Mildly hypothyroid patients do not possess unusual sensitivity to inhaled anesthetics, sedatives, or narcotics. Symptomatic or severe hypothyroidism in contrast should necessitate surgical delay for thyroid hormone replacement until the neurologic and cardiovascular abnormalities have resolved.

Thyroid Surgery

The most important perioperative considerations related to thyroid surgery involve physical or functional airway obstruction from tracheal compression or damage to the recurrent laryngeal nerves. Prior to surgery an enlarged thyroid gland may deviate or compress the trachea. This may cause patients with goiters to experience difficulty breathing, especially when sleeping supine or during the induction of general anesthesia. In terms of postoperative management, because a neck hematoma poses a risk of airway obstruction, the technique of extubating the trachea during a deep level of anesthesia may minimize coughing and straining, and thus reduce the likelihood of increased venous and arterial pressures in the neck.

Unilateral laryngeal nerve injuries from thyroid surgery produce voice impairment but are not a threat to airway function. Bilateral recurrent laryngeal nerve injury, in contrast, compromises the function of the posterior cricoarytenoid muscles, which are the muscles responsible for separating the cords during breathing. This can lead to life-threatening inspiratory airway obstruction that can only be relieved by intubation or tracheostomy. In such patients, the paralyzed vocal cords do not abduct during the respiratory cycle, and may appear apposed in the midline when seen during direct laryngoscopy.

Some surgeons request the use of a laryngeal nerve monitoring endotracheal tube during thyroid surgery as a putative safety measure to prevent inadvertent injury to the laryngeal nerves. These specialized endotracheal tubes have electrodes that are positioned in the immediate vicinity of the vocal cords and send an electromyographic signal to a receiver whenever the vocal cords contract. As a result, if the surgeon stimulates a laryngeal nerve either by retracting it or by using an electrocautery close to it, an audible signal provides a warning.

Pheochromocytoma and Paraganglioma

Tumor overproduction of any of the adrenal medullary hormones dopamine, norepinephrine, and epinephrine results in hypertension and tachycardia plus cardiovascular

IV

hyperresponsiveness to noxious stimulation. The cells that produce these hormones are of neural crest origin. When the tumor arises in the adrenal medulla, it is called a pheochromocytoma; when it arises from ganglia of the sympathetic nervous system, it is called a paraganglioma. The biologic behavior is the same in either case. Life-threatening hypertensive crises and tachyarrhythmias may occur, especially during surgery on a previously undiagnosed patient. Pheochromocytoma often goes unrecognized because its symptoms (headache, palpitations, sweating) are nonspecific and as many as 8% are asymptomatic. Its prevalence in the general population may be as high as 1 in 2000.[65]

Hypertension probably occurs because arteriolar smooth muscle has been exposed to norepinephrine, the neurotransmitter for sympathetic nervous system mediated vasoconstriction. According to this theory, tumor-secreted norepinephrine bathes the synapses directly. But if this were true, the production of norepinephrine by the sympathetic nerves should be suppressed and sympathetic nervous system activity should not be able to regulate arterial blood pressure; instead the circulating hormones would do so.[66] This theory has prompted the practice of preoperative α-adrenergic blockade with phenoxybenzamine prior to tumor resection as well as the unproven beliefs that blood catecholamine levels correlate with blood pressure levels and that hypertension occurs when the surgeon manipulates the tumor because this manipulation squeezes hormones out of the tumor and into the blood stream.

Other interpretations are likely. Catecholamine levels do not correlate with the time or magnitude of arterial blood pressure elevation,[67] and clinical experience is that 2 weeks of preoperative treatment with nonselective α-adrenergic blockade is commonly ineffective for prevention of intraoperative hypertension. An alternative approach to preoperative preparation should be considered.[68] Hypertension, if present, is controlled prior to surgery with any of a variety of drugs, and once arterial blood pressure is under reasonable control, the tumor is resected. There is, however, no basis to expect that arterial blood pressure and heart rate may not be labile during the surgery no matter what the pretreatment is.

An alternate theory of why adrenergic receptor blockade is not fully effective is that the effect of chronic catecholamine excess is to amplify the sympathetic nervous system's responses to all forms of physical stimulation. This would include hypertension and tachycardia from laryngoscopy and any surgical manipulations. These hemodynamic responses may be seen in any patient, but the effect is exaggerated under the influence of high catecholamine levels. Such a theory is supported by animal data[69] suggesting that, despite chronic catecholamine excess, sympathetic nerves remain active and continue to release mediators that influence or even control blood pressure. The failure of competitive receptor blockade might be explained by the ability of the sympathetic nervous system to overwhelm the competitive blockade by releasing norepinephrine in quantities that are much greater than normal.

PERIOPERATIVE CONSIDERATIONS

In theory, the nonspecific α-blocking drug phenoxybenzamine should not be chosen because it has $α_2$-blocking properties. Since $α_2$-agonists generally produce bradycardia, sedation, and decreased arterial blood pressure, blocking the $α_2$-receptor should increase arterial blood pressure and heart rate. Nevertheless, phenoxybenzamine is often recommended by authors and clinicians. For the chronic treatment of patients with unresectable catecholamine-secreting tumors, its long pharmacologic half-life is desirable. However, phenoxybenzamine is very expensive, and many less costly alternatives exist for preoperative blood pressure control. Each of the $α_1$-selective blockers (prazosin, doxazosin, terazosin), calcium channel blockers, angiotensin-converting enzyme (ACE) inhibitors and angiotensin receptor blockers, β-adrenergic blockers, and $α_2$-agonists has been used prior to adrenalectomy.[68] Intraoperative infusions of vasodilators and esmolol still may be required to treat hypertension or tachycardia, and infusions of magnesium[70] and the $α_2$-agonist dexmedetomidine[71] may be useful as well.

Multiple Endocrine Neoplasia and Neuroendocrine Tumors

There are two groups of multiple endocrine neoplasia (MEN) syndromes. These were originally called Wermer's syndrome and Sipple's syndrome, but are now known as MEN I and MEN II, respectively.

MEN I

This syndrome includes the triad of tumors of the pancreas, pituitary, and parathyroid glands and is inherited as an autosomal dominant trait.[72] The most common tumor is a parathyroid adenoma, which is present in 95% of MEN I patients and usually presents as hypercalcemia. All four parathyroid glands usually are removed surgically because all are involved by the disease.

Pancreatic tumors in MEN I patients are usually adenomas that secrete an excess of a specific hormone. Gastrin secretion is most common, occurring in approximately 50%, but insulin, glucagon, vasoactive intestinal polypeptide, and pancreatic polypeptide secreting tumors are seen. Pituitary tumors most commonly secrete prolactin (60%) or growth hormone (25%). A small number secrete adrenocorticotropic hormone, with the balance being nonfunctioning adenomas. Other tumors in MEN I include adrenal cortical adenomas, carcinoids and neuroendocrine tumors, lipomas, angiofibromas, and collagenomas. There are no specific anesthetic implications of MEN I.

MEN II

Medullary (solid) thyroid carcinomas (MTCs) are a component of two endocrine syndromes, which are now called MEN IIA and MEN IIB. MEN IIA, includes pheochromocytoma, MTC, and parathyroid adenoma. MEN IIB includes mucosal neuromas, pheochromocytoma, and MTC. These patients may have a marfanoid habitus and other mesodermal abnormalities. Unlike patients with MEN I, they do not develop parathyroid adenomas. A third subtype of MEN II is characterized only by familial MTC. All the MEN II subtypes are autosomal dominant conditions caused by germline activating mutations in the *RET* proto-oncogene on chromosome 10.[73] The overall prevalence is approximately 0.003%, or 1 in 35,000. The anesthetic implications of MEN II are related to its components and associated conditions.

Von Hippel–Lindau disease, which may include cerebellar tumors, is associated with MEN II and pheochromocytomas. MTC, which accounts for only 5% of all thyroid tumors, is commonly malignant and is the most common cause of death in MEN II patients. A patient of any age with MTC is therefore likely to undergo thyroidectomy, and may be at risk to have an undiagnosed pheochromocytoma at the time of surgery.

NEUROENDOCRINE TUMORS

Carcinoid and neuroendocrine tumors arise from dispersed cells of neural crest embryologic origin.[74] The normal function of these cells is to synthesize serotonin from the essential amino acid tryptophan. When these tumors arise in the midgut, they are called carcinoid tumors. When they arise elsewhere in the body, the current terminology is for them to be called neuroendocrine tumors.

The biochemical behavior of these tumors is to overproduce serotonin in preference to the normal products of tryptophan metabolism, including niacin (vitamin B_3). In rare instances, patients may therefore develop symptomatic niacin deficiency (pellagra), but this is rare. Most commonly, midgut carcinoid tumors are asymptomatic until they cause bowel obstruction or appendicitis because their venous drainage is via the portal vein to the liver, which detoxifies the excess serotonin they produce. When the tumors arise outside the drainage field of the hepatic portal venous system, or when metastatic disease has replaced so much of the liver as to compromise hepatic synthetic function, systemic symptoms of serotonin excess occur. This is known as the "carcinoid syndrome" and is characterized by diarrhea, flushing, palpitations, and bronchoconstriction. Medical management with octreotide may help ameliorate these symptoms.

PERIOPERATIVE CONSIDERATIONS

The direct hemodynamic effects of serotonin are not problematic in the context of perioperative anesthetic care, and an escalation of hemodynamic monitoring is seldom required as a consequence of the endocrine activity of the tumor. However, right-sided valvular heart disease should be suspected in these patients and echocardiography considered as a diagnostic tool. Right-sided heart failure, due to the sclerosing effect of serotonin on the tricuspid and pulmonary valves, ultimately may be the cause of death in 50% of patients with the carcinoid syndrome.

Adrenal Insufficiency and Steroid Replacement

The principal hormones secreted by the adrenal cortex are cortisol and aldosterone. Cortisol production is stimulated by blood concentrations of pituitary adrenocorticotropic hormone (ACTH), which is in turn secreted in response to hypothalamic corticotropin-releasing hormone (CRH). Stress stimulates the hypothalamus to release CRH, and blood cortisol levels exert negative feedback influence on the production of both CRH and ACTH.[75] Chronic insufficient cortisol production and secretion, with or without aldosterone insufficiency, is referred to as Addison's syndrome.

The symptoms of chronic adrenal insufficiency are nonspecific. They include fatigue, malaise, lethargy, weight loss, anorexia, arthralgias, myalgias, nausea, vomiting, abdominal pain, diarrhea, and fever. In primary adrenocortical insufficiency, due to nonfunction of the adrenal glands, hyponatremia and hyperkalemia due to concomitant aldosterone deficiency may be seen. In secondary or tertiary insufficiency, due to failure of the hypothalamus or pituitary to stimulate the adrenal glands, or when cortisol production is suppressed by exogenously administered steroid medications, aldosterone production is unimpaired. This is because the stimulus for aldosterone production is the renin-angiotensin system. Common etiologies of primary chronic adrenal insufficiency are immunologic (autoantibody), malignant (metastatic cancer, commonly from lung or breast), and infectious (such as tuberculosis).

Cortisol maintains homeostasis of the cardiovascular system, especially in the presence of stress. It maintains vascular tone, endothelial integrity, and the distribution of total body water in the vascular compartment. It reduces vascular permeability and it potentiates the vasoconstrictor effects of catecholamines. When cortisol levels are deficient, systemic vascular resistance and myocardial contractility are decreased.[76]

The term acute adrenal failure, or addisonian crisis, refers to circulatory shock due to cortisol deficiency. This generally occurs in the presence of primary adrenal insufficiency with a superimposed acute stress such as trauma, surgery, or infection and is characterized by hypovolemic shock with myocardial and vascular unresponsiveness to catecholamines. Treatment usually requires the intravenous infusion of several liters of isotonic saline and corticosteroid administration. In an adult, 100 mg of IV cortisol (or the equivalent every 6 to 8 hours) usually reverses the

Table 29-2 Relative Equivalent Potencies of Common Corticosteroid Drugs

Agent	Equivalent Dose (mg)	Relative Potency	Duration (hr)
Hydrocortisone	100	1	8-12
Cortisone	125	0.8	8-12
Prednisone; prednisolone	25	4	12-36
Methylprednisolone	20	5	12-36
Dexamethasone	4	25	>24

pathophysiology within the first day of treatment. Orally administered drugs can be started in 1 to 4 days. The equivalent doses of these drugs are expressed using hydrocortisone, the synthetic form of cortisol, with 100 mg as the standard for comparison (Table 29-2).

Critical illness-related corticosteroid insufficiency (CIRCI) applies to clinical situations in which 100 to 300 mg/day of IV hydrocortisone eliminates a preexisting need for vasopressors.[77] The implication is that the patient may not meet traditional criteria for adrenocortical dysfunction, but the adrenal response to critical illness and other stresses is inadequate. Prior steroid treatment is a potential cause of this condition. Signs and symptoms may include unexplained vasopressor-dependent refractory hypotension, a discrepancy between the anticipated severity of the patient's disease and the present state of the patient, high fever without apparent cause or not responding to antibiotics, hypoglycemia, hyponatremia, hyperkalemia, neutropenia, and eosinophilia.

PERIOPERATIVE CONSIDERATIONS

Etomidate (also see Chapter 9) is a relatively noncardiovascular depressant anesthetic that can suppress adrenal cortical function. This is a significant but transient effect (<24 hours) even after a single dose of the drug. It can be clinically significant in the setting of CIRCI. Perhaps an anesthetic can be developed with the advantages of etomidate but without its adrenal suppressing effects.[78]

Steroid replacement for the patient who has received exogenous steroids and may have adrenal insufficiency should be adequate but not excessive. The proper dose of replacement steroids is based on surgical research in primates[79] showing that ten times the normal cortisol production rate was not superior to simply replacing the normal daily production of cortisol.

Steroid-induced adrenal suppression is highly variable and its duration is unpredictable (days to perhaps years). The consequences of a short course of steroids are minimal, so anticipatory treatment is generally safe. Daily cortisol production rate is between 20 and 30 mg/day.[80] In surgical patients the recommended approach is to begin at the time of surgery with a dose between one and five times the daily production (no more than 100 to 150 mg of cortisol equivalent) per day and administer tapered replacement over 48 to 72 hours.[81]

Pituitary Apoplexy

Acute pituitary hemorrhage, swelling, and infarction (pituitary apoplexy) is an exception to the general rule that adrenal crisis is not usually associated with secondary adrenal hypofunction. Pituitary apoplexy is a potentially life-threatening condition that can lead to sudden total loss of all anterior and posterior pituitary hormonal secretion and severe hypoglycemia, hypotension, central nervous system hemorrhage, cerebral edema, and loss of vision (often bitemporal hemianopia).

Two well-known causes of spontaneous pituitary apoplexy are infarction of a large pituitary adenoma and postpartum hypotensive pituitary necrosis (Sheehan's syndrome). Other associations include diabetes, hypertension, sickle cell anemia, and acute shock. Acute pituitary hemorrhage into an unsuspected pituitary adenoma has also been reported following cardiopulmonary bypass.[82,83]

Signs and symptoms of pituitary apoplexy include severe headache, meningeal irritation, bitemporal hemianopia, ophthalmoplegia, cardiovascular collapse, and loss of consciousness. Computed tomography or magnetic resonance imaging most often confirms the diagnosis. Corticosteroid replacement is the first line of treatment, both for the resulting adrenal insufficiency and for brain swelling. If there is significant visual loss or mental status alteration, acute surgical decompression may be required.

Cushing's Syndrome

Cushing's syndrome is characterized by elevated cortisol levels in the blood. Primary Cushing's syndrome is independent of pituitary ACTH secretion, while secondary and tertiary disease is due to increased circulating levels of ACTH or an ACTH-like substance produced by a tumor. The primary condition is usually due to a hyperfunctioning adrenal gland or adenoma. The term Cushing's disease usually refers to one specific form of secondary Cushing's syndrome, that of adrenal cortical hyperfunction due to excess production of ACTH by a pituitary adenoma, which accounts for 60% to 70% of Cushing's syndrome patients.[84] The remainder of the patients with secondary or tertiary Cushing's syndrome have abnormal ACTH production from ectopic sources such as primary or metastatic cancers of the lung (usually small-cell), thyroid, or prostate,[85] tumors of the pancreas,[86] or intrathoracic neuroendocrine tumors[87] and have an elevated ACTH due to hypothalamic oversecretion of corticotropic releasing hormone. Cushing's syndrome may also be caused by exogenous administration of cortisol-like medications or synthetic ACTH.

Patients with Cushing's syndrome are often recognizable by a physical appearance that consists of rounding of the face, truncal obesity and thin extremities, an upper thoracic fat pad or "buffalo hump," purple abdominal striae, and thinning of the skin. The physiologic effects of chronic elevated corticosteroid levels include weight gain, hypertension, hypercoagulability, muscular weakness, glucose intolerance, gonadal dysfunction, and osteoporosis.[84,88] Biochemical diagnosis is made by measuring an elevated 24-hour urinary free cortisol.

There is no definitive medical treatment for Cushing's syndrome. Effective treatment requires removal of the source of the elevated hormone production, followed by corticosteroid replacement therapy if necessary. Anesthetic management of Cushing's patients may be associated with differences as compared to normal patients. For example, they may be more susceptible to the effects of muscle relaxants and subject to unanticipated postoperative respiratory failure, even after laparoscopic surgery.[89]

QUESTIONS OF THE DAY

1. What are the primary manifestations of the "metabolic syndrome"?
2. What are the risks and benefits of cricoid pressure and rapid sequence intubation in patients with gastroesophageal reflux disease (GERD)?
3. What are the potential adverse effects of perioperative hyperglycemia? What are the risks of "tight" glucose control in the perioperative period?
4. What are the signs and symptoms of thyrotoxicosis? How should a patient with thyrotoxicosis or thyroid storm be treated prior to urgent or emergent surgery?
5. What are the classic manifestations of carcinoid syndrome? What is the appropriate medical management?
6. What are the clinical findings in critical illness-related corticosteroid insufficiency?

ACKNOWLEDGMENTS

The editors and publisher would like to thank Dr. Ludwig Lin for contributing a chapter on this topic to the prior edition of this work. It has served as the foundation for the current chapter.

IV

REFERENCES

1. Buchwald H, Avidor Y, Braunwald E, et al: Bariatric surgery: A systematic review and meta-analysis, *JAMA* 292:1724–1737, 2004.
2. CDC: *Prevalence of overweight, obesity, and extreme obesity among adults: United States, trends 1960-1962 through 2005-2006.* Nov. 18, 2009. Available from http://www.cdc.gov/nchs/data/hestat/overweight/overweight_adult.htm.
3. Farrell TM, Haggerty SP, Overby DW, et al: Clinical application of laparoscopic bariatric surgery: An evidence-based review, *Surg Endosc* 23:930–949, 2009.
4. Colquitt JL, Picot J, Loveman E, et al: Surgery for obesity, *Cochrane Database Syst Rev* 2:CD003641, 2009.
5. Grundy SM, Brewer HB Jr, Cleeman JI, et al: Definition of metabolic syndrome: Report of the National Heart, Lung, and Blood Institute/American Heart Association conference on scientific issues related to definition, *Circulation* 109:433–438, 2004.
6. Saliba J, Wattacheril J, Abumrad NN: Endocrine and metabolic response to gastric bypass, *Curr Opin Clin Nutr Metab Care* 12:515–521, 2009.
7. Williams DB, Hagerdorn JC, Lawson EH, et al: Gastric bypass reduces

8. biochemical cardiac risk factors, *Surg Obes Relat Dis* 3:8–13, 2007.
8. Vaughan RW, Bauer S, Wise L: Volume and pH of gastric juice in obese patients, *Anesthesiology* 43:686–689, 1975.
9. Harter RL, Kelly WB, Kramer MG, et al: A comparison of the volume and pH of gastric contents of obese and lean surgical patients, *Anesth Analg* 86:147–152, 1998.
10. Lavi R, Segal D, Ziser A: Predicting difficult airways using the intubation difficulty scale: A study comparing obese and non-obese patients, *J Clin Anesth* 21:264–267, 2009.
11. Rocke DA, Murray WB, Rout CC, et al: Relative risk analysis of factors associated with difficult intubation in obstetric anesthesia, *Anesthesiology* 77:67–73, 1992.
12. Rose DK, Cohen MM: The airway: problems and predictions in 18,500 patients, *Can J Anaesth* 41:372–383, 1994.
13. Wilson ME, Spiegelhalter D, Robertson JA, et al: Predicting difficult intubation, *Br J Anaesth* 61:211–216, 1988.
14. Hagberg CA, Vogt-Harenkamp C, Kamal J: A retrospective analysis of airway management in obese patients at a teaching institution, *J Clin Anesth* 21:348–351, 2009.

15. Brodsky JB, Lemmens HJ, Brock-Utne JG, et al: Morbid obesity and tracheal intubation, *Anesth Analg* 94:732–736, 2002.
16. Scott HW Jr: Metabolic surgery for hyperlipidemia and atherosclerosis, *Am J Surg* 123:3–12, 1972.
17. Brill AB, Sandstead HH, Price R, et al: Changes in body composition after jejunoileal bypass in morbidity obese patients, *Am J Surg* 123:49–56, 1972.
18. Buchwald H: A bariatric surgery algorithm, *Obes Surg* 12:733–746, 2002 discussion 747–750.
19. Buchwald H, Estok R, Fahrbach K, et al: Weight and type 2 diabetes after bariatric surgery: Systematic review and meta-analysis, *Am J Med* 122:248–256, 2009.
20. Buchwald H, Fahrbach Estok RK, et al: Trends in mortality in bariatric surgery: A systematic review and meta-analysis, *Surgery* 142:621–632, 2007, discussion 632–635.
21. Chipkin SR, Goldberg RJ: Obesity surgery and diabetes: Does a chance to cut mean a chance to cure? *Am J Med* 122:205–206, 2009.
22. Picot J, Jones J, Colquitt JL, et al: The clinical effectiveness and cost-effectiveness of bariatric (weight loss) surgery for obesity: A systematic review and economic evaluation,

Health Technol Assess 13:1–190, 215–357, iii–iiv, 2009.

23. Esparza J, Boivin MA, Hartshorne MF, et al: Equal aspiration rates in gastrically and transpylorically fed critically ill patients, *Intensive Care Med* 27:660–664, 2001.

24. Pousman RM, Pepper C, Pandharipande P, et al: Feasibility of implementing a reduced fasting protocol for critically ill trauma patients undergoing operative and nonoperative procedures, *JPEN J Parenter Enteral Nutr* 33:176–180, 2009.

25. Podolsky DK: Inflammatory bowel disease, *N Engl J Med* 347:417–429, 2002.

26. Blumberg RS: Inflammation in the intestinal tract: Pathogenesis and treatment, *Dig Dis* 27:455–464, 2009.

27. Zaniboni A, Prabhu S, Audisio RA: Chemotherapy and anaesthetic drugs: Too little is known, *Lancet Oncol* 6:176–181, 2005.

28. Niemann CU, Stabernack C, Serkova N, et al: Cyclosporine can increase isoflurane MAC, *Anesth Analg* 95:930–934, 2002.

29. Cirella VN, Pantuck CB, Lee YJ, et al: Effects of cyclosporine on anesthetic action, *Anesth Analg* 66:703–706, 1987.

30. Dretchen KL, Morgenroth VH 3rd, Standaert FG, et al: Azathioprine: effects on neuromuscular transmission, *Anesthesiology* 45:604–609, 1976.

31. Triner L: Mechanism of action of azathioprine questioned, *Anesthesiology* 46:440, 1977.

32. Kostopanagiotou G, Smyrniotis V, Arkadopoulos N, et al: Anesthetic and perioperative management of adult transplant recipients in nontransplant surgery, *Anesth Analg* 89:613–622, 1999.

33. Sidi A, Kaplan RF, Davis RF: Prolonged neuromuscular blockade and ventilatory failure after renal transplantation and cyclosporine, *Can J Anaesth* 37:543–548, 1990.

34. Storr M, Meining A, Allescher HD: Pathophysiology and pharmacological treatment of gastroesophageal reflux disease, *Dig Dis* 18:93–102, 2000.

35. Richter JE: Review article: The management of heartburn in pregnancy, *Aliment Pharmacol Ther* 22:749–757, 2005.

36. Straathof JW, Lamers CB, Masclee AA: Effect of gastrin-17 on lower esophageal sphincter characteristics in man, *Dig Dis Sci* 42:2547–2551, 1997.

37. Cantu TG, Korek JS: Central nervous system reactions to histamine-2 receptor blockers, *Ann Intern Med* 114:1027–1034, 1991.

38. Neilipovitz DT, Crosby ET: No evidence for decreased incidence of aspiration after rapid sequence induction, *Can J Anaesth* 54:748–764, 2007.

39. Brimacombe JR, Berry AM: Cricoid pressure, *Can J Anaesth* 44:414–425, 1997.

40. Rice MJ, Mancuso AA, Gibbs C, et al: Cricoid pressure results in compression of the postcricoid hypopharynx: the esophageal position is irrelevant, *Anesth Analg* 109:1546–1552, 2009.

41. Lerman J: On cricoid pressure: "May the force be with you."*Anesth Analg* 109:1363–1366, 2009.

42. Ovassapian A, Salem MR: Sellick's maneuver: to do or not do, *Anesth Analg* 109:1360–1362, 2009.

43. Clements RH, Reddy S, Holzman MD, et al: Incidence and significance of pneumomediastinum after laparoscopic esophageal surgery, *Surg Endosc* 14:553–555, 2000.

44. Connery LE, Coursin DB: Assessment and therapy of selected endocrine disorders, *Anesthesiol Clin North America* 22:93–123, 2004.

45. Hall GM, Ruggier R: Diabetes mellitus and anaesthesia, *Curr Opin Anaesthesiol* 12:343–347, 1999.

46. Mangano DT, Layug EL, Wallace A, et al: Effect of atenolol on mortality and cardiovascular morbidity after noncardiac surgery. Multicenter Study of Perioperative Ischemia Research Group, *N Engl J Med* 335:1713–1720, 1996.

47. Poldermans D, Boersma E, Bax JJ, et al: The effect of bisoprolol on perioperative mortality and myocardial infarction in high-risk patients undergoing vascular surgery. Dutch Echocardiographic Cardiac Risk Evaluation Applying Stress Echocardiography Study Group, *N Engl J Med* 341:1789–1794, 1999.

48. Mercker SK, Maier C, Neumann G, et al: Lactic acidosis as a serious perioperative complication of antidiabetic biguanide medication with metformin, *Anesthesiology* 87:1003–1005, 1997.

49. Gowardman JR, Havill J: Fatal metformin induced lactic acidosis: case report, *N Z Med J* 108:230–231, 1995.

50. Salpeter SR, Greyber E, Pasternak GA, et al: Risk of fatal and nonfatal lactic acidosis with metformin use in type 2 diabetes mellitus, *Cochrane Database Syst Rev* 1:CD002967, 2010.

51. Sieber FE, Martin LJ, Brown PR, et al: Diabetic chronic hyperglycemia and neurologic outcome following global ischemia in dogs, *J Cereb Blood Flow Metab* 16:1230–1235, 1996.

52. Sieber FE, Traystman RJ: Special issues: Glucose and the brain, *Crit Care Med* 20:104–114, 1992.

53. Van den Berghe G, Schetz M, Vlasselaers D, et al: Clinical review: Intensive insulin therapy in critically ill patients: NICE-SUGAR or Leuven blood glucose target? *J Clin Endocrinol Metab* 94:3163–3170, 2009.

54. Akhtar S, Barash PG, Inzucchi SE: Scientific principles and clinical implications of perioperative glucose regulation and control, *Anesth Analg* 110:478–497, 2010.

55. Chiniwala NU, Woolf PD, Bruno CP, et al: Thyroid storm caused by a partial hydatidiform mole, *Thyroid* 18:479–481, 2008.

56. McCann SM, Emery SP, Vallejo MC: Anesthetic management of a parturient with fetal sacrococcygeal teratoma and mirror syndrome complicated by elevated hCG and subsequent hyperthyroidism, *J Clin Anesth* 21:521–524, 2009.

57. Nayak B, Burman K: Thyrotoxicosis and thyroid storm, *Endocrinol Metab Clin North Am* 35:663–686, vii, 2006.

58. Lee SM, Jung TS, Hahm JR, et al: Thyrotoxicosis with coronary spasm that required coronary artery bypass surgery, *Intern Med* 46:1915–1918, 2007.

59. Pimentel L, Hansen KN: Thyroid disease in the emergency department: A clinical and laboratory review, *J Emerg Med* 28:201–209, 2005.

60. Delikoukos S, Mantzos F: Thyroid storm induced by blunt thyroid gland trauma, *Am Surg* 73:1247–1249, 2007.

61. Adali E, Yildizhan R, Kolusari A, et al: The use of plasmapheresis for rapid hormonal control in severe hyperthyroidism caused by a partial molar pregnancy, *Arch Gynecol Obstet* 279:569–571, 2009.

62. Nishiyama K, Kitahara A, Natsume H, et al: Malignant hyperthermia in a patient with Graves' disease during subtotal thyroidectomy, *Endocr J* 48:227–232, 2001.

63. Cooper DS: Antithyroid drugs, *N Engl J Med* 352:905–917, 2005.

64. Bennett-Guerrero E, Kramer DC, Schwinn DA: Effect of chronic and acute thyroid hormone reduction on perioperative outcome, *Anesth Analg* 85:30–36, 1997.

65. McNeil AR, Blok BH, Koelmeyer TD, et al: Phaeochromocytomas discovered during coronial autopsies in Sydney, Melbourne and Auckland, *Aust N Z J Med* 30:648–652, 2000.

66. Bravo EL: Pheochromocytoma: An approach to antihypertensive management, *Ann N Y Acad Sci* 970:1–10, 2002.

67. Bravo EL, Tarazi RC, Gifford RW, et al: Circulating and urinary catecholamines in pheochromocytoma. Diagnostic and pathophysiologic implications, *N Engl J Med* 301:682–686, 1979.

68. Ulchaker JC, Goldfarb DA, Bravo EL, et al: Successful outcomes in pheochromocytoma surgery in the modern era, *J Urol* 161:764–767, 1999.

69. Johnson MD, Smith PG, Mills E, et al: Paradoxical elevation of sympathetic activity during catecholamine infusion in rats, *J Pharmacol Exp Ther* 227:254–259, 1983.

70. James MF, Cronje L: Pheochromocytoma crisis: The use of magnesium sulfate, *Anesth Analg* 99:680–686, 2004.

71. Wong AY, Cheung CW: Dexmedetomidine for resection of a large phaeochromocytoma with invasion into the inferior vena cava, *Br J Anaesth* 93:873, 2004.

72. Wermer P: Genetic aspects of adenomatosis of endocrine glands, *Am J Med* 16:363–371, 1954.

73. Shapiro SE, Cote GC, Lee JE, et al: The role of genetics in the surgical management of familial endocrinopathy syndromes, *J Am Coll Surg* 197:818–831, 2003.

74. Akerstrom G, Hellman P, Hessman O, et al: Management of midgut carcinoids, *J Surg Oncol* 89:161–169, 2005.

75. Lamberts SW, Bruining HA, de Jong FH: Corticosteroid therapy in severe illness, *N Engl J Med* 337:1285–1292, 1997.

76. de Herder WW, van der Lely AJ: Addisonian crisis and relative adrenal failure, *Rev Endocr Metab Disord* 4:143–147, 2003.

77. Marik PE, Pastores SM, Annane D, et al: Recommendations for the diagnosis and management of corticosteroid insufficiency in critically ill adult patients: Consensus statements from an international task force by the American College of Critical Care Medicine, *Crit Care Med* 36:1937–1949, 2008.

78. Cotten JF, Husain SS, Forman SA, et al: Methoxycarbonyl-etomidate: A novel rapidly metabolized and ultra-short-acting etomidate analogue that does not produce prolonged adrenocortical suppression, *Anesthesiology* 111:240–249, 2009.

79. Udelsman R, Ramp J, Gallucci WT, et al: Adaptation during surgical stress. A reevaluation of the role of glucocorticoids, *J Clin Invest* 77:1377–1381, 1986.

80. Purnell JQ, Brandon DD, Isabelle LM, et al: Association of 24-hour cortisol production rates, cortisol-binding globulin, and plasma-free cortisol levels with body composition, leptin levels, and aging in adult men and women, *J Clin Endocrinol Metab* 89:281–287, 2004.

81. Salem M, Tainsh RE Jr, Bromberg J, et al: Perioperative glucocorticoid coverage. A reassessment 42 years after emergence of a problem, *Ann Surg* 219:416–425, 1994.

82. Levy E, Korach A, Merin G, et al: Pituitary apoplexy and CABG: Should we change our strategy? *Ann Thorac Surg* 84:1388–1390, 2007.

83. Chen Z, Murray AW, Quinlan JJ: Pituitary apoplexy presenting as unilateral third cranial nerve palsy after coronary artery bypass surgery, *Anesth Analg* 98:46–48, 2004.

84. Bertagna X, Guignat L, Groussin L, et al: Cushing's disease, *Best Pract Res Clin Endocrinol Metab* 23:607–623, 2009.

85. McMahon GT, Blake MA, Wu CL: Case records of the Massachusetts General Hospital. Case 1-2010. A 75-year-old man with hypertension, hyperglycemia, and edema, *N Engl J Med* 362:156–166, 2010.

86. Illyes G, Luczay A, Benyo G, et al: Cushing's syndrome in a child with pancreatic acinar cell carcinoma, *Endocr Pathol* 18:95–102, 2007.

87. Salvatori R, Fintini D, Westra WH, et al: Cushing's syndrome attributable to ectopic secretion of corticotropin in a patient with two neuroendocrine tumors, *Endocr Pract* 12:656–659, 2006.

88. Boscaro M, Arnaldi G: Approach to the patient with possible Cushing's syndrome, *J Clin Endocrinol Metab* 94:3121–3131, 2009.

89. Kissane NA, Cendan JC: Patients with Cushing's syndrome are care-intensive even in the era of laparoscopic adrenalectomy, *Am Surg* 75:279–283, 2009.

IV

30 CENTRAL NERVOUS SYSTEM DISEASE

Pekka Talke and Alana Flexman

A nesthesia for neurosurgery requires an understanding of the physiology of the central nervous system (CNS). The anesthesia provider must control the physiologic and pharmacologic factors that influence cerebral blood flow (CBF), cerebral metabolic rate for oxygen consumption (CMRO$_2$), and intracranial pressure (ICP). The selection of drugs, ventilation techniques, and monitors have important implications in the care of patients with diseases of the CNS.

NEUROANATOMY

Conceptually, the cranium is divided into supratentorial and infratentorial compartments. The supratentorial compartment contains the cerebral hemispheres and diencephalon (thalamus and hypothalamus); the brainstem and cerebellum make up the infratentorial compartment. The location of intracranial pathology can have significant implications, particularly if eloquent areas such as the language centers and motor cortex of the brain are at risk.

The arterial blood supply to the brain is through the left and right internal carotid arteries and the vertebrobasilar system. Anastomoses between these vessels form the circle of Willis (Fig. 30-1) and create a collateral blood supply to protect against ischemia. The classic depiction of this ring is found in fewer than half of human brains and collateralization may not be complete in all individuals.

Many of the physiologic properties of the central nervous system are dependent on an intact blood-brain barrier. The blood-brain barrier is composed of capillary endothelial cells with tight junctions that prevent extracellular passage of macromolecules, such as proteins. In contrast, lipid-soluble substances (carbon dioxide, oxygen, anesthetics) cross the blood-brain barrier easily. The blood-brain barrier may be disrupted in the event of acute systemic hypertension, trauma, infection, arterial hypoxemia, severe hypercapnia, tumors, and sustained seizure activity.

Figure 30-1 Anatomy of the circle of Willis.

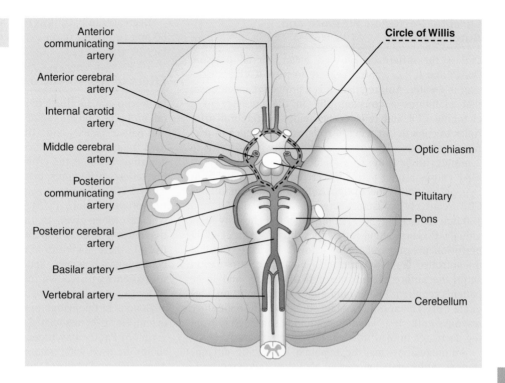

- Anterior communicating artery
- Anterior cerebral artery
- Internal carotid artery
- Middle cerebral artery
- Posterior communicating artery
- Posterior cerebral artery
- Basilar artery
- Vertebral artery
- Circle of Willis
- Optic chiasm
- Pituitary
- Pons
- Cerebellum

NEUROPHYSIOLOGY

Cerebral Blood Flow

Normal CBF is approximately 50 mL/100 g/min and represents 15% of cardiac output. The brain receives a disproportionately large share of cardiac output due to its high metabolic rate and inability to store energy. Determinants of CBF include (1) $CMRO_2$, (2) cerebral perfusion pressure (CPP) and autoregulation, (3) $PaCO_2$, (4) PaO_2, and (5) anesthetic drugs (Fig. 30-2). The impact of autonomic system innervation on CBF is small.

Cerebral Metabolic Rate

Cerebral blood flow in the brain is heterogeneous and directly influenced by $CMRO_2$ through cerebral flow-metabolism coupling. Increases or decreases in $CMRO_2$ result in a proportional increase or decrease in CBF. $CMRO_2$ is reduced by hypothermia and most anesthetic drugs and produces a coupled reduction in CBF in healthy brains (CBF decreases 7% for every 1° C decrease in body temperature below 37° C).[1] In contrast, $CMRO_2$ and CBF may be dramatically increased by seizure activity.

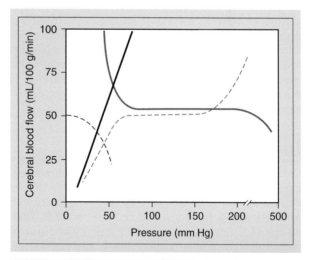

Figure 30-2 Schematic depiction of the impact of intracranial pressure (*dashed black line*), PaO_2 (*solid red line*), $PaCO_2$ (*solid black line*), and cerebral perfusion pressure (mean arterial pressure minus intracranial pressure or central venous pressure, whichever is greater) (*dashed red line*) on cerebral blood flow. Cerebral perfusion pressure less than 50 mm Hg (mean arterial pressure of 65 mm Hg, assuming an intracranial pressure of 15 mm Hg) does not necessarily produce cerebral ischemia, but the physiologic reserve is decreased. In the presence of decreased physiologic reserve, the addition of anemia may result in cerebral ischemia.

Cerebral Perfusion Pressure and Autoregulation

CPP is the difference between mean arterial pressure (MAP) and ICP or central venous pressure (CVP), whichever is greater. Autoregulation is a protective mechanism that maintains a constant CBF in the presence of a changing CPP and reflects the ability of cerebral arterioles to constrict or relax in response to changes in perfusion pressure. This response normally requires 1 to 3 minutes to develop, so a rapid increase or decrease in MAP causes a brief period of cerebral hyperperfusion or hypoperfusion, respectively. Autoregulation maintains CBF relatively constant between a CPP of 50 and 150 mm Hg (see Fig. 30-2) in normotensive, healthy individuals. Cerebral blood flow varies directly with cerebral perfusion pressures above or below this range. Chronic uncontrolled hypertension or sympathetic stimulation shifts the autoregulatory curve to the right, and these patients require a higher minimum CPP to maintain adequate CBF. The anesthetic state shifts the autoregulatory response to the left, which may provide some safety from the decreases in MAP that can occur intraoperatively.

Autoregulation may be impaired in specific circumstances. Autoregulation can be abolished following traumatic brain injury and intracranial surgery. As a result, CBF becomes directly proportional to MAP which has important clinical implications in the management of these patients. Autoregulation may also be impaired in the proximity of intracranial tumors. Inhaled anesthetics are potent cerebral vasodilators and impair autoregulation to varying degrees at high doses. Although autoregulation is maintained at anesthetic concentrations less than 1 minimum alveolar concentration (MAC),[2] higher concentrations abolish autoregulation, and CBF becomes proportional to MAP. In contrast, intravenous anesthetics do not disrupt autoregulation.

Effects of $PaCO_2$ and PaO_2 on CBF

Changes in $PaCO_2$ produce corresponding directional changes in CBF between a $PaCO_2$ of 20 to 80 mm Hg (see Fig. 30-2). CBF increases or decreases 1 mL/100 g/min for every 1–mm Hg increase or decrease in $PaCO_2$ from 40 mm Hg.[3] Such changes in CBF reflect the effect of carbon dioxide–mediated alterations in perivascular pH and lead to dilation or constriction of cerebral arterioles. These changes in CBF are transient because of an increase in cerebrospinal fluid (CSF) HCO_3 concentrations. CBF returns to normal in 6 to 8 hours, even if the altered $PaCO_2$ levels are maintained.[3] Aggressive or prolonged hyperventilation ($PaCO_2 < 30$ mm Hg) should be avoided because of the risk of cerebral ischemia. Prolonged aggressive hyperventilation following traumatic brain injury is probably associated with poorer neurologic outcome.[4]

Decreases in PaO_2 (less than a threshold value of about 50 mm Hg) result in an exponential increase in CBF (see Fig. 30-1).

Effect of Anesthetic on CBF

Intravenously administered anesthetics, such as thiopental, propofol, and etomidate, are cerebral vasoconstrictors and reduce $CMRO_2$ and CBF in parallel and are therefore used frequently for anesthesia for neurosurgery.[5] There is controversy about the effects of ketamine, which probably reflects differences in the conditions of the research study.[6] When ketamine is given on its own without control of ventilation, $PaCO_2$, CBF, and ICP all increase, whereas when given in the presence of another sedative/anesthetic drug in patients whose ventilation is controlled, these increases do not occur. Because of this controversy, however, ketamine is not usually selected for patients with known intracranial disease.

Benzodiazepines and opioids decrease $CMRO_2$ and CBF, analogous to thiopental and propofol, although to a lesser extent. However, associated respiratory depression and elevation of $PaCO_2$ may produce the opposite effect. Opioids should be used with caution in patients with intracranial disease because of their (1) depressant effects on consciousness, (2) production of miosis, and (3) depression of ventilation with associated increases in ICP from $PaCO_2$ increases.

α_2-Agonists (clonidine and dexmedetomidine) are unique sedatives in that they do not cause significant respiratory depression. They reduce arterial blood pressure, CBF, and CPP with minimal effects on ICP. α_2-Agonists can be used intraoperatively to reduce the dose of other anesthetics and analgesics or postoperatively as sedatives and to attenuate postoperative hypertension and tachycardia.

Volatile anesthetic drugs are potent cerebral vasodilators. When administered during normocapnia at concentrations higher than 0.5 MAC desflurane, sevoflurane, and isoflurane rapidly produce cerebral vasodilation and result in dose-dependent increases in CBF. CBF remains increased relative to $CMRO_2$ despite concomitant decreases in $CMRO_2$.[2] When used in isolation, nitrous oxide increases CBF and possibly $CMRO_2$, but these effects appear to be attenuated by co-administration of other anesthetics.

INTRACRANIAL PRESSURE

Intracranial Pressure-Volume Relationship

The intracranial compartment is composed of three substances: (1) brain matter, (2) cerebral spinal fluid, and (3) blood. Increases in any of the these substances can result in elevated intracranial pressure, defined as a sustained increase above 15 mm Hg. Marked increases in ICP can decrease CPP and thereby CBF to the point of producing cerebral ischemia. Pressure-volume elastance (change in pressure produced by a change in volume) curves reflect changes produced by expanding intracranial masses (Fig. 30-3). As the intracranial volume increases, CSF is initially translocated into the spinal canal. Once this compensation is maximized, ICP starts to rise and cerebral blood vessels are eventually compressed. A point is reached when even small increases in intracranial volume may result in marked increases in ICP. Ischemia will lead to cerebral edema and further increases in ICP. It is therefore critical to prevent sustained increases in ICP (Table 30-1).

Effect of Anesthetic on ICP

Most intravenous anesthetic drugs reduce $CMRO_2$ and CBF, and this decrease is associated with a reduction in ICP. The effects of ketamine are controversial and were discussed earlier. These drugs may be administered to patients with intracranial hypertension to decrease ICP. However, this must be done carefully as large doses of propofol or thiopental may decrease systemic blood pressure and CPP. An increased frequency of excitatory peaks on the electroencephalogram of patients receiving etomidate, as compared with thiopental, suggests caution in the administration of etomidate to patients with a history of epilepsy.[7] Opioids and benzodiazepines reduce ICP through reductions in

Table 30-1 Methods to Decrease Intracranial Pressure

Cerebrospinal Fluid Reduction
- External ventricular drain
- Lumbar drain
- Furosemide (Lasix)
- Acetazolamide (Diamox)

Cerebral Blood Volume Reduction
Decrease cerebral blood flow:
- Intravenous anesthetic drugs are preferred.
- Employ hyperventilation.
- Avoid cerebral vasodilators.
- Avoid extreme hypertension.

Increase venous outflow:
- Elevate head.
- Avoid constriction at the neck.
- Avoid PEEP and excess airway pressure.

Cerebral Edema Reduction
Mannitol
Decompressive craniectomy
Resection of space-occupying lesions
Prevention of ischemia and secondary edema

PEEP, Positive end-expiratory pressure.

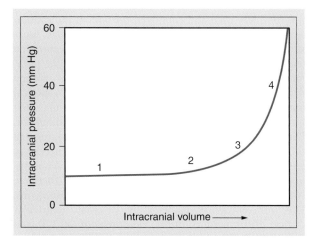

Figure 30-3 The pressure-volume compliance curve depicts the impact of increasing intracranial volume on intracranial pressure (ICP). As volume increases from point 1 to point 2 on the curve, ICP does not increase because cerebrospinal fluid is shifted from the cranium into the spinal subarachnoid space. Patients with intracranial tumors who are between point 1 and point 2 on the compliance curve are unlikely to manifest clinical symptoms of increased ICP. Patients who are on the rising portion of the pressure-volume curve (point 3) can no longer compensate for increases in intracranial volume, and ICP begins to increase. Clinical symptoms attributable to increased ICP are likely at this stage. Additional increases in volume at this point, as produced by increased CBF during anesthesia, can precipitate abrupt increases in ICP (point 4).

CBF and $CMRO_2$ although this benefit will be offset if respiratory depression and increases in $PaCO_2$ occur.

As discussed earlier, volatile anesthetic drugs are cerebral vasodilators and produce dose-dependent increases in ICP that parallel the increases in CBF and CBV. Hyperventilation to decrease $PaCO_2$ to less than 35 mm Hg attenuates the tendency for volatile anesthetics to increase ICP. In patients undergoing craniotomy for supratentorial tumors with evidence of a midline shift, neither isoflurane nor desflurane significantly affected lumbar CSF pressure when moderate hypocapnia ($PaCO_2$ of 30 mm Hg) was maintained.[8] However, these agents should be avoided in patients with abnormal intracranial compliance as evidenced by abnormal mental status, clinical signs, or radiologic imaging.

Neuromuscular blocking drugs (also see Chapter 12) do not usually affect ICP unless they induce release of histamine or hypotension. Histamine can cause cerebral vasodilation, leading to a small increase in ICP. Succinylcholine may increase ICP through stimulation of muscle spindles, which in turn either directly or indirectly results in increased $CMRO_2$.[9] Because CBF is coupled to $CMRO_2$, the increase in $CMRO_2$ is responsible for increasing CBF and thus ICP. However, the increases in ICP are not consistently observed and may be attenuated by a deep level of anesthesia.

NEUROPROTECTION

Many anesthetics may act as neuroprotectants given their potential to reduce cerebral metabolic rate and excitotoxicity during oxygen deprivation. In animal

IV

studies, many anesthetics, including barbiturates, volatile anesthetics, xenon, and propofol, provide neuroprotection although human outcome data are lacking. Hypothermia has been described as a method for cerebral protection during acute injury. Although numerous animal studies found that hypothermia reduces ischemic injury, this has not been confirmed in several large prospective, randomized trials of hypothermia in aneurysm surgery and traumatic brain injury.[1] Cooling of patients with return of spontaneous circulation after cardiac arrest improved neurologic outcome in one randomized controlled trial.[10] In contrast, hyperthermia worsens ischemic injury and should be avoided in patients vulnerable to cerebral ischemia.

NEUROPHYSIOLOGIC MONITORING

Neurophysiologic monitoring is employed during neurosurgery with increasing frequency due to minimal risk to patients and the potential to reduce neurologic deficits. An understanding of the effects of anesthetic agents on somatosensory and motor evoked potentials is critical in neuroanesthesia. In general, nitrous oxide and volatile anesthetics have a greater effect on motor and sensory evoked potentials than intravenous anesthetics (also see Chapter 20). Electrocorticography (ECoG) is another intraoperative mapping technique used to identify epileptic foci for resection and is sensitive to anesthetic drugs that change the seizure threshold (e.g., benzodiazepines and volatile anesthetic agents).

ANESTHESIA FOR NEUROSURGERY

Preoperative Assessment

Patients presenting for neurosurgical procedures can have a wide range of symptoms. Patients with intracranial mass lesions may present with seizures, altered level of consciousness, headaches, cranial nerve abnormalities, and motor or sensory deficits. Aneurysms and arteriovenous malformations (AVMs) can present with a severe ("thunderclap") headache if ruptured, and focal deficits or visual impairment from compression of the optic chiasm when unruptured.

Evidence of increased ICP should be elicited during the preoperative visit. Clinical signs may be consistent with, but do not reliably indicate, the level of ICP (Table 30-2). Imaging may reveal a midline shift of more than 0.5 cm, encroachment of expanding brain on cerebral ventricles, cerebral edema, hydrocephalus, or any combination of these signs. In symptomatic patients, preoperative medications that cause sedation or depression of ventilation are usually avoided. Drug-induced depression of ventilation

Table 30-2 Preoperative Evidence of Increased Intracranial Pressure

Positional headache
Nausea and vomiting
Hypertension and bradycardia
Altered level of consciousness
Altered patterns of breathing
Papilledema

can lead to increased $PaCO_2$ and subsequent increases in ICP. In alert patients, small doses of benzodiazepines may provide useful relief of anxiety.

Monitoring

In addition to standard monitors, continuous monitoring of arterial blood pressure via a peripheral arterial catheter is recommended because of hemodynamic perturbations occurring during induction of anesthesia, tracheal intubation, surgery, and emergence from anesthesia, all of which may compromise cerebral perfusion. These catheters also allow for arterial blood gas sampling and accurate determination of $PaCO_2$. Central venous catheters are not routinely used and employed for patient indications, such as anticipated need for vasoactive infusions. Measurement of the end-tidal carbon dioxide concentration (capnography) is used to determine ventilation parameters. The electrocardiogram (ECG) allows prompt detection of cardiac dysrhythmias caused by surgical manipulation of cardiovascular centers. Neuromuscular blockade is monitored with a peripheral nerve stimulator. Because of the length of these surgical procedures and the use of diuretics, a bladder catheter is often necessary and helps in guiding intravenous fluid therapy. A continuous monitor of ICP is helpful but rarely used. There are two main monitors for ICP inserted by neurosurgeons. The intraventricular catheter or external ventricular device (EVD) permits direct measurement of ICP and drainage of CSF. The subarachnoid or subdural bolt is placed through a burr hole and can be inserted quickly in an emergency setting, but it does not allow for CSF drainage.

Positioning (Also See Chapter 19)

Resection of supratentorial tumors and intracranial vascular lesions is typically accomplished with the patient in the supine or lateral position. Resection of posterior fossa/infratentorial tumors frequently requires placement of the patient in the sitting or prone position (Table 30-3). The sitting position facilitates surgical exposure of posterior fossa tumors, but because of the high risk for

Table 30-3 Management of Anesthesia for Patients with Intracranial Masses

Preoperative
- Avoid sedatives and opioids if ICP is elevated.
- Standard anxiolytics can be given if ICP is not elevated.

Monitors
Supratentorial masses
- Standard ASA monitors, arterial line, Foley catheter are used.

Infratentorial masses—depending on positioning:
- Prone or park bench position: Standard ASA monitors, arterial line, Foley catheter are adequate.
- Sitting position (associated with high frequency of VAE): Standard monitors plus CVP monitor, precordial Doppler, or TEE are required.

Induction
- Deep anesthesia and skeletal muscle paralysis are obtained before direct laryngoscopy/tracheal intubation to avoid increasing ICP while maintaining CPP.

Maintenance
- Minimize ICP and maintain adequate CPP.
- Opioid plus propofol and/or volatile anesthetic can be used with or without nitrous oxide.
- Mannitol (0.25-1g/kg IV) also can be given.
- Maintain euvolemia.

Postoperative
- Avoid coughing, straining, and systemic hypertension during tracheal extubation.
- Rapid awakening allows early neurologic assessment.

ASA, American Society of Anesthesiologists; CPP, cerebral perfusion pressure; CVP, central venous pressure; ICP, intracranial pressure; TEE, transesophageal echocardiography; VAE, venous air embolism.

venous air embolism (>25% incidence), many neurosurgeons prefer the prone position. Other risks associated with the sitting position include upper airway edema as a result of venous obstruction from excessive cervical flexion and quadriplegia from spinal cord compression and ischemia, especially in the presence of preexisting cervical stenosis. Another popular approach is the "park bench position" in which the patient is placed in a lateral position but rolled slightly forward with the head further rotated to "look" at the floor. This position allows the surgeon full access to the posterior fossa and minimizes the risk for venous air embolism.

The head is commonly fixed in a frame using pins (Mayfield head clamp). Caution must be used to avoid bucking or movement while the patient is fixed in the frame to avoid injury to the patient. Compression of the internal jugular veins resulting in excessive venous pressure should also be avoided to minimize increases in ICP.

Induction of Anesthesia

The goal of induction of anesthesia is to achieve a sufficient level of anesthesia to blunt the stimulation of direct laryngoscopy and tracheal intubation without compromising cerebral perfusion by increasing ICP or decreasing MAP. Intravenous induction with propofol (1.5 to 3 mg/kg), thiopental (3 to 6 mg/kg), or etomidate (0.2 to 0.5 mg/kg), produces reliable and prompt onset of unconsciousness and is unlikely to adversely increase ICP. Hemodynamic support with sympathomimetic drugs may be necessary and such drugs should be readily available, especially in cases in which CPP may already be compromised. A neuromuscular blocking drug (also see Chapter 12) is used to facilitate tracheal intubation, mechanical ventilation of the lungs, and patient positioning on the operating table. Increases in ICP may occur after the administration of succinylcholine, but the extent of the increase is quite variable and usually short-lived.[9] The trachea is intubated after a peripheral nerve stimulator confirms the establishment of skeletal muscle paralysis so that coughing is avoided, which may result in marked increases in ICP. Injection of additional intravenous doses of propofol, thiopental, opioids, or lidocaine 1 to 2 minutes before beginning direct laryngoscopy may be effective in attenuating the increase in arterial blood pressure and ICP that can accompany tracheal intubation.

After tracheal intubation, ventilation of the lungs is controlled at a rate and tidal volume sufficient to maintain $PaCO_2$ between 30 and 35 mm Hg. There is no evidence of additional therapeutic benefit when $PaCO_2$ is decreased below this range. Use of positive end-expiratory pressure is not encouraged because it could impair cerebral venous drainage and increase ICP, but it can usually be counteracted by raising the head 10 to 15 cm above the level of the chest.

Maintenance of Anesthesia

After tracheal intubation, measures should be taken to optimize CPP and minimize ICP. Maintenance of anesthesia is achieved with a combination of opioid (either bolus or infusion), continuous infusion of propofol, and inhalation of a volatile anesthetic with or without nitrous oxide. Volatile anesthetics must be used carefully because of their ability to increase ICP. Nevertheless, low concentrations of volatile anesthetics (<0.5 MAC) may be useful for blunting the increases in systemic blood pressure evoked by surgical stimulation. Direct-acting vasodilating drugs (hydralazine, nitroprusside, nitroglycerin, calcium channel blockers) increase CBF and ICP despite causing simultaneous decreases in systemic blood pressure; therefore, use of these drugs, particularly before the dura is open, is not encouraged.

Movement, coughing, or reacting to the presence of the tracheal tube during intracranial procedures is avoided

IV

because these responses can lead to increases in ICP, bleeding into the operative site, and a brain that bulges into the operative site and makes surgical exposure difficult. Thus, maintenance of an adequate depth of anesthesia is important. Skeletal muscle paralysis is often used to provide added insurance against movement or coughing. The choice of anesthetics is also determined in part by the use of intraoperative neurophysiologic monitoring.

If cerebral swelling occurs, administration of additional doses of diuretics can be given to decrease brain water. Mannitol (0.25 to 1 g/kg IV) is an osmotic diuretic and reduces cerebral water content. The onset of action is 5 to 10 minutes, maximum effects are seen in 20 to 30 minutes, and its effects last for about 2 to 4 hours. However, if administered rapidly, mannitol can also cause peripheral vasodilation (hypotension) and a short-term increase in intravascular volume, which could result in increased ICP. Acute mannitol toxicity, as manifested by hyponatremia, high measured serum osmolality, and a gap between the measured and calculated serum osmolality of greater than 10 mOsm/kg, can also occur when large doses of the drug (2 to 3 g/kg IV) are given. Furosemide (0.5 to 1 mg/kg IV) is effective in decreasing ICP, though less so than mannitol. Intermittent intravenous injections of thiopental or propofol may also be effective in decreasing ICP, and if surgically possible, placing the patient in a head-up position also helps. Other useful measures include hyperventilation and discontinuing the administration of volatile anesthetics.

Intravenous Fluid Management (Also See Chapter 23)

Maintaining euvolemia is recommended. Dextrose solutions are not recommended because they are rapidly distributed throughout body water, and if blood glucose concentrations decrease more rapidly than brain glucose concentrations, water crosses the blood-brain barrier and cerebral edema results. Furthermore, hyperglycemia augments ischemic neuronal cell damage by promoting neuronal lactate production, which worsens cellular injury. Therefore, crystalloid solutions such as normal saline and lactated Ringer's solution are recommended. Colloids, such as 5% albumin, are also an acceptable intravenous fluids, but no improvement in outcome has been shown as compared to crystalloids.

Postoperative Management

On awakening from anesthesia, coughing or straining by the patient should be avoided because these responses could increase the possibility of hemorrhage or edema formation. A prior intravenous bolus of lidocaine, opioid, or both may help decrease the likelihood of coughing during tracheal extubation. Postoperatively, assessing neurologic status frequently and providing adequate analgesia are important. Delayed return of consciousness postoperatively or neurologic deterioration in the postoperative period is evaluated by computed tomography (CT) or magnetic resonance imaging (MRI). Tension pneumocephalus as a cause of neurologic deterioration is a consideration, especially if nitrous oxide was administered during anesthesia. The postoperative stress response and resulting hyperdynamic events (e.g., hypertension, tachycardia) are attenuated with the use of hemodynamically active drugs and opioids. Labetalol is commonly used to treat hypertension prophylactically due to its ability to reduce MAP without cerebral vasodilation.

Venous Air Embolism

Neurosurgery that requires significant elevation of the head is associated with an increased risk for venous air embolism.[11] Not only is the operative site above the level of the heart but the venous sinuses in the cut edge of bone or dura may not collapse when transected. Air enters the pulmonary circulation and becomes trapped in the small vessels, thereby causing an acute increase in dead space. Massive air embolism may cause air to enter and be trapped in the right ventricle and lead to right ventricular failure. Microvascular bubbles may also cause reflex bronchoconstriction and activate the release of endothelial mediators causing pulmonary edema. Death is usually due to cardiovascular collapse and arterial hypoxemia. Air may reach the coronary and cerebral circulations (paradoxical air embolism) by crossing a patent foramen ovale (a probe-patent foramen ovale is present in 20% to 30% of adults) and may result in myocardial infarction or stroke. Furthermore, transpulmonary passage of venous air is possible in the absence of a patent foramen ovale.[12]

Transesophageal echocardiography (also see Chapter 20) is the most sensitive method to detect air embolism, but it is invasive and cumbersome. A precordial Doppler ultrasound transducer placed over the right side of the heart (over the second or third intercostal space to the right of the sternum to maximize audible signals from the right atrium) is the next most sensitive (detects amounts of air as small as 0.25 mL) and noninvasive indicator of the presence of intracardiac air. A sudden decrease in end-tidal concentration of carbon dioxide reflects increased dead space secondary to continued ventilation of alveoli no longer being perfused because of obstruction of their vascular supply by air bubbles. An increased end-tidal nitrogen concentration may reflect nitrogen from venous air embolism but is rarely available. Aspiration of air through a correctly positioned central venous catheter can also be used to diagnose air embolism. In this regard, a right atrial catheter with the tip positioned at the junction of the superior vena cava and the right atrium may provide the most rapid aspiration of air. During controlled ventilation of the lungs, sudden attempts (gasps) by patients to initiate spontaneous breaths may be the first indication of the occurrence of venous air embolism. Hypotension, tachycardia, cardiac dysrhythmias, cyanosis, and a "mill wheel" murmur are late signs of venous air embolism. A pulmonary artery catheter may provide additional evidence that venous air embolism has occurred because of increases in pulmonary artery pressure. Additional signs in awake patients include chest pain and coughing.

The surgeon should be notified immediately whenever a venous air embolism is suspected. Venous air embolism is treated by (1) irrigation of the operative site with fluid, as well as the application of occlusive material to all bone edges so that sites of venous air entry are occluded; (2) gentle compression of the internal jugular veins; and (3) placement of the patient in a head-down position. If nitrous oxide is being administered, it should be promptly discontinued to avoid the risk of increasing the size of venous air bubbles because of diffusion of this gas into the air bubbles. Despite the logic of positive end-expiratory pressure to decrease entrainment of air, the efficacy of this maneuver has not been confirmed. Furthermore, positive end-expiratory pressure could reverse the pressure gradient between the left and right atria and predispose to passage of air across a patent foramen ovale.

COMMON CLINICAL CASES

Intracranial Mass Lesions

Intracranial masses (tumors) requiring surgery occur most often in patients 40 to 60 years of age, and the initial signs and symptoms reflect increases in ICP. Seizures that appear in a previously asymptomatic adult suggest the presence of an intracranial tumor, and such tumors are usually confirmed by CT or MRI. Avoidance of abrupt increases in intracranial pressure is an important anesthetic goal when managing patients with intracranial tumors.

Posterior fossa masses have several additional considerations. In addition to an arterial line, monitoring for the sitting position should include a properly positioned central venous catheter and precordial Doppler given the high incidence of venous air embolism. Operations on posterior fossa tumors can injure vital brainstem respiratory and circulatory nuclei and result in intraoperative hemodynamic fluctuations and postoperative depression of ventilation. The cranial nerves can also be affected and lead to impairment of protective airway reflexes. Postoperatively, the patient should be assessed to determine whether the airway can be maintained, or whether tracheal intubation and mechanical ventilation should be continued in the intensive care unit.

Intracranial Aneurysms

Intracranial aneurysms are the most common cause of intracranial hemorrhage. They occur in 2% to 4% of the population, with 1% to 2% rupturing per year. Although aneurysms may be found incidentally or appear as a slowly enlarging mass, they are most frequently manifested as hemorrhage together with a sudden, severe headache, nausea, vomiting, focal neurologic signs, and depressed consciousness. Major complications of aneurysmal rupture include death, rebleeding, and vasospasm and they may be treated with either endovascular coiling or surgery. Short-term outcomes are similar in patients treated surgically versus endovascular insertion of platinum coils (see Chapter 38). Some patients are unsuitable candidates for insertion of platinum coils because of the anatomy and location of their aneurysms and they require surgery.

Early treatment is advocated for prevention of rebleeding, but surgery may be associated with more technical difficulty because of a swollen inflamed brain, whereas delaying treatment increases the risk for rebleeding. Vasospasm of the cerebral arteries is generally manifested clinically 3 to 5 days after subarachnoid hemorrhage and is the foremost cause of morbidity and death. Transcranial Doppler and cerebral arteriography can detect cerebral vasospasm before clinical symptoms (worsening headache, neurologic deterioration, loss of consciousness) occur. Treatment of vasospasm includes "triple H" therapy (hypervolemia, hypertension, hemodilution), which consists of the intravenous administration of fluids or inotropic drugs, or both. The intravenous administration of a calcium entry blocker, nimodipine, decreases the risk of morbidity and death from vasospasm. Other treatment modalities include selective intra-arterial injection of vasodilators and balloon dilation (angioplasty) of the affected cerebral vessels using interventional radiology.

Other complications of subarachnoid hemorrhage include seizures (10%), acute and chronic hydrocephalus, and intracerebral hematoma. Changes on the ECG (T-wave inversions, U waves, ST segment depressions, prolonged QT interval, and rarely Q waves) and mild elevation of cardiac enzymes are frequent but do not usually correlate with significant myocardial dysfunction or poor outcome. Hyponatremia is commonly seen after subarachnoid hemorrhage. Significant electrolyte imbalances, acid-base abnormalities, and hemodynamic derangements should be corrected if present, and a cardiac workup should ensue if Q waves are seen on the ECG.

Management of anesthesia for resection of an intracranial aneurysm is designed to (1) prevent sudden increases in systemic arterial blood pressure, which would increase the aneurysm's transmural pressure and could result in rupture, and (2) facilitate surgical exposure and access to the aneurysm (Table 30-4). Induction and maintenance of anesthesia must be designed to minimize the hypertensive responses evoked by noxious stimulation, such as

IV

Table 30-4 Anesthetic Management of Patients with Intracranial Aneurysms

Preoperative
- Neurologic evaluation is performed to look for evidence of increased intracranial pressure and vasospasm.
- Electrocardiogram changes frequently are present.
- HHH therapy is indicated if vasospasm is present.
- Calcium channel blockers.

Induction
- Avoid increases in systemic blood pressure.
- Maintain cerebral perfusion pressure to avoid ischemia.

Maintenance
- Opioid plus propofol and/or volatile anesthetic is recommended regimen.
- Mannitol (0.25-1 g/kg IV) also can be given.
- Maintain normal to increased systemic blood pressure to avoid ischemia during temporary clipping.

Postoperative
- Maintain normal to increased systemic blood pressure.
- Early awakening is recommended to facilitate neurologic assessment.
- HHH therapy is given as needed.

HHH, hypervolemia, hypertension, hemodilution.

direct laryngoscopy and placing the patient's head in immobilizing pins. Conversely, CPP must be maintained to prevent ischemia during retraction or temporary vessel occlusion or as a result of vasospasm.

Hemodynamic control is important during dissection of the aneurysm to prevent intraoperative rupture. Temporary occlusive clips applied to the major feeding artery of the aneurysm can create regional hypotension without the need for systemic hypotension and its inherent risks on multiple organ systems. As a result, normal or even increased systemic arterial blood pressure should be instituted to facilitate perfusion through the collateral circulation. In addition to maintaining collateral cerebral circulation via systemic hypertension, drugs such as thiopental may be administered in the hope that they can provide some protection from cerebral ischemia. Occasionally, hypothermic circulatory arrest may be used for very large complex aneurysms.

The patient's trachea is generally extubated at the completion of surgery unless there is significant neurologic impairment. Measures to prevent vasospasm and seizures while maintaining adequate CPP should be continued during care of these patients postoperatively.

Arteriovenous Malformations

The incidence of arteriovenous malformations (AVMs) in the general population and annual rate of rupture is similar to that for aneurysms at 2% to 4% and 2%, respectively. Up to 10% of patients diagnosed with an AVM have an

associated aneurysm.[13] Risk of hemorrhage is related to anatomic features of the AVM including size and characteristics of the feeding vessels. These patients may be treated several ways: expectantly, open resection, endovascular embolization, or with stereotactic radiosurgery (gamma knife). Preoperative embolization is frequently employed to reduce blood loss and facilitate surgical resection.

Anesthesia for resection or embolization of AVMs is similar to that for aneurysms with a few distinct considerations. Because their flow characteristics (low-pressure, high-flow shunts), AVMs are unlikely to rupture during acute systemic hypertension, such as occurs during laryngoscopy. Despite this, hypertension should still be avoided during induction of anesthesia, given the frequent rate of associated aneurysms. Finally, anesthesia for intracranial AVMs must include preparation for massive, persistent blood loss and postoperative cerebral swelling.

Carotid Disease

A significant proportion of strokes are due to stenosis of the carotid artery and may result in severe disability and death. Randomized controlled trials have confirmed the benefit of carotid endarterectomy (CEA) in symptomatic patients with 70% to 99% stenosis.[14] Although a perioperative risk of stroke and death (approximately 4% to 7%) must be taken into account, CEA may be beneficial in asymptomatic patients as well. Carotid stenting using interventional radiology is an alternative therapy for carotid stenosis and is increasing in popularity. CEA probably should be optimally performed within 2 weeks of the onset of symptoms given the presence of unstable atherosclerotic plaque.

Preoperative assessment of patients undergoing CEA should focus on assessment of perioperative risk of cardiac ischemia as these patients typically have atherosclerotic disease (Table 30-5). Either general or regional anesthesia (deep and superficial cervical plexus block) may be used for this procedure. Even though an awake patient may provide a more accurate intraoperative assessment of the patient's neurologic status and more stable hemodynamic profile, the procedure requires a cooperative and motionless patient. Controversy remains on whether CEA is best performed under regional or general anesthesia.

Goals of anesthesia for CEA include (1) prevention of cerebral ischemia through maintenance of adequate cerebral perfusion pressure and (2) prevention of myocardial ischemia through avoidance of acute peaks in arterial blood pressure and heart rate. Invasive hemodynamic monitoring with a peripheral arterial catheter is indicated to ensure adequate cerebral perfusion pressure. This is especially important during intraoperative clamping of the carotid artery. The anesthesiologist should ensure that the MAP is maintained above the patient's baseline pressure (within 20%) to ensure adequate collateral flow through the circle of Willis. Hypocarbia should be avoided given the risk of cerebral vasoconstriction and ischemia. Many methods have been

Table 30-5 Management of Anesthesia for Patients with Carotid Stenosis

Preoperative
- Neurologic examination is indicated to look for preoperative deficits.
- Screen for associated CAD.
- Anxiolytics may be useful.

Monitors
- Standard ASA monitors, arterial line, Foley catheter are used.

Induction
- Avoid increases in mean arterial pressure or heart rate if CAD is suspected.
- Maintain adequate CPP.

Maintenance
- Maintain adequate CPP (baseline to 20% above) during carotid clamping.
- Opioid plus propofol and/or volatile anesthetic can be used with or without nitrous oxide.

Postoperative
- Avoid coughing, straining, and systemic hypertension during tracheal extubation.
- Rapid awakening allows early neurologic assessment.
- Monitor for hyperperfusion syndrome and airway compromise.

ASA, American Society of Anesthesiologists; CAD, coronary artery disease; CPP, cerebral perfusion pressure.

employed to detect intraoperative cerebral ischemia and need for shunting during clamping including EEG, transcranial Doppler, and stump pressure, although none have been shown to definitively improve outcome.

Postoperative complications include cardiovascular ischemia and neurologic deficits secondary to intraoperative emboli. Hypertension may lead to neck hematoma with airway compromise and hyperperfusion syndrome and should be avoided.

QUESTIONS OF THE DAY

1. What is cerebral autoregulation? Under what circumstances is it altered? What is the impact of intravenous (IV) or inhaled anesthetics on cerebral autoregulation?
2. What are the effects of changes in $PaCO_2$ or PaO_2 on cerebral blood flow?
3. What are the effects of IV or inhaled anesthetics on cerebral blood flow?
4. What are the manifestations of venous air embolism in a patient undergoing craniotomy under general anesthesia? What is the appropriate management?
5. During craniotomy for tumor resection, the surgeon notes "brain swelling" in the operative field. What are the initial steps in management?
6. A patient with subarachnoid hemorrhage (SAH) presents for intracranial aneurysm clipping. What complications of SAH may develop in the perioperative period?

ACKNOWLEDGEMENT

The editors and publisher would like to thank Drs. Cheng Quah and Adrian Gelb for contributing a chapter on this topic to the prior edition of this work. It has served as the foundation for the current chapter.

IV

REFERENCES

1. Polderman KH: Mechanism of action, physiological effects and complications of hypothermia, *Crit Care Med* 37(Suppl 7):S186–202, 2009.
2. Cho S, Fujigaki T, Uchiyama Y, et al: Effects of sevoflurane with and without nitrous oxide on human cerebral circulation. Transcranial Doppler study, *Anesthesiology* 85:755–760, 1996.
3. Akca O: Optimizing the intraoperative management of carbon dioxide concentration, *Curr Opin Anaesthesiol* 19:19–25, 2006.
4. Guidelines for the management of severe traumatic brain injury. Brain Trauma Foundation; American Association of Neurological Surgeons; Congress of Neurological Surgeons, *J Neurotrauma* 24(Suppl 1):S1–106, 2007.
5. Pinaud M, Lelausque JN, Chetanneau A, et al: Effects of propofol on cerebral hemodynamics and metabolism in patients with brain trauma, *Anesthesiology* 73:404–409, 1990.

6. Albanese J, Arnaud S, Rey M, et al: Ketamine decreases intracranial pressure and electroencephalographic activity in traumatic brain injury patients during propofol sedation, *Anesthesiology* 87:1328–1334, 1997.
7. Reddy RV, Moorthy SS, Dierdorf SF, et al: Excitatory effects and electroencephalographic correlation of etomidate, thiopental, methohexital and propofol, *Anesth Analg* 77:1008–1011, 1993.
8. Muzzi D, Losasso T, Dietz N, et al: The effect of desflurane and isoflurane on cerebrospinal fluid pressure in humans with supratentorial mass lesions, *Anesthesiology* 76:720–724, 1992.
9. Kovarik WD, Mayberg TS, Lam AM, et al: Succinylcholine does not change intracranial pressure, cerebral blood flow velocity, or the electroencephalogram in patients with neurologic injury, *Anesth Analg* 78:469–473, 1994.

10. Bernard SA, Gray TW, Buist MD, et al: Treatment of comatose survivors of out of hospital cardiac arrest with induced hypothermia, *N Engl J Med* 346:557–563, 2002.
11. Muth CM, Shank ES: Gas embolism, *N Engl J Med* 342:476–482, 2000.
12. Byrick RJ, Korley RE, McKee MD, et al: Prolonged coma after unreamed, locked nailing of femoral shaft fracture, *Anesthesiology* 94:163–165, 2001.
13. Olgilvy CS, Stieg PE, Awak I, et al: Recommendations for the management of intracranial arteriovenous malformations: a statement for healthcare professionals from a special writing group of the Stroke Council, American Stroke Association, *Circulation* 103:2644–2657, 2001.
14. Benington S, Pichel AC: Anaesthesia for carotid endarterectomy, *Curr Anaesth Crit Care* 19:138–149, 2008.

31 OPHTHALMOLOGY AND OTOLARYNGOLOGY

Steven Gayer and Howard Palte

Surgical procedures of the head and neck present unique anesthesia challenges. Operative field isolation places the anesthesia provider at a distance from the airway and hampers access to the patient. The region's extensive parasympathetic innervations predispose patients to intraoperative bradycardia and asystole. Ophthalmic of- and otolaryngologic procedures require smooth induction and emergence from anesthesia because coughing and bucking raise venous and intraocular pressure, and may negatively impact surgical outcome.

OPHTHALMOLOGY

More than 2 million cataract operations are performed nationally each year. Most eye procedures are considered low risk for perioperative complications; however, ophthalmic patients are often at higher risk during surgery, because typically they include the elderly (also see Chapter 35) who frequently have multiple concomitant medical issues or pediatric (also see Chapter 34) patients who may be premature or have associated syndromes.[1] Additionally, most operations are conducted on an ambulatory basis (also see Chapter 37), emphasizing the importance of preoperative evaluation (also see Chapter 13).

The majority of ophthalmologic procedures are performed via monitored anesthesia care (MAC) and some form of regional eye anesthetic.[2] Aside from intraoperative analgesia and akinesia, advantages of ophthalmic regional blocks include suppression of the oculocardiac reflex (OCR) and provision of postoperative pain management. An understanding of regional block techniques and management of their complications is requisite. General anesthesia is reserved for operations of prolonged duration, more invasive orbital procedures, and those patients unable to remain relatively still such as neonates, infants, and children (also see Chapter 34).

Anesthetic drugs and maneuvers may affect ocular dynamics and surgical outcomes, and ophthalmic medications can cause adverse anesthesia reactions or may significantly impact systemic physiology. Appreciation of factors affecting intraocular pressure (IOP) and vigilance vis-à-vis the oculocardiac reflex are critical.

Intraocular Pressure

Adequate pressure within the eye serves to maintain refracting surfaces, corneal contour, and functionally correct vision. IOP is primarily derived from a balance between aqueous humor production and drainage. Aqueous humor is actively secreted from the posterior chamber's ciliary body and flows through the pupil into the anterior chamber where it is admixed with aqueous passively produced by blood vessels on the iris' forward surface. After washing over the avascular lens and corneal endothelium, aqueous humor filters through the spongy trabecular meshwork into the canal of Schlemm's tubules at the base of the cornea. From there, it exits the eye into episcleral veins and ultimately to the superior vena cava and right atrium. Therefore, any obstruction of venous return from the eye to the right side of the heart can increase IOP. Lesser factors that influence IOP include force transmitted to the globe by contraction of the orbicularis oculi or extraocular muscles as well as hardening of the lens, vitreous, and sclera that can occur with aging.

IOP ranges between 10 and 22 mm Hg in the intact normal eye. Typically, there is a 2 to 5 mm Hg diurnal variation. Small transient changes occur with each cardiac contraction as well as with eyelid closure, mydriasis, and postural changes. These changes are normal and have no bearing on the intact eye. A sustained increase in IOP during anesthesia, however, has the potential to produce acute glaucoma, retinal ischemia, hemorrhage, and permanent visual loss.

FACTORS THAT INFLUENCE INTRAOCULAR PRESSURE

Venous congestion resulting from obstruction at any point from the episcleral veins to the right atrium may cause substantive increase of IOP. Prior to induction of anesthesia, Trendelenburg positioning or presence of a tight cervical collar can increase intraocular blood volume, dilate orbital vessels, and inhibit aqueous drainage. Straining, retching, or coughing upon induction will markedly increase venous pressure and can readily precipitate an increase in IOP of 40 mm Hg or more. Should this occur while the globe is open during surgery, such as during corneal transplant, loss of vitreous, hemorrhage, and expulsion of eye contents may lead to permanent damage to the eye, or even blindness. Arterial hypertension can transiently increase IOP, but has much less impact than perturbations of venous drainage. External compression on the globe by a tightly applied face mask, laryngoscopy, and tracheal intubation also elevate IOP, but placement of a supraglottic airway has minimal impact. Hypoxemia and hypoventilation can increase IOP. Hyperventilation and hypothermia have the opposite effect.

ANESTHETIC DRUGS AND INTRAOCULAR PRESSURE

Inhaled and most intravenous anesthetics produce dose-related reductions in IOP. Although the exact mechanisms are not known, IOP is probably reduced by a combination of central nervous system depression, diminished aqueous humor production, enhanced aqueous outflow, and relaxation of extraocular muscles. There is controversy surrounding the effect of ketamine on IOP. While ketamine may not increase IOP, it does cause rotatory nystagmus and blepharospasm makes it not an ideal anesthetic for eye surgery.

In the absence of alveolar hypoventilation, nondepolarizing neuromuscular blocking drugs decrease IOP via relaxation of the extraocular muscles. In contrast, succinylcholine produces an increase of about 9 mm Hg in 1 to 4 minutes after intravenous administration with a subsequent diminution to baseline within 7 minutes. The increase in IOP is probably due to several mechanisms, including tonic contraction of extraocular muscles, relaxation of orbital smooth muscle, choroidal vascular dilation, and aqueous outflow-impeding cycloplegia. Pretreatment with a small dose of a nondepolarizing neuromuscular blocking drug, lidocaine, β-blocker, or acetazolamide may attenuate the increase in IOP associated with induction of anesthesia with succinylcholine, direct laryngoscopy, and endotracheal intubation. However, this approach for induction of anesthesia is rarely used.

Ophthalmic Medications

Systemic absorption of topical ophthalmic drugs from either the conjunctiva or via drainage through the nasolacrimal duct onto the nasal mucosa can produce untoward side effects. These drops include acetylcholine, anticholinesterases, cyclopentolate, epinephrine, phenylephrine, and timolol (Table 31-1). Phospholine iodide (echothiophate) is a miosis-inducing anticholinesterase that profoundly interferes with metabolism of succinylcholine. Prolonged paralysis following a single dose of succinylcholine may ensue. Phenylephrine drops are available in concentrations of 2.5% and 10%. Systemic absorption of the latter can induce transient malignant hypertension. Some systemic ophthalmic drugs, such as glycerol, mannitol, and acetazolamide, may also produce untoward side effects.

Oculocardiac Reflex

The oculocardiac reflex is a sudden profound decrease in heart rate in response to traction on the extraocular muscles or external pressure on the globe. There is a wide range of reported incidence, varying from approximately 15% to 80%. It occurs more commonly in young patients. The reflex arc has a trigeminal nerve afferent limb that generates an efferent vagal response that may precipitate a variety of dysrhythmias including junctional or sinus bradycardia, atrioventricular block, ventricular bigeminy,

IV

Table 31-1 Drugs Administered to Ophthalmic Surgery Patients

Ophthalmic Indication	Drug	Mechanism of Action	Systemic Effect
Miosis	Acetylcholine	Cholinergic agonist	Bronchospasm, bradycardia, hypotension
Glaucoma (increased intraocular pressure)	Acetazolamide	Carbonic anhydrase inhibitor	Diuresis, hypokalemic metabolic acidosis
	Echothiophate	Irreversible cholinesterase inhibitor	Prolongation of succinylcholine's effects Reduction in plasma cholinesterase activity up to 3-7 weeks after discontinuation Bradycardia, bronchospasm
	Timolol	β-Adrenergic antagonist	Atropine-resistant bradycardia, bronchospasm, exacerbation of congestive heart failure; possible exacerbation of myasthenia gravis
Mydriasis, ophthalmic capillary decongestion	Atropine	Anticholinergic	Central anticholinergic syndrome (*mad as a hatter*, delirium, agitation; *hot as a hare*, fever; *red as a beet*, flushing; *dry as a bone*, xerostomia, anhidrosis) Blurred vision (cycloplegia, photophobia)
	Cyclopentolate	Anticholinergic	Disorientation, psychosis, convulsions, dysarthria
	Epinephrine	α-, β-Adrenergic agonist	Hypertension, tachycardia, cardiac dysrhythmias; epinephrine paradoxically leads to decreased intraocular pressure and can also be used for glaucoma
	Phenylephrine	α-Adrenergic agonist, direct-acting vasopressor	Hypertension (one drop, or 0.05 mL, of a 10% solution contains 5 mg of phenylephrine)
	Scopolamine	Anticholinergic	Central anticholinergic syndrome (see atropine above)

multifocal premature ventricular contractions, ventricular tachycardia, and asystole.

The OCR is most often encountered during strabismus surgery but can occur during any type of ophthalmic surgery. It may also occur while performing an eye regional anesthetic nerve block. Hypercarbia, hypoxemia, and light planes of anesthetic depth augment the incidence and severity of OCR.

Prompt removal of the instigating surgical stimulus frequently results in rapid recovery. Unrelenting tension may induce cardiac arrest so heart rate must be continuously monitored during eye block and surgery. At the first sign of dysrhythmia, surgery must stop and all pressure on the eye or traction on eye muscles must be discontinued. The ventilatory status and depth of anesthesia should be reassessed. The reflex may extinguish itself after a few minutes, and also can be abated by administration of a parasympatholytic drug such as atropine or glycopyrrolate. The OCR can also be eradicated by inserting a regional anesthetic eye block, thereby abolishing its afferent arc.

The prophylactic use of intramuscular anticholinergics for adult ophthalmic surgery patients is not effective. In fact, tachycardia following atropine or glycopyrrolate may have significant consequence for geriatric patients with history of cardiac disease. In children, who are more dependent on heart rate to maintain cardiac output, prophylactic intravenous administration of atropine (0.01 to 0.02 mg/kg) or glycopyrrolate may be prudent prior to commencing eye surgery.

Preoperative Assessment (Also See Chapter 13)

Patients having eye surgery are often at the extremes of age—ranging from premature babies with retinopathy to the elderly. Hence, special age-related considerations such as altered pharmacokinetics and pharmacodynamics apply. The elderly, pediatric patients with various syndromes, and the premature infants frequently have multiple co-morbidities. Preoperative evaluation is vital. "Routine" laboratory testing is not adequate. Physician assessment and judgement determine the need for indicated laboratory testing.[3] Cessation of antiplatelet/anticoagulant drugs prior to eye surgery is controversial.[4] The risk of intraocular bleeding versus the risk of perioperative stroke, myocardial ischemia, and deep venous thrombosis must be assessed.[5]

One of the most important preoperative assessments is the likelihood of patient movement during surgery. Inability to remain supine and relatively still during intraocular surgery with monitored anesthesia care may result in eye injury and have devastating long-term visual consequences.[6]

Anesthetic Options (Table 31-2)

Anesthetic options for most ophthalmic procedures include general anesthesia, retrobulbar (intraconal) block, peribulbar (extraconal) anesthesia, sub-Tenon's block, and topical analgesia. Often, there is minimal exposure to regional anesthetic eye block techniques during

Table 31-2 Goals for Anesthesia Management of Ophthalmic Surgery

Safety
Analgesia
Akinesia (when indicated)
Control of intraocular pressure
Avoidance of the oculocardiac reflex
Awareness of possible drug interactions
Awakening without coughing, nausea, or vomiting

anesthesia training, creating a reluctance to perform such blocks. Professional societies dedicated to teaching safe ophthalmic regional anesthesia can provide valuable instruction.[7] There is recent widely adopted procedural requirement for a "time out" for all surgery. Of prime importance is confirmation of correct eye (i.e., right versus left) for anesthesia and surgery.

NEEDLE-BASED OPHTHALMIC REGIONAL ANESTHESIA

The anatomic foundation of needle-based eye blocks rests upon the concept of the orbital cone. This structure consists of the four ocular rectus muscles extending from their origin at the apex of the orbit to the globe anteriorly. These muscles and their surrounding connective tissue form a compartment behind the globe akin to the brachial plexus sheath in the axilla.

A retrobulbar block is performed by inserting a steeply angled needle from the inferotemporal orbital rim into this muscle cone such that the tip of the needle is behind (retro) the globe (bulbar).[8] A more descriptive term is intraconal block (Fig. 31-1).[9] Injection of a small volume of local anesthetics into this compartment will produce rapid onset of akinesia and analgesia.

The boundary separating the intraconal from extraconal space is porous, and thus local anesthetics injected outside the muscle cone diffuse inward. A peribulbar block can be achieved by directing a minimally angled needle to a shallow depth such that the tip remains outside the cone (see Fig. 31-1). This extraconal block is theoretically safer because the needle is not directed toward the apex of the orbit; hence the needle tip is ultimately situated further from key intraorbital structures. This distance minimizes the potential for optic nerve trauma, optic nerve sheath injection, orbital epidural, and brainstem anesthesia. Complications of needle-based eye blocks are listed in Table 31-3. These complications can lead to a variety of presentations and altered physiologic states (Table 31-4). Because local anesthetics are injected at a longer distance from the nerves, larger volumes and more time for diffusion

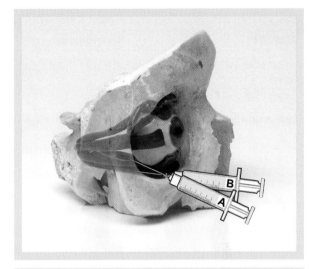

Figure 31-1 Needle-based regional anesthesia for ophthalmic surgery. **A,** An intraconal (retrobulbar) block is placed deeper and more steeply angled. **B,** An extraconal (peribulbar) block is shallower and minimally angled. Asterisk indicates needle entry point. A portion of the lateral orbital rim is removed. (Model courtesy of Dr. Roy Hamilton.)

Table 31-3 Complications of Regional Anesthesia for Ophthalmic Surgery

Superficial or retrobulbar hemorrhage
Elicitation of the oculocardiac reflex
Puncture of the globe
Intraocular injection
Optic nerve trauma
Seizures (intravenous injection of local anesthetic solution)
Brainstem anesthesia (spread of local anesthetic to the brainstem causing delayed-onset loss of consciousness, respiratory depression, paralysis of the contralateral extraocular muscles)
Central retinal artery occlusion
Blindness

are needed. Thus, intraconal versus extraconal anesthesia is somewhat analogous to subarachnoid versus epidural anesthesia in terms of volume, onset, and density of block.

Branches of the facial nerve that innervate the eyelid's orbicularis oculi muscle are blocked by the higher volume of local anesthetic used with extraconal injection. This prevents eyelid squeezing and is a distinct advantage during corneal transplantation. An intraconal block requires a separate facial nerve injection to limit blepharospasm.

Table 31-4 Differential Diagnosis of Altered Physiologic Status After Regional Anesthesia for Ophthalmic Surgery

Alteration	Oversedation	Brainstem Anesthesia	Intravascular Injection
Loss of consciousness	±	+	+
Apnea	±	+	±
Cardiac instability	±	+	±
Seizure activity	Ø	Ø	+
Contralateral mydriasis	Ø	±	Ø
Contralateral eye block	Ø	±	Ø

+, likely; ±, may or may not be present; Ø, not present.

CANNULA-BASED OPHTHALMIC REGIONAL ANESTHESIA

Ophthalmic anesthesia can also be achieved by instilling local anesthetics through a blunt cannula into the space between the globe's rigid sclera and sub-Tenon's capsule (Fig. 31-2).[10] The capsule consists of fascia that envelops the eye, providing a smooth friction-free interface in which to rotate. Anteriorly, it originates near the limbal margin where it is fused to the conjunctiva. As the capsule extends posteriorly, it surrounds the eye, with portions reflected onto the extraocular muscles. Local anesthetics injected into the sub-Tenon's space block cranial and ciliary nerves that penetrate the capsule as well as the optic nerve posteriorly.

Anesthesia Management of Specific Ophthalmic Procedures

RETINA SURGERY

The globe's posterior inner wall is lined by the retina, sensory tissue that converts incoming light into neural output and, ultimately, vision. The densely packed macula near its center provides fine detailed vision. Perfusion comes from the choroid layer situated between the sclera and the retina. The retina may break or detach from the choroid leading to ischemia and compromised vision. Diabetics and people with myopia are at particular risk. Surgical options include combinations of scleral buckle, vitrectomy, laser, cryotherapy, and injection of intravitreal gas.

Preoperative evaluation of diabetes and coexisting morbidities (also see Chapter 13) is important, and appropriate changes should be made to ensure that patients are in optimal medical condition for surgery. Retina surgery is often prolonged and associated with more extensive manipulation of the eye, therefore requiring general anesthesia or dense regional anesthetic block with MAC. Perfluorocarbons such as sulfur hexafluoride (SF6) and C_3F_8 are inert, relatively insoluble gases that are injected to internally tamponade the retina onto the choroid. Resorption can take 10 to 28 days depending on which drug is selected. As nitrous oxide is over 100-fold more diffusible than sulfur hexafluoride, it can expand the size of the gas bubble, increase IOP, and potentially cause retinal ischemia and permanent loss of vision.[11] Nitrous oxide should be discontinued 20 minutes prior to gas injection or omitted altogether.

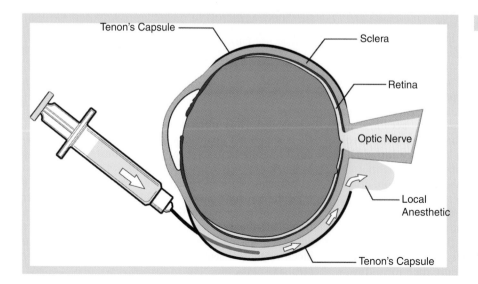

Figure 31-2 Sub-Tenon's block.

Tenon's Capsule
Sclera
Retina
Optic Nerve
Local Anesthetic
Tenon's Capsule

GLAUCOMA

Glaucoma is characterized by a sustained increase in IOP which leads to diminished perfusion of the optic nerve and eventual loss of vision. Closed angle (acute) glaucoma occurs when the angle between the iris and cornea narrows and obstructs outflow. Open angle (chronic) glaucoma results from sclerosis of trabecular meshwork and impaired aqueous drainage. Outflow is improved with constriction of the pupil by miotic drugs. Atropine drops into the eye produce mydriasis and are contraindicated. Intravenous atropine on the other hand is minimally absorbed by the eye and should be used when indicated during anesthesia. Infantile glaucoma may readily progress to blindness, making early surgery more urgent. Congenital glaucoma is often a component of many syndromes.

Many adult glaucoma procedures can be managed with regional anesthesia and MAC. General anesthesia is a requisite for pediatric glaucoma cases. Anesthesia implications include (1) avoiding mydriasis by continuing all miotic drops, (2) understanding the interactions of anti-glaucoma medications and anesthetics (see Table 31-1), and (3) preventing increases in IOP associated with induction, maintenance, and emergence from anesthesia.

STRABISMUS SURGERY

Strabismus surgery is performed to correct misalignment of extraocular muscles and realign the visual axis. Most patients are pediatric. Special considerations include (1) high incidence of intraoperative OCR, (2) increased risk for malignant hyperthermia, and (3) marked prevalence of postoperative nausea and vomiting.

Nausea and Vomiting

The incidence of postoperative nausea and vomiting (PONV) following strabismus surgery varies widely, but has been quoted as high as 85% (also see Chapter 39). PONV is the most common reason for pediatric inpatient admission after outpatient surgery and is probably a vagal-mediated response to surgical manipulation of extraocular muscles. Multimodal antiemetics with differing mechanisms of action may be more effective than individual medications for those patients at greatest risk of PONV following eye surgery.

Malignant Hyperthermia

Strabismus is a neuromuscular disorder that can be associated with other myopathies. The frequency of masseter muscle spasm after succinylcholine is fourfold greater than baseline. Suspect malignant hyperthermia if hypertension, tachycardia, hypercarbia, and increasing temperature occur.

TRAUMATIC EYE INJURIES

Eye injury occurs as a result of penetrating or blunt trauma. The anesthesia plan must balance specific risks. Increased IOP due to a tightly applied face mask, laryngoscopy, and endotracheal intubation, or due to coughing or bucking, can cause extrusion of globe contents and jeopardize vision. Additionally, in emergency situations, the patient may be nonfasting and at risk of aspiration upon induction of general anesthesia. Control of the airway can be achieved with a rapid sequence induction of anesthesia including succinylcholine; however, succinylcholine can also cause a transient increase in IOP.[12] Awake endotracheal intubation may be appropriate for patients with difficult airways; however, the resultant increases in IOP can be disastrous. The risks of succinylcholine or awake intubation on IOP must be weighed against the dangers imposed by a full stomach or difficult airway.

Inquire with the ophthalmologist if the operative repair can be delayed until the stomach is considered safe. If not, proceed after careful evaluation to rule out other issues. Administer appropriate drugs to decrease gastric acidity and volume. Place the patient in slight reverse Trendelenburg position and avoid any maneuvers that may increase IOP. If no airway problems are anticipated, consider a modified rapid sequence induction of anesthesia with a large dose of a nondepolarizing neuromuscular blocking drug (e.g., rocuronium, 1.0 mg/kg). If succinylcholine is selected, the IOP and systemic hypertension following laryngoscopy/intubation can be moderated by intravenous lidocaine, opioids, or a small pretreatment dose of nondepolarizing neuromuscular blocker prior to induction of anesthesia. Regional anesthesia may be an option for select injuries and patients at higher risk from general anesthesia.[13]

Postoperative Eye Issues

CORNEAL ABRASION

The most common cause of postoperative eye pain after general anesthesia is corneal abrasion. It manifests with conjunctivitis, tearing, and foreign body sensation. Damage may be mechanically incurred by dangling ID tags, the anesthesia mask, drapes, and more. During general anesthesia, abrasion may also occur owing to loss of the blink reflex, the drying effects of exposure to air, and diminished tear production. Preventive measures include gently taping the eyelids shut during mask ventilation, intubation, and thereafter. Ointments may cause allergic reaction or blurred postemergence vision. Protective goggles may be best. Antibiotic ointment and patching the eye usually result in healing of corneal abrasions within a day or two.

ACUTE GLAUCOMA

Acute glaucoma is also painful. Presence of a mydriatic pupil may be diagnostic. This is an urgent matter calling for consult with an ophthalmologist. Intravenous mannitol or acetazolamide can decrease IOP and relieve pain.

POSTOPERATIVE VISUAL LOSS

Painless loss of vision after surgery may be due to ischemic optic neuropathy (ION) or brain injury. Both are rare

IV

events. Risk is more frequent with spine surgery in the prone position and cardiac surgery.[14] Consultation with an ophthalmologist is mandatory as early funduscopic examination may aid in diagnosis.

OTOLARYNGOLOGY

Ear, nose, and throat (ENT) surgery can make the airway fairly inaccessible to the anesthesia provider. Preoperative planning with the surgeon and nursing staff is essential.[15] There is a distinct possibility of encountering a difficult airway due to anatomic factors, surgical issues, or underlying pathology. Attention should be directed to the establishment and firm anchoring of an endotracheal airway. The endotracheal tube (ETT) should be manually supported during patient repositioning such as turning of the head because movement can result in endobronchial intubation, tube occlusion, cuff leaks, disconnections, or even frank dislodgment of the ETT and inadvertent extubation. Prior to surgical preparation or placement of drapes, the neck position should be reassessed, and susceptible pressure points padded. During surgery, the airway may be compromised by often-undetected bleeding, edema, or surgical manipulation. The use of posterior pharyngeal packs can minimize the risk of aspiration of gastric contents. Operating room (OR) personnel should be alerted to their placement, and the anesthesia provider should confirm complete removal of all packs prior to extubation of the trachea.

Special Considerations for Head and Neck Surgery

THE DIFFICULT AIRWAY (Also See Chapter 16)
The anesthesia provider should address any airway concerns with surgical colleagues prior to patient entry into the operating room. Supplementary equipment must be readied in anticipation of a possible difficult airway, and expert assistance should be immediately available. Modified techniques to secure the airway include use of video-laryngoscopy, fiberoptic bronchoscopy, or even performance of a tracheostomy under local anesthesia. The placement of tracheal retention sutures with tracheostomy can facilitate recapture of airway access should it become compromised during or after surgery. Procedures within the airway can produce significant edema resulting in acute obstruction. In the postoperative period these patients may need to remain tracheally intubated, or if extubated, they may require treatment with humidified oxygen or nebulized bronchodilators.

LARYNGOSPASM
The laryngospasm reflex is mediated through vagal stimulation of the superior laryngeal nerve. Abrupt intense, prolonged closure of the larynx with compromise of

ventilation can occur upon instrumentation of the endolarynx, with blood or foreign body presence, and with inadequate depth of anesthesia. If the airway is completely obstructed, the anesthesia provider may be unable to ventilate the patient despite an adequate mask fit. The ensuing hypercarbia, hypoxia, and acidosis elicit an autonomic sympathetic response producing hypertension and tachycardia. A temporal reduction in brainstem firing to the superior laryngeal nerve eventually causes relaxation of the vocal cords. In small children even brief laryngospasm is particularly perilous as peripheral oxygen saturation decreases precipitously due to a small functional residual capacity and relatively high cardiac output (also see Chapter 34). Prompt recognition and intervention is essential. Treatment modalities include the administration of 100% oxygen via positive-pressure face mask ventilation, placement of an oral/nasal airway, and deepening of anesthesia with intravenously administered anesthetics. Small doses of succinylcholine (0.25 to 0.5 mg/kg) and tracheal intubation may be necessary in refractory cases. The likelihood of encountering laryngospasm may be reduced with use of intravenous or topical lidocaine (4% lidocaine spray) prior to laryngoscopy and endotracheal intubation.

UPPER RESPIRATORY INFECTIONS
Patients, especially children, scheduled for elective ENT surgery may present with an unresolved upper respiratory infection (URI) predisposing to airway hyperreactivity. They are at enhanced risk of intraoperative breath-holding, desaturation, and postoperative croup.[16] Postponing surgery for uncomplicated pediatric URI is controversial, and may not be required for brief nonairway ENT procedures such as myringotomy and tube placement (also see Chapter 34).

EPISTAXIS
After massive epistaxis, patients are often anxious, hypovolemic, and hypertensive. Rehydration and reassurance are essential. Because blood is being continuously swallowed, these patients are considered at high risk for regurgitation and aspiration of gastric contents and are managed accordingly. A large-bore peripheral intravenous cannula is vital because some blood loss is occult, and hypotension or continued hemorrhage is likely postinduction of anesthesia.

OBSTRUCTIVE SLEEP APNEA
This condition is characterized by upper airway obstruction and disordered breathing patterns during sleep. Symptoms include snoring, headache, sleep disturbance, daytime somnolence, and personality changes. Polysomnography (sleep study) establishes the diagnosis and severity of the disorder but is not routinely performed. Pediatric patients may have behavior and growth disturbances as well as poor school performance (also see Chapter 34). Patients are often obese with short, thick necks and large

tongues. These factors contribute to difficult airway management during mask ventilation, direct laryngoscopy, tracheal intubation, and extubation.[17] Patients with obstructive sleep apnea (OSA) are exquisitely sensitive to the effects of hypnotics and narcotics and may require prolonged recovery room stay.

AIRWAY FIRES

There are three elements essential to the creation of an airway fire: heat or an ignition source (laser or electrosurgical unit), fuel (paper drapes, ETT, or gauze swabs), and an oxidizer (O_2, air, or N_2O). The danger of an airway fire is not limited to general anesthesia. It can also occur during facial procedures under monitored anesthesia care via electrocautery used in close proximity to delivered supplemental oxygen.[18]

Anesthesia Management of Specific Otolaryngology Procedures

EAR SURGERY

There are several points to consider for anesthesia and ear surgery:

Nitrous Oxide

Nitrous oxide is more soluble than nitrogen in blood and diffuses into air-filled cavities quicker than nitrogen diffuses out. The ensuing increased middle ear pressure may be problematic, including potential dislodgment of tympanoplasty grafts. Furthermore, acute discontinuation of high concentrations of nitrous oxide markedly decreases cavity pressure and may cause serous otitis. Nitrous oxide should be avoided or used in moderate concentration (<50%) and discontinued approximately 15 to 30 minutes prior to graft application.

Facial Nerve Monitoring

The surgeon may elect to use a facial nerve monitor to prevent accidental incision of facial nerve branches during surgery. Complete paralysis by neuromuscular blocking drugs can inhibit facial nerve monitor function. The use of neuromuscular blocking drugs should be curtailed to either succinylcholine or small doses of nondepolarizing neuromuscular blocking drugs. Also, use of a neuromuscular monitor can be used to confirm a response to train-of-four stimulation of a peripheral nerve and absence of full paralysis prior to surgical dissection in the middle ear (also see Chapter 12).

Epinephrine

Epinephrine is frequently injected during ear microsurgery to decrease bleeding and improve the visual field. Systemic uptake may precipitate tachydysrhythmias. Hence, epinephrine concentration should be limited to a 1:200,000 solution.[19] Other means to control bleeding include moderate reverse Trendelenburg (head-up) positioning to decrease venous congestion and the use of

volatile anesthetics to decrease systolic arterial blood pressures within an acceptable range. The use of vasoactive drugs and controlled hypotension is controversial.

Emergence

Head and neck manipulation during the application of bandages at the conclusion of surgery produces movement of the ETT and airway irritation. Coughing and bucking increase venous pressure which can lead to graft disruption or acute bleeding. In the patient with an uncomplicated airway, extubation of the trachea at a deep plane of anesthesia may be beneficial.

Postoperative Nausea and Vomiting

Due to manipulation of the vestibular apparatus, PONV is common after middle ear surgery. Factors that may exacerbate PONV include anesthetic technique (use of nitrous oxide and narcotics), inadequate rehydration, and postoperative movement. The extent of prophylactic measures taken to prevent PONV is guided by a graded risk analysis.[20] Prophylactic interventions may include use of one or more antiemetics including corticosteroid, 5HT3-receptor antagonist, neurokinin-1 receptor antagonist, scopolamine patch, low-dose propofol, and gastric decompression. Scopolamine may cause confusion and probably should not be used in geriatric patients.

Myringotomy and Tube Insertion (Also See Chapter 34)

This procedure is performed for children with disorders of the middle ear who have a history of repeated ear infections with unsatisfactory response to antibiotic therapy. There may be residual inflammation of the middle ear and upper airway irritability. An inhaled induction and maintenance of anesthesia with ventilation via a face mask is preferred for this brief procedure. Postoperative pain is minimal, so premedication may not be needed and may result in residual postoperative sedative effects.

TONSILLECTOMY AND ADENOIDECTOMY

Most patients undergoing this procedure are young and healthy. Common surgical perioperative issues include airway obstruction, bleeding, cardiac arrhythmias, and croup (postextubation airway edema). Patients frequently have obstruction of the upper airway which only becomes apparent during sleep (OSA). In general, a comprehensive history and physical examination are sufficient for a preoperative workup but any history of sleep-disordered breathing, obesity, or a bleeding diathesis warrants further investigation. Sedative premedication is best avoided for children with OSA, obesity, intermittent airway obstruction, or significant tonsil hypertrophy.

In young children, an inhaled induction of anesthesia is preferred because preoperative establishment of an intravenous line may be difficult or traumatic. An intravenous line can be started once the child is anesthetized. Loss of pharyngeal muscle tone upon induction of anesthesia may lead

IV

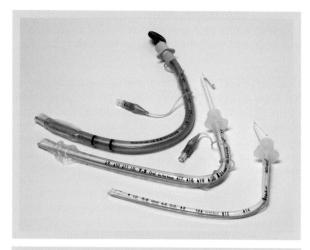

Figure 31-3 Armored and cuffed preformed curved oral endotracheal tubes.

to airway obstruction. Continuous positive airway pressure may relieve the problem. Placement of a cuffed preformed curved oral endotracheal tube optimizes field visualization and decreases the likelihood of accidental extubation (Fig. 31-3). An air leak at 20 cm H_2O peak airway pressure reduces the probability of tissue edema, a critical factor for pediatric patients who have narrower airway diameter than adults. A precordial stethoscope is useful to monitor breath sounds because ETT dislodgment can occur with movement of the head or mouth gag. The supraglottic area is occasionally packed with gauze to protect against aspiration. Prior to extubation of the trachea, the pack must be removed and the stomach should be decompressed. Tracheal extubation can be performed when the child is fully awake and actively responsive. Some anesthesia providers perform tracheal extubation when the patient is still anesthetized in order to minimize coughing and laryngospasm related to the presence of the ETT.

Intravenous dexamethasone may decrease edema and postoperative pain as well as PONV. Postoperative airway obstruction can occur for a variety of reasons ranging from secretions or blood on the vocal cords to a retained pharyngeal pack. Airway obstruction occasionally produces negative-pressure pulmonary edema. This manifests when the patient breathes against a closed glottis creating a marked negative intrathoracic pressure. This pressure is transmitted to interstitial tissue and promotes flow of fluid from the pulmonary circulation into the alveoli. Young children (less than 4 years old) are susceptible to airway obstruction as late as 24 hours postoperatively and may benefit from prolonged postoperative monitoring.

Bleeding Tonsils After Tonsillectomy and Adenoidectomy

Hemorrhage after tonsillectomy normally occurs within a few hours of surgery and presents with expectoration of red blood, repeated swallowing, tachycardia, and

PONV.[21] Blood loss is often underestimated because it is mostly swallowed. Intravenous fluid administration is critical prior to corrective urgent surgery. Patients are considered to have a full stomach, so precautions are taken during induction of anesthesia to avert regurgitation and pulmonary aspiration of blood and gastric contents. Features of a rapid sequence induction of anesthesia include application of cricoid pressure (Sellick's maneuver) until correct endotracheal tube positioning is confirmed, administration of intravenous anesthetics and neuromuscular blocking drugs in quick succession, and presence of a working suction catheter at the head of the table.

EPIGLOTTITIS (Also See Chapter 34)

Acute epiglottitis is an infectious disease caused by *Haemophilus influenzae* type B, most often affecting children between 2 and 7 years of age.[22] There is often a history of sudden onset of fever and dysphagia. Symptomatic progression from pharyngitis to airway obstruction and respiratory failure can be rapid (within hours). The child with epiglottitis appears agitated, drools, and leans forward holding the head in an extended position. Exhaustion may result from labored breathing against an almost fully occluded airway.

Direct visualization of the glottis should not be attempted because stimulation of the patient and struggling may result in complete airway obstruction. Anesthesia commences only when all emergency airway equipment is open and readied, with a surgeon adept at rigid bronchoscopy and tracheostomy present. An inhaled induction of anesthesia maintaining spontaneous ventilation is preferred. Atropine may be given to avoid bradycardia and also dry secretions. The edematous airway necessitates use of a small ETT. Because the degree of airway narrowing is unpredictable a range of ETT sizes should be available. In the event of any difficulty, the surgeon should intervene and secure the airway with a rigid bronchoscope or establish a surgical airway.

FOREIGN BODY IN AIRWAY

Tracheal aspiration of a foreign body is an emergency, especially in the pediatric population. Clinical manifestations include sudden dyspnea, dry cough, hoarseness, and wheezing. Mutual cooperation between the anesthesia provider and surgeon is vital to avoid inadvertent distal displacement of the foreign body and complete airway obstruction.

Removal of the foreign body is achieved either via direct laryngoscopy or rigid bronchoscopy, without application of positive airway pressure.[23] The surgeon should be present and ready to perform emergency cricothyrotomy or tracheostomy in the event of complete airway occlusion. Total intravenous anesthesia maintaining spontaneous respiration avoids exposing operating room personnel to volatile anesthetics. Postoperatively, the patient should breathe humidified oxygen and remain under close observation for airway edema.

NASAL AND SINUS SURGERY

Nasal surgery is performed for either cosmetic or functional purposes. Common surgical operations include polypectomy, septoplasty, functional endoscopic sinus surgery, and rhinoplasty. Patients having nasal surgery often also have significant nasal passage obstruction, which may hinder ventilation via face mask. Furthermore, nasal polyps are associated with allergy and reactive airway disease. The nose's rich vascular supply can result in substantial intraoperative blood loss that may be undetected as blood trickles backward into the pharynx. Many nasal procedures can be performed under regional anesthesia and sedation.

The anterior ethmoidal and sphenopalatine branches of the trigeminal nerve provide sensory innervation to the nasal septum and lateral walls. Topical anesthesia is achieved by packing the nose with 4% cocaine pledgets, which are left in situ for 15 minutes. The advantages of using cocaine include production of topical anesthesia, vasoconstriction of vascular tissue, and shrinking of the mucosa. Because cocaine's disadvantages include altered sensorium and deleterious cardiovascular effects, it is frequently substituted by a "pseudococaine" solution of a different local anesthetic mixed with a vasoconstrictor.[24] Anesthesia can be supplemented by submucosal local anesthetic infiltration. When general anesthesia is chosen the airway should be secured with a cuffed ETT. A posterior pharyngeal pack can prevent aspiration and decrease PONV due to swallowed blood. Extubation of the trachea should be performed only on return of protective airway reflexes.

ENDOSCOPIC SURGERY

Endoscopy includes esophagoscopy, bronchoscopy, laryngoscopy, and microlaryngoscopy (with or without laser surgery). Airway evaluation is performed for a variety of pathologic conditions, ranging from foreign body, gastroesophageal reflux, and papillomatosis to tumors or tracheal stenosis. The compromised and symptomatic airway needs careful preoperative assessment. Airway issues should be discussed with the surgeon and preoperative investigations such as blood gas analysis, flow-volume loops, radiographic studies, or magnetic resonance imaging may be warranted.

A proactive airway management plan is necessary. Consideration must be given to a fiberoptic endotracheal intubation in an unsedated patient if doubts exist about the efficacy of successful mask ventilation and direct laryngoscopy. Sedative premedication should be cautiously considered in the presence of upper airway obstruction. Administration of an anticholinergic drug will diminish secretions and facilitate airway visualization. If the patient exhibits stridor or inspiratory retractions, airway

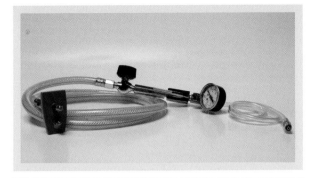

Figure 31-4 Sanders' injector apparatus. High flow oxygen insufflations through a small gauge catheter placed in the trachea.

obstruction probably exists. Although rarely done, a tracheostomy under local anesthesia can be performed.

Techniques can be employed to provide oxygenation and ventilation during endoscopy. The trachea can be intubated with a small diameter pediatric ETT but these are frequently too short for use in adults and offer high resistance to flow. Because an ETT impairs visualization of the posterior commissure, a technique using high-flow oxygen insufflations through a small-gauge catheter placed in the trachea is useful (Fig. 31-4).[25] Another alternative is a manual jet ventilator, which attaches to a side port of the laryngoscope. High-pressure oxygen (30 to 50 psi) is delivered during inspiration and concomitantly entrains air into the trachea via the Venturi effect. This technique carries risk of pneumothorax and pneumomediastinum from rupture of alveolar blebs.

An adequate degree of masseter relaxation is required for introduction of a suspension laryngoscope by the endoscopist. Even though a succinylcholine infusion provides the necessary relaxation, a phase II neuromuscular blockade can result, which often cannot be rapidly terminated. (also see Chapter 12).

LASER SURGERY

Laser (light amplification by stimulated emission of radiation) surgery affords precision in targeting lesions, provides hemostasis, causes minimal tissue edema, and promotes rapid healing. Its physical properties depend on the medium used to create the beam. Laser is used in the treatment of vocal cord papillomas, laryngeal webs, and resection of subglottic occlusive tissue. The use of a small-diameter ETT is necessary for maximum exposure.[26] Laser energy can cause retinal damage, and can produce a laser plume of toxic fumes, which has potential to transmit disease. An efficient smoke evacuator and special masks are necessary because small particles are readily inhaled. The patient's eyes should be taped, and operating room personnel must wear protective eyeglasses.

IV

Table 31-5 Operating Room Precautions for Laser Surgery

Preoperative Period

1. Arrange surgical drapes to avoid accumulation of combustible gases (O_2, N_2O).
2. Allow time for flammable skin preparations to dry.
3. Moisten gauze and sponges in vicinity laser beam.

Intraoperative Period

1. Alert surgeon and OR personnel about ignition risk.
2. Assign specific roles to each OR member in case of fire.
3. Use appropriate laser-resistant ETT.
4. Reduce inspired O_2 to minimal values (monitor Sp_{O_2}).
5. Replace N_2O with air.
6. Wait a few minutes after steps 3 to 5 before activating laser.

ETT, endotracheal tube; OR, operating room; Sp_{O_2}, oxygen saturation measured by pulse oximetry.

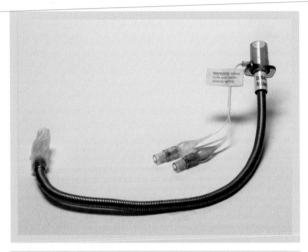

Figure 31-5 Laser endotracheal tube—stainless steel.

The greatest danger during laser surgery is ETT fire as described earlier, so suitable precautions should be taken (Table 31-5). Flexible stainless steel laser-resistant tubes are available for the specific type of laser employed (Fig. 31-5). In order to dissipate heat and detect cuff rupture, the tube cuff should be filled with saline and an indicator dye. Although polyvinylchloride tubes are flammable, they may be modified with a metallic tape wrap. Nonetheless, they may retain a risk of ignition and can reflect the laser beam onto nontargeted tissue. The tissue adjacent to the surgical field should be protected with moist packing. Postoperatively, patients should be monitored for laryngeal edema.

NECK DISSECTION SURGERY

Neck dissection may be complete, modified, or functional. Anatomically, the structures principally involved are (1) the sternocleidomastoid muscle, (2) cranial nerve XI, and (3) the internal and external jugular veins and carotid artery. Frequently, neck dissection is performed for removal of a tumor and may also involve partial or total glossectomy. Patients with such tumors may have a history of tobacco and alcohol abuse. Pulmonary disease is likely and is an indication for a preoperative pulmonary evaluation.

In many cases, the neck dissection may be bilateral, and a tracheostomy may be performed to maintain a patent airway. Upper airway management may be difficult in these patients, especially if there is a history of radiation treatment of the larynx and pharynx or if a mass is present in the oral cavity. Neuromuscular blocking drugs are avoided or the dose is markedly decreased if neuromonitoring is used. Traction or pressure on the carotid sinus can provoke prolongation of the QT interval, bradydysrhythmias, and even asystole. Treatment consists of early detection, cessation of surgical stimulus, and administration of atropine. The carotid sinus reflex can be blocked with local anesthetic infiltration. During dissection, open veins carry risk of venous air embolism.

Postoperative Complications

In the postoperative period the anesthesia provider should be aware of potential nerve injuries. Damage to the recurrent laryngeal nerve can cause vocal cord dysfunction and, if bilateral, results in airway obstruction. The phrenic nerve also traverses through the operative field, and injury to it can result in paralysis of the ipsilateral hemidiaphragm. Pneumothorax can also occur in the postoperative period. Excessive coughing or agitation can result in hematoma formation and airway compromise. If tracheostomy is not performed as part of the procedure, the patient should be monitored closely for signs of laryngeal or upper airway obstruction.

THYROID AND PARATHYROID SURGERY

Thyroid storm may be encountered in a patient who has inadequately controlled hyperthyroidism. It manifests with signs of massive catecholamine release including tachycardia, hypertension, and diaphoresis. Intraoperative anesthesia considerations again focus on airway management. Surgical manipulation of the head and neck can occlude a standard ETT, so an armored ETT may be beneficial (see Fig. 31-3). Airway obstruction after thyroid or parathyroid surgery can be caused by bleeding from the operative site compressing the trachea. Emergency measures include prompt incision and opening of the wound to release the accumulated hematoma. Surgical trauma to one or both recurrent laryngeal nerves can manifest as postextubation hoarseness or stridor. Some surgeons use

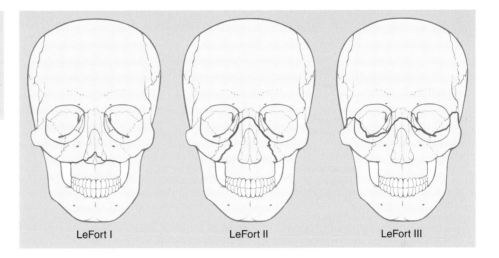

Figure 31-6 Facial injuries and the LeFort fracture classification. (From Myer CM. Trauma of the larynx and craniofacial structures: Airway implications. Paediatr Anaesth 2004;14:103-106, used with permission.)

LeFort I   LeFort II   LeFort III

electromyography (EMG) to monitor recurrent laryngeal nerve integrity, using a special endotracheal tube and EMG monitor. Parathyroid injury or removal may cause hypocalcaemia with clinical signs of tetany, cardiac dysrhythmias, and laryngospasm.

PAROTID SURGERY

The parotid gland may be excised in toto or surgery may be limited to the superficial portion of the gland. Because the parotid is traversed by the facial nerve, nerve function can be monitored with a facial nerve monitor in order to circumvent surgical trauma.[27] The facial nerve may need to be sacrificed during radical parotidectomy and reconstructed with a graft from the contralateral greater auricular nerve (branch of the superficial cervical plexus). Nasotracheal intubation is appropriate if a mandibular resection is planned.

FACIAL TRAUMA

Facial fractures are characterized by the LeFort classification of maxilla fractures (Fig. 31-6).[28] A LeFort I fracture extends across the lower portion of the maxilla but does not continue up into the medial canthal region. A LeFort II fracture also extends across the maxilla, but at a more cephalad level, and it continues upward to the medial

canthal region. A LeFort III fracture is a high-level transverse fracture above the malar bone and through the orbits. It is characterized by complete separation of the maxilla from the craniofacial skeleton. Orotracheal intubation is necessary when intranasal damage is a possibility. In orthognathic surgery, LeFort fractures are created for cosmetic repair.

QUESTIONS OF THE DAY

1. What are the effects of commonly administered anesthetic drugs on intraocular pressure?
2. Which topical ophthalmic medications can cause arterial hypertension? Which can cause bradycardia?
3. What are the manifestations of the oculocardiac reflex in a child undergoing strabismus surgery? How can the response be attenuated or prevented?
4. What are the complications of retrobulbar block? Which ones are life-threatening?
5. A patient is undergoing laser surgery of the vocal cords with an endotracheal tube in place. The surgeon suddenly notes an airway fire. What are the appropriate initial management steps?

IV

REFERENCES

1. Gayer S, Zuleta J: Perioperative management of the elderly undergoing eye surgery, *Clin Geriatr Med* 24(4):687–700, 2008.
2. Vann MA, Ogunnaike BO, Joshi GP: Sedation and anesthesia care for ophthalmologic surgery during local/regional anesthesia, *Anesthesiology* 107(3):502–508, 2007.
3. Schein OD, Katz J, Bass EB, et al: The value of routine preoperative medical testing before cataract surgery. Study of Medical Testing for Cataract Surgery, *N Engl J Med* 342:168–175, 2000.
4. Katz J, Feldman MA, Bass EB, et al: Risks and benefits of anticoagulant and antiplatelet medication use before cataract surgery, *Ophthalmology* 110(9):1784–1788, 2003.
5. Charles S, Rosenfeld PJ, Gayer S: Medical consequences of stopping anticoagulants prior to intraocular surgery or intravitreal injections, *Retina* 27(7):813–815, 2007.
6. Bhananker SM, Posner KL, Cheney FW, et al: Injury and liability associated with monitored anesthesia care. A closed claims analysis, *Anesthesiology* 104(2):228–234, 2006.

7. Ophthalmic Anesthesia Society: www.eyeanesthesia.org.

8. Fanning GL: Orbital regional anesthesia, *Ophthalmol Clin North Am* 19(2):221–232, 2006.

9. Gayer S: Ophthalmic anesthesia: More than meets the eye, ASA Refresher Courses in *Anesthesiology* 34(5):55–63, 2006.

10. Kumar CM, Dodds C: Sub-Tenon's anesthesia, *Ophthalmol Clin North Am* 19(2):209–219, 2006.

11. Wolf GL, Capuano C, Hartung J: Nitrous oxide increases intraocular pressure after intravitreal sulfur hexafluoride injection, *Anesthesiology* 59:547–548, 1983.

12. Vachon CA, Warner DO, Bacon DR: Succinylcholine and the open globe. Tracing the teaching, *Anesthesiology* 99:220–223, 2003.

13. Gayer S: Rethinking anesthesia strategies for patients with traumatic eye injuries: Alternatives to general anesthesia, *Curr Anaesth Crit Care* 17:191–196, 2006.

14. Shen Y, Drum M, Roth S: The prevalence of perioperative visual loss in the United States: A 10 year study from 1996 to 2005 of spinal, orthopedic, cardiac, and general surgery, *Anesth Analg* 109(5):1534–1545, 2009.

15. Satloff RT, Brown AC: Special equipment in the operating room for otolaryngology—head and neck surgery, *Otolaryngol Clin North Am* 14:669–686, 1981.

16. Tait AR, Malviya S, Voepel-Lewis T, et al: Risk factors for perioperative adverse respiratory events in children with upper respiratory tract infections, *Anesthesiology* 95:299–306, 2001.

17. Gross JB, Bachenberg KL, Benumof JL, et al: Practice guidelines for the perioperative management of patients with obstructive sleep apnea: a report by the American Society of Anesthesiologists (ASA) Task Force on Perioperative Management of patients with obstructive sleep apnea, *Anesthesiology* 104(5):1081–1093, 2006.

18. American Society of Anesthesiologists. Task Force on Operating Room Fires Caplan RA, Barker SJ, et al: Practice advisory for the prevention and management of operating room fires, *Anesthesiology* 108:786–801, 2008.

19. Dunlevy TM, O'Malley TP, Postma GN: Optimal concentration of epinephrine for vasoconstriction in neck surgery, *Laryngoscope* 106:1412–1414, 1996.

20. Apfel CC, Laara E, Koivuranta M, et al: A simplified risk score for predicting postoperative nausea and vomiting: Conclusions from cross-validations between two centers, *Anesthesiology* 91:693–700, 1999.

21. Randall DA, Hoffer ME: Complications of tonsillectomy and adenoidectomy, *Otolaryngol Head Neck Surg* 118:61–68, 1998.

22. Tanner K, Fitzsimmons G, Carrol ED, et al: *Haemophilus influenzae* type b epiglottitis as a cause of acute upper airways obstruction in children, *BMJ* 325:1099–1100, 2002.

23. Lam HC, Woo JK, van Hasselt CA: Management of ingested foreign bodies: A retrospective review of 5240 patients, *J Laryngol Otol* 115:954–957, 2001.

24. Lange RA, Cigarroa RG, Yancy CW Jr, et al: Cocaine-induced coronary-artery vasoconstriction, *N Engl J Med* 321:1557–1562, 1989.

25. Rajagopalan R, Smith F, Ramachandran PR: Anaesthesia for microlaryngoscopy and definitive surgery, *Can Anaesth Soc J* 19:83–86, 1972.

26. Rampil IJ: Anesthetic considerations for laser surgery, *Anesth Analg* 74:424–435, 1992.

27. Terrell JE, Kileny PR, Yian C, et al: Clinical outcome of continuous facial nerve monitoring during primary parotidectomy, *Arch Otolaryngol Head Neck Surg* 123:1081–1087, 1997.

28. Myer CM 3rd: Trauma of the larynx and craniofacial structures, Airway implications, *Paediatr Anaesth* 14:103–106, 2004.

32 ANESTHESIA FOR ORTHOPEDIC SURGERY

Andrew D. Rosenberg and Thomas J.J. Blanck

RHEUMATOLOGIC DISORDERS

Patients with rheumatoid arthritis (RA) and other rheumatologic disorders such as ankylosing spondylitis present for orthopedic surgery related to their disease state. Knowledge of these diseases and their underlying medical issues is essential for anesthesia and perioperative management.

Rheumatoid Arthritis

Rheumatoid arthritis is a chronic inflammatory disease, which initially destroys joints and adjacent connective tissue and then progresses to a systemic disease affecting major organ systems (Fig. 32-1). Implicated predisposing etiologies include genetic (gene loci have been identified), environmental, bacterial, viral, and hormonal factors. The role of T cells, autoimmunity, and inflammatory mediators are important in the progression of RA and may serve as sites for potential new treatments.[1-4]

Systemic manifestations of RA are widespread. They may include pulmonary involvement with interstitial fibrosis and cysts with honeycombing, gastritis and ulcers from aspirin and other analgesics, neuropathy, muscle wasting, vasculitis, and anemia. Ultimately the anatomy of the airway is damaged and altered in patients with RA.[1-4]

AIRWAY AND CERVICAL SPINE CHANGES

The patient must be carefully evaluated for both complexity and risk of endotracheal intubation because of difficulty in visualizing the airway, and normal intubation maneuvers may result in an increased risk of cervical spine injury. Many airway abnormalities may occur in patients with RA. Normal mouth opening may be decreased as a result of temporomandibular arthritis. This difficulty may be compounded by the presence of a hypoplastic mandible, which may fuse early in patients with juvenile RA. This results in the noticeable overbite in some patients with RA.[1-4]

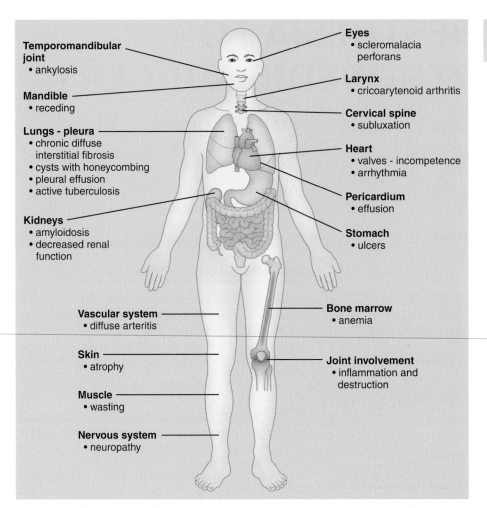

Figure 32-1 Systemic manifestations of rheumatoid arthritis.

Temporomandibular joint
• ankylosis

Mandible
• receding

Lungs - pleura
• chronic diffuse interstitial fibrosis
• cysts with honeycombing
• pleural effusion
• active tuberculosis

Kidneys
• amyloidosis
• decreased renal function

Vascular system
• diffuse arteritis

Skin
• atrophy

Muscle
• wasting

Nervous system
• neuropathy

Eyes
• scleromalacia perforans

Larynx
• cricoarytenoid arthritis

Cervical spine
• subluxation

Heart
• valves - incompetence
• arrhythmia

Pericardium
• effusion

Stomach
• ulcers

Bone marrow
• anemia

Joint involvement
• inflammation and destruction

As with other joints, the cricoarytenoid joint may be affected. Cricoarytenoid arthritis may result in shortness of breath and snoring. RA patients have been misdiagnosed as having sleep apnea as a result of this condition.[5] Patients with cricoarytenoid arthritis may present with stridor on inspiration, which may occur in the post-anesthesia care unit (PACU) after surgery while recovering from anesthesia. Acute subluxation of the cricoarytenoid joint as a result of tracheal intubation can cause stridor as well and it is not responsive to racemic epinephrine.[2]

The cervical spine is affected in up to 80% of patients with RA. Subluxation and unrestricted motion of the cervical spine can lead to impingement of the spinal cord and spinal cord injury.[6] Three anatomic areas of the cervical spine may become involved, resulting in atlantoaxial subluxation, subaxial subluxation, or superior migration of the odontoid (Fig. 32-2).

ATLANTOAXIAL SUBLUXATION

Atlantoaxial subluxation is the abnormal movement of the C1 cervical vertebra (the atlas) on C2 (the atlas). Normally, the transverse axial ligament (TAL) holds the odontoid

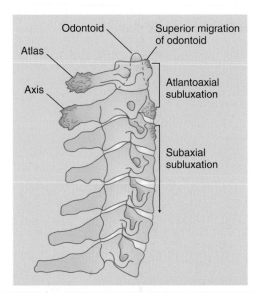

Figure 32-2 Sites of potential involvement of rheumatoid arthritis in the cervical spine.

process, also referred to as the dens, which is the superior projection of the vertebra of C2, in place directly behind the anterior arch of C1 (Fig. 32-3A). With an intact TAL, as the cervical spine is flexed and extended, the odontoid moves with the cervical arch of C1 and the movement between the two is minimal. With destruction of the TAL by RA, movement of the dens is no longer restricted and as the neck is flexed and extended, the C1 vertebra can sublux on the C2 vertebra as the dens and C1 cervical spine no longer move together (Fig. 32-3B). This can result in impingement of the spinal cord, placing it at risk for damage. Subluxation of C1 on C2, referred to as atlantoaxial subluxation, can be quantified by a measurement made between the back of the anterior arch of C1 and the front of the dens or odontoid. This distance is referred to as the atlas-dens interval (ADI). Flexion and extension radiographs of the cervical spine are obtained in order to determine the distance between the atlas and dens and the degree of subluxation (Fig. 32-4). If the ADI is 4 mm or more, atlantoaxial instability is present, the amount of subluxation is considered significant, and the patient is considered to be at risk for spinal cord injury. Because the ring of the cervical arch is an enclosed space, as the ADI increases, the safe area for the cord (SAC), that area left within the arch of C1, decreases and motion can lead to impingement of the cord. In a situation in which the TAL is disrupted, extension of the head minimizes the ADI and increases the SAC, whereas flexion increases the ADI (Fig. 32-5)

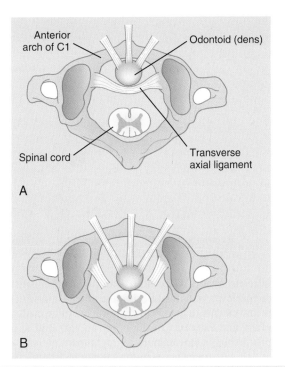

A

B

Figure 32-3 A, Cross-sectional view demonstrating intact TAL (transverse axial ligament) holding odontoid in place against the anterior arch of C1 vertebra. **B,** Rupture of TAL may result in spinal cord impingement.

IV

Figure 32-4 Radiograph of cervical spine in flexion and extension. Note significant atlantoaxial instability with flexion in left panel where odontoid and arch of C1 are outlined. Note contrast in right panel where in extension odontoid and arch of C1 are in close proximity.

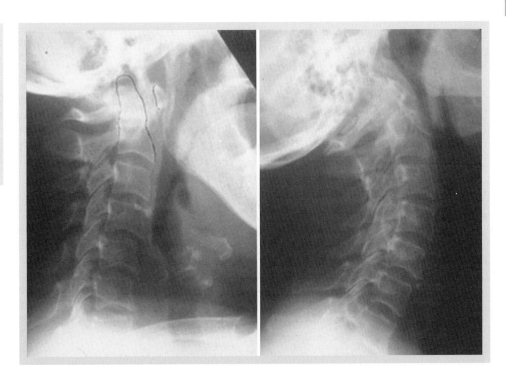

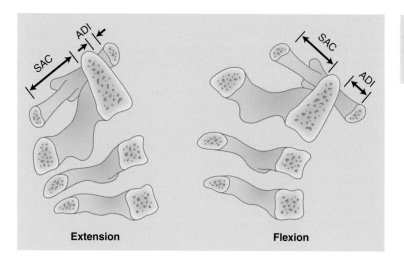

Figure 32-5 Flexion and extension views demonstrating how flexion increases ADI (atlas-dens interval) and decreases the SAC (safe area for the spinal cord). In extension the ADI is decreased and the SAC is increased.

and decreases the SAC, making flexion a more frequent risk position. However, as RA affects more than just the TAL, all neck movements in patients with RA have to be evaluated carefully and extension of the neck can also lead to problems. Although uncommon, asymptomatic patients can have ADI measurements as high as 8 mm to 10 mm. These asymptomatic patients are able to compensate for their cervical spine instability with use of local musculature while awake, but they will not be able to do so once anesthetized. Therefore, care must be taken to minimize neck motion after administration of sedation or general anesthesia in patients with atlantoaxial subluxation.[1–4,6–9]

SUBAXIAL SUBLUXATION
Subluxation of 15% or more of one cervical vertebra on another below the level of the axis (C2) is referred to as subaxial subluxation. This can result in significant spinal cord impingement and neurologic symptoms. The C5-C6 level is the most common area for subaxial subluxation.[8,9] In the presence of significant subaxial subluxation, neck motion can increase impingement and result in spinal cord injury. Therefore, minimal motion of the cervical spine is recommended in patients with this condition.

SUPERIOR MIGRATION OF THE ODONTOID
Inflammation and bone destruction can result in cervical spine collapse in patients with RA. As not all areas of the cervical spine are equally affected in any given patient, if the odontoid is spared, cervical spine collapse may actually result in an intact odontoid process projecting up through the foramen magnum and into the skull. The odontoid can impinge on the brainstem and patients may suffer neurologic symptoms including quadriparesis or paralysis (Fig. 32-6). This pathologic anatomic condition is referred

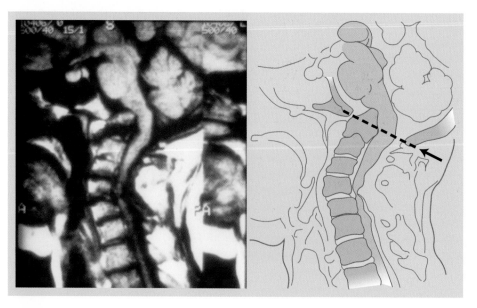

Figure 32-6 Magnetic resonance imaging (MRI) and reconstruction demonstrating superior migration of the odontoid through the foramen magnum and impingement on medulla and pons. Also note subaxial subluxation. (MRI courtesy of Malcolm Dobrow, MD.)

to as superior migration of the odontoid. The odontoid needs to be removed in order to decompress the spinal cord and brainstem. A complicated operative procedure, a transoral odontoidectomy, may be performed to accomplish this and involves an incision in the posterior pharyngeal wall, followed by removal of the arch of C1 and then removal of the odontoid, or pannus, or both, which is causing the neurologic symptoms. With completion of the transoral portion of the procedure, the cervical spine is very unstable, necessitating a posterior spinal fusion.

THE TRACHEA IN RHEUMATOID ARTHRITIS

Although the cervical spine is affected by RA and may collapse from bone destruction, the trachea is usually spared. This results in the trachea twisting in a characteristic manner as the cervical spine collapses, only serving to increase the difficulty of intubating these patients.[8] Tracheal intubation aids such as a fiberoptic bronchoscope, Glidescope, Airtraq, or intubating LMA should be available for assistance in intubating these patients should it be needed (also see Chapter 16).

Ankylosing Spondylitis

Ankylosing spondylitis is a rheumatologic disorder in which repetitive minute bone fractures followed by healing results in the characteristic bamboo spine, disease of the sacroiliac joint, fusion of the posterior elements of the spinal column, and fixed neck flexion that is characteristic in this patient population. There is an association between ankylosing spondylitis and HLA-B27, although not all HLA-B27 positive patients are affected with ankylosing spondylitis. Patients also develop thoracic and costochondral involvement, which may result in a rapid shallow breathing pattern.[2,10] The cervical spine becomes rigid, and direct laryngoscopy and airway manipulation should be performed only after careful assessment. An intubation assist device can help secure the airway. Return of the neck to the neutral position via cervical spine surgery involves removal of all the bony elements of the posterior portion of the spine followed by extension of the head back into a neutral position. This is a very complicated and dangerous procedure, especially at the time when the neck is extended back to the neutral position, which relies on spinal cord monitoring to assess neurologic function as the spine is manipulated.

SPINE SURGERY

Posterior spinal fusion, scoliosis correction, and combined anteroposterior spine procedures may be long complex operations associated with significant blood loss, marked fluid shifts, and major hemodynamic alterations. These factors necessitate adequate patient preparation for the perioperative period including a detailed preoperative evaluation (also see Chapter 13), anticipation regarding perioperative intravenous fluid administration, and appropriate monitoring requirements. Some patients have underlying neuromuscular disorders that could influence the timing of tracheal extubation. Preoperative pulmonary function testing will help in this patient population. Appropriate size and number of intravenous catheters, as well as hemodynamic and neurologic monitoring needs, should be determined. In addition, the blood bank needs to be advised that significant blood loss can occur requiring rapid administration of blood and blood products.

Anterior spine surgery may be performed via abdominal or thoracic approaches. Thoracic surgery may involve open thoracotomy or thoracoscopic techniques. Preoperative discussion with the surgeon is crucial to determine the surgical approach, as there may be a need to provide lung isolation and one-lung ventilation. High thoracic and thoracoscopic procedures frequently require one-lung ventilation to ensure adequate visualization. This can be accomplished with the use of a double-lumen tube or a bronchial blocker.

If the procedure is a combined anteroposterior procedure, a double-lumen endotracheal tube (ETT) can be used for the anterior component with the tube exchanged for a single-lumen ETT for the posterior portion of the surgery. While double-lumen ETTs are of great value, intraoperative exchange, or their removal after a long procedure in which airway edema can be an issue, is risky. Reintubation of the trachea can become difficult owing to airway edema and reintubation can be traumatic. Alternatively, a bronchial blocker can be used with a single-lumen ETT (Fig. 32-7) (also see Chapter 13).[3,11]

IV

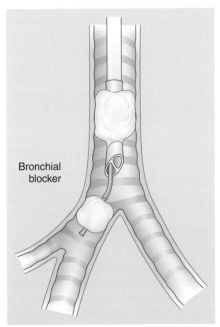

Bronchial blocker

Figure 32-7 Depiction of how bronchial blocker is placed to isolate lung for one-lung ventilation.

Advantages of the bronchial blocker include avoiding the issue of the need to change the tube between different stages of the procedure or at the end of the operation as deflating the cuff and withdrawing the catheter back into its casing and recapping the proximal end returns the endotracheal tube to its single-lumen tube characteristics. If extubation of the trachea at the end of the surgical procedure is not indicated, the endotracheal tube does not have to be changed at the end of the operation, thereby avoiding the issue of changing an endotracheal tube in the presence of potentially significant airway edema. Make certain that the PACU staff is properly educated as to the various ports of the bronchial blocker.[2,3,11]

Some surgeons are using CO_2 insufflation as the sole means of moving the lung away from the surgical field even in high thoracic spine surgical procedures. This allows for the use of a single-lumen ETT for the entire procedure, bypassing the need for either a double-lumen tube or a bronchial blocker.

Anesthetic Technique

Anesthetic technique is geared to provide anesthesia and analgesia for the procedure while avoiding drugs that may interfere with acquisition of the waveforms required for perioperative neurologic evaluation of the spine. Nitrous oxide/oxygen or air in oxygen is used in combination with opioids and an infusion of propofol or dexmedetomidine. If somatosensory evoked potentials (SSEPs) alone are being monitored, an inhaled anesthetic, equivalent to a small percentage of 1 MAC, can be administered. Volatile anesthetics may interfere with signal acquisition in patients monitored with transcranial motor evoked potentials (TCMEPs) and may have to be discontinued, if used at all, if adequate signals cannot be obtained. While neuromuscular blockade may be used to facilitate tracheal intubation, paralysis should not be maintained if TCMEPs are being continuously monitored. If the patient is having pedicle screws placed, then the neuromuscular blockade needs to be terminated before the EMGs (electromyograms) are obtained so that testing can be properly performed. A small dose of ketamine can be given in the perioperative period as an additional pain relief modality to provide analgesia for major surgery including spine surgery.[12,13]

Awareness (Also See Chapter 46)

Intraoperative awareness is a concern for patients and physicians. Patients undergoing spine surgery appear to be at increased risk for intraoperative awareness as a result of the requirement that the anesthetic technique administered to them be modified allowing for adequate intraoperative neurophysiologic monitoring waveforms to assess spinal cord function. Therefore, some advocate the use of brain function monitoring in these patients to help avoid intraoperative awareness. However, this is not a standard and, as noted in the Practice Advisory for Intraoperative Awareness and Brain Function Monitoring,[14] a decision should be made on a case-by-case basis by the individual practitioner for selected patients (e.g., light anesthesia). There was a consensus in the advisory that brain function monitoring is not routinely indicated for patients undergoing general anesthesia as the "general applicability of these monitors in the prevention of intraoperative awareness had not been established." In fact, Avidan and associates demonstrated that awareness is not decreased with use of brain function monitoring.[15] The need for brain monitoring is still not clear.

Blood Conservation during Spine Surgery (Also See Chapter 24)

Methods to decrease blood loss in spine surgery patients include predonation, hemodilution, wound infusion with a dilute epinephrine solution, hypotensive anesthesia techniques, cell salvage technique, positioning to diminish venous pressure, careful surgical hemostasis, and administration of antifibrinolytics. Medications to decrease blood loss during surgery include the antifibrinolytics aprotinin, tranexamic acid, and ε-aminocaproic acid. Aprotinin, a serine protease inhibitor, effectively decreases blood loss in cardiac patients and has been demonstrated to be efficacious in patients undergoing spine surgery as well.[16-18] The synthetic lysine analogs tranexamic acid and ε-aminocaproic acid have also been employed in spine surgery as well as in patients undergoing orthopedic surgery.[18] Tranexamic acid can be administered by an initial bolus injection of 10 mg/kg over 30 minutes followed by a continuous infusion of 1 mg/kg/hour.

Although apparently ε-aminocaproic acid can be helpful, a meta-analysis of the use of antifibrinolytics in orthopedic patients demonstrated that while both aprotinin and tranexamic acid are effective in decreasing blood loss, the data were not sufficient to demonstrate efficacy with ε-aminocaproic acid.[17] However, the negative side effects of aprotinin in cardiac patients include (1) increased risk of myocardial infarction (MI) or heart failure by approximately 55%, nearly double the risk of stroke, (2) increased risk of long-term mortality, and (3) a higher death rate in patients receiving aprotinin as demonstrated in a study over a 5-year period comparing aprotinin and lysine analogs in high-risk cardiac surgery. The study was terminated early and resulted in relabeling and ultimately withdrawing aprotinin from the market so that it is no longer available.[19-21]

Positioning (Also See Chapter 19)

Spine surgery is often performed with the patient in the prone position. Careful positioning is crucial to avoid patient injury. Movement to the prone position should be performed in a carefully coordinated manner with the surgical team. The neck should not be hyperextended or hyperflexed but placed in the neutral position, the endotracheal tube is positioned so it is not kinked, contact areas are padded, and the face and eyes are protected. Pressure and stretch on nerves is avoided by proper padding and avoiding any extension over 90 degrees. The abdomen needs to be hanging free to avoid increased venous pressure and thereby increased venous bleeding. The prone position alters pulmonary dynamics, so pulmonary function must be reassessed in this position.

Intraoperative Spinal Cord Monitoring (Also See Chapter 20)

Monitoring spinal cord function is an important component of major surgical procedures involving distraction and rotation of the spine such as occurs with major anteroposterior spinal fusions and scoliosis surgery. Spinal cord monitoring is employed in order to detect and hopefully reverse, in a timely manner, any adverse effects noted during the operative period. Spinal cord monitoring may include use of somatosensory evoked potentials (SSEPs), motor evoked potentials (MEPs), including transcranial motor evoked potentials, EMGs, or a wake-up test. The anesthetic technique must be adjusted appropriately when spinal cord monitoring is employed. Some anesthetics interfere with acquisition of the waveforms that are obtained intraoperatively and utilized to analyze spinal cord integrity.

SSEPs are sensory evoked potential waves generated in the extremities by repetitive stimulation that propagate up through the dorsum or sensory portion of the spinal cord and into the brain where these signals or waveforms are detected via electrodes placed over the scalp. Specific areas on the scalp coincide with the brain's sensory areas for the upper and lower extremities and proper signal acquisition obtained over these sites indicates an intact sensory or dorsal portion of the spinal cord. The SSEP waveform generated from multiple repetitive stimulations is analyzed for its latency and amplitude (Fig. 32-8). An increase in latency of greater than 10% or a decrease in amplitude of 60% or more, as well as inability to obtain a proper waveform or signal may be indicative of spinal cord dysfunction or disruption. Many factors can alter waveforms unrelated to surgery. These should be properly detected and eliminated. Surgically unrelated causes may include hypotension, hypothermia, high concentrations of volatile anesthetics, benzodiazepines, hyper- or hypocarbia, and anemia. Only a small concentration of volatile anesthetic (1% to 2%) should be employed when SSEP monitoring is used. Midazolam and other benzodiazepines are avoided as they may interfere with obtaining a waveform. Some physicians even avoid nitrous oxide and use a combination of air in oxygen.[2-4,12,13]

Surgically related conditions resulting in loss of SSEPs include direct injury or trauma to the cord or impairment of blood supply. Distraction, rotation, excessive bleeding, and severing or clamping of arterial blood supply can result in ischemia to the cord and neurologic injury. Unlike direct injury, which is demonstrated immediately by changes in SSEPs, ischemia may take time, up to half an hour, to manifest itself. Some areas of the spinal cord are more vulnerable and therefore more prone to ischemia as their blood supply is dependent on watershed blood flow. Surgical intervention as a result of either direct contact or stretching may impair blood supply and thus render the cord

IV

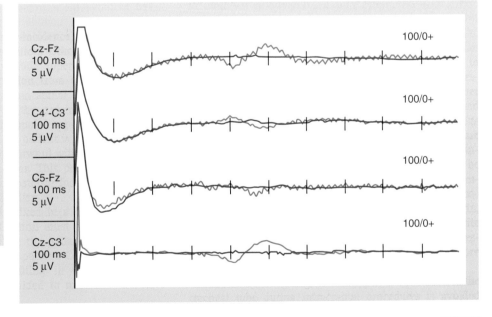

Figure 32-8 Somatosensory evoked potentials (SSEPs) of tibial nerve demonstrating loss of SSEP waveform. Note how the newly acquired waveforms (*purple color*) are flattened when compared to baseline tracings (*red color*) as amplitude of tracings are decreased and latency increased. Tracings returned to normal after retraction of cauda equina was released. (Courtesy of Department of Neurophysiology, NYU Hospital for Joint Diseases.)

Cz-Fz
100 ms
5 μV
100/0+

C4'-C3'
100 ms
5 μV
100/0+

C5-Fz
100 ms
5 μV
100/0+

Cz-C3'
100 ms
5 μV
100/0+

ischemic.[22] Once a significant change in SSEPs or other monitor is noted, specific maneuvers should be used such as releasing the rotation and distraction of the spine if it has occurred. In addition, as a result of distraction there may be insufficient blood supply to the spine, and therefore, the mean arterial blood pressure should be increased in an effort to restore adequate blood flow. All variables such as hemoglobin, temperature, CO_2, and arterial blood pressure should be considered. Once these are all evaluated, a wake-up test (see following discussion) may be necessary if the waveforms do not improve.

TRANSCRANIAL MOTOR EVOKED POTENTIALS

As SSEP monitoring only helps determine adequate status of the dorsal or sensory portion of the spinal cord, a method to monitor the motor or ventral aspect of the spinal cord became necessary.[23] Initially this was provided via neurogenic motor evoked potentials, but these waveforms could be obtained only while the surgical incision was open and the spinous processes available for insertion of electrodes. Thus, some vulnerable operative time periods remained unmonitored. Transcranial motor evoked potentials (TCMEPs) allow for monitoring the patient's motor pathways throughout the entire procedure. Stimulation over the motor cortex of the brain generates a waveform, which is propagated down the motor pathways and detected distally in the arm or leg. This stimulation results in a characteristic waveform (Fig. 32-9). Loss of the wave may be indicative of neurologic injury (see Fig. 32-9). As with SSEP waveforms, loss of the tracings requires an evaluation to determine the cause and may require a wake-up test as well.[24]

In order to generate TCMEP potentials, the patient cannot have a residual neuromuscular blockade. The electrical current causing the stimulus over the motor cortex also stimulates muscles directly in the area of the electrodes placed in the scalp—the masseter muscle and muscles of mastication. This muscle contraction may result in a strong bite, which can potentially injure the tongue, lip, and endotracheal tube. Instances of significant tongue lacerations and damage to endotracheal tubes can occur and can develop into emergency situations, especially with the patient in the prone position (also see Chapter 19).[25] The tongue should not protrude through the teeth. Placing a bite block made of tongue depressors and gauze in the back of the mouth along the teeth line bilaterally will help prevent injury. In the prone (facedown) position, any motion may allow for the tongue to slip and fall between the teeth, rendering it vulnerable to laceration. Each stimulus is associated with a masseter muscle contraction so the patient is at risk as long as waveforms are being generated.[24,25]

ELECTROMYOGRAMS

After pedicle screw placement, the surgeon may request EMGs to determine if the screw is in close proximity to a nerve root, as this can result in neurologic problems. An electric current is sent through the screw and EMGs are measured distally. If a low mA current can stimulate the nerve root, then the screw is too close to the nerve root. Therefore, in general, a current greater than 7 mA is sent to generate a response to know that screws are not too close to nerve roots. For accurate muscle EMGs, residual neuromuscular blockade must be terminated or reversed.

WAKE-UP TEST

The wake-up test was traditionally utilized to assess spinal cord integrity in many scoliosis cases. Development of sophisticated spinal cord monitoring is now standard in many hospitals and the wake-up test is generally reserved for those situations in which monitoring is unobtainable or a significant intraoperative change in spinal cord monitoring waveforms is noted. During the wake-up test the anesthetic is discontinued and the patient is asked to move the extremities. Potential complications of this approach include increased bleeding, venous air embolism, and even inadvertent extubation of the trachea in the prone position with the wound exposed. The

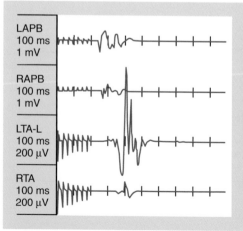
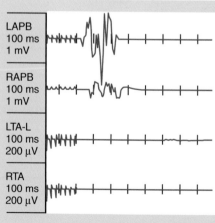

Figure 32-9 Normal transcranial motor evoked potentials (*left*) and loss of waveform (*right lower two panels*) indicating possible neurologic issue with motor component of spinal cord. (Courtesy of Department of Neurophysiology, NYU Hospital for Joint Diseases.)

wake-up test is performed as follows: turn off all inhaled anesthetics, reverse any muscle relaxant present, and stop infusions such as dexmedetomidine, propofol, or ketamine. If spontaneous respirations do not begin, inject naloxone, 0.04 mg at a time, to reverse any residual narcotic effect. The patient's head should be held to reduce the risk of self-extubation. Prior to assessing lower extremity function, confirm upper extremity function. Patient compliance denotes adequate recovery from general anesthesia. Then, while someone is observing the feet, ask the patient to wiggle his or her toes. A rapid-acting anesthetic such as propofol should be ready to be administered as soon as the assessment is complete, so the patient can rapidly be reanesthetized. If the wake-up test is not successful in demonstrating adequate motor movement, further surgical intervention may be warranted and the patient may require transport to the radiology suite for additional imaging studies.[2,4,26]

CONCLUSION OF THE CASE

At the conclusion of the operation, the patient is placed in the supine position. All lines and tubes are secured so that intravenous line, arterial line, and airway access are not lost at this crucial time. Carefully reassess the patient for hemodynamic status, intravascular volume status, hematocrit, blood loss, degree of fluid and blood replacement, temperature, and the potential for airway edema. Premature extubation must be avoided. Also, facial edema, respiratory effort, the amount of pain medication, and the presence of splinting and pain should be evaluated prior to extubating the trachea. After tracheal extubation, the patient may be transported to the PACU. Supplemental oxygen should be utilized in the PACU. Electrolytes, hemoglobin, and clotting studies should be ordered as indicated.

Postoperative pain management (also see Chapter 40) may prove complicated after spine surgery as some patients preoperatively may have been taking pain medications, particularly opioids. Patient controlled analgesia (PCA) may be effective, with the dose tailored to the patient's needs. Some centers utilize ketamine as an analgesic adjunct. The use of nonsteroidal anti-inflammatory drugs (NSAIDs), particularly ketorolac, needs careful consideration as it is a medication that interferes with bone formation and therefore should be avoided in patients who just underwent spinal fusion.[27] NSAIDs may be appropriate when bone healing is not a factor. Other oral medications that are helpful may include acetaminophen, anticonvulsants (e.g., gabapentin and pregabalin), antispasmodics that work at the spinal cord level (e.g., baclofen, tizanidine), anti-inflammatory medications, and opioids.

Vision Loss (Also See Chapter 31)

Postoperative visual loss (POVL) is a rare but significant complication occurring in patients undergoing spine surgery.[28-35] Although its etiology is unclear, patients undergoing prolonged spine surgery (>6 hours) in the prone position who have large blood loss (>1 L)are particularly at risk.[29] Yet, patients with small blood loss and short procedures also have had visual loss. Perioperative factors such as anemia, hypotension, prolonged surgery, blood loss, increased venous pressure from positioning in the prone position, edema, a compartment syndrome within the orbit, resistance to blood flow, such as direct pressure on the eye, as well as systemic diseases such as diabetes, hypertension, and vascular disease are all possible etiologic factors.[28-35]

Ischemic optic neuropathy is a major cause of POVL. Variations in blood supply to the optic nerve may play a role in the development of ischemic optic neuropathy including reliance on a watershed blood supply to critical areas of the optic nerve. The head-down position allows edema to develop in the orbit and this increase in venous pressure may impact arterial blood flow. Ocular perfusion pressure (OPP), or the blood pressure supplying blood flow to the optic nerve, is a function of the mean arterial pressure (MAP) and intraocular pressure (IOP) such that $OPP = MAP - IOP$. Increases in IOP or decreases in MAP can have a negative impact on OPP.[11] Increases in IOP can decrease OPP and lead to ischemia, and the prone position is associated with increases in IOP.[30]

A visual loss registry has been established by the American Society of Anesthesiologists (ASA) to facilitate establishing the etiology of POVL.[29] Also, an ASA Practice Advisory points to ischemic optic neuropathy as the most likely cause of POVL (Table 32-1).[28-35] Of the 93 cases reported in the registry publication, 83 resulted from ION, with the remainder attributed to central retinal artery occlusion (CRAO). CRAO may be embolic in nature or the result of direct pressure on the eyeball and tends to be unilateral. Most patients in the registry were healthy and placed in the prone position for spine surgery. Blood loss more than 1 L and procedures of 6 hours or longer were present in 96% of cases. Fifty-five of the POVL cases were bilateral, with 47 having total visual loss. A close examination of the registry publication reveals that blood loss in patients with POVL varied widely with a mean of 2 L but ranged from 0.1 to 25 L.[29,33,34] The advisory and registry publications promote a preoperative discussion with the patient and some suggest staged spine procedures for prolonged surgeries.[29,33,34]

SURGERY IN THE SITTING POSITION (Also See Chapter 19)

Shoulder surgery is frequently performed with patients in the sitting or "beach chair" position with the head and upper torso elevated 30 to 90 degrees from the supine position. Anesthesia in this position is associated with rare but significant and devastating neurologic complications including stroke, ischemic brain injury, and vegetative

IV

Table 32-1 Summary of the ASA Practice Advisory

- There is a subset of patients who undergo spine procedures in the prone position and receive general anesthesia. They are at increased risk for perioperative visual loss. These patients are scheduled to undergo procedures that are prolonged and have substantial blood loss.
- Consider informing high-risk patients that there is a small, unpredictable risk of perioperative visual loss.
- The use of deliberate hypotensive techniques during spine surgery is not associated with perioperative visual loss.
- In patients who have substantial blood loss, colloids should be administered along with crystalloids to maintain intravascular volume.
- There is no apparent transfusion "trigger" that would eliminate the risk of perioperative visual loss related to anemia.
- High-risk patients should be positioned such that the head level with or higher than the heart when possible. In addition, when possible, the head should be maintained in a neutral forward position (e.g., without significant neck flexion, extension, lateral flexion, or rotation).
- Staged spine procedures should be considered in high-risk patients.

ASA, American Society of Anesthesiologists.
From ASA. Practice Advisory for Perioperative Visual Loss Associated with Spine Surgery. Anesthesiology 2006;104:1319-1328.

states.[36,37] The cause is a decrease in cerebral perfusion pressure resulting with insufficient blood supply to the brain. This is due to the arterial blood pressure gradient that develops between the heart and brain in this position. For each centimeter of head elevation above the level of the heart there is a decrease in arterial blood pressure of 0.77 mm Hg. Therefore, arterial blood pressure measured at the level of the heart is not the blood and perfusion pressure at the brain. Measurements obtained at the level of the heart must be recalculated. A 20-cm height differential is not uncommon, which calculates to approximately a 15 to 16 mm Hg gradient. A convenient point for measuring height difference between the heart and brain is the external auditory meatus, which is at the same level as the circle of Willis (COW). Even so, there is still a significant amount of brain tissue above this level. If blood pressure decreases, or the surgeon's request for hypotensive anesthesia is followed, cerebral hypotension and therefore a significantly diminished cerebral perfusion pressure may occur at the level of the COW and the brain. Therefore, significant hypotension should be avoided in these patients especially those elderly, hypertensive patients whose autoregulatory curve is undoubtedly compromised.

FRACTURED HIP

Hip fractures occur frequently in elderly patients who often also suffer from multiple preexisting medical conditions or co-morbidities. Factors predisposing to fracture include medical co-morbidities, osteoporosis, lower limb dysfunction, visual impairment, increasing age, Parkinson's disease, previous fracture, stroke, female gender, dementia, institutionalized patients, excess alcohol or caffeine consumption, cold climate, and use of psychotropic medications.[38] Mortality rates can range up to 14% to 36% in the first year after fracture.[38] Medical status effects morbidity and mortality. One example is the number of co-morbidities from which the patient suffers, as in one study the presence of four to six co-morbidities is associated with increased mortality rate when compared to patients with less co-morbidity.[39] Roche and associates in studying 2448 patients reported that the presence of three or more co-morbidities was a strong preoperative risk factor with the postoperative development of chest infection or heart failure being associated with high mortality rate.[40] White and associates reported that ASA I and II patients had mortality rates equal to age-matched control subjects, but ASA III and IV patients had higher mortality rates (49% vs. 8%) after hip fracture.[41]

Generally, when significant co-morbidities that need correction exist, then patients benefit from delay in surgery while their medical status improves. Mortality rate in high-risk patients was decreased from 29% to 2.9% in one study when time was taken to correct physiologic abnormalities.[42] This was also demonstrated by Kenzora and coworkers, who noted a higher mortality rate (34% vs. 6.9%) in patients who went immediately into surgery as compared to those who were delayed 2 to 5 days to improve their medical status.[39] Moran and colleagues, in a study of 2660 hip fracture patients with an overall mortality rate of 9% at 30 days, 19% at 90 days, and 30% at 12 months, noted that healthy patients did well as long as surgery was performed within 4 days.[43] Patients with co-morbidities had a nearly 2.5 times increased mortality rate at 30 days as compared to healthy patients. Also, patients admitted to the hospital immediately after fracture did better than those admitted more than a day later.[43] Shiga and associates noted that operative delay over 48 hours after admission was associated with increased mortality rate and suggested that undue delay may be harmful to patients, especially young or low-risk patients.[44]

Preoperative evaluation (also see Chapter 13) is especially important. The diagnosis of a recent myocardial infarction (MI) illustrates how these evaluations have changed. Previously, surgery was delayed up to 6 months following an MI, but now, the tendency is to risk-stratify patients based on the severity of their MI to determine wait time until surgery.[45] The recent MI needs to be evaluated on a risk-benefit ratio comparing the risk of surgery after a recent MI with the negative side effects of keeping a patient bed bound with its attendant risks of pneumonia, pulmonary embolism, pain, loss of ability to walk, and decubitus ulcers. Factors to consider are the extent of the MI, additional myocardium that may be at risk, if the patient suffers from postinfarct angina, and the presence of congestive heart failure (CHF). Although ongoing angina or the presence of CHF may preclude early surgery, a small subendocardial MI with minimal increase in cardiac enzymes, normal echocardiogram and stress test would allow consideration for an earlier intervention. A fractured hip usually prevents the patient from undergoing a normal exercise stress test. Therefore, if indicated, a pharmacologic stress test may be needed.

Anesthetic Technique

There is no clear advantage of one anesthetic technique over another.[2,4,46,47] Therefore, choice of spinal or general anesthesia should be made on a case-by-case basis taking the patient's specific medical issues into consideration.

The anesthetic provider should consider the type of fracture when preparing for surgery. Intertrochanteric fractures are associated with larger blood losses and longer operations, because a plate and screw are inserted, than intracapsular fractures that may be repaired with cannulated screws or a hemiarthroplasty depending on the viability of the femoral head.

Although no one anesthetic technique has proved to be superior, the pros and cons of both spinal and general anesthesia must be considered when choosing the technique for a given patient. General anesthesia, although easy to administer, does not provide any thromboembolic protection for the patient that may be provided by a regional technique.[2,4]

Advantages of regional anesthesia, such as provided by a spinal anesthetic, are that (1) it avoids endotracheal intubation and airway manipulation and the medications that need to be administered to accomplish this, (2) it decreases the total amount of systemic medication the patient receives throughout the procedure, and (3) it may play a role in decreasing the risk of thromboembolism. The vasodilatory effect of the spinal anesthetic may help the patient with CHF. However, intravascular fluid still should be given cautiously because CHF may worsen as the intravascular vasodilatory effect of the spinal recedes.[2,4]

Preoperatively, intravascular volume status is a concern as fractures can result in significant blood loss, and a spinal anesthetic in the presence of hypovolemia can result in profound hypotension. An additional concern is time the patient must lay on the fracture table, especially in the elderly, as even small amounts of sedation can result in significant respiratory depression.

Peripheral nerve blocks including lumbar plexus, femoral, and lateral femoral cutaneous nerve blocks may also be used in selected situations. Chayen and coworkers demonstrated the effectiveness of lumbar plexus blocks in fractured hip patients.[48] This block can be performed with the nerve stimulator technique or use of ultrasound guidance. Fracture repair requiring only cannulated pins may be performed with combined femoral and lateral femoral cutaneous nerve blocks. The femoral nerve block provides analgesia in the region of the hip, and the lateral femoral cutaneous nerve (LFCN) block will anesthetize the region of cannulated pin insertion located on the lateral aspect of the thigh. An LFCN block is performed by administering a fan of local anesthetic in a cephalad direction from a point 1 cm medial and inferior to the anterior superior iliac spine. The LFCN is a sensory nerve and therefore not amenable to location with a nerve stimulator.

Intraoperative considerations for patients undergoing fractured hip repair include proper positioning and padding on the fracture table, maintaining adequate intravascular volume status as blood is lost, adequately maintaining body temperature, and observation for hemodynamic alterations and other unanticipated responses in the elderly patient as the procedure progresses.

At the conclusion of the procedure reassess hemodynamic status, ensuring that the patient has received adequate blood and fluid replacement. Determine if the dose of narcotic the patient received is going to have a prolonged effect, thereby resulting in respiratory depression once the patient is extubated. Check for hypothermia, anemia, and evaluate the patients end-tidal CO_2 as the elderly can be slow to awaken and can easily hypoventilate as a result of the opioids they received. Once the trachea is extubated, administer supplemental oxygen. The dose and frequency of pain medication should be given cautiously as increased circulation time and the cumulative effect of administered opioids may become evident when not expected.

TOTAL JOINT REPLACEMENT

Total hip, knee, and shoulder replacements are frequently performed in patients suffering from osteoarthritis, rheumatologic disorders, and trauma. Operations may include replacement of an entire joint, partial joint replacement, replacement of individual components, or resurfacing procedures. Major concerns include the patient's age, concurrent medical conditions, blood loss, proper positioning and padding, hemodynamic variations during the procedure, the response to methylmethacrylate cement, and the risk of fat and pulmonary emboli.

Total Hip Replacement

Total hip replacements (THRs) are performed with patients in either the supine or lateral decubitus position. A relatively new approach, the anterior approach to the hip, is frequently performed in the supine position on a

IV

special operating room. In the supine position, the arm that is on the same side as the hip needs to be flexed away from the side. In the lateral position an axillary roll is placed under the axilla to protect the axillary artery and brachial plexus from compression. Patients having procedures in the lateral position also have a lateral positioner placed to stabilize their pelvis. The positioner can push abdominal contents cephalad and interfere with respiratory function.

Total hip replacement can be performed with and without methylmethacrylate cement (MMC) to secure the prosthesis. Younger patients tend to receive noncemented joint replacements. The use of MMC is associated with cardiopulmonary side effects such as hypoxia, bronchoconstriction, hypotension, cardiovascular collapse, and even death. The etiology for the systemic reaction to MMC may result from the liquid MMC monomer itself, which is used in producing the cement for cementing the prosthesis, or may be due to air, fat, or bone marrow elements being forced into circulation. The higher the liquid content of the liquid monomer in the mix with the polymer MMC at the time of insertion, which occurs from not adequately mixing or not waiting long enough for mixing to occur, the more frequently side effects are noted. High-risk patients include those who are hypovolemic at the time of cementing, hypertensive patients, and patients with significant preexisting cardiac disease.[41,42]

Transesophageal echocardiographic evaluation of cardiac structure and function during reaming and cementing does indicate MMC and fat emboli flow centrally to the heart from the surgical site.[43,44] If a patient has a patent foramen ovale these emboli can theoretically cross the patent foramen into the left ventricle and then move into the arterial circulation. If the patient has a probe-patent foramen ovale it is also possible that an increase in pulmonary pressures as a result of bronchoconstriction, from methylmethacrylate cement, for example, can increase right atrial pressure and shunt blood flow directly across the probe-patent foramen ovale. Many patients may have a decreased PaO_2 during reaming and cementing. An increase in the FiO_2 of 1.0 may be necessary.

At the conclusion of surgery the patient is transferred to the PACU. Supplemental oxygen is administered, and a hemoglobin count should be obtained. Further testing is based upon the patient's underlying medical condition. Postoperative pain management may include epidural infusion with epidural PCA, PCA, oral medications, or peripheral nerve block including lumbar plexus block. The postoperative pain management the patient receives may be influenced by the thromboembolism prophylaxis administered.

Total Knee Replacements and Tourniquets

Total knee replacements (TKRs) are frequently performed with a tourniquet in place to provide a bloodless surgical field. The tourniquet should be carefully placed on the upper thigh over appropriate padding. The leg may be wrapped with an esmarch bandage to help exsanguinate the limb prior to tourniquet inflation. In the lower extremity the tourniquet is inflated to approximately 100 mm Hg above the systolic blood pressure, as this will prevent arterial blood from entering the exsanguinated limb.[2,3,49]

As tourniquets render the limb ischemic there is a limit to inflation time before the ischemia can result in permanent limb damage. The safe upper limit of ischemia time is considered to be 2 hours. The surgeon should be informed of tourniquet inflation time at 1 hour and then as the tourniquet approaches the 2-hour limit so it can be deflated in a timely manner. If the total tourniquet time will exceed the 2-hour limit, the tourniquet should be deflated at 2 hours for a period of at least 15 to 20 minutes before it is reinflated. This will allow for the "wash-out" of acidic metabolites from the ischemic limb as the limb is reperfused with oxygenated blood. Recirculation of the ischemic limb with release of the tourniquet is noted by a decrease in blood pressure and an increase in end-tidal CO_2 as the acid products recirculate.[2] The hypotension usually responds to intravascular fluid administration and vasopressors if necessary.[2,49]

Pain is noted as the duration of tourniquet inflation time increases, manifesting itself as an increase in blood pressure and heart rate. Overaggressively treating the increase in blood pressure with opioids and other medications can result in hypotension after the tourniquet is released. Animal models have determined the pain to occur as result of C-fiber firing. A regional block proximal to the tourniquet can prevent C-fibers from firing.[2,49,50]

Complications noted with tourniquet use include nerve damage, vessel damage especially in patients with atherosclerosis, pulmonary embolism, and skin damage. One source of skin damage is the antiseptic prep solution if it is allowed to seep under the tourniquet and tourniquet padding at the time of skin prep causing a chemical burn. Additional concerns at the time of tourniquet deflation are pulmonary embolism and a decrease in core temperature as the isolated extremity is reperfused.[2,45,46]

After deflating the tourniquet, the surgical field should be observed for evidence of bleeding. Occasionally the tourniquet is deflated at the tourniquet control box but there is no bleeding because the tubing to the tourniquet is kinked. This is a significant complication as the tourniquet is effectively still inflated and the patient is then at risk for prolonged tourniquet inflation time, limb ischemia, and complications. One method to ensure tourniquet deflation is to disconnect the tubing from the tourniquet box and observe the incision for bleeding.

Total knee replacements are frequently performed under regional anesthesia with intravenous sedation. As a tourniquet is used during the operation, in the operating room blood loss is usually not significant.

However, if much blood loss occurs into drains in the PACU, hypotension may result. Some surgeons do not deflate the tourniquet until the wound is closed and the dressing is on the patient. In this situation blood loss is usually less but there is a risk of bleeding.[51]

Debate exists as to whether bilateral total knee replacements should be performed in one setting. Many patients have undergone bilateral total knee replacements in one day or during one hospital admission.[52–56] If bilateral TKRs are scheduled, they should be performed after careful patient selection. Intraoperatively, be aware that drainage from the first total joint will be occurring into the wound drainage system, which may be "under the drapes," and if bleeding is significant, hypotension can occur for what might be "unrecognized" reasons.

TKR patients have more postoperative pain than patients receiving THR. A postoperative pain management plan should be delineated to address anticipated pain. This may include PCA, catheters, individual nerve blocks of the lower extremities, and oral medications.

Deep Venous Thrombosis and Thromboembolism Prophylaxis

The need for, and technique of, perioperative deep venous thrombosis (DVT) prophylaxis varies by surgeon and institution. Thromboembolism management should be coordinated with the anesthesia providers. Options for DVT prophylaxis include warfarin, low-molecular-weight heparin (LMWH), sequential compression boots, and aspirin, and although guidelines do exist as to which medications to use, there still remains variability in choice of DVT thromboprophylaxis. The surgeon's choice and timing of DVT prophylaxis will influence the choice of technique: spinal, combined spinal and epidural, epidural, peripheral block, or nerve block and catheter. At issue is concern that catheter manipulation while a patient is anticoagulated will result in bleeding, and if the catheter is in the epidural space, its removal can potentially result in epidural bleeding, epidural hematoma formation, and paralysis. Once an epidural hematoma develops, it must be removed expeditiously before irreversible paralysis occurs. While epidural hematomas classically present with severe pain and onset of numbness and weakness, in patients receiving epidural infusions of local anesthetics, these classic symptoms may be masked.

After introduction of the LMWH enoxaparin in the United States, the incidence of epidural hematomas increased. This did not occur to the same extent in Europe, where a once daily dosing schedule was employed in comparison to the twice-daily administration in the United States. Epidural hematoma formation probably resulted from a number of factors including performance of neuraxial anesthesia or removal of epidural catheters while the anticoagulation effect of LMWH was still present, the use of multiple medications at the same time that have anticoagulation properties, or lack of attention to dosing schedule. This prompted a warning from the Food and Drug Administration (FDA) noting "reports of epidural or spinal hematomas with concurrent use of low molecular weight heparin and spinal/epidural anesthesia or spinal puncture." Consensus statements from the American Society of Regional Anesthesia and Pain Medicine (ASRA) addressed the issue. Recommendations included waiting at least 10 to 12 hours before neuraxial needle placement in a patient who received a preoperative dose of enoxaparin; waiting 2 hours prior to dosing enoxaparin after an epidural catheter is removed; patients on warfarin should have their catheter removed only when the INR is below 1.5; avoiding other anticoagulants and antiplatelet medications when LMWH is being used and an epidural catheter is in place.[57]

The potent antiplatelet effect of clopidogrel also places a patient at risk for a neuraxial hematoma should a spinal or epidural anesthetic be performed while its effect is present. Current recommendations in the ASRA Practice Advisory, Anticoagulation, 3rd edition, 2010, suggest that clopidogrel be discontinued for 7 days prior to performing a neuraxial block. However, the article quotes labeling as recommending this while the PDR section for clopidogrel actually recommends that for elective surgery it only be discontinued for 5 days.[58] The Executive Summary for the Anesthetic Management of the Patient Receiving Antiplatelet Medication, as part of the third edition, states, "On the basis of labeling and surgical reviews, the suggested time interval between discontinuation of thienopyridine therapy and neuraxial blockade is 14 days for ticlopidine and 7 days for clopidogrel. If a neuraxial block is indicated between 5 and 7 days of discontinuation of clopidogrel, normalization of platelet function should be documented."[59] In patients who need to be maintained on clopidogrel or have not discontinued it for an adequate time period, other anesthesia techniques should be considered. The guidelines for some of the antiplatelet medications will probably undergo revision as physicians gain experience with the use of medications such as clopidogrel in the perioperative period.

QUESTIONS OF THE DAY

1. What abnormalities of the cervical spine and airway may be present in patients with rheumatoid arthritis?
2. What surgical conditions can lead to loss of somatosensory evoked potential (SSEP) signals during spine surgery?
3. What is the major cause of postoperative visual loss (POVL) after spine surgery? What factors may contribute to the development of POVL?
4. What findings are typically present after tourniquet release in the patient undergoing total knee replacement?

IV

REFERENCES

1. Klippel JH, Crofford LJ, Stone JH, Weyland CM: *Primer on Rheumatoid Diseases*, ed 12, Atlanta, GA, 2001, Arthritis Foundation, Chap. 9, Rheumatoid arthritis: Epidemiology, pathology and pathogenesis, pp 209–232.
2. Bernstein RL, Rosenberg AD: *Manual of Orthopedic Anesthesia and Related Pain Syndromes*, New York, 1993, Churchill Livingstone.
3. Rosenberg AD: Current issues in the anesthetic treatment of the patient for orthopedic surgery, ASA Refresher Courses in *Anesthesiology* 32:169–178, 2004.
4. Rosenberg AD: Anesthesia for major orthopedic surgery, ASA Refresher Courses in *Anesthesiology* 25:131–144, 1997.
5. Bienenstock H, Ehrlich GE, Freyberg RH: Rheumatoid arthritis of the cricoaretynoid joint: A clinicopathological study, *Arthritis Rheum* 6:48–63, 1963.
6. Skues MA, Welchew EA: Anaesthesia and rheumatoid arthritis, *Anaesthesia* 48:989–997, 1993.
7. Steel HH: Anatomical and mechanical considerations of the atlantoaxial articulations, *J Bone Joint Surg Am* 50:1481–1490, 1968.
8. Keenan MA, Stiles CM, Kaufman RL: Acquired laryngeal deviation associated with cervical spine disease in erosive polyarticular arthritis. Use of the fiberoptic bronchoscope in rheumatic disease, *Anesthesiology* 58:441–449, 1983.
9. Macarthur A, Kleiman S: Rheumatoid cervical joint disease—A challenge to the anesthetist, *Can J Anaesth* 40(2):154–159, 1993.
10. Klippel JH, Crofford LJ, Stone JH, et al: *Primer on Rheumatoid Diseases*, ed 12, Atlanta, GA, 2001, Arthritis Foundation, p 250.
11. Rosenberg AD: Annual Meeting 58th Refresher Course Lectures and Basic Science Review RCL American Society of Anesthesiology, *Anesthesiology*, 119, 2007.
12. Zakine J, Samarcq D, Lorne E, et al: Postoperative ketamine administration decreases morphine consumption in major abdominal surgery: A prospective, randomized, double-blind, controlled study, *Anesth Analg* 106(6):1856–1861, 2008.
13. Subramaniam K, Subramaniam B, Steinbrook RA: Ketamine as adjuvant analgesic to opioids: A quantitative and qualitative systematic review, *Anesth Analg* 99:482–495, 2004.
14. American Society of Anesthesiologists Task Force on Intraoperative Awareness: Practice advisory for intraoperative awareness and brain function monitoring: a report by the American Society of Anesthesiologists Task Force on Intraoperative Awareness, *Anesthesiology* 104:847–864, 2006.
15. Avidan MS, Zhang L, Burnside BA, et al: Anesthesia awareness and the bispectral index, *N Engl J Med* 358:1097–1108, 2008.
16. Urban MK, Jules-Elysee K, Urquhart B, et al: The efficacy of antifibrinolytics in the reduction of blood loss during complex adult reconstructive spine surgery, *Spine* (Phila Pa 1976) 26:1152–1156, 2001.
17. Zufferey P, Merquiol F, Laporte S, et al: Do antifibrinolytics reduce allogeneic blood in orthopedic surgery? Anesthesiology 105:1034–1046.
18. Neilipovitz DT, Murto K, Hall L, et al: A randomized trial of tranexamic acid to reduce blood transfusion for scoliosis surgery, *Anesth Analg* 93:82–87, 2001.
19. Mangano DT, Tudor IC, Dietzel C, et al: The risk associated with aprotinin in cardiac surgery, *N Engl J Med* 354:353–365, 2006.
20. Mangano DT, Miao Y, Vuylsteke A, et al: Mortality associated with aprotinin during 5 years following coronary bypass graft surgery, *JAMA* 297:471–479, 2007.
21. Fergusson DA, Hebert PC, Mazer CD, et al: A comparison of aprotinin and lysine analogues in high-risk cardiac surgery, *N Engl J Med* 358:2319–2331, 2008.
22. Pasternak BM, Boyd DP, Ellis FH: Spinal cord injury after procedures on the aorta, *Surg Gynecol Obstet* 135:29–34, 1972.
23. Owen JH, Laschinger J, Bridwell K, et al: Sensitivity and specificity of somatosensory and neurogenic motor evoked potentials in animals and humans, *Spine* (Phila Pa 1976) 13:1111–1118, 1988.
24. Hilibrand AS, Schwartz DM, Sethuraman V, et al: Comparison of transcranial electric motor and somatosensory evoked potential monitoring during cervical spine surgery, *J Bone Joint Surg Am* 86:1248–1253, 2004.
25. MacDonald D: Intraoperative motor evoked potential monitoring: overview and update, *J Clin Monit Comput* 20(5):347–377, 2006.
26. Vauzelle C, Stagnara P, Jouvinroux P: Functional monitoring of spinal cord activity during spinal surgery, *Clin Orthop Relat Res* 93:173–178, 1973.
27. Glassman SD, Rose SM, Dimar JR, et al: The effect of postoperative nonsteroidal anti-inflammatory drug administration on spinal fusion, *Spine* (Phila Pa 1976) 23:834–838, 1998.
28. Williams EL: Postoperative blindness, *Anesthiol Clin North America* 20:605–622, 2002.
29. Lee L, Roth S, Posner K, et al: The American Society of Anesthesiologists Postoperative Visual Loss Registry: Analysis of 93 spine surgery cases with postoperative visual loss, *Anesthesiology* 105:652–659, 2006.
30. Cheng MA, Todorov A, Tempelhoff R, et al: The effect of prone positioning on intraocular pressure in anesthetized patients, *Anesthesiology* 95:1351–1355, 2001.
31. Lee L, Lam A: Unilateral blindness after position lumbar spine surgery, *Anesthesiology* 95:793–795, 2001.
32. Roth S, Barach P: Postoperative visual loss: Still no answers—yet, *Anesthesiology* 95:575–577, 2001.
33. Warner MA: Postoperative visual loss: experts, data and practice, *Anesthesiology* 105:641–642, 2006.
34. American Society of Anesthesiologists Task Force on Perioperative Blindness: Practice advisory for perioperative visual loss associated with spine surgery: a report by the American Society of Anesthesiologists Task Force on Perioperative Blindness, *Anesthesiology* 104:1319–1328, 2006.
35. Roth S: Perioperative Visual Loss: What do we know, what can we do? *Br J Anaesth* 103(Suppl)1:i31–i40, 2009.
36. Pohl A, Cullen DJ: Cerebral ischemia during shoulder surgery in the upright position: A case series, *J Clin Anesth* 17:463–469, 2005.
37. Cullen DJ, Kirby RB: Beach chair position may decrease cerebral perfusion pressure. Catastrophic outcomes have occurred, *APSF Newsl* 22(2):25, 2007.
38. Zuckerman J: Hip fracture, *N Engl J Med* 334:1519–1525, 1996.
39. Kenzora JE, McCarthy RE, Lowell JD, et al: Hip fracture mortality: Relation to age, treatment, preoperative illness, time of surgery, and complications, *Clin Orthop Relat Res* 186:45–56, 1984.
40. Roche JJ, Wenn RT, Sahota O, et al: Effect of comorbidities and postoperative complications on mortality after hip fracture in elderly people: Prospective observational cohort study, *BMJ* 331(7529):1374, 2005.
41. White BL, Fisher WD, Laurin CA: Rate of mortality for elderly patients after fracture of the hip in the 1980s, *J Bone Joint Surg Am* 69(A):1335–1340, 1987.

42. Schultz RJ, Whitfield GF, LaMura JJ, et al: The role of physiologic monitoring in patients with fractures of the hip, *J Trauma* 25:309–316, 1985.

43. Moran CG, Wenn RT, Sikand M, et al: Early mortality after hip fracture: Is delay before surgery important? *J Bone Joint Surg Am* 87:483–489, 2005.

44. Shiga T, Wajimaa Z, Ohe Y: Is operative delay associated with increased mortality of hip fracture patients? Systematic review, meta-analysis, and meta-regression, *Can J Anaesth* 55:146–154, 2008.

45. Shah KB, Kleinman BS, Sami H, et al: Reevaluation of perioperative myocardial infarction in patients with prior myocardial infarction undergoing noncardiac operations, *Anesth Analg* 71:231–235, 1990.

46. Valentin N, Lomholt B, Jensen JS, et al: Spinal or general anaesthesia for surgery of the fractured hip? A prospective study of mortality in 578 patients, *Br J Anaesth* 58:284–291, 1986.

47. Davis FM, Woolner DF, Frampton C, et al: Prospective multi-centre trial of mortality following general or spinal anesthesia for hip fracture surgery in the elderly, *Br J Anaesth* 59:1080–1088, 1987.

48. Chayen D, Nathan H, Chayen M: The psoas compartment block, *Anesthesiology* 45:95–99, 1976.

49. Odinsson A, Finsen V: Tourniquet use and its complications in Norway, *J Bone Joint Surg* 88:1090–1092, 2006.

50. Chabel C, Russell LC, Lee R: Tourniquet-induced limb ischemia: A neurophysiologic animal model, *Anesthesiology* 72:1038–1044, 1990.

51. Rama KR, Apsingi S, Poovali S, et al: Timing of tourniquet release in knee arthroplasty. Meta-analysis of randomized, controlled trials, *J Bone Joint Surg Am* 89:699–705, 2007.

52. Memtsoudis SG, Ma Y, Gonzalez Della Valle A, et al: Perioperative outcomes after unilateral and bilateral total knee arthroplasty, *Anesthesiology* 111:1206–1216, 2009.

53. Chan WC, Musonda P, Cooper AS, et al: One-stage versus two-stage bilateral unicompartmental knee replacement: a comparison of immediate post-operative complications, *J Bone Joint Surg* 91:1305–1309, 2009.

54. Ritter MA, Harty LD, Davis KE, et al: Simultaneous bilateral, staged bilateral, and unilateral total knee arthroplasty: A survival analysis, *J Bone Joint Surg Am* 85:1532–1537, 2003.

55. Restrepo C, Parvizi J, Dietrich T, et al: Safety of simultaneous bilateral total knee arthroplasty. A meta-analysis, *J Bone Joint Surg Am* 89:1220–1226, 2007.

56. Chan WC, Musonda P, Cooper AS, et al: One-stage versus two-stage bilateral unicompartmental knee replacement: a comparison of immediate post-operative complications, *J Bone Joint Surg (Br)* 91:1305–1309, 2009.

57. Horlocker TT, Wedel DJ, Benzon H, et al: Regional anesthesia in the anticoagulated patient: defining the risks (the second ASRA Consensus Conference on Neuraxial Anesthesia and Anticoagulation), *Reg Anesth Pain Med* 28:172–197, 2003.

58. Horlocker TT, Wedel D, Rowlingson JC, et al: Regional anesthesia in the patient receiving antithrombotic or thrombolytic therapy: American Society of Regional Anesthesia and Pain Medicine Evidence-Based Guidelines (Third Edition), *Reg Anesth Pain Med* 35:64–101, 2010.

59. Horlocker TT, Wedel DJ, Rowlingson JC, et al: Executive summary: regional anesthesia in the patient receiving antithrombotic or thrombolytic therapy: American Society of Regional Anesthesia and Pain Medicine Evidence-Based Guidelines (Third Edition), *Reg Anesth Pain Med* 35(1):102–105, 2010.

IV

OBSTETRICS

Jennifer M. Lucero and Mark D. Rollins

Providing peripartum analgesia and anesthesia requires an understanding of the physiologic changes during pregnancy and labor; the effects of anesthetics on the mother, fetus, and neonate; and the benefits and risks associated with various techniques. Furthermore, peripartum analgesia and anesthesia demand an understanding of the course of labor and delivery, knowledge of high-risk maternal conditions, ability to provide a variety of neuraxial techniques, and preparation for potential obstetric emergencies and complications requiring immediate intervention, such as fetal distress and maternal hemorrhage.

PHYSIOLOGIC CHANGES IN PREGNANT WOMEN

During pregnancy, labor, and delivery, women undergo significant changes in anatomy and physiology as a result of (1) altered hormonal activity; (2) biochemical changes associated with increasing metabolic demands of a growing fetus, placenta, and uterus; and (3) mechanical displacement by an enlarging uterus.[1,2]

Cardiovascular System Changes

Changes in the cardiovascular system during pregnancy can be summarized as (1) an increase in intravascular fluid volume; (2) an increase in cardiac output; (3) a decrease in systemic vascular resistance; and (4) the presence of supine aortocaval compression (Table 33-1).

INTRAVASCULAR FLUID AND HEMATOLOGY

Maternal intravascular fluid volume begins to increase in the first trimester. At term, the plasma volume has increased about 45% above the nonpregnant state, while the erythrocyte volume has increased only about 20%. This disproportionate increase in plasma volume accounts for the relative anemia of pregnancy. The hemoglobin normally remains at 11 g/dL or greater. This expanded intravascular fluid volume of 1000 to 1500 mL at term offsets the 300 to 500 mL blood loss that accompanies vaginal delivery and the average 800 to 1000 mL blood loss that accompanies cesarean delivery. In addition, the contracted uterus following delivery causes an autotransfusion often in excess of 500 mL of blood.

The total plasma protein concentration is decreased as a result of the dilutional effect of the increased intravascular fluid volume. Pregnancy is a hypercoagulable state with concentration increases in factors I, VII, VIII, IX, X, and XII, and decreases in factors XI, XIII, and antithrombin III. This results in an approximately 20% decrease in prothrombin time (PT) and partial thromboplastin time (PTT). Platelet count may remain normal or decrease 10% by term, and leukocytosis is common.

Table 33-1 Changes in the Cardiovascular and Pulmonary Systems during Pregnancy

Cardiovascular System	Value Near Term Compared with Nonpregnant Value
Intravascular fluid volume	Increased 35%
Plasma volume	Increased 45%
Erythrocyte volume	Increased 20%
Cardiac output	Increased 40%-50%
Stroke volume	Increased 25%-30%
Heart rate	Increased 15%-25%
Peripheral Circulation	
Systemic vascular resistance	Decreased 20%
Pulmonary vascular resistance	Decreased 35%
Central venous pressure	No change
Femoral venous pressure	Increased 15%
Pulmonary System	
Minute ventilation	Increased 50%
Tidal volume	Increased 40%
Breathing frequency	Increased 15%
Lung volumes	
Expiratory reserve volume	Decreased 20%
Residual volume	Decreased 20%
Functional residual capacity	Decreased 20%
Vital capacity	No change
Total lung capacity	Decreased 0-5%
Arterial blood gases and pH	
pH	No change or minimal alkalosis
$Paco_2$	Decreased 10 mm Hg
Pao_2	Normal or slightly increased
Oxygen consumption	Increased 20%

CARDIAC OUTPUT

Cardiac output increases about 10% by the tenth week of gestation and increases 40% to 50% by the third trimester. This augmentation of cardiac output is due to increases in both stroke volume (25% to 30%) and heart rate (15% to 25%). The onset of labor is associated with further increases in cardiac output with increases above prelabor values of 10% to 25% during the first stage and 40% in the second stage. The largest increase occurs immediately after delivery, when cardiac output is increased by as much as 80%. This presents a unique postpartum risk for patients with cardiac disease, such as fixed valvular stenosis. Cardiac output returns toward prelabor values by about 24 hours post partum, and decreases substantially toward prepregnant values by 2 weeks post partum.

SYSTEMIC VASCULAR RESISTANCE

Although cardiac output and plasma volume increase, systemic blood pressure decreases in an uncomplicated

IV

pregnancy secondary to a 20% reduction in systemic vascular resistance at term. Systolic, mean, and diastolic blood pressure may all decrease 5% to 15% by 20 weeks' gestational age and gradually increase slightly toward prepregnant values as the pregnancy progresses further. There is no change in central venous pressure during pregnancy despite the increased plasma volume because venous capacitance increases.

AORTOCAVAL COMPRESSION

When supine, the gravid uterus can compress the aorta and vena cava. Compression of the vena cava can decrease preload, cardiac output, and systemic blood pressure (Fig. 33-1). At term there is almost full occlusion of the inferior vena cava when supine, with venous return of blood from the lower extremities through the epidural, azygos, and vertebral veins. In addition, significant aortoiliac artery compression occurs in 15% to 20% of pregnant women. Nearly 15% of pregnant women at term experience significant hypotension in the supine position. Diaphoresis, nausea, vomiting, and changes in cerebration often accompany the hypotension. This constellation of symptoms is termed *supine hypotension syndrome*. Vena cava compression decreases cardiac output 10% to 20% and may also contribute to lower extremity venous stasis and thereby result in ankle edema, varices, and increased risk of venous thrombosis.

Compensatory Responses and Risks

In the supine position, most pregnant women do not experience significant arterial hypotension because they compensate for the reduction in preload by reflex increases in systemic vascular resistance. This compensatory increase in systemic vascular resistance is impaired by regional anesthesia. Consequently, supine positioning is avoided during neuraxial anesthetic administration in

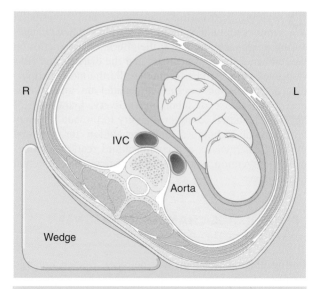

Figure 33-2 Schematic diagram depicting left uterine displacement by elevation of the right hip with a wedge. This position deflects the gravid uterus off the inferior vena cava (IVC) and aorta.

the second and third trimesters. Significant lateral tilt is frequently used during labor analgesia and cesarean deliveries to reduce hypotension and preserve fetal circulation by displacing the gravid uterus leftward and off the inferior vena cava (Fig. 33-2). Left uterine displacement can be accomplished by placing the patient in a left lateral position or by elevation of the right hip 10 to 15 cm with a blanket, wedge, or table tilt.

The gravid uterus can also compress the lower abdominal aorta. Such compression leads to arterial hypotension in the lower extremities, but maternal symptoms or decreases in systemic blood pressure as measured in the arms are often not reflective of this decrease. The significance of aortocaval compression is the associated decrease in uterine and placental blood flow. Even with a healthy uteroplacental unit, prolonged maternal hypotension (more than 25% decrease for an average patient) for longer than 10 to 15 minutes can significantly decrease uterine blood flow and lead to progressive fetal acidosis.

Another compensatory mechanism is increased venous pressure below the level of inferior vena caval compression, which serves to divert blood return from the lower half of the body via the paravertebral venous plexuses to the azygos vein. Flow from the azygos vein enters the superior vena cava and cardiac venous return is maintained. Dilation of the epidural veins may make unintentional intravascular placement of the epidural catheter more likely. This could lead to accidental intravascular injection of the local anesthetic solution. This systemic bolus of local anesthetic can have profound consequences on the cardiovascular and central nervous

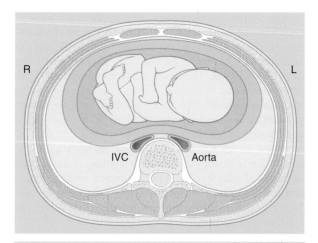

Figure 33-1 Schematic diagram showing compression of the inferior vena cava (IVC) and abdominal aorta by the gravid uterus in the supine position.

systems with potential for complete hemodynamic collapse, seizures, and death. A "test dose" is employed before dosing an epidural catheter in order to decrease the likelihood of an unintended intravascular placement before initiating neuraxial blockade. This technique is described later in the section "Epidural Analgesia."

Pulmonary System Changes

The most significant changes in the pulmonary system during pregnancy include alterations in (1) the upper airway, (2) minute ventilation, (3) arterial oxygenation, and (4) lung volumes (see Table 33-1).

UPPER AIRWAY

During pregnancy there is significant capillary engorgement of the mucosal lining of the upper respiratory tract and increased tissue friability. As a result, there is increased risk of obstruction from tissue edema and bleeding with instrumentation of the upper airway. Additional care is needed during suctioning, placement of airways (avoid nasal instrumentation if possible), direct laryngoscopy, and intubation. It may be prudent to select a smaller cuffed tracheal tube (6.0 to 6.5 mm internal diameter) because the vocal cords and arytenoids are often edematous. The presence of preeclampsia, upper respiratory tract infections, and active pushing with associated increased venous pressure further exacerbate airway tissue edema, making both endotracheal intubation and ventilation more challenging. In addition, the weight gain associated with pregnancy, particularly in women of short stature or with coexisting obesity, can result in difficulty placing the laryngoscope because of a shorter neck and increased breast tissue.

MINUTE VENTILATION AND OXYGENATION

Minute ventilation is increased about 50% above prepregnant levels during the first trimester and is maintained for the remainder of the pregnancy. This increased minute ventilation is achieved primarily by a greater tidal volume, with small increases in the respiratory rate (see Table 33-1). Increased circulating levels of progesterone and increased CO_2 production are probably the stimulus for the increased minute ventilation. Resting maternal Pa_{CO_2} decreases from 40 mm Hg to approximately 30 or 32 mm Hg during the first trimester as a reflection of the increased minute ventilation. Arterial pH, however, remains only mildly alkalotic (7.42 to 7.44) because of increased renal excretion of bicarbonate ions.

Early in gestation, maternal Pa_{O_2} while breathing room air is normally above 100 mm Hg because of the presence of hyperventilation and the associated decrease in alveolar CO_2. Later, Pa_{O_2} becomes normal or even slightly decreased, most likely reflecting airway closure and intrapulmonary shunt. Maternal hemoglobin is right-shifted with the P-50 increasing from 27 to approximately 30 mm Hg which should facilitate downloading oxygen to the tissues.

At term, oxygen consumption is increased by 20%. The added work of labor results in further increases in both minute ventilation and oxygen consumption. During labor, oxygen consumption increases above prelabor rates by 40% during the first stage and 75% during the second stage. The pain of labor can result in severe hyperventilation with Pa_{CO_2} less than 20 mm Hg. This pain-associated hyperventilation and alkalosis can be attenuated by neuraxial analgesic techniques.

LUNG VOLUMES

The expiratory reserve volume (ERV) and residual lung volume (RV), in contrast to the early appearance of increased minute ventilation, do not begin to change until about the third month of pregnancy (see Table 33-1). With increasing enlargement of the uterus, the diaphragm is forced cephalad, which is primarily responsible for the 20% decrease in functional residual capacity (FRC) present at term. This change is created by approximately equal decreases in the ERV and RV. As a result, FRC can be less than closing capacity for many small airways and may give rise to atelectasis in the supine position. Vital capacity is not significantly changed with pregnancy. The combination of increased minute ventilation and decreased FRC results in a faster rate at which changes in the alveolar concentration of inhaled anesthetics can be achieved.

ANESTHETIC IMPLICATIONS

During induction of general anesthesia in a pregnant patient, Pa_{O_2} decreases more rapidly than in a nonpregnant patient because of decreased oxygen reserve (decreased FRC) and increased oxygen uptake (increased metabolic rate). For these reasons, the administration of supplemental oxygen or "preoxygenation" prior to general anesthesia is critical for patient safety. The pregnant patient should breathe oxygen for 3 minutes before any period of anticipated apnea (such as induction of anesthesia), or take four maximal breaths over the 30 seconds just prior to induction if emergent general anesthesia is needed. In addition, the increased airway edema makes both ventilation and endotracheal intubation more difficult and further increases the potential for complications and morbidity.

Gastrointestinal Changes

Gastrointestinal changes during pregnancy make women beyond 20 weeks' gestation significantly vulnerable to regurgitation, aspiration of gastric contents, and the development of acid pneumonitis. Displacement of the stomach and pylorus cephalad by the enlarged uterus repositions the intra-abdominal portion of the esophagus into the thorax and decreases the competence of the esophageal sphincter. Higher progesterone and estrogen levels of pregnancy further reduce esophageal sphincter tone. Gastric pressure is increased by both the gravid uterus and the lithotomy position during vaginal delivery. Gastrin, which is secreted by the placenta, stimulates gastric hydrogen ion secretion such that the pH of gastric fluid is predictably low in pregnant women. For these reasons, gastric fluid reflux into the esophagus with subsequent esophagitis (heartburn) is common and increases with the pregnancy gestational age. In addition, gastric emptying is delayed with the onset of labor or administration of opioids, further increasing the risk of aspiration.

ANESTHETIC IMPLICATIONS

Regardless of the time interval since the ingestion of food, women in labor must be treated as having a full stomach and an increased risk for pulmonary aspiration of gastric contents. This includes the routine use of non-particulate antacids, rapid sequence induction, cricoid pressure, and intubation with a cuffed endotracheal tube as part of general anesthesia induction sequence in a pregnant woman after approximately 20 weeks gestational age. Pain, anxiety, and opioids administered during labor can further slow gastric emptying beyond an already prolonged transit time. Epidural analgesia using local anesthetics does not delay gastric emptying, but using epidural boluses of fentanyl does.[3] The low pH of aspirated gastric fluid is important in the production and severity of acid pneumonitis and is the basis for the administration of antacids to pregnant women before induction of anesthesia. The use of a nonparticulate antacid such as sodium citrate (30 mL) is recommended prior to induction of general anesthesia. Metoclopramide is useful for decreasing the gastric fluid volume of pregnant women in active labor who require general anesthesia. It decreases gastric volume in as little as 15 minutes, although gastric hypomotility associated with prior opioid administration reduces the effectiveness of metoclopramide.[4] Often recommended, H_2 receptor antagonists increase gastric fluid pH in pregnant women approximately 1 hour after administration without producing adverse effects.

Nervous System Changes

Volatile anesthetic requirements (minimum alveolar anesthetic concentration, or MAC) decrease up to 40% during pregnancy. The sedative activity of progesterone may be partially responsible. The important clinical implication of decreased MAC is that alveolar anesthetic concentrations that would not routinely produce unconsciousness may approximate anesthetizing concentrations in pregnant women. This degree of central nervous system depression can impair protective upper airway reflexes and subject pregnant women to increased risk of pulmonary aspiration that is already elevated secondary to gastrointestinal changes detailed previously. Furthermore, the reduced FRC increases the rate at which potential excessive alveolar concentrations of anesthetics can be achieved.

Pregnant patients are more sensitive to the local anesthetics used during neuraxial blockade. There is a decrease in local anesthetic dose needed for epidural or spinal anesthesia in pregnant women at term. The observation of decreased neuraxial local anesthetic doses as early as the first trimester suggests a role for biochemical changes causing increased nerve sensitivity. This decreased requirement is occurring before significant aortocaval compression and decreases in the volume of the epidural space from dilated veins. Although this increased sensitivity is likely based on hormonal changes, there may be some role for mechanical changes as well. Engorgement of epidural veins as intra-abdominal pressure increases with progressive enlargement of the uterus results in a decrease in both the size of the epidural space and volume of cerebrospinal fluid (CSF) in the subarachnoid space. The decreased volume of these spaces facilitates the spread of local anesthetics. However, CSF pressure itself does not increase with pregnancy.

Renal Changes

Renal blood flow and the glomerular filtration rate are increased about 50% to 60% by the third month of pregnancy and do not return to prepregnant levels until 3 months postpartum. Therefore, the normal upper limits in blood urea nitrogen and serum creatinine concentrations are decreased about 50% in pregnant women. There is decreased tubular resorption of both protein and glucose, and excretion of these in the urine is common. A 24-hour urine collection of less than 300 mg protein or 10 g glucose are considered the upper limits of normal in pregnancy.

Hepatic Changes

Liver blood flow does not change significantly with pregnancy. Plasma protein concentrations are reduced during pregnancy because of dilution, similar to the physiologic anemia of pregnancy. These decreased serum albumin levels can result in increased free blood levels of highly protein-bound drugs. Slightly increased liver function tests are common in the third trimester. Plasma cholinesterase (pseudocholinesterase) activity is decreased about 25% from the tenth week of gestation up to 6 weeks post partum. This decreased activity is insufficient to significantly prolong the neuromuscular blockade from succinylcholine. In addition, incomplete gallbladder emptying and changes in bile composition increase the risk of gallbladder disease during pregnancy.

PHYSIOLOGY OF THE UTEROPLACENTAL CIRCULATION

The placenta is the interface of maternal and fetal tissue for the purpose of physiologic exchange. Maternal blood is delivered to the placenta by two uterine arteries, and fetal blood arrives via two umbilical arteries. Nutrient-rich and waste-free blood is returned from the placenta to the fetus through a single umbilical vein.

Uterine Blood Flow

Uterine blood flow (UBF) increases throughout gestation from about 100 mL/min before pregnancy to 700 mL/min (about 10% of cardiac output) at term gestation. About 80% of the uterine blood flow perfuses the intervillous space (placenta) and 20% supports the myometrium. The uterine vasculature has limited autoregulation and remains essentially maximally dilated under normal pregnancy conditions. UBF decreases because of either reduced uterine perfusion pressure or increased umbilical arterial resistance. Decreased perfusion pressure can result from systemic hypotension secondary to hypovolemia, aortocaval compression, or decreased systemic resistance from either general or neuraxial anesthesia. Uterine blood flow also decreases with increased uterine venous pressure. This can result from vena caval compression (supine position), uterine contractions (particularly uterine tachysystole, as may occur with oxytocin administration), or significant abdominal musculature contraction (Valsalva maneuver during pushing). Additionally, extreme hypocapnia ($Paco_2 < 20$ mm Hg) associated with hyperventilation secondary to labor pain can reduce UBF to the point of fetal hypoxemia and acidosis.

Epidural or spinal anesthesia does not alter UBF as long as maternal hypotension is avoided. Endogenous catecholamines induced by stress or pain and exogenous vasopressors have the capability of increasing uterine arterial resistance and decreasing UBF. In animal models, α-adrenergic stimulation produced by methoxamine and metaraminol increased uterine vascular resistance and decreased UBF, whereas administration of ephedrine was not accompanied by significant decreases in UBF despite drug-induced increases in maternal arterial blood pressure. Consequently, ephedrine was considered to be the drug of choice for the treatment of hypotension caused by the administration of regional anesthesia in pregnant women. However, phenylephrine (α-adrenergic agonist) is currently recommended to correct maternal hypotension because it is not associated with adverse effects on indices of fetal well-being. Phenylephrine administration results in less fetal acidosis and base deficit compared to ephedrine (primarily β-adrenergic) in clinical trials.[5–7]

Placental Exchange

Transfer of oxygen from the mother to the fetus is dependent on a variety of factors including the ratio of maternal UBF to fetal umbilical blood flow, the oxygen partial pressure gradient, the respective hemoglobin concentrations and affinities, the placental diffusing capacity, and the acid-base status of the fetal and maternal blood (Bohr effect). The fetal oxyhemoglobin dissociation curve is left-shifted (greater oxygen affinity) while the maternal hemoglobin dissociation curve is right-shifted (decreased oxygen affinity), resulting in facilitated oxygen transfer to the fetus. The fetal Pao_2 is normally 40 mm Hg and never more than 60 mm Hg, even if the mother is breathing 100% oxygen, because the placental exchange to the fetus from the mother represents venous rather than arterial blood.

Placental exchange of most drugs and other substances less than 1000 daltons occurs principally by diffusion from the maternal circulation to the fetus and vice versa. Diffusion of a substance across the placenta to the fetus depends on maternal-to-fetal concentration gradients, maternal protein binding, molecular weight, lipid solubility, and the degree of ionization of that substance. Minimizing the maternal blood concentration of a drug is the most important method of limiting the amount that ultimately reaches the fetus.

The high molecular weight and poor lipid solubility of nondepolarizing neuromuscular blocking drugs result in limited ability of these drugs to cross the placenta. Succinylcholine has a low molecular weight but is highly ionized and therefore does not readily cross the placenta. Thus, during administration of a general anesthetic for cesarean delivery, the fetus/neonate is not paralyzed. Additionally, both heparin and glycopyrrolate have significantly limited placental transfer. Placental transfer of barbiturates, local anesthetics, and opioids is facilitated by the relatively low molecular weights of these substances. In general, drugs that readily cross the blood-brain barrier also cross the placenta.

FETAL UPTAKE

Fetal uptake of a substance that crosses the placenta is facilitated by the lower pH (0.1 unit) of fetal blood compared to maternal. The lower fetal pH means that weakly basic drugs (local anesthetics, opioids) that cross the placenta in the nonionized form will become ionized in the fetal circulation. Because an ionized drug cannot readily cross the placenta and then return to the maternal circulation, this drug will accumulate in the fetal blood against a concentration gradient. Therefore, in an acidotic fetus, higher concentrations of local anesthetic can accumulate (ion trapping), especially during periods of fetal distress. Increased concentrations of local anesthetics in the fetus result in decreased neonatal neuromuscular tone similar to that seen with magnesium.

IV

If direct maternal intravascular local anesthetic injection occurs, significant fetal toxicity can result in bradycardia, ventricular arrhythmia, acidosis, and severe cardiac depression. Placental transfer and fetal uptake of specific analgesic and anesthetics drugs are detailed in the upcoming sections on "Methods of Labor Analgesia" and "Anesthesia for Cesarean Delivery."

CHARACTERISTICS OF THE FETAL CIRCULATION

The fetal circulation protects the vital fetal organs from exposure to high concentrations of drugs initially present in umbilical venous blood. For example, about 75% of umbilical venous blood passes through the fetal liver such that significant portions of drugs can be metabolized before reaching the fetal arterial circulation for delivery to the heart and brain. Despite decreased liver enzyme activity in comparison to adults, fetal/neonatal enzyme systems are adequately developed to metabolize most drugs. Moreover, drugs in the portion of umbilical venous blood entering the inferior vena cava via the ductus venosus will be diluted by drug-free blood returning from the lower extremities and pelvic viscera of the fetus. These circulatory characteristics markedly decrease the fetal plasma drug concentrations compared to maternal following an intravenous drug bolus.

STAGES OF LABOR

The stages of labor and the point at which labor can become dysfunctional requiring more intervention from the obstetrician are often unpredictable. A patient may adopt a particular birth plan only to have it change at the outset of labor or after many hours. Labor can occur spontaneously or may be induced based on maternal or fetal indications.

Labor is a continuous process divided into three stages. The *first stage* refers to the onset of labor until the cervix is fully dilated. The first stage is further divided into two phases: latent phase and active phase. The latent phase can persist for many hours and in some cases days. The active phase begins at the point when the rate of cervical dilation increases. This usually occurs between 3 and 5 cm of dilation. The *second stage* of labor begins when the cervix is fully dilated and ends when the neonate is born. This stage is referred to as the "pushing and expulsion" stage. Once the neonate is delivered, the *third and final stage* begins and is completed when the placenta is delivered. If progression of labor through the stages is halted or delayed, there is concern for dysfunctional labor and potential for obstetric intervention.

If a woman's cervix fails to dilate or dilates slowly in the active phase despite pharmacologic interventions, this is defined as an active phase arrest and will result in a cesarean delivery. During the second stage of labor, the patient may not be able to "push" the neonate out of the pelvis. This is termed arrest of descent. The mode of delivery depends on what pelvic level the arrest of descent occurred. If the neonate is low enough in the pelvis, the obstetrician can perform an instrumented vaginal delivery via vacuum or forceps. If the neonate remains too high in the pelvis, then the patient will need to undergo a cesarean delivery. In addition to the potential labor dysfunction, the fetal condition can dictate a change in labor course and delivery mode based on the fetal heart rate tracing.

The anesthesia provider can be consulted at any time throughout the labor to aid in a safe delivery. The labor course and mode of delivery can dictate which analgesic or anesthetic technique is most appropriate.

ANATOMY OF LABOR PAIN

Contraction of the uterus, dilatation of the cervix, and distention of the perineum cause pain during labor and delivery. Somatic and visceral afferent sensory fibers from the uterus and cervix travel with sympathetic nerve fibers to the spinal cord (Fig. 33-3). These fibers pass through the paracervical tissue, and course with the hypogastric nerves and the sympathetic chain to enter the spinal cord at T10 to L1. During the first stage of labor (cervical dilation), the majority of painful stimuli are the result of afferent nerve impulses from the lower uterine segment and cervix, with contributions from the uterine body causing visceral pain (poorly localized, diffuse, and usually described as "a dull but intense aching"). Theses nerve cell bodies are located in the dorsal root ganglia of levels T10 to L1. During the second stage of labor (pushing and expulsion), afferents innervating the vagina and perineum cause somatic pain (well localized and described as "sharp"). These somatic impulses travel primarily via the pudendal nerve to dorsal root ganglia of levels S2 to S4. Pain during this stage of labor is caused by distention and tissue ischemia of the vagina, perineum, and pelvic floor muscles. When descent of the fetus into the pelvis occurs, delivery is imminent. Neuraxial analgesic techniques that block levels T10 to L1 during the first stage of labor must be extended to include S2 to S4 for efficacy during the second stage of labor.

Labor pain can have significant physiologic effects on the mother, fetus, and the course of labor. Pain stimulates the sympathetic nervous system, increases plasma catecholamine levels, creates reflex maternal tachycardia and hypertension, and can reduce uterine blood flow. In addition, changes in uterine activity can occur with the rapid decrease in plasma epinephrine concentrations associated with onset of neuraxial analgesia. Oscillations in epinephrine can result in a range of uterine effects from a transient period of uterine tachysystole to a period

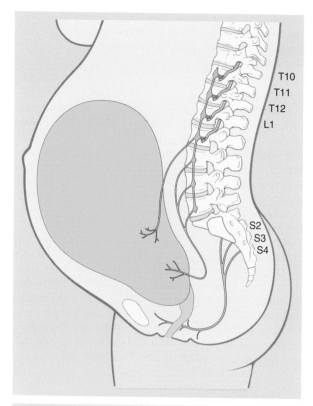

Figure 33-3 Schematic diagram of pain pathways during pregnancy. Visceral pain during the first stage of labor is due to uterine contraction and cervical dilation. Afferent sensory fibers from the uterus and cervix travel with sympathetic nerve fibers and enter the spinal cord at T10-L1. Somatic afferents from the vagina and perineum travel via the pudendal nerve to levels S2-S4.

of uterine quiescence. Alternatively, these epinephrine changes can convert dysfunctional uterine activity patterns associated with poorly progressive cervical dilation to more regular patterns associated with normal cervical dilation.[8]

METHODS OF LABOR ANALGESIA

Nonpharmacologic Techniques

The nonpharmacologic techniques for labor analgesia include hypnosis, the breathing techniques described by Lamaze, acupuncture, acupressure, the LeBoyer technique, transcutaneous nerve stimulation, massage, hydrotherapy, vertical positioning, presence of a support person, intradermal water injections, biofeedback, and many others. A meta-analysis reviewing the effectiveness of a support individual (e.g., doula, family member) noted that women with a support individual used less pharmacologic analgesia, had a decreased length of labor, and

had a lower incidence of cesarean delivery.[9] In a 2006 retrospective national survey of women's childbearing experiences, although neuraxial methods of pain relief were rated as the most helpful and effective, nonpharmacologic methods of tub immersion and massage were rated more or equally helpful in relieving pain when compared to the use of opioids.[10] Although many nonpharmacologic techniques seem to reduce labor pain perception, most published studies lack the rigorous scientific methodology for useful comparison of these techniques to pharmacologic methods.

Systemic Medications

Systemic analgesics are utilized on labor and delivery, but normally limited by bolus intravenous doses, dosing interval, and 24-hour cumulative dose. Although the use of systemic opioid analgesics is quite common, the use of sedatives, anxiolytics, and dissociative agents is rare. The potential for maternal sedation, respiratory compromise, loss of airway protection, and proximity to time of delivery dictate judicious use of systemic opioids. In women who are in early spontaneous labor or beginning induction of labor, systemic opioid analgesia can be beneficial.

OPIOIDS

Although there are individual differences among opioids, all readily cross the placental barrier and exert neonatal effects in typical clinical doses, including decreased fetal heart rate variability and dose-related neonatal respiratory depression. All opioids can have maternal side effects, including nausea, vomiting, pruritus, and decreased stomach emptying.

Meperidine is one of the most frequently used opioids worldwide. It can be given in doses of 12.5 to 25 mg IV or 25 to 50 mg IM. Maternal half-life of meperidine is 2 to 3 hours; half-life in the fetus and newborn is significantly longer (13 to 23 hours) and more variable. In addition, meperidine is metabolized to an active metabolite (normeperidine) that can significantly accumulate in the patient after repeated doses. With increased dosing and shortened time interval between dose and delivery, there is increased neonatal risk of decreased Apgar scores, lowered oxygen saturation, and prolonged time to sustained respiration.[11]

Morphine was used more frequently in the past, but currently is rarely used. Like meperidine it has an active metabolite (morphine 6-glucuronide) and a prolonged duration of analgesia; the half-life is longer in neonates compared to adults, and the drug produces significant maternal sedation. In latent labor, obstetric providers may use intramuscular morphine combined with phenergan for analgesia, sedation, and rest termed "morphine sleep." This produces analgesia for approximately 2.5 to 4 hours with an onset of 10 to 20 minutes.

IV

Fentanyl is commonly used for labor analgesia. It has a short duration and no active metabolites. When given in small IV doses of 50 to 100 μg/hour there are no significant differences in neonatal Apgar scores and respiratory effort compared to newborns of mothers not receiving fentanyl.[12]

Remifentanil PCA has been considered for women who have contraindications to neuraxial blockade. Although pain was improved with remifentanil, a randomized control trial comparing epidural analgesia to remifentanil PCA had overall pain scores that were lower in the epidural group.[13] More sedation and hemoglobin desaturation were noted during remifentanil analgesia, but there was no difference between groups in fetal and neonatal outcomes. In a more recent study, remifentanil PCA was compared with other opioids (fentanyl and meperidine) and demonstrated better analgesia in the first hour, but in all groups pain scores returned to pretreatment values after 3 hours.[14]

ANXIOLYTICS

Although used in obstetrics, *diazepam* readily crosses the placenta and yields roughly equal maternal and fetal blood levels. Because neonates have a limited ability to excrete the active metabolites, use of diazepam can cause neonatal respiratory depression. *Midazolam* is a shorter acting anxiolytic, but it also rapidly crosses the placenta, and large doses (≥5 mg during labor) are associated with low Apgar scores. Use of midazolam during labor is controversial. Although it is an effective anxiolytic, it will cause amnesia that is not desired by most women. If midazolam is chosen, smaller doses (1 to 2 mg) should be used.

DISSOCIATIVE ANALGESIA

Ketamine is a "dissociative analgesic" and can be administered in divided IV doses (10 to 20 mg) totaling less than 1 mg/kg and will provide analgesia, useful for vaginal delivery and episiotomy. It has a rapid onset (30 seconds) and minimal duration of action (<5 minutes). When given with opioids, it reduces the amount of opioid necessary to produce adequate analgesia in a synergistic manner. The use of ketamine during labor should be reserved for acute urgent situations where other preferential techniques cannot be employed given the urgency and need for rapid control of maternal pain.

Neuraxial (Regional) Analgesia

Neuraxial analgesia (e.g., epidural, spinal, combined spinal-epidural [CSE]) is currently the most widely used method of labor analgesia in the United States. Paracervical and pudendal blocks, currently are rarely performed. Neuraxial analgesia typically involves the administration of local anesthetics, and often the coadministration of opioid analgesics. In addition, adjuvant drugs such as clonidine or neostigmine have been shown to decrease the dose of local anesthetics or opioids required for analgesia.[15-17] However, they are currently not in routine clinical use.

LOCAL ANESTHETICS (Also See Chapter 11)

The ester-linked local anesthetics (e.g., 2-chloroprocaine, procaine, tetracaine) are rapidly metabolized by plasma cholinesterase, decreasing the risk of maternal toxicity and placental drug transfer. Amide-linked local anesthetics (e.g., lidocaine, bupivacaine, ropivacaine) are degraded by P-450 enzymes in the liver. Vascular absorption of local anesthetics limits the safe dose that can be administered. Bupivacaine and ropivacaine are the most commonly used local anesthetics for labor analgesia and both are extremely safe when appropriately dosed for epidural or intrathecal administration. An accidental, large intravascular dose of any local anesthetic can result in significant maternal morbidity (seizures, loss of consciousness, severe arrhythmias, and cardiovascular collapse) or death and the potential for fetal accumulation (ion trapping) (see "Physiology of Uteroplacental Circulation"). Immediate recognition and treatment is essential (see "Systemic Toxicity and Excessive Blockade").

NEURAXIAL OPIOIDS

Neuraxial opioids are commonly used in obstetric anesthesia. Lipid-soluble opioids such as fentanyl and sufentanil are frequently used to augment the neuraxial analgesia of local anesthetics. The administration of opioids alone in the epidural space can provide moderate analgesia, but is not nearly as effective as even dilute solutions of local anesthetic. Intrathecal opioids are more potent than epidural or systemic administration, but are of limited duration (less than 2 hours) and also less effective than using neuraxial local anesthetics. Coadministration of opioids with local anesthetics prolongs and improves the quality of analgesia and has local anesthetic-sparing effects. The addition of neuraxial opioids is associated with dose-related maternal side effects including pruritus, sedation, and nausea. In addition, administration of intrathecal opioids can result in fetal bradycardia independent of hypotension.[18] The mechanism is unclear, but fetal bradycardia may result from uterine hyperactivity following the rapid onset of analgesia.[19]

ADJUVANT NEURAXIAL DRUGS

Clonidine and neostigmine are being evaluated as potential adjuncts for labor analgesia.[17] *Neostigmine* (acetylcholinesterase inhibitor) prevents the breakdown of acetylcholine within the spinal cord. Acetylcholine binds to muscarinic and nicotinic receptors of the spinal cord and stimulates nitric oxide synthesis to produce analgesia.

Clonidine (α_2-adrenergic agonist) inhibits the release of substance P in the dorsal horn and produces analgesia. It also increases the level of acetylcholine in the CSF. Intrathecal clonidine can produce excellent analgesia; however, sedation and hypotension are common, making its suitability questionable as a labor analgesic. Intrathecal neostigmine alone has poor efficacy but, in combination with intrathecal opioids, may prolong labor analgesia.[17] Unfortunately, it is associated with severe refractory nausea.

As epidural adjuncts, clonidine and neostigmine have local anesthetic-sparing effect and augment labor analgesia. Adjuvant analgesics may have a future role in early labor and the transition to active labor. Currently these adjuvant neuraxial drugs are being evaluated in clinical trials and are not recommended as standard practice.[15]

NEURAXIAL TECHNIQUES

Neuraxial techniques represent the most effective form of labor analgesia, and achieve the highest rates of maternal satisfaction.[10] The patient remains awake and alert without sedative side effects, maternal catecholamine concentrations are reduced, hyperventilation is avoided, cooperation and capacity to participate actively during labor are facilitated, and excellent, predictable analgesia can be achieved, superior to the analgesia provided by all other techniques.

Preoperative Assessment

Prior to initiation of any neuraxial blockade, anesthesia providers should assess the woman's pregnancy and health history; perform a focused physical examination; discuss the risks, benefits, and alternatives; and obtain consent. In otherwise healthy women, routine laboratory tests are not required.[20] Resuscitation equipment and drugs must be immediately available to manage serious complications secondary to initiation of epidural or spinal blocks (see "Contraindications to Neuraxial Anesthesia" and "Complications of Regional Anesthesia"). During initiation of the neuraxial blockade, mother and fetus are closely monitored (maternal vital signs and fetal heart rate monitoring). Current recommendations allow otherwise healthy laboring women to have modest amounts of clear liquids. However in complicated labors (e.g., complicated by morbid obesity, difficult airway, factors concerning fetal status), the decision to restrict oral intake should be determined by the individual anesthesia provider.[20]

Timing and Placement of Epidural

The decision of when to place an epidural was previously controversial over the concern of adversely affecting the progress of labor. This belief has been long debated and

the subject of many studies. Current American Society of Anesthesiologists (ASA) guidelines recommend that a maternal request for labor pain relief is sufficient justification for epidural placement, and the decision should not depend on an arbitrary cervical dilation.[20] Randomized controlled clinical trials comparing women receiving either systemic opioids or neuraxial analgesia in early labor (both spontaneous and induced) demonstrated no difference in rates of cesarean delivery.[21,22] A Cochrane Review based on studies up to 2005 comparing neuraxial and systemic opioid labor analgesia noted no difference in rates of cesarean delivery, but women with neuraxial analgesia did have an increased rate of instrumented vaginal delivery.[23]

Epidural Technique (Also See Chapter 17)

Epidural analgesia is a catheter-based technique used to provide continuous pain relief during labor. The technique involves insertion of a specialized needle (Tuohy) between vertebral spinous processes in the back, into the epidural space (Fig. 33-4). This needle has a slightly curved blunt tip to minimize dural puncture. The patient can either be in the sitting or lateral position based on both the experience of the anesthesia provider and optimal exposure to critical anatomic landmarks. Based on ASA task force recommendations regarding neuraxial infectious complications, aseptic techniques should always be used during placement of neuraxial needles and catheters, including (1) removal of jewelry (e.g., rings and watches), hand washing, and wearing of caps, masks, and sterile gloves; (2) use of individual packets of antiseptics for skin preparation; (3) use of chlorhexidine (preferred) or povidone-iodine (preferably with alcohol) for skin preparation, allowing for adequate drying time; (4) sterile draping of the patient; and (5) use of sterile occlusive dressings at the catheter insertion site.[24] The needle is normally inserted between L1 and L4. The needle traverses the skin and subcutaneous tissues, supraspinous ligament, interspinous ligament, the ligamentum flavum and is advanced into the epidural space (Fig. 33-5). The tip of the Tuohy needle should not penetrate the dura, which forms the boundary between the intrathecal or subarachnoid space and the epidural space. To locate the epidural space, a tactile technique called "loss of resistance" is used. The tactile resistance noted with pressure on the plunger of an air- or saline-filled syringe dramatically decreases as the tip of the needle is advanced through the ligamentum flavum (dense resistance) into the epidural space (no resistance), which has an average depth of approximately 5 cm from the skin. Once the needle is properly positioned, a catheter is inserted through the needle. The catheter remains in the epidural space and the needle is removed. The catheter is secured with tape and adhesives, and used for intermittent or continuous injections. Once the catheter is in place,

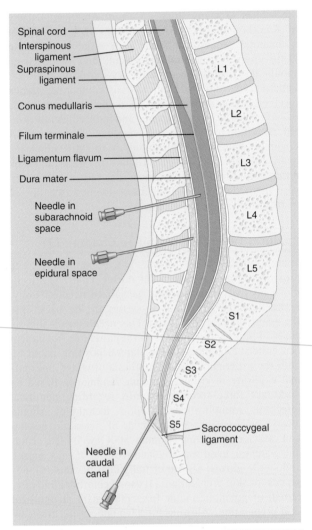

Spinal cord
Interspinous ligament
Supraspinous ligament
Conus medullaris
Filum terminale
Ligamentum flavum
Dura mater
Needle in subarachnoid space
Needle in epidural space
Needle in caudal canal
Sacrococcygeal ligament

L1
L2
L3
L4
L5
S1
S2
S3
S4
S5

Figure 33-4 Schematic diagram of lumbosacral anatomy showing needle placement for subarachnoid, lumbar, epidural, and caudal blocks.

analgesia is achieved by administration of local anesthetics or opioids (see earlier discussion) and maintained throughout the course of labor and delivery. The catheter can also be used for instrumented or cesarean delivery as well as postoperative analgesia, when necessary.

Combined Spinal-Epidural Technique

The combined spinal-epidural (CSE) technique follows the epidural technique as above but after the "loss of resistance" a spinal needle (24- to 26-gauge, pencil-point) is inserted into the epidural needle, using a needle through needle technique. Once CSF is visualized, an intrathecal dose of local anesthetic or opioid is given. The spinal needle is removed and the epidural catheter is threaded as described with the epidural technique.

The benefit of the CSE technique is quicker onset of analgesia and no motor blockade if opioids alone are placed intrathecally. A systematic review of CSE versus epidural literature found no major difference in maternal benefit or fetal risks, except for an increased rate of maternal pruritus.[25] Additionally, use of opioid-only "walking epidurals" showed no increase in the amount of walking compared to epidurals with local anesthetic.

Epidural and Combined Spinal-Epidural Dosing and Delivery Techniques

During labor, an epidural catheter allows continuous infusion of local anesthetic with or without opioid drugs. In addition, anesthesia providers can administer a bolus of either the same or a more concentrated solution of local anesthetic. Programmable infusion pumps allow the patient to self-bolus the chosen anesthetic mixture with or without a background infusion. This method of delivery allows for a decrease in medical personnel, improved patient satisfaction, and smaller local anesthetic consumption.[20] Comparison of PCEA (patient-controlled epidural analgesia) settings noted that the presence of a background infusion improved analgesia, increased maternal satisfaction, and reduced need for anesthetic intervention, but there were no differences in mode of delivery, frequency of motor block, or Apgar scores compared to settings without a background infusion.[20] Concentrations of labor epidural local anesthetics have decreased over time as dense motor blockade may adversely affect vaginal delivery rate. Typical infusion concentrations for epidural bupivacaine (0.0625% to 0.125%) or ropivacaine (0.08% to 0.2%) are both effective. Opioids such as fentanyl (1 to 3 μg/mL) or sufentanil (0.1 to 0.5 μg/mL) may be added to the infusion mixture to augment analgesia and decrease local anesthetic requirements, but these drugs increase the side effects of pruritis, nausea, and sedation. Opioids can also be bolused through the epidural catheter with typical doses of fentanyl 50 to 100 μg or sufentanil 5 to 10 μg to improve analgesia. Dilute concentrations of epinephrine (1:400,000 or 1:800,000) can also be added to the epidural mixture to augment analgesia, but are associated with increased motor blockade.

For CSEs the initial intrathecal dose can include opioid, local anesthetic, or a combination of the two. Typical intrathecal doses for opioids are fentanyl (10 to 20 μg) or sufentanil (1.5 to 5 μg), and local anesthetic doses include bupivacaine (1.25 to 3.5 mg) and ropivacaine (2.5 to 5 mg). Use of high-dose opioids (sufentanil 7.5 μg) is associated with increased risk of fetal bradycardia and severe pruritis even without the presence of hypotension.[26] Prior to initiation of the epidural, a *test dose* should be performed to evaluate the possibility of unintended intravenous or intrathecal catheter placement. Commonly, 3 mL of 1.5% lidocaine containing

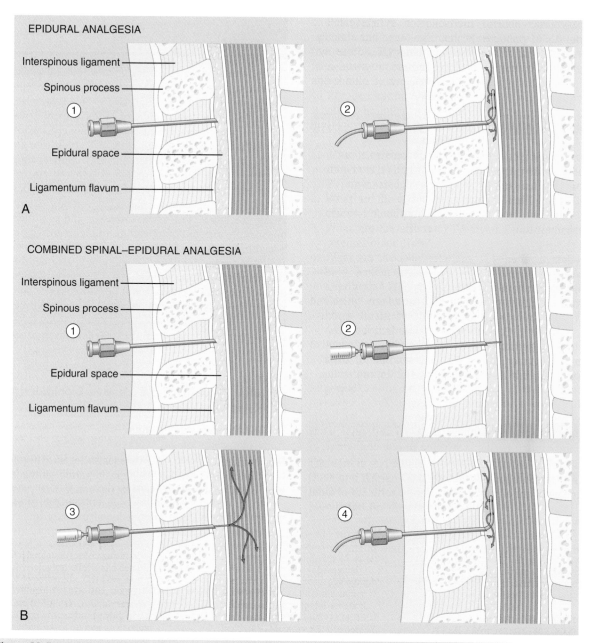

Figure 33-5 Technique of epidural and combined spinal-epidural analgesia. **A,** Epidural catheter placement for labor analgesia: (1) The desired epidural space L2-L4 is identified. Following infiltration with local anesthetic a Tuohy needle is seated in the intervertebral ligaments. A syringe is connected to the epidural needle for confirmation of degree of resistance using constant or periodic pressure on the plunger. As the needle tip is passed from the high resistance of the ligaments to the low resistance in the epidural space, a sudden loss of resistance is recognized by the anesthesia provider and advancement is stopped. (2) An epidural catheter is advanced through the needle into the space. Analgesic medications are administered through the catheter following a "test dose." **B,** Combined spinal-epidural analgesia: (1) Following Tuohy needle placement into the epidural space, (2) a spinal needle (24- to 26-gauge) is introduced through the epidural needle into the subarachnoid space. (3) Proper placement is confirmed by free flow of the cerebrospinal fluid. A bolus of local anesthetic or opioid is given through the spinal needle. (4) Following spinal needle removal, an epidural catheter is advanced through the Tuohy needle into the epidural space. The epidural catheter can be used for continuation of labor analgesia. (From Eltzschig HK, Lieberman ES, Camann WR. Regional anesthesia and analgesia for labor and delivery. N Engl J Med 2003; 348:319-332, used with permission)

1:200,000 epinephrine is used. Increases in heart rate and arterial blood pressure greater than 20% (intravascular placement) or rapid analgesia and motor block (intrathecal placement) indicate epidural catheter misplacement. Whenever a bolus is given in the epidural for initiation or breakthrough pain, the anesthetic mixture should be given incrementally through the epidural catheter (5 mL) while monitoring maternal arterial blood pressure and fetal heart rate (FHR) continuously.

Instrumented vaginal delivery (forceps/vacuum) may become necessary for arrest of descent or fetal indications. This procedure requires a denser block with perineal anesthesia. Supplementation of 5 to 10 mL of local anesthetic in the epidural (lidocaine 1% to 2% or 2-chloroprocaine 2% to 3%) is usually necessary.

Spinal Labor Analgesia

Spinal analgesia can be administered just before vaginal delivery. This technique is useful for advanced second stage analgesia, instrumented (forceps/vacuum) delivery, evaluation/evacuation of retained placenta, or repair of high-degree perineal lacerations. Placement of spinal block (3 to 5 mg bupivacaine with or without 10 to 20 μg of fentanyl) allows the rapid onset of analgesia, which is important in these situations. This dose is significantly less than that needed for a cesarean delivery. The duration of this type of spinal analgesia is approximately 90 minutes. A 24- to 26-gauge "pencil-point" spinal needle is selected to reduce the risk of post–dural puncture headache. If mainly perineal anesthesia is needed (i.e., forceps delivery, perineal laceration repair), the patient may be left in the sitting position for 2 to 3 minutes following use of hyperbaric local anesthetic in order to concentrate the sensory block in the perineal region ("saddle block"). A true saddle block anesthetic (requiring more time in the sitting position) does not produce complete uterine pain relief because the afferent fibers (extending to T10) from the uterus are not blocked.

CONTRAINDICATIONS TO NEURAXIAL ANESTHESIA

Certain conditions contraindicate neuraxial procedures. These conditions include (1) patient refusal, (2) infection at the needle insertion site, (3) significant coagulopathy, (4) hypovolemic shock, (5) increased intracranial pressure from mass lesion, and (6) inadequate provider expertise. Other conditions such as systemic infection, neurologic disease, and mild coagulopathies are relative contraindications should be evaluated on a case-by-case basis. Human immunodeficiency virus (HIV) and hepatitis infection are not contraindications to neuraxial technique in pregnant women.

COMPLICATIONS OF REGIONAL ANESTHESIA

The retrospective rates of inadequate epidural analgesia or inadequate CSE analgesia requiring catheter replacement were 7% and 3%, respectively, at a U.S. academic center.[27] The rate of accidental dural puncture during epidural catheter placement is approximately 1% to 2%, and about half of these punctures will result in a severe headache, which is typically managed with analgesics, hydration, rest, caffeine, or blood patch if necessary. Other potential side effects from neuraxial blockade include pruritus, nausea, shivering, urinary retention, motor weakness, low back soreness, and a prolonged block. More serious complications of meningitis, epidural hematoma, and nerve or spinal cord injury are extremely rare. A retrospective Swedish study of severe neurologic complications from neuraxial blockade included 200,000 obstetric epidurals and 50,000 obstetric spinals. Rates of serious neurologic events (i.e., neuraxial hematoma or abscess, nerve or cord damage) were 1:29,000 for obstetric epidurals and 1:25,000 for obstetric spinal procedures.[28]

Systemic Toxicity and Excessive Blockade (Also See Chapters 11 and 17)

Life-threatening complications can infrequently result from administration of neuraxial anesthesia. The most serious complications are from accidental IV or intrathecal injections of local anesthetics. An unintended bolus of IV local anesthetic causes dose-dependent consequences ranging from minor side effects (e.g., tinnitus, perioral tingling, mild arterial blood pressure and heart rate changes) to major complications (seizures, loss of consciousness, severe arrhythmias, cardiovascular collapse). The severity depends on the dose, type of local anesthetic, and preexisting condition of the patient. Bupivacaine has more affinity for sodium channels than lidocaine and dissociates more slowly. In addition, its high protein affinity makes cardiac resuscitation more difficult and prolonged. Measures that minimize the likelihood of accidental intravascular injection include careful aspiration of the catheter before injection, test dosing, and incremental administration of therapeutic doses. Successful resuscitation and support of the mother will reestablish uterine blood flow. This will provide adequate fetal oxygenation and allow time for excretion of local anesthetic from the fetus. The neonate has an extremely limited ability to metabolize local anesthetics and may have prolonged convulsions if emergent delivery is required.

A high spinal (total spinal) can result from an unrecognized epidural catheter placed subdural, migration of the catheter during its use, or an overdose of local anesthetic in the epidural space (i.e., high epidural). Both high spinals and high epidurals can result in severe maternal hypotension, bradycardia, loss of consciousness, and blockade of the motor nerves to the respiratory muscles.

TREATMENT

Treatment of complications resulting from both intravascular injection and high spinal block are directed at restoring maternal and fetal oxygenation, ventilation, and circulation. Intubation, vasopressors, fluids, and advanced cardiac life support (ACLS) algorithms are often required (ACLS-Pregnancy). Changes to ACLS guidelines for pregnancy include use of left uterine displacement, avoidance of lower extremity vessels for drug delivery, chest compressions positioned slightly higher on the sternum, and no modifications to the defibrillation protocol except removal of fetal and uterine monitors prior to shock. If a local anesthetic overdose occurs, consider use of a 20% IV lipid emulsion to bind the drug and decrease toxicity (also see Chapter 11). In any situation of maternal cardiac arrest with unsuccessful resuscitation, the fetus should be emergently delivered if the mother is not resuscitated within 4 minutes of the arrest. This guideline for emergent cesarean delivery increases the chances of survival for both the mother and neonate.[20]

Hypotension

Hypotension (decrease in systolic blood pressure > 20%) secondary to sympathetic blockade is the most common complication of neuraxial blockade for labor analgesia with rates between 10% and 24%.[25] Prophylactic measures include left uterine displacement and hydration. Although a standard for timing, amount, and hydration fluid remain controversial, all agree dehydration should be avoided. Prehydration with up to 1 L IV crystalloid does not appear to significantly decrease rates of hypotension from low-dose labor epidurals,[29] although use of colloid preload appears to reduce rates of hypotension in low-dose spinal anesthesia.[30] Treatment of hypotension consists of further uterine displacement, IV fluids, and vasopressor administration. Small boluses of either phenylephrine or ephedrine can be used to treat hypotension. As indicated previously, phenylephrine (primarily α-adrenergic) is preferred because of less fetal acidosis than with ephedrine.[5-7] If treated promptly, maternal hypotension does not lead to fetal depression or neonatal morbidity.

Increased Core Temperature

An increase in core maternal body temperature is associated with labor epidural analgesia and may be influenced by several factors, including duration, ambient temperature, administration of systemic opioids, and the presence of shivering. During the first 5 hours of epidural analgesia, there is no significant increase in body temperature. Temperature increases at a rate of about 0.1° C/hour, and may reach 38° C in as many as 15% of women with a labor epidural compared with 1% without an epidural. Although the etiology of the increased maternal temperature remains uncertain, it need not affect neonatal septic workup. Labor epidural analgesia does not increase the incidence of neonatal sepsis. Such a fever is not associated with a change in white blood cell count or with an infectious process, and treatment is not necessary.

OTHER NERVE BLOCKS FOR LABOR

Paracervical Block

A paracervical block is infrequently used to provide pain relief during the first stage of labor. The technique consists of submucosal administration of local anesthetics immediately lateral and posterior to the uterocervical junction, which blocks transmission of pain impulses at the paracervical ganglion. Complications from systemic absorption can occur as well as the possibility of direct fetal trauma or injection. Paracervical block is associated with a 15% rate of fetal bradycardia.[31] The mechanism of this phenomenon is unclear, and close fetal monitoring is warranted. The bradycardia is usually limited to less than 15 minutes, and treatment is mainly supportive.

Pudendal Block

The obstetrician performs a pudendal block with a transvaginal technique, guiding a sheathed needle to the vaginal mucosa and sacrospinous ligament just medial and posterior to the ischial spine. It primarily blocks sensation of the lower vagina and perineum, and is typically placed just prior to vaginal delivery. Although the technique provides analgesia for vaginal delivery or uncomplicated instrumented vaginal delivery, the rate of failure is high. In many centers, this technique is used when an epidural or spinal technique is unavailable. Complications in addition to failure include systemic local anesthetic toxicity, ischiorectal or vaginal hematoma, and rarely, fetal injection of local anesthetic.

INHALED ANALGESIA FOR VAGINAL DELIVERY

Some birthing centers provide nitrous oxide as an analgesic option, usually administered by a device that delivers 50% nitrous oxide in oxygen. With this mixture, nitrous oxide is a weak analgesic, and provides satisfactory analgesia in some pregnant women. Without coadministration of opioids, it is safe and does not result in hypoxia,

IV

unconsciousness, or loss of protective airway reflexes.[32] Maternal cardiovascular and respiratory depression is minimal, uterine contractility is not affected, and neonatal depression does not occur regardless of the duration of nitrous oxide administration. Appropriate equipment and fully trained personnel are essential to ensure safety when delivering this gas mixture because effects of opioids and sedatives are additive.

ANESTHESIA FOR CESAREAN DELIVERY

The majority of cesarean deliveries are performed with neuraxial anesthesia. Use of regional anesthesia (1) avoids the risks of maternal aspiration and difficult airway associated with general anesthesia, (2) allows less anesthetic exposure to the neonate, (3) has the benefit of an awake mother, and (4) allows placement of neuraxial opioids to decrease postoperative pain. Sometimes the severity of the fetal condition and emergent nature of the situation (fetal bradycardia or uterine rupture) necessitates the use of general anesthesia for its rapidity, and at other times it is required when regional anesthesia is contraindicated (coagulopathy or severe hemorrhage). Benefits of general anesthesia over regional include rapid and dependable onset, secure airway, controlled ventilation, and potential for less hemodynamic instability. Regardless of method planned, all pregnant women being prepared for a cesarean delivery should receive an oral antacid (nonparticulate such as sodium citrate) to reduce gastric fluid pH. In addition, some anesthesia providers routinely administer a drug to accelerate gastric emptying (metoclopramide) or an H_2 receptor antagonist (ranitidine) to reduce gastric acid production.

Spinal Anesthesia

For a pregnant woman without an epidural catheter, spinal anesthesia is the most common regional anesthetic technique used for cesarean delivery. The block is technically easier than an epidural anesthetic, more rapid in onset, does not carry the risk of systemic drug toxicity due to the smaller dose, and is more reliable in providing surgical anesthesia from the midthoracic level to the sacrum. The incidence of post–dural puncture headache has become low (<5%) with the introduction of smaller diameter, noncutting, "pencil-point" spinal needles. However, maternal hypotension is more likely and more profound with spinal anesthesia than with epidural anesthesia because the onset of sympathectomy is more rapid. Avoidance of aortocaval compression, providing hydration, and appropriate use of vasopressors may minimize the risk for hypotension. Colloid is significantly more effective than crystalloid.[30] As indicated previously a phenylephrine infusion given at the time of spinal placement is preferred to ephedrine in preventing hypotension.[6]

Spinal anesthesia can be safely used for patients with pre-eclampsia. A typical spinal anesthetic could consist of bupivacaine (10 to 15 mg) with preservative-free morphine (150 to 250 µg) added to decrease postoperative pain. A large variety of other combinations of local anesthetics and opioids are also used. A hyperbaric solution of local anesthetic is often used to facilitate anatomic and gravitational control of the block distribution. The medication will flow with the spinal curvature to a position near T4. The duration of a single-shot spinal anesthetic is variable, but normally provides adequate surgical anesthesia for 90 minutes. A continuous spinal anesthetic technique with deliberate catheter placement approximately 3 cm subdural is a rarely used alternative, but sometimes is chosen in cases of accidental dural puncture during attempts to place an epidural catheter. This allows the advantage of a titratable, reliable, dense anesthetic, but carries the risks of high spinal block if the intrathecal catheter is mistaken for an epidural catheter, or the provider is unfamiliar with the technique. The rates of rare complications such as meningitis or neurologic impairment from local anesthetic toxicity with use of a spinal catheter may be somewhat higher than with the other neuraxial techniques, but remain unknown. Some data suggest that leaving the spinal catheter in place for 24 hours decreases the risk of post–dural puncture headache.[33]

Epidural Anesthesia

Epidural anesthesia is an excellent choice for surgical anesthesia when an indwelling, functioning epidural catheter has been placed for labor analgesia. It allows titration to the desired level of anesthesia and ability to extend the block time if needed. It is also ideal for patients who cannot tolerate the sudden onset of sympathectomy, such as some patients with severe cardiac disease. Some disadvantages include a slower onset compared to spinal anesthesia and a greater risk of maternal systemic drug toxicity. The volume and concentration of local anesthetic drugs used for surgical anesthesia are larger than those used for labor analgesia; however, the technique of catheter placement, test dosing, and potential complications are similar. A standard dosing regimen for epidural anesthesia for cesarean delivery could include approximately 20 mL of 2% lidocaine or 3% 2-chloroprocaine in divided doses. The addition of epinephrine (1:200,000) or fentanyl (50 to 100 µg) can enhance the intensity and duration of the block. Typically, the anesthesia provider attempts to provide sensory anesthesia from the T4 level to the sacrum. This level of anesthesia may not always alleviate the visceral pain associated with peritoneal manipulation, and adjuvant drugs such as intravenous ketamine (10-mg boluses) may be needed. Epidural morphine (3 to 5 mg) is typically given near the end of the procedure to decrease postoperative pain for up to 24 hours.

Combined Spinal-Epidural Anesthesia

In selected circumstances, use of a CSE technique offers the advantage of a spinal anesthetic with rapid, reliable onset of a dense block, as well as the ability to administer additional local anesthetic through the epidural catheter. This allows titration of the block level or extension of the block duration if the procedure lasts for a longer period. One disadvantage is the delay in verification of a functioning epidural catheter.

General Anesthesia

General anesthesia is used in obstetric practice for cesarean delivery, typically when neuraxial anesthesia is contraindicated or for emergencies because of its rapid and predictable action. The main causes of maternal morbidity and death with general anesthesia are an increased risk of failed endotracheal intubation (approximately 1 in 500) and of pulmonary aspiration of gastric contents (1 in 650) compared to nonpregnant patients undergoing general anesthesia.[34] Appropriate airway examination, preparation, and familiarity with techniques and an algorithm for the difficult airway are critical for providing a safe anesthetic (Fig. 33-6). The sequence of events for general anesthesia for cesarean delivery are detailed in Table 33-2.

After administration of a nonparticulate antacid, administration of oxygen, and confirmation of surgical readiness, a rapid-sequence induction of anesthesia is typically performed and a cuffed endotracheal tube placed. Surgical incision is made after confirmation of tracheal intubation and adequate ventilation. Anesthesia is maintained by administration of a combination of inhaled nitrous oxide and a volatile anesthetic, as well as benzodiazepines, opioid analgesics, and additional muscle relaxant if needed. During typical general anesthesia for cesarean delivery, opioids and benzodiazepines are administered after the baby is delivered to avoid placental transfer of these drugs to the neonate. Prior to delivery of the baby, the primary anesthetic for the incision and delivery is an intravenously administered anesthetic, as there is little time for uptake and distribution of the inhaled anesthetic into either the mother or fetus. If endotracheal intubation attempts fail, the cesarean delivery may proceed if the anesthesia provider communicates that she or he can reliably ventilate the mother with either face mask or laryngeal mask airway (see Fig. 33-6).[20]

ANESTHETICS USED TO INDUCE GENERAL ANESTHESIA (Also See Chapter 9)

A number of different drugs are used by anesthesia providers to rapidly induce general anesthesia.

Thiopental

Sodium thiopental (4 to 6 mg/kg IV) was the most common intravenous anesthetic for cesarean delivery under general anesthesia, rendering the patient unconscious within 30 seconds. It peaks in the umbilical vein blood in 1 minute and in the umbilical artery blood in 2 to 3 minutes, and has no significant clinical effect on neonatal well-being. The lack of neonatal effects in standard doses is unclear, but may be due to first-pass metabolism by the neonatal liver, rapid redistribution into maternal vascular-rich tissue beds, additional dilution by the fetal circulation, and higher fetal brain water content. However, doses of 8 mg/kg can result in neonatal depression.

Propofol

This highly lipid-soluble drug results in rapid onset of action similar to thiopental. Compared to thiopental, it has a more complete recovery with less residual sedative effect, but is preservative free and must be drawn up only hours before use. Other differences are that propofol decreases the incidence of nausea and vomiting and it is currently not a controlled substance. However, it may soon become a controlled substance. Propofol is not superior to thiopental in maternal or neonatal outcome. Propofol administration has no significant effect on neonatal behavior scores with induction doses of 2.5 mg/kg, but larger doses (9 mg/kg) are associated with newborn depression.

Etomidate

Like thiopental, etomidate has a rapid onset of action because of its high lipid solubility, and redistribution results in a relatively short duration of action. At typical induction doses (0.3 mg/kg), unlike thiopental and propofol, etomidate has minimal effects on the cardiovascular system, but it is painful on injection, can cause involuntary muscle tremors, has higher rates of nausea and vomiting, and can increase risk of seizures in patients with decreased thresholds.

Ketamine

Ketamine produces a rapid onset of anesthesia, but unlike thiopental, ketamine's sympathomimetic characteristics increase arterial pressure, heart rate, and cardiac output through central stimulation of the sympathetic nervous system, making it an ideal choice for a pregnant woman in hemodynamic compromise. Doses above those appropriate for induction of general anesthesia (1 to 1.5 mg/kg) can increase uterine tone, reducing uterine arterial perfusion, lower seizure threshold. In low doses (0.25 mg/kg), ketamine has profound analgesic effects, unlike barbiturates, but has been associated with undesirable psychomimetic side effects (bad dreams), which can be lessened by coadministration of benzodiazepines. Many anesthesia providers consider ketamine the appropriate drug for induction of anesthesia in a pregnant woman who is actively hemorrhaging, has uncertain blood volume, and is at risk for profound hypotension.

MAINTENANCE OF ANESTHESIA

Maintenance of anesthesia for cesarean delivery often includes the inhalation of 50% nitrous oxide in

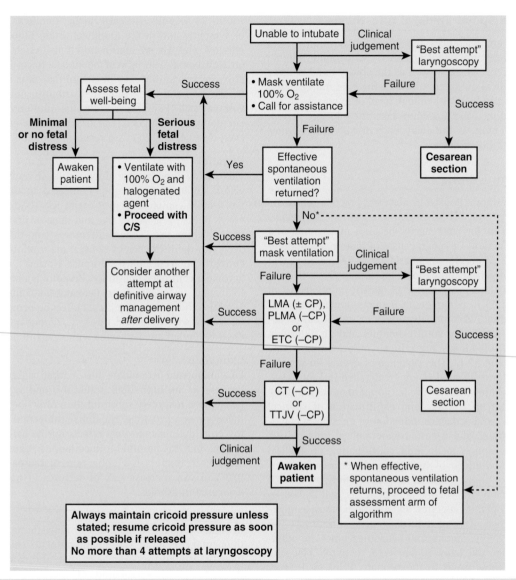

Figure 33-6 Algorithm for difficult airway management with failed intubation in obstetrics. CP, cricoid pressure; C/S, cesarean section; CT, cricothyrotomy; ETC, esophageal tracheal combitube; LMA, laryngeal mask airway (Laryngeal Mask Company, Henley-on-Thames, U.K.); TTJV, transtracheal jet ventilation. (From Hughes S, Levinson G, Rosen M. Shnider and Levinson's Anesthesia for Obstetrics, 4th ed. Philadelphia, Lippincott, Williams & Wilkins, used with permission.)

combination with a low concentration (<0.75 MAC) of volatile anesthetic. Because awareness can occur with a cesarean delivery (see Chapter 46), the addition of a volatile anesthetic will decrease that risk. Placental transfer of volatile anesthetics is rapid because they are nonionized, highly lipid-soluble substances of low molecular weight. Fetal concentrations depend on the concentration and duration of anesthetic administered to the mother. During a typical general anesthetic for cesarean delivery, opioids are administered after the baby is delivered to avoid the concern of placental transfer to the neonate.

There may be confusion regarding the presence of fetal distress, the use of general anesthesia, and subsequent delivery of a depressed neonate. A depressed fetus is likely to be associated with a depressed neonate, and general anesthesia is selected because it is the most rapidly acting anesthetic technique to allow cesarean delivery. A Cochrane Review of 16 studies comparing neuraxial blockade versus general anesthesia in otherwise uncomplicated cesarean deliveries found no significant difference in neonatal Apgar scores or the need for neonatal resuscitation."[35] The authors concluded that there was no evidence to show that neuraxial anesthesia

Table 33-2 General Anesthesia for Cesarean Section: A Suggested Technique

- Administer a nonparticulate oral antacid (sodium citrate) prior to induction of anesthesia.
- Place standard monitors and maintain left uterine displacement.
- Start an infusion of crystalloid solution through a large-bore intravenous catheter.
- Preoxygenate for 3 minutes, or 4 maximal breaths over 30 seconds.
- When the surgeon is ready and patient prepped, an assistant should apply cricoid pressure (and maintain until the position of the endotracheal tube is verified).*
- Administer induction agent and paralytic in rapid sequence, wait 30 to 60 seconds, and then initiate direct laryngoscopy for tracheal intubation.
- After confirming endotracheal tube placement, communicate to surgeon to begin incision.
- Administer 50% nitrous oxide in oxygen plus 0.5 to 0.75 MAC of a volatile anesthetic.
- After delivery, anesthesia may be augmented by administering opioids, barbiturates, or propofol while continuing the volatile anesthetic.
- Extubate the trachea when the patient is fully awake and strong.

*Not all agree that cricoid pressure is efficacious or required in every patient.
MAC, minimal alveolar concentration.

was superior to general anesthesia for neonatal outcome. The induction to delivery interval is not as important to neonatal outcome as the interval from uterine incision to delivery, when uterine blood flow may be compromised and fetal asphyxia may occur. A long time from induction to delivery may result in a lightly anesthetized, but not an asphyxiated neonate. If excessive concentrations of volatile anesthetics are administered for prolonged periods, neonatal effects of these drugs, as evidenced by flaccidity, cardiorespiratory depression, and decreased tone, may be anticipated. If neonatal depression is due to transfer of anesthetic drugs, the infant is merely anesthetized and should respond easily to simple treatment measures such as assisted ventilation of the lungs to facilitate excretion of the volatile anesthetic. Rapid improvement of the infant should be expected, and if it does not occur, it is important to search for other causes of depression. For these reasons, it is critical that clinicians experienced with neonatal ventilation are present at cesarean deliveries under general anesthesia in which the time from incision to delivery may be longer (i.e., known percreta, large fibroids) or when the maternal condition necessitates an atypical induction and maintenance of anesthesia. A discussion of the operative and anesthetic plan by the neonatologist, obstetrician, and anesthesia provider is crucial for optimizing the outcome of neonates in these situations.

NEUROMUSCULAR BLOCKING DRUGS (Also See Chapter 12)

Succinylcholine (1 to 1.5 mg/kg IV) remains the neuromuscular blocking drug of choice for obstetric anesthesia because of its rapid onset (30 to 45 seconds) and short duration of action. Because it is highly ionized and poorly lipid soluble, only small amounts cross the placenta. It is normally hydrolyzed in maternal blood by the enzyme pseudocholinesterase and does not generally interfere with fetal neuromuscular activity. If large doses are given (2 to 3 mg/kg) it results in detectable levels in umbilical cord blood, and extreme doses (10 mg/kg) are needed for the transfer to result in neonatal neuromuscular blockade. If the hydrolytic enzyme is present either in low concentration or in a genetically determined atypical form, prolonged maternal paralysis can occur and the return of neuromuscular strength should always be determined before additional muscle relaxants are given or extubation is performed.

Rocuronium is an acceptable alternative to succinylcholine. It provides adequate endotracheal intubating conditions in approximately 90 seconds at doses of 0.6 mg/kg and under 60 seconds at doses of 1.2 mg/kg. Unlike succinylcholine it has a much longer duration of action, decreasing maternal safety in the event the anesthesia provider is unable to intubate or ventilate the patient. Uterine smooth muscle is not affected by neuromuscular blockade. Under normal circumstances, the poorly lipid-soluble, highly ionized, nondepolarizing neuromuscular blockers (i.e., rocuronium, vecuronium, cisatracurium, pancuronium) do not cross the placenta in amounts significant enough to cause neonatal muscle weakness. This placental impermeability is only relative and when large doses are given over long periods, neonatal neuromuscular blockade can occur. A paralyzed neonate will have normal cardiovascular function and good color but no spontaneous ventilatory movements or reflex responses, and skeletal muscle flaccidity is present. Treatment consists of respiratory support until the neonate excretes the drug, which may take up to 48 hours. Antagonism of nondepolarizing neuromuscular blocking drugs with cholinesterase inhibitors may be attempted, but adequate respiratory support is the mainstay of treatment.

ABNORMAL PRESENTATIONS AND MULTIPLE BIRTHS

Multiple Gestations

The United States is seeing an increase in multiple gestations with the expanded use of artificial reproductive technologies.[36] In 2006 twin pregnancy accounted for 3.4% of the live births.[37] The vast majority of multiple

IV

gestations are twin (97% to 98%). Higher order multiples account for 0.1 to 0.03% of the births. Multiple pregnancies account for a significant risk to both the mother and the fetuses. Antepartum complications may develop in up to 80% of the multiple gestations. These complications include a higher rate of preterm labor, preeclampsia, gestational diabetes, preterm premature rupture of membranes, intrauterine growth restriction, and intrauterine fetal demise. Pregnancies with multiple gestations account for 9% to 12% of the perinatal deaths.[38] The majority of twin pregnancies are vertex-vertex positioning of the fetuses. If the second twin is breech, it is important to discuss the mode of delivery with the obstetricians and perinatologists. If vaginal delivery is attempted, an emergent cesarean delivery might be required if (1) the second twin changes position after delivery of the first twin or (2) fetal bradycardia is present in the second twin. In cases of vaginal delivery, women are strongly advised to undergo placement of an epidural to facilitate delivery and extraction of the second twin. The epidural provides both analgesia and optimal perineal relaxation during the delivery of the fetal head of the second twin. The obstetrician may need to perform an instrumented delivery of the second twin. At the late second stage of delivery, a more concentrated local anesthetic will provide optimal perineal anesthesia and relaxation during this critical portion of the delivery. At this time, the potential for head entrapment or fetal bradycardia is the most likely and a denser block allows for possible transition to cesarean delivery.

Abnormal Presentations

BREECH PRESENTATION

Singleton breech presentation occurs in about 3% to 4% of all pregnancies. External cephalic version (ECV) has a mean success rate of approximately 60%. The procedure involves rotating the fetus via external palpation and pressure of the fetal parts. The use of ultrasound and fetal heart rate monitoring is useful in assessing position and fetal distress during this procedure. Throughout the procedure, maternal relaxation of abdominal muscles is beneficial. Neuraxial analgesia reduces pain and may improve success of the ECV. The risks of ECV include placental abruption, fetal bradycardia, and rupture of membranes. These risks are low, but the anesthesia provider should be immediately available if an ECV is being performed in case an urgent or emergent cesarean delivery is needed.

Few centers perform singleton vaginal breech delivery. Only recently, obstetric practice guidelines allow individual obstetricians the flexibility of performing these deliveries based on their experience and comfort level.[39] Institutions offering a singleton vaginal breech delivery should have clear guidelines for performing the procedure. Women should undergo pelvimetry, an ultrasound to determine fetal weight, and counseling by the obstetrician to review the risks of the procedure. The patient is strongly encouraged to have an epidural placed during labor as the anesthetic management and risks are similar to a breech extraction of the second twin.

SHOULDER DYSTOCIA

A shoulder dystocia is an obstetric emergency analogous to a difficult airway in anesthesia. The diagnosis is made after the delivery of the fetal head when further expulsion of the infant is prevented by impaction of the fetal shoulders with the maternal pelvis. It occurs in approximately 1% to 1.5% of all deliveries. Risk factors include macrosomia, diabetes, obesity, history of dystocia, labor induction, and instrumented delivery. Among deliveries with shoulder dystocia, the risk of postpartum hemorrhage is increased 11% and fourth-degree laceration increased 3.8%.[40] Once shoulder dystocia is diagnosed by the obstetrician, a set of maneuvers are performed to deliver the infant. Fetal pH declines 0.04 units/min between delivery of the head and trunk. Cases of shoulder dystocia 7 minutes or longer have a significant increase in risk of neonatal brain injury. The final maneuver in a failed shoulder dystocia delivery requires pushing the fetus back up and proceeding to emergent cesarean delivery. Among the fetal injuries and sequelae of shoulder dystocia are brachial plexus injury, neurologic injury from asphyxia, and broken clavicle. Often these neurologic injuries improve over time with roughly less than 10% resulting in permanent Erb's palsy.[41]

HYPERTENSIVE DISORDERS OF PREGNANCY

Gestational Hypertension

The clinical spectrum of hypertensive diseases during pregnancy has varying maternal and fetal effects. The most benign is *gestational hypertension*. It is diagnosed in previously normotensive women who develop elevated blood pressure (SBP > 140 mm Hg or DBP > 90 mm Hg) after 20 weeks' gestation without evidence of proteinuria. If these levels of increased blood pressure are present prior to 20 weeks' gestational age or persist through 12 weeks post partum the patient is considered a chronic hypertensive. Often the diagnosis of gestational hypertension can become more specific with time, as the patient may develop signs and symptoms of preeclampsia or if the elevated blood pressure continues past 12 weeks post partum.[42]

Preeclampsia

A more ominous hypertensive disorder in pregnancy is preeclampsia, affecting 3% to 4% of pregnant women. Risk factors include primigravida, chronic hypertension, gestational/preexisting diabetes, obesity, preeclamptic

Table 33-3	Peeclampsia Definitions

Criteria for Preeclampsia

For preeclampsia, both of the following must be present:

- Blood pressure of 140 mm Hg systolic or higher or 90 mm Hg diastolic or higher that occurs after 20 weeks of gestation in a patient with previously normal blood pressure
- Proteinuria defined as urinary excretion of 0.3 g protein or higher in a 24-hour urine specimen ($\geq$1+ on urine dipstick testing)

Criteria for Severe Preeclampsia

Preeclampsia is considered severe if one or more of the following criteria is present:

- Blood pressure of 160 mm Hg systolic or higher or 110 mm Hg diastolic or higher on two occasions at least 6 hours apart while the patient is on bed rest
- Proteinuria of 5 g or higher in a 24-hour urine specimen or 3+ or greater on two random urine samples collected at least 4 hours apart
- Oliguria of less than 500 mL in 24 hours
- Cerebral or visual disturbances
- Pulmonary edema or cyanosis
- Epigastric or right upper quadrant pain
- Impaired liver function
- Thrombocytopenia
- Fetal growth restriction

Data from the Report of the National High Blood Pressure Education Program Working Group Report on High Blood Pressure in Pregnancy. Am J Obstet Gynecol 2000;S1-S22.

family history, multiple gestation, and use of assisted reproductive technology. Preeclampsia is a systemic disease affecting every organ system with both maternal and fetal manifestations. Diagnostic criteria are detailed in Table 33-3. Preeclampsia is a syndrome. The clinical spectrum of preeclampsia ranges from mild to severe. A subcategory of severe preeclampsia is *HELLP syndrome*, which is a constellation of *h*emolysis, *e*levated *l*iver enzymes, and *l*ow platelet count. In most cases the progression through the preeclampsia spectrum is slow and often never progresses to severe. However, in some cases the progression can be more rapid and occur within days. Given that the cause of preeclampsia is still unknown there is no way to predict who will remain mild, slowly progress, or rapidly become severe. In addition, it is also difficult to determine who will become eclamptic (presence of seizures).

Preeclampsia begins with the pathogenic maternal/fetal interface. During placental formation there is failure of complete trophoblast cell invasion of the uterine spiral arteries. The failure of spiral artery remodeling creates decreased placental perfusion, which may ultimately lead to early placental hypoxia. Ultimately there is up-regulation of cytokines and inflammatory factors as seen in sepsis.[43]

Currently, the definitive treatment of preeclampsia is delivery. If the pregnancy is remote from term in the presence of severe preeclampsia, a determination must be made whether to deliver or expectantly manage. This requires repeated evaluation of the mother and fetus. It is critical for the anesthesia provider on labor and delivery to be aware of these patients and their clinical course, as they can rapidly deteriorate and require urgent or emergent delivery.

MANAGEMENT

Normally, invasive monitoring is not required and central venous lines may increase risk without known benefit. However, in certain cases of severe preeclampsia and HELLP an invasive pressure line or central venous catheter may be beneficial. These clinical situations might include the need for (1) management of labile hypertension, (2) frequent blood gas/laboratory studies (severe pulmonary edema), (3) rapid central acting vasoactive medications, or (4) estimation of intravascular volume status (oliguria).[42] The use of judicious volume expansion is generally supported before initiation of neuraxial blockade.

Magnesium

Magnesium sulfate is used for seizure prophylaxis in preeclamptic women. Although a magnesium sulfate infusion reduces seizure rates among severe preeclamptic women, it is unclear whether women with mild preeclampsia similarly benefit.[44] Magnesium reduces central nervous system irritability by decreasing activity at the neuromuscular junction. Consequently, it can potentiate the action of both depolarizing and nondepolarizing muscle relaxants. Magnesium sulfate also provides uterine and smooth muscle relaxation. Magnesium toxicity is important to consider in preeclamptic women with worsening renal function and oliguria, as it is renally excreted. Women are monitored for magnesium toxicity with evaluation of deep tendon reflexes, respiratory depression, and neurologic compromise. The infusion usually is performed by loading 4 to 6 g over 20 to 30 minutes followed by continued magnesium sulfate infusion of 1 to 2 g/hour until 12 to 24 hours after delivery. Therapeutic range for seizure prophylaxis is between 6 to 8 mg/dL. Loss of deep tendon reflexes occurs at 10 mg/dL with prolonged PQ intervals and widening QRS complex on electrocardiogram (ECG). Respiratory arrest occurs at 15 to 20 mg/dL, and asystole occurs when the level exceeds 20 to 25 mg/dL. If toxicity occurs, IV calcium chloride (500 mg) or calcium gluconate (1 g) should be administered.

Antihypertensive Drugs

During the intrapartum management of preeclampsia, women often have additional increases in arterial blood pressure from pain. Arterial blood pressure management may require antihypertensive agents. Current guidelines recommend treating SBP greater than 160 mm Hg for

IV

prevention of intracerebral hemorrhage.[42] Initial therapy normally includes hydralazine and labetalol. In refractory severe hypertension, nitroglycerin and sodium nitroprusside may be used in the acute situation. Increases in maternal arterial blood pressure and fetal heart rate are important as drug-induced decreases in maternal perfusion pressure can result in uteroplacental insufficiency and fetal bradycardia.

NEURAXIAL ANALGESIA CONSIDERATIONS

The American College of Obstetricians and Gynecologists (ACOG) considers neuraxial analgesia the preferred analgesic method for labor in preeclamptics, but careful titration of the local anesthetic is needed to prevent the reduction in uteroplacental perfusion pressure.[45] Prior to placement of any neuraxial block a thorough evaluation of the patient's current status should be performed including hemoglobin and platelet levels. Given the potential for thrombocytopenia in severe preeclampsia and HELLP, most anesthesia providers recommend neuraxial block not be performed with platelet levels below 50,000, and for some the threshold is somewhat higher. The decision to place a neuraxial block should be evaluated for risk versus benefit and requires frank discussion with the patient regarding the risks of epidural hematoma. When removing the epidural catheter, one should be aware of possible platelet concentrations that are often decreased further after delivery. Bleeding time has not been demonstrated to be of clinical value. If hypotension occurs following initiation of neuraxial analgesia, prompt but judicious titration of phenylephrine or ephedrine should be given, keeping in mind the presumed hypersensitivity to catecholamines in preeclamptics.

Given the potential for placental insufficiency with preeclampsia, the anesthesia provider must be prepared for urgent delivery. Exaggerated upper airway edema is frequent in preeclamptics and increases the risk of difficult intubation if an emergent general anesthetic is required. Tracheal intubation may produce further hypertension during laryngoscopy and a small amount of nitroglycerin can be beneficial. If there is concern for a difficult airway, appropriate alternatives such as direct video laryngoscopy at the outset should be considered. Postpartum uterine atony is common with magnesium sulfate infusion and accentuated if inhaled anesthetic is given. Pitocin and prostaglandins are safe for uterine atony, but methylergonovine (methergine) should be used cautiously as it can precipitate a hypertensive crisis.

HEMORRHAGE IN PREGNANT WOMEN

Hemorrhage in pregnant women is one of the leading causes of maternal death. Placenta previa, abruptio placentae, and uterine rupture are the major causes of bleeding and uncontrolled hemorrhage during the third trimester and labor. Postpartum hemorrhage occurs in 3% to 5% of all vaginal deliveries and is typically due to uterine atony, retained placenta, placenta accreta, or lacerations involving the cervix or vagina. Common problems identified with hemorrhages leading to significant morbidity and mortality rates in obstetrics include (1) poor quantification of blood loss, (2) unrecognized associated risk factors for hemorrhage, (3) delayed initiation of treatment, and (4) inadequate transfusion of blood products in a massive hemorrhage situation.

Placenta Previa

Placenta previa is an abnormal uterine implantation of the placenta in front of the presenting fetus. The incidence is approximately 1 in 200 pregnancies. Risk factors include advanced age, multiparity, assisted reproductive techniques, prior hysterotomy, and prior placenta previa. The cardinal symptom of placenta previa is painless vaginal bleeding that typically occurs preterm in the third trimester. This first episode is normally self-limited. When this diagnosis is suspected, the position of the placenta should be confirmed by ultrasonography. Cesarean delivery is required unless the placental margin is further than 2 cm from the internal os.[46] Neuraxial anesthesia is an appropriate choice if there is no active bleeding or hypovolemia. The use of two large-bore intravenous lines with fluid warmers is suggested for rapid infusion of fluids or blood products. Invasive monitoring should also be available.

MASSIVE HEMORRHAGE

For emergency situations with active hemorrhage, general anesthesia may be required. *Ketamine* (1 to 1.5 mg/kg IV) and *etomidate* (0.3 mg/kg) are useful drugs for induction of anesthesia. If a massive hemorrhage occurs, aggressive use of fresh frozen plasma and platelets in addition to packed red blood cells may be needed for transfusion in ratios similar to those used for a trauma resuscitation, as a dilutional coagulopathy can quickly result in such a situation. In these cases of uncontrolled rapid hemorrhage, there is often not time to wait for the return of laboratory studies before transfusion of appropriate blood products. In rare occasions, cryoprecipitate and recombinant activated factor VII may be needed. Neonates delivered from pregnant women in hemorrhagic shock are likely to be acidotic and hypovolemic, and may need resuscitation. If hemorrhage is not controlled with standard measures, the obstetric team can consider (1) uterine artery ligation, (2) B-Lynch sutures, (3) an intrauterine balloon, (4) use of arterial embolization by interventional radiology if the patient is stable for transport, or (5) hysterectomy.

Abruptio Placentae

Abruptio placentae is separation of the placenta after 20 weeks of gestation, but before delivery. The incidence is approximately 1 in 100 pregnancies. Risk factors include advanced age, hypertension, trauma, smoking, cocaine use, chorioamnionitis, premature rupture of membranes, and history of prior abruption. When the separation involves only the placental margin, the escaping blood can appear as vaginal bleeding often associated with uterine tenderness. Alternatively, large volumes of blood loss (>2 L) can remain entirely concealed in the uterus. Chronic bleeding and clotting between the uterus and placenta can cause maternal disseminated intravascular coagulopathy (DIC). Ultrasound is specific if abruption is noted, but has poor sensitivity and a normal examination does not exclude abruption. Definitive treatment of abruptio placentae is to deliver the pregnancy. The anesthetic plan is based on both the delivery urgency and the abruption severity. If there are no signs of maternal hypovolemia, active bleeding, clotting abnormalities, or fetal distress, epidural analgesia can be used for labor and vaginal delivery. However, severe hemorrhage necessitates emergency cesarean delivery and the use of a general anesthetic similar to that described for placenta previa. It is predictable that neonates born under these circumstances will be acidotic and hypovolemic.

Uterine Rupture

Uterine rupture is poorly defined and includes cases ranging from scar dehiscence to those with catastrophic uterine wall rupture. In addition to prior uterine scar, uterine rupture is associated with rapid spontaneous delivery, motor vehicle trauma, trauma from instrumented vaginal delivery, large or malpositioned fetus, and excessive oxytocin stimulation. After previous cesarean delivery, vaginal birth is associated with a 0.4% to 1% incidence of uterine rupture.[47] Spontaneous rupture of an unscarred uterus is far more rare. The presentation is variable but may include vaginal bleeding, cessation of contractions, FHR deceleration, and abdominal pain normally not masked by neuraxial analgesia. Unfortunately, pain is not always a diagnostic finding. Immediate evaluation, aggressive resuscitation, and general anesthesia for emergent cesarean delivery are normally required for management. Often uterine repair by the obstetrician can occur following an emergent cesarean delivery if a minor scar dehiscence is present, but hysterectomy is needed for most cases of uterine wall rupture of an unscarred uterus. When vaginal birth is planned after a previous cesarean delivery, it is required that a surgical team, including an obstetrician, anesthesia provider, and nursing staff members, be immediately available so that an emergency delivery can be initiated without delay should uterine rupture occur.

Retained Placenta

Retained placenta occurs in about 1% of all vaginal deliveries and usually necessitates manual exploration of the uterus. If a lumbar epidural or spinal anesthetic was not used for vaginal delivery, manual removal of the placenta may be initially attempted with analgesia provided by intravenous administration of opioids or the inhalation of nitrous oxide. If uterine relaxation is necessary, nitroglycerin (50 to 150 µg IV) is normally effective. Additionally relocation to the operating room and placement of neuraxial analgesia may be beneficial for thorough evaluation. Rarely, induction of general anesthesia with tracheal intubation and administration of a volatile anesthetic to provide uterine relaxation will be necessary. An effort to obtain accurate blood loss is critical in determining an appropriate anesthetic and resuscitation plan.

Uterine Atony

Uterine atony is a common cause of postpartum hemorrhage and can occur immediately after delivery or several hours later. Risk factors for postpartum uterine atony include retained products, long labor, high parity, macrosomia, polyhydramnios, excessive oxytocin augmentation, and chorioamnionitis. Following bimanual massage, uterine atony is initially treated with oxytocin (20 to 40 units/L). This dilute solution of oxytocin exerts minimal cardiovascular effects, but rapid intravenous injection is associated with tachycardia, vasodilation, and hypotension. Other drugs can be used if oxytocin alone is not effective. Methylergonovine (0.2 mg IM) is an ergot derivative given to improve uterine tone. Owing to the significant vasoconstriction, it is relatively contraindicated in preeclamptics and patients with cardiac disease. The prostaglandin $F_{2\alpha}$ (0.25 mg IM) is another uterotonic used to treat refractory atony. It is associated with nausea, tachycardia, pulmonary hypertension, desaturation, and bronchospasm. It should be avoided in asthmatics. Prostaglandin E_1 (600 µg oral/sublingual/rectal) can be effective in treating atony if other drugs are not. It has no significant cardiac effects but may cause hyperthermia. If postpartum hemorrhage is not controlled with these initial methods, more invasive techniques and blood product transfusion will be urgently needed.

Placenta Accreta

Placental implantation beyond the endometrium gives rise to (1) *placenta accreta vera*, which is implantation and adherence onto the myometrium; (2) *placenta increta*, which is implantation into the myometrium; and (3) *placenta percreta*, which is penetration through the full thickness of the myometrium (Fig. 33-7). With placenta percreta, implantations may occur onto bowel,

IV

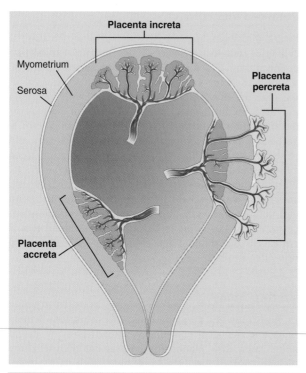

Figure 33-7 Classification of placenta accreta based on the degree of penetration of myometrium. (From Kamani AAS, Gambling DR, Chritlaw J, et al. Anesthetic management of patients with placenta accreta. Can J Anaesth 1987;34:613-617, used with permission.)

bladder, ovaries, or other pelvic organs and vessels. Any of these placental implantations can produce a markedly adherent placenta that cannot be removed without tearing the myometrium and producing a life-threatening severe hemorrhage.

These abnormal placental implantations occur more frequently in association with placenta previa. In the general obstetric population, placenta accreta occurs in approximately 1 in 2500, and although the sensitivity of ultrasonography in diagnosis is improving, anesthetic management should not be exclusively guided by the result. In patients with placenta previa and no previous cesarean delivery, the incidence of accreta is approximately 3%. However, the risk of placenta accreta associated with placenta previa increases with the number of previous cesarean deliveries. With one previous uterine incision, the incidence of placenta accreta is 11%, and with two previous uterine incisions the rate is 40%, and with three or more prior uterine incisions the incidence increases to above 60%.[48]

In patients with both placenta previa and accreta, massive and rapid intraoperative blood loss is common with reported average blood loss ranging from 2000 to 5000 mL, and in some the loss is substantially more. Coagulopathies develop in approximately 20% of these patients, and a significant portion require hysterectomies. Placenta accreta is not reliably diagnosed until the uterus is open. The anesthesia provider must keep in mind this possibility and be prepared to treat sudden massive blood loss. The decision of anesthetic technique can be individualized by case and provider. In cases in which there is a preoperative diagnosis, or high suspicion, preparations for massive hemorrhage are needed and intraoperative cell salvage should be considered.[20]

AMNIOTIC FLUID EMBOLISM

The incidence of amniotic fluid embolism (AFE) is estimated between 1:20,000 and 1:80,000. Clinical features of AFE include the sudden onset of hypotension, respiratory distress, hypoxia, disseminated intravascular coagulopathy, altered mental status, and eventual maternal collapse. These signs must be differentiated from other more common morbidities of pregnancy and delivery. The exact cause and pathogenesis of AFE remain uncertain, but it is no longer believed to be an embolic disease and is thought instead to be a type of anaphylactoid reaction.[49] The diagnosis of AFE is a clinical diagnosis of exclusion. Although in the past it had been believed that aspirating amniotic fluid debris such as fetal squamous cells from the maternal pulmonary circulation was diagnostic, the presence of fetal squames has been demonstrated in asymptomatic pregnant women, and no diagnostic laboratory test for AFE currently exists.

Treatment of AFE is supportive and directed toward cardiopulmonary resuscitation with inotropic support and correction of arterial hypoxemia. Tracheal intubation and mechanical support of ventilation are almost always required. Rapid onset of coagulopathy may occur and result in life-threatening hemorrhage. Conditions that mimic AFE include venous air embolism, pulmonary embolism, and inhalation of gastric contents. Definitive diagnosis is extremely difficult or impossible, even with postmortem examination.

ANESTHESIA FOR NONOBSTETRIC SURGERY DURING PREGNANCY

The overall incidence of nonobstetric surgery during pregnancy is 1 in 50 to 1 in 100, with trauma, appendicitis, and cholecystitis being the most frequent causes.[50] The anesthesia management objectives for pregnant women undergoing nonobstetric surgery include avoidance of teratogenic drugs and prevention of intrauterine fetal hypoxia and acidosis. In addition there is concern for prevention of spontaneous abortion with procedures early in pregnancy and premature labor with surgery later in pregnancy. Elective procedures should be delayed until 6 weeks post partum. When possible, nonelective operations should be delayed until after the first trimester in order to minimize teratogenic effects on the fetus. The second trimester is considered the optimal time for intervention as the risk of preterm labor is lowest. In the case of acutely urgent surgical procedures, their timing should mimic that of nonpregnant patients.

For operations that are necessary during pregnancy, the anesthesia provider should (1) determine an anesthetic plan that optimizes the maternal and fetal condition; (2) consult an obstetrician and perinatologist in order to optimize plans for unexpected events; (3) determine a plan for fetal monitoring if appropriate; and (4) discuss a plan in the event of a cesarean delivery or maternal arrest. There is always the possibility that anesthesia will be unknowingly administered to women with an early undiagnosed pregnancy. For this reason, routine pregnancy testing may be recommended by some before elective surgery for women of childbearing age.

Avoidance of Teratogenic Drugs

Most drugs, including anesthetics, have been demonstrated to be teratogenic in at least one animal species. In humans, the critical period of organogenesis is between 15 and 56 days of gestation. Nevertheless, there is no evidence that any of the currently used anesthetics, administered during pregnancy, are teratogenic with the exception of cocaine. Neurodegeneration and widespread apoptosis following exposure to anesthetics has been clearly established in developing animals, and a few studies demonstrate cognitive impairment in adult animals after neonatal anesthetic exposure. Currently there are no data to extrapolate these animal findings to humans, and this phenomenon is difficult to study in humans as clinical evidence is still scarce and amounts to an associative and not causal relationship.[51]

Avoidance of Intrauterine Fetal Hypoxia and Acidosis

Avoidance of decreased uterine blood flow and oxygenation is critical to fetal well-being as both hypercapnia and hypocapnia result in reduced uterine blood flow and fetal acidosis. The development of intrauterine fetal hypoxia and acidosis is minimized by avoiding maternal hypotension with left uterine displacement after the twentieth week of gestation, as well as by preventing arterial hypoxemia and excessive changes in Pa_{CO_2}. High inspired concentrations of oxygen do not increase the risk for in utero retrolental fibroplasia (retinopathy) because the high oxygen consumption of the placenta plus the uneven distribution of maternal and fetal blood flow in the placenta prevent fetal Pa_{O_2} from exceeding about 60 mm Hg (even if maternal Pa_{O_2} exceeds 500 mm Hg).

Fetal heart rate (FHR) monitoring via Doppler is possible at 16 to 18 weeks' gestational age (GA), but variability as a marker of well-being is not established until 25 to 27 weeks of gestation. ACOG states that the use of intraoperative "fetal monitoring should be individualized, and each case warrants a team approach for optimal safety of the patient and her baby."[52] The greatest value of fetal monitoring is that by displaying fetal compromise, maternal and fetal conditions can be treated effectively. Currently there is no evidence for the efficacy of FHR monitoring. In addition, interpretation is difficult because most anesthetics reduce FHR variability, placement and signal acquisition may be challenging, and a trained person is needed to interpret the strip.

Prevention of Preterm Labor

The underlying pathology requiring surgery, and not the anesthetic technique, has been associated with an increased risk for preterm delivery. Intra-abdominal procedures have more risk than minor peripheral procedures. After successful completion of surgery, both the fetal heart rate and maternal uterine activity should be monitored. Preterm labor can be treated with tocolytics (e.g., magnesium, nifedipine, or indomethacin) in consult with an obstetrician. Postoperative analgesics can alter the perception of contractions, stressing the need for external monitoring.

Management of Anesthesia

Elective surgery for pregnant women should be deferred until 6 weeks after delivery. When surgery is necessary, it is best to delay the operation until the second trimester. Before proceeding, a plan for fetal monitoring, potential maternal arrest, and implications of a cesarean delivery should be discussed with an obstetrician and perinatologist. When feasible, neuraxial anesthetic techniques should be considered given appropriate provider experience and circumstance as they limit fetal drug exposure and maternal risks associated with general anesthesia. When a general anesthetic is chosen, aspiration prophylaxis and left uterine displacement should be used. Induction technique should be similar to that for cesarean delivery under general anesthesia as previously discussed. Eucarbia should be maintained (30 mm Hg end-tidal CO_2), as well as adequate uterine perfusion with fluids and appropriate vasopressors use such as phenylephrine. Regardless of the anesthetic technique selected, inhaled concentrations of oxygen should be at least 50%. Postoperatively, deep venous thrombosis prophylaxis should be instituted, FHR and uterine activity monitored (often at least 24 hours), and a plan for postoperative analgesia determined.

IV

Laparoscopic Surgery

Laparoscopy is considered as safe as open approaches during any trimester, and the indications for its use are the same as for nonpregnant patients.[53] A recent systematic review noted that trimester did not influence the complication rate, the conversion to open was low (1%), there was a slightly higher fetal loss rate, but the lower preterm delivery rate was noted compared to open approaches.[54] Most investigations comparing laparoscopic to open techniques note no difference in fetal or maternal outcomes. If a laparoscopic technique is used, in addition to considerations discussed above, end-tidal CO_2 should be monitored throughout surgery and low pneumoperitoneum pressures (10 to 15 mm Hg) should be used if feasible.

DIAGNOSIS AND MANAGEMENT OF FETAL DISTRESS

Overview

The evolution of FHR monitoring began with the question, How was hypoxia and metabolic acidosis detected in the fetus? Intrapartum fetal monitoring was designed to detect hypoxia in labor and allow the clinicians to intervene prior to acidosis and long-term fetal CNS damage. The fetal brain responds to peripheral and central stimuli: (1) chemoreceptors, (2) baroreceptors, and (3) direct effects of metabolic changes within the CNS. FHR monitoring was developed as a crude, nonspecific method of tracking fetal oxygenation and distress. Excellent external FHR monitors are available, but it is often necessary to apply an internal fetal scalp electrode to obtain accurate continuous FHR monitoring.

Key Evaluation Components

Based on a 2008 National Institutes of Health (NIH) report, the assessment of FHR interpretation involves evaluation of (1) uterine contractions, (2) baseline FHR, (3) baseline FHR variability, (4) presence of accelerations, (5) periodic or episodic decelerations, and (6) changes or trends of FHR patterns over time.[55]

UTERINE CONTRACTIONS

Uterine contractions can be monitored externally or internally. External monitors only relay contraction frequency, but internal monitoring allows for both frequency and measurement of intrauterine pressure (in Montevideo units). Uterine activity and definitions are detailed in Table 33-4. If a tonic contraction or period of tachysystole occurs during labor, treatment with either sublingual or IV nitroglycerin can briefly relax the uterus and restore fetal perfusion. In addition, the obstetrician can give subcutaneous terbutaline.

Table 33-4 Uterine Activity Terminology

A. Normal: ≤5 contractions in 10 minutes, averaged over a 30-minute window

B. Tachysystole: >5 contractions in 10 minutes, averaged over a 30-minute window

C. Characteristics of uterine contractions: Tachysystole should be always qualified as to presence or absence of associated fetal heart rate decelerations.
- Tachysystole applies to either spontaneous or stimulated labor. The clinical response to tachysystole may differ depending on whether contractions are spontaneous or stimulated.
- Hyperstimulation and hypercontractility are not defined and should be abandoned.

Data from Macones GA, Hankins GD, Spong CY, et al. The 2008 National Institute of Child Health and Human Development workshop report on electronic fetal monitoring: update on definitions, interpretation, and research guidelines. J Obstet Gynecol Neonatal Nurs 2008;37(5):510-515.

BASELINE FETAL HEART RATE

Baseline FHR is determined by approximating the mean FHR rounded to increments of 5 beats/min during a 10-minute window excluding accelerations, decelerations, and periods of marked FHR variability (change > 25 beats/min). Abnormal baseline includes bradycardia (<110 beats/min) and tachycardia (>160 beats/min).

VARIABILITY

Baseline variability is also determined by examining fluctuations that are irregular in amplitude and frequency during a 10-minute window excluding accelerations and decelerations. Variability is classified as follows:

Absent FHR variability: amplitude range undetectable

Minimal FHR variability: amplitude range greater than undetectable and 5 beats/min or less

Moderate FHR variability: amplitude range 6 to 25 beats/min

Marked FHR variability: amplitude range above 25 beats/min

ACCELERATIONS

An acceleration is an abrupt increase in FHR defined as an increase from the acceleration onset to the peak in greater than 30 seconds. In addition, the peak must be 15 beats/min or greater, and last 15 seconds or longer from the onset to return. Before 32 weeks of gestation, accelerations are defined as having a peak 10 beats/min or more and a duration of 10 seconds or longer.

DECELERATIONS

Decelerations are classified as variable or late based on specific criteria described in Table 33-5 and displayed

Table 33-5 Fetal Heart Rate (FHR) Tracing Criteria for Decelerations

Characteristics of Late Deceleration

- Visually apparent, usually symmetrical gradual decrease and return of the FHR associated with a uterine contraction
- A gradual FHR decrease is defined as from the onset to the FHR nadir of $\geq$ 30 seconds
- The decrease in FHR is calculated from the onset to the nadir of the deceleration
- The deceleration is delayed in timing, with the nadir of the deceleration occurring after the peak of the contraction
- In most cases, the onset, nadir, and recovery of the deceleration occur after the beginning, peak, and ending of the contraction, respectively

Characteristics of Variable Deceleration

- Visually apparent abrupt decrease in FHR
- An abrupt FHR decrease is defined as from the onset of the deceleration to the beginning of the FHR nadir of < 30 seconds
- The decrease in FHR $\geq$15 bpm, lasting $\geq$15 seconds, and <2 minutes in duration
- When the variable decelerations are associated with uterine contractions, their onset, depth, and duration commonly vary with successive uterine contractions

Data from Macones GA, Hankins GD, Spong CY, et al. The 2008 National Institute of Child Health and Human Development workshop report on electronic fetal monitoring: update on definitions, interpretation, and research guidelines. J Obstet Gynecol Neonatal Nurs 2008;37(5):510-515.

in Figure 33-8. A prolonged deceleration is present when there is a visually apparent decrease in the FHR from the baseline that is greater than or equal to 15 beats/min, lasting 2 minutes or longer.

Late decelerations are a result of uteroplacental insufficiency causing relative fetal brain hypoxia during a contraction. The change results in sympathetic response and increased peripheral vascular resistance, increasing the fetal blood pressure which is detected by the fetal baroreceptors and results in slowing in the FHR. This response is termed a "reflex" late. A second type of late deceleration is caused by myocardial depression in the presence of worsening hypoxia. A moderate decrease in FHR indicates some uteroplacental insufficiency, but a more severe decrease in the FHR can indicate near total insufficiency. The term "early" deceleration is controversial. Although often associated with head compression, it is more likely a variant of the "reflex" late deceleration that mirrors the uterine contraction, is considered benign, but might evolve into a more typical late deceleration.[56] *Variable decelerations* are generally synonymous with umbilical cord compression. An ominous sinusoidal

FHR pattern is defined as having a smooth sine wave–like pattern with a cycle frequency of 3 to 5/min that persists for 20 minutes or longer and can be associated with placental abruption.[55]

Minimal to undetectable FHR variability in the presence of decelerations is associated with fetal acidemia. Severe decelerations (<70 beats/min for > 60 sec) are associated with fetal acidemia, and extremely ominous with the absence of variability.[57]

The FHR tracing is a nonspecific assessment of fetal acidosis and should be interpreted over the course of time in relation to the clinical context and fetal and maternal factors. A normal fetus will experience episodes of hypoxia during labor and should tolerate these periods without long-term neurologic sequelae.

EVALUATION OF THE NEONATE AND NEONATAL RESUSCITATION

The transition from fetal to neonate life involves major physiologic changes in the pulmonary and circulatory systems. The importance of the intrapartum and antepartum events can predict how safe and successful the transition to neonate will be. Umbilical cord gases are frequently sent at delivery as a measure of fetal assessment. Typical values are shown in Table 33-6.

Assessment of neonates immediately after birth is important to promptly identify depressed infants who require active resuscitation. The Apgar score assigns a numerical value (0, 1, or 2) to five vital signs measured or observed at 1 and 5 minutes after delivery (Table 33-7). It still is the best method of facilitating recognition of the need for and guiding resuscitation management of a newborn. Most newborns (Apgar $\geq$ 8) require little treatment other than suctioning of the nose and mouth, tactile stimulation to promote breathing, and avoiding hypothermia. The neonate's skin should be wiped dry and the baby placed on a radiantly heated bed, covered with warm blankets, or placed in skin-to-skin contact with mother. Apgar scores of 10 are rare because the acrocyanosis persists in a normal newborn well past 5 minutes of life.

Cardiopulmonary Resuscitation

Management of neonates in the delivery room falls into 30-second evaluations and interventions as detailed in Figure 33-9. At delivery, once the infant is placed under a radiant warmer and drying and stimulation have occurred, the first 30-second evaluation begins. This evaluation starts with the determination of tone, breathing, or crying. If breathing and crying do not occur, then clearing of the airway (mouth, then nose) and repeated stimulation should be performed; this is the next 30-second evaluation. Following this, the 1-minute Apgar score is determined with evaluation of the

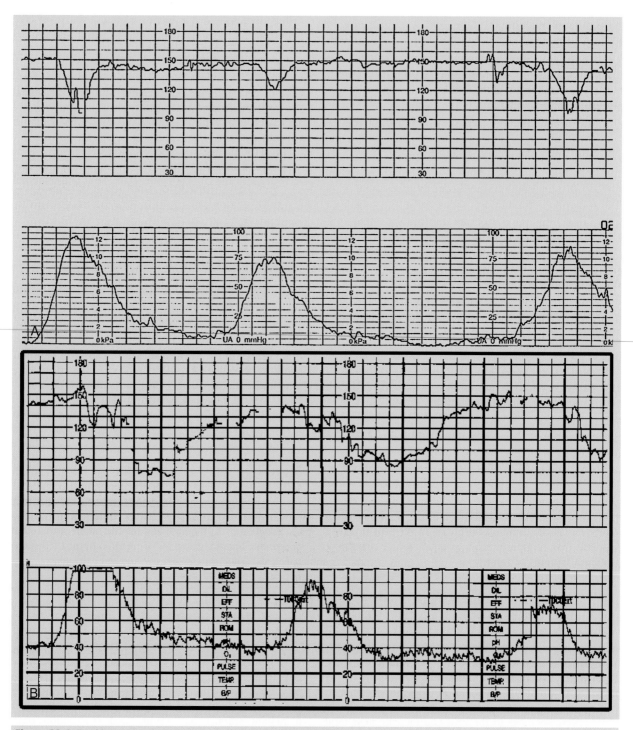

Figure 33-8 Fetal heart rate decelerations. **A,** Variable deceleration with minimal variability. **B,** Late deceleration with minimal variability.

Table 33-6 Normal Blood Gas Values of Umbilical Artery and Vein

	Mean Value	
	Artery	Vein
pH	7.27	7.34
Pco$_2$ (mm Hg)	50	40
Po$_2$ (mm Hg)	20	30
Bicarbonate (mEq/L)	23	21
Base excess (mEq/L)	−3.6	−2.6

Data derived from Thorp JA, Rushing RS. Umbilical cord blood gas analysis. Obstet Gynecol Clin North Am 1999;26(4):695-709.

Table 33-7 Evaluation of a Neonate with the Apgar Score

	Score		
Criterion	2	1	0
Heart rate (beats/min)	>100	<100	Absent
Breathing	Irregular, crying	Slow	Absent
Reflex irritability	Cry	Grimace	No response
Muscle tone	Active	Flexion of the extremities	Limp
Color	Pink	Body pink, extremities cyanotic	Cyanotic

respirations, heart rate, and color. In the event of apnea or heart rate below 100 beats/min, positive-pressure hand ventilation should be provided with 21% or up to 100% oxygen using a properly fitted face mask (avoiding excessive inspiratory pressure > 30 cm H$_2$O).[58,59] Based on the current 2005 neonatal resuscitation guidelines, if the clinician begins with room air it is recommended that supplemental oxygen be given if no improvement is seen within 90 seconds after birth.[59] Proper neonatal head positioning for airway management is neutral with the neck slightly extended. Ventilation of the lungs is controlled at a rate of about 40 breaths/min. A positive end-expiratory pressure of 3 to 5 cm H$_2$O is often useful.

Evaluate the heart rate again if less than 60 beats/min and continue positive-pressure ventilation. At this point, the third 30-second evaluation will begin. If the heart rate is persistently less than 60 beats/min, chest compressions should be instituted with continued positive-pressure ventilation. Epinephrine should be administered if there is no

improvement. Throughout the resuscitation, endotracheal intubation is always considered if ventilation is not adequate by mask.

The recommended sternal compression technique involves positioning both thumbs one fingerbreadth below the nipple line with hands encircling the neonate's thorax or by using the middle and ring fingertips. Firm support of the neonate's back is necessary. The sternum is compressed to 1 to 2 cm depth. The ratio of compressions to ventilation should be 3:1 with 90 compressions and 30 breaths per minute.[59]

EPINEPHRINE

Epinephrine should be given for a heart rate that continues to stay less than 60 beats/min despite positive-pressure ventilation and chest compressions or immediately if asystole is present. The dose is 0.1 to 0.3 mL/kg of a 1:10,000 solution given rapidly intravenously through an umbilical artery catheter inserted just below the abdominal skin (preferred) or via the trachea. The dose may be repeated every 3 to 5 minutes, if necessary.

HYPOVOLEMIA

In certain circumstances blood loss in the neonate may lead to hypovolemia, such as placental abruption, placenta previa, or vasa previa, although arrest secondary to hypovolemia is rare. Intravascular volume expansion should be instituted in a newborn who appears to have suffered blood loss or is in shock and has not responded to other resuscitation measures discussed previously.[60] In the absence of blood (the preferred volume expander) an appropriate alternative is isotonic crystalloid given in 10 mL/kg aliquots. In three clinical trials isotonic crystalloid was found to be as effective as albumin for the treatment of perinatal hypotension.[61]

BICARBONATE

In a neonate with a metabolic acidosis, administration of bicarbonate or THAM might be appropriate. Early animal experiments suggested that bicarbonate assisted with resuscitation in cases of asphyxia, although the accumulation of generated carbon dioxide and hyperosmolality properties might impair the myocardial and cerebral function. Use of bicarbonate in newborn resuscitation has not demonstrated a significant effect on survival or neurologic outcomes and remains controversial.[62]

GLUCOSE

During deliveries in which the newborn is suspected to have severe asphyxia, intrauterine growth restriction, or maternal diabetes, hypoglycemia should be suspected. During the resuscitation, a heel stick can

IV

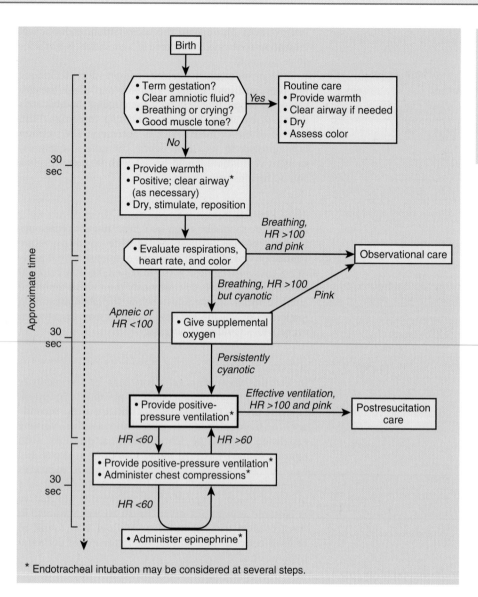

Figure 33-9 NRP resuscitation flow diagram (From Rajani AK, Chitkara R, Halamek LP. Delivery room management of the newborn. Pediatr Clin North Am 2009;56:515-535, used with permission.) American Academy of Pediatrics and American Heart Association, 2006.

* Endotracheal intubation may be considered at several steps.

determine the blood glucose level. In addition, administration of glucose should be considered in a preterm newborn who is unresponsive with bradycardia or asystole.[60]

NALOXONE

Naloxone is no longer recommended for use in newborns in the delivery room. Should the newborn manifest respiratory depression in the delivery room, appropriate ventilation should be maintained until the neonate is transported to the intensive care nursery. Continued stabilization and evaluation can be performed in the nursery and administration of naloxone considered once the mother's history is reviewed to evaluate for prenatal exposure to chronic opioids.[63]

Pulmonary Aspiration of Meconium-Stained Amniotic Fluid

Meconium-stained amniotic fluid (MSAF) is encountered in 7% to 20% of live births with 2% to 9% of infants born through MSAF acquiring meconium aspiration syndrome (MAS).[63] Currently, neonates at delivery with MSAF who are at term should not be suctioned vigorously at the perineum, and once delivered do not require endotracheal intubation.[63] Intubation and suctioning should be performed in MSAF neonates if they are not vigorous (heart rate < 100 beats/min, decreased muscle tone, and ineffectual respirations).[59] The most significant advance in the prevention of MAS is improved estimation of gestational age and use of post-dates induction at 41 weeks' gestational age instead of 42 weeks.

QUESTIONS OF THE DAY

1. What is the time course of changes in maternal cardiac output during pregnancy? What are the cardiac output changes during labor and delivery?
2. What are the most significant changes in lung volumes during pregnancy? What are the anesthetic implications?
3. How do the requirements for inhaled anesthesia and local anesthesia change during pregnancy?
4. Which commonly administered anesthetic drugs cross the placental barrier and reach the fetus? What are the characteristics of drugs that do not cross the placenta?
5. What is the likely impact of epidural analgesia on the rate of cesarean delivery?
6. A patient receiving epidural analgesia for labor develops fever. What are the possible mechanisms?
7. What is HELLP syndrome? What are the implications for providing epidural labor analgesia in a patient with HELLP?
8. What are the major causes of obstetric hemorrhage during the third trimester and labor? How can the specific cause be determined?

REFERENCES

1. Cheek TG, Gutsche BB: Maternal physiologic alterations. In Hughes SC, Levinson G, Rosen MA, editors: *Shnider and Levinson's Anesthesia for Obstetrics*, ed 4, Philadelphia, 2002, Lippincott Williams & Wilkins, pp 3–18.
2. Gaiser R: Physiologic changes of pregnancy. In Chestnut DH, Polley LS, Tsen LC, Wong CA, editors: *Chestnut's Obstetric Anesthesia: Principles and Practice*, ed 4, Philadelphia, 2009, Elsevier, pp 15–36.
3. Ewah B, Yau K, King M, et al: Effect of epidural opioids on gastric emptying in labour, *Int J Obstet Anesth* 2(3):125–128, 1993.
4. Hey VM, Ostick DG, Mazumder JK, et al: Pethidine, metoclopramide and the gastro-oesophageal sphincter. A study in healthy volunteers, *Anaesthesia* 36(2):173–176, 1981.
5. Lee A, Ngan Kee WD, Gin T: A quantitative, systematic review of randomized controlled trials of ephedrine versus phenylephrine for the management of hypotension during spinal anesthesia for cesarean delivery, *Anesth Analg* 94(4):920–926, 2002.
6. Ngan Kee WD, Khaw KS, Tan PE, et al: Placental transfer and fetal metabolic effects of phenylephrine and ephedrine during spinal anesthesia for cesarean delivery, *Anesthesiology* 111(3):506–512, 2009.
7. Smiley RM: Burden of proof, *Anesthesiology* 111(3):470–472, 2009.
8. Leighton BL, Halpern SH, Wilson DB: Lumbar sympathetic blocks speed early and second stage induced labor in nulliparous women, *Anesthesiology* 90(4):1039–1046, 1999.
9. Hodnett ED, Gates S, Hofmeyr GJ, et al: Continuous support for women during childbirth, *Cochrane Database Syst Rev* (3):CD003766, 2007.
10. Declercq ER, Sakala C, Corry MP, et al: Listening to Mothers II: Report of the Second National U.S. Survey of Women's Childbearing Experiences: Conducted January-February 2006 for Childbirth Connection by Harris Interactive in partnership with Lamaze International, *J Perinat Educ* 16(4):15–17, 2007.
11. Nissen E, Widstrom AM, Lilja G, et al: Effects of routinely given pethidine during labour on infants' developing breastfeeding behaviour. Effects of dose-delivery time interval and various concentrations of pethidine/norpethidine in cord plasma, *Acta Paediatr* 86(2):201–208, 1997.
12. Rayburn W, Rathke A, Leuschen MP, et al: Fentanyl citrate analgesia during labor, *Am J Obstet Gynecol* 161(1):202–206, 1989.
13. Volmanen P, Sarvela J, Akural EI, et al: Intravenous remifentanil vs. epidural levobupivacaine with fentanyl for pain relief in early labour: A randomised, controlled, double-blinded study, *Acta Anaesthesiol Scand* 52(2):249–255, 2008.
14. Douma MR, Verwey RA, Kam-Endtz CE, et al: Obstetric analgesia: A comparison of patient-controlled meperidine, remifentanil, and fentanyl in labour, *Br J Anaesth* 104(2):209–215, 2010.
15. Eisenach JC: Epidural neostigmine: Will it replace lipid soluble opioids for postoperative and labor analgesia? *Anesth Analg* 109(2):293–295, 2009.
16. Parker RK, Connelly NR, Lucas T, et al: Epidural clonidine added to a bupivacaine infusion increases analgesic duration in labor without adverse maternal or fetal effects, *J Anesth* 21(2):142–147, 2007.
17. Roelants F: The use of neuraxial adjuvant drugs (neostigmine, clonidine) in obstetrics, *Curr Opin Anaesthesiol* 19(3):233–237, 2006.
18. Mardirosoff C, Dumont L, Boulvain M, et al: Fetal bradycardia due to intrathecal opioids for labour analgesia: A systematic review, *BJOG* 109(3):274–281, 2002.
19. Eisenach JC: Combined spinal-epidural analgesia in obstetrics, *Anesthesiology* 91(1):299–302, 1999.
20. American Society of Anesthesiologists Task Force on Obstetric Anesthesia: Practice guidelines for obstetric anesthesia: An updated report by the American Society of Anesthesiologists Task Force on Obstetric Anesthesia, *Anesthesiology* 106(4):843–863, 2007.
21. Wong CA, McCarthy RJ, Sullivan JT, et al: Early compared with late neuraxial analgesia in nulliparous labor induction: A randomized controlled trial, *Obstet Gynecol* 113:1066–1074, 2009.
22. Wong CA, Scavone BM, Peaceman AM, et al: The risk of cesarean delivery with neuraxial analgesia given early versus late in labor, *N Engl J Med* 352:655–665, 2005.
23. Anim-Somuah M, Smyth R, Howell C: Epidural versus non-epidural or no analgesia in labour, *Cochrane Database Syst Rev* (4):CD000331, 2005.
24. American Society of Anesthesiologists Task Force on Infectious Complications Associated with Neuraxial Techniques: Practice advisory for the prevention, diagnosis, and management of infectious complications associated with neuraxial techniques: A report by the American Society of Anesthesiologists Task Force on infectious complications associated with neuraxial techniques, *Anesthesiology* 112:530–545, 2010.
25. Simmons SW, Cyna AM, Dennis AT, et al: Combined spinal-epidural versus epidural analgesia in labour, *Cochrane Database Syst Rev* (3):CD003401, 2007.
26. Van de Velde M, Teunkens A, Hanssens M, et al: Intrathecal sufentanil and fetal heart rate abnormalities: A double-blind, double placebo-controlled trial comparing two

forms of combined spinal epidural analgesia with epidural analgesia in labor, *Anesth Analg* 98:1153–1159, 2004.

27. Pan PH, Bogard TD, Owen MD: Incidence and characteristics of failures in obstetric neuraxial analgesia and anesthesia: A retrospective analysis of 19,259 deliveries, *Int J Obstet Anesth* 13:227–233, 2004.

28. Moen V, Dahlgren N, Irestedt L: Severe neurological complications after central neuraxial blockades in Sweden 1990–1999, *Anesthesiology* 101:950–959, 2004.

29. Hofmeyr G, Cyna A, Middleton P: Prophylactic intravenous preloading for regional analgesia in labour, *Cochrane Database Syst Rev* (4): CD000175, 2004.

30. Ko JS, Kim CS, Cho HS, et al: A randomized trial of crystalloid versus colloid solution for prevention of hypotension during spinal or low-dose combined spinal-epidural anesthesia for elective cesarean delivery, *Int J Obstet Anesth* 16:8–12, 2007.

31. Rosen MA: Paracervical block for labor analgesia: A brief historic review, *Am J Obstet Gynecol* 186(Suppl 5): S127–S130, 2002.

32. Yentis MY, Cohen SE: Inhalational analgesia and anesthesia for labor and vaginal delivery. In Hughes SC, Levinson G, Rosen MA, editors: *Shnider and Levinson's Anesthesia for Obstetrics*, ed 4, Philadelphia, 2002, Lippincott Williams & Wilkins, pp 189–197.

33. Ayad S, Demian Y, Narouze SN, et al: Subarachnoid catheter placement after wet tap for analgesia in labor: Influence on the risk of headache in obstetric patients, *Reg Anesth Pain Med* 28:512–515, 2003.

34. Cheek TG, Gutsche BB: Pulmonary aspiration of gastric contents. In Hughes SC, Levinson G, Rosen MA, editors: *Shnider and Levinson's Anesthesia for Obstetrics*, ed 4, Philadelphia, 2002, Lippincott Williams & Wilkins, pp 391–407.

35. Afolabi BB, Lesi FE, Merah NA: Regional versus general anaesthesia for caesarean section, *Cochrane Database Syst Rev* (4):CD004350, 2006.

36. Sunderam S, Chang J, Flowers L, et al: Assisted reproductive technology surveillance—United States, 2006, *MMWR Surveill Summ* 58:1–25, 2009.

37. National Center for Health Statistics: *Final natality data: Multiple Deliveries: U.S. 1996–2006.* Available at www.marchofdimes.com/peristats/. Accessed January, 2010.

38. Norwitz ER, Edusa V, Park JS: Maternal physiology and complications of multiple pregnancy, *Semin Perinatol* 29:338–348, 2005.

39. ACOG Committee on Obstetric Practice: ACOG Opinion No. 340: Mode of term singleton breech delivery, *Obstet Gynecol* 108(1):235–237, 2006.

40. Sokol RJ, Blackwell SC, American College of Obstetricians and Gynecologists. Committee on Practice Bulletins-Gynecology: ACOG Practice Bulletin. Shoulder dystocia. No. 40, Nov. 2002 (Replace practice pattern number 7, Oct. 1997), *Int J Gynaecol Obstet* 80(1):87–92, 2003.

41. Gottlieb AG, Galan HL: Shoulder dystocia: An update, *Obstet Gynecol Clin North Am* 34:501–531, 2007.

42. Report of the National High Blood Pressure Education Program Working Group on High Blood Pressure in Pregnancy, *Am J Obstet Gynecol* 183(1):S1–S22, 2000.

43. Taylor RN, Davidge ST, Roberts JN: Endothelial cell dysfunction and oxidative stress. In Lindheimer MD, Roberts JM, Cunningham FG, editors: *Chesley's Hypertensive Disorders in Pregnancy*, ed 3, San Diego, 2009, Elsevier, pp 143–168.

44. Sibai BM: Magnesium sulfate prophylaxis in preeclampsia: Evidence from randomized trials, *Clin Obstet Gynecol* 48:478–488, 2005.

45. ACOG Committee on Practice Bulletins–Obstetrics: ACOG Diagnosis and management of preeclampsia and eclampsia. No. 33, Jan. 2002, *Obstet Gynecol* 99(1):159–167, 2002.

46. Oyelese Y, Smulian JC: Placenta previa, placenta accreta, and vasa previa, *Obstet Gynecol* 107:927–941, 2006.

47. Kaczmarczyk M, Sparen P, Terry P, et al: Risk factors for uterine rupture and neonatal consequences of uterine rupture: A population-based study of successive pregnancies in Sweden, *BJOG* 114:1208–1214, 2007.

48. Silver RM, Landon MB, Rouse DJ, et al: Maternal morbidity associated with multiple repeat cesarean deliveries, *Obstet Gynecol* 107:1226–1232, 2006.

49. Moore J, Baldisseri MR: Amniotic fluid embolism, *Crit Care Med* 33(Suppl 10): S279–S285, 2005.

50. Chames MC, Pearlman MD: Trauma during pregnancy: Outcomes and clinical management, *Clin Obstet Gynecol* 51:398–408, 2008.

51. Istaphanous GK, Loepke AW: General anesthetics and the developing brain, *Curr Opin Anaesthesiol* 22:368–373, 2009.

52. ACOG Committee on Obstetric Practice: ACOG Opinion No. 284, Aug. 2003: Nonobstetric surgery in pregnancy, *Obstet Gynecol* 102(2):431, 2003.

53. Guidelines Committee of the Society of American Gastrointestinal and Endoscopic Surgeons, Yumi H: Guidelines for diagnosis, treatment, and use of laparoscopy for surgical problems during pregnancy: this statement was reviewed and approved by the Board of Governors of the Society of American Gastrointestinal and Endoscopic Surgeons (SAGES), September 2007. It was prepared by the SAGES Guidelines Committee.

54. Walsh CA, Tang T, Walsh SR: Laparoscopic versus open appendicectomy in pregnancy: A systematic review, *Int J Surg* 6:339–344, 2008.

55. Macones GA, Hankins GD, Spong CY, et al: The 2008 National Institute of Child Health and Human Development workshop report on electronic fetal monitoring: Update on definitions, interpretation, and research guidelines, *J Obstet Gynecol Neonatal Nurs* 37:510–515, 2008.

56. Parer JT: Fetal heart rate patterns: Basic and variant. In Parer JT, editor: *Handbook of Fetal Heart Rate Monitoring*, ed 2, Philadelphia, 1997, WB Saunders, pp 145–195.

57. Parer JT, King T, Flanders S, et al: Fetal acidemia and electronic fetal heart rate patterns: Is there evidence of an association? *J Matern Fetal Neonatal Med* 19:289–294, 2006.

58. Saugstad OD, Ramji S, Vento M: Resuscitation of depressed newborn infants with ambient air or pure oxygen: A meta-analysis, *Biol Neonate* 87:27–34, 2005.

59. American Heart Association, American Academy of Pediatrics: 2005 AHA guidelines for cardiopulmonary resuscitation (CPR) and emergency cardiovascular care (ECC) of pediatric and neonatal patients: Neonatal resuscitation guidelines, *Pediatrics* 117:e1029–e1038, 2006.

60. Wyllie J, Niermeyer S: The role of resuscitation drugs and placental transfusion in the delivery room management of newborn infants, *Semin Fetal Neonatal Med* 13:416–423, 2008.

61. Niermeyer S: Volume resuscitation: Crystalloid versus colloid, *Clin Perinatol* 33:133–140, 2006.

62. Beveridge CJ, Wilkinson AR: Sodium bicarbonate infusion during resuscitation of infants at birth, *Cochrane Database Syst Rev* (1): CD004864, 2006.

63. Rajani AK, Chitkara R, Halamek LP: Delivery room management of the newborn, *Pediatr Clin North Am* 56:515–535, 2009.

Recommended Reading

Breivik H, et al: Nordic guidelines for neuraxial blocks in disturbed haemostasis from the Scandinavian Society of Anaesthesiology and Intensive Care Medicine, *Acta Anaesthesiol Scand* 54(1):16–41, 2010. Epub 2009 Oct 19.

Hawkins JJ: Epidural analgesia for labor and delivery, *N Engl J Med* xx:1503–1510, 2010.

IV

34 PEDIATRICS

Erin A. Gottlieb and Dean B. Andropoulos

Providing anesthesia care for infants and children poses unique challenges because of the profound differences in physiology, pharmacokinetics, and pharmacodynamics of anesthetic drugs, and the wide variety of procedures that these patients undergo, which are often very different from the adult population. This chapter will address the developmental physiology of pediatric patients, as well as pharmacology, fluid and transfusion therapy, and the pediatric airway. Then anesthetic considerations and techniques in pediatric patients will be reviewed, followed by the anesthetic management of medical and surgical diseases affecting the neonate, which is the most unique group of pediatric patients. The new field of fetal surgery will be addressed, and finally, the growing area of anesthesia in remote locations for pediatric patients and anesthetic neurotoxicity in the developing brain will briefly be discussed.

DEVELOPMENTAL PHYSIOLOGY

Respiratory System

LUNG DEVELOPMENT

Lung development begins in the fourth week of gestation, but extrauterine survival only becomes possible when terminal air sacs begin to form and the capillary network surrounding them is sufficient for pulmonary gas exchange around the twenty-sixth week. Alveolar formation begins by the thirty-sixth postconceptual week, but most alveoli form postnatally. Type II pneumocytes begin producing surfactant around the twenty-fourth week of gestation, and production of this mixture of phospholipids and surfactant proteins is critical for reducing surface tension and facilitating the inflation of alveoli.

CHEST WALL AND RESPIRATORY MUSCLES

The ribs extend from the vertebral column horizontally in infants compared to a caudad angle in adults. This configuration renders the accessory muscles of respiration ineffective in infants. The rib cage also tends to move inward during inspiration due to the high cartilage content in the ribs of neonates and infants. This paradoxical chest wall movement occurs commonly under general anesthesia and is due to decreased tone of the intercostal muscles and upper airway obstruction. The diaphragm increases its work to maintain tidal volume, which can lead to fatigue.

The mature diaphragm has a low content of type I (slow twitch, high oxidative capacity) muscle fibers. Prior to 37 weeks postconceptual age, less than 10% of the diaphragmatic fibers are type I. A term infant has approximately 25% type I fibers, and an adult has approximately 50%. This means that the diaphragm is more likely to become fatigued in premature and term infants, leading to earlier respiratory failure.

Chest wall compliance decreases throughout childhood and adolescence due to the ossification of the ribs and development of thoracic muscle mass. The elastic recoil pressure of the lung increases throughout this time due to an increase in pulmonary elastic fibers.

RESPIRATORY VARIABLES

There are some major differences in static lung volumes and respiratory variables between children of different ages and adults. Table 34-1 illustrates the major differences in static lung volumes and other variables between infants and adults. Total lung capacity (TLC) is much larger per kilogram in adults compared with infants. This is largely due to the relative efficiency and strength of adult muscles of inspiration and effort.

Functional residual capacity (FRC) is similar on a per kilogram basis among age groups, but the mechanical reasons for this differ. The FRC in adults is defined as the volume at which passive elastic forces of the chest wall are balanced by the recoil of the lung. This is the volume at end exhalation. In infants, both the elastic recoil of the chest and the recoil pressure of the lung are very small. This would predict an FRC of about 10% of TLC. However, the FRC is about 40% of TLC owing to a prolongation of the expiratory time constant by a process known as laryngeal braking.

In an apneic infant, the lung volume is less than the FRC. Thus, an apneic infant has a disproportionately smaller store of intrapulmonary oxygen than an adult, and hypoxia will develop rapidly if the airway is poorly maintained.

The closing capacity (CC) also differs with age. In infants, the CC is larger than the FRC, so during exhalation, small airways start to collapse and trap air. In adults, the closing capacity is smaller than the FRC.

FACTORS AFFECTING RESPIRATION

In both infants and adults, Pao_2, $Paco_2$, and pH control ventilation. An increase in $Paco_2$ leads to an increase in minute ventilation by increasing respiratory rate and tidal volume. This response to hypercapnia is not enhanced by hypoxemia. In fact, hypoxia may depress the hypercapnic ventilatory response.

High inspired oxygen concentrations depress newborn respiratory drive, and low inspired oxygen concentrations stimulate it. However, continued hypoxia will eventually lead to respiratory depression. Hypoglycemia, anemia, and hypothermia also decrease respiratory drive.

Metabolic demand drives minute ventilation. As oxygen consumption increases, alveolar minute ventilation increases. Although tidal volume also increases, the increase in respiratory rate is the predominant variable that increases minute ventilation in infants.

IV

Table 34-1 Age-Dependent Respiratory Variables

Variable	Units	Neonate	6 mo	12 mo	3 yr	5 yr	9 yr	12 yr	Adult
Approx. weight	kg	3	7	10	15	19	30	50	70
Respiratory rate	Breaths/min	50 ± 10	30 ± 5	24 ± 6	24 ± 6	23 ± 5	20 ± 5	18 ± 5	12 ± 3
Tidal volume	mL	21	45	78	112	170	230	480	575
	mL/kg	6-8	6-8	6-8	6-8	7-8	7-8	7-8	6-7
Minute ventilation	mL/min	1050	1350	1780	2460	4000		6200	6400
	mL/kg/min	350	193	178	164	210		124	91
Alveolar ventilation	mL/min	665		1245	1760	1800		3000	3100
	mL/kg/min	222		125	117	95		60	44
Dead space–tidal volume ratio		0.3	0.3	0.3	0.3	0.3	0.3	0.3	0.3
Oxygen consumption	mL/kg/min	6-8							3-4
Vital capacity	mL	120			870	1160		3100	4000
	mL/kg	40			58	61		62	57
Functional residual capacity	mL	80			490	680		1970	3000
	mL/kg	27			33	36		39	43
Total lung capacity	mL	160			1100	1500		4000	6000
	mL/kg	53			73	79		80	86
Closing volume as percentage of vital capacity	%					20		8	4
Number of alveoli	Saccules × 10^6	30	112	129	257	280			300
Specific compliance	C$_L$/FRC:mL/cm H$_2$O/L	0.04	0.038			0.06			0.05
Specific conductance of small airways	mL/sec/cm H$_2$O/g	0.02		3.1	1.7	1.2		8.2	13.4
Hematocrit	%	55 ± 7	37 ± 3	35 ± 2.5	40 ± 3	40 ± 2	40 ± 2	42 ± 2	43-48
Arterial pH	pH units	7.30-7.40		7.35-7.45					7.35-7.45
Pa$_{CO_2}$	mm Hg	30-35		30-40					30-40
Pa$_{O_2}$	mm Hg	60-90		80-100					80-100

Adapted and reproduced with permission from O'Rourke PP, Crone RK. The respiratory system. In Gregory GA (ed). Gregory's Pediatric Anesthesia, 2nd ed. New York, Churchill Livingstone, 1989, pp 63-91.

BREATHING PATTERNS

Normal newborn breathing is periodic. There are pauses of less than 10 seconds and periods of increased respiratory activity. Periodic breathing is different from apnea, a ventilatory pause associated with desaturation and bradycardia. Apnea is associated with prematurity and is treated with respiratory stimulants and with tactile stimulation such as stroking or rocking. Postoperative apnea in former premature infants is an important consideration in the planning of outpatient surgery.

Cardiovascular System

FETAL CIRCULATION

The fetal circulation is characterized by (1) increased pulmonary vascular resistance (PVR) with very little pulmonary blood flow, (2) decreased systemic vascular resistance (SVR) with the placenta as the major low resistance vascular bed, and (3) right-to-left blood flow through the ductus arteriosus and foramen ovale (Fig. 34-1). At birth, three events change the circulation into its postnatal configuration. First, the alveolar oxygen concentration increases, and the alveolar carbon dioxide concentration decreases

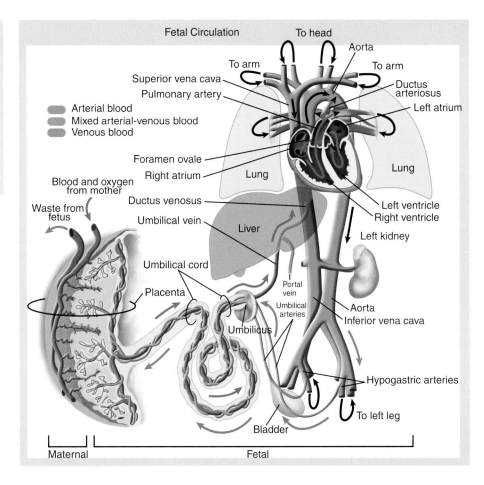

Figure 34-1 Course of the fetal circulation in late gestation. Note the selective blood flow patterns across the foramen ovale and the ductus arteriosus. (From Greeley WJ, Steven JM, Nicolson SC, et al. Anesthesia for pediatric cardiac surgery. In Miller RD [ed]. Anesthesia, 5th ed. Philadelphia, Churchill Livingstone, 2000, vol. 2, pp 1805-1847.)

with the expansion of the lungs. This results in a decrease in PVR. Second, the low resistance placental bed is removed from the circulation when the umbilical cord is clamped. This results in an increase in SVR. The decrease in PVR leads to an increase in pulmonary blood flow and therefore an increase in blood return to the left side of the heart. The increase in left atrial pressure functionally closes the foramen ovale.

The three fetal channels that close after birth are the ductus arteriosus, ductus venosus, and foramen ovale. The ductus arteriosus is functionally closed in 98% of neonates at 4 days of life. It constricts due to an increase in arterial oxygen tension and a decrease in prostaglandins released from the placenta. Later, the constricted duct becomes fibrotic becoming the ligamentum arteriosum. The ductus venosus closes with the clamping of the umbilical vein. The portal pressure decreases, and the ductus venosus closes. It is through the ductus venosus that an umbilical venous catheter enters the inferior vena cava and becomes "central." The foramen ovale is patent in many infants and is probe patent in 30% of adults.

If pulmonary artery vasoconstriction occurs in the first few days of life due to hypoxemia, acidosis, or pulmonary hypertension, blood can shunt right to left through the previously functionally closed foramen ovale or the ductus arteriosus, resulting in profound hypoxemia and acidosis. This is termed "persistent fetal circulation" and can be life-threatening. Treatment is directed towards decreasing PVR.

THE NEONATAL MYOCARDIUM

The neonatal myocardium is characterized by poorly organized myocytes that contain fewer contractile elements than the adult myocardium, in which the myocytes are well organized in a parallel arrangement. The sarcoplasmic reticulum in the neonatal heart is immature with disorganized T-tubules. The neonatal myocardium depends heavily on the concentration of free ionized calcium for contractility. Administration of citrated blood products to neonates may cause hypocalcemia and depressed cardiac function, which can be treated with calcium administration.

Although the stroke volume of neonates is usually fixed and the cardiac output usually increases by increasing heart rate only, the neonate can increase stroke volume up to a point according to the Frank-Starling relationship if the afterload is kept low.[1]

AUTONOMIC INNERVATION OF THE HEART

The parasympathetic nervous system predominates early in life, while the sympathetic nervous system is still developing. This imbalance is clinically relevant and can be seen as marked bradycardia or even asystole during laryngoscopy, orogastric tube placement, or tracheal suctioning in the neonate or infant. Many practitioners will pretreat with an anticholinergic, atropine or glycopyrrolate, prior to airway instrumentation.

NEWBORN CARDIOVASCULAR ASSESSMENT

The newborn cardiovascular examination should focus on the hemodynamics, including heart rate and four extremity blood pressure and oxygen saturation measurements. Capillary refill, pulses, and respiratory status should be assessed as well as the presence or absence of a murmur or third or fourth heart sound on auscultation. Urine output trends should be investigated. Arterial, venous, or capillary blood gas measurement should be made if acidosis is suspected. If performed, results of a chest radiograph, electrocardiogram, or echocardiogram should be reviewed. Normal cardiovascular variables are displayed in Table 34-2.

The Renal System

Postnatally, the kidneys take over the role of the placenta in maintaining metabolic homeostasis. The glomerular filtration rate (GFR) is 15% to 30% of adult values at birth and increases to 50% at 5 to 10 days of life. Adult values are reached by 1 year of age. The low GFR affects the neonate's ability to excrete saline, water loads and some drugs. Tubular function develops after 34 weeks of gestation. The tubules are immature and have a reduced threshold at which bicarbonate is no longer completely reabsorbed by the kidney. This is associated with the inability of young infants to respond to an acid load and the slightly reduced values of pH (7.37) and plasma bicarbonate (22 mEq/L) in this age group compared with older children and adults. Infants also have decreased concentrating ability and a low level of production and excretion of urea. Blood urea nitrogen (BUN) remains normal because less urea is being produced. Creatinine immediately postnatally equals the maternal value and decreases in the first 48 hours to levels of 0.5 mEq/L or lower if renal function is normal.

The Hematologic System

The blood volume in the newborn ranges from 82 to 93 mL/kg for the term newborn to 90 to 105 mL/kg for the preterm newborn. After the first year of life, blood volume declines to approximately 70 to 80 mL/kg. The normal newborn hemoglobin is 14 to 20 g/dL. Fetal hemoglobin (HgF) makes up 70% to 80% of the hemoglobin at birth. Fetal hemoglobin has a higher affinity for oxygen than does adult hemoglobin. The higher affinity of HgF for oxygen shifts the oxyhemoglobin dissociation curve to the left. The P_{50} of HgF is 18 to 20 mm Hg, and the P_{50} of adult hemoglobin is 27 mm Hg. The difference in P_{50} between the two types of hemoglobin facilitates the uptake of oxygen by the fetus at the placental interface.

The physiologic nadir in hemoglobin occurs at 9 to 12 weeks of life and is 10 to 11 g/dL in the term infant. The reduction in hemoglobin does not affect oxygen delivery due to a shift in the oxyhemoglobin dissociation curve to the right. The rightward shift is caused by an increase in 2,3-diphosphoglycerate (2,3-DPG) and the replacement of HgF by adult hemoglobin and facilitates the unloading of oxygen in the tissues. The hemoglobin concentration settles at 11.5 to 12 g/dL until 2 years of age, after which it increases gradually to adult values in puberty.

At birth, the vitamin K–dependent coagulation factors (II, VII, IX, X) are present at 20% to 60% of adult levels. This may lead to a prolonged prothrombin time. It can take several weeks for these factors to reach normal values due to synthesis in an immature liver. Prophylactic intramuscular vitamin K is given to all newborns. In addition, maternal ingestion of some drugs including anticonvulsants and warfarin can cause vitamin K deficiency in the newborn.

PHARMACOLOGIC DIFFERENCES

Pharmacokinetics

Protein binding of drugs is different between infants and adults. Some of this difference is due to a lower concentration of serum protein/albumin in younger children.

Table 34-2 Normal Heart Rate and Systolic Blood Pressure as Functions of Age

Age Group	Normal Range	
	Heart Rate (beats/min)	Systolic Blood Pressure* (mm Hg)
Neonate (<30 days)	120-160	60-75
1-6 months	110-140	65-85
6-12 months	100-140	70-90
1-2 years	90-130	75-95
3-5 years	80-120	80-100
6-8 years	75-115	85-105
9-12 years	70-110	90-115
13-16 years	60-110	95-120
>16 years	60-100	100-125

*As measured using oscillometric blood pressure device.

There is also a lower affinity of protein-bound drugs for serum proteins in neonates compared with adults. With decreased protein binding, the concentration of free drug is increased, resulting in an increase in drug effect. The effect of decreased protein binding is most apparent in highly protein-bound drugs such as phenytoin, bupivacaine, barbiturates, and diazepam.

The difference in body composition also has an effect on pharmacokinetics. Preterm and term neonates have a larger percentage of total body water compared with older children and adults. This is reflected in an increase in the volume of distribution (Vd). A larger initial dose of drug is needed to reach the same therapeutic serum level and pharmacologic effect when the Vd is increased. Larger initial doses are required for digoxin, succinylcholine, and antibiotics in neonates. Fentanyl is an important example of a commonly used anesthetic in neonates which requires larger initial doses. Also, neonates and infants may be more sensitive to the effects of certain drugs and need lower serum blood levels to achieve the same effects. Medications should be given slowly and titrated to predetermined effects.

There is also a decreased percentage of fat and muscle in small infants compared with older children and adults. Drugs that rely on redistribution to these tissues for the termination of clinical effects may last longer in small infants. Thiopental, for example, depends on redistribution for awakening after a single dose.

Hepatic Metabolism

Hepatic metabolism of drugs changes lipid-soluble, pharmacologically active drugs into usually inactive, non-lipid-soluble drugs for excretion. The activity of most hepatic enzymes is reduced in neonates, as is blood flow to the liver. This can result in a longer duration of effect of some pharmacologic agents. Again, fentanyl is an important example.

Renal Excretion

Neonatal kidneys become more efficient with age. Owing to immature glomerular and tubular function, drugs that depend on the kidney for excretion such as aminoglycosides have prolonged elimination half-times in neonates. Glomerular and tubular function is nearly mature at 20 postnatal weeks and is fully mature at 2 years.

Pharmacology of Inhaled Anesthetics

F_A/F_I is the ratio of concentration of alveolar to inspired anesthetic. At the beginning of an inhaled induction, F_A is zero, and F_I is large. As the F_A/F_I increases toward 1, induction of anesthesia occurs. The F_A/F_I ratio increases faster in neonates compared to adults, and, therefore, induction of anesthesia via inhalation is more rapid.[2] There is a higher alveolar ventilation to functional residual capacity ratio (V_A/FRC) in neonates compared to adults, and thus a more rapid increase in F_A/F_I. The ratio is 5:1 in neonates and 1.5:1 in adults.

Infants and small children may have an increased cardiac output during an inhaled induction via a mask because of preoperative anxiety. Increased cardiac output is associated with increased pulmonary blood flow and higher uptake of anesthetic from the lungs which decreases F_A and slows the increase in F_A/F_I. Therefore, as a result of uptake, the rate of anesthetic induction would be slowed. However, the increased cardiac output also increases anesthetic delivery to the vessel-rich group (VRG), and the partial pressure of anesthetic in the VRG equilibrates with F_A. The partial pressure of anesthetic in the venous blood approaches the partial pressure in the alveoli and speeds the increase in F_A/F_I.

In neonates, there are also reduced tissue/blood solubility and reduced blood/gas solubility. Blood solubilities of the higher solubility agents (isoflurane) are 18% less in neonates. Therefore, there is less uptake from the alveoli, and the increase in F_A/F_I is more rapid. The blood solubility of the less soluble agents such as sevoflurane and desflurane does not differ between infants and adults, and F_A/F_I does not rise as rapidly. The reduced tissue solubility of isoflurane also contributes to a faster increase in F_A/F_I in neonates compared with adults.

EFFECT OF SHUNT ON AN INHALED INDUCTION OF ANESTHESIA

Left-to-right shunts are mostly intracardiac (ventricular or atrial septal defects) and are associated with increased pulmonary blood flow. These have no real effect on the rate at which induction of anesthesia occurs. Right-to-left shunts involve a portion of the systemic venous return that bypasses gas exchange in the lungs and is pumped systemically. Right-to-left shunts can be either intracardiac (tetralogy of Fallot) or intrapulmonary (endobronchial intubation, atelectasis). Right-to-left shunts slow the rise in F_A/F_I and delay induction of anesthesia. This is more pronounced with less soluble anesthetics such as sevoflurane and desflurane.

MINIMUM ALVEOLAR CONCENTRATION

Minimum alveolar concentration (MAC) varies with age. The MAC of inhaled anesthetic agents is highest in infants 1 to 6 months old. The MAC is 30% less in full-term neonates for isoflurane and desflurane. Sevoflurane MAC at term is the same as at age 1 month.[2] The presence and degree of prematurity cause decreases in MAC. This may be due to immaturity of the central nervous system or neurohumoral factors. Cerebral palsy and mental retardation also reduce the MAC by 25%.

IV

FLUIDS AND ELECTROLYTES

Intraoperative Fluid Administration

Intravenous fluid given to children in the operating room serves one of four purposes: replacement of a deficit, maintenance, balancing ongoing losses, and treatment of hypovolemia. Although hypotonic solutions such as 0.2% normal saline with added potassium are used outside the operating room for maintenance fluid administration, generally, non-glucose-containing isotonic solutions are given in the operating room in order to avoid hyponatremia and abnormalities of serum potassium. Lactated Ringer's solution and Plasmalyte A are the most commonly used isotonic solutions in pediatric patients. Administration of 5% albumin is the most common colloid used in pediatric patients, but disagreement exists as to the efficacy of this therapy versus isotonic crystalloid administration.

REPLACEMENT OF PREOPERATIVE DEFICIT

The preoperative deficit is the number of hours that a patient has had no oral intake (NPO) multiplied by the hourly maintenance fluid requirement of the patient (Table 34-3). Generally, 50% of the deficit is replaced in the first hour of the anesthetic, and the remaining 50% is replaced over the following 2 hours.[3]

Patients presenting for emergency surgery may have larger fluid deficits due to vomiting, fever, third-space loss, or blood loss that need to be taken into account. The use of warmed fluids should be considered to avoid hypothermia with administration of large amounts of intravascular volume replacement.

MAINTENANCE FLUIDS

The hourly maintenance rate should be calculated using the "4-2-1 rule" and should be administered in the form of isotonic solution throughout the case.

ONGOING FLUID LOSSES

Ongoing losses can be characterized as whole blood loss, third space loss, and evaporation. When blood or colloid is used to replace blood loss, a ratio of 1:1 is used. When crystalloid is used to replace blood loss, a ratio of 3:1 is used, just as with adults. Third-space and evaporative losses vary with the invasiveness of the procedure from noninvasive such as a strabismus repair to very invasive such as an exploratory laparotomy for necrotizing enterocolitis (see Table 34-3). Third-space losses are replaced with isotonic crystalloid.

TREATMENT OF HYPOVOLEMIA

Intravascular volume can be monitored in pediatric patients by assessing the hemodynamic variables for the age group. Tachycardia and decreased blood pressure suggest hypovolemia. Monitoring of urine output or central venous pressure can provide other information about volume status. If hypovolemia is suspected, a 10 to 20 mL/kg bolus of crystalloid or colloid can be given.

Glucose Administration

Glucose-containing solutions should not be used routinely in pediatric patients intraoperatively.[3] They should not be used to replace deficits, third-space losses, or blood loss. In children more than 1 year of age, the stress and catecholamine release associated with surgery usually prevent hypoglycemia. Glucose is commonly given to patients who are younger than 1 year of age or less than 10 kg. Pediatric patients at greater risk for developing hypoglycemia include premature and term neonates and any patient who is critically ill or who has hepatic dysfunction. Patients receiving hyperalimentation with high dextrose concentrations preoperatively can either be continued on a reduced rate of the same infusion or can be converted to a 5% or 10% dextrose-containing

Table 34-3 Fluid Replacement in Children		
	Fluid Requirements	
Basis for Replacement	*Hourly*	*24 Hours*
Maintenance		
Weight (kg)		
<10	4 mL/kg	100 mL/kg
11-20	40 mL + 2 mL/kg >10 kg	1000 mL + 50 mL/kg >10 kg
>20	60 mL + 1 mL/kg >20 kg	1500 mL + 20 mL/kg >20 kg
Replacement of Ongoing Losses*		
Type of surgery		
Noninvasive (e.g., inguinal hernia repair, clubfoot repair)	0-2 mL/kg/hr	
Mildly invasive (e.g., ureteral reimplantation)	2-4 mL/kg/hr	
Moderately invasive (e.g., elective bowel reanastomosis)	4-8 mL/kg/hr	
Significantly invasive (e.g., bowel resection for necrotizing enterocolitis)	≥10 mL/kg/hr	

*Replacement for ongoing losses with crystalloid must always be integrated with the patient's current cardiorespiratory status, status as evaluated during the surgical procedure, estimated blood loss with plans for blood product replacement, and baseline medical problems.

infusion to maintain the administration of glucose. An infusion pump should be used for high-concentration dextrose solutions to avoid bolus administration. Blood glucose concentration should be monitored closely in patients with risk of glucose instability.

TRANSFUSION THERAPY
(Also See Chapter 24)

Maximum Allowable Blood Loss

Before anesthesia, the maximum allowable blood loss (MABL) should be calculated for a given case and to prepare for possible transfusion of red blood cells. The estimated blood volume (EBV) is dependent on the age of the child:

$$MABL = EBV \times (patient\ Hct - minimum\ acceptable\ Hct)/patient\ Hct$$

Initial treatment for blood loss is to maintain intravascular volume by administering crystalloid or colloid solution. When the hematocrit reaches the threshold, red blood cells should be transfused. The minimum acceptable hematocrit depends on patient age and co-morbidities. For example, a higher hematocrit (e.g., 30% to 40% is desired in patients with congenital heart disease, those with significant pulmonary disease, and infants with apnea and bradycardia or tachypnea and tachycardia.

Transfusion of Blood Products

PACKED RED BLOOD CELLS
Transfusion of 10 to 15 mL/kg of packed red blood cells (PRBCs) should increase the hemoglobin concentration by 2 to 3 g/dL. The estimated volume of transfusion of PRBCs should be predicted in advance in order to split units of cells in the blood bank into 10 to 15 mL/kg aliquots. This reduces the waste of a residual unit when only 60 mL, for example, is required for transfusion. It also allows the blood bank to reserve the remaining unit for later administration to the same patient, reducing donor exposure for the patient.

Special processing of PRBCs including leukocyte reduction and irradiation is warranted in some settings, including young infants less than 4 months of age, immunosuppressed patients, or transplant patients. Leukocyte reduction is achieved by removing white blood cells by filtration to a maximum concentration of 5×10^6. White blood cells are responsible for febrile, nonhemolytic transfusion reactions, HLA allosensitization, and transmission of cytomegalovirus.

Irradiation of blood products is necessary to reduce the risk of transfusion-associated graft-versus-host disease, a potentially fatal condition in which transfused lymphocytes engraft and proliferate in the bone marrow of the recipient. Irradiated blood should be given to immunocompromised children and to children with normal immunity who share an HLA haplotype with the donor. For this reason, all directed donor blood from family members is irradiated.

PLATELETS
Platelet concentrates are either derived from whole blood or collected by apheresis. They are suspended in plasma, which contains coagulation factors. Administration of 5 to 10 mL/kg of platelet concentrate should increase the platelet count by 50,000 to 100,000 per dL. Indications for platelet transfusion are dependent on platelet number, function, and the presence or absence of bleeding. Platelets are a cellular component of blood and may require irradiation using the same criteria noted above for PRBC.

FRESH FROZEN PLASMA
Fresh frozen plasma (FFP) is administered to correct coagulopathy due to insufficient coagulation factors. It contains all coagulation factors and regulatory proteins. Administration of 10 to 15 mL/kg will increase factor levels by 15% to 20%.

CRYOPRECIPITATE
Cryoprecipitate is primarily used as a source of fibrinogen, factor VIII, and factor XIII. It is ideal for administration to infants due to high levels of these factors in a small volume. Administration of 1 unit (10 to 20 mL) for every 5 kg to a maximum of 4 units is usually adequate for correcting coagulopathy due to insufficient fibrinogen.

Antifibrinolytics

Antifibrinolytics include aprotinin, a serine protease inhibitor, and tranexamic acid and ε-aminocaproic acid, lysine analogs. These drugs have been used to decrease bleeding and the transfusion requirements during pediatric cardiac, spine, and cranial reconstructive surgery. Aprotinin is not available for use at this time owing to concerns about adverse effects in adults.

Recombinant Factor VIIa

Recombinant factor VIIa is indicated for the treatment and prevention of bleeding in patients with factor VII deficiency and hemophiliacs with inhibitors to factors VIII and IX. Over the last 10 years, there have been multiple reports of off-label use of the drug in nonhemophiliac pediatric patients in a variety of situations including postcardiopulmonary bypass bleeding and trauma with a reduction in transfusion of blood products and normalization of coagulation studies. Concerns remain about the potential for thromboembolic complications.[4]

IV

PEDIATRIC AIRWAY (Also See Chapter 16)

Airway Assessment

There is no valid airway assessment in children that is similar to the Mallampati classification in adults. Children are often uncooperative with examination. Care should be taken to inspect for micrognathia, midface hypoplasia, or other craniofacial anomalies that can predict difficult laryngoscopy. The patient and parents should be questioned about the presence of loose teeth or orthodontic appliances that may be dislodged or broken during airway manipulation.

Airway Management Techniques

Airway management techniques in children are similar to those in adult patients, although the anatomy differs. Infants and young children have larger craniums and thus it is unnecessary to place a pillow under the occiput to achieve the "sniffing position" for airway management. The tongue is often relatively large in young infants and can more easily obstruct the airway. The cricoid ring is thought to be the narrowest part of the airway of the infant and young child, instead of the laryngeal aperture at the vocal cords as in adults. However, recent magnetic resonance imaging (MRI) and bronchoscopic data indicate that the pediatric airway is cylindrical, and the narrowest part is the glottis, as in adults.[5] The larynx is positioned relatively higher, at C4 in the neonate rather than C6 as in the adult. The epiglottis is omega-shaped and soft in the infant, rather than U-shaped and stiff in the adult. Management of the airway using a face mask is more common in children. An appropriately sized mask should be selected, and care should be taken to optimally position the patient to avoid airway obstruction. If obstruction is encountered, continuous positive airway pressure of 5 to 10 cm H_2O, or an oral airway can be introduced to restore airway patency.

Laryngeal mask airways (LMA) are also made in pediatric sizes and can be used for routine cases or as part of a difficult airway algorithm. The LMA allows the patient to breathe spontaneously with no upper airway obstruction and without instrumentation of the trachea. The LMA can also be used with pressure control mechanical ventilation safely in children.

Endotracheal tubes are used for a large percentage of anesthetics in children. Historically, uncuffed tubes were the standard of care in children younger than 8 years of age owing to concerns about subglottic stenosis and postextubation stridor. However, with the introduction of tubes with high volume–low pressure cuffs, recent studies suggest that there is no increased risk of airway edema with cuffed tubes and that the use of cuffed tubes may decrease the number of laryngoscopies and intubations due to inappropriate tube size. As a result of

Table 34-4 Oral Endotracheal Tube (ETT) Size for Age

Age Group	Uncuffed ETT Size (ID mm)	Cuffed ETT Size (ID mm)
Preterm	2.5-3.0	NA
Term	3.0-3.5	3.0-3.5
1-6 months	3.5	3.5
7-12 months	4.0	3.5-4.0
1-2 years	4.5	4.0-4.5
3-4 years	4.5-5.0	4.5
5-6 years	5.0-5.5	4.5-5.0
7-8 years	NA	5.0-5.5
9-10 years	NA	5.5-6.0
11-12 years	NA	6.0-6.5
13-14 years	NA	6.5-7.0
14+ years	NA	7.0-7.5

Depth of Insertion
Multiplying the ID of the ETT by 3 yields the proper depth of insertion to the lips, in cm. *Example:* 4.0 mm ETT × 3 = 12 cm for depth of insertion.

ID, inner diameter.

innovation in material and design, cuffs are now very thin and do not enlarge the outer diameter of the tube, and downsizing inner diameter tube size to compensate for the bulk of the cuff is no longer recommended.[6] A comparison of classic sizing for uncuffed and cuffed tubes and the new recommendations for cuffed tubes is shown in Table 34-4.

Difficult Pediatric Airway

The difficult airway in children can be challenging because of lack of patient cooperation in most age groups, which makes awake endotracheal intubation virtually impossible. Most techniques are performed under deep sedation or general anesthesia. A difficult airway should be anticipated in patients with craniofacial abnormalities or syndromes including Pierre Robin, Treacher Collins, and Goldenhar. A plan for management of the airway and equipment should be prepared.

Anesthesia can be induced intravenously or via inhalation. Adequacy of mask ventilation should be determined. At this point, the airway can be visualized or managed with a variety of airway adjuncts including the optical stylet, video laryngoscope, flexible fiberoptic bronchoscope, and the laryngeal mask airway, all of which are made in one or more pediatric sizes.[7] Prenatally diagnosed difficult airways (e.g., large cystic hygroma) are occasionally delivered as an ex utero intrapartum therapy (EXIT) procedure during which the fetus is partially delivered via cesarean section and the airway is secured while oxygenation is achieved via placental exchange (see later discussion).

ANESTHETIC CONSIDERATIONS

Preoperative Evaluation and Preparation (Also See Chapter 13)

The preoperative evaluation of a pediatric patient differs from that of an adult in a number of respects. Age and weight of the child are extremely important as equipment such as laryngoscopes, endotracheal tubes, masks, and intravenous fluid setups are based on the age and size of the child. Pharmacologic drugs are dosed based on weight, and accuracy is critical to avoid under- and overdosage. A history of prematurity is important, including the gestational age at which the patient was delivered and any sequelae of prematurity such as cerebral palsy, chronic lung disease and apnea and bradycardia. If the child has a genetic or dysmorphic syndrome, distinguishing features should be reviewed for potential impact on the anesthetic including craniofacial or cervical spine abnormalities that may lead to a difficult endotracheal intubation.

The family should be questioned about risk factors for malignant hyperthermia (MH) including family history of MH, patient history of MH, and congenital myopathies such as central core disease or King-Denborough syndrome. The parents should also be questioned about the presence of muscular dystrophies. Although possibly not associated with true MH, exposure to succinylcholine and inhaled anesthetics can result in hyperkalemia and rhabdomyolysis, and a nontriggering anesthetic (e.g., propofol) should be used.

A review of systems should be performed, and any pertinent positive findings should be explored. The patient and parent should be questioned about the presence or recent history of congestion, cough, fever, vomiting or diarrhea, which may impact the decision to proceed with an elective procedure. Vital signs, including pulse, respiratory rate, temperature, and blood pressure, should be measured. In addition, a room air pulse oximeter check is important to screen for occult cardiac or pulmonary disease.

Physical examination should include a general assessment of the patient's growth and development. The airway should be examined as thoroughly as possible with attention to craniofacial abnormalities, presence of micrognathia, and tonsillar size. The heart and lungs should be auscultated to evaluate for murmurs and wheezing or decreased breath sounds. The patient should be examined for any signs of infectious process including rhinorrhea, tonsillar exudate, fever and cough. Extremities should be examined for potential sites for intravenous access.

PREOPERATIVE LABORATORY TESTING

Routine preoperative laboratory testing for healthy children is probably not indicated except in the case of urine pregnancy testing (see later discussion). However, preoperative testing may be indicated in children with organ system dysfunction. For example, BUN, creatinine, and potassium levels should be tested preoperatively in patients with renal disease. Hemoglobin should be measured in former premature infants at risk for anemia having procedures associated with significant blood loss. Radiologic examination is not routinely performed. However, if recent radiographs, computed tomography (CT) scans, or MRIs are available, they should be reviewed. If echocardiogram results or subspecialist notes are available, they should also be reviewed.

Preoperative urine pregnancy testing (UPT) of pediatric patients is a controversial topic. Adolescent females are unlikely to admit that they are sexually active or if there is a chance that they might be pregnant. Parents are reluctant to believe that their child might be pregnant. Asking the parent and child about the possibility of pregnancy can be uncomfortable for all parties. For these reasons, most hospitals have a policy on preoperative UPT and will test all female patients beginning at menarche, or at an arbitrary age (e.g., 10 years old). Occasionally, a UPT will be positive, and there must be a process for verification. There must also be a process for revealing the results to the patient and parents and for counseling, based on local institutional considerations and individual state law.[8]

RECENT UPPER RESPIRATORY TRACT INFECTION

The presence or recent history of upper respiratory tract infection (URI) is another controversial topic. Whereas cancellations for URI were quite common in the past, the present view is that the risks associated with anesthetizing a child with URI are manageable with little morbidity. Still, there is a slightly increased risk of airway hyperreactivity with associated bronchospasm, laryngospasm, and postoperative arterial desaturation due to atelectasis. Parents should be questioned about the presence of a URI. The patient should be examined for nasal congestion, cough, wheezing, and fever, and if a decision is made to proceed with the anesthetic, care should be taken to minimize chances of an adverse respiratory event occurring.[9] Signs of lower respiratory tract infection require cancellation of elective surgery. Practical considerations usually result in minor surgery being performed in the face of URI, especially ear, nose, and throat (ENT) procedures when URI is frequent and the surgery will often decrease the frequency of these infections. Elective major surgery (i.e., intra-abdominal, intrathoracic, cardiac) is usually postponed for 2 to 6 weeks.

PREOPERATIVE FASTING GUIDELINES

It is difficult for both the parents and the patient to keep a child without oral intake for an extended period of time, and fasting can lead to significant perioperative stress. However, adherence to fasting guidelines minimizes the risk of aspiration of gastric contents. In the absence of bowel obstruction, gastroesophageal reflux, or other conditions leading to delayed gastric emptying, NPO guidelines in children are as follows: Solid foods allowed until 6 to 8 hours before anesthesia; milk, fortified breast milk, and infant formula until 6 hours before; unfortified breast milk until 4 hours before; and clear liquids until 2 hours before anesthesia.[10] Forethought in scheduling and giving preoperative instructions about NPO times can minimize the time without oral intake, and children who are scheduled later in the day are often able to ingest clear liquids until 2 hours prior to the beginning of the anesthetic.

PREMEDICATION

Both parental and patient anxiety can lead to significant perioperative stress and dissatisfaction. Attempts should be made to allay anxiety during the preoperative interview. If it appears that the family and child are significantly anxious, premedication may be required to calm and sedate the child. This may, in turn, improve parental anxiety.

The most widely used premedication in North America is midazolam. It can be administered via oral, intranasal, rectal, and intramuscular routes. Midazolam 0.5 to 0.75 mg/kg, provides adequate anxiolysis and sedation approximately 20 minutes after oral administration. Rarely, a child will experience a paradoxical reaction to midazolam characterized by agitation. Diazepam and lorazepam are most often used in older children and also produce sedation and amnesia.

Ketamine, a phencyclidine derivative, can also be used as an oral, nasal, rectal, or intramuscular premedication. It produces sedation, amnesia, and analgesia, but it is also associated with excessive salivation, nystagmus, postoperative nausea and vomiting and hallucinations. It does not depress airway reflexes, and airway tone is preserved. Intramuscular ketamine may be administered to agitated or developmentally delayed children who refuse a mask or premedication.

The α₂-agonist clonidine, given orally, provides preoperative sedation that is similar to that produced by benzodiazepines. It acts centrally and peripherally to decrease blood pressure. It also decreases anesthetic requirements so that a lower concentration of volatile anesthetic is required to produce the same effect. Clonidine does not cause airway obstruction and reduces requirements for postoperative pain medication. Clonidine has a longer onset of effect than most other premedications, and must be given at least 1 hour prior to the anesthetic. This reduces its utility in most busy, high turnover settings.

Parental presence at induction of anesthesia (PPIA) is another technique used to allay both patient and parental anxiety. The parent accompanies the child to either the operating room or an induction room for the induction of anesthesia. It is usually comforting for both the parent and child. However, occasionally PPIA increases parental anxiety and can lead to increased patient anxiety and physiologic changes in the parent, including syncope. The temperament of both the child and the parent should be considered prior to the suggestion of PPIA.[11]

Perioperative Considerations

THERMOREGULATION AND HEAT LOSS
Because of a larger surface area to weight ratio, small infants tend to lose heat more rapidly than adults when placed in a cold environment, by both radiation and convection. Small infants are unable to shiver and rely on nonshivering thermogenesis by metabolizing brown fat for heat production. Heat loss can also be limited by thermoregulatory vasoconstriction. The warming of the operating room environment and the use of radiant warmers, warmed intravenous fluids, airway humidification, and forced air warming can help to preserve normothermia in children.

Perioperative hyperthermia can also be encountered; it may be due to infection, inflammatory states, or overzealous warming. Hyperthermia is a late sign in malignant hyperthermia; the first signs are usually tachycardia, hypercarbia, and acidosis.

MONITORING
Standard American Society of Anesthesiologists' monitors include electrocardiography (ECG), blood pressure monitoring, pulse oximetry, and capnography, and they should be utilized in every pediatric anesthetic situation. A nerve stimulator is recommended for monitoring neuromuscular blockade. The continuous auscultation of breath sounds via esophageal or precordial stethoscope is also recommended, but recent surveys demonstrate that this monitor is being utilized less in favor of other monitors.[12] The monitoring of temperature is mandatory to detect malignant hyperthermia or, more commonly, hypothermia.

Invasive arterial blood pressure and central venous pressure monitoring are indicated for invasive surgery and with significant cardiopulmonary co-morbidities. It is often useful to monitor cerebral oxygenation via near-infrared spectroscopy during cardiac surgery and other cases in which cerebral perfusion may be compromised. Monitoring of processed electroencephalogram is also available for children to estimate anesthetic depth, although there is some controversy over the reliability of this modality in children.[13]

ROUTES OF INDUCTION OF ANESTHESIA
General anesthesia can be induced via inhalation or through the administration of intravenous or intramuscular (IM) drugs in children. An inhaled induction of

anesthesia with sevoflurane in oxygen with or without nitrous oxide is a common method used in children because it does not require intravenous access. The child is taken to the operating or induction room, monitors are placed, and a face mask is applied. The concentration of inhaled anesthetic should be increased slowly in a cooperative child. As induction progresses, the child will usually go through stage 2, the excitement phase. During this phase, coughing, vomiting, involuntary movement, and laryngospasm are possible. Attention should be devoted to the adequacy of the mask airway and the extent of obstruction. After the patient has passed through stage 2, an intravenous catheter can be placed. If laryngospasm occurs prior to placement of the peripheral IV catheter, treatment with continuous positive airway pressure or intramuscular succinylcholine may be required.

Intravenous induction is selected in children who already have intravenous access, who request an intravenous induction, or for whom an intravenous induction is indicated (a full stomach, persistent gastroesophageal reflux disease). In some centers, a peripheral intravenous catheter is placed in all children presenting for surgery. Common induction agents in children include propofol 2 to 3 mg/kg and sodium thiopental 4 to 6 mg/kg.

Intramuscular inductions of anesthesia are used most commonly in developmentally delayed or severely uncooperative children, and can be achieved with intramuscular administration of ketamine (5 mg/kg). IM atropine or glycopyrrolate can be given with the ketamine to decrease excess salivation. An IM ketamine induction may also be utilized in burned children with poor peripheral veins and a difficult airway due to extensive scarring for whom an inhaled induction of anesthesia may result in loss of both airway tone and the ability to ventilate the lungs via a mask.

MAINTENANCE OF ANESTHESIA

Anesthesia is maintained with inhaled anesthetic or intravenous administration of drugs or a combination of the two. A muscle relaxant can be used to facilitate endotracheal intubation and operative exposure. However, muscle relaxant is probably used less frequently in children than in adults.

EMERGENCE

In pediatric anesthetic practice, the decision to extubate the trachea while deeply anesthetized, or after emergence, must be made on a case-by-case basis. In some circumstances, children are allowed to regain their airway reflexes and are extubated "awake." However, extubation during deep anesthesia and emergence without an endotracheal tube in place is a common practice in pediatric anesthesia. Advantages to awake extubation include the ability to protect against aspiration of stomach contents or blood/secretions from the airway, and the relative safety of passing through stage 2 with an endotracheal tube in place. Advantages of extubation during deep anesthesia include no coughing or straining against suture lines or incisions and removal of the endotracheal tube before it leads to airway reactivity, both of which lead to a smoother emergence. The child then emerges in the operating room or in the recovery room, and meticulous attention is needed to ensure that laryngospasm or airway obstruction does not go undetected during or after transfer to the postanesthesia care unit.

PAIN MANAGEMENT (Also See Chapter 40)

Analgesic drugs used for pain control in children include acetaminophen, nonsteroidal anti-inflammatory drugs (NSAIDs), and opioids, and they can be administered by an oral, intramuscular, or intravenous route. The most common opioids used in pediatric anesthesia are fentanyl and morphine. Side effects include sedation, respiratory depression, pruritus, and nausea/vomiting.

Acetaminophen carries the risk of hepatotoxicity, and daily dosages must be calculated to avoid potential liver injury. Intravenous acetaminophen is currently available in Europe and Australia, but is not yet available in the United States. Rectal acetaminophen given after anesthesia induction can be an important adjunct to other analgesics. NSAIDs including ketorolac can be associated with platelet dysfunction, gastrointestinal bleeding, and renal dysfunction. Therefore, it is important to consider patient co-morbidities such as renal impairment and risk of bleeding (tonsillectomy, cardiac surgery) prior to administration of NSAIDs for pain control. Advantages of acetaminophen and NSAIDs include lack of excessive sedation and respiratory depression, common side effects of opioids.

REGIONAL ANESTHESIA (Also See Chapters 17 and 18)

Regional anesthesia for intraoperative and postoperative pain control provides excellent analgesia with minimal side effects and decreases the requirement for opioid and nonopioid pain relievers. The single-shot caudal injection with local anesthetic is most commonly used for surgery on or below the umbilicus. Alternatively, a catheter can be advanced into the caudal epidural space for delivery of an infusion of local anesthetic, which can be continued into the postoperative period. In children younger than 5 years of age, the catheter can usually be advanced to any spinal level and deliver local anesthetic to the associated dermatomes. In addition, the epidural space can be accessed relatively easily from the lumbar or thoracic level with subsequent placement of a catheter.

Other commonly performed regional blocks include brachial plexus, ilioinguinal nerve, femoral nerve, lateral femoral cutaneous nerve, sciatic and popliteal nerve, ankle, and penile blocks. These blocks are either performed using landmark technique or with the aid of a nerve stimulator or ultrasound guidance.

IV

When performing regional blocks in children, the child is commonly under a general anesthetic, and therefore unable to communicate the elicitation of a paresthesia or extreme pain on injection, possible perineural injection. For this reason, guidance with ultrasound is extremely helpful.

Spinal anesthesia has also been used as the sole anesthetic or in combination with a general anesthetic for a variety of cases. The technique gained popularity as an alternative to general anesthesia in former preterm infants having inguinal hernia repair that were high risk for perioperative apnea. Spinal anesthesia has also been used in older infants and children with and without increased risk for a general anesthetic.[14]

The Postanesthesia Care Unit (Also See Chapter 39)

AIRWAY MONITORING

The postanesthesia care unit (PACU) is a critical part of the perioperative experience where many problems may arise. Many patients are transferred deeply anesthetized without an endotracheal tube from the operating room and will emerge from general anesthesia there. As the patient regains airway reflexes, there is an increased risk for airway obstruction. The airway must be monitored closely for signs of obstruction, laryngospasm, and hypoxemia, and a self-inflating or Jackson-Rees style ventilating circuit and mask must be available to provide oxygen, continuous positive airway pressure, and ventilation. In addition, succinylcholine should be available. The airway should also be monitored for stridor/postintubation croup due to swelling. Treatment with dexamethasone, humidified oxygen, or nebulized racemic epinephrine may be warranted. Patients should also be monitored closely for apnea and hypoventilation in the recovery area.

POSTOPERATIVE NAUSEA AND VOMITING

Postoperative nausea and vomiting (PONV) is ranked by parents as the most unwanted side effect from anesthesia. A recent study identified four risk factors that predict PONV in children: age 3 years and older, strabismus surgery, duration of surgery, and previous history of postoperative vomiting in the patient or in a parent or sibling. If the patient has a high risk of PONV, avoiding opioids and nitrous oxide and the prophylactic administration of antiemetics will decrease the incidence of PONV. Two-drug pharmacologic prophylaxis with ondansetron and dexamethasone has an expected relative risk reduction of approximately 80%.[15]

EMERGENCE DELIRIUM

Emergence delirium is another issue frequently encountered in the PACU that is troublesome to families, recovery room nurses, and anesthesia care providers. It is often encountered after sevoflurane or desflurane. The incidence is the most frequent after sevoflurane. The Pediatric Anesthesia Emergence Delirium (PAED) scale was developed to assist in the diagnosis of emergence delirium. Though many drugs including propofol, fentanyl, clonidine, and dexmedetomidine may decrease the incidence of emergence delirium, only low-dose ketamine and nalbuphine decrease the incidence without prolonging emergence.

PAIN CONTROL (Also See Chapter 40)

The adequacy of pain control must be assessed frequently for pediatric patients of all ages from neonates to adolescents. The patients are recovering from a wide spectrum of procedures with differing amounts of associated pain. The children may be preverbal, nonverbal, or developmentally delayed and unable to communicate their pain level. There are several scales for assessing pain in children, including the FLACC (face, legs, activity, cry, consolability) and Wong-Baker Faces Pain Scale, along with evaluating vital signs. However, pain can be confused with anxiety, emergence delirium, and anger in children. Opioids can be titrated to effectively treat moderate to severe postoperative pain. NSAIDs or acetaminophen can also be administered, and if an epidural catheter is in place, it can be assessed for functionality and re-dosed.

DISCHARGE CRITERIA

PACUs are often structured in two stages. Patients are transferred from the operating room directly to first stage of recovery where the airway is assessed continuously and acute postoperative pain and PONV are treated. After the patient is awake with a stable airway and pain under control, he/she may be moved to a second stage to complete recovery. The modified Aldrete scoring system is the most frequently used scoring system to determine discharge readiness. In the outpatient setting, patients may go directly from the operating room to second stage recovery, known as "fast-tracking" (also see Chapter 37).

BEHAVIORAL RECOVERY

Children can develop maladaptive behavioral changes after surgery including sleep and eating disturbances, separation anxiety, new-onset enuresis, and other behavioral issues. Parental anxiety, parental presence at induction, parental presence in the PACU, and the use of premedication have been shown to influence the incidence of these behavioral changes. Most of these behavioral changes do not persist beyond 3 days postoperatively. However, avoidance of negative behavior changes is associated with higher patient/parent satisfaction and a better overall perioperative experience.[11]

MEDICAL AND SURGICAL DISEASES AFFECTING THE NEONATE

Necrotizing Enterocolitis

Necrotizing enterocolitis (NEC) is a common surgical emergency in the neonate. This condition is primarily seen in premature infants, with over 90% of affected patients born before 36 weeks of gestation. The incidence of NEC among premature and low-birth-weight infants is 3% to 7% and is inversely proportional to gestational age. Twenty percent to 40% of infants with NEC will require surgery, with a surgical mortality rate of 23% to 36%.[16]

Pathophysiology of NEC involves intestinal mucosal ischemic injury secondary to reduced mesenteric blood flow, often in conjunction with a patent ductus arteriosus (PDA) with its resultant "steal" of blood flow away from the systemic circulation. Bacterial infection is also an important component, and signs of abdominal sepsis are prominent. Ischemia, infection, and inflammation may result in full-thickness necrosis of small intestine, particularly in the ileocolic region, with resultant intestinal perforation.

CLINICAL MANIFESTATIONS

The patient presenting for surgery for NEC is most often a preterm infant, with other complications of prematurity such as respiratory distress syndrome, PDA, a history of birth asphyxia, or other cardiorespiratory instability. Clinical signs include abdominal distention, bloody stools, dilated intestinal loops and pneumatosis intestinalis on abdominal radiograph, temperature instability, and signs of sepsis including thrombocytopenia, hemodynamic instability, and disseminated intravascular coagulopathy (DIC). Intestinal perforation is evident on abdominal radiography and is a surgical emergency; these patients are often critically ill or unstable with hypotension, DIC, metabolic acidosis, and worsening respiratory status.

MEDICAL AND SURGICAL TREATMENT

Initial treatment of NEC without intestinal perforation or other signs of extensive bowel necrosis is usually medical, with broad-spectrum antibiotics, gastric decompression, serial abdominal examination and radiographs, and careful monitoring for signs of cardiorespiratory decompensation. Originally, surgery for NEC with perforation was by laparotomy, resection of necrotic intestine, and creation of ostomies. This necessitated later reconstructive surgery and often resulted in resection of extensive lengths of small intestine, resulting in short-gut syndrome. In more recent years, primary peritoneal drainage, whereby a small incision is made and a surgical drain is left in place, has gained popularity for smaller, sicker infants, who may then have definitive surgery later when their medical condition has improved. Some patients may not require further treatment at all, and survival using this more conservative approach is comparable in many series.[16]

MANAGEMENT OF ANESTHESIA

Surgery for NEC is most often emergent, and preoperative preparation should focus on assessment and correction of fluid and electrolyte abnormalities, hemodynamic and respiratory instability, providing broad-spectrum antibiotics, and correcting coagulation abnormalities. Surgery for NEC can be done at the bedside in the neonatal intensive care unit, necessitating a mobile surgical and anesthesia team and equipment. Most patients are already tracheally intubated. Monitoring often includes a peripheral arterial catheter; umbilical artery catheters are often removed because of concern over further mesenteric ischemia. Central venous access is often desirable, but attempts to secure invasive monitors should not delay emergent surgery.

Anesthesia with synthetic opioids such as fentanyl is the regimen best tolerated in the critically unstable neonate. Doses are titrated, starting at 2 to 5 µg/kg, but additional doses are added to provide 20 to 50 µg/kg fentanyl if tolerated. Volatile anesthetics are often not tolerated owing to vasodilatory effects, and small doses of benzodiazepines such as midazolam 0.05 to 0.1 mg/kg, or ketamine 0.5 mg/kg, may be added. Muscle relaxation with pancuronium, vecuronium, or another nondepolarizing neuromuscular blocking drug, is necessary. Because of large fluid losses from exposed intestine undergoing resection, intravenous fluid requirements are often very high, at 10 to 20 mL/kg/hour, and 5% albumin, packed red blood cells, fresh frozen plasma, and platelets are often infused in the face of DIC and significant blood loss. Inotropic support in the form of dopamine, 5 to 10 µg/kg/min, or epinephrine, 0.03 to 0.05 µg/kg/min, is often needed and should be instituted early, rather than infusing excessive amounts of intravenous fluid to maintain blood pressure in unstable patients. Calcium chloride or gluconate bolus is often necessary to maintain normal ionized calcium levels to preserve myocardial contractility and vascular tone, particularly with infusion of significant volumes of citrated blood products. Frequent analysis of arterial blood gases to measure acid-base status and oxygenation, as well as serum electrolytes, glucose, ionized calcium, and lactate, is often desirable to direct therapy. Mechanical ventilation is adjusted to maintain Pao_2 50 to 70 mm Hg and Spo_2 90% to 95% in the premature infant; however, in the extremely ill patient it is preferable to maintain somewhat higher oxygen tensions to allow for a margin of safety. Hemoglobin should be maintained at 10 to 15 g/dL to preserve oxygen-carrying capacity. Temperature management is critical, and these surgeries are often performed on the patient's overhead warming bed. The operating room temperature must be 85° F to 90° F or higher, and forced air warming as well as warmed blood products must be used in an effort to maintain core temperature at 36° C or higher. Postoperatively, mechanical ventilation, inotropic and fluid support, and antibiotics are continued, and

IV

a full report of the operation and anesthetic is given to the NICU (neonatal intensive care unit) team.

Abdominal Wall Defects: Gastroschisis and Omphalocele

Gastroschisis is an abdominal wall defect whereby the intestines protrude, usually to the right of the umbilical cord, without a covering sac, with the umbilical cord not part of the defect (Fig. 34-2).[17] These infants most often do not have associated congenital or chromosomal anomalies. An omphalocele is a midline defect with the intestines covered by a peritoneal sac and the umbilical cord incorporated into the defect (Fig. 34-3). These neonates frequently have other associated anomalies.

MEDICAL AND SURGICAL TREATMENT

These diagnoses may be made prenatally, and presurgical management includes covering the exposed bowel with plastic or other synthetic material, attention to fluid replacement, and prevention of volvulus and bowel ischemia. Nasogastric decompression is important to minimize fluid and air accumulation. The size of the defects varies greatly; formerly even large defects were candidates for primary surgical reduction of the viscera and fascial closure, as this was thought to prevent later intestinal complications. However, with excessive increases in intra-abdominal pressure, an abdominal compartment syndrome can arise resulting in intestinal ischemia and renal failure. In addition, the sudden increase in intra-abdominal pressure may lead to increased ventilatory requirements, often necessitating days of sedation, muscle

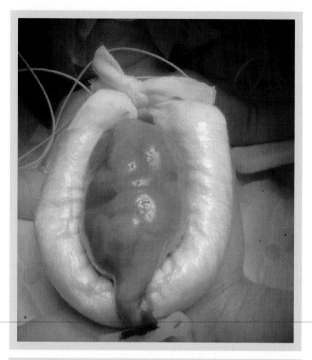

Figure 34-3 A giant omphalocele supported with dressing collar. Note the midline position, covering with peritoneal sac, and inclusion of the umbilical cord. (Reproduced and used with permission from Marven S, Owen A. Contemporary postnatal surgical management strategies for congenital abdominal wall defects. Semin Pediatr Surg 2008;17:223.)

relaxation, and careful monitoring of ventilatory and hemodynamic status. Now a staged approach is often used, which involves containing the viscera in a Silastic silo with its edges sutured to the peritoneum around the defect. Then, using gravity, compression of the bowel, traction, and expansion of the abdominal cavity, the viscera are gradually reduced into the peritoneal cavity over a period of days to weeks. Surgical closure of the peritoneum and skin are undertaken at the end of this period. Some small to moderate-sized defects can be managed with a similar staged reduction strategy, with the peritoneum and skin defects healing by secondary intention.

MANAGEMENT OF ANESTHESIA

Because of the modern staged approach, the challenges of providing anesthesia for a one-stage reduction and closure are rarely encountered. Still, the initial surgery is often to suture the Silastic silo and partially reduce the viscera. Preoperative preparation includes maintaining adequate fluid replacement to account for losses from the exposed viscera. These infants may be premature, but are often full term and have a stable cardiorespiratory status. The general considerations noted earlier for NEC surgery concerning temperature management and fluid

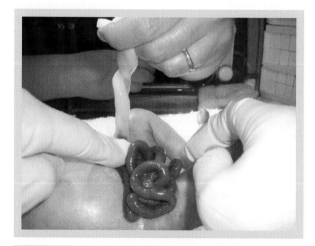

Figure 34-2 Gastroschisis. Note position to right of umbilical cord, which is not included in the defect. It is also not covered with a peritoneal sac. (Reproduced and used with permission from Marven S, Owen A. Contemporary postnatal surgical management strategies for congenital abdominal wall defects. Semin Pediatr Surg 2008;17:224.)

replacement apply to surgery for abdominal wall defects. Induction of anesthesia and tracheal intubation can be accomplished with a variety of agents, with precautions to prevent aspiration of gastric contents. The umbilical vessels are not available, so secure large-bore venous access should be obtained, and possibly arterial catheter monitoring for patients with very large defects or unstable cardiorespiratory status. Intravenous fluid replacement of 10 to 20 mL/kg/hour is important, along with administration of 5% or 10% dextrose at maintenance rates. Anesthesia can be maintained with volatile anesthetics or benzodiazepines, with opioids, with dose depending on plans for tracheal extubation at the end of the procedure. If the primary procedure is silo placement without primary reduction, the tracheas of full-term infants can often be extubated at the end of the procedure, and subsequent reductions can be done at the bedside with small-dose sedation. The final fascial and skin closure will require a full general anesthetic. If a full reduction and closure of a major defect is planned, arterial and central venous pressure monitoring are important, along with bladder catheterization and careful management of cardiorespiratory status. This often requires significant increases in positive end-expiratory pressure, additional fluid administration, and inotropic support with dopamine, as well as prolonged postoperative ventilation, sedation, and muscle relaxation.

Tracheoesophageal Fistula

Tracheoesophageal fistula (TEF) is seen in five different anatomic configurations (Fig. 34-4), with the most common being type C, with esophageal atresia, and a distal TEF. Diagnosis is made when the neonate experiences choking and cyanosis when attempting oral feeds. The chest and abdominal radiograph reveal inability to pass an orogastric tube, which lodges in the blind esophageal pouch, and the presence of gas-filled intestines from the distal TEF. Infants with TEF often have other anomalies, and many have VACTERL association: V for vertebral defects; A for imperforate anus, C for cardiac defects, TE for TE fistula, R for renal anomalies, and L for limb anomalies. A thorough evaluation for these additional defects, especially cardiac, should be undertaken in these infants. The severity of illness can be mild (e.g., feeding difficulties in a full-term neonate with no respiratory distress), but some patients are critically ill. Severe respiratory failure can result from continuous aspiration of gastric contents via the distal TEF, exacerbated by respiratory distress syndrome as well as massive abdominal distention from filling of the stomach with gas from the TEF.

SURGICAL APPROACHES

Earlier approaches were usually staged, often first performing a gastrostomy under local anesthesia to decompress the stomach and allow some recovery of pulmonary function. Then, a right thoracotomy would be done to ligate the TEF, and possibly to reconstruct the esophageal atresia. Other approaches included a cervical esophagostomy to drain the upper esophageal pouch and prevent aspiration. In recent years, the staged approach has largely been abandoned. In the current era a one-stage ligation of the TEF with primary esophageal repair, without a gastrostomy, is the preferred strategy and is possible in 80% to 90% of patients.[18] Critically ill premature infants may still require gastrostomy before thoracotomy and TEF ligation, and if the gap between esophageal

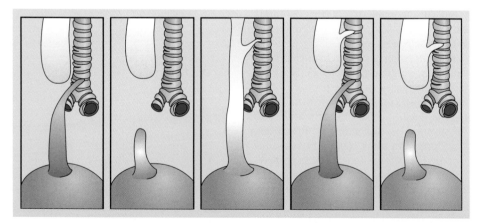

Figure 34-4 Classification of tracheoesophageal anomalies in descending order of incidence. Type C (86%) is esophageal atresia with a distal tracheoesophageal fistula. Type A (8%) is esophageal atresia without a tracheoesophageal fistula. Type E (4%) is an H-type fistula without esophageal atresia. Type D (1%) is esophageal atresia with both proximal and distal tracheoesophageal fistulas. Type B (1%) is esophageal atresia with a proximal tracheoesophageal fistula. (From Gross RE. The Surgery of Infancy and Childhood. Philadelphia, WB Saunders, 1953.)

segments is too long, gastrostomy followed by esophageal dilation and stretching may be required after the initial thoracotomy. Outcomes of neonatal TEF surgery vary; the critically ill premature infant or neonate with multiple anomalies has a higher mortality and morbidity rate; the full-term neonate without other problems has an operative survival rate approaching 100%.

ANESTHETIC MANAGEMENT

The critically ill neonate with high ventilation pressures and gastric distention will emergently undergo anesthesia for right thoracotomy and ligation of the TEF. These infants may present in extremis due to a large TEF with most of the tidal volume being lost through the TEF, severely compromising pulmonary ventilation. Manual ventilation, inotropic support, sodium bicarbonate, and vasoactive bolus drugs such as epinephrine and atropine may be needed until the TEF is ligated and the stomach decompressed. More commonly the trachea is intubated and there are varying degrees of difficulty with ventilation. The patient is transported carefully to the operating room, anesthesia is carefully induced with intravenous or inhaled anesthetics and muscle relaxants, and the patient is positioned for right thoracotomy. An arterial catheter is essential for monitoring of blood pressure and gas exchange. Very careful attention is paid to adequacy of ventilation during the entire case, as the endotracheal tube may migrate into the TEF and preclude ventilation. End-tidal CO_2, careful observation of lung inflation and chest movement, and a precordial stethoscope in the left axillary area are important monitors. Periods of difficult ventilation and hypoxemia during lung retraction and TEF ligation should be expected. Normally, after the TEF is ligated, ventilation improves dramatically.

In the patient whose trachea is not intubated, awake tracheal intubation was classically considered to be the best technique, but in the modern era this is rarely practiced. Instead, either intravenous or inhaled induction of anesthesia, with muscle relaxation, can be achieved after suctioning the upper esophageal pouch and administration of oxygen. Then, an endotracheal tube is passed into the distal trachea, and gentle positive-pressure ventilation is accomplished with careful assessment of effectiveness of ventilation. Endotracheal tube migration into the TEF should be suspected with ventilation difficulties. Bronchoscopy is performed in some centers to assess the size and position of the TEF before surgery and to properly position the ET tube; only in the presence of a large TEF (>3 mm) which is located near the carina is there likely to be difficulty with ventilation.[19] After ligation of the TEF the esophagus is usually repaired primarily. Some centers are performing TEF repair via video-assisted thoracoscopy approach, which itself can cause difficulty with ventilation secondary to the CO_2 insufflation. Although it is possible to extubate the trachea in the operating room in a vigorous full-term infant without complications, a more prudent approach is to leave the trachea intubated to allow adequate analgesic administration in the NICU. If the patient requires reintubation, the subsequent airway manipulation could disrupt the esophageal repair. A nasogastric tube is placed by the surgeon in the operating room for early gastric decompression and feeding.

Congenital Diaphragmatic Hernia

Congenital diaphragmatic hernia (CDH) is a defect in the diaphragm evident early in gestation, which results in the herniation of the intestines, spleen, and sometimes stomach or liver, into the thorax. Most commonly this is on the left side through the foramen of Morgagni, and results in severe restriction of lung development (Fig. 34-5). This lesion is often diagnosed prenatally, and with significant defects the neonate presents with respiratory failure, requiring mechanical ventilation. These neonates present with a scaphoid abdomen, bowel sounds in the chest, and respiratory distress and cyanosis of varying degrees. Pulmonary hypertension from lung hypoplasia and immediate postnatal elevation in pulmonary vascular resistance cause right-to-left shunting through patent foramen ovale and ductus arteriosus, often resulting in severe cyanosis from persistent fetal circulation. In these cases, surgical treatment, which consists of an abdominal or thoracoabdominal incision to reduce the viscera into the abdominal cavity and repair the diaphragm either primarily or with a synthetic mesh material, must be delayed while therapy is instituted to stabilize the medical condition of the infant.

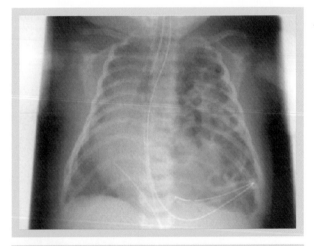

Figure 34-5 Left-sided congenital diaphragmatic hernia. Note bowel loops filling the left hemithorax, and nasogastric tube in the stomach, which is also herniated through the defect. The heart is shifted to the right side of the chest. (Reproduced and used with permission from de Buys Roessingh AS, Dinh-Xuan A. Congenital diaphragmatic hernia: Current status and review of the literature. Eur J Pediatr 2009;168:398.)

Laparoscopic repair has also been described. High-frequency oscillatory ventilation (HFOV) to improve gas exchange in hypoplastic lungs, inhaled nitric oxide (iNO) to treat the pulmonary hypertension, or extracorporeal membrane oxygenation (ECMO) to stabilize the cardiorespiratory status in the most severely affected neonates may be necessary. Surgical repair is then undertaken several days later, sometimes while on ECMO, which results in reduction of the abdominal viscera but does not solve the problem of lung hypoplasia and pulmonary hypertension, which may require days or weeks of support until they improve sufficiently.[20]

MANAGEMENT OF ANESTHESIA

These infants are often critically ill. Transport to the operating room is achieved carefully, and the patient may need to be transitioned from HFOV to conventional ventilation as surgery with HFOV may not be possible. iNO should be continued throughout the operating room course. Anesthesia is provided with high-dose synthetic opioids such as fentanyl, 25 to 50 µg/kg or more, to provide analgesia and blunt the pulmonary hypertensive response to painful stimuli. Volatile anesthetics are often not tolerated, so small doses of benzodiazepines or ketamine may be used as drugs to provide amnesia. Monitoring of arterial and central venous pressures via umbilical route is essential, and inotropic support with dopamine or epinephrine is continued. Frequent arterial blood gases are analyzed and changes in ventilation are made to maximize oxygenation, and reduce $Paco_2$ and increase pH to lower pulmonary artery pressures. After left thoracoabdominal incision at the costal margin, the abdominal contents are reduced out of the thorax, which may acutely improve ventilation. The diaphragm is reconstructed with a synthetic mesh material. Manual ventilation, or ventilation with an ICU ventilator may be necessary throughout the case as standard anesthesia machine ventilators are often not capable of delivering the high inspired gas flows and small tidal volumes necessary to ventilate such patients. The patient is transported back to the NICU where HFOV may need to be reinstated and iNO should be continued.

The most severely ill neonates with CDH receive ECMO support, and surgery may be done while on ECMO, which is problematic because of bleeding secondary to heparinization. Adequate blood products, including packed red blood cells, platelets, and fresh frozen plasma, must be available if the repair is done on ECMO. Anesthesia is provided with high-dose opioids, benzodiazepines, or ketamine.

Patent Ductus Arteriosus (Also See Chapter 26)

The patent ductus arteriosus (PDA) is most often seen in the premature neonate and can result in pulmonary edema, reduced ventilatory compliance, and ventilator dependence worsened by concurrent respiratory distress syndrome (RDS) or pneumonia. The PDA may prevent weaning from the ventilator and result in secondary complications such as feeding intolerance or NEC. Clinical presentation includes persistent pulmonary edema, bounding pulses and wide pulse pressure from diastolic runoff from the aorta to the pulmonary artery through the PDA, and sometimes hypotension and cardiac failure from the large left-to-right shunt via the PDA, requiring inotropic support. Diagnosis is made with transthoracic echocardiography. Attempts at medical closure with indomethacin may be successful, but this therapy may adversely effect renal and platelet function, and this is important to evaluate if the neonate presenting for surgery has recently failed medical therapy.[21]

MANAGEMENT OF ANESTHESIA

The patient is often a small premature neonate weighing 500 to 1000 g, ventilator dependent, and possible hemodynamically unstable. Surgery may be done at the bedside in the NICU in some centers. Transport to the operating room must be done carefully with continuous monitoring. Anesthesia is normally provided with synthetic opioids such as fentanyl, 25 to 50 µg/kg, muscle relaxation with pancuronium, and small doses of benzodiazepines or ketamine, as volatile agents are usually not tolerated. Arterial monitoring is important for frequent assessment of hemodynamics and arterial blood gases. A left thoracotomy is done and the PDA is approached via a retropleural dissection. Careful monitoring of ventilation with visual inspection, capnography, and a precordial or esophageal stethoscope, are performed as ventilation is easily compromised. Because of the risk of worsening retinopathy of prematurity (ROP), target Pao_2 is normally 50 to 80 mm Hg and Spo_2 90% to 95%, so high inspired Fio_2 is avoided unless absolutely necessary. Because the PDA is often larger than the descending thoracic aorta, monitoring with a pulse oximeter on the lower extremity is important to ensure that the surgeon identifies and ligates the correct structure. The PDA can be ligated with sutures or surgical clips. Packed red blood cells must be immediately available in case there is bleeding from damage to the paper-thin PDA. Maintenance of normothermia and provision of glucose is critically important during PDA ligation in the premature infant. Most infants will remain mechanically ventilated for some period of time after PDA ligation.

In contrast to the premature infant with otherwise normal cardiac anatomy in whom the PDA must be closed, infants with congenital heart disease may be dependent on the PDA to provide pulmonary blood flow in the case of pulmonary atresia or stenosis, or systemic blood flow in the case of hypoplasia of left-sided cardiac structures such as severe coarctation of the aorta or hypoplastic left-sided heart syndrome. Prostaglandin E_1 is infused in these cases at 0.025 to 0.05 µg/kg/min and must be maintained until corrective cardiac surgery can be performed.

IV

Retinopathy of Prematurity

Retinopathy of prematurity (ROP) is a vasoproliferative disease affecting premature or low-birth-weight infants. Five stages of ROP exist, and in stages 4 and 5, retinal detachment occurs, which can result in permanent visual loss.[22] The pathophysiology is complex, with the more premature infants at higher risk, but one of the main causes is excessive oxygen tensions in the vessels of the retina, accompanied by wide swings in oxygen tension such as those seen in cardiopulmonary instability with ventilated premature infants with RDS, PDA, sepsis, apnea/bradycardia, and other problems associated with prematurity. Thus, Spo_2 is maintained at 88% to 93% in many premature infants, with resulting oxygen tensions of 50 to 70 mm Hg targeted. Excessive oxygen tensions, as may be seen with general endotracheal anesthesia, are to be avoided, even if short-lived. The challenge for the anesthesiologist caring for such infants is to manage oxygenation with these restrictions in mind.

Premature infants hospitalized in the NICU receive regular retinal examinations, and if high-risk type I or greater ROP is diagnosed, urgent surgical therapy is undertaken within 24 to 72 hours to maximize visual outcomes. This often results in the urgent scheduling of treatment during evening and weekend hours. Retinal ablative therapy with indirect laser photocoagulation of proliferating vessels in one or both eyes is the treatment of choice. Cryotherapy may also be used, and at more severe stages a vitrectomy may be required.

MANAGEMENT OF ANESTHESIA

Due to the urgent or emergent nature of ROP surgery, the patient may not have feeding withheld. If the patient is still ventilated, any anesthetic technique, usually in conjunction with muscle relaxation, may be used. If the patient is not ventilated, any technique for induction, followed by muscle relaxation and endotracheal intubation, may be used. As these cases may last several hours, especially with extensive disease in both eyes, attention must be paid to patient temperature and provision of glucose during the surgery. Because of the often prolonged nature of the anesthetic, the risk of postanesthetic apnea in the premature infant, and the eye discomfort necessitating analgesia after the procedure, mechanical ventilation should be controlled after ROP surgery for 12 to 24 hours. Regardless of airway management after surgery, the patient must be carefully monitored in the NICU setting for postanesthetic problems.

Myelomeningocele

Myelomeningocele is a developmental defect of the neural tube, resulting in an open neural placode covered only by a thin membrane and cerebrospinal fluid. The defect is often diagnosed prenatally, varies in size, and may be located in the thoracolumbar, or lumbosacral spine areas. The most common presentation is a lumbosacral myelomeningocele in a full-term infant. Preoperatively, it is critical not to allow the sac covering the spinal defect to rupture, which will result in a high risk of meningitis. These infants are nursed prone, with a moist gauze covering the defect. Surgery is scheduled emergently, and consists of dissection of nerve roots and covering the defect with fascia and skin. In addition, over 75% of infants have hydrocephalus and many have Arnold-Chiari malformation of the spinal cord and brainstem and will require a ventriculoperitoneal shunt, usually done after the initial repair. Long-term outcome depends on early repair to prevent infection, and level of spinal cord dysfunction.[23]

MANAGEMENT OF ANESTHESIA

Great care must be taken to prevent rupture of the sac covering the myelomeningocele during transport and positioning for induction of anesthesia and surgery. The infant cannot lie directly supine for this reason. Anesthetic induction and endotracheal intubation can be performed with the infant in the left lateral decubitus position. An alternative approach is to carefully place the infant supine in a doughnut-shaped padded foam bolster so that the myelomeningocele defect is in the center but not touching the operating room bed. After confirmation of endotracheal tube position, the infant is positioned prone for surgery. Any technique can be used for induction and maintenance of anesthesia, but the surgeon usually performs the repair under the microscope, and requests that no muscle relaxant be used during the repair portion of the surgery so that motor function can be assessed. In addition, as patients with myelomeningocele repair at birth are at highest risk for developing latex allergy, all surgical gloves and all other materials in contact with the patient must be latex free. After surgery the trachea can be extubated, using the same positioning techniques as for intubation. The patient then is turned prone and is kept in this position in which the infant will be nursed for several days.

Pyloric Stenosis

Pyloric stenosis is hypertrophy of the pyloric muscle leading to a gastric outlet obstruction. A typical presentation is a young infant between 2 and 8 weeks of age with persistent projectile vomiting. This results in weight loss, dehydration, and electrolyte imbalance consisting of a hypochloremic, hypokalemic metabolic alkalosis from loss of hydrogen and chloride ions from stomach contents. These infants may develop severe dehydration, lethargy, poor skin turgor, sunken eyes and fontanel, poor urine output, and plasma chloride concentrations as low as 65 to 70 mEq/dL. Diagnosis is by clinical history; there is a

5:1 male predominance and average age at presentation is 5 to 6 weeks. An olive-shaped and -sized mass may be palpable in the epigastrium; definitive diagnosis is made by ultrasound. Repair of pyloric stenosis is *not* a surgical emergency; the patient must be rehydrated, starting with a bolus of 10 to 20 mL/kg of normal saline or lactated Ringer's solution, and then more than maintenance IV fluids usually consisting of 5% dextrose in half normal saline with potassium chloride. The fluid and electrolyte status is followed carefully and laboratory values rechecked periodically. When the patient has been rehydrated to normal vascular volume status and normal or near-normal electrolytes, he is ready for surgery. This preparation may require 12 to 72 hours, depending on the severity at presentation.[24]

MANAGEMENT OF ANESTHESIA

After adequate rehydration the patient is brought to the operating room, and gastric contents are evacuated with a large-bore orogastric suction catheter before induction of anesthesia. Although awake tracheal intubation has been the preferred technique, this is rarely practiced in the modern era. After adequately breathing 100% oxygen, an intravenous induction of anesthesia is accomplished with propofol 2 to 2.5 mg/kg, which is preferable to short-acting barbiturates because of its shorter terminal half-life. Cricoid pressure is applied, and paralysis is achieved with succinylcholine 1 to 2 mg/kg (after pretreatment with atropine), or preferably, a nondepolarizing muscle relaxant such as rocuronium. A modified rapid sequence technique, with rapid small tidal volume mask ventilation through cricoid pressure, is utilized to prevent arterial desaturation in a young infant whose oxygen consumption is two to three times that of the adult. After successful confirmation of tracheal intubation, maintenance of anesthesia proceeds with a volatile anesthetic. Opioids are best avoided because of the risk of postanesthetic apnea in pyloric stenosis, and instead local anesthetic infiltration of the incision by the surgeon, and rectal acetaminophen are utilized for postoperative analgesia. Surgery proceeds either via small open epigastric incision, or via laparoscopy with CO_2 insufflation of the abdomen. After conclusion of the surgery a nasogastric tube may be left in place. The trachea is extubated after reversal of nondepolarizing muscle relaxant and full return of airway reflexes and a regular breathing pattern without pauses or apnea. Because of the metabolic alkalosis seen in many pyloric stenosis patients, CSF pH may be increased, causing a reduction in respiratory drive which is not corrected for 12 to 48 hours. This, in conjunction with respiratory drive that may not be fully mature until 44 weeks' postconceptual age, may place even full-term infants undergoing pyloromyotomy at risk for postanesthetic apnea. These patients should be monitored for 12 to 24 hours after anesthesia for this complication.[25]

SPECIAL ANESTHETIC CONSIDERATIONS

Anesthesia for the Former Premature Infant

Many former premature infants present for surgery, either during their initial hospitalization, or later as outpatients. The most common procedures include inguinal herniorraphy, circumcision, eye examination, and strabismus surgery. Although many infants have recovered well without sequelae, many have chronic conditions such as bronchopulmonary dysplasia (need for supplemental oxygen beyond 30 days of life after a diagnosis of RDS), apnea and bradycardia, anemia, hydrocephalus from intraventicular hemorrhage, visual disturbances, and developmental delay. It is also important to understand the infant's postconceptual age; an infant born at 28 weeks' gestation who presents at 12 weeks for surgery is now 40 weeks' postconceptual age and is equivalent in many respects to only a full-term infant, not an infant at 3 months of age. The major risk in this regard is postanesthetic apnea, which in some cases is fatal. The risk of postanesthetic apnea increases with increasing prematurity at birth and younger age at the time of the anesthetic.[26] Although the time at which the risk of apnea is eliminated is not clear, 50 weeks' postconceptual age or less is commonly used as the cutoff point for admitting former premature infants after an anesthetic for 24 hours of apnea monitoring.

Anesthesia for Remote Locations (Also See Chapter 38)

Anesthesia and sedation for diagnostic and therapeutic procedures are increasing for children in locations remote from the operating room. These procedures include MRI and CT scans, interventional radiology procedures, bone marrow aspirations, gastrointestinal endoscopy, auditory brainstem evoked response testing, and cardiac catheterization. Techniques vary widely and include moderate or deep sedation, general anesthesia with intravenous agents, volatile agents with mask or laryngeal mask airway, or full general endotracheal anesthesia. Frequently used anesthetics include propofol, ketamine, barbiturates, benzodiazepines, and opioids. The central α_2-agonist dexmedetomidine is increasingly being used for nonpainful diagnostic studies such as MRI.[27] The same standards for preoperative evaluation, monitoring, and recovery must be maintained for anesthesia in remote locations.

Ex Utero Intrapartum Therapy Procedure and Fetal Surgery

The ex utero intrapartum therapy (EXIT) procedure was first performed in 1989. The purpose is to secure the neonatal airway while the fetus is still being oxygenated via the placenta. The mother is placed under general anesthesia, a hysterotomy is made, and the fetus is partially

IV

delivered. The airway is then secured by direct laryngoscopy, rigid bronchoscopy, or tracheostomy while on placenta bypass. Indications include large neck masses, congenital airway obstruction, and previous tracheal occlusion for congenital diaphragmatic hernia. The EXIT procedure has also been used for patients with fetal anomalies in whom neonatal resuscitation may be difficult including large thoracic masses, congenital diaphragmatic hernia, unilateral pulmonary agenesis, and some complex cardiac lesions. Maintenance of placental bypass provides time to establish intravenous access and an airway, give resuscitative drugs, and cannulate for ECMO when necessary in a controlled manner.[28]

The anesthesiologist caring for the mother administers inhaled agent for both anesthesia and to promote uterine relaxation. While the placenta is still part of the fetal circulation, the inhaled agent also anesthetizes the fetus. Opioids, muscle relaxant, and atropine may also be administered intramuscularly or intravenously to the baby.

Fetal interventions have been performed via open hysterotomy, through hysteroscopy, and by a percutaneous approach to treat congenital diaphragmatic hernia, myelomeningocele, congenital cystic adenomatoid malformation, hypoplastic left-sided heart syndrome, obstructive uropathy due to posterior urethral valves, and other congenital anomalies with varied success. For cases done under general anesthesia and monitored anesthesia care with sedation, the fetus can be anesthetized via the mother either with inhaled anesthetic agent or through intravenous drug delivery. Maternal administration of an intravenous infusion of remifentanil is a popular choice for sedation that crosses the placenta to the fetus. The fetus may also be given muscle relaxant, atropine, and fentanyl intravenously via the umbilical vein or intramuscularly to prevent fetal movement, bradycardia, and pain.[28]

Anesthetic Neurotoxicity and Neuroprotection in the Developing Brain

Neonatal rodent models of prolonged anesthesia with γ-aminobutyric acid agonists (isoflurane, midazolam, propofol) or N-methyl-D-aspartate antagonists (ketamine) produce accelerated apoptosis, or programmed cell death, of neurons in the developing brain.[29] This data raised concern that commonly used anesthetic agents could be having similar effects in the developing human brain, generating intense interest and a number of new research avenues to determine if this effect applies to human neonates and infants. Criticism of the animal studies includes the fact that most were conducted in the absence of a surgical stimulus, and that the exposure periods were quite prolonged compared to the corresponding exposure of a human infant during anesthesia and surgery. Other animal models have demonstrated that anesthetics such as ketamine and desflurane are neuroprotective in animal models that include surgery or painful stimuli. Currently there is insufficient evidence to change the current approach to anesthesia in the infant.

QUESTIONS OF THE DAY

1. What are the differences in thermoregulation between infants and adults? Why are infants more prone to the development of hypothermia?
2. What are the risk factors for postoperative nausea and vomiting (PONV) in children? What interventions can reduce the incidence of PONV?
3. What is the typical presentation of an infant with necrotizing enterocolitis? What are the most important aspects of anesthesia management?
4. What are the expected electrolyte abnormalities in a child with pyloric stenosis?
5. What should be the goal for arterial P_{O_2} in a premature infant at risk for retinopathy of prematurity (ROP)?
6. What are the major anesthetic risks in the former premature infant? How should these patients be monitored postoperatively?

ACKNOWLEDGMENTS

The editors and publisher would like to thank Dr. Claire Brett for contributing a chapter on this topic to the prior edition of this work. It has served as the foundation for the current chapter.

REFERENCES

1. Andropoulos DB: Physiology and molecular biology of the developing circulation. In Andropoulos DB, editor: *Anesthesia for Congenital Heart Disease*, ed 2, Oxford, UK, 2010, Wiley Blackwell, pp 55–76.
2. Lerman J: Inhalation agents in pediatric anaesthesia—An update, *Curr Opin Anaesthesiol* 20:221–226, 2007.
3. Bailey AG, McNaull PP, Jooste E, et al: Perioperative crystalloid and colloid fluid management in children: Where are we and how did we get here? *Anesth Analg* 110:375–390, 2010.
4. Alten JA, Benner K, Green K, et al: Pediatric off-label use of recombinant factor VIIa, *Pediatrics* 123:1066–1072, 2009.
5. Dalal PG, Murray D, Messner AH, et al: Pediatric laryngeal dimensions: An age-based analysis, *Anesth Analg* 108:1475–1479, 2009.
6. Salgo B, Schmitz A, Henze G, et al: Evaluation of a new recommendation for improved cuffed tracheal tube size selection in infants and small children, *Acta Anaesthesiol Scand* 50:557–561, 2006.

7. Fiadjoe J, Stricker P: Pediatric difficult airway management: Current devices and techniques, *Anesthesiol Clin* 27:185–195, 2009.

8. Wheeler M, Coté CJ: Preoperative pregnancy testing in a tertiary care children's hospital: A medico-legal conundrum, *J Clin Anesth* 11:56–63, 1999.

9. Tait AR, Malviya S: Anesthesia for the child with an upper respiratory tract infection: Still a dilemma? *Anesth Analg* 100:59–65, 2005.

10. Practice guidelines for preoperative fasting and the use of pharmacologic agents to reduce the risk of pulmonary aspiration: Application to healthy patients undergoing elective procedures: A report by the American Society of Anesthesiologists Task Force on Preoperative Fasting, *Anesthesiology* 90:896–905, 1999.

11. Sadhasivam S, Cohen LL, Szabova A, et al: Real-time assessment of perioperative behaviors and prediction of perioperative outcomes, *Anesth Analg* 108:822–826, 2009.

12. Watson A, Visram A: Survey of the use of oesophageal and precordial stethoscopes in current paediatric anaesthetic practice, *Paediatr Anaesth* 11:437–442, 2001.

13. Davidson AJ: Monitoring the anaesthetic depth in children—An update, *Curr Opin Anaesthesiol* 20:236–243, 2007.

14. Tobias JD: Spinal anaesthesia in infants and children, *Paediatr Anaesth* 10:5–16, 2000.

15. Engelman E, Salengros JC, Barvais L: How much does pharmacologic prophylaxis reduce postoperative vomiting in children? Calculation of prophylaxis effectiveness and expected incidence of vomiting under treatment using Bayesian meta-analysis, *Anesthesiology* 109:1023–1035, 2008.

16. Henry MC, Moss RL: Neonatal necrotizing enterocolitis, *Semin Pediatr Surg* 17:98–109, 2008.

17. Marven S, Owen A: Contemporary postnatal surgical management strategies for congenital abdominal wall defects, *Semin Pediatr Surg* 17:222–235, 2008.

18. Orford J, Cass DT, Glasson MJ: Advances in the treatment of oesophageal atresia over three decades: The 1970's and the 1990's, *Pediatr Surg Int* 20:402–407, 2004.

19. Andropoulos DB, Rowe RW, Betts JM: Anaesthetic and surgical airway management during tracheo-oesophageal fistula repair, *Paediatr Anaesth* 8:313–319, 1998.

20. de Buys Roessingh AS, Dinh-Xuan A: Congenital diaphragmatic hernia: Current status and review of the literature, *Eur J Pediatr* 168:393–406, 2009.

21. Malviya MN, Ohlsson A, Shah SS: Surgical versus medical treatment with cyclooxygenase inhibitors for symptomatic patent ductus arteriosus in preterm infants (review), *Cochrane Database Syst Rev* 1:CD003951, 2008.

22. Sylvester CL: Retinopathy of prematurity, *Semin Ophthalmol* 23:318–323, 2008.

23. Thompson DN: Postnatal management and outcome for neural tube defects including spina bifida and encephalocoeles, *Prenat Diagn* 29:412–419, 2009.

24. Bissonnette B, Sullivan PJ: Pyloric stenosis, *Can J Anaesth* 38:668–676, 1991.

25. Andropoulos DB, Heard MB, Johnson KL, et al: Postanesthetic apnea in full-term infants after pyloromyotomy, *Anesthesiology* 80:216–219, 1994.

26. Cote CJ, Zaslavsky A, Downes JJ, et al: Postoperative apnea in former preterm infants after inguinal herniorrhaphy: A combined analysis, *Anesthesiology* 82:809–822, 1995.

27. Mason KP: Sedation trends in the 21st century: The transition to dexmedetomidine for radiological imaging studies, *Paediatr Anaesth* 20:265–272, 2010.

28. De Buck F, Deprest J, Van de Velde M: Anesthesia for fetal surgery, *Curr Opin Anaesthesiol* 21:293–297, 2008.

29. Loepke AW, Soriano SG: An assessment of the effects of general anesthetics on developing brain structure and neurocognitive function, *Anesth Analg* 106:1681–1707, 2008.

IV

35 ELDERLY PATIENTS

Sheila Ryan Barnett

The change in demographics of the United States and world population has lead to a significant shift in the age of the population and the absolute numbers of geriatric patients. Between 2005 and 2030, the percentage of individuals over 65 years of age probably will increase from 12% to 20% of the U.S. population—an increase of almost 30 million individuals—from 37 million to over 70 million individuals. The increase in those elderly people older than 80 years of age will create anesthetic challenges to most anesthetic providers. At present there are approximately 11 million and this number is expected to increase to over 20 million in the next 20 years. The increase in population is due to the combined effect of the aging baby boomers and the increase in longevity. The increase in population of older patients will place a burden on health care systems and this will be reflected in an increase in the numbers of older patients with multiple co-morbidities undergoing surgery and invasive procedures outside the operating room. Anesthesia providers must have a clear understanding of fundamental geriatric issues and the challenges inherent in caring for this segment of the population.[1]

WHY GERIATRIC ANESTHESIOLOGY IS IMPORTANT

About one third of geriatric patients undergo at least one surgery prior to death; however, the explosion of new procedures requiring anesthesia will probably lead to an increase in this number. Concomitant with the increasing number of patients, the associated anesthetic and surgical morbidity and mortality rates in the elderly will also be increased.[2,3] The increase in risk to these patients is largely due to the presence of co-morbid conditions versus age per se. Advanced age by itself should not be considered a contraindication for surgery but should take into consideration the patient's actual health and function.[4] Certain conditions are associated

Table 35-1 Challenges in Management of the Geriatric Patient

- Population is heterogeneous.
- Wide disparity between physiologic and chronologic age is common.
- Advancing age is associated with a steady decline in organ function.
- Preoperative reserve organ function is unknown.
- Multiple acute and chronic co-morbid conditions are typical.
- Common conditions may have atypical clinical presentations.
- Emergency procedures are associated with increased mortality and morbidity rates.
- Patients often have complex medication regimens.
- Potential diminished mental capacity makes history taking difficult.

with increased risk from anesthesia and surgery and these include emergency surgery, a high ASA physical status (classification greater than II), partial or complete immobility, intracavitary surgery, congestive heart failure, and trauma. Overall the presence of significant medical conditions indicated by a high ASA score is more important than chronologic age (Table 35-1) (Fig. 35-1).[5–9]

MORBIDITY AND MORTALITY RATES

Morbidity and mortality rates in older patients probably range from 3% to 10% following noncardiac surgery. The highest mortality rate follows emergency surgery; the lower mortality rates accordingly reflect nonemergent, less invasive procedures. For example, patients older than 80 years have a significantly higher mortality rate than those younger than 80 years for noncardiac surgery. Mortality rates vary widely depending on the type of procedure. For elective noninvasive surgeries such as transurethral resection of the prostate (TURP), hernia repair, knee replacement, and carotid endarterectomy, the mortality rate is less than 2%. However, in the oldest patients the development of a complication greatly influences the outcome. In patients over 80 years who developed one or more complications, the 30-day mortality rate was 26% versus 4% in patients without a complication. Death occurred most frequently following a cardiac arrest (88%), acute renal failure (52%), and myocardial infarction (48%).[10] In an analysis of surgical outcomes for patients 80 years of age and older, for every year above 80 there is an associated 5% increase in mortality rate; thus, a 90-year-old had a 50% higher risk of death compared to an 80-year-old.[10]

MEDICATIONS TO AVOID IN THE GERIATRIC POPULATION

An important aspect of risk reduction in geriatric patients is the avoidance of iatrogenic complications from medication side effects. Although it is rarely used, anesthesia

IV

Figure 35-1 Mortality rates. (Redrawn from Li G, Warner M, Lang BH, et al. Epidemiology of anesthesia-related mortality in the United States, 1999-2005. Anesthesiology 2009;110:759-765.)

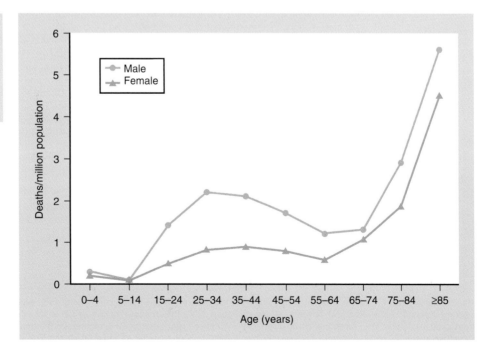

providers need to remember that meperidine should be avoided in elderly patients, except for the small doses commonly administered for shivering postoperatively. Geriatric patients have decreased cholinergic reserve and are at risk from developing side effects from central anticholinergic medications. The most prominent side effects include cognitive decline and delirium, and patients with Alzheimer's dementia or other types of dementia, such as multi-infarct and vascular dementia, are particularly sensitive. Perioperatively, antihistamines such as chlorpheniramine, promethazine, and the antiemetic scopolamine are the most commonly encountered anticholinergic medications to be avoided. Haloperidol also has anticholinergic properties, but in the small doses commonly prescribed for agitation and nausea, it is usually not an issue.

AGE-RELATED PHYSIOLOGIC CHANGES

Although the high mortality rate observed in older patients is mostly due to co-morbid conditions, age-related deterioration in organ function is observed in all body systems, leading to reduced reserve capacity. The addition of multiple co-morbid conditions further reduces reserve capacity, increasing the risk from anesthesia and surgery (Table 35-2).[8]

Table 35-2 Age-Related Changes in Selected Organ Systems

Organ System	Structural Changes	Functional Changes
Body composition	Decreased skeletal muscle mass Increased percentage of body fat Decreased total body water	Increased storage size for lipid-soluble drugs Decreased O_2 consumption and heat production
Central nervous system	Loss of neural tissue Decreased number of serotonin, acetylcholine, and dopamine receptors	Reduction in cerebral blood flow Decline in memory, reasoning, perception Disturbed sleep/wake cycle
Cardiovascular system	LV hypertrophy and decreased compliance Increase in vascular rigidity Decreased compliance of venous vessels	Decreased parasympathetic nervous system tone Increased sympathetic neuronal activity Desensitization of β-adrenergic receptors Increase in SVR and SBP Decrease in stroke volume and cardiac output Diastolic LV dysfunction Decreased maximally attainable HR
Pulmonary system	Increase in central airway size Decrease in small-airway diameter Decrease in elastic tissue, reorientation of elastic fibers, increased amount of collagen Decrease in respiratory muscle strength Increased chest wall stiffness Decrease in chest wall height and increase in AP diameter	Decreased respiratory center sensitivity Decreased effectiveness of coughing and swallowing Increase in lung compliance and decrease in chest wall compliance Decreased function alveolar surface area Decrease in DL_{CO_2} Decrease in PI_{max} and PE_{max} Decrease in ERV and VC Increase in RV and FRC with no change in TLC Increase in RV/TLC and FRC/TLC ratios Increase in closing volume and closing capacity Decrease in FVC, FEV_1, FEV_1/VC, and FEF at low lung volumes Increased A-a gradient and decrease in Pa_{O_2}
Renal system	Loss of tissue mass Decreased perfusion	Decreased GFR Reduced ability to dilute and concentrate urine and conserve sodium Decreased drug clearance
Hepatic system	Decrease in tissue mass Decrease in blood flow	Possible decrease in affinity for substrate Possible decrease in intrinsic activity Decreased first-pass metabolism of some drugs

A-a, alveolar-arterial; AP, anteroposterior; DL_{CO}^2, single-breath carbon monoxide diffusion capacity; ERV, expiratory reserve volume; FEF, peak expiratory flow rate—the peak flow rate during expiration; FEV_1, the amount that can be forcefully exhaled in the first second from a full inspiration; FRC, functional residual capacity; FVC, forced vital capacity; GFR, glomerular filtration rate; HR, heart rate; LV, left ventricle; RV, residual volume; SBP, systolic blood pressure; SVR, systemic vascular resistance; TLC, total lung capacity; VC, vital capacity.

Cardiovascular Changes

Aging leads to progressive stiffening and loss of compliance in the vasculature and the myocardium. This results from the collective effects of a gradual loss of elastin, increases in collagen, and damage to collagen through glycosylation and the deposition of free radicals in connective tissue. Systolic arterial blood pressure and pulse wave velocity increase, and the left ventricle faces greater impedance to outflow and subsequent myocardial hypertrophy, further reducing ventricular compliance. Diastolic dysfunction refers to the reduction of left ventricular relaxation during diastole. The impaired relaxation of the ventricle leads to a decrease in early diastolic filling; in the elderly this may be reduced as much as 50% compared to younger patients.[11-13] These alterations render the older patient very dependent on adequate atrial pressures and active atrial contraction to complete diastolic filling. Preoperatively diastolic dysfunction may be underestimated because patients frequently have vague symptoms. Approximately, one third of patients with normal preoperative left ventricular function have diastolic dysfunction.[14] Older patients with diastolic dysfunction may not tolerate even brief periods of atrial fibrillation and readily develop congestive heart failure in the setting of intravascular volume overload (Fig. 35-2).[15,16]

Aging also alters cardiovascular autonomic function. Vagal or parasympathetic tone is decreased and at the same time there is an increase in sympathetic nerve activity and plasma levels of noradrenaline. β-Adrenergic receptors are less responsive to stimulation with a lesser increase in heart rate and less arterial and venous relaxation with direct stimulation. α-Adrenergic receptor activity appears largely preserved. The reduction in baroreflex function and overall vascular stiffening leads to more labile blood pressure and predisposes elderly patients to orthostatic hypotension. This condition may be exaggerated during anesthesia, especially in volume-depleted patients. The impaired β-adrenergic receptor responsiveness reduces an older patient's ability to respond to an increase in demand through increased heart rate alone, and the elderly patient becomes very reliant on vascular tone and preload.

Myocardial fibrosis and fatty infiltration of pacemaker cells lead to conduction abnormalities such as sick sinus syndrome, atrial fibrillation, and frequent premature atrial contractions. The changes in the conduction system may lead to exaggerated bradycardia following the administration of opioids, such as remifentanil.

Cardiac function in the older patient is frequently compromised further by the development of cardiac disease. Cardiovascular disease occurs in over 75% of the U.S. population over the age of 75 years. The incidence of hypertension increases dramatically in older individuals and is a leading cause of congestive heart failure. Congestive heart failure is one of the most significant risk factors for death following anesthesia and surgery.[15]

Pulmonary Changes

In the perioperative period, 40% of deaths in patients older than 65 years are due to postoperative pulmonary complications.[17,18] Several predictable changes occur during aging, including a reduction in respiratory muscle strength, a decrease in chest wall compliance, and a decrease in the elastic recoil.

With aging the chest wall becomes stiffer and at the same time muscle strength is diminished, leading to an increase in the work of breathing. The aging chest is more barrel-shaped and the diaphragm can become flattened, negatively impacting chest wall dynamics. The combined impact of these changes can lead to diaphragmatic fatigue and a predisposition to respiratory failure in the postoperative period and difficulty weaning from a ventilator, especially in frail older patients. Pulmonary changes with aging are similar to those that occur with smoking-induced emphysema. They both have increased size of central airways and anatomic-physiologic dead space. The lack of elastic recoil in smaller airways can result in air-trapping with positive-pressure ventilation. Closing capacity is increased, and by the age of 65 years it exceeds functional residual capacity (FRC), leading to closure of small airways and increase in shunt fraction, predisposing older patients to hypoxemia.

In addition to structural changes with the lungs, alveolar gas exchange is also impacted by an age-related increase in ventilation-perfusion mismatch, decreased diffusing capacity, and an increase in dead space. There is a gradual decrease in resting arterial oxygen tension, leaving the older patient vulnerable to the development of significant hypoxemia with even minimal residual weakness or sedation.

Central nervous system changes also occur, leading to a decrease in hypoxemic and hypercapnic ventilatory drive

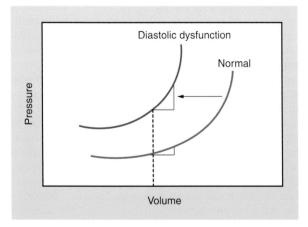

Figure 35-2 Depiction of the diastolic function.

IV

by 50% or more. The elderly patient has an increased susceptibility to narcotic-induced apnea, potentially leading to hypoxemia and hypercapnia.

Metabolic and Renal Changes

Metabolic and renal changes lead to significant changes in pharmacokinetics of anesthetic and analgesic drugs. Overall there is a decrease in the total body water and an increase in percentage of body fat, accompanied by a reduction of protein and muscle mass. Both plasma volume and intracellular water decline by 20% to 30% by the age of 75. This can lead to a significant increase in the initial volume of distribution and thus an increase in plasma concentration of an anesthetic drug. This can have important hemodynamic consequences. For example, following the administration of propofol, older patients have an exaggerated and prolonged hypotensive reaction. The effect is due to the combined effect of a higher initial plasma concentration and probably to an age-related delay in the redistribution of propofol from the central compartment. These and other age-related changes have led to the broad recommendation to reduce the initial drug dose and increase the intervals between boluses in elderly patients. As total body water declines, the percentage of fat increases, which can lead to increases in drug deposition of lipid-soluble drugs and delayed elimination.

Renal changes include a 20% to 25% decrease in renal cortical mass by the age of 80 years that may be exacerbated by co-morbid conditions such as hypertension and diabetes mellitus. Other renal changes include a decrease in renal blood flow with the number of functioning glomeruli and remaining glomeruli exhibiting an increase in sclerosis. There is a progressive reduction in glomerular filtration rate (GFR) from an average of 125 mL/min in a young adult to only 60 mL/min by age 80 years. As aging leads to significant reduction in protein, the serum creatinine in the older patient will not accurately reflect the degree of renal insufficiency in the geriatric patient.

Several changes predispose the older patient to fluid and electrolyte abnormalities, especially hypo- and hypernatremia. These changes include a reduction in tubular function and limited ability to concentrate urine appropriately and a reduction in the renin-angiotensin system and the secretion of antidiuretic hormone (ADH), impacting the geriatric patient's ability to regulate sodium appropriately. These changes predispose older patients to hyponatremia. Renal failure accounts for 20% of all perioperative deaths, and acute renal failure in elderly patients in the postoperative period has a more frequent mortality rate.[19]

Hepatic blood flow decreases and the size of the liver and enzyme systems decrease in the elderly patients. Both qualitative and quantitative reductions in protein binding occur, potentially leading to an increase in free fraction of protein-bound drugs.[20] Owing to the significant hepatic reserve, the impact on metabolism is less than on other systems, and hepatic aging has less clinical impact compared to age-related changes in renal function.

Changes in Basal Metabolic Rate

Metabolic rate and the effectiveness of peripheral vasoconstriction decrease in the elderly, making it more difficult for them to maintain body temperature during surgery and anesthesia. Hypothermia can lead to significant negative effects such as slowed metabolism of medications, shivering with subsequent increased oxygen demand, and potential myocardial ischemia, as well as increased coagulation. Active warming is an important component for most patients, and especially for geriatric patients undergoing procedures.[21]

Central Nervous System Changes

A gradual decrease in brain size occurs in aging, most likely secondary to a decrease in neuronal size. The loss in brain size is associated with an increase in ventricular volume and widening of sulci. Normal aging can be accompanied by cognitive changes such as mild memory difficulty and a decrease in speed of processing; however, the extent of these changes among individuals is widely variable. The number of neuroreceptors and neurotransmitters decrease even in the absence of dementia or recognized neurodegenerative diseases. The most significant declines are observed in acetylcholine and serotonin receptors in the cortex, dopamine receptors in the neostriata, and dopamine levels in substantia nigra and neostriata.

PERIOPERATIVE CARE IN THE ELDERLY

The preoperative evaluation (also see Chapter 13) in the older patient is challenging but remains an important aspect of the anesthetic. In all patients, there is an increasing emphasis on decreasing or even eliminating routine preoperative tests unless there is a specific medical indication. The challenge is what preoperative evaluations would specifically be required in elderly patients that may not be the case in younger patients. As for all preoperative assessments the overall goal is to minimize the risk of anesthesia through assessment of the patient, the existing co-morbidities, and related testing. In the older patient, the past medical history can be especially complex, and ultimately the functional assessment of the patient is one of the most important aspects of the preoperative evaluation. Excellent medical fitness, as described by activity level, is associated with a reduction in postoperative complications. Thus, in addition to the standard preoperative questions about the patient's past medical history, an assessment of function using activity scores, activities of daily living (ADLs), and

Table 35-3 Activities of Daily Living and Instrumental Activities of Daily Living*

Activities of Daily Living
Bathing
Dressing
Toileting
Transferring
Eating

Instrumental Activities of Daily Living
Use of telephone
Use of public transportation
Shopping
Preparation of meals
Housekeeping
Taking medications properly
Managing personal finances

*The ability of the patient to perform the listed tasks independently, partially independently, or with complete assistance required is recorded.

instrumental activities of daily living (IADLs) is recommended for frail older patients (Table 35-3).

As questioned previously, routine laboratory testing should not be performed just because a patient is elderly alone. All laboratory testing should be based on the patient's medical history and the anticipated surgery.[22–24] Most recommendations are no longer using age-based criteria for electrocardiograms (ECGs) and other testing.[25] Older patients with a cardiac history or a history of active cardiac disease will need a preoperative ECG. The preoperative ECG may reveal significant abnormalities and confirm the presence of preexisting cardiac disease such as left ventricular hypertrophy and prior myocardial infarction. Comparison with a prior ECG is recommended to establish the timing of a possible cardiac event, yet preoperative abnormalities on ECGs have a low specificity for predicting postoperative complications. Furthermore, an older patient may have a normal ECG and still have significant occult cardiac dysfunction.[26,27] A routine chest radiograph is not indicated preoperatively in the absence of pulmonary symptoms or abnormalities on physical examination. A chest radiograph may be indicated to assess cardiopulmonary status such as pulmonary congestion or the presence of pneumonia.

Patients with preexisting preoperative cognitive difficulties probably carry an increased risk of postoperative delirium and possibly postoperative cognitive dysfunction (POCD), which is discussed later.[28] Preoperative cognitive function assessment should be considered in patients at risk from the development of postoperative delirium. The cognitive testing scales include the mini-mental status examination, but this is not a sensitive screen for dementia and a normal score does not rule out underlying dysfunction.

The preoperative evaluation of institutionalized elderly patients can be especially challenging. These patients often have significant co-morbid conditions that may make the preoperative interview challenging. In addition, a separate trip to a hospital for a preoperative evaluation may not be feasible. In these patients a history and list of medications may be reviewed prior to the day of surgery anesthetia. This approach may also be useful for cataract patients, who carry an intense burden of disease, but are undergoing a very low risk noninvasive procedure.[23] For all patients with cognitive dysfunction from dementia or neurologic disease, the person who can provide consent for the patient must be identified and how that person can be reached. The preoperative assessment also provides an opportunity to initiate a discussion on advanced health care directives.

Medications

The preoperative examination should include a complete history of all medications including over-the-counter drugs. More than 90% of persons older than 65 years of age use at least one drug, 40% take five or more drugs per week, and 12% used 10 or more drugs per week on average.[29,30] These numbers increase in very old patients, especially those that are hospitalized. In general, most medications, especially cardiac and antihypertensive medications, should be continued through the morning of surgery, with the exception of angiotensin-converting enzyme (ACE) inhibitors and Angiotensin II Receptor Blockers (ARBs).[31,32] Continuation of ACE inhibitors has been associated with increased hypotension immediately following induction of anesthesia, which means that these drugs should not be taken for at least 12 hours prior to anesthesia. Decisions regarding platelet antagonists and anticoagulants should be made with the patient's primary care doctor and the surgeon (Table 35-4).

Intraoperative Monitoring (See Chapter 20)

Standard ASA monitoring is required during the administration of any anesthetic. In the older patient additional hemodynamic monitoring is often required for invasive and prolonged surgeries and in patients with significant co-morbid conditions.

Choice of Anesthesia

As with all anesthetics, the choice of general versus regional anesthesia or sedation will depend on the surgical requirements, the patient's physical status and the patient's preferences. In elderly patients, there is no evidence that one type of anesthesia is safer than another, although regional anesthesia may confer certain benefits such as improved postoperative pain control, decreased blood intraoperative loss during hip surgery, and decreased postoperative venous thrombosis.[33–35]

Table 35-4 Drugs Often Taken by Elderly Patients That May Contribute to Adverse Effects or Drug Interactions

Drug/Drug Class	Response
Diuretics	Hypokalemia Hypovolemia
Centrally acting antihypertensives	Decreased autonomic nervous system activity
β-Adrenergic antagonists	Decreased autonomic nervous system activity Decreased anesthetic requirements Bronchospasm Bradycardia
Cardiac antidysrhythmics	Potentiation of neuromuscular blocking drugs
Digitalis	Cardiac dysrhythmias Cardiac conduction disturbances
Tricyclic antidepressants	Anticholinergic effects
Antibiotics	Potentiation of neuromuscular blocking drugs
Oral hypoglycemics Alcohol	Hypoglycemia Increased anesthetic requirements Delirium tremens

Table 35-5 Adjustments to Anesthetic and Adjuvant Drug Administration in Elderly Patients

Drug/Drug Class	Adjustment
Volatile anesthetics	Decrease inspired concentration
Intravenous induction drugs (thiopental, propofol)	Small to moderate decreases in initial dose Decreased maintenance infusion
Opioids	Decrease initial dose* Increased incidence of skeletal muscle rigidity Increased duration of systemic and neuraxial effects Increased incidence of depression of ventilation
Local anesthetics (spinal and epidural)	Small to moderate decrease in segmental dose requirements Anticipate prolonged effects
Benzodiazepines	Modest decrease in initial dose Anticipate marked increase in duration of action
Atropine	Increased dose needed for comparable heart rate response Anticipate possible central anticholinergic syndrome
Isoproterenol	Increased dose needed for comparable heart rate response

*Supportive data not available.

General Anesthesia

Elderly patients are more likely to be edentulous compared with young patients. Thus, laryngoscopy may be easier, but difficulty during ventilation via a mask may necessitate the use of an oral or nasopharangeal airway to maintain a patent airway (also see Chapter 16). Reduced extension of the neck secondary to advanced arthritis may limit head and neck manipulation during laryngoscopy, and vertebrobasilar disease may predispose older patients to cerebral ischemia with neck manipulation. Older patients present in more advanced stages of disease (for example, with end-stage rheumatoid arthritis), which may increase the frequency of a difficult airway. Elderly patients frequently exhibit exaggerated hemodynamic responses to laryngoscopy, which is an obvious concern in patients with underlying cardiac conditions. A small dose of lidocaine (e.g., 50 mg) intravenously or short-acting β-adrenergic blockade with induction of anesthesia can attenuate this response. An age-related decrease in pharyngeal reflexes predisposes older patients to pulmonary aspiration of gastric contents. Prolonged periods of intraoperative hypotension may lead to an increase in postoperative morbidity in older patients. Hypotension should be avoided in older patients and arterial blood pressure probably should arbitrarily be maintained within 10% of starting levels.

ANESTHETIC DRUGS

Pharmacokinetic and pharmacodynamic changes with aging necessitate dosing adjustments for most anesthetic drugs. In general "start low, go slow" remains a valid axiom when taking care of elderly patients (Table 35-5).

INTRAVENOUS ANESTHETICS (Also See Chapter 9)

Propofol is commonly used to induce general anesthesia. The mechanism of action appears to be mediated through the central γ-aminobutyric acid A ($GABA_A$) receptors. Propofol produces a rapid loss of consciousness, apnea in sufficient doses, and a dose-dependent reduction in vascular resistance and preload. The hemodynamic effects of propofol can be greatly exaggerated in older patients, especially if their intravascular volumes are depleted possibly leading to significant cardiac or cerebral ischemia. The initial dose of propofol should be reduced and the time interval between repeated doses increased to prevent an exaggerated and potentially prolonged hypotension. Propofol does allow for rapid recovery with minimal delayed cognitive effects. Given in smaller total doses than in younger adults, propofol infusions probably provide a more stable hemodynamic course, but the dose required for sedation should be reduced.

Etomidate, a carboxylated imidazole ring, has the disadvantage of producing some disinhibitory effects leading to development of myoclonus, which has been observed in 30% to 60% of patients. Yet its minimal cardiovascular effects make it preferred in patients in whom a decrease in blood pressure may not be tolerated. It is an excellent anesthetic for an emergency situation. The volume of distribution for etomidate is reduced with aging and a 50% reduction in dose is recommended in patients 80 years of age or older.

The anxiolytic and sedative properties of midazolam make it an excellent premedication for anesthesia, and the short duration, and absence of significant active metabolites or cardiovascular effects increases the utility in the elderly population. Although pharmacokinetic changes can prolong elimination, especially in obese elderly patients, the increase in sensitivity observed in geriatric patients appears to be due mainly to a pharmacodynamic change within the benzodiazepine GABA receptor unit.[36] In general the dose of midazolam should be reduced by 50% and repeat doses administered in increments of 0.5 mg or less. Older patients are susceptible to midazolam-induced apnea, and when administered during spinal anesthesia there may be an increased risk of respiratory depression. Unwanted effects of midazolam can be reversed with flumazenil. Long-acting benzodiazepines have been associated with delirium in the elderly due to prolonged clearance and active metabolites. For these reasons, diazepam and lorazepam are not recommended in elderly patients.

INHALED ANESTHETICS (Also See Chapter 8)
The minimum alveolar concentration (MAC) of inhaled anesthetics decreases predictably by 6% every decade after age 20 years. Thus, the MAC at age 90 years is reduced by 30% compared to a 40-year-old. This change most likely reflects a combination of age-related cerebral atrophy and alterations in neurotransmitter balance.[37]

MUSCLE RELAXANTS (Also See Chapter 12)
Aging does not increase sensitivity to muscle relaxants at the neuromuscular junction. Of course, age-related diseases (e.g., kidney dysfunction) may increase sensitivity. Furthermore, decreases in hepatic metabolism and renal clearance may lead to delayed elimination of nondepolarizing agents. This is most prominent for pancuronium, for which 85% is eliminated through renal clearance, and the drug probably should be avoided in elderly patients. Vecuronium and rocuronium are less dependent on renal excretion and their effects are less likely to be significantly prolonged. Cisatracurium and atracurium are dependent on Hoffman elimination that is not impacted by aging or renal or hepatic function. To ensure complete recovery from neuromuscular blockade, monitoring of neuromuscular blockade should be done to assure that successive doses are appropriate and complete reversal from neostigmine or sugammadex has occurred prior to extubation of the trachea. In the older patient, even a small degree of

weakness can result in a clinically significant respiratory incident during transport to and while in the postanesthesia care unit (PACU).

OPIOIDS
Pharmacodynamic changes in elderly patients account for the increase in the sensitivity of the brain to opioids, and pharmacokinetic changes impacting elimination and distribution of opioids are less significant. Opioid doses should be reduced by 50% in older patients. Interindividual variability of opioid response is common among older patients and it is important to titrate these drugs to desired effect. Fentanyl is a popular short-acting lipid-soluble opioid with a large volume of distribution. The dose should be reduced by 50%, largely due to pharmacodynamic changes. Remifentanil is an ultrashort-acting mu receptor agonist that is metabolized by plasma esterases. The bolus dose and the infusion rates should be reduced in the elderly and titrated to effect. Morphine is one of the most popular postoperative analgesics administered. In elderly patients there is a reduction in the volume of distribution and a potential accumulation of active metabolites morphine 3-glucuronide and morphine 6-glucuronide that are eliminated via the kidneys.[38-40]

Meperidine has been a popular opioid for sedation and analgesia with nonanesthesia providers. In older patients, administration of meperidine causes delirium, possibly through anticholinergic mechanism and accumulation of active metabolite normeperidine. It is not recommended for elderly patients for sedation or analgesia.

Monitored Anesthesia Care (Also See Chapters 37 and 38)

Assistance from anesthesiology is more frequently requested for nonsurgical procedures such as endoscopic retrograde cholangiopancreatography (ERCP), advanced gastrointestinal procedures, bronchoscopy, and radiologic interventions. Elderly patients with complex medical conditions are frequent candidates for these noninvasive procedures and administration of anesthesia can be especially challenging. In general, geriatric principles should be applied, and reduction of the dose, infusion, and an increase in bolus interval are recommended. Due to age-related heightened sensitivity to narcotics and benzodiazepines, as well as pulmonary changes, older patients are particularly susceptible to developing hypoventilation and apnea during procedures. Supplemental oxygen and monitoring of ventilation through end-tidal CO_2 is recommended. Standard intravenously administered anesthetics that can be used for MAC include benzodiazepines, midazolam, short-acting fentanyl, and remifentanil. In addition, small doses of ketamine, 10 mg to 30 mg intravenously, can be a valuable adjunct for procedures, especially if associated with painful stimuli. At these small doses the positive hemodynamic

IV

effects of ketamine are less pronounced and can be treated with low doses of labetalol. Dexmedetomidine, a relatively new, centrally acting α_2-agonist, has no adverse respiratory effects and can provide both analgesia and sedation. Side effects that may preclude its use are prolonged sedation, bradycardia, and hypotension.

Neuraxial Anesthesia (Also See Chapter 17)

Spinal and epidural anesthesia compared to general anesthesia do not alter the 30-day mortality rate in elderly patients. However, these techniques may be particularly useful for a wide range of orthopedic procedures such as hip fracture repair, lower extremity joint replacement, transurethral resection of the prostate, and gynecologic and lower extremity vascular procedures. Age-related changes including calcification of the interspinous ligaments and ligamentum flavum and narrowing of the intervertebral foramina, combined with a reduction in flexibility and difficulty positioning, may make the placement of the needle for a spinal or epidural block more challenging. Age-related changes can also lead to exaggerated spread of the local anesthetic within the epidural space and a higher than expected anesthetic level. Similarly for spinal anesthesia, the cephalad spread may be wider than expected and the dose of local anesthetic should be reduced in older patients. Hypotension is the most likely hemodynamic consequence of neuraxial anesthesia. Hypotension is due to vasodilation from the sympathetic blockade, causing a decrease in systemic vascular resistance and central venous pressure and a redistribution of blood volume to the extremities from central splanchnic and mesenteric vascular beds. Hypotension is of particular concern in very elderly patients with limited cardiac reserve, and may be exaggerated in patients with baseline hypertension. Pretreatment with crystalloid does not consistently offset the hypotension following a spinal block. Treatment of hypotension with vasopressors, such as ephedrine and phenylephrine, is frequently required.[41-43]

POSTOPERATIVE CARE

Pain

The treatment of intraoperative and postoperative pain in the elderly patient is an important part of the anesthetic plan.[44-46] Age-related reduction in nerve conductivity and receptors may lead older patients to experience less pain following surgery,[47,48] but untreated pain can have significant adverse consequences. Postoperative pain has been associated with increased length of stay, increased morbidity, pulmonary complications, and delirium. The longer a patient stays in the hospital, the more the risks of complications increase. Generational and cultural issues may lead older patients to complain less about pain, and elderly patients frequently have lower expectations for successful treatment. For cognitively intact elders patient-controlled analgesia (PCA) is the preferred method for administering postoperative intravenous narcotics.[49] Treatment of pain in patients with significant dementia is challenging both to assess and treat. If possible, pain should be assessed using a specially designed pain scale such as the PAINAD. For demented and nonverbal elders, pain medication should be offered on a regularly scheduled interval as opposed to an as-needed basis.

Opioid use can be reduced by concomitant administration of acetaminophen.[50] Nonsteroidal anti-inflammatory drugs (NSAIDs) in older patients cause renal failure and gastrointestinal hemorrhage, and medications such as ibuprofen and ketorolac should be administered cautiously. When administered, the dose of ketorolac should be reduced to 15 mg IV every 6 hours, with a 60 mg 24-hour dose maximum.

Gabapentin, originally released for its antiepileptic properties, is another useful opioid adjunct for postoperative pain control. Although most commonly used to treat chronic neuropathic pain, it has been used preemptively before surgery as well as following surgery. It is an oral medication excreted renally, and in elderly patients a reduction in dose is recommended; larger doses are associated with sedation.

The role of nerve blocks for postoperative pain control in elderly patients is increasingly important (see Chapter 40). Adequate, but safe, postoperative analgesia is very important in the elderly. The total dose of local anesthetic should be reduced as the metabolism and clearance of local anesthetics is delayed in advanced age. Postoperative epidural analgesia with local anesthetics or opioids probably improves postoperative pulmonary outcomes including (1) improved postoperative pain control, (2) decline in atelectasis, (3) improved tracheal extubation variables, and (4) shorter intensive care unit stays.[51]

Postoperative Neurologic Events

The most common postoperative neurologic events in the elderly are postoperative delirium and postoperative cognitive dysfunction (POCD).[52] Delirium refers to an acute state of confusion that generally occurs within 1 to 3 days following surgery. It can persist for weeks or months after surgery. Delirium is not unique to surgery patients; it also commonly develops in hospitalized elderly patients, especially those admitted to the intensive care unit. Delirium is a significant source of morbidity and occurs in 15% to 60% of elderly patients who have a hip fracture.[53,54] POCD can increase length of hospital stay, require discharge to rehabilitation facilities as opposed to home, and is associated with an increased mortality rate. There are multiple causes of delirium in the postoperative patient. The more common ones include acute metabolic derangements such as hypo- or hypernatremia, hypoxemia, anemia, uremia, sepsis, uncontrolled pain, disorientation, depression, residual effects of anticholinergic medications, and alcohol withdrawal. Treatment of delirium should start with a search for an underlying reversible condition such as hypoxemia or pain; unfortunately often there is no single factor that is easily reversed. Agitated patients may benefit from intravenously administered small doses of haloperidol.

POCD is a distinct cognitive disorder found in patients after anesthesia.[52] It is diagnosed through neuropsychological testing and results in subtle changes in mental ability; unlike patients with delirium, POCD patients are not acutely confused or agitated. In some studies 10% of older patients developed POCD 3 months after major noncardiac surgery. In most cases it resolved by 6 to12 months, although its occurrence has been associated with an increased mortality rate. The role of anesthetics in the development of POCD is a current focus of significant research.

Perioperative stroke is an uncommon event following general surgery; it occurs more frequently after head and neck, vascular, and cardiac surgery. Risk factors for a postoperative stroke include advanced age and predisposing co-morbidities such as hypertension and reduced ejection fraction of less than 40%. The most frequent incidence of stroke occurs after cardiac and aortic surgery. Most perioperative strokes are embolic and ischemic. A perioperative stroke is associated with prolonged hospitalization, increased disability, and death following surgery.

REDUCTION OF PERIOPERATIVE RISK

Elderly patients have high mortality and morbidity rates after surgery, especially after major and emergent surgery. Reduction of risk should be aimed at avoiding complications and limiting risk. The patient should be in optimal condition preoperatively. Unfortunately it is not always possible to delay surgery, especially in emergent situations. Administration of perioperative β-adrenergic blockers may reduce postoperative cardiac events through a reduction in sympathetic tone, improved oxygen myocardial supply/demand, and reduction in ventricular arrhythmias as well as decreasing shear stress surrounding atherosclerotic plaque. Perioperative β-adrenergic blockade should be continued for the entire perioperative period; abrupt discontinuation can increase the incidence of adverse events. Patients with AHA Class 1 or 2a indications should receive β-adrenergic blockers; more data are still needed to establish the most effective use of perioperative β-blockade for elderly patients.[55] As mentioned previously, appropriate pain control is

Table 35-6 Guidelines for Treating Geriatric Patients

1. Advanced chronologic age is not a contraindication to surgery.
2. Clinical presentation of disease may have been atypical, leading to delays and errors in diagnosis.
3. Assume interindividual variability and titrate medications to physiologic effect when possible.
4. Expect complexity: Multiple medications and illnesses are common, and persons older than 65 years of age have on average 3.5 medical diseases.
5. Diminished organ reserve can be unpredictable and difficult to measure preoperatively; limitations may become apparent only during stress.
6. A disproportionate increase in perioperative risk may occur without adequate preoperative optimization—for example, after emergent procedures.
7. Meticulous attention to detail can help avoid minor complications, which in elderly patients can rapidly escalate into major adverse events.
8. Impact of extrinsic factors, such as smoking or those related to the environment or socioeconomic status, is difficult to quantify.

also important, and epidural analgesia may have a significant role in preventing pulmonary complications. Other measures that may be used to limit pulmonary complications include using positive end-expiratory pressure (5 to 10 cm H_2O) to maintain FRC above closing capacity. Maintaining a higher inspired oxygen concentration ($>30\%$) during surgery may reduce surgical infections and lead to a reduced incidence of nausea and vomiting (Table 35-6).[18,51,56]

SUMMARY

In summary, aging is associated with significant physiologic changes and an increase in co-morbid conditions that influence the administration and choice of anesthetics. In the future there will be even larger numbers of elderly patients undergoing surgical procedures. Anesthetic plans must be designed to reduce or minimize postoperative complications.

QUESTIONS OF THE DAY

1. What are the lung structural changes expected with aging? What is the impact on gas exchange?
2. What are the expected changes in the minimum alveolar concentration (MAC) of inhaled anesthetics for each decade after 20 years of age?

IV

3. What changes in neuraxial anesthesia technique should be made in elderly patients?
4. What is the incidence of delirium in elderly postoperative patients? What factors can contribute to the development of delirium?

ACKNOWLEDGMENT

The editors and publisher would like to thank Dr. Jacqueline M. Leung for contributing a chapter on this topic to the prior edition of this work. It has served as the foundation for the current chapter.

REFERENCES

1. Cook DJ, Rooke GA: Priorities in perioperative geriatrics, *Anesth Analg* 96:1823–1836, 2003.
2. Li G, Warner M, Lang BH, et al: Epidemiology of anesthesia-related mortality in the United States, 1999–2005, *Anesthesiology* 110:759–765, 2009.
3. Fleisher LA, Pasternak LR, Herbert R, et al: Inpatient hospital admission and death after outpatient surgery in elderly patients, *Arch Surg* 139:67–72, 2004.
4. Hosking MP, Warner MA, Lobdell CM, et al: Outcomes of surgery in patients 90 years of age and older, *JAMA* 261:1909–1915, 1989.
5. Liu LL, Leung JM: Predicting adverse postoperative outcomes in patients aged 80 years or older, *J Am Geriatr Soc* 48:405–412, 2000.
6. Kheterpal S, O'Reilly M, Englesbe MJ, et al: Preoperative and intraoperative predictors of cardiac adverse events after general, vascular, and urological surgery, *Anesthesiology* 110:58–66, 2009.
7. Turrentine FE, Wang H, Simpson VB, et al: Surgical risk factors, morbidity, and mortality in elderly patients, *J Am Coll Surg* 203:865–877, 2006.
8. Leung JM, Dzankic S: Relative importance of preoperative health status versus intraoperative factors in predicting postoperative adverse outcomes in geriatric surgical patients, *J Am Geriatr Soc* 49:1080–1085, 2001.
9. Chung F, Mezei G, Tong D: Adverse events in ambulatory surgery. A comparison between elderly and younger patients, *Can J Anaesth* 46:309–321, 1999.
10. Hamel MB, Henderson WG, Khuri SF, et al: Surgical outcomes for patients aged 80 and older: Morbidity and mortality from major noncardiac surgery, *J Am Geriatr Soc* 53:424–429, 2005.
11. Rooke GA: Cardiovascular aging and anesthetic implications, *J Cardiothorac Vasc Anesth* 17:512–523, 2003.
12. Silvay G, Castillo JG, Chikwe J, et al: Cardiac anesthesia and surgery in geriatric patients, *Semin Cardiothorac Vasc Anesth* 12:18–28, 2008.
13. Groban L: Diastolic dysfunction in the older heart, *J Cardiothorac Vasc Anesth* 19:228–236, 2005.
14. Phillip B, Pastor D, Bellows W: The prevalence of preoperative diastolic filling abnormalities in geriatric surgical patients, *Anesth Analg* 97:1214–1221, 2003.
15. Hammill BG, Curtis LH, Bennett-Guerrero E, et al: Impact of heart failure on patients undergoing major noncardiac surgery, *Anesthesiology* 108:559–567, 2008.
16. Groban L, Butterworth J: Perioperative management of chronic heart failure, *Anesth Analg* 103:557–575, 2006.
17. Sprung J, Gajic O, Warner DO: Review article: Age related alterations in respiratory function-anesthetic considerations, *Can J Anaesth* 53:1244–1257, 2006.
18. Warner DO: Preventing postoperative pulmonary complications, *Anesthesiology* 92:1467–1472, 2000.
19. Novis BK, Roizen MF, Aronson S, et al: Association of preoperative risk factors with postoperative acute renal failure, *Anesth Analg* 78:143–149, 1994.
20. Schmucker DL: Age related changes in liver structure and function: Implications for disease? *Exp Gerontol* 40:650–659, 2005.
21. Kenney WL, Munce TA: Invited review: Aging and human temperature regulation, *J Appl Physiol* 95:2598–2603, 2003.
22. Narr BJ: Outcomes of patients with no laboratory assessment before anesthesia and a surgical procedure, *Mayo Clin Proc* 72:505–509, 1997.
23. Schein OD, Katz J, Bass EB, et al: The value of routine preoperative medical testing before cataract surgery: Study of medical testing for cataract surgery, *N Engl J Med* 342:168–175, 2000.
24. Dzankic S, Pastor D, Gonzalez C, et al: The prevalence and predictive value of abnormal preoperative laboratory tests in elderly surgical patients, *Anesth Analg* 93:301–308, 2001.
25. Smetana GW, Macpherson DS: The case against routine preoperative laboratory testing, *Med Clin North Am* 87:7–40, 2003.
26. Liu L, Dzankic S, Leung JM: Preoperative electrocardiogram abnormalities do not predict postoperative cardiac complications in geriatric surgical patients, *J Am Geriatr Soc* 50:1186–1191, 2002.
27. Noordzij PG, Boersma E, Bax JJ, et al: Prognostic value of routine preoperative electrocardiography in patients undergoing noncardiac surgery, *Am J Cardiol* 97:1103–1106, 2006.
28. Silverstein JH, Timberger M, Reich DL, et al: Central nervous system dysfunction after noncardiac surgery and anesthesia in the elderly, *Anesthesiology* 106:622–628, 2007.
29. Qato DM, Alexander GC, Conti RM, et al: Use of prescription and over-the-counter medications and dietary supplements among older adults in the United States, *JAMA* 300:2867–2878, 2008.
30. Gurwitz JH, Field TS, Harrold LR, et al: Incidence and preventability of adverse drug events among older persons in the ambulatory setting, *JAMA* 289:1107–1116, 2003.
31. Kheterpal S, Khodaparast O, Shanks A, et al: Chronic angiotensin-converting enzyme inhibitor or angiotensin receptor blocker therapy combined with diuretic therapy is associated with increased episodes of hypotension in noncardiac surgery, *J Cardiothorac Vasc Anesth* 22:180–186, 2008.
32. Rosenman DJ, McDonald FS, Ebbert JO, et al: Clinical consequences of withholding versus administering renin-angiotensin-aldosterone system antagonists in the preoperative period, *J Hosp Med* 3:319–325, 2008.
33. Rodgers A, Walker N, Schug S, et al: Reduction of postoperative mortality and morbidity with epidural or spinal anesthesia: Results from overview of randomized trials, *BMJ* 321:1493–1501, 2000.
34. Urwin SC, Parker MJ, Griffiths R: General versus regional anaesthesia for hip fracture surgery: A meta-analysis of randomized trials, *Br J Anaesth* 84:450–455, 2000 (erratum in *Br J Anaesth* 88:619, 2002).
35. Rasmussen LS, Johnson T, Kuipers HM, et al: Does anaesthesia cause postoperative cognitive dysfunction? A randomized study of regional versus

general anaesthesia in 438 elderly patients, *Acta Anaesthesiol Scand* 47:260–266, 2003.

36. Jacobs JR, Reves JG, Marty J, et al: Aging increases pharmacodynamic sensitivity to the hypnotic effects of midazolam, *Anesth Analg* 801:143–148, 1995.

37. Nickalls RW, Mapleson WW: Age-related iso-MAC charts for isoflurane, sevoflurane and desflurane in man, *Br J Anaesth* 91:170–174, 2003.

38. Minto CF, Schnider TW, Egan TD, et al: Influence of age and gender on the pharmacokinetics and pharmacodynamics of remifentanil. I. Model development, *Anesthesiology* 86:10–23, 1997.

39. Cepeda MS, Farrar JT, Baumgarten M, et al: Side effects of opioids during short-term administration: Effect of age, gender, and race, *Clin Pharmacol Ther* 74:102–112, 2003.

40. Bentley JB, Borel JD, Nenad RE Jr, et al: Age and fentanyl pharmacokinetics, *Anesth Analg* 61:968–971, 1987.

41. Simon MJ, Veering BT, Stienstra R, et al: The effects of age on neural blockade and hemodynamic changes after epidural anesthesia with ropivacaine, *Anesth Analg* 94:1325–1330, 2002.

42. Pitkanen M, Haapaniemi L, Tuominen M, et al: Influence of age on spinal anaesthesia with isobaric 0.5 percent bupivicaine, *Br J Anaesth* 56:279–284, 1984.

43. Critchley LA: Hypotension, subarachnoid block and the elderly patient, *Anaesthesia* 51:1139–1143, 1996.

44. Aubrun F: Management of postoperative analgesia in elderly patients, *Reg Anesth Pain Med* 30:363–379, 2005.

45. Aubrun F, Monsel S, Langeron O, et al: Postoperative titration of intravenous morphine in the elderly patient, *Anesthesiology* 96:17–23, 2002.

46. Vaurio LE, Sands LP, Wang Y, et al: Postoperative delirium: The importance of pain and pain management, *Anesth Analg* 102:1267–1273, 2006.

47. Verdu E, Ceballos D, Vilches JJ, et al: Influence of aging on peripheral nerve function and regeneration, *J Peripher Nerv Syst* 5:191–208, 2000.

48. Gibson SJ, Farrell M: A review of age differences in the neurophysiology of nociception and the perceptual experience of pain, *Clin J Pain* 20:227–239, 2004.

49. Gagliese L, Jackson M, Ritvo P, et al: Age is not an impediment to effective use of patient-controlled analgesia by surgical patients, *Anesthesiology* 93:601–610, 2000.

50. Remy C, Marret E: Bonnet F. Effects of acetaminophen on morphine side-effects and consumption after major surgery: Meta-analysis of randomized controlled trials, *Br J Anaesth* 94:505–513, 2005.

51. Rigg JR, Jamrozik K, Myles PS, et al: Epidural anesthesia and analgesia and outcome of major surgery: A randomized trial, *Lancet* 359:1276–1282, 2002.

52. Moller JT, Cluitmans P, Rasmussen LS, et al: Long-term postoperative cognitive dysfunction in the elderly ISPOCD1 study. ISPOCD investigators. International Study of Post-Operative Cognitive Dysfunction, *Lancet* 351:857–861, 1998.

53. Marcantonio ER, Flacker JM, Michaels M, et al: Delirium is independently associated with poor functional recovery after hip fracture, *J Am Geriatr Soc* 48:618–624, 2000.

54. Inouye SK: Delirium in older persons, *N Engl J Med* 354:1157–1165, 2006.

55. Fleisher LA, Beckman JA, Brown KA, et al: ACC/AHA 2007 guidelines on perioperative cardiovascular evaluation and care for noncardiac surgery: A report of the American College of Cardiology/American Heart Association Task Force on Practice Guidelines (Writing Committee to Revise the 2002 Guidelines on Perioperative Cardiovascular Evaluation for Noncardiac Surgery). Developed in collaboration with the American Society of Echocardiography, American Society of Nuclear Cardiology, Heart Rhythm Society, Society of Cardiovascular Anesthesiologists, Society for Cardiovascular Angiography and Interventions, Society for Vascular Medicine and Biology, and Society for Vascular Surgery, *Circulation* 116: e418–e499, 2007.

56. Lawrence VA, Cornell JE, Smetana GW: Strategies to reduce postoperative pulmonary complications after noncardiothoracic surgery: Systematic review for the American College of Physicians, *Ann Intern Med* 144:596–608, 2006.

IV

36 ORGAN TRANSPLANTATION

Randolph H. Steadman and Victor W. Xia

Patients waiting for a transplantable organ share a hope for the future that is predicated on the availability of a donor. Donor death must be declared prior to organ procurement. Donation after brain death (DBD) is the most common setting in which donation occurs.[1] Organ shortages have led to donation after cardiac death (DCD).[2] The ethical considerations related to DCD donation are challenging, yet DCD donation is increasing in response to the national organ shortage.[3,4]

CONSIDERATIONS FOR ORGAN TRANSPLANTATION

Because of the shortage of available organs not all potential recipients on the waiting list survive long enough to undergo a transplant. Those who do, wait a year or more. Prelisting assessments may be outdated by the time an organ is identified, and supplemental testing may be indicated. This testing may necessitate a deferral of the scheduled transplant, which must be weighed against the risk of further deterioration that can preclude transplantation.

Untreated systemic infection, incurable malignancy, untreated substance abuse, and the lack of sufficient social support to comply with post-transplant care can preclude transplantation.

Once the decision is made to proceed with transplantation, coordination between the donor procedure and multiple recipient hospitals may be involved. Because not all donor organs are suitable for transplantation, the recipient operation should not begin until visual or biopsy-based confirmation of organ suitability has been made. During the time between the identification of the donor and the procurement surgery, the recipient's latest laboratory values are ascertained. If necessary, dialysis can be performed. The anesthetic plan is reviewed with the patient and the family, questions and concerns are addressed, and the patient's consent is obtained.

KIDNEY TRANSPLANTATION

Kidney transplantation confers a survival advantage over dialysis for the management of renal failure.[5] The best organ survival occurs from transplantation with grafts from living donors, but even marginal deceased donor grafts confer a survival advantage over dialysis.[6] Marginal, or extended criteria donor (ECD) grafts have lower graft survival rates than standard grafts. Criteria for ECD grafts include older and diabetic donors, and grafts with a prolonged duration of cold or warm ischemia, as seen with long preservation times and DCD donors, respectively.

Transplant recipients who undergo a prolonged period of dialysis before transplantation have decreased post-transplant survival compared to patients who do not require pretransplant dialysis (Table 36-1).[7] Exposure to uremic toxins may affect myocardial contractility and cardiovascular risk.

Preoperative Assessment (Also See Chapter 13)

Because of the shortage of deceased donor grafts, the average time on the waiting list in the United States is longer than 3 years for recipients of deceased donor grafts. This makes it challenging to maintain an up-to-date pretransplant assessment.

Diabetes is the most common cause of end-stage renal disease, followed by hypertension (Table 36-2). These two causes alone account for over two thirds of the cases of renal failure. Patients with these conditions should be medically managed to achieve treatment goals while on the waiting list.

Cardiovascular disease is responsible for over 50% of deaths in patients receiving dialysis. After transplant, the cardiovascular risk diminishes from a tenfold to a twofold increase compared to that of normal patients. Accordingly, the preoperative assessment should focus on screening for ischemic heart disease and congestive

Table 36-1 Kidney Transplantation Facts

- The kidney is the most frequently transplanted solid organ.
- More than 10,000 deceased donor and 6000 live donor kidney transplant procedures are performed annually in the United States.
- Five-year post-transplantation survival rates are 91% for recipients of live donor grafts, 83% for standard (non-ECD) deceased donor recipients, and 70% for recipients of grafts from ECDs.
- Transplantation improves survival over that achieved with dialysis, which carries a 20% annual mortality risk.

ECD, extended criteria donor.
From 2008 OPTN/SRTR Annual Report 1998-2007. HHS/HRSA/HSB/DOT.[7]

Table 36-2 Kidney Transplant Recipient: Preoperative Assessment

Cardiovascular
  Ischemic heart disease
  Congestive heart failure
  Hypertension
Diabetes
  Hyperkalemia
  Acidosis
  Anemia
  Dialysis history

heart failure. Ischemic heart disease may be silent, particularly in diabetic patients. Stress echocardiography is probably superior to thallium imaging in predicting postoperative cardiac events.[8] Coronary angiography, accompanied by therapeutic intervention for significant lesions, should be considered in patients with reversible ischemia or in those with significant risk.

Congestive heart failure is prevalent in dialysis patients but, in the absence of ischemic heart disease, does not preclude safe transplantation. Ejection fraction typically improves after transplantation. The preoperative focus is on optimal medical management of heart failure and maintenance of intravascular fluid balance.

Cardiac risk factors prevalent in patients who present for kidney transplant are dyslipidemia, hyperphosphatemia, and hyperhomocysteinemia. Anemia may increase cardiovascular risk, particularly in patients with ischemic heart disease. A hemoglobin of 12 g/dL is sufficient; higher hemoglobin concentrations may increase the risk of thrombotic events. Erythropoietin, when used to correct anemia to levels of 12 g/dL or less, lessens the risk of blood transfusion (see Chapter 24).

Hyperkalemia is common in patients with renal insufficiency and may be associated with increased risks during transplant surgery, particularly during reperfusion. However, mild increases in potassium may reflect normal homeostasis for renal failure, and potassium levels of 5.0 to 5.5 mEq/L are acceptable in this population. Dialysis-dependent patients may benefit from dialysis immediately prior to transplantation; however, a reduced intravascular central volume may offset the benefits of reduced potassium levels.

Intraoperative Management

Donor kidneys are usually implanted in the iliac fossa. Vascular anastomoses are most frequently to the external iliac artery and vein, and the ureter is anastomosed directly to the bladder (Fig. 36-1). Chronic renal disease can affect drug excretion via the kidney but also through changes in plasma protein binding or hepatic metabolism. When the protein binding is diminished the free

IV

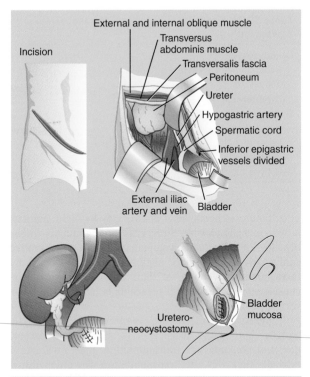

Figure 36-1 Kidney recipient operation. (From Townsend CM Jr, Beauchamp RD, Evers BM, Mattox KL (eds). Sabiston Textbook of Surgery, 18th ed. Philadelphia, Saunders Elsevier, 2007, used with permission.)

fraction of the drug is increased. This results in an apparent increase in the volume of distribution and the clearance. The net effect for the unbound fraction is similar to that in normal patients.

Some drugs require particular caution when administered in patients with renal failure.[9] These include neuromuscular blocking (NMB) drugs, and certain opioids. Long-acting NMB drugs, which are excreted via the kidneys (e.g., pancuronium), are best avoided. Vecuronium and rocuronium may have a prolonged action in renal failure patients. Cisatracurium's duration of action is more predictable because of spontaneous breakdown (also see Chapter 12). Although atracurium undergoes similar elimination, it is less potent than cisatracurium, so its breakdown product, laudanosine, is found in higher concentrations. Laudanosine's theoretical potential to cause seizures has never been clinically realized.

The 6-glucuronide metabolite of morphine has clinical activity that can result in a prolonged duration of action. Meperidine should be avoided because of the seizure-inducing potential of its metabolite, normeperidine.

Inhaled anesthetics can be used in renal failure patients. Although sevoflurane's metabolite, compound A, is nephrotoxic in rats, similar effects have not been seen in humans. Serum fluoride concentrations of 30 μmol occur in humans after sevoflurane, but do not produce renal damage. Isoflurane is metabolized to fluoride, but the extent of metabolism is so small that fluoride levels are negligible. Desflurane is not contraindicated in renal failure; but like the other volatile anesthetics, it produces a decrease in renal blood flow and glomerular filtration rate in a dose-dependent manner.

Intravascular fluid balance should be maintained in patients undergoing kidney transplantation. Typically normal saline is used for this purpose with colloids preferred by some centers. Albumin is the typical colloid of choice, but hydroxyethyl starch is acceptable in volumes up to 15 mL/kg/day, which minimizes the likelihood of bleeding complications. Central venous pressure monitoring is sometimes used to guide intra- and postoperative intravascular fluid management.

Postoperative Management (Also See Chapter 39)

Maintaining renal perfusion is an important consideration and is best accomplished by maintaining intravascular volume status. Renally effective doses of dopamine, large-dose diuretics, and osmotic diuretics are of no proven benefit. Postoperative analgesia can be achieved by epidural infusion, though many centers prefer intravenous patient-controlled analgesia with fentanyl or morphine. Nonsteroidal anti-inflammatory drugs should be avoided.

LIVER TRANSPLANTATION

The liver is second to the kidney as the most frequently transplanted solid organ. Patients with liver failure have no alternatives to liver transplantation.[10] The median time to transplant for waiting list candidates is approximately 1 year. The model for end-stage liver disease (MELD) score is used to allocate grafts based upon the urgency of the recipient's condition (the 90-day mortality risk in the absence of transplantation). International normalized ratio of prothrombin time (INR), creatinine, and bilirubin are used to derive the MELD score. Over a 30-day period approximately 30% of the highest MELD score group (>30) are removed from the waiting list because they are too sick to transplant or have died. The most common indication for liver transplantation in the United States is noncholestatic cirrhosis (73% of waiting list candidates). Noncholestatic cirrhosis includes the diagnosis of hepatitis C, which accounts for 30% of waiting list candidates.

Preoperative Assessment (Also See Chapter 13)

Liver transplant candidates have many symptoms ranging from fatigue to multiple organ failure (Table 36-3). Encephalopathy is common in end-stage liver disease

Table 36-3 Liver Transplant Recipient: Preoperative Assessment

Neurologic
  Encephalopathy
  Cerebral edema (acute liver failure)

Cardiovascular
  Hyperdynamic circulation
  Cirrhotic cardiomyopathy
  Portopulmonary hypertension

Pulmonary
  Restrictive lung disease
  Ventilation-perfusion mismatch
  Intrapulmonary shunts
  Hepatopulmonary syndrome

Gastrointestinal
  Portal hypertension
  Variceal bleeding
  Ascites

Renal/metabolic
  Hepatorenal syndrome
Acid-base abnormalities
  Hematology
  Coagulopathy
  Anemia

Musculoskeletal
Muscle atrophy

(ESLD). In acute liver failure (ALF), encephalopathy and resulting cerebral edema is the most common cause of death in ALF.[11] Cerebral edema is managed similarly to other causes of increased intracranial pressure (also see Chapter 30). The etiology of ALF often predicts whether spontaneous recovery without transplant is likely. In ALF patients unlikely to recover, urgent identification of a suitable donor can be life-saving. Approximately 25% of ALF patients undergo liver transplantation; survival in those receiving transplants is similar to post-transplant survival in patients with ESLD.

The pretransplant cardiac evaluation includes an assessment for ischemic heart disease and screening for portopulmonary hypertension. Over two thirds of deceased donor transplant recipients are older than 50 years, and many are sedentary due to debilitation from liver disease. Dobutamine stress echocardiography and nuclear scans are appropriate screening tests to rule out coronary artery disease. In older patients with diabetes, multiple risk factors or a history of coronary disease, left-sided heart catheterization may be indicated. Over two thirds of ESLD patients have a hyperdynamic circulation characterized by a high cardiac output and low systemic vascular resistance, most likely due to circulating vasoactive substances not cleared by the liver. This hyperdynamic state can be confused with sepsis, and is exacerbated with graft reperfusion.

Resting echocardiography is the test of choice in screening for portopulmonary hypertension (PPHTN). An estimated right ventricular systolic pressure less than 50 mm Hg by echocardiography rules out significant PPHTN. Right-sided heart catheterization is indicated if estimated right ventricular pressure exceeds 50 mm Hg. The definitive diagnosis of PPHTN is made when the mean pulmonary artery (PA) pressure is higher than 25 mm Hg in the presence of a normal pulmonary artery occlusion pressure and an increased pulmonary vascular resistance (>3 Wood units, or >240 dynes/sec/cm^5). Mean PA pressures higher than 35 mm Hg are associated with a perioperative mortality rate of 50%, and treatment prior to transplant should be considered. Hepatopulmonary syndrome (resting, room air P_{O_2} <70 mm Hg in the presence of an intrapulmonary shunt on bubble echocardiography) resolves after transplantation; however, Pa_{O_2} levels less than 50 mm Hg while breathing room air are associated with more frequent perioperative mortality rates.

Renal disease is common in patients who present for liver transplantation. If not long standing, hepatorenal syndrome may resolve after transplantation. Prior to transplantation, excessive intravascular volume, acidosis or hyperkalemia may necessitate renal replacement therapy. The coagulopathy of ESLD is multifactorial and requires correction in the presence of active bleeding.

Intraoperative Management

Intraoperative management requires a consideration of the effects of liver failure on drug metabolism. Preoperative amnestic doses should be reduced in patients with a history of encephalopathy. The chosen anesthetic should maintain systemic vascular resistance. The intermediate duration neuromuscular blocking drugs metabolized by the liver can have a prolonged duration of action; however, after reperfusion, evidence of liver function typically occurs and metabolism of these drugs improves. Alternatively cisatracurium, which undergoes Hofmann elimination, can be selected to avoid these concerns. Seizures can also be caused by an accumulation of normeperidine, so meperidine should be avoided. The metabolite of morphine, 6-glucuronide morphine, can accumulate and cause a prolonged effect. Fentanyl and the other synthetic opioids are safe choices. Volatile anesthetics have similar, mild effects on hepatic blood flow. Sevoflurane undergoes metabolism by the liver, but the metabolite, compound A, is not toxic to the liver or kidneys in humans.

Intraoperative monitoring varies among centers (Table 36-4). An arterial line is placed, followed by a central venous catheter (CVC) and pulmonary artery catheter (PAC), or CVC alone. Many centers use transesophageal echocardiography, which may obviate the need for PAC monitoring in the operating room. Venovenous bypass is

IV

Table 36-4 Liver Transplantation: Unique Aspects of Case Preparation

Transfusion
Red blood cells: 10 units for adults
Fresh frozen plasma: 10 units for adults
Rapid infusion device

Medication
Vasopressors: phenylephrine, epinephrine (10 and 100 µg/mL), vasopressin
Calcium chloride: for infusion and bolus

Monitors
Arterial line
Central venous pressure catheter
Pulmonary artery catheter
Transesophageal echocardiography

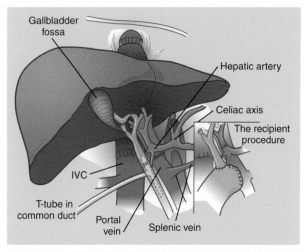

Figure 36-2 Liver recipient operation. IVC, inferior vena cava. Illustrated are the anastomoses of the donor and recipient suprahepatic IVC, infrahepatic IVC, portal vein, hepatic artery, and duct-to-duct biliary anastomosis, which can be performed with or without T tube placement. Alternatively (*inset*), in the presence of pathology of the bile duct biliary drainage is via a choledochojejunostomy. (From Townsend CM Jr, Beauchamp RD, Evers BM, Mattox KL (eds). Sabiston Textbook of Surgery, 18th ed. Philadelphia, Saunders Elsevier, 2007, used with permission.)

Table 36-5 Liver Transplantation: Treatment for the Physiologic Changes of Reperfusion

- *Hyperkalemia*: calcium, bicarbonate, insulin, and glucose
- *Acidosis*: bicarbonate, other buffers such as tris (hydroxymethyl) aminomethane
- *Decreased SVR*: α-agonists
- *Hypothermia*: warm saline peritoneal lavage

SVR, systemic vascular resistance.

used in some centers to attenuate the effects of inferior vena caval (IVC) clamping on intravascular volume; however, it has risks and adds to the length of the procedure.

The operation is divided into three phases: preanhepatic, anhepatic, and neohepatic. In the preanhepatic phase dissection and preparation for the native hepatectomy occur. This phase is associated with blood loss, particularly in the presence of varices and prior abdominal surgery. Vascular isolation of the native liver (cross-clamping of the inferior vena cava, portal vein, and hepatic artery) begins the anhepatic phase. Excision of the native liver occurs next, and is followed by implantation of the donor graft. The implantation involves anastomoses of the suprahepatic inferior vena cava, the infrahepatic inferior vena cava, and the portal vein (Fig. 36-2). An alternative "piggy back" technique involves anastomosis of the donor hepatic veins to the recipient vena cava, followed by portal anastomosis. The anhepatic period is typically quiescent from a hemodynamic perspective. Reperfusion follows portal anastomoses and begins the neohepatic period. Reperfusion is the most precarious event during the procedure due to the release of cold, acidotic effluent from the graft and lower extremities (Table 36-5). The portal effluent contains vasoactive peptides that reduce systemic vascular resistance (SVR) and can increase pulmonary resistance. Hyperkalemia can be life-threatening. If hyperkalemia is a concern, dialysis is helpful if started early in the preanhepatic period. Insulin is effective if given 10 to 15 minutes prior to reperfusion. Calcium given immediately prior to reperfusion blunts the effect of hyperkalemia on the myocardium. α-Adrenergic agonists and alkalizing drugs may be required to maintain SVR and pH, respectively.

During the neohepatic phase fibrinolysis can occur, resulting in ongoing oozing. If fibrinolysis is prolonged, antifibrinolytic drugs can be administered. The metabolic acidosis, which worsens during the anhepatic phase and peaks after reperfusion, should improve when the liver starts functioning. Additional signs of liver function include increased core temperature and decreasing calcium requirement (indicating citrate metabolism by the liver). On occasion oliguric patients with hepatorenal syndrome may show an increase in urine output in the operating room.

Postoperative Management (Also See Chapter 39)

Adjusted patient survival is 87% at 1 year and 73% after 5 years. Recipients of grafts from living donors have the most success with 1- and 5-year post-transplant survival. Thrombosis of the hepatic artery in the early postoperative period usually necessitates retransplantation. Infection is a major threat to survival in the initial months after transplant.

HEART TRANSPLANTATION

Heart transplantation is the definitive treatment for patients with end-stage heart disease. The most common indications for heart transplantation are idiopathic dilated cardiomyopathy and ischemic heart disease, which account for approximately 90% of the transplants. Other less common indications include valvular and congenital heart disease, life-threatening arrhythmia, an unresectable cardiac tumor, and repeat transplantation.[12]

Preoperative Evaluation (Also See Chapter 13)

Although patients undergo extensive multidisciplinary evaluation before being listed, a detailed preanesthetic evaluation is often challenging owing to the urgent nature of the operation, the complex clinical presentation and multiple co-morbidities.[13] Many patients require inotropic drugs or mechanical support at the time of heart transplantation. Preoperative evaluation should focus on current cardiac status, medications (particularly the need for inotropic and anticoagulant drugs), and mechanical support such as intra-aortic balloon pump or ventricular assist device. The patients should not have severe, irreversible pulmonary hypertension and active infectious disease. For patients with multiple organ failure, combined heart transplantation with other organs (lung, kidney, liver, etc.) may be considered.

Intraoperative Management (Also See Chapter 25)

In addition to standard monitors, invasive hemodynamic monitors (arterial, central venous, and pulmonary artery catheters) are routinely inserted for heart transplantation.[14] The right internal jugular vein remains a preferred site despite a concern that it may jeopardize postoperative biopsies. The pulmonary artery catheter needs to be withdrawn to the jugular vein before the native heart is excised. Alternatively, the pulmonary artery catheter is inserted at the central venous position and is advanced after the donor heart is implanted. In some institutions, a pulmonary artery catheter with capability of continuous monitoring of mixed venous O_2 saturation and cardiac output is also used. Transesophageal echocardiography plays an important role in assessing intravascular volume status, contractility, and valvular function, while monitoring for thromboembolism.

Heart transplant patients often have a full stomach due to the urgency of the procedure; therefore, a rapid sequence induction of anesthesia is needed. The choice of anesthetic is dictated by the patient's cardiac status. A failing heart is dependent on preload and sensitive to afterload. Even small changes in venous return, vascular resistance, rhythm, heart rate, and contractility can lead to hemodynamic collapse. Anesthetics with minimal hemodynamic impact are often chosen to induce anesthesia. Etomidate is a reasonable selection. Maintenance of anesthesia is often achieved with a combination of a volatile anesthetic and an opioid. A high-dose opioid technique can be used as well. Nitrous oxide is usually avoided as cardiac suppression can be seen in heart transplant patients presumably due to catecholamine store depletion and β-adrenergic receptors down-regulation.

Management goals during heart transplantation are dictated by the underlying congestive heart failure and the need to avoid conditions that increase pulmonary artery pressure (Table 36-6). Before weaning from cardiopulmonary bypass, patients should be warm, acid-base and electrolytes should be in the normal range, the lungs are ventilated, and the cardiac chambers are free of air.

Several intraoperative issues are unique to heart transplantation. First, the transplanted heart is denervated and bradycardia can occur following reperfusion. The heart rate response to hemodynamic changes is absent and drugs acting indirectly on the heart are ineffective. Bradycardia can be treated by pacing (usually 90 to 110 beats/min) or chronotropic drugs such as isoproterenol. Second, failure to wean from cardiopulmonary bypass is often caused by right-sided heart failure. Several possible mechanisms are related to right-sided heart failure during heart transplantation: preexisting pulmonary hypertension can be worsened during reperfusion of the donor heart and the right ventricle is particularly prone to ischemia/reperfusion injury. The primary treatment goals for right-sided heart failure during heart transplantation are to increase contractility of the right ventricle and decrease pulmonary artery resistance. Failure to respond may necessitate mechanical right ventricular support. Worsening pulmonary hypertension during heart transplantation is multifactorial. An increase in cardiac output, pulmonary vessel spasm, and blood or air embolism are all possible causes. Adequate ventilation and oxygenation, with avoidance of hypoxia and hypercarbia, can prevent an increase in pulmonary vasculature

---

Table 36-6 Heart Transplantation: Perioperative Goals

- Maintain systemic blood pressure to maintain coronary filling
- Optimize preload
- Reduce afterload to improve ejection fraction
- Avoid pulmonary vasoconstriction
  - Maintain oxygenation
  - Avoid hypercapnia
  - Avoid high tidal volumes
  - Correct acid-base abnormalities
- Support contractility
  - Pharmacologic drugs
  - Intra-aortic balloon pump
  - Assist devices

resistance. Treatment of pulmonary hypertension with nonselective vasodilators such as nitroglycerin and sodium nitroprusside can decrease systemic vascular resistance and result in systemic hypotension. Selective drugs such as inhaled nitric oxide, aerosolized iloprost (a carbacyclin analog of prostaglandin I_2) and sildenafil (inhaled or infused) may be helpful.

Postoperative Management (Also See Chapter 39)

Postoperative management targets adequate oxygenation, ventilation, intravascular volume, pulmonary and systemic pressures, coagulation, and body temperature. Extubation of the trachea is considered when stable hemodynamics and adequate spontaneous ventilation have been achieved. Up to 25% of patients require permanent pacemaker implantation to treat post-transplant bradycardia. Most patients require inotropic and chronotropic support in the first few days following heart transplant. Post-transplant bleeding and a nonfunctional graft are life-threatening and need to be diagnosed and managed emergently.

LUNG TRANSPLANTATION

Chronic obstructive lung disease is the most common indication for adult lung transplant.[15] In children, cystic fibrosis is the most common indication for lung transplantation. The choice of transplant type (single, sequential, double lung) is dependent on the surgeon's preference and the nature and severity of disease. Each operative type requires slightly different anesthetic setup and intraoperative management.

Preoperative Evaluation

Preoperative evaluation should focus on the severity of lung disease, the baseline function of other vital organs, the airway, and interval changes since the last examination.[16,17] Preoperative anxiolytic drugs should be used with caution, as too much sedation or uncontrolled anxiety can worsen pulmonary hypertension. Supplemental oxygen is used with care because most lung transplant patients depend on their hypoxic drive. Epidural analgesia should be considered in lung transplant patients for postoperative pain control and may actually improve outcome.

Intraoperative Management

In addition to standard monitors, arterial, central venous, and pulmonary artery catheters are usually placed. In some institutions, a pulmonary artery catheter with continuous mixed venous O_2 saturation and cardiac output monitoring is used. Endobronchoscopy is necessary

during lung transplantation. In addition to assessing the position of the double-lumen endotracheal tube, endobronchoscopy can examine the airway anastomoses for stenosis, bleeding, and obstruction secondary to blood or sputum. Transesophageal echocardiography is usually used during lung transplantation.

Anesthetic induction needs to balance the risk of aspiration of gastric contents with hypoxia and hemodynamic instability. Positive-pressure ventilation can cause a decreased venous blood return. Patients with severe pulmonary hypertension are at risk of cardiac arrest during induction of anesthesia. Emergent cardiopulmonary bypass is established in this situation. Positive-pressure ventilation can cause further damage to diseased lungs and worsen hypoxia and hypercarbia. Air trapping and barotrauma should be avoided. Ventilation with small tidal volume should be instituted.

The most challenging intraoperative issues associated with lung transplant involve ventilation-reperfusion mismatch and pulmonary artery hypertension. Strategies to treat hypoxemia during lung transplant are similar to those seen in thoracic surgery. At the time of pulmonary artery clamping, increased pulmonary artery pressure is often encountered. Methods to reduce pulmonary artery pressure include intravascular fluid restriction, and nonselective and selective pulmonary vasodilators in both intravenous and inhaled forms. Excessive intravascular fluid administration should be avoided because noncardiogenic pulmonary edema is a frequent development in lung transplant patients.

Postoperative Management (Also See Chapter 39)

Special care for lung transplant patients in the postoperative period is provided to avoid barotrauma, volutrauma, and anastomotic dehiscence during positive-pressure mechanical ventilation.

PANCREAS TRANSPLANTATION

Pancreas transplantation is a surgical therapy for patients with type 1 diabetes mellitus.[18] The transplanted pancreas can provide endogenous insulin and restore normoglycemia and the glucagon response. Diabetes mellitus affects cardiovascular, autonomic, nervous, renal, gastrointestinal, and metabolic systems. Preoperative evaluation should focus on functional status of the vital organs. Ischemic heart disease is a primary cause of perioperative death. Diagnosis of coronary artery disease in this patient population is difficult in the presence of neuropathy and silent ischemia. If coronary artery disease is suspected, a preoperative stress test or coronary artery angiogram should be performed. Preoperative evaluation should also include examination of renal function, acid-base status electrolytes, and hemoglobin. Most pancreas transplants

(65%) are performed simultaneously with kidney transplantation. Compared with pancreas alone or pancreas after kidney (PAK) transplant, simultaneous pancreas and kidney transplants (SPK) experience the best graft survival rates: 86% at 1 year and 53% at 10 years.

Pancreas transplantation can be performed under general or regional anesthesia. Invasive monitors should be considered if there is cardiovascular disease. The choice of anesthetic drugs should take into account the possibility of severe postinduction hypotension due to diabetic autonomic nervous system dysfunction. Muscle relaxants not dependent on renal excretion are preferred if renal function is impaired. Severe intraoperative hyperglycemia should be avoided because it may adversely affect islet function and promote post-transplant infection.

CONCLUSIONS

Successful transplantation reverses end-stage organ failure, and promotes the recovery of organ systems beyond the transplanted organ. Examples include improvement of cardiac function after renal transplant and improved renal function, reversal of hepatopulmonary syndrome, and resolution of encephalopathy after liver transplant. Nutritional status, muscle mass, and quality of life improve with successful transplantation.

The most common life-threatening complications of transplantation are cardiovascular and infectious. Vigilant anesthetic care, both before and after the transplant, can have a profound impact on minimizing these complications and improving post-transplant outcomes.

QUESTIONS OF THE DAY

1. What is the most common cause of death in a patient with end-stage renal disease receiving dialysis?
2. What is the MELD score? What laboratory tests are used to calculate the MELD score?
3. What are the three phases of the liver transplant procedure?
4. What are the principles of managing acute right-sided heart failure during heart transplantation?

ACKNOWLEDGMENT

The editors and publisher would like to thank Drs. Claus U. Niemann and C.S. Yost for contributing a chapter on this topic to the prior edition of this work. It has served as the foundation for the current chapter.

IV

REFERENCES

1. Yost CS, Niemann CU: Anesthesia for abdominal organ transplantation. In Miller RD, editor: *Miller's Anesthesia*, ed 7, Philadelphia, 2010, Elsevier, pp 2155–2184, Chap. 67.
2. Centers for Medicare and Medicaid Services, Department of Health and Human Services: Medicare and Medicaid programs, conditions for coverage for organ procurement organizations (OPOs), final rule, *Fed Regist* 71:30981–31054, 2006. Available at http://www.ustransplant.org/annual_reports/current/. Accessed March 7, 2010.
3. Bernat JL, D'Alessandro AM, Port FK, et al: Report of a National Conference on Donation after cardiac death, *Am J Transplant* 6:281–291, 2006.
4. Verheijde JL, Rady MY, McGregor JL: The United States Revised Uniform Anatomical Gift Act (2006): New challenges to balancing patient rights and physician responsibilities, *Philos Ethics Humanit Med* 2:19, 2007.
5. Lemmens HJ: Kidney transplantation: Recent developments and recommendations for anesthetic management, *Anesthesiol Clin North America* 22:651–662, 2004.
6. Ojo AO, Hanson JA, Meier-Kriesche H, et al: Survival in recipients of marginal cadaveric donor kidneys compared with other recipients and wait-listed transplant candidates, *J Am Soc Nephrol* 12:589–597, 2001.
7. *Annual Report of the U.S. Organ Procurement and Transplantation Network and the Scientific Registry of Transplant Recipients: Transplant Data 1998–2007*, Rockville, MD, 2008, U.S. Department of Health and Human Services, Health Resources and Services Administration, Healthcare Systems Bureau, Division of Transplantation.
8. Beattie WS, Abdelnaem E, Wijeysundera DN, et al: A meta-analytic comparison of preoperative stress echocardiography and nuclear scintigraphy imaging, *Anesth Analg* 102:8–16, 2006.
9. Koehntop DE, Beebe DS, Belani KG: Perioperative anesthetic management of the kidney-pancreas transplant recipient, *Curr Opin Anaesthesiol* 3:341–347, 2000.
10. Steadman RH: Anesthesia for liver transplant surgery, *Anesthesiol Clin North America* 22:687–711, 2004.
11. Stravitz RT, Kramer AH, Davern T, et al: Intensive care of patients with acute liver failure: Recommendations of the U.S. Acute Liver Failure Study Group, *Crit Care Med* 35:2498–2508, 2007.
12. Hunt SA, Haddad F: The changing face of heart transplantation, *J Am Coll Cardiol* 52:587–598, 2008.
13. Ramakrishna H, Jaroszewski DE, Arabia FA: Adult cardiac transplantation: A review of perioperative management. Part I, *Ann Card Anaesth* 12:71–78, 2009.
14. Shanewise J: Cardiac transplantation, *Anesthesiol Clin North America* 22:753–765, 2004.
15. Baez B, Castillo M: Anesthetic considerations for lung transplantation, *Semin Cardiothorac Vasc Anesth* 12:122–127, 2008.
16. Rosenberg AL, Rao M, Benedict PE: Anesthetic implications for lung transplantation, *Anesthesiol Clin North America* 22:767–788, 2004.
17. Myles PS, Snell GI, Westall GP: Lung transplantation, *Curr Opin Anaesthesiol* 21:21–26, 2007.
18. Larson-Wadd K, Belani KG: Pancreas and islet cell transplantation, *Anesthesiol Clin North America* 22:663–674, 2004.

37 OUTPATIENT ANESTHESIA

Douglas G. Merrill

Until a few hundred years ago, all surgery and anesthesia procedures were performed on an "outpatient" basis. Trephination was performed in the Andes thousands of years ago.[1] The Hindus performed outpatient tonsillectomy 4000 years ago, and Egyptians used regional anesthesia to perform circumcision over 2500 years ago.[2,3] Then, as now, convenience and speed were undoubtedly valued aspects of surgical practice.

In 1917, after 100 years of hospital-based surgery made that venue the norm, Dr. Ralph Waters opened the first modern ambulatory surgery center in downtown Sioux City, Iowa. Of note, the name of his center emphasized the value of its practice to both patients and surgeons: "The Downtown Anesthesia Clinic."[4] His work brought anesthesia to the fore as a commodity of comfort and his location allowed surgeons and dentists to operate close to their offices on patients who could be taken home that day. Despite remarkable success there and later in Kansas City, surgery remained an exclusively inpatient practice until 1970 when inpatient medicine became increasingly expensive. Dr. Wallace Reed and Dr. John Ford opened the modern era of ambulatory surgery centers with their Phoenix Surgery Center, with the primary goal of decreasing the cost of surgery for patients.[5] For Drs. Waters, Reed, and Ford, the reasons to open these sites describe the value that surgery centers and office-based practices still provide today: convenience and cost savings to patients, their families, and the surgeons. Timeliness and excellent outcomes in patient comfort are fundamental to that convenience. This chapter will review some unique aspects of outpatient anesthesia practice, which—more than other anesthesia subspecialties—is defined by its focus on customer and community service, rather than by a specific set of statistics based on morbidities, organ systems, age groups, or disease types.

PATIENT GOALS AND EXPECTATIONS

In order to provide the best service, the expectations of the customer should be fulfilled. Patients undergoing surgery in the ambulatory setting ask that they be safe, be provided excellent pain relief, not be nauseated, and be able to return to their normal daily routines as quickly as possible.[6-8] They expect that they will be safe during anesthesia and that no severe harm will occur during their surgical experience. They also hope that they will be comfortable in the hours and days after surgery, and not be a burden to their families or friends.

FOUR KEY FOCUS POINTS FOR SUCCESS IN OUTPATIENT ANESTHESIA

To achieve the goals desired by patients, families, and surgeons, the anesthesia provider (and the facility medical director) must focus on four factors:

I. Selection criteria for cases and patients that create a predictable environment
II. Attention to safety that exceeds that applied in the hospital setting, which has more redundant support systems
III. Careful monitoring of patient outcomes and the literature to discover the "best practices," the techniques and medications that consistently leave postoperative patients clear-headed and as free of nausea and pain as possible
IV. Codification of best practices into "standard work," directive care plans that leverage the predictability of the ambulatory anesthesia to create consistently excellent outcomes and service for patients and families

Patient, Procedure, and Practitioner Selection

Careful selection of patients, with regard to co-morbidities and social structure, will allow providers to correctly predict the likely durations of the admission process, anesthesia preparation, surgical period, and recovery that define the families' and surgeons' experiences at the facility. Procedures and practitioners must be chosen with equal care. The ability to avoid wasting either the family's or surgeon's time is a key component of a successful outpatient anesthesia provider's profile. The team that works in an operating suite is a primary determinant of the duration and the predictability of operative room time.[9]

In order to achieve such predictability, consistent and directive guidelines for management of patient co-morbidity should be agreed upon by surgeon, facility, and anesthesia providers. These guidelines will vary by venue (e.g., a hospital-based outpatient surgery suite can be more aggressive in accepting patients with cardiopulmonary disease than can a small free-standing ambulatory surgery center [ASC]) as well as by community resources (e.g., a free-standing surgery center one block distant from a tertiary care pediatric hospital may be preferable to provide care for younger children than a center in a small community with no pediatrician). Thus, no single list of acceptable patients or case types will work for all venues, but further discussion is provided in Appendix C at the end of this chapter.

Patient Safety Outside the Hospital

Historically, ASCs have been the safest location to undergo surgery, with the office-based safety record not appearing to be quite as good.[10] The reasons for this safety profile may be the careful attention to preoperative case and patient selection as well as on-site preparation practiced by free-standing ASCs.[11] In an office or free-standing ambulatory surgery center, the on-site support systems must be more replete than those found in an outpatient

IV

surgical department located within a tertiary care hospital (Hospital Outpatient Department, or HOPD). For instance, an office or free-standing ASC must have all items required to follow each step of the ASA Guideline on the Management of the Difficult Airway,[12] whereas an HOPD may not require such equipment, having the resources of the inpatient operating room only steps away.

Nursing and anesthesia support personnel are often trained in emergency care to a greater degree in the free-standing or office setting because of their facility's relative isolation. ASC operating room nurses often complete Advanced Cardiac Life Support (ACLS) and Pediatric Advanced Life Support (PALS) training, because they will have to serve as primary caregivers in an emergency situation for a longer period of time than will an operating room nurse in a tertiary care inpatient operating room.

Because of this isolation, ASCs and offices must create a schedule of recurrent on-site simulation exercises (e.g., cardiac arrest, tonsil bleed, malignant hyperthermia, emergency transfusion) to enhance system and provider readiness for emergency situations. These events are typically stressful and should be followed by debriefings that emphasize the potential improvements in system design and teamwork, rather than individual failings.[13,14] Patient and procedure selection aimed at avoiding unexpected events are undoubtedly significant reasons that ASCs are historically safe venues.[15] Yet, more needs to be known about patient characteristics that lead to quality and safety failures.[16] Consequently, preparation for unanticipated emergency situations must also be meticulous.

Monitoring Outcomes

Outcome measurement and use of that data to create standard work plans has successfully improved safety and service delivery in a variety of industries, including health care.[17-20] A recognized tenet of evidence-based medicine is to reference past patient outcomes when selecting appropriate therapies.[21] Individual anesthesia providers should routinely call their patients the day after the procedure and discover the successes and failures of their care. Providers should collect that information in a relational database or a spreadsheet so they can discern any associations between technique and outcomes.

Anesthesia providers who contact patients after discharge will improve care and safety, as they provide an additional access point for a patient or family if there are problems postoperatively.

Creating Standard Work: Local Outcomes Monitoring and Literature Review

Unnecessary variation and an hierarchical culture that fosters a lack of transparency and teamwork care are the sources of unsafe, inefficient, and high-cost practices in the delivery of health care.[22] An effective response is for health care delivery teams to integrate published studies and guidelines with analysis of local outcome and process data to develop and use algorithm-driven care policies and processes ("standard work") in an effort to eliminate unnecessary variation.[23-28] The ambulatory surgery center or office provides a uniquely suitable location for this work. It is a more homogeneous environment in which fewer providers perform a smaller set of procedures when compared to the inpatient operating suite.[29] Admittedly, genetic heterogeneity (and our increasing knowledge about it) will inevitably challenge attempts to use standard approaches to perioperative care, making the effort to create and track such efforts all the more important.[30] Patient care decisions in the most stable clinical environments are of particular value, therefore, as their results reveal the best outcomes, and therefore best practice.[31]

The most effective means to develop these standard care plans is to create multidisciplinary teams of physicians and nurses to assay the literature, create "best guess" protocols, measure the clinical outcomes of practitioners who do and do not adopt the protocols, and report those outcomes to the entire team. When the results are posted with names attached (connecting each patient's outcomes with all providers whose work was involved) in a secure staff area (e.g., medication room), then everyone can clearly see which providers and techniques were associated with the highest quality outcomes. The small teams can then reassess the value of their protocols and refine them so that each center creates algorithms of care tailored to maximize and replicate its own successes. Algorithms are printed, collated on-line, and made easily accessible to clinicians for guidance, and are reevaluated quarterly. The expectation should be that providers follow these guidelines, unless their alternative approach induces equal or better results than the "best practice."

CLINICAL ISSUES

Preoperative Considerations (Also See Chapter 13)

PREOPERATIVE EVALUATION AND TESTING

The American Society of Anesthesiologists (ASA) has determined that a review of the patient's medical and social history and a physical examination by an anesthesiologist is of value in the preparation of patients for anesthesia and surgery.[32] It is easy to be lulled into hurried complacency by a long list of "minor" surgeries on "healthy" patients, but the simple act of reviewing past anesthesia experiences, exercise tolerance, snoring, allergies, and similar details cannot be skipped. Anesthesia providers uncover significant perturbations in patient health that can affect postoperative and long-term health.[33,34] This clinical history drives the preoperative evaluation.

LABORATORY DATA REQUIRED PREOPERATIVELY
(Also See Chapter 13)

Practice in ASC and office settings has reduced the cost of care delivery in part by the elimination of much of the routine preoperative testing that marked inpatient surgical care for so many years. No value accrues to testing that is not specifically indicated by patient co-morbidities or procedural characteristics, and some "indicated" testing might be safely abandoned.[35] For instance, routine electrocardiogram (ECG) orders made prior to performing a clinical assessment that elicits an indication for the test increases costs and patient inconvenience usually without value. The only patients who should have an ECG performed prior to outpatient surgery are those who are older than 65 years or who have a history of congestive heart failure, previous myocardial infarction, angina, high cholesterol, significant valvular disease, or a family history of sudden death.[36-38] In the absence of acutely unstable chronic disease, an unusual family history (e.g., sudden death),[39] potential for blood loss[40] (a good reason not to perform elective surgery in a free-standing ASC or office), expected use of injected contrast medium, or potential pregnancy (creatinine level and pregnancy testing, respectively) there is no indication for laboratory testing.[41,42] Pregnancy testing remains controversial, with some facilities requiring it for all women of childbearing age and others offering it only to those women who feel they may be pregnant. In one study, mandating that all women undergo testing resulted in a cost of over $3000 per positive test, a particularly troubling price in view of an unknown level of benefit.[43]

Should We Proceed with Surgery for This Patient Today?

The anesthesia provider asks this untimely question when patients fall acutely ill, or preoperative evaluation is not sufficient to catch significant chronic disease states, or patients are noncompliant with previous recommendations for consultation, testing, or therapy. What are some appropriate "stop signs" on the day of surgery? Some particularly notable considerations in outpatient anesthesia will be discussed here.

CARDIAC DISEASE (Also See Chapter 25)

Elective surgery can proceed in a nonhospital environment, particularly if the procedure will not require entry into the thoracic, peritoneal, or vascular spaces,[46] if a patient with cardiac disease is stable, meaning that the patient does *not* have any of the following:

1. Unstable angina, labile hypertension, or severe valvular disease

2. Cardiac dysrhythmias (i.e., Mobitz II atrioventricular [AV] block, supraventricular arrhythmias with rapid or erratic ventricular response, third-degree AV block, symptomatic bradycardia or ventricular arrhythmias, or new ventricular tachycardia)[44]

3. Myocardial infarction within the past 3 months with either ongoing pain or evidence of at-risk myocardium

4. A drug-eluting coronary stent placed within the last year or a bare-metal stent within 1 month[45]

5. Three or more of the following conditions: ischemic heart disease, a history of congestive heart failure, insulin-dependent diabetes, chronic renal insufficiency (creatinine greater than 2.0 mg/dL), a transient ischemic attack, or cerebrovascular accident (stroke)

Some free-standing centers and offices do not admit patients with implantable cardioverter-defibrillators or pacemakers (unless pacemaker interrogation services are immediately available perioperatively).

PULMONARY DISEASE (Also See Chapter 27)

If a patient has been given therapy sufficient to achieve his or her optimal condition (e.g., medications have been reviewed by the primary physician and no other therapy is believed to be appropriate), but is still symptomatic (e.g., wheezing at rest, a bedside forced expiratory time of less than 6 seconds, unable to climb a flight of stairs because of dyspnea), or has pulmonary hypertension, then surgery should be performed in the hospital environment, where respiratory therapy services are ideal.[47-50] Invasive pediatric airway surgery is not appropriate for a free-standing center but may be appropriate for a hospital-based center if it is easily accessible (walking indoors) to pediatric intensivists and respiratory therapists with pediatric expertise. See later discussion of an upper respiratory infection (URI) in the presence of chronic pulmonary disease.

RENAL DISEASE (Also See Chapter 28)

The presence of an elevated creatinine level may impact the outcome of outpatient surgery if other co-morbidities are present, as noted previously. However, arteriovenous fistula surgery (creation or revision) and unstable renal failure are each associated with a high morbidity rate and these patients are not good candidates for surgery in a free-standing outpatient facility.[51,52]

TECHNIQUES OF ANESTHESIA FOR OUTPATIENT SURGERY

Goals

The overall goals of outpatient anesthesia today are unchanged from those espoused by Waters, Reed and Ford: convenience, low-cost, and provision of care in alignment with the patient's and surgeon's goals.

IV

Therefore, the techniques of anesthesia should be chosen to most optimally provide safety and to diminish or eliminate pain, postoperative nausea and vomiting (PONV), and postoperative prolonged cognitive impairment.

Monitored Anesthesia Care (Also See Chapter 20)

Monitored anesthesia care (MAC) is an anesthetic technique that can allow a patient to be sedated and to transition in and out of general anesthesia, if that is required by changes in patient or surgical conditions. Only anesthesia practitioners can provide MAC. MAC thus differs from sedation (conscious sedation, moderate sedation), a technique practiced by nonanesthesia practitioners, the performance of which must ensure that patients maintain airway patency throughout the procedure.

MAC is typically chosen when general anesthesia or regional anesthesia are considered too invasive either for the anesthetic requirements of the procedure or for the health of the patient. However, the use of MAC carries finite risk. In fact, the potential for catastrophic outcome with MAC may be equal to that associated with the use of general anesthesia, with particular risk for oversedation and operating room fires.[53] Vigilance and adequate monitoring are just as important during MAC, since events such as hypoventilation and relative hypoxemia may occur.[54] When deciding whether to provide MAC versus general anesthesia, the anesthesia provider should factor in the need for oxygen supplementation. If the procedure will be so uncomfortable that obtundation will be needed, a resulting need for high levels of oxygen will also be present. If these conditions are present, and if the procedure is going to occur in proximity to the airway, and if electrocautery will be in use, the author recommends that MAC not be used. In that case, a general anesthetic should be employed so that a closed system may be used for oxygen delivery.

Regional and Neuraxial Anesthesia (Also See Chapters 17 and 18)

The use of regional anesthesia—alone or in conjunction with general anesthesia or sedation—has significant benefits for patients and facilities.[55,56] Performing regional nerve blocks in a preoperative area for patients undergoing orthopedic procedures decreases overall anesthesia time and does not increase the duration of turnover time, when compared to general anesthesia.[57] Additionally, postanesthesia care unit (PACU) discharge time can be shortened and the immediate postoperative period made more pleasant for the patient.[58,59] The use of regional catheters, in the presence of safe postdischarge conditions, has been associated with reductions in pain for days after surgery and improved rehabilitation.[60–62]

The use of paravertebral regional block can be valuable for hernia repair[63] and breast surgery,[64] decreasing required opioid, PONV, urinary retention, and acute and chronic pain ratings, as compared to general or neuraxial anesthetics.[65,66] In addition, paravertebral block for patients undergoing mastectomy may decrease the incidence of tumor recurrence or metastasis via an immunologic damping process.[67]

Neuraxial blockade with or without sedation has been an effective means to manage anesthesia for lower extremity surgery as well as abdominal surgery, with significant benefits in the reduction of PONV and pain,[68] and for patients with chronic respiratory disease.[69] In small doses (bupivacaine 4 mg with 20 µg fentanyl), spinal anesthesia can provide effective but very short acting coverage for transurethral procedures in elderly males, without delaying discharge.[70] The use of 2-chloroprocaine in the subarachnoid space provides superb anesthesia for procedures of less than 1 hour in duration (e.g., knee arthroscopies, inguinal hernia repairs) at a dose of 40 to 50 mg.[71,72] For outpatient knee arthroscopy, 7.5 mg of 0.5% hyperbaric ropivacaine is also a useful spinal dose, but the ranges of duration of surgical anesthesia (up to 2.5 hours) and time to discharge (up to 3.5 hours) are wider than with 2-chloroprocaine.[73,74]

General Anesthesia

General anesthesia (GA) is associated with a more frequent risk of PONV, postdischarge nausea and vomiting (PDNV), airway injury, postoperative hypothermia, postoperative cognitive dysfunction (POCD), and delayed discharge when compared to MAC or regional anesthesia (see previous discussion). However, GA may be provided effectively with low perioperative morbidity rate if total intravenous anesthesia (TIVA) techniques or the use of desflurane or sevoflurane is employed, when endotracheal intubation is avoided, low-dose propofol infusions are used, and multimodal analgesia and preemptive antinausea methods are employed (please see later discussions under "Postoperative Nausea and Vomiting" and "Opioids and Pain in the Care of Surgical Outpatients").[75–79]

Five Principles of Outpatient Anesthesia

No single approach to anesthesia is best for all patients. The decisions made among the many choices must be based upon the need for muscle relaxation or positioning, and patient characteristics: psychology, co-morbidities, and history. A shoulder procedure may be well managed with an interscalene block and only light sedation, but the use of lateral decubitus positioning, patient anxiety, language barrier, or a contralateral missing lung or phrenic nerve palsy may each rule out that choice.

These choices should be based upon the evidence in the literature, then routinely checked and validated by careful assessment of local patient outcomes. Following that practice has yielded these five principles:

I. Active and intentional management of preoperative evaluation, patient and case selection, anesthesia delivery decisions, and postoperative recovery room care is required to provide optimal patient outcomes.[80–82]

II. Avoidance of opioids prior to the postoperative period and the use of multimodal analgesia is the most effective means of decreasing postoperative pain and nausea, providing the least impact on cognitive function and the highest patient satisfaction.[83,84]

III. Avoidance of general anesthesia alone in favor of only regional anesthesia (peripheral nerve block) or a combined regional-general technique, when possible, improves patient satisfaction.[85]

IV. Avoidance of some inhaled anesthetics for general anesthesia in favor of TIVA may improve patient outcomes.[86]

V. It is appropriate to use preemptive antiemetic therapy for the majority of patients receiving a general anesthetic.[87–89]

SOME TOPICS OF IMPORTANCE IN OUTPATIENT ANESTHESIA

Diabetes Mellitus (Also See Chapter 29)

In the outpatient surgery setting, three decisions are critical regarding the care of a patient with diabetes mellitus:

1. Whether or not long-term control is adequate to decrease the risk of perioperative morbidity sufficiently for surgery to proceed
2. Whether or not a given blood sugar level is acceptable as "safe" and whether or not treating it acutely may positively impact the patient's perioperative morbidity
3. How best to manage glucose on-site: pre-, intra- and postoperatively

Unfortunately, finding guidance in the literature and among professional guidelines is difficult. Guidelines have not addressed perioperative care in the outpatient venue but instead attend only to the care of inpatients.[90] However, Society for Ambulatory Anesthesia (SAMBA) will soon publish consensus guidelines for outpatient perioperative management of the diabetic patient at http://www.sambahq.org/. The literature supports the following approach:

A. Adult patients with diabetes who have a HbA_{1c} value less than 7% are considered to be in excellent control. Consequently, in the absence of other significant co-morbidities, such patients are good candidates for elective surgery as outpatients. Those with higher glycosylated hemoglobin values may be at increased risk for perioperative morbidity, such as postoperative infections.[91] The range of acceptable levels of HbA_{1c} for pediatric patients is wider and reaches higher levels, with variation depending upon age.[92] If there is any value in assessment of the HbA_{1c} in the preoperative period (and there are no studies that reveal a "safe level"), it is to alert the anesthesia provider that a high value may indicate a need to aggressively pursue further evaluation regarding chronic cardiac and renal health prior to surgical intervention.[93] If an elevated HbA_{1c} result is obtained as soon as the patient is scheduled, then the medical director has some time to obtain any needed testing or appropriate consults prior to surgery. The need for testing (e.g., ECG or creatinine) will also be guided by the frequency of the patient's interaction with a primary care provider or endocrinologist.

B. Fasting blood glucose levels obtained on the day of surgery are less valuable as a means of detecting a patient's overall diabetic control, in part because different patients strive for tighter or less control, based upon life-style.[94] Postponement of elective surgery based upon a specific fasting or random glucose level obtained on the day of surgery is not supported by controlled trials or retrospective data. Typically, diabetic patients are given half or more of their normal morning dose prior to outpatient surgery, but this practice is subject to scheduling. Ideally, patients with diabetes should have surgery early in the day, so as to provide the least disruption in their dosing. Patients on indwelling pumps do not normally have to adjust these (certainly they should not be told to "hold" the infusion) if surgery is scheduled early. They should be advised to either wait until arrival at the facility before giving themselves bolus insulin doses, or to travel with their hypoglycemic rescue treatment (clear liquid oral glucose source) if they are going to take their medication at home before arrival.[95]

C. On-site treatment of hyperglycemia should be done with subcutaneous dosing of insulin, rather than intravenous dosing, to avoid wide swings in glucose levels. Achieving normal glucose levels should not be sought in patients with poor control before, during, or after surgery. Patients with poor control have an altered "set-point" and may suffer the hypoglycemic symptoms and impairment at normal glucose levels.[96] Insulin may be used to treat hyperglycemia in insulin-dependent patients, with the "rule of 1800" being a good approach to dosing. In this paradigm, the number 1800 is divided by the patient's normal daily insulin dose (that is, the *total* daily dose of all forms of insulin),

IV

including basal and boluses, or long- and shorter-acting taken in a typical 24-hour period) of insulin to determine the probable change in glucose level (mg/dL) that would be anticipated by the use of a single unit of regular insulin. An appropriate serum glucose goal is the patient's typical morning baseline fasting glucose. Practitioners are referred to the cited references for a full discussion of perioperative insulin dosing.[97,98]

Other considerations in the outpatient diabetic surgical patient:

- Intravenous fluids should be given liberally (e.g., 20 mL/kg or more) prior to induction of anesthesia to diminish the risk of nausea and vomiting. However, patients with diabetes may be at risk for congestive heart failure, and the risk is heightened in patients with type II diabetes on oral thiazolidinediones.
- Dexamethasone, in doses typically chosen to avoid PONV, may be given to diabetic patients safely, but elevated blood glucose readings should be expected and the patient instructed to manage home insulin dose adjustments accordingly.
- Finally, the most significant aspect of managing the perioperative experience for diabetic patients is to disrupt their lives as little as possible. This includes using all means available to avoid changing medication and dietary regimens, and preventing PONV, PDNV, and pain. Such alterations can wreak havoc on a diabetic patient's glycemic control and potentially lead to significant complications, such as postoperative infection.

Fast-Tracking

Ambulatory anesthesia and surgery conditions allow the discharge of a high percentage of patients from the operating room directly to a "second stage" of the PACU, bypassing the "first stage." Second-stage patients do not require airway support and have stable cardiopulmonary indices and good analgesia. "Fast-tracking" bypass provides a more pleasant experience for the patient and family (who can be more rapidly reunited) and may decrease cost in the outpatient facility, depending upon personnel management practices.[99] Some anesthetic decisions are important to this process (e.g., regional or local anesthesia versus GA), but others do not typically have such impact (e.g., desflurane versus sevoflurane).[100,101] The use of multimodal analgesia and preemptive interventions to reduce PONV are key means of achieving fast-tracking even with general anesthesia, as is monitoring with either a Bispectral Index (BIS) monitor or using an auditory evoked potential monitor, which provides an electroencephalographic-derived index (AAI).[102,103] However, the use of standard criteria, chosen by local practitioners (anesthesiologists, nurse anesthetists, and PACU RNs) and based upon published recommendations, can avoid inappropriate admissions to second-stage recovery (where resources are limited and not designed to manage patients with airway issues or significant pain).[104] These criteria should be reevaluated by the local team on a quarterly basis to discover how they affected patient care (i.e., how many patients were returned to stage I, after bypass? How many were deemed stage I by the anesthesia team, but were graded stage II on arrival in the PACU?) and amended as needed.

Hypertension (and Antihypertensive Medications) (Also See Chapter 13)

Patients with treated hypertension who undergo surgery have as much as a 50% increased risk of myocardial infarction (MI), cardiac arrest, or a significant new dysrhythmia in the first 30 days after their procedure.[105] Although angiotensin-converting enzyme (ACE) inhibitors have provided significant improvement in the chronic care of hypertension, they have been associated with profound hypotension after induction of general anesthesia.[106,107] However, at least one study has questioned this conclusion.[108] The question is significant, as the same authors found that patients who experience such postinduction hypotension have a significant increase in postoperative morbidity and mortality rates. Probably patients should not take ACE inhibitors (ACEIs) and angiotensin II receptor subtype-1 antagonists (ARA) within 10 hours of induction for general surgery cases.[109] However, an informal poll by this author found that fewer than half of ambulatory surgery centers associated with academic medical centers asked their patients to stop these medications prior to surgery.

In fact, perhaps patients scheduled to undergo surgery under MAC should take these medications. In our experience in two ASCs, several patients who have not taken their ACEI or ARA medications required on-site intravenous antihypertensive medication administration, and some required cancellation of eye surgery because of extreme hypertension.

Malignant Hyperthermia

All facilities that provide anesthesia must be able to manage the immediate and definitive care of patients experiencing malignant hyperthermia (MH). A recent study of the North American MH Registry by Larach and associates shows that these events occurred even in healthy patients undergoing typical outpatient procedures and having a "nontriggering" anesthetic, in the absence of a family history, and who had undergone previous anesthetics without problem.[110] Thus, facilities must be prepared for the unexpected MH event. However, it is another question entirely as to whether patients with a known history of or at high risk for malignant hyperthermia should be cared for in the free-standing ambulatory surgery facility or office. Although controversial, some thoughtful experts believe the answer to that question is "yes."[111-113]

Another possible response is, "why try?" Because the disease is rare, it is reasonable to provide anesthesia to patients without a known susceptibility to MH if a facility has the ability to cool via Foley/bladder irrigation, can provide "clean" airway equipment and oxygen delivery systems, and has a minimum of 36 vials of dantrolene in the facility (although the growing average BMI (body mass index) and requirement for more than 36 vials to treat a substantial number of these cases has led to Larach group's recommendation that more than 36 vials be on hand, if possible).

However, to purposefully admit patients with a known or suspected personal history of malignant hyperthermia, or first-degree relatives with the disease, potentially requires that free-standing facilities replicate exactly the standard of capability for definitive care found in any other operating location in the community, including a hospital. For instance, after initial care is provided, blood gases are recommended to guide therapy, and few free-standing sites currently own and maintain arterial blood gas analysis equipment. The availability of pediatric and adult intensivists, and respiratory therapists, who could make the difference of a positive outcome in the definitive care of a severe case of MH episode, cannot be replicated in the ASC. Therefore, every free-standing facility should carefully assess the potential cost and benefit attendant to the decision to electively admit patients with known MH or MH-associated diagnoses.[114]

Morbid Obesity (Also See Chapter 29)

Morbidly obese patients seek outpatient surgical intervention in increasing numbers, as incisions grow ever smaller while patients grow larger. Patients with morbid obesity have a proclivity for higher perioperative risk, due to a frequent incidence of co-morbidities,[115] as well as for difficult airway management.[116,117] Thus, anesthesia providers and medical directors must educate surgeons and their office staffs to refer these patients for airway, pulmonary, and sleep disorder evaluations as soon as surgery is contemplated.[118,119] Scrupulous evaluation of the airway and cardiopulmonary and endocrine systems is necessary once the anesthesia provider has been apprised of a patient to be scheduled whose BMI is greater than 35 kg/m^2. An on-site evaluation to rule out a difficult endotracheal intubation is important.

A difficult endotracheal intubation recognized prior to the day of surgery may lead to the procedure. Maybe this patient should be redirected to a hospital, because many free-standing facilities do not accept patients with recognized difficult airways to manage. This approach is due to limited on-site equipment or airway expertise, including an otolaryngologist (ENT) surgeon with the ability to perform a tracheotomy. Although such policies may allow a free-standing ASC or office to avoid dealing with a known difficult airway instrumentation, preparation for management of the unanticipated difficult airway management and intubation is always necessary in all facilities.

The decision to electively care for morbidly or supramorbidly obese patients in a typical ambulatory surgery center is based on more than airway management capability. Consideration must be given to factors such as the number of caregivers available to manage patient transfers and the rated weight capacities of wheelchairs, stretchers and OR tables. Some free-standing facilities are buying equipment and staffing sufficiently to perform bariatric surgery, although the data is not yet sufficient to judge the success or safety of that trend. Even if the facility has a policy of not accepting patients over 300 pounds who require general or neuraxial anesthesia, the medical director may admit even supramorbidly obese patients if they are healthy and undergoing peripheral extremity surgery that can be managed with local or regional anesthesia and will not incur severe postoperative pain.

Obstructive Sleep Apnea in Adults (Also See Chapter 27)

Obstructive sleep apnea (OSA) creates sympathetic neural activation and leads to hypertension and cardiovascular abnormalities that can cause morbidity and sudden death during or after the perioperative period.[120] The majority of patients with OSA remain undiagnosed.[121] The increased potential for cerebrovascular events, myocardial infarction, bleeding, and the association with perioperative respiratory events, difficult intubation, and death makes this diagnosis critical to establish prior to surgery.[122,123] The value of preoperative evaluation is that patients can benefit from even a few days or weeks of treatment with continuous positive airway pressure (CPAP), decreasing their risk for airway obstruction and cardiovascular morbidity in the postoperative period.[124] A simple screening test can be applied over the phone and can direct evaluation (need for a sleep study).[125] The patient is best served by a sleep study and, if indicated, at least a few weeks of CPAP therapy. This will improve cardiovascular function, potentially decrease the size of the tongue and hypopharyngeal muscles, and diminish hypertension, thereby leading to easier airway management and less bleeding in the postoperative period.[126-130] As well, the use of postoperative opioids at home in the untreated OSA patient introduces additional risk, in view of the potential for increased respiratory depression.[131] Therefore, if a patient

IV

appears to, or is known to have moderate or severe OSA, is untreated, and will require general anesthesia or moderate doses of opioids to manage postoperative pain, then the hospital setting with respiratory monitoring is a more appropriate location for surgery than an outpatient facility.

Office-Based Anesthesia and Safety

Dental surgery, plastic surgery, and an ever-widening variety of surgical procedures are now being performed in offices, rather than ambulatory surgery facilities or hospitals. Excellent reviews published elsewhere provide full recommendations as to the facility requirements and appropriate case selection and anesthesia methodologies for the office location.[132-135] The outcomes of office-based procedures have generally been excellent, albeit with some notably high-profile tragedies occurring in offices, which highlights the need for superb anesthesia care in those settings.[136] The exact risk associated with anesthesia and surgery in the office setting in comparison to that of ASCs or hospitals is difficult to assess, because reporting mechanisms are insufficient.[137]

As is true for all outpatient surgical venues, the office-based anesthesia provider should be attentive to patient and case selection, as prolonged cases (longer than 2 hours), general anesthesia, and advancing age appear to be independent factors for increased morbidity after surgery.[138] However, most remote-site injuries related to anesthesia occur as a result of inadequate monitoring, not errors in patient selection.[139]

Notable factors associated with increased risk in the office setting include the use of unqualified providers of surgery or anesthesia, a lack of appropriate equipment and training for resuscitation and other emergencies, and a lack of appropriate access to hospitals.[140] If these factors and concerns are properly addressed, office-based anesthetic provided by careful anesthesia providers in an accredited facility appears to be safe, in comparison to outpatient anesthetics provided in other venues.[141]

Opioids and Pain in the Care of Surgical Outpatients (Also See Chapter 40)

As with all medications, the use of opioids should be restricted to those situations for which they are specifically indicated. In surgical outpatients, opioids should be titrated to alleviate experienced pain, which is to say very rarely in the preoperative setting, almost never in the intraoperative setting, and only occasionally in the postoperative setting. Opioids should be avoided prior to the postoperative period, in an effort to avoid the PONV, sedation and induction of higher opioid requirements associated with pre- and intraoperative opioid use.[142-146] Preoperatively, unless a patient is being seen with new acute pain (e.g., a new fracture) or is on long-term opioids (which should be managed by having them take their regularly scheduled opioids rather than using intravenous or intramuscular injections on-site to achieve their regular baseline), there is no need for opioid administration. The use of opioid as a routine sedative or to manage discomfort for placement of regional anesthesia can impair the value of that regional anesthesia (decreased PONV and postoperative opioid requirement). Judicious use of local anesthetic and gentle management of the patient relationship as well as sedation with midazolam or propofol are far better means of managing pain related to placement of needles.

Intraoperatively, management of pain should be accomplished with multimodal preemptive analgesics, because the use of opioid in the operating room induces PONV and PDNV as well as increased need for opioid in the PACU, while neither improving patient satisfaction nor pain ratings.[147] The use of multimodal analgesia techniques, including nonopioid medications, local anesthetic infiltration, and regional anesthetics can greatly decrease pain for patients (long and short term) and thereby produce high patient satisfaction and rapid throughput, or fast-tracking.[148-150] Studies support that preoperative gabapentin[151] and COX-2 inhibitors,[152,153] or intraoperative β-blockers,[154-157] ketorolac,[158] subanesthetic doses (0.15 mg/kg in one dose)[159] of ketamine,[160-162] magnesium (50 mg/kg over 15 minutes, then 15 mg/kg until surgery is completed),[163,164] dexamethasone,[165] methylprednisolone,[166] and intravenous lidocaine infusion[167] all diminish the need for postoperative opioids, alleviate acute postoperative pain and some postsurgical chronic pain, and reduce PONV and time to discharge.[168] As well, use of β adrenergic-blockers, COX-2 inhibitors, and paravertebral blocks may reduce immune suppression and tumor metastasis, perhaps an ultimate positive outcome of reduced stress due to reduced pain.[169,170] In the PACU, use of opioid should also be relatively infrequent if appropriate multimodal analgesia techniques were employed prior to arrival. PACU nurses should be discouraged from using opioid as sedation for the emerging general anesthetic patient with dysphoria. Pain scores in recovery can predict the length of stay there and are decreased by the use of nonopioids in the operating room.[171]

The anesthesia provider must determine a plan for adequate management of postdischarge pain before the decision is made to proceed with surgery, because pain is the cause for a significant number of hospital admissions following outpatient surgery.[172] If the postoperative analgesic plan for any patient or procedure depends upon significant amounts of intravenous or oral opioid administration, the outpatient venue should be reconsidered, as those patients will be at high risk for the complications (PDNV, pain) that lead to unplanned health care contacts and admission that increase the cost of health care without viable benefit.

Pediatric Patients: Airway Surgery and Obstructive Sleep Apnea (Also See Chapter 34)

Obstructive sleep apnea is a frequent finding in many pediatric patients undergoing outpatient surgery, particularly adenotonsillectomy. The presence (but not the severity) of OSA in children is associated with an increase in frequency of airway and respiratory events during the induction and postanesthesia period.[173] The ideal is to identify in advance those patients who could undergo surgery and be safely discharged home. However, in children particularly, the onerous process of polysomnography deters appropriate preoperative testing.[174] Simpler modalities such as home oximetry and screening questionnaires have not been reliable.[175–178]

Consequently, efforts have centered on retrospective evaluations of associations between significant outcomes with particular co-morbidities, generating guidelines that identify markers (e.g., age less than 36 months, failure to thrive, craniofacial abnormalities, morbid obesity, cor pulmonale, relative hypoxemia in the preoperative period, concomitant uvulopalatoplasty) that recommend planned inpatient care, with postoperative oximetry and apnea monitoring.[179,180] Notably, since OSA alters function in multiple organ systems, both blood testing and the altered profile of urinary proteins may offer a future means of delineating risk for pediatric patients without requiring invasive and inconvenient sleep laboratory testing.[181,182] Immediate and late complications of outpatient pediatric airway surgery (e.g., airway obstruction due to tissue swelling, laryngospasm, pulmonary edema) can be avoided at least in part by the surgeon's careful intraoperative management of tissues.[183] However, the outpatient anesthesia provider must be aware that any child undergoing tonsillectomy for moderate or severe obstructive symptoms may have increased obstruction, not improvement, in the 24 hours following surgery.[184]

Children undergoing adenotonsillectomy older than age 36 months with craniofacial abnormalities or obesity, and who have severe obstructive sleep apnea, are at high risk for respiratory complications and should be admitted to the hospital overnight.[185] Every child age 36 months or younger who undergoes adenotonsillectomy should be admitted and monitored overnight, owing to an unacceptably high (5% to 25%) incidence of respiratory complications, which cannot be predicted by the presence of co-morbidities.[186]

Postoperative Nausea and Vomiting: Prevention and Treatment

Patients place a high value on the prevention of PONV, ranking it equivalent to prevention and treatment of pain.[187,188] PONV and PDNV interfere with recovery of daily function after surgery and are therefore incompatible with the goals of anesthesia care and perioperative medicine.[189,190] In recent years, the Apfel predictive scoring system has been used to direct effective prophylaxis against PONV.[191] This approach is effective in preventing PONV in the PACU and first 24 hours after discharge, but the system is a poor predictor of nausea and vomiting 24 to 72 hours after discharge (PDNV).[192] As well, although PONV occurs in up to 74% of untreated at-risk outpatients,[193] and PDNV in up to one third,[194] some practitioners do not provide prophylaxis in accordance with recommendations of the literature and professional society guidelines. For most patients, practitioner adherence to guidelines that dictate multimodal management, such as those developed by ASPAN,[195] SAMBA,[196] or ASA,[197] will reduce the incidence of PONV early in the discharge period.[189,198] However, a regimen of both IV dexamethasone 8 mg and ondansetron 4 mg intraoperatively, followed by oral tablets of 8 mg ondansetron at discharge and on postoperative days 1 and 2, can virtually eliminate early and late PONV/PDNV in even the highest risk patients.[199] Also, a scopolamine patch applied prior to transfer to the operating room is as effective as droperidol or ondansetron in prevention of PONV in adults, although dry mouth is a problem for some patients.[200]

Intravenous hydration is also important. During the immediate preoperative period, adult patients should receive 2 mL/kg of sodium lactate solution (lactated Ringer's solution) for each hour fasted, infused over 20 minutes. This will decrease both PONV and pain.[201] Most pediatric patients should also be aggressively hydrated and given dual prophylaxis (dexamethasone and ondansetron) as this approach decreases their risk of PONV by as much as 80%.[202] If nausea or vomiting occurs in the PACU despite intraoperative use of ondansetron, rescue with repeated use of ondansetron is not as effective as is a small dose of promethazine, 6.25 mg IV.[203]

Preoperative Medication (Also See Chapter 13)

A long-held approach in the outpatient surgery facility has been to allow patients to walk to the operating room, thereby de-emphasizing the sense of "illness" patients have long associated with any and all surgical intervention. Such a technique precludes the use of preoperative sedation outside the operating room and many patients express satisfaction with the lack of routine use of sedation. However, for the occasional patient who portrays significant anxiety, premedication with midazolam IV can alleviate those symptoms in adults without delay of discharge, and may also improve some outcomes, including improved satisfaction with needle procedures and reduced pain.[204] In children, use of 0.5 mg/kg oral midazolam in the preoperative area may attenuate separation anxiety, improve induction of anesthesia conditions, and even decrease negative behavior disturbances in the first 7 days after surgery.[205] However, there may be a

IV

delay in discharge with the use of premedication, a possibility that may increase with age of the patient and if the preoperative sedation was profound.[206,207]

Upper Respiratory Infection

Present or recent upper respiratory infection (URI) has been considered by some practitioners to be sufficient reason for cancellation of cases, due to concern about potential increased pulmonary morbidity in the perioperative period. Supraglottic edema, stridor, laryngospasm, desaturation, and coughing have all been associated with provision of general anesthesia to patients with URI, particularly when endotracheal intubation has been performed.[208] Although the use of the laryngeal mask airway (LMA) may be associated with fewer problems in these patients, there is still an opportunity for severely negative outcomes, such as laryngeal edema, after use of an LMA in a patient with a recent URI.[209] The choice of a particular type of anesthetic or technique, the value of glycopyrrolate, or the decision to extubate the trachea while the patient is deeply or lightly anesthetized is not clear.[210,211]

Recent studies do support the decision to proceed with elective surgery in patients with a current or recent mild URI if the procedure can be safely performed without endotracheal intubation, the patient has no other cardiac or pulmonary problems (i.e., congenital heart disease, asthma, or chronic obstructive pulmonary disease [COPD]) and the surgical procedure will not impact the airway.[212] On the other hand, surgery should probably be postponed for those patients who have current, severe URIs (severe defined as the presence of systemic symptoms such as fever and malaise, or focal pulmonary symptoms of wheezing and dyspnea) or are within 4 weeks of a severe URI and whose elective surgery will require intubation or will directly affect the airway.

POSTOPERATIVE ISSUES

PACU Management (Also See Chapter 39)

Achievement of excellent throughput and outcomes in the PACU requires active and intentional management of its care systems, personnel, and individual patients. Deliberate attention to preoperative optimization of congestive heart failure, avoidance of prolonged cases, and aggressive management of pain and PONV are necessary to avoid prolonged stays in PACU or readmissions to either the emergency department (ED) or hospital inpatient wards.

Availability of anesthesia personnel to manage airway or cardiopulmonary emergencies is usually limited in a fast-paced ambulatory surgery unit or office. The importance of this factor is not always clear to those surgeons or administrators who wish to trial longer, more invasive case types or to accept less healthy patients. This need

makes the anesthesia care team model (CRNAs directed by an anesthesiologist) the ideal approach for a busy ambulatory surgery center or office. In the absence of such a model, the solo provider should remain available (i.e., not begin the next induction) to care for any patient who has not yet awakened sufficiently to maintain his or her own airway.

Postdischarge Issues

Some outpatient anesthesia providers cannot describe the outcomes of the outpatients for whom they care, because they do not contact those patients or discuss the findings of those nurses who make calls to those patients. They do not know their own "batting average" for PONV, PDNV, or postdischarge ED visits. These same practitioners are nonetheless often quite certain that they provide an above-average anesthetic experience for their patients. Yet, after discharge a significant number of patients suffer moderate to severe pain, cognitive impairment, PDNV, and take more than 3 days to return to normal activity.[213] This suggests that we do not really know the impact of our care choices. For instance, many of us do not know if our decisions regarding PONV prevention—based upon studies of on-site PONV only—are useful in preventing nausea and vomiting that occurs after discharge (PDNV), even though the factors that cause PDNV are likely different from those that cause PONV.[88] Thus, it is important that anesthesia providers contact their patients in the days following surgery, or ask for the findings of those facilities that make these contacts. This is the only way providers can monitor the outcomes of their care and improve it.

UNIQUE ROLES OF THE ANESTHESIOLOGIST AND MEDICAL DIRECTOR (Also See Chapter 45)

It is clear that significant differences exist between the practices of outpatient anesthesia in different outpatient venues: hospital-based, free-standing ASCs, or offices. Providers who move along the spectrum from hospital to office practice quickly become aware that oxygen and suction don't always "come out of the wall," opioid security isn't vouched for by an unseen pharmacy director, and that poorly crafted gas scavenging systems can have a direct impact on your sense of well-being at the end of a long day. More than one ASC or office anesthesia provider has had to postpone or cancel Monday cases because someone left an oxygen flowmeter open on the preceding Friday afternoon.

Nonetheless, ASC and office anesthesia providers find that their roles expand and provide new opportunities as they become aware of state, payer, and DEA requirements for medication records, facility size, emergency equipment, sterilizing systems, personnel to patient ratio minimums, costs of medications, and scarcity of labor. As anesthesia providers are often the physicians present for the longest periods at ASCs and offices, they eventually migrate to the position of providing advice and direction to the administrative teams who manage the facility. This role can be quite fulfilling, but brings with it the need to shift from a mindset of independent physician to a physician-manager who can provide a unique skill-set and expertise to the facility. The physician will learn about personnel issues: how to manage anesthesia shortages, professionals with substance abuse, quirky accreditation inspectors with peculiar axes to grind, profit and loss statements, and how to use data to choose which providers to welcome back and what equipment to buy. There are no courses that provide a curriculum specific to becoming a medical director for an ambulatory surgery facility. However, the author strongly recommends membership in and attendance at the annual spring meetings of SAMBA as well as the meetings of the ambulatory track at the annual meeting of the ASA. These meetings, combined with the expertise borne of daily immersion in the ambulatory anesthesia and surgery environment, will serve the reader well in growing through the challenges and opportunities of medical directorship.

CONCLUSION

The future of outpatient anesthesia is not murky. The volumes of patients will continue to increase, the venues will continue to grow more experientially distant from medical center operating rooms, and the technology of surgical intervention will continue to advance the invasiveness of the procedures on the daily list. The choices we will make about anesthesia techniques will be made easier by data generated by nascent local and national outcome registries, while we wait for the era when patients arrive at the front door with their genetic profiles in hand, as containers of their dose-specific and phenotypically appropriate anesthetic drugs are delivered at the back loading dock.

We know more now than ever before about what we don't know. We recognize that our future therapies will be guided by yet-to-be established principles of pharmacogenetics. In the meantime, our subspecialty benefits from the fact that greater than 90% of our patients have the same set of procedures performed by the same surgeons and dentists, in the same ways, day in and day out. Owing to the nature of ambulatory surgery, outpatient anesthesia providers don't have to anticipate many outliers, either among patients or procedures. As a result, we can rely on the trends and associations identified by clinical registries of outcome data derived from the experiences of similar patients undergoing similar procedures. Registries have begun to extend lives and save

them, when their findings have been applied to guide therapy for patients with similar diagnoses.[214] It is reasonable to expect they will have the same impact on the homogeneous patient and procedural populations that make up outpatient surgery. In fact, such peer review audits have significantly lowered surgical mortality rates in elective surgery.[215]

Outpatient anesthesia providers should lead the way in tracking the real outcomes of all their patients. Each anesthesia provider today can create a small database from the many spreadsheet or relational database software programs present today to link the characteristics of their practice's patients with the anesthetic management and the few salient outcomes that matter to patients. Until the lessons of national ambulatory anesthesia registries are commonly available, our best decision guides will be driven not by our individual memories of anecdotal outcome, but by our use of standard care pathways derived from our own participation in local registries. While we wait for national experience to delineate best practices, we can provide "better practice," if we discontinue our dependence on faith-based anesthesia (i.e., "this is what I always do and my patients do fine") and instead base our decisions on techniques based upon the best outcomes to be found among all the patients for whom our partners provide care.

Be eager to join the national registries now being built, but build locally while you wait.

QUESTIONS OF THE DAY

1. Under what conditions should laboratory tests be performed prior to outpatient surgery?
2. What manifestations of cardiac disease should preclude a patient from undergoing outpatient surgery in a nonhospital environment?
3. How should perioperative hyperglycemia be managed in a diabetic patient undergoing outpatient surgery?
4. What measures can be taken to reduce the incidence of postoperative and postdischarge nausea and vomiting after outpatient surgery?
5. How should the availability of 23-hour stay facilities affect patient selection for outpatient surgery?

ACKNOWLEDGMENTS

The author wishes to thank Drs. Lucy Everett and Mary Ann Vann and Ms. Deborah Ann Davis for their advice in preparation of this manuscript.

The editors and publisher would like to thank Dr. Martin Bogetz for contibuting a chapter on this topic to the prior edition of this work. It has served as the foundation for the current chapter.

IV

REFERENCES

1. Stone JL, Miles ML: Skull trepanation among the early Indians of Canada and the United States, *Neurosurgery* 26:1015–1020, 1990.

2. Júnior JFN, Hermann DR, Américo RR, et al: A brief history of tonsillectomy, *Arch Int Otorhinolaryngol* 10(4):314–317, 2006.

3. http://www.nysora.com/regional_anesthesia/sub-specialties/pediatric_anesthesia/3082-regional_anesthesia_in_pediatric_ patients.html (downloaded 02/15/2010).

4. Waters RM: The Downtown Anesthesia Clinic, *Am J Surg* 33(7):71–77, 1919.

5. Personal communication. My memory is of a story that Dr. Reed told. He and Dr. Ford had a mutual barber and one day the man told one of them that one of his children had just undergone a myringotomy and tube placement in the hospital, with two nights' stay, and notable expense. The two anesthesiologists mused, "How many haircuts should it take to pay for ear tubes?" From that idle conjecture was born the Phoenix Surgery Center.

6. Macario A, Weinger M, Carney S, et al: Which clinical anesthesia outcomes are important to avoid? The perspective of patients, *Anesth Analg* 89:652–658, 1999.

7. Macario A, et al: Which clinical anesthesia outcomes are both common and important to avoid? The perspective of a panel of expert anesthesiologists, *Anesth Analg* 88(5):1085–1091, 1999.

8. Gan J, Sloan F, Dear G, et al: How much are patients willing to pay to avoid postoperative nausea and vomiting? *Anesth Analg* 92:393–400, 2001.

9. Eijkemans MJC, van Houdenhoven M, Nguyen T, et al: Predicting the unpredictable: A new prediction model for operating room times using individual characteristics and the surgeon's estimate, *Anesthesiology* 112:41–49, 2010.

10. Fleisher LA, Pasternak LR, Herbert R, Anderson GF: Inpatient hospital admission and death after outpatient surgery in elderly patients: Importance of patient and system characteristics and location of care, *Arch Surg* 139(1):67–72, 2004.

11. Grisel J, Arjmand E: Comparing quality at an ambulatory surgery center and a hospital-based facility: Preliminary findings, *Otolaryngol Head Neck Surg* 141(6):701–709, 2009.

12. ASA: Practice guidelines for management of the difficult airway, *Anesthesiology* 98:1269–1277, 2003. Accessed at http://www2.asahq.org/publications/pc-177-4-practice-guidelines-for-management-of-the-difficult-airway.aspx (downloaded 02/10/2009).

13. Salas E, Wilson KA, Burke CS, et al: Using simulation-based training to improve patient safety: What does it take? *Jt Comm J Qual Patient Saf* 31(7):363–371, 2005.

14. Rosen MA, Salas E, Wilson KA, et al: Measuring team performance in simulation-based training: Adopting best practices for healthcare, *Simul Healthcare* 3(1):33–41, 2008.

15. Fleisher LA, Pasternak LR, Lyles A: A novel index of elevated risk of inpatient hospital admission immediately following outpatient surgery, *Arch Surg* 142(3):263–268, 2007.

16. Menachemi N, Chukmaitov A, Brown LS, et al: Quality of care differs by patient characteristics: Outcome disparities after ambulatory surgical procedures, *Am J Med Qual* 22(6):395–401, 2007.

17. Laffel G, Blumenthal D: The case for using industrial quality management science in health care organizations, *JAMA* 262(20):2869–2873, 1989.

18. Spear S: Learning to Lead at Toyota, *Harv Bus Rev* 82(5):78–86, 2004.

19. Spencer FC: Human error in hospitals and industrial accidents: Current concepts, *J Am Coll Surg* 191(4):410–418, 2000.

20. Uhlig P: Interview with a quality leader: Paul Uhlig on transforming healthcare. Interviewed by Jason Trevor Fogg, *J Health Care Qual* 31(3):5–9, 2009.

21. Jamtvedt G, Young JM, Kristoffersen DT, et al: Audit and feedback: Effects on professional practice and health care outcomes, *Cochrane Database Syst Rev* 19(2): CD000259, 2001; downloaded 01/24/2010.

22. Leape L, Berwick D, Clancy C: Transforming healthcare: A safety imperative, *Qual Saf Health Care* 18:424–428, 2009.

23. Blumenthal D: Quality of care—What is it? Part one of six, *N Engl J Med* 335:891–1194, 1996.

24. Manuel DG, Mao Y: Avoidable mortality in the United States and Canada, 1980-1996, *Am J Public Health* 92(9):1481–1484, 2002.

25. Berwick DM: The clinical process and the quality process, *Qual Manag Health Care* 1:1–8, 1992.

26. Eitan-Naveh ZS: *How quality improvement programs can affect general hospital performance*. http://www.emeraldinsight.com/10.1108/09526860510602532.

27. Brown EC, Kros J: Reducing room turnaround time at a regional hospital, *Qual Manag Health Care* 19(1):90–100, 2010.

28. Carlhed R, Bojestig M: Improved clinical outcome after acute myocardial infarction in hospitals participating in a Swedish quality improvement initiative, *Circ Card Qual Outcomes* 2(3):458–464, 2009.

29. Macario A: Truth in scheduling: Is it possible to accurately predict how long a surgical case will last? *Anesth Analg* 108(3):681–685, 2009.

30. Kim JH, Schwinn DA, Landau R: Pharmacogenomics and perioperative medicine: Implications for modern clinical practice, *Can J Anaesth* 55(12):799–806, 2008.

31. Merrill D: Management of outcomes in the ambulatory surgery center: The role of standard work and evidence-based medicine, *Curr Opin Anaesthesiol* 21:743–747, 2008.

32. ASA: Practice Advisory for Preanesthesia Evaluation, *Anesthesiology* 96:485–496, 2002. http://www.asahq.org/publicationsAndServices/preeval.pdf; downloaded 01/24/2010.

33. Chung F, Yegneswaran B, Herrera F, Shenderey A: Patients with difficult intubation may need referral to sleep clinics, *Anesth Analg* 107:915–920, 2008.

34. Van Klei WA, Moons KG, Rutten CL, et al: The effect of outpatient preoperative evaluation of hospital inpatients on cancellation of surgery and length of hospital stay, *Anesth Analg* 94:644–649, 2002.

35. Narr BJ, Hansen TR, Warner MA: Preoperative laboratory screening in healthy Mayo patients: Cost-effective elimination of tests and unchanged outcomes, *Mayo Clin Proc* 66:155–159, 1991.

36. Correll DJ, Hepner DL, Chang C, et al: Preoperative electrocardiograms: Patient factors predictive of abnormalities, *Anesthesiology* 110:1217–1222, 2009.

37. Alexoudis A, Spyridonidou A, Vogiatzaki T, Iatrou C: Preoperative electrocardiograms (letter), *Anesthesiology* 112:255, 2010.

38. Chung F: Elimination of preoperative testing in ambulatory surgery, *Anesth Analg* 108:467–475, 2009.

39. Apostolos A, Spyridonidou A, Voglatzaki T, Iatrou C: Preoperative electrocardiograms (letter), *Anesthesiology* 112:255, 2010.

40. Goodnough LT, Shander A, Spivak JL, et al: Detection, evaluation, and

management of anemia in the elective surgical patient, *Anesth Analg* 101:1858–1861, 2005.

41. Sweitzer BJ: To test or not to test, *SAMBA Newsletter* 24(2):8–10, 2009.

42. Olson RP, Stone A, Lubarsky D: The prevalence and significance of low preoperative hemoglobin in ASA 1 or 2 outpatient surgery candidates, *Anesth Analg* 101:1337–1340, 2005.

43. Kahn RL, Stanton MA, Tong-Ngork S, et al: One-year experience with day-of-surgery pregnancy testing before elective orthopedic procedures, *Anesth Analg* 106:1127–1131, 2008.

44. Fleisher LA: Cardiac risk stratification for noncardiac surgery. Update from the American College of Cardiology/ American Heart Association 2007 guidelines, *Cleve Clin J Med* 76(Suppl 4): S9–S15, 2009.

45. Grines CL, Bonow RO, Casey DE Jr, et al: Prevention of premature discontinuation of dual antiplatelet therapy in patients with coronary artery stents: A science advisory from the American Heart Association, American College of Cardiology, Society for Cardiovascular Angiography and Interventions, American College of Surgeons, and American Dental Association, with representation from the American College of Physicians, *J Am Coll Cardiol* 49(6):734–739, 2007.

46. Ford MK, Beattie WS, Wijeysundera DN: Systematic review: Prediction of perioperative cardiac complications and mortality by the revised cardiac risk index, *Ann Intern Med* 152(1):26–35, 2010.

47. Woods BD, Sladen RN: Perioperative considerations for the patient with asthma and bronchospasm, *Br J Anaesth* 103(Suppl 1):i57–i65, 2009.

48. Licker M, Schweizer A, Ellenberger C: Perioperative medical management of patients with COPD, *Int J Chron Obstruct Pulm Dis* 2(4):493–515, 2007.

49. Carmosino MJ, Friesen RH, Doran A: Perioperative complications in children with pulmonary hypertension undergoing noncardiac surgery or cardiac catheterization, *Anesth Analg* 104:521–527, 2007.

50. Lai HC, Lai HC, Wang KY, et al: Severe pulmonary hypertension complicates postoperative outcome of noncardiac surgery, *Br J Anaesth* 99:184–190, 2007.

51. Solomonson MD, Johnson ME, Ilstrup D: Risk factors in patients having surgery to create an arteriovenous fistula, *Anesth Analg* 79:694–700, 1994.

52. Sladen RN: Anesthetic considerations for the patient with renal failure, *Anesthesiol Clin North America* 18(4):863–882, 2000.

53. Bhananker SM, Posner KL, Cheney FW, et al: Injury and liability associated with monitored anesthesia care: A closed claims analysis, *Anesthesiology* 104:228–234, 2006.

54. Metzner J, Posner KL, Domino KB: The risk and safety of anesthesia at remote locations: The US closed claims analysis, *Curr Opin Anaesthesiol* 22:502–508, 2009.

55. Liu SS, Strodtbeck WM, Richman JM, et al: A comparison of regional versus general anesthesia for ambulatory anesthesia: A meta-analysis of randomized controlled trials, *Anesth Analg* 101(6):1634–1642, 2005.

56. O'Donnell BD, Iohom G: Regional anesthesia techniques for ambulatory orthopedic surgery, *Curr Opin Anaesthesiol* 21(6):723–728, 2008.

57. Mariano ER, Chu LF, Peinado CR, Mazzei WJ: Anesthesia-controlled time and turnover time for ambulatory upper extremity surgery performed with regional versus general anesthesia, *J Clin Anesth* 21:253–257, 2009.

58. Hadzic A, Williams BA, Karaca PE, et al: For outpatient rotator cuff surgery, nerve block anesthesia provides superior same-day recovery over general anesthesia, *Anesthesiology* 102:1001–1007, 2005.

59. Hadzic A, Alris J, Kerimoglu B, et al: A comparison of infraclavicular nerve block versus general anesthesia for hand and wrist day-case surgeries, *Anesthesiology* 101:127–132, 2004.

60. Klein SM, Pietrobon R, Nielsen KC, et al: Peripheral nerve blockade with long-acting local anesthetics: A survey of the Society for Ambulatory Anesthesia, *Anesth Analg* 94:71–76, 2002.

61. Ilfeld BM, Morey TE, Enneking FK: Continuous infraclavicular brachial plexus block for post-operative pain control at home: A randomized, double-blinded, placebo-controlled study, *Anesthesiology* 96:1297–1304, 2002.

62. Swenson JD, Bay N, Loose E, et al: Outpatient management of continuous peripheral nerve catheters placed using ultrasound guidance: An experience in 620 patients, *Anesth Analg* 103:1436–1443, 2006.

63. Hadzic A, Kerimoglu B, Loreio D, et al: Paravertebral blocks provide superior same-day recovery over general anesthesia for patients undergoing inguinal hernia repair, *Anesth Analg* 102:1076–1081, 2006.

64. Iohom G, Abdalla H, O'Brien J, et al: The associations between severity of early post-operative pain, chronic post-surgical pain and plasma concentration

of stable nitric oxide products after breast surgery, *Anesth Analg* 103:995–1000, 2006.

65. Naja Z, Lonnqvist PA: Somatic paravertebral nerve blockade. Incidence of failed block and complications, *Anaesthesia* 56:1181–1201, 2001.

66. Eid H: Paravertebral block: An overview, *Curr Anesth Crit Care* 20:65–70, 2009.

67. Exadaktylos AK, Buggy DJ, Moriarty DC, et al: Can anesthetic technique for primary breast cancer surgery affect recurrence or metastasis? *Anesthesiology* 105:660–664, 2006.

68. Korhonen AM, Valanne JV, Jokela RM, et al: A comparison of selective spinal anesthesia with hyperbaric bupivacaine and general anesthesia with desflurane for outpatient knee arthroscopy, *Anesth Analg* 99:1668–1673, 2004.

69. Kodeih MG, Al-alami AA, Atiyeh BS, et al: Combined spinal epidural anesthesia in an asthmatic patient undergoing abdominoplasty, *Plast Reconstr Surg* 123(3):118e–120e, 2009.

70. Zohar E, Noga Y, Rislick U, et al: Intrathecal anesthesia for elderly patients undergoing short transurethral procedures: A dose-finding study, *Anesth Analg* 104(3):552–554, 2007.

71. Yoos JR, Kopacz DJ: Spinal 2-chloroprocaine for surgery: An initial 10-month experience, *Anesth Analg* 100:553–558, 2005.

72. Casati A, Danelli G, Berti M, et al: Intrathecal 2-chloroprocaine for lower limb outpatient surgery: A prospective, randomized, double-blind, clinical evaluation, *Anesth Analg* 103:234–238, 2006.

73. Cappelleri G, Aldegheri G, Danelli G, et al: Spinal anesthesia with hyperbaric levobupivacaine and ropivacaine for outpatient knee arthroscopy: A prospective, randomized, double-blind study, *Anesth Analg* 101:77–82, 2005.

74. Smith KN, Kopacz DJ: Spinal 2-chloroprocaine: A dose-ranging study and the effect of added epinephrine, *Anesth Analg* 98:81–88, 2004.

75. Fredman B, Nathanson MH, Smith I, et al: Sevoflurane for outpatient anesthesia: A comparison with propofol, *Anesth Analg* 81:823–828, 1995.

76. Nathanson MH, Fredman B, Smith I, et al: Sevoflurane vs. desflurane for outpatient anesthesia: A comparison of maintenance and recovery profiles, *Anesth Analg* 81:1186–1190, 1995.

77. Song D, Whitten CW, White PF, et al: Antiemetic activity of propofol after sevoflurane and desflurane anesthesia for outpatient laparoscopic cholecystectomy, *Anesthesiology* 89:838–843, 1998.

IV

78. Gupta A, Steirer T, Zukerman R, et al: Comparison of recovery profile after ambulatory anesthesia with propofol, isoflurane, sevoflurane and desflurane: A systematic review, *Anesth Analg* 98:632–641, 2004.

79. Higgins PP, Chung F, Mezei G: Postoperative sore throat after ambulatory surgery, *Br J Anaesth* 88(4):582–584, 2002.

80. Colye KC, Williams BA, DaPos SV, et al: Retrospective evaluation of unanticipated admissions and readmissions after same day surgery and associated costs, *J Clin Anesth* 14(5):349–353, 2002.

81. Pavlin DJ, Rapp SE, Polissar NL, et al: Factors affecting discharge time in adult outpatients, *Anesth Analg* 87:816–826, 1998.

82. Chung F, Mezei G: Factors contributing to a prolonged stay after ambulatory surgery, *Anesth Analg* 89:1352–1359, 1999.

83. Pavlin JD, Horvarth KD, Pavlin EG, et al: Preincisional treatment to prevent pain after ambulatory hernia surgery, *Anesth Analg* 97:1627–1632, 2003.

84. White PF: The changing role of non-opioid analgesic techniques in the management of postoperative pain, *Anesth Analg* 101:S5–S22, 2005.

85. Liu SS, Strodtbeck WM, Richman JM, Wu CLA: comparison of regional versus general anesthesia for ambulatory anesthesia: A meta-analysis of randomized controlled trials, *Anesth Analg* 101:1634–1642, 2005.

86. Visser K, Hassingk EA, Bonsel GJ, et al: Randomized controlled trial of total intravenous anesthesia with propofol versus inhalation anesthesia with isoflurane-nitrous oxide: Postoperative nausea with vomiting and economic analysis, *Anesthesiology* 95:616–626, 2001.

87. Apfel CC, Laara E, Koivuranta M, et al: A simplified risk score for predicting postoperative nausea and vomiting: Conclusions from cross-validations between two centers, *Anesthesiology* 91:693–700, 1999.

88. Kolodzie K, Apfel CC: Nausea and vomiting after office-based anesthesia. *Curr Opin Anaesthesiol* 22:532–538, 2009.

89. Gan TJ, Meyer TA, Apfel CC, et al: Society for Ambulatory Anesthesia guidelines for the management of postoperative nausea and vomiting, *Anesth Analg* 105:1615–1628, 2007.

90. Moghissi ES, Korytkowski MT, Dinardo M, et al: American Association of Clinical Endocrinologists and American Diabetes Association consensus statement on inpatient glycemic control, *Diabetes Care* 32:1119–1131, 2009.

91. Drange AS Perkal MF, Kancir S, et al: Long-term glycemic control and postoperative infectious complications, *Arch Surg* 141:375–380, 2006.

92. Rhodes ET, Ferrari LR, Wolfsdorf JL: Perioperative management of pediatric surgical patients with diabetes mellitus, *Anesth Analg* 101:986–999, 2005.

93. American Diabetes Association: Standards of medical care in diabetes 2009, *Diabetes Care* 32:S13–S61, 2009.

94. Nathan DM, Buse JB, Davidson MB, et al: Medical management of hyperglycemia in type 2 diabetes: A consensus algorithm for the initiation and adjustment of therapy: A consensus statement of the American Diabetes Association and the European Association for the Study of Diabetes, *Diabetes Care* 32:193–203, 2009.

95. Clement S, Brithwaite SS, Magee MF, et al: Management of diabetes and hyperglycemia in hospitals, *Diabetes Care* 27(2):553–591, 2004.

96. Cryer PE, Axelrod L, Grossman AB, et al: Evaluation and management of adult hypoglycemic disorders: An Endocrine Society Clinical Practice Guideline, *J Clin Endocrinol Metab* 94:709–728, 2009.

97. Vann MA: Perioperative management of ambulatory surgical patients with diabetes mellitus, *Curr Opin Anaesthesiol* 22:718–724, 2009.

98. Rhodes ET, Ferrari LR, Wolfsdorf JL: Perioperative management of pediatric surgical patients with diabetes mellitus, *Anesth Analg* 101:986–999, 2005.

99. Lubarsky DA: Fast-track in the postanesthesia care unit: Unlimited possibilities, *J Clin Anesth* 8:70–72, 1996.

100. White PF, Tang J, Wender RH, et al: Desflurane versus sevoflurane for maintenance of outpatient anesthesia: The effect on early versus late recovery and perioperative coughing, *Anesth Analg* 109(2):387–393, 2009.

101. Gupta A, Stierer T, Zuckerman R, et al: Comparison of recovery profile after ambulatory anesthesia with propofol, isoflurane, sevoflurane and desflurane: A systematic review, *Anesth Analg* 98(3):632–641, 2004.

102. White PF: The changing role of non-opioid analgesic techniques in the management of post-operative pain, *Anesth Analg* 101:S5–S22, 2005.

103. White PF, Ma H, Tang J, et al: Does the use of electroencephalographic bispectral index or auditory evoked potential index monitoring facilitate recovery after desflurane anesthesia in the ambulatory setting? *Anesthesiology* 100:811–817, 2004.

104. White PF, Song D: New criteria for fast-tracking after outpatient anesthesia: A comparison with the modified Aldrete's scoring system, *Anesth Analg* 88(5):1069–1072, 1999.

105. Kheterpal S, O'Reilly M, Englesbe MJ, et al: Preoperative and intraoperative predictors of cardiac adverse events after general, vascular and urological surgery, *Anesthesiology* 110:58–66, 2009.

106. Coriat P, Richer C, Douraki T, et al: Influence of chronic angiotensin-converting enzyme inhibition on anesthetic induction, *Anesthesiology* 81:299–307, 1994.

107. Colson P, Saussine M, Seguin JR, et al: Hemodynamic effects of anesthesia in patients chronically treated with angiotensin-converting enzyme inhibitors, *Anesth Analg* 74:805–808, 1992.

108. Reich DL, Hossain S, Krol M, et al: Predictors of hypotension after induction of general anesthesia, *Anesth Analg* 101:622–628, 2005.

109. Comfere T, Sprung J, Kumar MM, et al: Angiotensin system inhibitors in a general surgical population, *Anesth Analg* 100:636–644, 2005.

110. Larach MG, Gronert G, Allen GC, et al: Clinical presentation, treatment, and complications of malignant hyperthermia in North America from 1987 to 2006, *Anesth Analg* 110:498–507, 2010.

111. Yentis SM, Levine MF, Hartley EJ: Should all children with suspected or confirmed malignant hyperthermia susceptibility be admitted after surgery? A ten year review. *Anesth Analg* 75:345–350, 1992.

112. Everett LL, Fuzaylov G: Pediatric clinical challenges. In Twersky RS, Philip BK, editors: *Handbook of Ambulatory Anesthesia*, ed 2, New York, 2008, Springer Science & Business Media, pp 108–109.

113. White PF, Eng MR: Ambulatory (outpatient) anesthesia. In Miller RD, editor: *Miller's Anesthesia*, ed 7, Philadelphia, 2010, Churchill Livingstone, p 2423.

114. Klingler W, Rueffert H, Lehmann-Horn F, et al: Core myopathies and risk of malignant hyperthermia, *Anesth Analg* 109:1167–1173, 2009.

115. De Lusignan S, Hague N, Van Vlymen J, et al: A study of cardiovascular risk in overweight and obese people in England, *Eur J Gen Pract* 12(1):19–29, 2006.

116. Brodsky JB, Lemmens HJ, Brock-Utne JG, et al: Morbid obesity and tracheal intubation, *Anesth Analg* 94:732–736, 2002.

117. Gonzalez H, Minville V, Delanoue K, et al: The importance of increased neck circumference to intubation

118. difficulties in obese patients, *Anesth Analg* 106:1132–1136, 2008.

119. Kaw R, Aboussuan L, Auckley D, et al: Challenges in pulmonary risk assessment and perioperative management in bariatric surgery patients, *Obes Surg* 18:134–138, 2008.

119. Gonzalez H, Minville V, Delanoue K, et al: The importance of increased neck circumference to intubation difficulties in obese patients, *Anesth Analg* 106:1132–1136, 2008.

120. Dincer HE, O'Neill W: Deleterious effects of sleep-disordered breathing on the heart and vascular system, *Respiration* 73:124–130, 2006.

121. Young T, Evans L, Finn L, Palta M: Estimation of the clinically diagnosed proportion of sleep apnea syndrome in middle-aged men and women, *Sleep* 20:705–706, 1997.

122. Siyam MA, Benhamou D: Difficult endotracheal intubation in patients with sleep apnea syndrome, *Anesth Analg* 95:1098–1102, 2002.

123. Chung S, Yuan H, Chung F: A systematic review of obstructive sleep apnea and its implications for anesthesiologists, *Anesth Analg* 107:1543–1563, 2008.

124. Bonsignore MR, Parati G, Insalaco G, et al: Baroreflex control of heart rate during sleep in severe obstructive sleep apnea: Effects of acute CPAP, *Eur Respir J* 27:128–135, 2006.

125. Chung F, Yegneswaran B, Liao P, et al: Stop questionnaire: A tool to screen patients for obstructive sleep apnea, *Anesthesiology* 108:812–821, 2008.

126. Dursunoglu N, Dursunoglu D, Ozkurt S, et al: Effects of CPAP on left ventricular structure and myocardial performance index in male patients with obstructive sleep apnea, *Sleep Med* 8(1):51–59, 2007.

127. Bayram NA, Ciftci B, Keles T, et al: Endothelial function in normotensive men with obstructive sleep apnea before and 6 months after CPAP treatment, *Sleep* 32(10):1257–1263, 2009.

128. Christou K, Kostikas K, Pastaka C, et al: Nasal continuous positive airway pressure treatment reduces systemic oxidative stress in patients with severe obstructive sleep apnea, *Sleep Med* 10(1):87–94, 2009.

129. Ryan CF, Lowe AA, Li D, et al: Magnetic resonance imaging of the upper airway in obstructive sleep apnea before and after chronic nasal continuous positive airway pressure, *Am Rev Respir Dis* 144(4):939–944, 1991.

130. Collop NA, Block AJ, Hellard D: The effect of nightly nasal CPAP treatment on underlying obstructive sleep apnea and pharyngeal size, *Chest* 99:855–860, 1991.

131. Catley DM, Thornton C, Jordan C, et al: Pronounced, episodic oxygen desaturation in the postoperative period: Its association with ventilatory pattern and analgesic regimen, *Anesthesiology* 63:20–28, 1985.

132. Vila H Jr, Desai MS, Miguel RV: Office-based anesthesia. In Twersky RS, Philip BK, editors: *Handbook of Ambulatory Anesthesia*, ed 2, New York, 2008, Springer Science & Business Media, pp 283–324.

133. Twersky RS: ASA Committee on Ambulatory Surgical Care and ASA Task Force on Office-Based Anesthesia. Office-based anesthesia: Considerations for anesthesiologists in setting up and maintaining a safe office anesthesia environment. http://www2.asahq.org/publications/p-319-office-based-anesthesia-considerations-for-anesthesiologists-in-setting-up-and-maintaining-a-safe-office-anesthesia-environment-2nd-edition-november-2008.aspx.

134. Evron S, Ezri T: Organizational prerequisites for anesthesia outside the operating room, *Curr Opin Anaesthesiol* 22:514–518, 2009.

135. ASA: *Guidelines for Office Based Anesthesia*, 2004. http://www.asahq.org/publicationsAnd Services/office.pdf (downloaded 02/07/2010).

136. Vila H Jr, Soto R, Cantor AB, Mackey D: Comparative outcomes analysis of procedures performed in physicians' offices and ambulatory surgery centers, *Arch Surg* 138(9):991–995, 2003.

137. Li G, Warner M, Lang BH, et al: Epidemiology of anesthesia-related mortality in the United States, 1999-2005, *Anesthesiology* 110(4):759–765, 2009.

138. Fleischer LA, Pasternak LR, Lyles A: A novel index of elevated risk of inpatient hospital admission immediately following outpatient surgery, *Arch Surg* 142(3):263–268, 2007.

139. Metzner J, Posner KL, Domino KB: The risk and safety of anesthesia at remote locations: The US closed claims analysis, *Curr Opin Anaesthesiol* 22:502–508, 2009.

140. Vila H Jr, Desai MS, Miguel RV: Office-based anesthesia. In Twersky RS, Philip BK, editors: *Handbook of Ambulatory Anesthesia*, ed 2, New York, 2008, Springer Science & Business Media, p 285.

141. Keyes GR, Singer R, Iverson RE, et al: Mortality in outpatient surgery, *Plast Reconstr Surg* 122(1):245–250, 2008.

142. White PF: The role of non-opioid analgesic techniques in the management of pain after ambulatory surgery, *Anesth Analg* 94:577–585, 2002.

143. Lentschener C, Tostivint P, White PF, et al: Opioid-induced sedation in the postanesthesia care unit does not insure adequate pain relief: A case-control study, *Anesth Analg* 105:1143–1147, 2007.

144. Angst MS, Clark JC: Opioid-induced hyperalgesia: A qualitative systematic review, *Anesthesiology* 104:570–587, 2006.

145. White PF: Prevention of postoperative nausea and vomiting: A multimodal solution to a persistent problem, *N Engl J Med* 350:2511–2512, 2004.

146. Crawford MW, Hickey C, Zaarour C: Development of acute opioid tolerance during infusion of remifentanil for pediatric scoliosis surgery, *Anesth Analg* 102(6):1662–1667, 2006.

147. Kehlet H, Dahl JB: The value of "multimodal" or "balanced analgesia" in post-operative pain treatment, *Anesth Analg* 77:1048–1056, 1993.

148. Chung F, Mezei G: Factors contributing to a prolonged stay after ambulatory surgery, *Anesth Analg* 89:1352–1359, 1999.

149. White PF, Kehlet H, Neal JM, et al: The role of the anesthesiologist in fast-track surgery: from multimodal analgesia to perioperative medical care, *Anesth Analg* 104:1380–1396, 2007.

150. Fung D, Cohen MM, Stewart S, et al: What determines patient satisfaction with cataract care under topical local anesthesia and monitored sedation in a community hospital setting? *Anesth Analg* 100:1644–1650, 2005.

151. Turan A, White PF, Karamanlioglu B, et al: Premedication with gabapentin: The effect on tourniquet pain and quality of intravenous regional anesthesia, *Anesth Analg* 104(1):97–101, 2007.

152. White PF: Changing role of COX-2 inhibitors in the perioperative period, Is parecoxib really the answer? *Anesth Analg* 100:1306–1308, 2005.

153. Kaye AD, Baluch A, Kaye AJ, et al: Pharmacology of cyclooxygenase-2 inhibitors and preemptive analgesia in acute pain management. *Curr Opin Anaesthesiol* 21:439–445, 2008.

154. Coloma M, Chiu JW, White PF: The use of esmolol as an alternative to remifentanil during desflurane anesthesia for fast-track outpatient

IV

gynecologic laparoscopic surgery, *Anesth Analg* 92:352–357, 2001.

155. Collard V, Mistraletti G, Taqi A, et al: Intra-operative esmolol infusion in the absence of opioids spares postoperative fentanyl in patient undergoing ambulatory laparoscopic cholecystectomy, *Anesth Analg* 105:1255–1262, 2007.

156. White PF, Wang B, Tang J, et al: The effect of intraoperative use of esmolol and nicardipine on recovery after ambulatory surgery, *Anesth Analg* 97:1633–1638, 2003.

157. Johansen JW, Flaishon R, Sebel PS: Esmolol reduces anesthetic requirement for skin incision during propofol/nitrous oxide/morphine anesthesia, *Anesthesiology* 86:364–371, 1997.

158. Norman PH, Daley MD, Lindsey RW: Preemptive analgesic effects of ketorolac in ankle fracture surgery, *Anesthesiology* 94(4):599–603, 2001.

159. Menigaux C, Guignard B, Fletcher D, et al: Intra-operative small-dose ketamine enhances analgesia after outpatient knee arthroscopy, *Anesth Analg* 93:606–612, 2001.

160. Conceicao MJ, Condeicao DB, Leao CC: Effect of an intravenous single dose of ketamine on postoperative pain in tonsillectomy patients, *Paediatr Anaesth* 16:962–967, 2006.

161. Schmid RL, Sandler AN, Katz J, et al: Use and efficacy of low-dose ketamine in the management of acute postoperative pain: A review of current techniques and outcomes, *Pain* 82:111–125, 1999.

162. Bell RF, Dahl JB, Moore RA, Kalso EA: Perioperative ketamine for acute postoperative pain, *Cochrane Database Syst Rev* 1: CD004603, 2006.

163. Ryu JH, Kang MH, Park KS, et al: Effects of magnesium sulphate on intraoperative anaesthetic requirements and postoperative analgesia in gynaecology patients receiving total intravenous anaesthesia, *Br J Anaesth* 100(3):397–403, 2008.

164. Hwang JY, Na HS, Jeon YT, et al: I.V. infusion of magnesium sulphate during spinal anaesthesia improves postoperative analgesia, *Br J Anaesth* 104(1):89–93, 2010.

165. Coloma M, Duffy LL, White PF, et al: Dexamethasone facilitates discharge after outpatient anorectal surgery, *Anesth Analg* 92:85–88, 2001.

166. Romundstad L, Breivik H, Roald H, et al: Methylprednisolone reduces pain, emesis, and fatigue after breast augmentation surgery: A single-dose, randomized, parallel-group study with methylprednisolone 125 mg, parecoxib 40 mg and placebo, *Anesth Analg* 102(2):418–425, 2006.

167. Lauwick S, Kim DJ, Michelagnoli G, et al: Intraoperative infusion of lidocaine reduces postoperative fentanyl requirements in patients undergoing laparoscopic cholecystectomy, *Can J Anaesth* 55:754–760, 2008.

168. Rasmussen ML, Mathiesen O, Dierking G, et al: Multimodal analgesia with gabapentin, ketamine and dexamethasone in combination with paracetamol and ketorolac after hip arthroplasty; a preliminary study. *Eur J Anaesthesiol* 2009. Accessed at http://journals.lww.com/ejanaesthesiology/pages/results.aspx?k=multimodal%20analgesia%20with%20gabapentin&Scope=AllIssues&txtKeywords=multimodal%20analgesia%20with%20gabapentin (downloaded 02/08/2010).

169. Benish M, Bartal I, Goldfarb Y, et al: Perioperative use of beta-blockers and COX-2 inhibitors may improve immune competence and reduce the risk of tumor metastasis, *Ann Surg Oncol* 15(7):2042–2052, 2008.

170. Exadaktylos AK, Buggy DJ, Moriarty DC, et al: Can anesthetic technique for primary breast cancer surgery affect recurrence or metastasis? *Anesthesiology* 105(4):660–664, 2006.

171. Pavlin DJ, Chen C, Penaloza DA, et al: Pain as a factor complicating recovery and discharge after ambulatory surgery, *Anesth Analg* 95:627–634, 2002.

172. Coley KC, Williams BA, DaPos SV, et al: Retrospective evaluation of unanticipated admissions and readmissions after same day surgery and associated costs, *J Clin Anesth* 14(5):349–353, 2002.

173. Sanders JC, King MA, Mitchell RB, Kelly JP: Perioperative complications of adenotonsillectomy in children with obstructive sleep apnea syndrome, *Anesth Analg* 103:1115–1121, 2006.

174. Hoban TF: Polysomnography should be required both before and after adenotonsillectomy for childhood sleep disordered breathing, *J Clin Sleep Med* 3(7):675–677, 2007.

175. Kirk VG, Bohn SG, Flemons WW, Remmers JE: Comparison of home oximetry monitoring with laboratory polysomnography in children, *Chest* 124(5):1702–1708, 2003.

176. Chervin RD, Weatherly RA, Garetz, et al: Pediatric sleep questionnaire: Prediction of sleep apnea and outcomes, *Arch Otolaryngol Head Neck Surg* 133:216–222, 2007.

177. Lamm C, Mandeli J, Kattan M: Evaluation of home audiotapes as an abbreviated test for obstructive sleep apnea syndrome (OSAS) in children, *Pediatr Pulmonol* 27:267–272, 1999.

178. Brouillette RT, Morelli A, Leimanis A, et al: Nocturnal pulse oximetry as an abbreviated testing modality for pediatric obstructive sleep apnea, *Pediatrics* 105:405–412, 2000.

179. Rosen GM, Muckle RP, Mahowald MW, et al: Pediatrics. Postoperative respiratory compromise in children with obstructive sleep apnea syndrome: Can it be anticipated? *Pediatrics* 93(5):784–788, 1994.

180. ASA: Practice guidelines for the perioperative management of patients with obstructive sleep apnea, *Anesthesiology* 104:1081–1093, 2006.

181. Polotsky VY, O'Donnell CP: Genomics of sleep-disordered breathing, *Proc Am Thorac Soc* 4(1):121–126, 2007.

182. Krishna J, Shah ZA, Merchant M, et al: Urinary protein expression patterns in children with sleep-disordered breathing: Preliminary findings, *Sleep Med* 7(3):221–227, 2006.

183. Isaacson G: Avoiding airway obstruction after pediatric adenotonsillectomy, *Int J Pediatr Otorhinolaryngol* 73(6):803–806, 2009.

184. Mehta VM, Har-El G, Goldstein NA: Postobstructive pulmonary edema after laryngospasm in the otolaryngology patient, *Laryngoscope* 116(9):1693–1696, 2010.

185. Ye J, Liu H, Zhang G: Postoperative respiratory complications of adenotonsillectomy for obstructive sleep apnea syndrome in older children: Prevalence, risk factors and impact on clinical outcome, *J Otolaryngol Head Neck* 38(1):49–58, 2009.

186. Statham MM, Elluru RG, Buncher R: Adenotonsillectomy for obstructive sleep apnea syndrome in young children: Prevalence of pulmonary complications, *Arch Otolaryngol Head Neck Surg* 132(5):476–480, 2006.

187. Gan TJ, Sloan F, Dear GL, et al: How much are patients willing to pay to avoid postoperative nausea and vomiting? *Anesth Analg* 92:393–400, 2001.

188. Lee A, Gin T, Lau AS, et al: A comparison of patients' and health care professionals' preferences for symptoms during immediate postoperative recovery and the management of postoperative nausea and vomiting. *Anesth Analg* 100:87–93, 2005.

189. White PF, O'Hara JF, Roberson CR, et al: The impact of current antiemetic

practices on patient outcomes: A prospective study on high-risk patients. *Anesth Analg* 107:452–458, 2008.

190. Lichtor JL, Glass PSA: We're tired of waiting, *Anesth Analg* 107(2):353–355, 2008.

191. Apfel CC, Laara E, Koivuranta M, et al: A simplified risk score for predicting postoperative nausea and vomiting: Conclusions from cross-validations between two centers, *Anesthesiology* 91:693–700, 1999.

192. White PF, Sacan O, Nuangchamnong N, et al: The relationship between patient risk factors and early versus late postoperative emetic symptoms. *Anesth Analg* 107:459–463, 2008.

193. Candiotti KA, Kovac AL, Melson TI, et al: A randomized, double-blind study to evaluate the efficacy and safety of three different doses of palonosetron versus placebo in preventing postoperative nausea and vomiting, *Anesth Analg* 107:445–451, 2008.

194. Gupta A, Wu CL, Elkassabany N, et al: Does the routine prophylactic use of antiemetics affect the incidence of postdischarge nausea and vomiting following ambulatory surgery? A systematic review of randomized controlled trials, *Anesthesiology* 99:488–495, 2003.

195. American Society of Peri-Anesthesia Nurses PONV/PDNV Strategic Work Team: ASPAN's evidence-based clinical practice guideline for the prevention and/or management of PONV, *J Perianesth Nurs* 21:230–250, 2006.

196. Gan TJ, Meyer TA, Apfel CC, et al: Society for Ambulatory Anesthesia guidelines for the management of postoperative nausea and vomiting, *Anesth Analg* 105:1615–1628, 2007.

197. American Society of Anesthesiologists Task Force on Postanesthetic Care: Practice guidelines for postanesthetic care, *Anesthesiology* 96:742–752, 2002.

198. Scuderi PE, James RL, Harris L, et al: Multimodal antiemetic management prevents early postoperative vomiting after outpatient laparoscopy, *Anesth Analg* 91:1408–1414, 2000.

199. Pan PH, Lee SC, Harris LC: antiemetic prophylaxis for postdischarge nausea and vomiting and impact on functional quality of living during recovery in patients with high emetic risks: A prospective, randomized, double-blind comparison of two prophylactic antiemetic regimens, *Anesth Analg* 107:429–438, 2008.

200. White PF, Tang J, Song D: Transdermal scopolamine: An alternative to ondansetron and droperidol for the prevention of postoperative and postdischarge emetic symptoms, *Anesth Analg* 104:92–96, 2007.

201. Maharaj CH, Kallam SR, Malik A: Preoperative intravenous fluid therapy decreases postoperative nausea and pain in high risk patients, *Anesth Analg* 100:675–682, 2005.

202. Engelman E, Salengros J, Barvais L: How much does pharmacologic prophylaxis reduce postoperative vomiting in children? *Anesthesiology* 109:1023–1035, 2008.

203. Habib AS, Reuveni J, Taguchi A, et al: A comparison of ondansetron with promethazine for treating postoperative nausea and vomiting in patients who received prophylaxis with ondansetron: A retrospective database analysis, *Anesth Analg* 104:548–551, 2007.

204. Van Vlymen JM, Sa Rego MM, White PF: Benzodiazepine premedication: Can it improve outcome in patients undergoing breast biopsy procedures? *Anesthesiology* 90(3):740–747, 1999.

205. Kain ZN, Mayes LC, Wang SM, et al: Postoperative behavioral outcomes in children: Effects of sedative premedication, *Anesthesiology* 90(3):758–765, 1999.

206. Fredman B, Lahav M, Zohar, et al: The effect of midazolam premedication on mental and psychomotor recovery in geriatric patients undergoing brief surgical procedures, *Anesth Analg* 89:1161–1166, 1999.

207. Brosius KK, Bannister C: Oral midazolam premedication in preadolescents and adolescents, *Anesth Analg* 94:31–36, 2002.

208. Tait AR, Pandit UA, Voepel-Lewis T, et al: Use of the laryngeal mask airway in children with upper respiratory tract infections: A comparison with endotracheal intubation, *Anesth Analg* 86:706–711, 1998.

209. Chin KJ, Chee VW: Laryngeal edema associated with the ProSeal laryngeal mask airway in upper respiratory tract infections, *Can J Anaesth* 53(4):389–392, 2006.

210. Tait AR, Burke C, Voepel-Lewis T, et al: Glycopyrrolate does not reduce the incidence of perioperative adverse events in children with upper respiratory tract infections, *Anesth Analg* 104:265–270, 2007.

211. Tait AR, Malviya S, Voepel-Lewis T, et al: Risk factors for perioperative adverse respiratory events in children with upper respiratory tract infections, *Anesthesiology* 95:299–306, 2001.

212. Tait AR, Malviya S: Anesthesia for the child with an upper respiratory tract infection: Still a dilemma? *Anesth Analg* 100:59–65, 2005.

213. Wu CL, Berenholtz SM, Provonost PJ: Systematic review and analysis of postdischarge symptoms after outpatient surgery, *Anesthesiology* 96:994–1003, 2002.

214. Freudenheim M: *Tool in Cystic Fibrosis Fight: a Registry.* http://www.nytimes.com/2009/12/22/health/22cyst.html?_r=1.

215. Thompson AM, Ashraf Z, Burton H, Stonebridge PA: Mapping changes in surgical mortality over 9 years by peer review audit, *Br J Surg* 92:1449–1452, 2005.

216. Mattila K, Toivonen J, Janhunen L: Postdischarge symptoms after ambulatory surgery: first-week incidence, intensity, and risk factors, *Anesth Analg* 101:1643–1650, 2005.

217. Fortier J, Chung F, Su J: Unanticipated admission after ambulatory surgery: A prospective study, *Can J Anaesth* 45:612–619, 1998.

218. Goldhill D: Preventing surgical deaths: Critical care and intensive care out-reach services in the postoperative period, *Br J Anaesth* 95:88–94, 2005.

219. Chung F, Chan V: A post-anesthetic discharge scoring system for home readiness after ambulatory surgery, *J Clin Anesth* 7:500–506, 1995.

IV

C GUIDELINES FOR CASE AND PATIENT SELECTION

Cases and patients should be chosen in a manner that supports the "predictability dictum." For instance, if not in a dental office (i.e., if in a mixed-specialty center) initial management of restorative dental procedures in patients with developmental delay is rarely a good match for the goal of predictability. Usually the dentist or oral surgeon has not been able to evaluate the patient either via physical examination of the mouth or by x-rays, due to a lack of cooperation. Therefore, no exact plan— or time estimate—for the case can be formulated, beyond "EUA and possible . . . ." As such, these cases can last 30 minutes or 4 hours (or more) and it is not reasonable to try to fit them into a schedule in which following patients, families and surgeons could be forced to wait for an uncertain or long period.

Case selection should also avoid procedures that engender large fluid shifts, or potential blood loss that could require blood or component transfusions. Such patients will have unpredictable courses in the PACU and should be monitored overnight for cardiopulmonary embarrassment.

A maximum case duration (e.g., 2 hours, 4 hours, 6 hours) that is appropriate will be different for each facility. However, it should be noted that postdischarge morbidity of all types (pain, nausea, dizziness, sore throat, etc.)[216] and unanticipated admission[217] increases with increasing duration of procedures beyond 1 hour. However, most cases in an academic center and many in private practice go longer than 1 hour. A good rule is that cases that are to go longer than 3 hours must be reviewed and approved by the Medical Director.

The patient's health and the invasiveness of the surgery, as well as the postoperative pain plan, should be assessed prior to planning to perform long procedures in the outpatient setting. The author rarely accepts cases in the outpatient facility that are planned to go more than 3½ hours, but recognizes that some practitioners in specialized centers (e.g., dental reconstruction) do perform longer cases frequently and successfully.

The impact of availability of a 23-hour stay facility on case selection can be significant, since access to a facility with excellent nursing and even physicians on site overnight allows the surgical facility to schedule cases in which surgical uncertainty requires overnight monitoring. However, no matter how clinically excellent the overnight stay facility and personnel are, it is not appropriate to use 23-hour care for medical indications outside a hospital. Thus, pain relief, fluid management, or drain management after surgery (e.g., surgical indications) are appropriate drivers of overnight care. On the other hand, if a patient has a potential airway problem (e.g., severe obstructive sleep apnea combined with difficult to manage pain) or an underlying cardiopulmonary instability, then the surgery should be performed in a hospital and the patient monitored there. In the same vein, "emergency" add-on cases in the ambulatory surgery facility can be accepted if the facility has the expertise to provide the service, but should not be taken if the patient's medical stability is in question. Thus, a fractured wrist in a healthy patient is appropriate. An ectopic pregnancy that has ruptured but "isn't bleeding right now" is not.

In some facilities, ASA health status is considered in the decision to admit a patient. It is true that for all surgical procedure types, risk for morbidity of ASA III patients is twice that of ASA I or II patients.[218] However, among the procedures that are typically done in outpatient scenarios, the impact of the difference between ASA classifications may be attenuated, due to the typically less invasive nature of outpatient surgery. This author has only used the ASA classification of IV and above as "no-go" for the outpatient facility, allowing patients who meet ASA III classification to undergo surgery in that setting if their health status is optimized and the procedure and anesthesia contemplated are not so invasive or of a duration such that the stability of their health would be likely to be negatively affected.

D AN ALLOCATION OF MEDICATIONS TO ANESTHESIA CONTROLLED DEVICES, EMERGENCY BOXES, AND ANESTHESIA CARTS

Here is a list of medications for stocking in controlled medication devices and for medications to be kept in the OR carts as well as in emergency tackle boxes.

Medications to be kept adjacent to the operating rooms, ideally in a controlled access device:

1. Clonidine (50 µg/0.5 mL) 50-µg syringe
2. Dexmedetomidine 200-µg injection
3. Fentanyl 100 µg/2 mL in a 2-mL amp
4. Hydromorphone 2 mg/1 mL in a 2-mg amp
5. Ketamine 200 mg/20 mL, 200-mg vial
6. Ketamine 500 mg/5 mL in a 500-mg vial
7. Meperidine 100 mg/1 mL in a 100-mg amp
8. Midazolam 10 mg/5 mL in a syrup container
9. Midazolam 2 mg/2 mL in a 2-mg vial
10. Methohexital
11. Thiopental, 500 mg, syringe
12. Insulin
13. Sodium citrate

A separate tackle box for rarely used; high-risk medications (on each anesthesia OR cart, but sealed)

This segregation of low-use, high-risk medications will avoid the negative outcomes of some inadvertent administration (syringe swaps).

1. Epinephrine injectors
2. CaCl
3. Amiodarone
4. D50
5. Albuterol Inhaler
6. Adenosine
7. NaHCO$_3$
8. Nitroglycerin sublingual tablets

9. Heparin 1000 U/mL 2-mL vial
10. Atropine injectors
11. Hydrocortisone
12. Methylprednisolone
13. Benadryl
14. Dopamine
15. Dobutamine
16. IV nitroglycerin
17. Hydralazine

Medications to be stocked in each OR anesthesia cart (stocked in sufficient quantities to avoid restocking during the day)

1. Propofol (20-mL and 100-mL vials)
2. 1% lidocaine for IV or SQ use (20-mL vial)
3. Dexamethasone 4 mg/mL
4. Labetalol
5. Metoprolol
6. Esmolol
7. Ketorolac
8. Phenylephrine (Neosynephrine) nasal spray
9. Neostigmine (1 mg/mL)
10. Glycopyrrolate 0.2 mg/mL, 5-mL vial
11. Atropine 0.4 mg/mL, 1-mL vial
12. Succinylcholine
13. Rocuronium
14. Vecuronium
15. Preservative free Bupivacaine 0.5%
16. Preservative free Ropivacaine 0.5%
17. Preservative free 2-Chloroprocaine (3%)
18. Metoclopramide (Reglan)
19. Droperidol
20. Acetaminophen suppositories (low and high dose)
21. Preservative free normal saline (10-mL vials)
22. Etomidate
23. Ondansetron

IV

E AN OUTCOMES MANAGEMENT PROGRAM

Since 2000, the author's ambulatory surgery centers (ASCs) have used a "patient diary" to collect data points for measuring outcomes. These data have provided guidance to discern best practice as well as to support incentive programs. Each worker fills in only a small portion of the diary as the patient moves through the facility, and again notes are added by the clerk who calls the patient in the days after discharge. An electronic health record would eventually replace the need for the extra work required of staff in order to collect the data in this fashion. However, the extra work will be accepted and the process valued by staff if they are provided with the data and management is open to using the data to improve outcomes.

Patient diary (single sheet, printed on both sides) (Fig. 37-1)

Report I: a typical "report card" with surgeon names attached to their metrics, which are posted in the ASC to allow recognition of best practice (Fig. 37-2A)

Report II: a report of anesthesia providers combined with surgeons to portray which anesthesia providers obtain the best outcomes when compared to other anesthesia providers doing work with the same surgeon (a simple method of risk adjustment) (Fig. 37-2B)

Surgery includes or procedure is

Scalpel incision through skin with

  No injection of local anesthetic/other substance

  Injection prior to incision and <u>before</u> prep

  Injection prior to incision, but <u>after</u> prep

BMT, or airway surgery (e.g. TGA)

Intra-ocular eye surgery

Procedure start

Time of incision

Time of incision

Time of injection

Time of table turn

Time surgeon first
   looks into positioned
   microscope

Procedure _____

Admitting clerk _____

Scheduled arrival   : _____

I. PreOp

Admitting NA _____ Primary PreOp RN _____

Passport defects?   Yes   No   If yes, specify:

  ☐ Anesthesia update   ☐ Surgical consent   ☐ Surgical H and P

  ☐ Antibiotic orders   ☐ Meds/equip orders   ☐ Ride/escort

Was the patient marked at time nursing ready for OR?   Yes   No

Any other delays or problems? _____

24-hour clock

ASC desk
Arrival   : _____

PreOp
Arrival   : _____

Nursing ready
for OR   : _____

II. ANESTHESIA

Regional Type: (check all that apply)

  ☐ None

Brachial plexus

    ☐ Cervical para-vertebral w/wo catheter/infusion

    ☐ Infraclavicular w/wo catheter/infusion

    ☐ Interscalene w/wo catheter/infusion

    ☐ Axillary w/wo catheter/infusion

    ☐ Supraclavicular w/wo catheter/infusion

☐ Other peripheral

☐ Other _____

☐ Spinal

☐ Epidural/Caudal

☐ Para-vertebral (Thoracic/Lumbar)

☐ Femoral

☐ Sciatic

☐ Popliteal

☐ Saphenous

☐ IV regional (Bier)

If multiple regional blocks, record earliest start and latest finish

Regional
start   : _____

Regional
finish   : _____

Drug(s) given (Check all that apply)

☐ None	☐ Ephedrine	☐ Lorazepam	☐ Pancuronium
☐ Alfentanil	☐ Esmolol	☐ Mepivacaine	☐ Phenylephrine
☐ 2-Chloroprocaine	☐ Fentanyl	☐ Meperidine	☐ Procaine
☐ Atracurium	☐ Glycopyrrolate	☐ Metoclopramide	☐ Propofol
☐ Atropine	☐ Heparin	☐ Metoprolol	☐ Rapacuronium
☐ Bupivacaine	☐ Hydralazine	☐ Midazolam	☐ Rocuronium
☐ Desflurane	☐ Isoflurane	☐ Morphine	☐ Ropivacaine
☐ Dexamethasone	☐ Ketamine	☐ N2	☐ Sevoflurane
☐ Diphenhydramine	☐ Ketorolac	☐ Naloxone	☐ Succinylcholine
☐ Dolasetron	☐ Labetalol	☐ Neostigmine	☐ Thiopental
	☐ Lidocaine	☐ Ondansetron	☐ Vecuronium
☐ Other _____			

Induction
start   : _____

Anesthetic Technique(s):

  ☐ Local/Topical (no IV meds)

  ☐ MAC

  ☐ Regional only

  ☐ Regional with sedation

  ☐ Regional with general

  ☐ General anesthesia only

  ☐ TIVA

  ☐ Volatile anesthetic

Primary Airway Techniques(s)

  ☐ None

  ☐ O2 Nasal Cannula/Mask

  ☐ Oral/Nasal Airway

  ☐ General with Mask

  ☐ LMA

  ☐ Endotracheal

Did anesthesia induction delay surgical start?

☐ Yes   ☐ No

Difficult intubation?   Yes   No   If yes, recognized pre-op?   Yes   No

Intubation technique	Success		Attempts			
Direct laryngoscopy	Yes	No	☐ 1	☐ 2	☐ 3	☐ 4 or more
Flexible fiberoptic	Yes	No	☐ 1	☐ 2	☐ 3	☐ 4 or more
Rigid fiberoptic	Yes	No	☐ 1	☐ 2	☐ 3	☐ 4 or more
Intubating LMA	Yes	No	☐ 1	☐ 2	☐ 3	☐ 4 or more

Describe ANY anesthesia NEAR MISSES:

Antibiotic
initiated   : _____

Antibiotic
finished   : _____

III. OR NURSING

Nurse IV Sedation?   Yes   No

Circulator RN   1 _____   2 _____

Scrub Tech   1 _____   2 _____

Were there delays/problems?   Yes   No   ☐ Operative   ☐ Equipment   ☐ Tissue

_____

Ready
for prep   : _____

Prep
complete   : _____

Procedure
starts   : _____

IV

Figure 37-1 Patient diary.

Continued

IV. PACU	Stage I	Stage II	Stage I
RN name	_____	_____	Arrival _____ : _____
Was pt. transported w/O2?	Yes No	Yes No	
Lowest SPO2 in PACU?	_____ %	_____ %	Ready for
Unexpected urinary cath?	Yes No	Yes No	departure _____ : _____
First pain score	0 1 2 3 4 5 6 7 8 9 10	0 1 2 3 4 5 6 7 8 9 10	
Final pain score	0 1 2 3 4 5 6 7 8 9 10	0 1 2 3 4 5 6 7 8 9 10	Actual
Nausea	Yes No	Yes No	departure _____ : _____
Vomiting	Yes No	Yes No	

PADSS score	Arrival 1st stage PACU	Arrival 2nd stage PACU	Regional start _____ : _____
Level of consciousness	0 1 2	0 1 2	
Physical activity	0 1 2	0 1 2	Regional
Hemodynamic stability	0 1 2	0 1 2	finish _____ : _____
Oxygen saturation	0 1 2	0 1 2	
Pain	0 1 2	0 1 2	**Stage II**
Emetic symptoms	0 1 2	0 1 2	Arrival _____ : _____

Problems in PACU I? _____

Problems in PACU II? _____

Reason for any delayed discharge from ASC?

Ready for departure _____ : _____

Actual departure _____ : _____

☐ Nausea/Vomiting   ☐ Hospital (escort/bed/etc.)   ☐ Anesthesia delay
☐ Drowsiness   ☐ Pharmacy delay   ☐ Patient needs
☐ Urinary retention   ☐ Surgery delay   (clothing/restroom/etc.)
☐ Ride   ☐ Other: _____

Anesthesia post-operative Block (PACU):

☐ Brachial plexus   ☐ Sciatic   ☐ Para-vertebral   ☐ Femoral   ☐ Other

---

V. Call back   Phone #: _____
Nurse recording responses: _____   Message left 1: ____ / ____ / ____
Date of call back: ____ / ____ / ____   Message left 2: ____ / ____ / ____

Person spoken to: ☐ Patient   ☐ Spouse   ☐ Parent   ☐ Other: _____

Patient outcomes **after discharge**:
Highest pain score? 0 1 2 3 4 5 6 7 8 9 10   Unplanned urinary catheter? Yes   No
Nausea?   Yes   No   Unplanned admission to ED or hospital? Yes   No
Vomiting? Yes   No   Problem that required they call the doctor? Yes   No

How would you rate how you were treated at check-in?
☐ No opinion   ☐ Poor   ☐ Fair   ☐ Good   ☐ Excellent

How would you rate the care you received at the UI ASC?
☐ No opinion   ☐ Poor   ☐ Fair   ☐ Good   ☐ Excellent

If the patient had a nerve block, ask: (Circle one)
When did the numbness in your (arm, leg) begin to wear off (xx/xx)? ____ : ____   **Same Day** or **Next Day**
If you have a similar surgery in the future, will you want to have a nerve block again?   Yes   No

Are there any particular things the patient would have liked done differently? _____

Was anything or anyone particularly helpful? _____
Would the patient have a procedure done here again if doctor recommended it?   Yes   No
Would the patient recommend a loved one or friend have a procedure here if their doctor recommended it?   Yes   No
Was the pain medication strong enough to take care of their pain and did they have enough?   Yes   No
Any other comments: _____

Figure 37-1, cont'd

Surgeon Classification	Staff Surgeon Name	ASC Case Volume	Average Turnover Time (Min.)	% Pts Rating Care Excellent	% Pts Recommending ASC	Passport Accuracy %	Case Time Accuracy	% Nausea in PACU	% Vomiting in PACU	% Nausea at Callback	% Vomiting at Callback
ORT – General		4	12	100.00%	100.00%	66.70%	100.00%	0.00%	0.00%	33.00%	00.00%
ORT – General		6	26.75	100.00%	100.00%	66.70%	50.00%	0.00%	0.00%	33.00%	33.30%
ORT – General		12	15.75	100.00%	100.00%	83.30%	50.00%	0.00%	0.00%	0.00%	0.00%
ORT – General		9	10.8	71.40%	100.00%	66.70%	77.80%	0.00%	0.00%	0.00%	0.00%
ORT – General		11	16.5	87.50%	100.00%	70.00%	36.40%	25.00%	0.00%	33.00%	25.00%
ORT – General		1				100.00%	100.00%				
ORT – General		1				100.00%	0.00%				
ORT – General		44	16.81	89.30%	100.00%	72.50%	56.80%	6.10%	0.00%	16.10%	9.70%
ORT – Hand		80	16.38	86.50%	98.10%	90.00%	82.50%	0.00%	0.00%	19.20%	5.80%
ORT – Hand		59	18.54	89.20%	100.00%	91.20%	76.30%	0.00%	0.00%	15.40%	7.90%
ORT – Hand		84	23.79	87.50%	98.30%	89.90%	71.40%	1.50%	0.00%	17.20%	5.20%
ORT – Hand		223	19.82	87.60%	98.70%	90.30%	76.70%	0.60%	0.00%	17.50%	6.10%
ORT – Sports		33	16.82	73.10%	100.00%	78.10%	63.60%	3.60%	3.60%	14.80%	3.70%
ORT – Sports		97	13.36	79.70%	96.80%	91.20%	71.10%	2.50%	1.20%	21.20%	15.20%
ORT – Sports		37	12.82	92.00%	100.00%	82.40%	67.60%	3.20%	0.00%	7.70%	0.00%
ORT – Sports		26	15.2	83.30%	100.00%	66.70%	61.50%	5.90%	0.00%	16.70%	8.30%
ORT – Sports		70	26.1	85.10%	100.00%	87.00%	61.40%	4.80%	0.00%	15.70%	4.10%
ORT – Sports		263	16.96	82.30%	98.90%	85.00%	66.20%	3.70%	0.90%	16.50%	7.80%

Surgeon	Anesthesiologist	Cases	Diaries	Average TO	N PACU%	V PACU %	PDN %	PDV %	% Rated Excellent	Recommend ASC %	% Passport Defect
A	1	39	32	11.12	0.00%	0.00%	16.67%	8.00%	85.19%	95.65%	43.75%
AA	2	36	36	12.62	3.13%	0.00%	26.09%	21.74%	69.57%	90.48%	50.00%
AA	3	43	42	12.66	5.41%	2.70%	25.71%	14.29%	82.86%	100.00%	28.57%
B	4	25	25	18.81	0.00%	0.00%	6.67%	0.00%	93.75%	100.00%	68.00%
C	5	25	22	11.17	0.00%	0.00%	0.00%	0.00%	88.89%	100.00%	54.55%
D	5	26	24	17.37	0.00%	0.00%	5.00%	5.00%	85.00%	100.00%	25.00%
EE	6	27	22	23.27	0.00%	0.00%	7.69%	7.69%	85.71%	100.00%	31.82%
EE	7	25	21	21.29	0.00%	0.00%	8.33%	8.33%	78.57%	87.50%	38.10%
F	4	106	95	15.85	6.02%	3.61%	6.06%	5.88%	84.06%	100.00%	33.68%
F	8	45	43	12.83	0.00%	0.00%	8.70%	8.70%	66.67%	100.00%	27.91%
G	4	62	51	17.83	2.00%	4.00%	21.43%	17.86%	85.71%	100.00%	50.98%
G	6	25	25	20.1	0.00%	0.00%	0.00%	10.53%	72.22%	91.67%	44.00%
G	8	79	79	14.14	0.00%	0.00%	3.92%	3.92%	87.76%	100.00%	46.84%
H	3	27	26	33.25	0.00%	0.00%	22.73%	18.18%	68.18%	100.00%	46.15%

IV

Figure 37-2 Reports I and II.

F SOME POLICIES AND PROCEDURES

1. Preoperative Evaluation Systems

Many of the systems that an office or ambulatory surgery center (ASC) will create are based on community norms. One approach is to provide surgeons' offices with a health status assessment form that the patient fills out while on site for his or her preoperative evaluation. That form is then faxed or scanned and e-mailed by the surgeon's office to the ASC with the booking for the case. At the ASC, it is used by a licensed practitioner (RN, CRNA, MD) to decide that either the patient doesn't need a phone call (healthy, low-invasive surgery) or should get a phone call, during which the form is used to direct review of systems and past medical history questions. If the patient needs any consultations or studies done, then the ASC staff set that up, generally within 24 hours of receiving the booking. The patient's appointment with the ASC is confirmed at that time and information about an escort and ride is given (see item 3). Patients are contacted again within 72 hours of their surgery by an RN, who provides information about timing of arrival, appropriate oral fluid and medication intake, and reiterates the information about the escort and the ride. Finally, within 24 hours of surgery a clerk will confirm the information about arrival time and need for an escort and ride.

2. Example of a Patient Health Status Assessment Form (Fig. 37-3A and B)

3. Rides, Escorts, and Home Care

The author requires every patient to have an escort on site throughout the time the patient is on site, as well as a driver and a signed attestation by the patient that he or she will have a caregiver for the first night after surgery. The escort must be present for the patient to be admitted and prepared for surgery. If they are not able to bring an escort, get a driver, or have someone stay with them the night after surgery, then the procedure is canceled for that day. Since putting this requirement in place in 2001, there has been the virtual elimination of the formerly frequently occurring problem of abandoned patients (phantom drivers) and late-staying RNs, making phone calls to arrange for a friend or relative to come get the patient. These requirements are not popular with a small minority of patients, but we try to identify those patients for whom these requirements will be problematic when the case is first booked and redirect them to the hospital for their care at that time, if they truly cannot find a driver, escort, or home care provider.

4. Discharge Criteria and Postdischarge Requirements

The author uses a PADSS (Post-Anesthetic Discharge Scoring System) scale to allow discharge.[219] We do not have minimum stay requirements at the ASC. We also do not require a patient to void prior to discharge except after adult inguinal hernia cases and urethropexy procedures.

Questions for the parent or guardian:
If your child has had surgery before, please check any of these that happened:

☐ Problem putting a breathing tube in
☐ Got sick to stomach
☐ Had an allergic reaction
☐ Took a long time to wake up in the recovery room
☐ Had to be in the hospital overnight when that wasn't the plan

Has anyone related by blood to your child had a problem with anesthesia, or been told that he or she has "malignant hyperthermia"?

☐ No   ☐ Yes   If yes to either, please explain: _____

How old is your child? _____

If any of the following apply to your child, please check the box:

☐ Does anyone smoke in your home?
☐ Was your child born prematurely?

   ☐ If **yes**, was he or she less than 37 weeks gestational age or premature at birth?
   ☐ If **yes**, was oxygen or a ventilator needed?

☐ Does your child have any congenital problems, syndromes or genetic defects?

   ☐ If **yes**, please tell us what these are: _____

☐ Has your child been sick in the past week?
☐ Has your child been admitted to the hospital in the last three months?
☐ Does your child use an inhaler to take asthma medicine?
☐ Can your child sleep on his or her back without having severe difficulty with breathing?
☐ Does your child snore at night AND have episodes where he or she stops breathing?
☐ Has your child been diagnosed as having developmental delay?
☐ Does your child have autism?
☐ Has your child had any organ (or bone marrow) transplant?
☐ Has your child been diagnosed with metabolic disease?
☐ Does your child have muscular dystrophy?
☐ Does your child have cerebral palsy?
☐ Does your child have sickle cell disease?
☐ Has your child had acute illness or been seen in the emergency room in the past week?
☐ Has your child been diagnosed with diabetes?
☐ Has your child had 2 or more episodes of croup?

Parent or guardian escort on day of surgery:

I understand as the parent or guardian of the patient that for the child's safety and the safety of others, I must:

• Drive my child to the Outpatient Surgery Center on the day of his/her procedure
• Stay on-site at the Outpatient Surgery Center for the entire time my child is having the procedure done and is in recovery, and take my child home after surgery
• Stay with my child for at least 24 hours after surgery

I understand that if my child comes to the Outpatient Surgery Center for surgery without these arrangements in place that my child's surgery will not be performed.

Parent/guardian signature _____

Figure 37-3 A, Pediatric preoperative health assessment form.

Continued

IV

Parent/guardian signature _____

Date ____ / ____ / ____

For surgeon's office use only: Patient weight _____ (kg)

Planned procedure _____

Planned date for procedure ____ / ____ / ____

Date of birth ____ / ____ / ____   Patient height _____

Patient BMI _____

Anesthesia Provider: I have reviewed this information. The plan is:

☐ Okay for OSC or Main with no further work up needed.
☐ Okay for OSC or Main but needs the following tests or consults:
☐ PAT consult   ☐ PCP consult   ☐ LABs   ☐ Other _____
☐ Okay for Main OR ONLY (not OSC) Reason _____

  ☐ and needs no further work up
  ☐ and needs the following work up _____

Figure 37-3, cont'd

Questions for the patient:
If you have had surgery before, please check any of these that happened:

☐ Problem putting a breathing tube in
☐ Got sick to my stomach
☐ Had an allergic reaction
☐ Took a long time to wake up in the recovery room
☐ Had to be in the hospital overnight when that wasn't the plan

Has anyone in your family had a problem with anesthesia or been told that he or she has "malignant hyperthermia"?

☐ No   ☐ Yes

If yes to either, please explain: ————————————————————

Please check any of the following that apply to you (or the patient):

☐ I have high blood pressure
☐ I have diabetes–taking insulin
☐ I have diabetes–**not** taking insulin
☐ I have congestive heart failure
☐ I have angina/coronary artery disease
☐ I have had a heart attack
☐ I have had a stroke or a "temporary stroke" (transient ischemic attack or TIA)
☐ I have a heart valve problem
☐ I have a coronary stent
☐ I have a pacemaker or defibrillator
☐ I have seizures
☐ I have acid reflux/GERD or a hiatal hernia (or both)
☐ I take blood thinners (name ————————————————)
☐ I have a blood disease
☐ I have or have had cancer
☐ I have had radiation or surgery for head or neck cancer
☐ I get car sick or motion sick
☐ I have a problem opening my mouth
☐ I snore so loud that people can hear me through the wall
☐ I have been told that I sometimes stop breathing in my sleep
☐ I fall asleep during the day when I don't plan to
☐ I often feel tired, fatigued, or sleepy during the daytime
☐ I have been told that I have obstructive sleep apnea and that I should use CPAP
         If yes, do you use CPAP?   ☐ Yes   ☐ No
☐ I smoke cigarettes or cigars
☐ I use home oxygen
☐ I have to stop to catch my breath when I climb one set of stairs or if I walk one level block
☐ I have lung problems (asthma, emphysema, or COPD)
☐ I have had an organ transplant
☐ I have sickle cell disease
☐ I have kidney disease
☐ I have liver disease
☐ I am or could be pregnant
☐ I have muscular dystrophy or a nerve disease
☐ I drink more than 2 glasses of wine or beer, or 1 "hard" drink on most days
☐ I have a birth or genetic defect
☐ I have a living will that says I should not be revived
☐ I am a male and the neck size for my button up shirts is over 17 inches

Figure 37-3, cont'd B, Adult preoperative health assessment form.

Continued

<u>**Adult escort on day of surgery:**</u>

I understand that for my own safety and the safety of others, I must arrange to have a responsible adult:
- drive me to the Outpatient Surgery Center on the day of my procedure
- stay on-site at the Outpatient Surgery Center for the entire time I am having my procedure done and in recovery
- take me home after surgery
- care for children, and stay with me for at least 24 hours after surgery

I understand that if I come to the Outpatient Surgery Center for my surgery without having made these arrangements that my surgery will not be performed.

Patient signature _____ Date _____ / _____ / _____

For surgeon's office use only:

Planned procedure _____
Planned date of procedure _____ / _____ / _____
Date of birth _____ / _____ / _____ Patient height _____ Patient weight _____ (kg)
Patient BMI _____

Anesthesia Provider: I have reviewed this information. The plan is:

☐ Okay for OSC or Main with no further work up needed
☐ Okay for OSC or Main but needs the following tests or consults:
☐ PAT CONSULT ☐ PCP CONSULT ☐ LABs ☐ OTHER _____
☐ Okay for Main OR ONLY (not OSC) REASON _____
   ☐ and needs no further work up
   ☐ and needs the following work up _____

Figure 37-3—cont'd

38 PROCEDURES PERFORMED OUTSIDE THE OPERATING ROOM

Lawrence Litt and William L. Young

The types of diagnostic and therapeutic medical procedures, listed in Table 38-1, that require specialized environments such that they must be performed away from traditional hospital and outpatient operating room suites is increasing. In addition to "remote locations" in medical centers there are off-site medical offices established by surgeons who choose to perform outpatient surgery in private settings that they find more convenient and economical. Office-based anesthesia has become a primary mode of practice for many anesthesiologists.

Table 38-1 Remote Locations That Commonly Require Anesthesia Services

Radiology and Nuclear Medicine
Diagnostic radiology and nuclear medicine
  Computed tomography
  Fluoroscopy
Therapeutic radiology
  Interventional body angiography (can involve
    embolization or stent placement)
  Interventional neuroangiography (can involve
    embolization or stent placement)
Magnetic resonance imaging
Ultrasound imaging

Radiation Therapy
Standard x-ray therapy with collimated beams
GammaKnife x-ray surgery for brain tumors and AV malformations
CyberKnife x-ray surgery for central nervous system and body tumors and AV malformations
Electron beam radiation therapy (usually intraoperative)

Cardiology
Cardiac catheterization with or without electrophysiologic studies
Cardioversion

Gastroenterology
Endoscopy
Colonoscopy
Endoscopic retrograde cholangiopancreatography

Pulmonary Medicine
Tracheal and bronchial stent placement
Bronchoscopy
Pulmonary lavage

Psychiatry
Electroconvulsive therapy

Urology
Extracorporeal shock wave lithotripsy

General Dentistry and Oral and Maxillofacial Surgery
Dental surgery

AV, arteriovenous.

CHARACTERISTICS OF REMOTE LOCATIONS

Remote locations are much different from self-contained operating rooms. Anesthesia providers should have a basic understanding of logistic arrangements between the anesthesia department and the various medical and nursing departments that host the remote location. Within the anesthesia department, detailed arrangements must be in place regarding immediate contacts that can be established between remote locations and centrally located anesthesia colleagues and technicians, especially when help is required or vital information needs to be transmitted. There should also be clear policies for dealing with remote equipment problems and unexpected escalations of medical problems.

An anesthetic provider working in an unfamiliar remote location must keep track of the identity and role of personnel who participate in the surgical procedure or patient care. During times when the anesthetic provider may need experienced medical assistance (tracheal intubation, placement of a central venous catheter), the availability of such qualified staff members must be identified. Readily available preoperative documents for all patients in remote locations must include the attending surgeon's history and physical examination. Arrangements for patient arrival and check-in should be similar to those for outpatients and inpatients undergoing procedures in a traditional operating room setting.

Remote locations must provide for the same basic anesthesia care that is possible in any operating room. There must be adequate monitoring capabilities, the means to deliver supplemental oxygen via a face mask with positive pressure ventilation, the availability of suction, equipment for providing controlled mechanical ventilation, an adequate supply of anesthetic drugs and ancillary equipment, and supplemental lighting for procedures that involve darkness. Although portable anesthesia machines (Fig. 38-1) can sometimes be placed very close to the patient to facilitate gas connections, often an anesthesia machine cannot be as close to the patient as in the operating room (Fig. 38-2). The use of sedation, as for insertion of a nerve block, should take place in an area (block room) where adequate equipment, drugs, and support personnel are available for immediate intervention. Remote locations for anesthesia care should also keep pace with the increasing use of automated anesthesia records and advanced information technology hardware and software (see Chapter 2).

If anesthetic gases are to be used, scavenging must be sufficient to ensure that trace amounts are below the upper limits set by the Occupational Safety and Health Administration (OSHA). Remote locations frequently involve additional hazards, such as exposure to radiation, high sound levels, and heavy mechanical equipment. Advance preparation should be made to have all needed

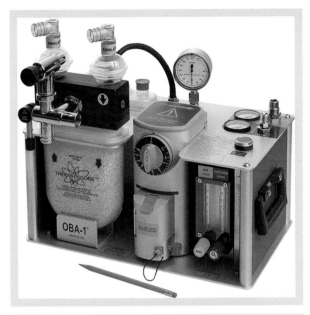

Figure 38-1 The OBA-1, a 14-kg, MRI-compatible, portable anesthesia machine that may also be taken to a physician's office, a hospital block room, a bedside, or a field location. MRI, magnetic resonance imaging. (Courtesy of OBAMED, Inc., Louisville, KY.)

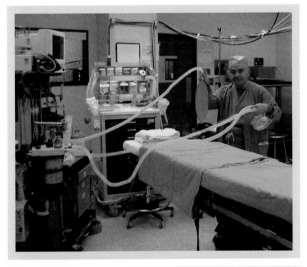

Figure 38-2 Example of an operating room setup for use when it is not possible to locate equipment in close proximity to the patient.

equipment available, such as lead aprons, portable lead-glass shields, and earplugs. At the end of the procedure one must often travel distances that are typically longer than the usual distance to the postanesthesia care unit or other patient units. So that patients can be safely and expeditiously taken to a recovery area, remote

locations should always have available sufficient supplies of supplemental oxygen, appropriate transport monitoring equipment, and elevator and passageway keys. The anesthesia provider should always know the location of the nearest defibrillator, fire extinguisher, gas shutoff valves, and exits.

RADIATION SAFETY

Safety Practices

Ionizing radiation and radiation safety issues may be present in remote locations.[1,2] Radiation intensity and exposure decrease with the inverse square of the distance from the emitting source. Frequently, the anesthesia provider can be located immediately behind a movable lead-glass screen. Regardless of whether this is possible, the anesthesia provider should wear a lead apron and a lead thyroid shield and remain at least 1 to 2 m from the radiation source. Clear communication between the radiology and anesthesia teams is crucial for limiting radiation exposure.

Monitoring the Radiation Dose

Anesthesia providers, like all other health care workers who are at risk for radiation exposure, can monitor their monthly dosage by wearing radiation exposure badges. The physics unit of measurement for a biologic radiation dose is the sievert (Sv); 100 rem = 1 Sv. Because some types of ionizing radiation are more injurious than others, the biologic radiation dose is obtained by multiplying together a "quality factor" and the ionizing energy absorbed per gram of tissue. Radiation exposure can be monitored with one or more film badges. In the United States, the average annual dose from cosmic rays and naturally occurring radioactive materials is about 3 mSv (300 mrem). Patients undergoing a chest radiograph receive a dose of 0.04 mSv, whereas those undergoing a computed tomography (CT) scan of the head receive 2.00 mSv. Federal guidelines give a limit of 50 mSv for the maximum annual occupational dose.

ALLERGIC REACTIONS

Contrast agents are used in more than 10 million diagnostic radiology procedures performed each year. In 1990, fatal adverse reactions after the intravenous administration of contrast media were estimated to occur approximately once for every 100,000 procedures, whereas serious adverse reactions were estimated to occur 0.2% of the time with ionic agents and 0.4% of the time with low osmolarity agents. Radiocontrast agents can produce anaphylactoid reactions in sensitive patients, and such reactions necessitate aggressive intervention, including the administration of oxygen, intravenous fluids, and epinephrine, with epinephrine being the essential component of therapy.[3]

Adverse drug reactions are more common after the injection of iodinated contrast agents (used for x-ray examinations such as CT) than after gadolinium contrast agents (used for magnetic resonance imaging [MRI]).[4] The signs and symptoms of anaphylactoid reactions can be mild (nausea, pruritus, diaphoresis), moderate (faintness, emesis, urticaria, laryngeal edema, bronchospasm), or severe (seizures, hypotensive shock, laryngeal edema, respiratory distress, cardiac arrest). Prophylaxis against anaphylactoid reactions is directed against the massive vasodilatation that results from mast cell and basophil release of inflammatory cytokines such as histamine, serotonin, and bradykinin. The main approach to prophylaxis is steroid and antihistamine administration on the night before and the morning of the procedure. A typical regimen for a 70-kg adult is 40 mg prednisone, 20 mg famotidine, and 50 mg diphenhydramine. Patients undergoing contrast procedures usually have an induced diuresis from the intravenous osmotic load presented by the contrast agent. In this regard, adequate hydration of these patients is important to prevent aggravation of coexisting hypovolemia or azotemia. Chemotoxic reactions to contrast media are typically dose dependent (unlike anaphylactoid and anaphylactic reactions) and related to osmolarity and ionic strength.

NONINVASIVE X-RAY PROCEDURES

Sedation and General Anesthesia

Radiology departments commonly use remote locations where anesthesia services are required for patient immobility, maintenance of adequate oxygenation and perfusion, and minimization of pain and anxiety. Most adult patients, when provided with adequate instructions and preparation, do not need sedation or general anesthesia for noninvasive radiologic procedures. For many other adults, conscious sedation can be provided by qualified nurses. In contrast, sedation or general anesthesia is often required to enable children to cooperate.

PHYSIOLOGIC MONITORING

Normal physiologic monitoring is essential, as is supplemental oxygen, which is usually supplied by nasal cannula attached to a capnograph. Capnography provides the respiratory rate and pattern, as well as the end-tidal CO_2 concentration. Anesthesia providers commonly use specially constructed nasal cannulas that have a sample line for a capnograph. If capnography is not possible, ventilation must be assessed by continuous visual inspection or auscultation, or both.

SUPPLEMENTAL OXYGEN

It is preferable to have nasal cannula oxygen come from a separate flowmeter instead of from the common gas outlet of the anesthesia machine to permit more rapid deployment of the anesthesia machine's breathing circuit for delivering oxygen via a face mask. For long procedures it is best to administer humidified oxygen through the nasal cannula to avoid leaving the patient with an uncomfortably dry mouth and throat. Certain patients, including infants and small children, will not tolerate a nasal cannula but will do well with an oxygen "blow-by" technique.

PHARMACOLOGICALLY INDUCED SEDATION

Conscious sedation can usually be managed successfully with a continuous propofol infusion, with or without supplemental intravenous opioids or benzodiazepines (or both). Often a small dose of a rapid-onset, short-acting opioid such as remifentanil or alfentanil is also an appropriate selection. Dexmedetomidine is another useful drug, primarily in procedures lasting more than an hour.[5] This anesthetic is especially useful for patients who cannot tolerate CO_2 retention, such as those with severe pulmonary hypertension, or those who require frequent assessment of mental status. Dexmedetomidine should be used cautiously in patients who require strict arterial blood pressure control at or above their baseline levels.[5] Because dexmedetomidine tends to decrease systemic arterial pressure, its use might require intravenous vasopressor support or even be inappropriate in patients at risk for hypoperfusion of vital organs or tissues. For example, patients with atherosclerotic lesions in cerebral, cardiac, or renal arteries, as well as patients with brain or spinal cord compression from tumors, are particularly vulnerable.

COMPUTED TOMOGRAPHY

CT is often used for intracranial imaging and for studies of the thorax and abdomen. Because CT is painless and noninvasive, adult patients undergoing elective scans rarely require more than emotional support. CT scanning is a crucial diagnostic tool in several acute settings, including traumatic injury (head and abdominal) and stroke (hemorrhagic and nonhemorrhagic). It is also used for urgent assessments of gastrointestinal integrity in very sick ICU patients who require complex care during transport to and from the scanner, as well as for rapid assessment of expanding intracranial masses when an increase in intracranial pressure may be a concern. Sedation or general anesthesia is often essential for such patients, as well as for children and adults who have difficulty remaining motionless.

Airway management and adequate oxygenation are the anesthesia provider's primary concerns when providing sedation or general anesthesia to patients undergoing CT. During CT scanning the anesthesiologist steps behind radiation shielding as a controlled, mechanized table moves the patient. Airway hoses, intravenous delivery tubing, and monitors can become kinked or disconnected as the table moves the patient.

MAGNETIC RESONANCE IMAGING

MRI is a standard diagnostic tool and is likely to supplant or replace conventional x-ray techniques. Patient immobility is the primary indication for sedation or general anesthesia, which is routinely needed for children, adults who are claustrophobic or in pain, and critical care patients. Although ionizing radiation is not a safety issue because no x-rays or radioactive substances are involved, other important safety issues pertain to the magnet suite. For example, missile injuries can occur if ferromagnetic objects are brought near the magnet. In addition, hearing loss may occur from high sound levels during a scan, as can electrical burns if incompatible monitoring equipment is attached to the patient. Patients with implanted devices or ferromagnetic material should never be inside a large magnetic field.

Safety Considerations

Objects in the magnet room need to be both MRI safe and MRI compatible. Before an MRI scan is started, the anesthesiologist should be sure that the patient has been screened and cleared by MRI technicians responsible for knowing that the patient's body does not contain susceptible metal objects, such as incompatible orthopedic hardware, cardiac pacemakers, wire-reinforced epidural catheters, or a pulmonary artery catheter with a temperature wire. Pulse oximetry is essential during MRI scans, and only an MRI-compatible fiberoptic pulse oximeter should be used. (Patient burns can result at the point of attachment if one uses a standard pulse oximeter.) Similar concerns pertain to any other monitoring or management devices that make actual or potential patient contact.

Intravenous contrast material is often administered for radiologic imaging. A serious adverse reaction called nephrogenic systemic fibrosis (NSF) can occur after exposure to gadolinium-based MRI contrast agents.[6] In NSF there is fibrosis of the skin, of connective tissue, and sometimes of internal organs. The severity of NSF can range from mild to severe and can also be fatal. However, NSF apparently occurs only when severe renal impairment (e.g., dialysis-dependent renal failure) also exists. Anesthesia providers should not casually administer gadolinium-containing MRI contrast agent to patients with renal problems.

MISSILE INJURY

Missile injury in an MRI suite is a serious and life-threatening risk. The superconducting electrical currents that generate an MRI scanner's large magnetic field are always "on." Therefore, MRI scanners are also always surrounded by large magnetic field gradients (up to 6 m away). Magnetic field gradients can pull magnetic objects into the magnet with alarming speed and force.[7]

Whereas certain metals (nickel, cobalt) are dangerous because they are magnetic, other metals (aluminum, titanium, copper, silver) do not pose a missile danger. These metals are used to make MRI-compatible intravenous poles, fixation devices, and nonmagnetic anesthesia machines. MRI-compatible intravenous infusion pumps are clinically available. If one must bring susceptible metal items such as infusion pumps into the MRI magnet room, they should be safely located and fixed, preferably bolted to a wall or floor, with everything being done and checked before the patient enters the MRI scanner. Anesthesia providers should know that if a missile does fly into the magnet and cause injury while pinning the patient to the inside of the scanner, there is a way that the superconducting magnet can be turned off immediately and this should be done only by MRI technicians. The patient should be removed from the scanner as soon as possible because it can become extremely cold during magnet shutdown.

Monitoring Issues

Many anesthesia providers prefer to be outside the magnet room during the scan. This would seem to be acceptable if in addition to having monitor displays of vital signs, sufficient simultaneous vigilance can also take place via video cameras and windows.

INVASIVE BLOOD PRESSURE MONITORING

Critically ill patients undergoing MRI may require invasive systemic blood pressure monitoring. Long lengths of pressure tubing are added so that pressure transducers and their electrical cables can be far from the magnet, preferably outside the magnet room. All arterial catheter stopcocks should be capped so that hemorrhage is impossible in the event of accidental perturbations in the stopcock setting. Radiofrequency pulsing can sometimes cause the pressure transducer to generate artifactual spikes, which in turn cause the monitoring equipment to falsely calculate an erroneously high blood pressure and possibly mislead the anesthesia provider. Visual inspection of the waveform can lead to rapid detection of this type of artifact.

Compatible Equipment

The MRI-compatible equipment that goes into the magnet room is really a second anesthesia station.[8] Although suction, physiologic monitoring, and mechanical ventilation must be possible inside the magnet room, it is nevertheless crucial that a primary anesthesia station be located just outside the magnet room. If a potentially life-threatening problem arises, it must be possible to promptly remove the patient from the scanner for transfer to the primary

IV

anesthesia station so that optimal care and additional help can be provided more efficiently.

Management of Anesthesia (See Chapter 34)

An inhaled induction of anesthesia with sevoflurane plus subsequent establishment of intravenous access for infusion of propofol is a useful technique for pediatric patients requiring anesthesia for MRI.[9] Mechanical ventilation via an endotracheal tube may be needed (concern about aspiration risk, presence of increased intracranial pressure); alternatively, a laryngeal mask airway may be placed after sevoflurane induction for continued maintenance of anesthesia. General anesthesia for adults undergoing MRI brain scans usually requires an endotracheal tube, although a laryngeal mask airway will sometimes suffice. Upper airway obstruction during an MRI brain scan results in motion artifact that is unacceptable. Because hyperoxia can increase signal intensity in brain cerebrospinal fluid, the radiologist must consider this possibility when interpreting the MRI scan.[10]

INVASIVE X-RAY PROCEDURES

Interventional Radiology—Neuroangiography and Body Angiography

Interventional neuroradiology (endovascular neurosurgery) mixes traditional neurosurgery with neuroradiology while also including certain aspects of head and neck surgery. Body angiography mixes general surgery with general radiology. In angiographic procedures, the relevant blood vessel trees are imaged, after which a decision is made to advance to one or more therapeutic interventions via drugs or devices (or both). Patients undergoing placement of a transjugular intrahepatic portosystemic shunt (TIPS) can be especially sick. The procedure can take several hours to complete, and commonly involves placement of an intrahepatic stent. Although the liver disease of many TIPS patients might not yet be end stage, such patients often have significant co-morbidities related to hepatic dysfunction, including coagulopathy, anemia, ascites, hepatic encephalopathy, hepatorenal syndrome, cardiomyopathy, and pulmonary hypertension. Patients undergoing endoscopic retrograde cholangiopancreatography (ERCP) can also present with serious hepatic dysfunction.

MANAGEMENT OF ANESTHESIA

Anesthesia-related concerns include (1) maintenance of patient immobility and physiologic stability, (2) perioperative management of anticoagulation, (3) readiness for sudden unexpected complications during the procedure, (4) provision of smooth and rapid emergence from anesthesia and sedation at appropriate times (may be required during the procedure), and (5) appropriate monitoring and management during transport after completion of

the procedure, particularly for critically ill patients, who may require continuous evaluation of breathing and systemic blood pressure.[11]

Physiologic Stability

Maintenance of arterial blood pressure at predetermined values is particularly important in patients with cerebrovascular disease. Arterial blood pressure targets should always be discussed preoperatively with the surgical team. Maintaining a higher than normal arterial blood pressure is important in cases in which the patient has occlusive cerebrovascular disease. Such cases include patients undergoing emergency thrombolysis and patients with aneurysmal subarachnoid hemorrhage in whom vasospasm has developed. Maintaining normal or higher blood pressure is also essential in patients having tumor compression that can compromise blood for to the spinal cord, kidneys, and other organs. Conversely, prevention of blood pressure increases may be critical in certain groups. Examples include patients with recently ruptured intracranial aneurysms or recently obliterated intracranial arteriovenous malformation and patients who have undergone cerebrovascular angioplasty and stent placement in extracranial conductance vessels such as the carotid artery. These patients are also susceptible to posttreatment cerebral hyperperfusion injury and require careful control of systemic blood pressure after the procedure.

TIPS procedures should be performed under general anesthesia, obviously with an effort to avoid as much as possible drugs that are metabolized principally by the liver. Complications of TIPS can involve bleeding at multiple sites, for example, via capsular tears, hepatic vein tears, and disruption of the portal vein. Worsening of hepatic encephalopathy is another commonly reported complication, along with shunt stenosis and right-sided heart failure, with the latter occurring as a result of the augmented right-sided heart filling that occurs via increased shunt flow from the portal vein. Such augmented filling can also cause serious hemodynamic deterioration that requires that complex postoperative monitoring. Although diagnostic ERCP can often be performed under conscious sedation, general anesthesia is indicated for all patients when the procedure will involve placement of catheters and devices that must be advanced well beyond the ampulla of Vater, as is often the case for removing stones in the biliary tree.

Anticoagulation (Also See Chapters 25 and 26)

Anticoagulation is often needed during intracranial catheter navigation to prevent thromboembolic complications. Heparin (70 U/kg) is commonly used to prolong the baseline activated clotting time (ACT) by a factor of 2 to 3. Hourly monitoring of the ACT is performed to assess the need for additional heparin, which can be given continuously or as intermittent boluses.

Hemorrhagic complications during the procedure may necessitate emergency reversal of anticoagulation. If heparin has been administered, a full reversal dose of protamine (1 mg for each 100 units of heparin activity) should always be available for immediate injection. At the completion of uneventful procedures, heparin can be reversed with protamine, if deemed appropriate.

Antiplatelet drugs (aspirin, ticlopidine, and antagonists to glycoprotein IIb/IIIa receptors) are often used together with heparin, particularly when placing intra-arterial stents. Although antiplatelet drugs decrease the incidence of serious thromboembolic complications, emergency reversal of their anticoagulant effects is difficult. The only practical approach to antagonism of these drugs is empirical provision of exogenous platelets.

Patient Transport

During transport from the imaging suite, airway management equipment, including a face mask and an Ambu bag or a Jackson-Rees circuit, should be immediately available for providing positive-pressure ventilation. Maintaining an intravenous sedation regimen (propofol infusion) is increasingly common during transport or to have given additional medications just before transport.

RADIATION THERAPY

Patient immobility during radiation therapy is the primary goal of sedation or general anesthesia so that the delivered radiation can be precisely targeted. Radiation therapy may involve daily treatments for several weeks. Treatments frequently take very little time, and patients want to quickly resume normal daily activities. In such instances, sedation or general anesthesia should be achieved with fast-onset, short-acting drugs appropriate for brief duration and rapid emergence while keeping in mind that sedation or anesthesia will be repeated daily. Anesthesia may also be required for lengthy or complex cases.

Devices to Deliver Large Targeted Doses of Radiation

Radiation therapy for cancer delivers large radiation doses to target tissues. In some patients, radiation is used to kill vulnerable cancer cells while only minimally injuring noncancer cells. In others, radiation is used to kill all cells in the target region (these radiation devices may be referred to as a "knife"). Such radiation therapy is known as stereotactic because three-dimensional MRI and CT images are used by the radiation instrument to target specific tissue volumes. For example, the GammaKnife simultaneously directs multiple carefully aligned, pencil-thin gamma-ray beams into the targeted area. The Cyber-Knife is also characterized by delivery of a large number of overlapping pencil-thin gamma-ray beams to provide lethal radiation. In contrast to the GammaKnife, which exposes the patient to the gamma rays as a simultaneous single dose, the CyberKnife exposes the patient to a sequence of several hundred gamma-ray beams, each being delivered from a computer-controlled robot arm that moves around the patient and shoots the beams at cancer regions from different directions.

ANESTHESIA REQUIREMENTS

Anesthesia for GammaKnife procedures can involve general anesthesia or sedation for placement of a head frame, subsequent MRI or CT (or both), transport to the recovery room where anesthesia or sedation is maintained as one waits for generation of the computer data needed by the GammaKnife, and finally transport of the anesthetized or sedated patient to the GammaKnife room for the treatment. CyberKnife procedures require prior surgical implantation of radiopaque markers. The anesthesia provider must keep the anesthesia machine, the drug cart, and all tubes and hoses away from all locations that will be occupied by the robot arm. Robot motions can be monitored closely by a remote video connection to verify that one's setup is appropriate. Scattered gamma radiation during therapy reaches high enough levels in the treatment room to require that all health care personnel be outside. Treatments occur in a heavily shielded room with health care personnel typically waiting on the other side of a large lead or iron door that takes 30 to 60 seconds to open. Physiologic monitoring is accomplished via two or more remote video connections.

Alternative Radiation Therapy Delivery Devices

Other external beam radiation therapy modalities for cancer include electron beam radiation and heavy particle ion beam radiation. The "heavy particles" are nuclei from atoms larger than helium. This treatment mode has limited availability, but has significant advantages because the energy deposition of a heavy ion beam is very concentrated and can be targeted with millimeter precision. Intraoperative use of particle beams has become popular in cancer surgery. During intraoperative radiation therapy (IORT), a giant linear accelerator is placed in the operating room, and the depth and width of the electron beam are adjusted according to the patient's needs. Adjacent organs and tissues are shielded with lead. All personnel must leave the room during the radiation treatment, but thick shielding walls are not necessary. A single IORT session will typically provide as much therapy as 10 to 20 daily gamma-ray treatments.

In some instances the patient cannot receive IORT in the operating room when an intraoperative gamma-ray treatment is needed. In such cases, the anesthesia provider must transport the anesthetized patient to the alternative treatment area.

IV

ELECTROCONVULSIVE THERAPY

Electroconvulsive therapy (ECT) is used primarily after failure of pharmacotherapy for affective disorders, most notably severe depression, but also bipolar syndrome and schizophrenia. Because the ECT effect is evident within only a few treatments, it has been proposed for the treatment of psychiatric disorders of high acuity, such as suicidal patients or those unable to take food. There is little doubt about the short-term effectiveness of ECT for depression, but controversies remain regarding its place in long-term management, as well as the definition of failed pharmacotherapy. ECT's therapeutic effects are thought to result from the release of neurotransmitters during the electrically induced grand mal seizure or, perhaps, from the reestablishment of neurotransmitter levels that occurs after seizure activity.

Characteristics of Electrically Induced Seizures

An electrically induced seizure must be of sufficient duration (>20 seconds) for optimal therapeutic effect. In this regard, the anesthesia provider must consider the impact of selected anesthetic drugs on the duration of seizure activity. Electrically induced seizures are characterized by an initial tonic phase (lasts 10 to 15 seconds), followed by a second myoclonic phase (lasts 30 to 60 seconds). Seizure duration is monitored by motor activity and usually a single-channel electroencephalogram. Needs for adjustments in seizure length should be discussed with the anesthesia provider before ECT.

Management of Anesthesia

The two goals of anesthetic management are to (1) provide partial neuromuscular blockade because unmitigated motor activity can result in long bone fractures and skeletal muscle injury and (2) render the patient briefly unconscious for application of the electrical stimulus.[12] Seizures are generally associated with a profound amnestic response and are not painful if motor activity is blocked. However, because of case reports involving awareness and recall in instances where the patient awakened just prior to the ECT shock,[13] careful timing of drug administration and proper dose selection are crucial. In the past the anesthetics most often used for ECT were the short-acting barbiturates methohexital (0.5 to 1.0 mg/kg IV) and thiopental (1.0 to 2.0 mg/kg IV). More recently, propofol (1 mg/kg IV) and etomidate (0.3 mg/kg IV) have become popular.[14]

PROPOFOL

Although studies have found that systemic hemodynamics during ECT is more stable under propofol than under barbiturate anesthesia, propofol tends to shorten seizure duration.[14] In this regard, reducing the propofol dose while adding a short-acting opioid (alfentanil or remifentanil) increases seizure duration by about 50% without causing significant differences in hemodynamics or recovery time.[15]

ETOMIDATE

Etomidate may be preferred over propofol because of its association with longer electrically induced seizures and minimal cardiovascular and respiratory depression. However, a 50% to 80% incidence of myoclonus occurs with etomidate. Although myoclonus is quickly terminated by the succinylcholine dose given immediately following the etomidate injection, the skeletal muscle response to succinylcholine (fasciculations) can produce myalgias. Large doses of etomidate cause adrenocortical suppression, and after a single dose some suppression occurs at 6 hours, with responses being normal at 24 hours. The adrenocortical effects of daily doses of etomidate as administered for ECT are not known.

Psychotropic Medications

In many instances, patients selected for ECT will have had their psychotropic medications tapered for 1 or 2 weeks before a series of 10 to 20 ECT treatments delivered over a period of several weeks. However, patients undergoing ECT usually take one or more psychotropic drugs. Such drugs include monoamine oxidase inhibitors, serotonin reuptake inhibitors, tricyclic antidepressants, lithium, and benzodiazepines. Hypothyroidism occurs in patients who have been taking lithium for a long time (15 years or more).

Delivery of Electroconvulsive Therapy

ECT treatments are usually performed in a procedure room that is fully equipped for general anesthesia, typically in or close to the postanesthesia care unit. Patients should be NPO during the preceding night. Preoperative evaluation of ECT patients should follow the guidelines for other surgical patients, including a current medical history and physical examination.

On the morning of the procedure, the anesthesia provider should document any interval change in the patient's medical condition. Such changes can occur during a course of several ECT treatments, with anesthesia having been provided by multiple personnel. Generally, ECT should not be performed on patients with intracranial mass lesions. If a pregnant patient undergoes ECT, the fetus should be monitored. Although the overall risk of aspiration of gastric contents in ECT cases is very small (less than 1 per 2000 cases), esophageal reflux and hiatal hernia are common findings in ECT patients. Some centers use drugs before the procedure to increase gastric fluid pH or decrease gastric fluid volume, or both.

However, the efficacy of this approach has not been established. External cardiac pacemaker function should not be affected by ECT because the current path is far from the heart. Patients with a history of coronary artery disease, congestive heart failure, and valvular heart disease may benefit from invasive monitoring to assess myocardial function and permit aggressive hemodynamic control.

PREPARATION FOR ANESTHESIA

Anesthesia for ECT begins with attachment of all monitors, administration of 100% oxygen by face mask, and acquisition of vital signs. Supplemental oxygen is continued during and after ECT. A second blood pressure cuff is placed on the lower part of the leg or forearm. This cuff is inflated before administration of the neuromuscular blocking drug to allow monitoring of motor activity during the seizure. Standard neuromuscular blockade monitoring may be performed distal to the cuff, if desired.

INDUCTION OF ANESTHESIA

After administration of oxygen, anesthesia is induced by the administration of propofol (1 to 1.5 mg/kg IV) or etomidate (0.15 to 0.30 mg/kg IV), alone or in combination with esmolol or a rapidly acting opioid such as remifentanil or alfentanil. After the patient loses consciousness, the blood pressure cuff on the leg or arm is inflated above arterial pressure so that it functions as a tourniquet to prevent distal perfusion. During this time, ECT electrodes are applied by the psychiatrist to one or both sides of the head, and an oral airway, if placed previously, is removed and replaced with a bite block to protect the tongue. Because hypercapnia can increase a patient's seizure threshold, the anesthesia provider often provides ventilatory support via the mask just before the therapist energizes the electrodes. Indeed, ECT therapists often prefer that the patient's lungs be hyperventilated to generate hypocapnia and a decrease seizure threshold.

PREVENTION OF EXCESS SKELETAL MUSCLE ACTIVITY

Succinylcholine (0.5 to 1 mg/kg IV) is injected just before application of the electrical current. Full relaxation is not required to prevent seizure-induced skeletal muscle and bone injury. Succinylcholine can increase intragastric pressure, and suction must be available to treat possible regurgitation. When succinylcholine is contraindicated or its side effects not tolerated, rocuronium with its rapid onset can be used. The resultant neuromuscular blockade can be reversed by sugammadex, which hopefully will be approved in the United States by 2011 or 2012 (see Chapter 12).

AIRWAY MANAGEMENT AND MONITORING

Endotracheal intubation is rarely required, but all necessary equipment needs to be present should unexpected airway problems arise. Monitoring with pulse oximetry is used to guide the need for continued administration of supplemental oxygen. The use of a second peripheral nerve stimulator, placed anywhere proximal to the leg tourniquet, will confirm the degree of neuromuscular blockade produced by the neuromuscular blocking drug and will also identify unexpected prolonged neuromuscular blockade, which will occur from succinylcholine in patients with previously unrecognized cholinesterase deficiency (see Chapter 12). The electrocardiogram (ECG) is a necessary monitor because cardiac dysrhythmias can occur during ECT.

PRODUCTION OF THE SEIZURE

Visual monitoring of the seizure is possible by observing the tonic contractions and myoclonus distal to the previously inflated tourniquet (blood pressure cuff) that has been placed on an extremity (serves to isolate this portion of the body from the circulation and the effects of the neuromuscular blocking drug). The electrodes are energized by the psychiatrist once it is clear from fasciculations or the neural blockade monitor that succinylcholine has acted throughout the body (except below the inflated blood pressure cuff). Just before the ECT shock, a few breaths of supplemental oxygen can be given to the patient via the anesthesia mask, which serves to reduce end-tidal CO_2, denitrogenate the functional residual capacity (FRC), and help prevent airway collapse during apnea. During the ECT shock, it is safe for the anesthesia provider to be using gloved hands to gently displace the mandible forward to ensure that the tonic phase of the seizure does not displace the bite block.

PHYSIOLOGIC RESPONSES TO THE SEIZURE

The two phases of the electrically induced seizure (tonic and clonic) have characteristic and highly predictable effects on the vital signs. The initial tonic phase is characterized by profound stimulation of the parasympathetic nervous system that results in a consistent brief period of bradycardia. Blood pressure may decrease as well. This phase quickly converts to a state of sympathetic nervous system stimulation as the seizure enters the clonic phase. Systemic hypertension and tachycardia are often observed but usually abate at or soon after the conclusion of the seizure. During this time cardiac dysrhythmias may be visible on the ECG, as well as changes indicative of myocardial ischemia. Because the maximum arterial blood pressure and heart rate occur and end so quickly, medications to reduce these self-limited changes must be used with great caution. If used, they are most effective when given before the seizure is induced. In appropriate patients, esmolol (0.15 to 1.50 mg/kg IV) or labetalol (0.13 mg/kg IV) may be administered 30 to 60 seconds before the seizure is induced.[16] Similarly, remifentanil or alfentanil may also be administered just before seizure induction. However, routine blunting of sympathetic nervous system responses by β-adrenergic antagonists is not recommended because severe bradycardia can occur.

IV

ANALYSIS OF RESPONSES TO SEIZURES

Because patients undergo a series of ECT sessions, after the first treatment one can evaluate previous cardiovascular responses to the electrical shocks and revise whatever decision one made before about the use of esmolol and other drugs. One can similarly assess the dose used to produce neuromuscular blockade. On rare occasion a seizure will not abate. Seizures that last longer than 90 seconds should generally be terminated with a repeat dose of propofol or an equivalent drug (e.g., thiopental).

CARDIAC CATHETERIZATION— ANGIOGRAPHY, INTERVENTION, ELECTROPHYSIOLOGY

Pediatric cardiac catheterization (also see Chapter 26) is usually performed for the diagnosis and evaluation of congenital heart disease. However, septal defects can sometimes be repaired. Intravenous sedation or general anesthesia must be adequate to prevent stress-induced changes in heart rate and systemic blood pressure without interfering with existing intracardiac shunts as reflected by arterial blood gas measurements. Excess myocardial depression or changes in preload as a result of fluid imbalance must be avoided. Normocapnia is a goal of ventilation during anesthesia for cardiac catheterization. A high hematocrit may be associated with an increased risk for thrombosis, whereas decreasing the hematocrit may jeopardize tissue oxygen delivery. Cardiac dysrhythmias and heart block are important causes of morbidity, thus emphasizing the need for prompt access to a defibrillator and resuscitation drugs.

Premedication and sedation (often combinations of midazolam and a short-acting opioid) may be sufficient to allay the anxiety that could exacerbate coexisting cardiopulmonary problems. Atropine premedication is sometimes useful, particularly if cyanotic congenital heart disease is present. The onset of action of injected or inhaled drugs (or both) may be influenced by the presence of a left-to-right or right-to-left intracardiac shunt, as well as by coexisting congestive heart failure and associated low cardiac output. Patient monitoring during cardiac catheterization may include analysis of arterial blood gases. Access to the patient can be limited by fluoroscopy and the presence of surgical equipment on all sides of the patient during the procedure.

Adult cases (also see Chapter 25) can be extremely challenging, particularly in patients with advanced myocardial disease, whose ejection fraction (EF) generally is less than 20% and who come for installation of a programmable pacemaker that is also an implanted cardioverter/defibrillator (ICD). Such pacemakers often provide right and left dual-chamber pacing. Timing parameters are adjusted during the electrophysiology session, and the session is concluded with repeated defibrillator

tests during which the cardiologist induces fibrillation and the device automatically delivers a rescue shock. Conscious sedation with spontaneous respiration is best in such cases. Before starting the procedure the anesthesia provider should be sure to check the filter setting on the ECG monitoring setup. Many ECG monitors routinely filter out sharp pulses, thus making pacemaker spikes invisible unless "HIDE" is changed to "SHOW" under the setting for pacemakers. Using a minidrip intravenous set can be very helpful in avoiding inadvertent administration of intravenous fluids. A primary element in the anesthesia plan is avoidance of positive-pressure ventilation whenever possible because it will increase pulmonary vascular resistance, decrease left ventricular filling, and decrease arterial pressure. Systemic blood pressure in cardiomyopathy patients with a low EF should be monitored continuously via an arterial catheter; if necessary, the pressure can often be increased with small-dose boluses of phenylephrine (e.g., 25 to 50 µg per bolus), but response is slower than in patients with normal cardiac output. In rare cases phenylephrine can cause an increase in systemic vascular resistance that is not tolerated by a cardiomyopathic heart. If such is the case when dangerous hypotension exists, gentle inotrope administration is needed, as sometimes occurs when inducing anesthesia for cardiac transplantation. Although patients with ICDs have many indwelling catheters and lie on a narrow table, brief neuromuscular blockade is rarely needed to avoid adverse sudden muscle movements at the time of ICD testing. At that time a small dose of propofol after breathing oxygen and voluntary hyperventilation is usually sufficient for patients undergoing conscious sedation with spontaneous ventilation. Once ICD testing is complete, gentle hand-assisted ventilation via a mask can be used if needed to maintain oxygenation until spontaneous respirations return. Cases will occur in which general anesthesia, endotracheal intubation, and mechanical ventilation are all unavoidable. Small doses of etomidate can be used to induce anesthesia in such instances. Supplementation with midazolam is helpful in minimizing the likelihood of awareness (also see Chapter 46). However, spontaneous ventilation will be reduced by midazolam. During general anesthesia, maintenance typically consists of 50% or more nitrous oxide and a small amount of vapor. Arterial blood pressure is often improved when dual-chamber cardiac pacing is initiated by the cardiologist.

CARDIOVERSION

Elective cardioversion requires a brief period of sedation and amnesia for the discomfort produced by the electric shock. After monitors are attached and emergency drugs and equipment have been checked, including the availability of suction, the patient breathes oxygen and the desired level of sedation is typically produced by the intravenous administration of a short-acting drug such as propofol. After loss of consciousness, the electrical charge is delivered to the patient, and gentle assisted ventilation of the lungs with 100% oxygen is provided as needed, with a bag and mask used until consciousness has returned. Hypotension, especially after the administration of propofol, can be minimized by the use of a small dose at a reduced rate of injection. Etomidate is an unlikely selection despite its reduced cardiac depression because the myoclonus that it often induces can make airway management and ECG analysis difficult. Because of slower onset, a less profound degree of central nervous system depression, and duration of action, benzodiazepines are not as useful for cardioversion.

EXTRACORPOREAL SHOCK WAVE LITHOTRIPSY

Extracorporeal shock wave lithotripsy (ESWL) uses focused shock waves (high-intensity pressure waves of short duration) to pulverize renal and ureteral calculi into very small fragments, which are then washed out by normal urine flow. Modern lithotripters deliver several precisely focused, simultaneous shock waves that have been generated in water-filled cushions at the surface of a special table on which the patient lies. Pain at the skin is usually tolerable or amenable to short-acting drugs. Patient immobility during lithotripsy is very important.

Ureteroscopic Lithotripsy

Ureteroscopic lithotripsy (also referred to as "endoscopic lithotripsy") is needed for the disintegration of complex upper urinary tract calculi. A powerful yttrium-aluminum-garnet (YAG) laser is aimed directly at the stones. ESWL and ureteroscopic lithotripsy are routinely performed on an outpatient basis.

Immersion Lithotripsy

ESWL was initially possible only by immersing the patient from the neck down in a water bath. Modern ESWL machines do not require immersion in water, and these have largely replaced immersion lithotripsy, and thus have also eliminated numerous concerns unique to patient immersion, which produces effects similar to those of a G-suit. For example, immersion causes peripheral venous compression, thereby increasing central intravascular volume and central venous pressure—typically by 8 to 11 mm Hg. Immersion lithotripsy also increases the work of breathing, and breathing in awake patients often becomes shallow and rapid. Extrinsic pressure on the abdomen and chest results in a decrease in vital capacity and FRC. Patients with preexisting pulmonary disease may experience impaired ventilation and oxygenation during water immersion. Despite the increased central venous pressure, some patients will exhibit hypotension secondary to vasodilatation as a result of the effects of warm water. Hypotension may also occur during removal from the water bath. During immersion or emersion, cardiac dysrhythmias can occur, presumably reflecting abrupt changes in right atrial pressure and rapid changes in central venous return. Because placement in a water bath puts patients with marginal cardiovascular reserve at greater risk for congestive heart failure or myocardial ischemia, such patients should undergo lithotripsy only in modern units that do not involve immersion.

Risk for Cardiac Dysrhythmias

To minimize the risk of initiating cardiac dysrhythmias (especially ventricular tachycardia), shock waves are triggered from the ECG to occur 20 msec after the R wave, which corresponds to the absolute refractory period of the heart. The concern that shock waves could interfere with functioning of external cardiac pacemakers has not been validated, and the presence of such a device is not considered a contraindication to ESWL, assuming that the external cardiac pacemaker is not positioned in the path of the shock waves.

Side Effects

Hematuria occurs in nearly all patients, presumably from renal parenchymal damage or dislodgment of calculi. In very rare instances, calcifications in blood vessels near the kidney can unintentionally be disintegrated by shock waves aimed at renal stones. Thus, vigilance must always be maintained for bleeding, hematoma formation, and emboli. Other very rare side effects of shock wave damage include pulmonary contusions and pancreatitis. Flank pain may persist for several days after ESWL, and petechiae and soft tissue swelling are common at the shock wave entry site.

Management of Anesthesia

Shock waves cause cutaneous pain as they traverse the water-skin interface. With modern lithotripters the pain is minimal, and intravenous sedation and analgesia are usually sufficient. Supplemental oxygen should be administered during the procedure. It is often possible to avoid endotracheal intubation and use a laryngeal mask, an ordinary face mask, or simply nasal prongs. The pain is more intense with immersion lithotripsy, and general or regional anesthesia is needed. If an epidural technique is used, air should never be injected because it can create a significant density difference just outside the dura. Midline back pain often develops postoperatively in patients who have had air injected into their epidural space during immersion lithotripsy. Adequate intravenous fluid administration is essential during lithotripsy to facilitate the passage of disintegrated stones and maintenance of systemic blood pressure.

IV

DENTAL SURGERY

Anesthesia for dental surgery is commonly needed for patients who are very young as well as for mentally handicapped patients. Special considerations must often be incorporated into the anesthetic plan for a patient with developmental delay as associated with congenital heart disease. Because the teeth and gums are highly innervated, the ECG may reveal cardiac dysrhythmias during periods of intense stimulation.

Management of Anesthesia

Management goals include rapid induction and prompt emergence from anesthesia. Ketamine injected intramuscularly is commonly used for induction of anesthesia. After onset of the effects of ketamine, intravenous access should be done and short-acting drugs (thiopental, etomidate, propofol) administered. Inhaled induction of anesthesia with sevoflurane is also commonly used. Tracheal intubation, often via a nasal route, is recommended for lengthy or unusually bloody procedures. Because tracheal suction through a nasal tube can sometimes be difficult, consideration should be given to the preoperative or intraoperative use of atropine to reduce secretions. A cuffed endotracheal tube is preferred. If an esophageal stethoscope cannot be used, a precordial stethoscope can be placed to monitor breath and heart sounds. The choice of maintenance anesthesia drugs depends on the probable duration of the planned dental surgery. Combinations of inhaled and intravenous anesthetics can be used. The antiemetic properties of propofol may be useful in this setting. Short-acting opioids such as remifentanil and alfentanil may also be considered. Bleeding and the use of oropharyngeal packing during dental procedures emphasize the need for close observation and maintenance of airway patency during emergence, as well as the immediate availability of appropriate personnel and equipment (airways, drugs, suction).

QUESTIONS OF THE DAY

1. What are the signs and symptoms of adverse reactions to iodinated intravenous contrast agents? What are the initial steps in management?
2. What are the risks of providing anesthesia care for magnetic resonance imaging (MRI)? Which risks can be immediately life-threatening?
3. What are the expected physiologic responses to a seizure induced by electroconvulsive therapy (ECT)?
4. What is the risk of cardiac dysrhythmias during extracorporeal shock wave lithotripsy (ESWL)? How can the risk be minimized?

REFERENCES

1. Brateman L: Radiation safety considerations for diagnostic radiology personnel, *Radiographics* 19:1037–1055, 1999.
2. Miller KL: Operational health physics, *Health Phys* 88:1–15, 2005.
3. Robertson PS, Rhoney DH: Prophylaxis for anaphylactoid reactions in high risk patients receiving radiopaque contrast media, *Surg Neurol* 48:292–293, 1997.
4. Ketkar M, Shrier D: An allergic reaction to intraarterial nonionic contrast material, *AJNR Am J Neuroradiol* 24:292, 2003.
5. Nichols DP, Berkenbosch JW, Tobias JD: Rescue sedation with dexmedetomidine for diagnostic imaging: A preliminary report, *Paediatr Anaesth* 15:199–203, 2005.
6. Marckmann P, Skov L: Nephrogenic systemic fibrosis: Clinical picture and treatment, *Radiol Clin North Am* 47:833–840, 2009.
7. Litt L, Cauldwell C: Being extra safe when providing anesthesia for MRI examinations, *ASA Newsl* 66:17–18, 2002.
8. Miyasaka K, Kondo Y, Tamura T, Sakai H: Anesthesia-compatible magnetic resonance imaging, *Anesthesiology* 102:235, 2005, author reply 235–236, discussion 236.
9. Gooden CK, Dilos B: Anesthesia for magnetic resonance imaging, *Int Anesthesiol Clin* 41:29–37, 2003.
10. Frigon C, Shaw DW, Heckbert SR, et al: Supplemental oxygen causes increased signal intensity in subarachnoid cerebrospinal fluid on brain FLAIR MR images obtained in children during general anesthesia, *Radiology* 233:51–55, 2004.
11. Hashimoto T, Gupta DK, Young WL: Interventional neuroradiology—Anesthetic considerations, *Anesthesiol Clin North America* 20:347–359, 2002.
12. Ding Z, White PF: Anesthesia for electroconvulsive therapy, *Anesth Analg* 94:1351–1364, 2002.
13. Litt L, Li D: Awareness without recall during anesthesia for electroconvulsive therapy, *Anesthesiology* 106:871–882, 2007.
14. Avramov MN, Husain MM, White PF: The comparative effects of methohexital, propofol, and etomidate for electroconvulsive therapy, *Anesth Analg* 81:596–602, 1995.
15. Recart A, Rawal S, White PF, et al: The effect of remifentanil on seizure duration and acute hemodynamic responses to electroconvulsive therapy, *Anesth Analg* 96:1047–1050, 2003.
16. Castelli I, Steiner LA, Kaufmann MA, et al: Comparative effects of esmolol and labetalol to attenuate hyperdynamic states after electroconvulsive therapy, *Anesth Analg* 80:557–561, 1995.

RECOVERY PERIOD

The postanesthesia care unit (PACU) is designed and staffed to monitor and care for patients who are recovering from the immediate physiologic effects of anesthesia and surgery. PACU care spans the transition from delivery of anesthesia in the operating room to the less acute monitoring on the hospital ward and, in some cases, independent function of the patient at home. Also, PACUs provide critical care to patients for whom there is no intensive care unit bed in busy medical centers. To serve this unique transition period, the PACU must be equipped to monitor and resuscitate unstable patients while simultaneously providing a tranquil environment for the "recovery" and comfort of stable patients. The proximity of the unit to the operating room facilitates rapid access to postoperative patients by anesthesia and surgical caregivers.

ADMISSION TO THE POSTANESTHESIA CARE UNIT

Upon arrival in the unit, the anesthesia provider informs the PACU nurse of pertinent details on the patient's history, medical condition, anesthesia, and surgery. Particular attention is directed to monitoring oxygenation (pulse oximetry), ventilation (breathing frequency, airway patency, capnography), and circulation (systemic arterial blood pressure, heart rate, electrocardiogram [ECG]).

Vital signs are recorded as often as necessary but at least every 15 minutes while the patient is in the unit. The American Society of Anesthesiologists has adopted Standards for Postanesthesia Care that delineate the minimal requirements for PACU monitoring and care (see Appendix 39-1). More specific recommendations addressing clinical evaluation and therapeutic intervention can be found in the ASA Practice Guidelines for Postanesthesia Care.[1,2]

EARLY POSTOPERATIVE PHYSIOLOGIC DISORDERS

A variety of physiologic disorders affecting multiple organ systems must be diagnosed and treated in the PACU during emergence from anesthesia and surgery (Table 39-1). Nausea and vomiting, the need for upper airway support, and systemic hypertension are among the most frequently encountered complications. Not surprisingly, serious outcomes are the result of airway, respiratory, or cardiovascular compromise.[3] In 2002 airway problems and cardiovascular events accounted for the majority (67%) of 419 recovery room incidents reported to the Australian Incident Monitoring Study (AIMS).[4] Similar data were collected by the U.S. closed claims database, in which critical respiratory incidents accounted for more than half of the PACU malpractice claims.[5] In addition,

Table 39-1 Physiologic Disorders Manifested in the Postanesthesia Care Unit

Upper airway obstruction
Arterial hypoxemia
Hypoventilation
Hypotension
Hypertension
Cardiac dysrhythmias
Oliguria
Bleeding
Decreased body temperature
Agitation (emergence delirium)
Delayed awakening
Nausea and vomiting
Pain

transport of the patient from the operating room to the PACU is also a time when patients are especially vulnerable to airway obstruction, as discussed next.

UPPER AIRWAY OBSTRUCTION (Also See Chapter 16)

Loss of Pharyngeal Muscle Tone

Airway obstruction is a common and potentially devastating complication in the postoperative period. The most frequent cause of airway obstruction in the PACU is the loss of pharyngeal tone in a sedated or obtunded patient. The residual depressant effects of inhaled and intravenous anesthetics and the persistent effects of neuromuscular blocking drugs (also see Chapter 12) contribute to the loss of pharyngeal tone in the immediate postoperative period.

In an awake patient, the pharyngeal muscles contract synchronously with the diaphragm to pull the tongue forward and tent the airway open against the negative inspiratory pressure generated by the diaphragm. This pharyngeal muscle activity is depressed during sleep, and the resulting decrease in tone promotes airway obstruction. With the collapse of compliant pharyngeal tissue during inspiration, a vicious circle may ensue in which a reflex compensatory increase in respiratory effort and negative inspiratory pressure promotes further airway obstruction.[6] This effort to breathe against an obstructed airway is characterized by a paradoxic breathing pattern consisting of retraction of the sternal notch and exaggerated abdominal muscle activity. Collapse of the chest wall plus protrusion of the abdomen with inspiratory effort produces a rocking motion that becomes more prominent with increasing airway obstruction.

Obstruction secondary to loss of pharyngeal tone can be relieved by simply opening the airway with the "jaw thrust maneuver" or continuous positive airway pressure (CPAP) applied via a face mask (or both). Support of the airway is needed until the patient has adequately recovered from the effects of drugs administered during anesthesia. In selected patients, placement of an oral or nasal airway, laryngeal mask airway, or endotracheal tube may be required (also see Chapter 16).

Residual Neuromuscular Blockade (Also See Chapter 12)

When evaluating upper airway obstruction in the PACU, the possibility of residual neuromuscular blockade must be considered in any patient who received neuromuscular blocking drugs during anesthesia. Residual neuromuscular blockade may not be evident on arrival in the PACU because the diaphragm recovers from neuromuscular blockade before the pharyngeal muscles do. With an endotracheal tube in place, end-tidal carbon dioxide concentrations and tidal volumes may indicate adequate ventilation while the ability to maintain a patent upper airway and clear upper airway secretions remain compromised. The stimulation associated with tracheal extubation, followed by the activity of patient transfer to the gurney and subsequent mask airway support, may keep the airway open during transport. Only after the patient is calmly resting in the PACU does upper airway obstruction become evident. Even patients treated with intermediate- and short-acting neuromuscular blocking drugs may manifest residual paralysis in the PACU despite what was deemed clinically adequate pharmacologic reversal in the operating room (OR).

Measurement of the train-of-four (TOF) ratio is commonly used to assess reversal of neuromuscular blockade at the end of surgery. Subjective measurement of the TOF ratio, however, may not accurately reflect recovery of pharyngeal tone because a decline in the TOF ratio may not be appreciated until it reaches a value less than 0.4 to 0.5. Significant clinical weakness may persist to a ratio of 0.7, and pharyngeal function does not return to baseline until an adductor pollicis TOF ratio is greater than 0.9.[7,8]

When patients with residual neuromuscular blockade are awake in the PACU, their struggle to breathe may manifest as agitation. In an awake patient, clinical assessment of reversal of neuromuscular blockade is preferred to the application of painful TOF or tetanic stimulation. Clinical evaluation includes grip strength, tongue protrusion, the ability to lift the legs off the bed, and the ability to lift the head off the bed for a full 5 seconds. Of these maneuvers, the 5-second sustained head lift is considered the gold standard because it reflects not only generalized motor strength but, more important, the patient's ability to maintain and protect the airway. In patients whose tracheas have been extubated, the ability to strongly oppose the incisor teeth against a tongue depressor is another reliable indicator of pharyngeal muscle tone in the awake patient. This maneuver correlates with an average TOF ratio of 0.85. Inadequate ventilation or airway obstruction is less likely if the neuromuscular blockade has been reversed with neostigmine or sugammadex (also see Chapter 12).

If persistence or return of neuromuscular weakness in the PACU is suspected, prompt review of possible etiologic factors is indicated (Table 39-2). Common factors include respiratory acidosis and hypothermia, alone or in combination. Residual depressant effects of volatile anesthetics or opioids (or both) may result in progressive respiratory acidosis only after the patient is admitted to the PACU and external stimulation is minimized. Similarly, a patient who becomes hypothermic during anesthesia and surgery may show signs of weakness in

Table 39-2 Prolonged Neuromuscular Blockade
Factors Contributing to Prolonged Nondepolarizing Neuromuscular Blockade
Drugs
Inhaled anesthetic drugs
Local anesthetics (lidocaine)
Cardiac antidysrhythmics (procainamide)
Antibiotics (polymyxins, aminoglycosides, lincosamines [clindamycin], metronidazole [Flagyl], tetracyclines)
Corticosteroids
Calcium channel blockers
Dantrolene
Furosemide
Metabolic and Physiologic States
Hypermagnesemia
Hypocalcemia
Hypothermia
Respiratory acidosis
Hepatic/renal failure
Myasthenia syndromes
Factors Contributing to Prolonged Depolarizing Neuromuscular Blockade
Excessive dose of succinylcholine
Reduced plasma cholinesterase activity
Decreased levels
Extremes of age (newborn, old age)
Disease states (hepatic disease, uremia, malnutrition, plasmapheresis)
Hormonal changes
Pregnancy
Contraceptives
Glucocorticoids
Inhibited activity
Irreversible (echothiophate)
Reversible (edrophonium, neostigmine, pyridostigmine)
Genetic variant (atypical plasma cholinesterase)

V

the PACU that were not noted on extubation in the operating room. Simple measures such as warming the patient, airway support, and correction of electrolyte abnormalities can facilitate recovery from neuromuscular blockade.

Laryngospasm

Laryngospasm refers to a sudden spasm of the vocal cords that completely occludes the laryngeal opening. It typically occurs in the transitional period when the extubated patient is emerging from general anesthesia. Although it is most likely to occur in the operating room at the time of tracheal extubation, patients who arrive in the PACU asleep after general anesthesia are also at risk for laryngospasm on awakening.

Jaw thrust with CPAP (up to 40 cm H_2O) is often sufficient stimulation to "break" the laryngospasm. If jaw thrust and CPAP maneuvers fail, immediate skeletal muscle relaxation can be achieved with succinylcholine (0.1 to 1.0 mg/kg IV or 4 mg/kg IM). A tracheal tube should not be passed forcibly through a glottis that is closed because of laryngospasm.

Airway Edema

Airway edema is a possible operative complication in patients undergoing prolonged procedures in the prone or Trendelenburg position and in procedures with large amounts of blood loss requiring aggressive fluid resuscitation. Surgical procedures on the tongue, pharynx, and neck, including thyroidectomy, carotid endarterectomy, and cervical spinal procedures, can result in upper airway obstruction because of tissue edema or hematoma, or both. Although facial and scleral edema are important physical signs that can alert the clinician to the presence of airway edema, significant edema of pharyngeal tissue is often not accompanied by visible external signs. If tracheal extubation is to be attempted in these patients in the PACU, evaluation of airway patency must precede removal of the endotracheal tube (ETT). The patient's ability to breathe around the ETT can be evaluated by suctioning the oral pharynx and deflating the ETT cuff. With occlusion of the proximal end of the ETT, the patient is then asked to breathe around the tube. Good air movement suggests that the patent's airway will remain patent after tracheal extubation. Alternative methods include (1) measuring the intrathoracic pressure required to produce an audible leak around the ETT when the cuff is deflated, or (2) measuring the exhaled tidal volume before and after ETT cuff deflation in a patient receiving volume control ventilation. Though helpful, none of these cuff leak "tests" take the place of sound clinical judgment when deciding when to safely extubate the patient with an airway compromise.[9]

Sleep Apnea

Special consideration must be given to patients with obstructive sleep apnea (OSA) in the PACU.[10] Because patients with OSA are particularly prone to airway obstruction, their tracheas should not be extubated until they are fully awake and following commands. Any redundant compliant pharyngeal tissue in these patients not only increases the incidence of airway obstruction but also makes intubation by direct laryngoscopy difficult or at times impossible. Once in the PACU, a patient with OSA whose trachea has been extubated is exquisitely sensitive to opioids, and when possible, continuous regional anesthesia techniques should be used to provide postoperative analgesia. Benzodiazepines can have a more intense effect on pharyngeal muscle tone than opioids and, therefore, can contribute to airway obstruction in the PACU.

When caring for a patient with OSA, plans should be made preoperatively to provide CPAP in the immediate postoperative period. Patients are often asked to bring their CPAP machines with them on the day of surgery so that the equipment can be set up before the patient's arrival in the PACU. Patients who do not routinely use CPAP at home or who do not have their machines with them may require additional attention from the respiratory therapist to ensure proper fit of the CPAP delivery device (mask or nasal airways) and to determine the amount of positive pressure needed to prevent upper airway obstruction. Finally, because the majority of patients with mild to moderate OSA are undiagnosed at the time of surgery, care should be taken to identify at-risk patients based on preoperative clinical suspicion, a history of snoring, and daytime sleepiness.

Management of Airway Obstruction

An obstructed upper airway requires immediate attention. Efforts to open the airway by noninvasive measures should be attempted before reintubation of the trachea. Jaw thrust with CPAP (5 to 15 cm H_2O) is often enough to tent the upper airway open in patients with decreased pharyngeal muscle tone. If CPAP is not effective, an oral, nasal, or laryngeal mask airway can be inserted rapidly. After successfully opening the upper airway and ensuring adequate ventilation, the cause of the upper airway obstruction should be identified and treated. The sedating effects of opioids and benzodiazepines can be reversed with persistent stimulation or small titrated doses of naloxone (0.3 to 0.5 µg/kg IV) or flumazenil, respectively. Residual effects of neuromuscular blocking drugs can be reversed pharmacologically or by correcting contributing factors such as hypothermia.

It may not be possible to mask-ventilate a patient with severe upper airway obstruction as a result of edema or hematoma. In the case of hematoma after thyroid or carotid surgery, an attempt can be made to decompress the airway by releasing the clips or sutures on the wound and evacuating the hematoma. This maneuver is recommended as a temporizing measure, but it will not effectively decompress the airway if a significant amount of fluid or blood (or both) has infiltrated the tissue planes of the pharyngeal wall. If emergency tracheal intubation is required, it is important to have ready access to difficult airway equipment and, if possible, surgical backup for performance of an emergency tracheostomy. If the patient is able to move air by spontaneous ventilation, an awake endotracheal intubation technique is preferred because visualization of the cords by direct laryngoscopy may not be possible.

Monitoring Airway Patency During Transport

Upper airway patency and the effectiveness of the patient's respiratory efforts must be monitored during transportation from the operating room to the PACU. Hypoventilation in a patient receiving supplemental oxygen will not be reliably detected by monitoring with pulse oximetry during transport.[11] Adequate ventilation must be confirmed by watching for the appropriate rise and fall of the chest wall with inspiration, listening for breath sounds, or simply feeling for exhaled breath with the palm of one's hand over the patient's nose and mouth. As indicated previously, this can be a critically dangerous time in the immediate postoperative period.

HYPOXEMIA IN THE PACU

Atelectasis and alveolar hypoventilation are the most common causes of transient postoperative arterial hypoxemia in the immediate postoperative period. Filling the patient's lungs with oxygen at the conclusion of anesthesia, as well as the administration of supplemental oxygen, should blunt any effect of diffusion hypoxia as a contributor to arterial hypoxemia. Clinical correlation should guide the workup of a postoperative patient who remains persistently hypoxic. Review of the patient's history, operative course, and clinical signs and symptoms will direct the workup to rule in possible causes (Table 39-3).

Alveolar Hypoventilation (Table 39-4)

Postoperative ventilatory failure can result from a depressed drive to breathe or generalized weakness from either residual neuromuscular blockade or underlying neuromuscular disease. Restrictive pulmonary conditions such as preexisting chest wall deformity, postoperative abdominal binding, or abdominal distention can also contribute to inadequate ventilation.

Review of the alveolar gas equation demonstrates that hypoventilation alone is sufficient to cause arterial

Table 39-3 Postoperative Hypoxemia

Right-to-left shunt
  Pulmonary: atelectasis
  Intracardiac: congenital heart disease

Mismatching of ventilation to perfusion
Congestive heart failure
Pulmonary edema—fluid overload, postobstructive
Alveolar hypoventilation—residual effects of anesthetics and/or neuromuscular blocking drugs
Diffusion hypoxia—unlikely if patient is receiving supplemental oxygen
Aspiration of gastric contents
Pulmonary embolus
Pneumothorax
Posthyperventilation hypoxia
Increased oxygen consumption—as from shivering

Acute lung injury
  Sepsis
  Transfusion-related acute lung injury

Advanced age
Obesity

Table 39-4 Factors Leading to Postoperative Hypoventilation

Drug-induced central nervous system depression (volatile anesthetics, opioids)
Residual effects of neuromuscular blocking drugs
Suboptimal ventilatory muscle mechanics
Increased production of carbon dioxide
Coexisting chronic obstructive pulmonary disease

hypoxemia in a patient breathing room air (Fig. 39-1). At sea level, a normocapnic patient breathing room air will have an alveolar oxygen pressure of 100 mm Hg. Thus, a healthy patient without a significant alveolar-arterial (A-a) gradient will have a Pa_{O_2} near 100 mm Hg. In the same patient, a rise in Pa_{CO_2} from 40 to 80 mm Hg (alveolar hypoventilation) results in an alveolar oxygen pressure ($P_{A_{O_2}}$) of 50 mm Hg. This exercise demonstrates that even a patient with normal lungs will become hypoxic if allowed to significantly hypoventilate while breathing room air.

Normally, minute ventilation increases by approximately 2 L/min for every 1 mm Hg increase in arterial P_{CO_2}. This linear ventilatory response to carbon dioxide can be significantly depressed in the immediate

V

$$PAO_2 = FIO_2(PB - PH_2O) - \frac{PaCO_2}{RQ}$$

$PaCO_2 = 40$ mm Hg
$$PAO_2 = 0.21(760 - 47) - \frac{40}{0.8} = 150 - 50 = 100 \text{ mm Hg}$$

$PaCO_2 = 80$ mm Hg
$$PAO_2 = 0.21(760 - 47) - \frac{80}{0.8} = 150 - 100 = 50 \text{ mm Hg}$$

PAO_2 = alveolar oxygen pressure
FIO_2 = fraction of inspired oxygen concentration
PB = barometric pressure
PH_2O = vapor pressure of water
RQ = respiratory quotient

Figure 39-1 Hypoventilation as a cause of arterial hypoxemia.

postoperative period by the residual effects of drugs (inhaled anesthetics, opioids, sedative-hypnotics) administered during anesthesia.

Arterial hypoxemia secondary to hypercapnia alone can be reversed by the administration of supplemental oxygen or by normalizing the $PaCO_2$, or both (Fig. 39-2).[12] In the PACU, $PaCO_2$ can be returned to normal by external stimulation of the patient to wakefulness, pharmacologic reversal of opioid or benzodiazepine effect, or controlled mechanical ventilation. Figure 39-2 demonstrates why pulse oximetry is an unreliable marker of hypoventilation in a patient receiving supplemental oxygen.

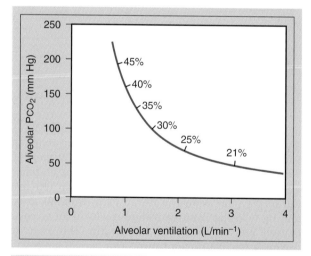

Figure 39-2 Alveolar P_{CO_2} as a function of alveolar ventilation at rest. The percentages indicate the inspired oxygen concentration required to restore alveolar P_{O_2} to normal. (Adapted from Lumb AB, ed. Nunn's Applied Respiratory Physiology, 6th ed. Philadelphia, Elsevier/Butterworth-Heinemann, 2005, used with permission.)

Decreased Alveolar Partial Pressure of Oxygen

Diffusion hypoxia refers to the rapid diffusion of nitrous oxide into alveoli at the end of a nitrous oxide anesthetic. Nitrous oxide dilutes the alveolar gas and produces a transient decrease in PAO_2 and $PACO_2$. In a patient breathing room air, the resulting decrease in PAO_2 can produce arterial hypoxemia. In the absence of supplemental oxygen administration, diffusion hypoxia can persist for 5 to 10 minutes after a nitrous oxide anesthetic and thus contribute to arterial hypoxemia in the initial moments as the patient is admitted to the PACU.

When providing supplemental oxygen to a patient during transport to the PACU, care should be taken to avoid the relative decrease in FIO_2 that can result from an unrecognized disconnection of the oxygen source or empty oxygen tank.

Ventilation-to-Perfusion Mismatch and Shunt

Hypoxic pulmonary vasoconstriction (HPV) is an attempt of normal lungs to optimally match ventilation and perfusion. This response constricts vessels in poorly ventilated regions of the lung and directs pulmonary blood flow to well-ventilated alveoli. The HPV response is inhibited by a number of conditions and medications, including pneumonia, sepsis, and vasodilators. In the PACU, the residual effects of inhaled anesthetics and vasodilators such as nitroprusside and dobutamine used to treat systemic hypertension or improve hemodynamics will blunt HPV and contribute to arterial hypoxemia.

Unlike a ventilation-to-perfusion mismatch, a true shunt will not respond to supplemental oxygen. Causes of postoperative pulmonary shunt include atelectasis, pulmonary edema, gastric aspiration, pulmonary emboli, and pneumonia. Of these, atelectasis is probably the most common cause of pulmonary shunting in the immediate postoperative period. Mobilization of the patient to the sitting position, incentive spirometry, and positive airway pressure by face mask can be effective in treating atelectasis.

Increased Venous Admixture

Increased venous admixture typically refers to low cardiac output states. It is due to mixing of desaturated venous blood with oxygenated arterial blood. Normally, only 2% to 5% of cardiac output is shunted through the lungs, and this small amount of shunted blood with a normal mixed venous saturation has a minimal effect on PaO_2. In low cardiac output states, blood returns to the heart severely desaturated. Additionally, the shunt fraction increases significantly in conditions that impede alveolar oxygenation, such as pulmonary edema and atelectasis. Under these conditions, mixing of desaturated shunted blood with saturated arterialized blood decreases PaO_2.

Decreased Diffusion Capacity

A decreased diffusion capacity suggests the presence of underlying lung disease such as emphysema, interstitial lung disease, pulmonary fibrosis, or primary pulmonary hypertension. In this regard, the differential diagnosis of arterial hypoxemia in the PACU must include the contribution of any preexisting pulmonary condition.

PULMONARY EDEMA IN THE PACU

Pulmonary edema in the immediate postoperative period is often cardiogenic in nature, the result of intravascular volume overload or cardiac dysfunction. Noncardiogenic edema may occur in the PACU as a result of pulmonary aspiration or sepsis. Rarely, postoperative pulmonary edema is the result of airway obstruction (postobstructive pulmonary edema) or transfusion of blood products (transfusion-related acute lung injury).

Postobstructive Pulmonary Edema

Postobstructive pulmonary edema and the resulting arterial hypoxemia are rare, but significant consequences of upper airway obstruction, as may follow tracheal extubation at the conclusion of anesthesia and surgery. It is a transudative edema produced by the exaggerated negative pressure generated by inspiration against a closed glottis. This exaggerated negative intrathoracic pressure increases venous return, which further promotes the transudation of fluid. Muscular healthy patients are at increased risk because of their ability to generate significant inspiratory force.

Laryngospasm is the most common cause of upper airway obstruction leading to postobstructive pulmonary edema, but it may result from any condition that occludes the upper airway. Arterial hypoxemia is usually manifested within 90 minutes after development of postobstructive pulmonary edema and is accompanied by bilateral fluffy infiltrates on the chest radiograph. The diagnosis depends on clinical suspicion once other causes of pulmonary edema are ruled out. Treatment is supportive and includes supplemental oxygen, diuresis, and in severe cases, positive-pressure ventilation.[13]

Transfusion-Related Acute Lung Injury (Also See Chapter 24)

The differential diagnosis of pulmonary edema in the PACU should include transfusion-related acute lung injury (TRALI) in any patient who received blood, coagulation factor, or platelet transfusions intraoperatively. TRALI is typically manifested within 1 to 2 hours after the transfusion of plasma-containing blood products, including packed red blood cells, whole blood, fresh frozen plasma, or platelets. Because reactions can occur up to 6 hours after transfusion, the syndrome may develop during the patient's stay in the PACU after a transfusion in the operating room. The resulting noncardiogenic pulmonary edema is often associated with fever and systemic hypotension. If a complete blood count is obtained with the onset of symptoms, an acute decrease in the white blood cell count (leukopenia) reflecting the sequestration of granulocytes within the lung and exudative fluid can be documented. The diagnosis is made clinically with the appearance of bilateral pulmonary infiltrates and an increased alveolar-to-arterial oxygen difference that is temporally related to the transfusion. Initially it may be difficult distinguishing TRALI from TACO (transfusion-associated circulatory overload) caused by the volume of blood products transfused. In either case treatment is supportive and includes supplemental oxygen and diuresis. Rarely, TRALI results in a prolonged course of adult respiratory distress syndrome (ARDS).

Historically, the lack of specific diagnostic criteria has led to the under diagnosis and reporting of TRALI. The recent increased awareness of the syndrome is due largely to the adoption of diagnostic criteria by the American European Consensus Conference.[14] Most recently, elimination of female donors of fresh frozen plasma has decreased the incidence of TRALI.

OXYGEN SUPPLEMENTATION

Although there is common sense agreement that the delivery of supplemental oxygen in the immediate postoperative period is indicated to correct the hypoxemia associated with the recovery from anesthesia and surgery, the "optimal" perioperative oxygenation remains controversial. Whether increased oxygenation delivery results in a reduction in the incidence of postoperative nausea and vomiting (PONV) and promotion of surgical wound healing is not clear. Though initial studies produced positive results, not all studies are in agreement, and the extent to which supplemental oxygen improves PONV and wound healing is not clear.[15]

Oxygen Delivery

The choice of oxygen delivery systems in the PACU is determined by the degree of hypoxemia, the surgical procedure, and patient compliance. Patients who have undergone head and neck surgery may not be candidates for face mask oxygen due to the risk of pressure necrosis of incision sites and microvascular flaps, while nasal packing prohibits the use of nasal cannulas in others.

Delivery of oxygen by traditional nasal cannula is limited to 6 L/min flow to minimize discomfort and complications that result from inadequate humidification. As a general rule each L/min of oxygen flow through nasal cannula increases FiO_2 by 0.04, with 6 L/min resulting in approximately 0.44 FiO_2.

Until recently maximum oxygen delivery to patients whose tracheas have been extubated required a non-rebreather mask or high-flow nebulizer. Delivery by mask can be inefficient, however, because of inadequate mask fit or high minute ventilation requirements that result in significant entrainment of room air. Alternatively, oxygen can be delivered up to 40 L/min by high-flow nasal cannulas. These high-flow nasal cannula delivery systems humidify and warm the gas to 99.9% relative humidity and 37° C. Unlike non-rebreather masks, these devices deliver oxygen directly to the nasopharynx throughout the respiratory cycle. The efficacy of these systems may be enhanced by a CPAP effect produced by the high gas flow.

Continuous Positive Airway Pressure and Noninvasive Positive-Pressure Ventilation

A reported 8% to 10% of patients who undergo abdominal surgery subsequently require endotracheal intubation and mechanical ventilation for hypoxemia. Application of CPAP in the PACU reduces the incidence of intubation, pneumonia, infection, and sepsis in this population.[16]

Even with the application of CPAP in the PACU, many patients will require additional ventilatory support. Ventilatory failure in the immediate postoperative period may result from a number of conditions including excessive intravascular volume, splinting due to pain, diaphragmatic dysfunction, muscular weakness, and pharmacologically depressed respiratory drive.

Although the use of noninvasive positive-pressure ventilation (NPPV) in both chronic and acute respiratory failure is well established, there is limited experience with its application in the PACU. NPPV is often avoided in the immediate postoperative period because of the potential for gastric distention, aspiration, and wound dehiscence, especially in patients who have undergone gastric or esophageal surgery. Thus, the decision to use noninvasive modes of ventilation in the PACU must be guided by careful consideration of both patient and surgical factors. Contraindications include hemodynamic instability or life-threatening arrhythmias, altered mental status, high risk of aspiration, inability to use a nasal or face mask (head and neck procedures), and refractory hypoxemia. In the appropriate patient population, NPPV is effective in avoiding endotracheal intubation in the PACU.[17]

HEMODYNAMIC INSTABILITY

Hemodynamic instability in the immediate postoperative period can have a negative impact on outcome. Surprisingly, postoperative systemic hypertension and tachycardia are more predictive of unplanned admission to the critical care unit and mortality rate than are hypotension and bradycardia.[18]

Systemic Hypertension

Patients with a history of essential hypertension are at greatest risk for significant systemic hypertension in the PACU. Additional factors include pain, hypoventilation and associated hypercapnia, emergence excitement, advanced age, a history of cigarette smoking, and preexisting renal disease (Table 39-5). Surgical procedures that predispose the patient to postoperative hypertension include craniotomy and carotid endarterectomy.

Systemic Hypotension

Postoperative hypotension may be characterized as (1) hypovolemic (2) cardiogenic, or (3) distributive (Table 39-6).

HYPOVOLEMIA (DECREASED PRELOAD)

Systemic hypotension in the PACU is usually due to decreased intravascular fluid volume and preload, and as such, responds favorably to intravenous fluid administration. The most common causes of decreased intravascular volume in the immediate postoperative period include ongoing third-space translocation of fluid, inadequate intraoperative fluid replacement (especially in patients who undergo major intra-abdominal procedures or preoperative bowel preparation), and loss of sympathetic nervous system tone as a result of neuraxial (spinal or epidural) blockade.

Persistent bleeding should be ruled out in hypotensive patients who have undergone a surgical procedure in which significant blood loss is possible. This is true regardless of the estimated intraoperative blood loss. If the patient is unstable, hemoglobin can be measured at the bedside to eliminate laboratory turnover time. It is also important to remember that tachycardia may not be a reliable indicator of hypovolemia or anemia (or both) if the patient is taking β-adrenergic or calcium channel blockers.

Table 39-5 Factors Leading to Postoperative Hypertension
Arterial hypoxemia
Preoperative essential hypertension
Enhanced sympathetic nervous system activity—hypercapnia from hypoventilation, pain, gastric distention, bladder distention
Hypervolemia
Emergence excitement
Shivering
Drug withdrawal—clonidine, β-blockers, narcotics
Increased intracranial pressure

Table 39-6 Causes of Hypotension in the Postanesthesia Care Unit

Intravascular fluid volume depletion
  Ongoing fluid losses—bowel preparation,
  gastrointestinal losses, surgical bleeding
  Increased capillary permeability—sepsis, burns,
  transfusion-related lung injury

Decreased cardiac output
  Myocardial ischemia/infarction
  Cardiomyopathy
  Valvular disease
  Pericardial disease
  Cardiac tamponade
  Cardiac dysrhythmias
  Pulmonary embolus
  Tension pneumothorax
  Drug-induced—β-blockers, calcium channel blockers

Decreased vascular tone
  Sepsis
  Allergic reactions—anaphylactic, anaphylactoid
  Spinal shock—cord injury, iatrogenic: spinal or epidural
  anesthesia

Adrenal insufficiency

CARDIOGENIC HYPOTENSION (INTRINSIC PUMP FAILURE)

Significant cardiogenic causes of postoperative systemic hypotension include myocardial ischemia and infarction, cardiomyopathy, and cardiac dysrhythmias. The differential diagnosis depends on the surgical procedure, intraoperative course, and the patient's preoperative medical condition. To determine the cause of the hypotension, central venous pressure monitoring or echocardiography may be required.

DISTRIBUTIVE HYPOTENSION (DECREASED AFTERLOAD)

Iatrogenic Sympathectomy

Iatrogenic sympathectomy secondary to regional anesthetic techniques is an important cause of hypotension in the PACU. A high sympathetic block (to T4) will decrease vascular tone and block the cardioaccelerator fibers. If not treated promptly, the resulting bradycardia in the presence of severe hypotension can lead to cardiac arrest, even in young healthy patients. Vasopressors, including phenylephrine and ephedrine, are pharmacologic treatments of hypotension caused by residual sympathetic nervous system blockade.

Critically Ill Patients

Critically ill patients may rely on exaggerated sympathetic nervous system tone to maintain systemic blood pressure and heart rate. In these patients even minimal doses of inhaled anesthetics, opioids, or sedative-hypnotics can decrease sympathetic nervous system tone and produce marked systemic hypotension.

Allergic Reactions

Allergic (anaphylactic or anaphylactoid) reactions may be the cause of hypotension in the PACU. Anaphylaxis should be considered in all cases of sudden refractory extreme hypotension even when not accompanied by the classic sequelae of bronchospasm and rash. Increased serum tryptase concentrations confirm the occurrence of an allergic reaction, but this change does not differentiate anaphylactic from anaphylactoid reactions. The blood specimen for tryptase determination must be obtained within 30 to 120 minutes after the allergic reaction, but the results may not be available for several days. Neuromuscular blocking drugs are the most common cause of anaphylactic reactions in the operative setting. Epinephrine is the drug of choice to treat anaphylaxis.[19]

Sepsis

If sepsis is suspected as the cause of hypotension in PACU, blood should be obtained for culture, after which empiric antibiotic therapy should be initiated before transfer of the patient to the ward. Urinary tract manipulations and biliary tract procedures are examples of interventions that can result in a sudden onset of severe systemic hypotension in the PACU. In these cases hypotension is often accompanied by fever and rigor.

Myocardial Ischemia

Detection of myocardial ischemia in the PACU can be challenging because of the patient's inability to identify or communicate symptoms related to cardiac ischemia. Postoperative patients with myocardial infarction complain of typical chest pain only 8% to 20% of the time. Additionally ST-segment changes on cardiac monitors are visually difficult to interpret and therefore often inaccurate. Because of this, the American College of Cardiology recommends computed ST-segment analysis (if available) be used to monitor high-risk patients in the PACU.

LOW-RISK PATIENTS

Interpretation of ST-segment changes on the ECG in the PACU should be interpreted in light of the patient's cardiac history and risk index. In low-risk patients (<45 years of age, no known cardiac disease, only one risk factor), postoperative ST-segment changes on the ECG do not usually indicate myocardial ischemia. Relatively benign causes of ST-segment changes in these low-risk patients include anxiety, esophageal reflux, hyperventilation, and hypokalemia. In general, low-risk patients require only routine PACU observation unless associated signs and symptoms warrant further clinical evaluation. A more aggressive evaluation is indicated if the changes

V

are accompanied by cardiac rhythm disturbances, hemodynamic instability, or both.

HIGH-RISK PATIENTS

In contrast to low-risk patients, ST-segment and T-wave changes on the ECG in high-risk patients can be significant even in the absence of typical signs or symptoms. In this patient population, any ST-segment or T-wave changes that are compatible with myocardial ischemia should prompt further evaluation to rule out myocardial ischemia. Determination of serum troponin levels is indicated when myocardial ischemia or infarction is suspected in the PACU. Once blood samples for measurement of troponin and the MB fraction of creatine phosphokinase are obtained and a 12-lead ECG is completed, arrangements must be made for the appropriate cardiology follow-up.

ROUTINE POSTOPERATIVE 12-LEAD ELECTROCARDIOGRAM

A routine postoperative 12-lead ECG is recommended only for patients with known or suspected coronary artery disease who have undergone high- or intermediate-risk surgery. High-risk surgery includes major emergency surgery, aortic and other major vascular surgery, peripheral vascular surgery and unanticipated prolonged procedures associated with large fluid shifts or blood loss. Intermediate-risk procedures include intra-abdominal and thoracic surgery, carotid endarterectomy, head and neck surgery, orthopedic surgery, and prostate surgery.[20,21]

Cardiac Dysrhythmias

Perioperative cardiac dysrhythmias are frequently transient and multifactorial in cause (Table 39-7). Reversible causes of cardiac dysrhythmias in the perioperative period include hypoxemia, hypoventilation and associated hypercapnia, endogenous or exogenous catecholamines, electrolyte abnormalities, acidemia, fluid overload, anemia, and substance withdrawal.

TACHYDYSRHYTHMIAS

Common causes of sinus tachycardia in the PACU include postoperative pain, agitation (rule out arterial hypoxemia), hypoventilation with associated hypercapnia, hypovolemia (continued postoperative bleeding), shivering, and the presence of a tracheal tube. Additional causes include cardiogenic or septic shock, pulmonary embolism, thyroid storm, and malignant hyperthermia.

ATRIAL DYSRHYTHMIAS

The incidence of new postoperative atrial dysrhythmias may be as frequent as 10% after major noncardiothoracic surgery. The incidence is even more frequent after

Table 39-7 Factors Leading to Postoperative Cardiac Dysrhythmias
Hypoxemia
Hypercarbia
Intravasuclar volume shifts
Pain, agitation
Hypothermia
Hyperthermia
Anticholinesterases
Anticholinergics
Myocardial ischemia
Electrolyte abnormalities
Respiratory acidosis
Hypertension
Digitalis intoxication
Preoperative cardiac dysrhythmias

cardiac and thoracic procedures where the cardiac dysrhythmia is often attributed to atrial irritation. These new-onset atrial dysrhythmias are not benign because they are associated with a longer hospital stay and increased mortality.

Atrial Fibrillation

Control of the ventricular response rate is the immediate goal in the treatment of new-onset atrial fibrillation. Hemodynamically unstable patients may require prompt electrical cardioversion, but most patients can be treated pharmacologically with intravenous β-blocker or calcium channel blocker. Diltiazem is the calcium channel blocker of choice for patients in whom β-blockers are contraindicated. Rate control with these drugs is often enough to chemically cardiovert the postoperative patient whose arrhythmia may be catecholamine driven. If the goal of therapy is chemical cardioversion, an amiodarone load can be initiated in the PACU.

VENTRICULAR DYSRHYTHMIAS

Ventricular tachycardia is uncommon, whereas premature ventricular contractions (PVCs) and ventricular bigeminy are common. PVCs most often reflect increased sympathetic nervous system stimulation, as many accompany tracheal intubation and transient hypercapnia. True ventricular tachycardia is indicative of underlying cardiac disease, and in the case of torsades de pointes, QT-interval prolongation on the ECG may be intrinsic or drug related (amiodarone, procainamide, or droperidol).

BRADYDYSRHYTHMIAS

Bradycardia in the PACU is often iatrogenic. Drug-related causes include β-blocker therapy, anticholinesterase reversal of neuromuscular blockade, opioid administration, and treatment with dexmedetomidine. Procedure- and patient-related causes include bowel distention, increased intracranial or intraocular pressure, and spinal anesthesia. A high spinal block of cardioaccelerator fibers originating from T1 through T4 can produce severe bradycardia. The resulting sympathectomy, bradycardia, and possible intravascular fluid volume depletion and associated decreased venous return can produce sudden bradycardia and cardiac arrest, even in young healthy patients.

TREATMENT

The urgency of treatment of a cardiac dysrhythmia depends on the physiologic consequences (principally systemic hypotension and myocardial ischemia) of the dysrhythmia. Tachydysrhythmia decreases diastolic and coronary perfusion time and increases myocardial oxygen consumption. Its impact depends on the patient's underlying cardiac function and it is most harmful in patients with coronary artery disease. Bradycardia has a more deleterious effect in patients with a fixed stroke volume, such as infants and patients with restrictive pericardial disease or cardiac tamponade.

DELIRIUM

Approximately 10% of adult patients older than 50 years who undergo elective surgery will experience some degree of postoperative delirium within the first 5 postoperative days. The incidence is much more frequent for certain procedures, such as repair of a hip fracture and bilateral knee replacement (Table 39-8).

Risk Factors

Persistent postoperative delirium is generally a condition of elderly patients. It is a costly complication in both human and monetary terms because it increases the length of hospital stay, pharmacy costs, and mortality rate. In adults, patients at risk for postoperative delirium can be identified before surgery. The most significant preoperative risk factors include (1) advanced age, (2) preoperative cognitive impairment, (3) decreased functional status, (4) alcohol abuse, and (5) a previous history of delirium.

In addition to iatrogenic factors, including inadequate hydration and medications, the workup for postoperative delirium must exclude arterial hypoxemia, hypercapnia, pain, sepsis, and electrolyte abnormalities. Intraoperative factors that are predictive of postoperative delirium include surgical blood loss, hematocrit less than 30%, and the number of intraoperative blood transfusions. Intraoperative hemodynamic derangements and the

Table 39-8 Differential Diagnosis of Postoperative Delirium in the Postanesthesia Care Unit

Arterial hypoxemia
Preexisting cognitive disorder—Parkinson disease, baseline dementia
Hypoventilation with hypercapnia
Metabolic derangements—renal, hepatic, endocrine
Drugs—anticholinergics, benzodiazepines, opioids, β-blockers
Drug or ETOH withdrawal
Electrolyte abnormalities
Incomplete muscle relaxant reversal
Acute CNS event—hemorrhage, ischemic stroke
Infection
Seizures

CNS, central nervous system; ETOH, ethanol.

anesthetic technique do not seem to be predictors of postoperative delirium. Clinical evaluation of a delirious patient in the PACU includes a thorough evaluation of any underlying disease and metabolic derangements, such as hepatic- and renal-related encephalopathy.[22,23]

Management

A high-risk patient should be identified before admission to the PACU. Severely agitated patients may require restraints and additional personnel to control their behavior and avoid self-inflicted injury or dislodgment of intravascular catheters and the endotracheal tube. Early identification of patients at risk for delirium can also guide pharmacologic therapy postoperatively. Patients with tolerance to alcohol or opioids will probably require increased opioid doses to treat pain and anxiety and avoid the onset of alcohol withdrawal. Conversely, in the elderly population drug therapy and doses should be limited as much as possible to avoid further exacerbation of drug-induced delirium.

Emergence Excitement

Delirium may mimic a transient confusional state ("emergence excitement") that is associated with emergence from general anesthesia. Emergence excitement is common in children, with more than 30% experiencing agitation or delirium at some period during their PACU stay. The peak age of emergence excitement in children is between 2 and 4 years.

Unlike delirium, emergence excitement typically resolves quickly and is followed by uneventful recovery. Emergence excitement is more frequent with rapid "wake up" from inhalational anesthesia. In children, preoperative medication with midazolam has been associated with an increase in the incidence and duration of postoperative delirium, but

V

whether midazolam is an independent factor or merely a reflection of other preoperative variables remains unclear.

RENAL DYSFUNCTION

The differential diagnosis of postoperative renal dysfunction includes preoperative, intraoperative, and postoperative causes (see Chapter 28). Frequently, the cause is multifactorial, with a preexisting renal insufficiency that is exacerbated by an intraoperative insult. For example, preoperative or intraoperative angiography can result in ischemic injury secondary to renal vasoconstriction and direct renal tubular injury. Intravascular volume depletion can exacerbate hepatorenal syndrome or acute tubular necrosis caused by sepsis. In the PACU, diagnostic efforts should focus on identification and treatment of the readily reversible causes of oliguria (urine output <0.5 mL/kg/hour). For example, urinary catheter obstruction or dislodgment is easily remedied and often overlooked (Table 39-9).

Oliguria

POSTOPERATIVE URINARY RETENTION
The reported incidence of urinary retention in the PACU is between 5% and 70%. Clinical studies define postoperative urinary retention (POUR) as the inability to void despite a bladder volume of more than 500 to 600 mL. Risk factors include age older than 50 years, male gender, volume of intraoperative fluid infusion, duration of surgery, and bladder volume on admission. Type of surgery is also predictive, with the highest incidence reported in anorectal and joint replacement surgery. Commonly

Table 39-9 Postoperative Oliguria
Prerenal
Hypovolemia (bleeding, sepsis, third-space fluid loss, inadequate volume resuscitation)
Hepatorenal syndrome
Low cardiac output
Renal vascular obstruction or disruption
Intra-abdominal hypertension
Renal
Ischemia (acute tubular necrosis)
Radiographic contrast dyes
Rhabdomyolysis
Tumor lysis
Hemolysis
Postrenal
Surgical injury to the ureters
Obstruction of the ureters with clots or stones
Other
Mechanical (urinary catheter obstruction or malposition)

used perioperative medications such as anticholinergics, β-blockers and narcotics also contribute to urinary retention. Diagnosis can be made by clinical examination, bladder catheterization, or ultrasound assessment. Bladder volumes measured by ultrasound imaging correlate well with volumes obtained by urinary catheterization, an uncomfortable procedure that can be complicated by catheter-related infections and urethral trauma. Bladder ultrasound is an efficient and accurate method to evaluate oliguric high-risk patients.[24]

INTRAVASCULAR VOLUME DEPLETION
The most common cause of oliguria in the immediate postoperative period is depletion of intravascular volume. In this regard, a fluid challenge (500 to 1000 mL of crystalloid) is usually effective in restoring urine output. A hematocrit measurement is indicated when surgical blood loss is suspected and repeated volume boluses are required to maintain urine output. Volume resuscitation to maximize renal perfusion is particularly important in order to prevent ongoing ischemic injury and the development of acute tubular necrosis.

If an intravascular fluid challenge is contraindicated or oliguria persists, assessment of intravascular volume or cardiac function is indicated to differentiate hypovolemia from sepsis and low cardiac output states. Fractional excretion of sodium can be useful in determining the adequacy of renal perfusion (assuming that diuretics have not been given), but the diagnosis of prerenal azotemia will not differentiate between hypovolemia, congestive heart failure, or hepatorenal syndrome. In these cases evaluation with central venous monitoring or echocardiography may facilitate the diagnosis.

Intra-abdominal Hypertension

Intra-abdominal hypertension should be considered as a cause of oliguria in any patient with a tense abdomen after surgery. An intra-abdominal pressure higher than 30 cm H_2O can impede renal perfusion and lead to renal ischemia and postoperative renal dysfunction. Bladder pressure should be measured in patients in whom intra-abdominal hypertension is suspected so that prompt intervention can be initiated to relieve intra-abdominal pressure and restore renal perfusion.[25]

Rhabdomyolysis

Rhabdomyolysis is a possible cause of postoperative renal insufficiency in patients who have suffered major crush or thermal injury. The incidence is also increased in morbidly obese patients, particularly those who have undergone gastric bypass procedures. Risk factors include the degree of elevated body mass index (BMI) and duration of surgery. Patient history and the operative course should guide the decision to measure creatine phosphokinase in the PACU. Volume loading, mannitol, and alkalinization of urine to flush the renal tubules can prevent ongoing renal tubular damage and subsequent acute renal failure. Loop diuretics can be used to maintain urine output and avoid fluid overload.

Contrast Nephropathy

Angiography with intravascular stent placement is replacing open procedures to treat carotid stenosis, aortic aneurysms, and peripheral vascular disease. Patients undergoing these procedures often have chronic renal insufficiency and are at risk for developing renal failure secondary to intravenous contrast infusion. Management of these patients in the PACU includes particular attention to intravascular volume status in order to prevent subsequent renal failure. While aggressive hydration with normal saline provides the single most effective protection against contrast nephropathy, alkalinization with bicarbonate has been shown to provide additional protection. If bicarbonate is used for renal protection in this setting, 154 mEq/L should be infused at a rate of 1 mL/kg/hour for 6 hours after the procedure. Mucomyst can be given and is a relatively inexpensive and easily administered medication (single oral dose pre- and postprocedure) that may also provide renal protection.[26]

BODY TEMPERATURE AND SHIVERING

Postoperative shivering is a dramatic consequence of general and epidural anesthesia. The incidence of postoperative shivering may be as frequent as 65% (range 5% to 65%) after general anesthesia and 33% after epidural anesthesia. Identified risk factors include male gender and the choice of drug (propofol more likely than thiopental) for induction of anesthesia.

Mechanism

Postoperative shivering is usually, but not always, associated with a decrease in the patient's body temperature. Although thermoregulatory mechanisms can explain shivering in a hypothermic patient, a separate mechanism has been proposed to explain shivering in normothermic patients. The proposed mechanism is based on the observation that the brain and spinal cord do not recover simultaneously from general anesthesia. The more rapid recovery of spinal cord function is thought to result in uninhibited spinal reflexes manifested as clonic activity. This theory is supported by the fact that doxapram, a central nervous system stimulant, is somewhat effective in abolishing postoperative shivering.

Treatment

Intervention includes the identification and treatment of hypothermia if present. In addition to shivering, mild to moderate hypothermia (33° to 35° C) inhibits platelet function, coagulation factor activity, and drug metabolism. It exacerbates postoperative bleeding, prolongs neuromuscular blockade, and may delay awakening. Accurate core body temperatures can be most easily obtained at the tympanic membrane. Axillary, rectal, and nasopharyngeal temperature measurements are less accurate and may underestimate core temperature. Forced air warmers are used to actively warm the hypothermic patient. A number of opioids and clonidine are effective in abolishing shivering once it starts, but meperidine (12.5 to 25 mg IV) is the most effective treatment.[27]

POSTOPERATIVE NAUSEA AND VOMITING

The consequences of nausea and vomiting in the PACU include delayed discharge from the PACU, unanticipated hospital admission, increased incidence of pulmonary aspiration, and significant postoperative discomfort. Therefore, the ability to identify high-risk patients for prophylactic intervention can significantly improve the quality of patient care and satisfaction in the PACU.

High-Risk Patients

Risk factors for PONV can be grouped into three categories: patient factors, type of anesthetic drug, and surgery-related factors. Although the literature supports a number of independent risk factors in each of these categories, a subset of factors have been established. The most significant patient-related factors include female gender (postpuberty), nonsmoking status, childhood (past infancy), and history of motion sickness or PONV. Anesthesia-related factors include the use of volatile anesthetics or nitrous oxide, the administration of large doses of neostigmine and perioperative opioids. The most significant surgical risk factor is duration of surgery (Table 39-10).

High-risk patients can be identified by a simplified risk score consisting of four mostly patient-related factors: (1) female gender, (2) history of motion sickness or

Table 39-10 Factors Associated with Increased Incidence of Postoperative Nausea and Vomiting (PONV)
History of PONV or motion sickness
Female gender
Postoperative opioid requirement
Nonsmoking status
Type of surgery—eye muscle surgery, middle ear surgery, laparoscopic surgery
Duration of surgery
Anesthetic drugs—opioids, nitrous oxide (?)
Gastric distention—swallowed blood

PONV, (3) nonsmoking, and (4) the use of postoperative opioids. The incidence of PONV correlates with the number of these factors present: zero, one, two, three, or four factors correspond to an incidence of 10%, 21%, 39%, 61%, and 79%, respectively.

Cost-effective management of PONV takes into consideration the patient's underlying risk. A single intervention in a patient with four risk factors will result in an absolute risk reduction of 21% compared with a 3% risk reduction in a patient with an initial risk of only 10%. These numbers correlate to a number of 5 and 40, respectively, needed to treat.[28]

Prevention and Treatment

Prophylactic measures against PONV include modification of the anesthetic technique and pharmacologic intervention. Although prophylactic measures to prevent PONV are clearly more effective than rescue, a subset of patients will require treatment in the PACU even after receiving appropriate prophylactic treatment. When choosing an antiemetic for these patients, both the class of drug and the timing of administration are factors (Table 39-11). For instance, dexamethasone is effective when given prophylactically at the start of surgery, whereas serotonin receptor antagonists are effective when given 30 minutes before the end of anesthesia.

Upon admission to the PACU, the patient's risk profile and anesthetic technique should be noted, along with whether a prophylactic antiemetic was administered intraoperatively. If an adequate dose of antiemetic given at the appropriate time proves ineffective, simply giving more of the same class of drug in the PACU is unlikely to be of significant benefit. If no prophylactic drug was given, the recommended treatment is a low dose 5-HT3 antagonist.

DELAYED AWAKENING

Even after prolonged surgery and anesthesia, a response to stimulation in 60 to 90 minutes should be expected. When delayed awakening occurs, the vital signs (systemic blood pressure, arterial oxygenation, ECG, body temperature) should be evaluated and a neurologic examination performed. Monitoring with pulse oximetry and analysis of arterial blood gases should be used to rule out hypoxemia and hypoventilation. Additional studies may be indicated to evaluate possible electrolyte derangements, metabolic disturbances and hypoglycemia. Rarely computed tomographic imaging is indicated to rule out an acute intracerebral event.

Treatment

Residual sedation from drugs used during anesthesia is the most frequent cause of delayed awakening in the PACU. If residual effects of opioids are a possible cause of delayed awakening, carefully titrated doses of IV

Table 39-11 Commonly Used Antiemetics, with Adult Doses

Anticholinergics
Scopolamine: 0.3-0.65 mg IV, IM
Scopolamine: transdermal patch, 1.5 cm^2
    Apply to a hairless area behind the ear before surgery; remove 24 hours postoperatively

Antihistamines
Hydroxyzine: 12.5-25 mg IM

Phenothiazines
Promethazine: 12.5-25 mg IM

Butyrophenones
Droperidol: 0.625-1.25 mg IV
    See black box warning regarding torsades de pointes: monitor the ECG for prolongation of the QT interval for 2-3 hours after administration—preoperative 12-lead ECG recommended

Prokinetic
Metoclopramide: 10-20 mg IV
    Avoid in patients with any possibility of gastrointestinal obstruction

Serotonin Receptor Antagonists
Ondansetron: 4 mg IV 30 minutes before conclusion of surgery
Dolasetron: 12.5 mg IV 15-30 minutes before conclusion of surgery

Vasopressors
Ephedrine: 25 mg IM with hydroxyzine 25 mg

Corticosteroids
Dexamethasone: 4-8 mg IV with induction of anesthesia

ECG, electrocardiogram; IM, intramuscularly; IV, intravenously.

naloxone (20- to 40-µg increments in adults) should be given, while keeping in mind that this treatment will also antagonize opioid-induced analgesia. Physostigmine may be effective in reversing the central nervous system sedative effects of anticholinergic drugs (especially scopolamine). Flumazenil is a specific antagonist for the residual depressant effects of benzodiazepines. In the absence of pharmacologic effects to explain delayed awakening, other causes, such as hypothermia (especially <33° C) and hypoglycemia, should be considered.

DISCHARGE CRITERIA

Specific PACU discharge criteria may vary, but certain general principles are universally applicable (Table 39-12). For example, a mandatory minimum stay in the PACU is not required. Patients must be observed until they are no longer at risk for ventilatory depression and their mental status is clear or has returned to baseline. Hemodynamic

Table 39-12 Criteria for Determination of Discharge Score for Release from the Postanesthesia Care Unit

Variable Evaluated	Score
Activity	
Able to move four extremities on command	2
Able to move two extremities on command	1
Able to move no extremities on command	0
Breathing	
Able to breathe deeply and cough freely	2
Dyspnea	1
Apnea	0
Circulation	
Systemic blood pressure:	
Within 20% of the preanesthetic level	2
20% to 49% of the preanesthetic level	1
≥50% of the preanesthetic level	0
Consciousness	
Fully awake	2
Arousable	1
Not responding	0
Oxygen saturation (pulse oximetry)	
>92% while breathing room air	2
Needs supplemental oxygen to maintain saturation >90%	1
<90% even with supplemental oxygen	0

Adapted from Aldrete JA. The post anaesthesia recovery score revisited. J Clin Anesth 1995;7:89-91.

criteria are based on the patient's baseline hemodynamics without specific systemic blood pressure and heart rate requirements (Table 39-13).[1,2] Additionally, an assessment and written documentation of the patient's peripheral nerve function on discharge from the PACU may become useful information should a new peripheral neuropathy develop in the later postoperative period (Table 39-14).

To facilitate PACU discharge, discharge scoring systems have been developed and modified over time to reflect current technology and anesthesia practice (Table 39-15).[29-32]

Table 39-13 General Principles for Discharge from the Postanesthesia Care Unit

- Patients should be routinely required to have a responsible person accompany them home.
- Requiring patients to urinate before discharge should not be part of a routine discharge protocol and may be necessary only in selected patients.
- The demonstrated ability to drink and retain clear fluids should not be part of a routine discharge protocol but may be appropriate for selected patients.
- A minimum mandatory stay in the unit should not be required.
- Patients should be observed until they are no longer at increased risk for cardiorespiratory depression.

Table 39-14 Neurologic Examination before Discharge from the Postanesthesia Care Unit

Ulnar nerve	Normal sensation on the palmar surface of the fifth finger
Medial nerve	Normal sensation on the palmar surface of the second finger
Radial nerve	Ability to abduct the thumb
Sciatic nerve	Ability to flex the leg at the knee
Peroneal nerve	Ability to dorsiflex the first toe
Tibial nerve	Ability to plantar-flex the first toe

The ASA Standards of Care require that a physician accept responsibility for discharge of patients from the unit (Standard V). This is the case even when the decision to discharge the patient is made by the bedside nurse in accordance with the hospital-sanctioned discharge criteria or scoring

Table 39-15 Criteria for Determination of Discharge Score for Release Home to a Responsible Adult

Variable Evaluated	Score*
Vital signs (stable and consistent with age and preanesthetic baseline)	
Systemic blood pressure and heart rate within 20% of the preanesthetic level	2
Systemic blood pressure and heart rate 20% to 40% of the preanesthetic level	1
Systemic blood pressure and heart rate >40% of the preanesthetic level	0
Activity level	
Steady gait without dizziness or meets the preanesthetic level	2
Requires assistance	1
Unable to ambulate	0
Nausea and vomiting	
None to minimal	2
Moderate	1
Severe (continues after repeated treatment)	0
Pain (minimal to no pain, controllable with oral analgesics)	
Yes	2
No	1
Surgical bleeding (consistent with that expected for the surgical procedure)	
Minimal (does not require dressing change)	2
Moderate (up to two dressing changes required)	1
Severe (more than three dressing changes required)	0

*Patients achieving a score of at least 9 are ready for discharge.
Modified from Marshall SI, Chung F. Discharge criteria and complications after ambulatory surgery. Anesth Analg 1999;88: 508-517.

V

system. If discharge scoring systems are to be used in this way, they must first be approved by the department of anesthesia and the hospital medical staff. A responsible physician's name must be noted on the record.

QUESTIONS OF THE DAY

1. What are the most common causes of upper airway obstruction in the PACU? What are the initial steps in management of upper airway obstruction?

2. A patient who just arrived in the PACU develops ST-segment changes on ECG. What are the potential causes? How should the patient be managed?

3. What are the risk factors for postoperative urinary retention? How can the diagnosis be confirmed?

4. What is the incidence of shivering after general anesthesia or epidural anesthesia? What is the mechanism of postanesthesia shivering?

5. What are the principles used to determine PACU discharge criteria? What are the components of the "Aldrete Score"?

REFERENCES

1. Standards of the American Society of Anesthesiologists: Standards for Postanesthesia Care, approved by the House of Delegates on Oct. 12, 1988, and last amended on Oct. 23, 2004. Copyright © 1999, American Society of Anesthesiologists.

2. American Society of Anesthesiologists Task Force on Post Anesthetic Care: Practice guidelines for postanesthetic care: A report by the American Society of Anesthesiologists Task Force on Post Anesthetic Care, *Anesthesiology* 96:742–752, 2002.

3. Hines RR, Barash PG, Watrous G, et al: Complications occurring in the postanesthesia care unit: A survey, *Anesth Analg* 74:503–509, 1992.

4. Kluger MT, Bullock MF: Recovery room incidents: A review of 419 reports from the Anaesthetic Incident Monitoring Study (AIMS), *Anaesthesia* 57:1060–1066, 2002.

5. Zeitlin GL: Recovery room mishaps in the ASA Closed Claim Study, *ASA Newsl* 53:28–30, 1989.

6. Benumof JL: Obstructive sleep apnea in the adult obese patient: Implications for airway management, *J Clin Anesth* 13:144–156, 2001.

7. Kopman AF, Yee PS, Neuman GG: Relationship on the train-of-four fade ratio to clinical signs and symptoms of residual paralysis in awake volunteers, *Anesthesiology* 86:765–771, 1997.

8. Eriksson LI, Sundman E, Olsson R, et al: Functional assessment of the pharynx at rest and during swallowing in partially paralyzed humans: Simultaneous videomanometry and mechanomyography of awake human volunteers, *Anesthesiology* 87:1035–1043, 1997.

9. DeBast Y, De Backer D, Moraine JJ, et al: The cuff leak test to predict failure of tracheal extubation for laryngeal edema, *Intensive Care Med* 28:1267–1272, 2002.

10. American Society of Anesthesiologists Task Force on Perioperative Management of Patients with Obstructive Sleep Apnea: Practice guidelines for the perioperative management of patients with obstructive sleep apnea: A report of the American Society of Anesthesiologists Task Force on Perioperative Management of Patients with Obstructive Sleep Apnea, *Anesthesiology* 104:1081–1093, 2006.

11. Fu EU, Downs JB, Schweiger JW, et al: Supplemental oxygen impairs detection of hypoventilation by pulse oximetry, *Chest* 126:1552–1558, 2004.

12. Lumb AB: *Nunn's Applied Respiratory Physiology*, ed 6, Philadelphia, 2005, Butterworth-Heinemann.

13. Herrick IA, Mahendran B, Penny FJ: Postoperative pulmonary edema following anesthesia, *J Clin Anesth* 2:116–120, 1990.

14. Moore SB: Transfusion-related acute lung injury (TRALI): Clinical presentation, treatment, and prognosis, *Crit Care Med* 34(5 Suppl):S114–S117, 2006.

15. Kabon B, Kurz A: Optimal perioperative oxygen administration, *Curr Opin Anaesthesiol* 19:11–18, 2006.

16. Squadrone V, Coha M, Cerutti E, et al: Continuous positive airway pressure for treatment of postoperative hypoxemia: A randomized controlled trial, *JAMA* 293:589–595, 2005.

17. Albala MZ, Ferrigno M: Short-term noninvasive ventilation in the postanesthesia care unit: A case series, *J Clin Anesth* 17:636–639, 2005.

18. Rose DK, Cohen MM, DeBoer DP: Cardiovascular events in the postanesthesia care unit: Contribution of risk factors, *Anesthesiology* 84:772–781, 1996.

19. Hepner DL, Castells MC: Anaphylaxis during the perioperative period, *Anesth Analg* 97:1381–1395, 2003.

20. Wright DE, Hunt DP: Perioperative surveillance for adverse myocardial events, *South Med J* 101:52–58, 2008.

21. Fleisher LA, Beckman JA, Brown KA, et al: ACC/AHA 2007 Guidelines on Perioperative Cardiovascular Evaluation and Care for Noncardiac Surgery: Executive Summary. A Report of the American College of Cardiology/American Heart Association Task Force on Practice Guidelines (Writing Committee to Revise the 2002 Guidelines on Perioperative Cardiovascular Evaluation for Noncardiac Surgery) Developed in Collaboration with the American Society of Echocardiography, American Society of Nuclear Cardiology, Heart Rhythm Society, Society of Cardiovascular Anesthesiologists, Society for Cardiovascular Angiography and Interventions, Society for Vascular Medicine and Biology, and Society for Vascular Surgery, *J Am Coll Cardiol* 50:1707–1732, 2007.

22. Mercantonio ER, Goldman L, Orav EJ, et al: The association of intraoperative factors with the development of postoperative delirium, *Am J Med* 105:380–384, 1998.

23. Leung JM, Sands LP, Vaurio LE, et al: Nitrous oxide does not change the incidence of postoperative delirium or cognitive decline in elderly surgical patients, *Br J Anaesth* 96:754–760, 2006.

24. Baldini G, Bagry H, Aprikian A, et al: Postoperative urinary retention, *Anesthesiology* 110:1139–1157, 2009.

25. Sugrue M, Jones F, Deane SA, et al: Intra-abdominal hypertension is an independent cause of postoperative renal impairment, *Arch Surg* 134:1082–1085, 1999.

26. Merten GJ, Burgess WP, Gray LV, et al: Prevention of contrast induced nephropathy with sodium bicarbonate: A randomized controlled led trial, *JAMA* 291:2328–2334, 2004.

27. Buggy DJ, Crossley AW: Thermoregulation, mild perioperative hypothermia and post-anaesthetic shivering, *Br J Anaesth* 84:615–628, 2000.

28. Apfel C, Korttila K, Abdalla M, et al: A factorial trial of six interventions for the prevention of postoperative nausea

and vomiting, *N Engl J Med* 350:2441–2451, 2004.

29. Society for Ambulatory Anesthesia: Guidelines for the Management of Postoperative Nausea and Vomiting, *Anesth Analg* 105:1615–1628, 2007.

30. Aldrete JA: The post anaesthesia recovery score revisited, *J Clin Anesth* 7:89–91, 1995.

31. Marshall SI, Chung F: Discharge criteria and complications after ambulatory surgery, *Anesth Analg* 88:508–517, 1999.

32. Brown I, Jellish WS, Kleinman B, et al: Use of postanesthesia discharge criteria to reduce discharge delays for inpatients in the postanesthesia care unit, *J Clin Anesth* 20:175–179, 2008.

V

G STANDARDS FOR POST ANESTHESIA CARE COMMITTEE OF ORIGIN: STANDARDS AND PRACTICE PARAMETERS†

These standards apply to postanesthesia care in all locations. These standards may be exceeded based on the judgment of the responsible anesthesiologist. They are intended to encourage quality patient care, but cannot guarantee any specific patient outcome. They are subject to revision from time to time as warranted by the evolution of technology and practice.

STANDARD I

ALL PATIENTS WHO HAVE RECEIVED GENERAL ANESTHESIA, REGIONAL ANESTHESIA, OR MONITORED ANESTHESIA CARE SHALL RECEIVE APPROPRIATE POST ANESTHESIA MANAGEMENT.[1]

1. A postanesthesia care unit (PACU) or an area which provides equivalent postanesthesia care (for example, a surgical intensive care unit) shall be available to receive patients after anesthesia care. All patients who receive anesthesia care shall be admitted to the PACU or its equivalent **except** by specific order of the anesthesiologist responsible for the patient's care.
2. The medical aspects of care in the PACU (or equivalent area) shall be governed by policies and procedures which have been reviewed and approved by the Department of Anesthesiology.
3. The design, equipment, and staffing of the PACU shall meet requirements of the facility's accrediting and licensing bodies.

STANDARD II

A PATIENT TRANSPORTED TO THE PACU SHALL BE ACCOMPANIED BY A MEMBER OF THE ANESTHESIA CARE TEAM WHO IS KNOWLEDGEABLE ABOUT THE PATIENT'S CONDITION. THE PATIENT SHALL BE CONTINUALLY EVALUATED AND TREATED DURING TRANSPORT WITH MONITORING AND SUPPORT APPROPRIATE TO THE PATIENT'S CONDITION.

STANDARD III

UPON ARRIVAL IN THE PACU, THE PATIENT SHALL BE REEVALUATED AND A VERBAL REPORT PROVIDED TO THE RESPONSIBLE PACU NURSE BY THE MEMBER OF THE ANESTHESIA CARE TEAM WHO ACCOMPANIES THE PATIENT.

1. The patient's status on arrival in the PACU shall be documented.
2. Information concerning the preoperative condition and the surgical/anesthetic course shall be transmitted to the PACU nurse.
3. The member of the anesthesia care team shall remain in the PACU until the PACU nurse accepts responsibility for the nursing care of the patient.

STANDARD IV

THE PATIENT'S CONDITION SHALL BE EVALUATED CONTINUALLY IN THE PACU.

1. The patient shall be observed and monitored by methods appropriate to the patient's medical condition. Particular attention should be given to monitoring oxygenation, ventilation, circulation, level of consciousness, and temperature. During recovery from all anesthetics, a quantitative method of assessing oxygenation such as pulse oximetry shall be employed in the initial phase of recovery.* This is not intended

---

[1]Refer to Standards of Perianesthesia Nursing Practice 2008-2010, published by ASPAN, for issues of nursing care.

*Under extenuating circumstances, the responsible anesthesiologist may waive the requirements marked with an asterisk (*); it is recommended that when this is done, it should be so stated (including the reasons) in a note in the patient's medical record.

for application during the recovery of the obstetrical patient in whom regional anesthesia was used for labor and vaginal delivery.

2. An accurate written report of the PACU period shall be maintained. Use of an appropriate PACU scoring system is encouraged for each patient on admission, at appropriate intervals prior to discharge and at the time of discharge.

3. General medical supervision and coordination of patient care in the PACU should be the responsibility of an anesthesiologist.

4. There shall be a policy to assure the availability in the facility of a physician capable of managing complications and providing cardiopulmonary resuscitation for patients in the PACU.

STANDARD V

A PHYSICIAN IS RESPONSIBLE FOR THE DISCHARGE OF THE PATIENT FROM THE POSTANESTHESIA CARE UNIT.

1. When discharge criteria are used, they must be approved by the department of anesthesiology and the medical staff. They may vary depending upon whether the patient is discharged to a hospital room, to the intensive care unit, to a short stay unit or home.

2. In the absence of the physician responsible for the discharge, the PACU nurse shall determine that the patient meets the discharge criteria. The name of the physician accepting responsibility for discharge shall be noted on the record.

[†]From Standards for Postanesthesia Care. Approved by the House of Delegates on October 27, 2004, and last amended on October 21, 2009. Printed with permission of the American Society of Anesthesiologists, 520 N. Northwest Highway, Park Ridge, Ill. 60068-2573.

V

40 PERIOPERATIVE PAIN MANAGEMENT

Robert W. Hurley and Meredith C.B. Adams

Postoperative pain is a complex physiologic reaction to tissue injury. Commonly, a patient's primary concern about surgery is how much pain they will experience following the procedure. Postoperative pain produces acute adverse physiologic effects with manifestations on multiple organ systems that can lead to significant morbidity (Table 40-1).[1] For example, pain after upper abdominal or thoracic surgery often leads to hypoventilation from splinting. This promotes atelectasis, which impairs ventilation-to-perfusion relationships, and increases the likelihood of arterial hypoxemia and pneumonia. Pain that limits postoperative ambulation, combined with a stress-induced hypercoagulable state, may contribute to an increased incidence of deep vein thrombosis.[2] Catecholamines released in response to pain may result in tachycardia and systemic hypertension, which may induce myocardial ischemia in susceptible patients.

Factors that positively correlate with severity of postoperative pain include preoperative opioid intake, anxiety, depression, pain level, and the duration of surgical operation. Factors that are negatively correlated include the patient's age and the level of the surgeon's operative experience. A perioperative plan should be developed that encompasses these factors in order to lessen the severity of the patient's postoperative pain. Elderly patients and patients receiving preoperative opioid regimens can represent management challenges (also see Chapter 35). Elderly patients are at higher risk than younger patients for cognitive dysfunction in the perioperative period due to various factors, including increased sensitivity to drugs and other medical co-morbidities. Patients taking opioids for pain relief preoperatively have higher pain scores and lower pain thresholds in the immediate postoperative period. Perioperative management plans that incorporate these variables may favor the use of regional anesthesia because of the decreased mortality rate and infrequent incidence of postoperative cognitive dysfunction and pain (also see Chapters 17 and 18).[3] Preemptive regional analgesia may enhance pain

Table 40-1 Adverse Physiologic Effects of Postoperative Pain

Pulmonary System (decreased lung volumes)
Atelectasis
Ventilation-to-perfusion mismatching
Arterial hypoxemia
Hypercapnia
Pneumonia

Cardiovascular System (sympathetic nervous system stimulation)
Systemic hypertension
Tachycardia
Myocardial ischemia
Cardiac dysrhythmias

Endocrine System
Hyperglycemia
Sodium and water retention
Protein catabolism

Immune System
Decreased immune function

Coagulation System
Increased platelet adhesiveness
Decreased fibrinolysis
Hypercoagulation
Deep vein thrombosis

Gastrointestinal System
Ileus

Genitourinary System
Urinary retention

control, decrease adverse cognitive effects, and improve postoperative recovery overall.[4] Well-controlled pain postoperatively will enhance postoperative rehabilitation, which may improve short- and long-term recovery, as well as the quality of life after surgery.

Postoperative pain also may have long-term consequences as well. Poorly controlled postoperative pain may be an important predictive factor for the development of chronic postsurgical pain (CPSP),[5] defined as pain after a surgery lasting longer than the normal recuperative healing time. CPSP is a largely unrecognized problem that may occur in 10% to 65% of postoperative patients, with 2% to 10% of these patients experiencing severe CPSP.[6] Transition from acute to chronic pain occurs very quickly, and long-term behavioral and neurobiologic changes occur much earlier than previously anticipated.[7] CPSP is relatively common after surgical procedures, such as limb amputation (30% to 83%), thoracotomy (22% to 67%), sternotomy (27%), breast surgery (11% to 57%), and gallbladder surgery (up to 56%).[8]

Improved understanding of the epidemiology and pathophysiology of postoperative pain has created the utilization of multimodal management of pain in an effort to improve patient comfort, decrease perioperative morbidity, and reduce cost by shortening the time spent in postanesthesia care units, intensive care units, and hospitals. Multimodal approaches involve the use of multiple, mechanistically distinct medications with the application of peripheral nerve or neuraxial analgesia. The added complexity of a true multimodal approach to perioperative pain requires the formation of perioperative pain management services, most often directed by an anesthesiologist or pain medicine physician.

COMMON TERMINOLOGY (Also See Chapter 43)

- *Pain (nociception):* Pain is described as an unpleasant sensory and emotional experience caused by actual or potential tissue damage, or described in terms of such damage.[9]
- *Acute pain:* Acute pain follows injury to the body, and generally disappears when the bodily injury heals. It is often, but not always, associated with objective physical signs of autonomic nervous system activity (eg. increased heart rate).
- *Chronic (persistent) pain:* Chronic pain is pain that has persisted beyond the time of healing.[9] This length of time is determined by common medical experience. In the first instance, it is the time needed for inflammation to subside, or for acute injuries, such as lacerations or incisions, to repair with the union of separated tissues. In these circumstances, chronic pain is recognized when the process of repair is complete.
- *Pain medicine:* Pain medicine is the clinical practice of relieving acute and chronic (persistent) pain through the implementation of psychological, physical, therapeutic, pharmacologic, and interventional methods. Pain medicine is practiced in the inpatient and outpatient settings.
- *Perioperative pain medicine:* The perioperative pain medicine service is a team of highly specialized members who practice acute pain medicine and regional analgesic interventions for the patient who is about to undergo surgery or is in the recovery process from surgery. This team often manages the trauma-induced pain as well. The role of the perioperative pain physician is to reduce the pain resulting from surgery and minimize the period of recuperation, and to inhibit the development of chronic (persistent) pain through early intervention.
- *Chronic (persistent) pain medicine* (also see Chapter 43): The persistent pain medicine service is a team of highly specialized members who treat chronic (persistent pain) and cancer pain using regional analgesic and chronic pain interventions. The patient population served includes the perioperative patient with preoperative chronic/persistent pain issues, the nonoperable patient with chronic/persistent pain

V

issues, and patients who have undergone surgery by the persistent pain service. The role of the persistent pain physician is to attenuate the patient's pain, provide rationalized pain medication care, and transition the patient to outpatient pain care.

NEUROPHYSIOLOGY OF PAIN

Nociception

Nociception involves the recognition and transmission of painful stimuli. Stimuli generated from thermal, mechanical, or chemical tissue damage may activate nociceptors, which are free afferent nerve endings of myelinated Aδ and unmyelinated C fibers. These peripheral afferent nerve endings send axonal projections into the dorsal horn of the spinal cord, where they synapse with second-order afferent neurons. Axonal projections of second-order neurons cross to the contralateral side of the spinal cord, and ascend as afferent sensory pathways (e.g., spinothalamic tract) to the level of the thalamus.[10] Along the way, these neurons divide and send axonal projections to the reticular formation and periaqueductal gray matter. In the thalamus, second-order neurons synapse with third-order neurons, which send axonal projections into the sensory cortex.

Modulation of Nociception

Surgical incision produces tissue injury, with consequent release of histamine and inflammatory mediators, such as peptides (e.g., bradykinin), lipids (e.g., prostaglandins), neurotransmitters (e.g., serotonin), and neurotrophins (e.g., nerve growth factor).[11] The release of inflammatory mediators activates peripheral nociceptors, which initiate transduction and transmission of nociceptive information to the central nervous system (CNS). Noxious stimuli are transduced by peripheral nociceptors and transmitted by Aδ and C nerve fibers from peripheral visceral and somatic sites to the dorsal horn of the spinal cord, where integration of peripheral nociceptive and descending inhibitory modulatory input (i.e., serotonin, norepinephrine, γ-aminobutyric acid [GABA], and enkephalin) or descending facilitatory input (i.e., cholecystokinin, excitatory amino acids, dynorphin) occurs. Further transmission of nociceptive information is determined by complex modulating influences in the spinal cord. Some impulses pass to the ventral and ventrolateral horns to initiate spinal reflex responses. These segmental responses may be associated with increased skeletal muscle tone, inhibition of phrenic nerve function, or even decreased gastrointestinal motility. Other signals are transmitted to higher centers through the spinothalamic and spinoreticular tracts, where they produce cortical responses to ultimately generate the perception of pain.

The question of how chronic pain develops from acute pain remains unanswered. The traditional dichotomy between acute and chronic pain is arbitrary, as animal and clinical studies demonstrate that acute pain may transition into chronic pain.[7] Noxious stimuli can produce expression of new genes (the basis for neuronal sensitization[12]) in the dorsal horn of the spinal cord within 1 hour, and that these changes are sufficient to alter behavior within the same time frame.[13] Also, the intensity of acute postoperative pain is a significant predictor of chronic postoperative pain.[8]

Continuous release of inflammatory mediators in the periphery sensitizes functional nociceptors and activates dormant nociceptors (Table 40-2).[7] Sensitization of peripheral nociceptors results in a decreased threshold for activation, increased discharge rate with activation, and increased rate of spontaneous discharge. Intense noxious input from the periphery may also produce central sensitization and hyperexcitability. Central sensitization is the development of "persistent post-injury changes in the CNS that result in pain hypersensitivity."[14] (Hyperexcitability is the "exaggerated and prolonged responsiveness of neurons to normal afferent input after tissue damage."[14]) Noxious input can trigger the cascade that leads to functional changes in the dorsal horn of the spinal cord and other sequelae. Ultimately, these changes may later cause postoperative pain to be perceived as more painful than would otherwise have been experienced. The neural circuitry in the dorsal horn is extremely complex, and we are just at the beginning of understanding the specific role of the various neurotransmitters and receptors in the process of nociception.[11,13]

Key receptors (e.g., N-methyl-d-aspartate [NMDA]) may play a significant role in the development of chronic pain after an acute injury. Neurotransmitters or second messenger effectors (e.g., substance P, protein kinase C-γ) may also play important roles in spinal cord sensitization and chronic pain (Table 40-3).[12] Our understanding of the neurobiology of nociception includes the dynamic integration and modulation of nociceptive transmission at several levels. Still, the specific roles of various receptors, neurotransmitters, and molecular structures in the process of nociception are not fully understood.

Table 40-2 Endogenous Mediators of Inflammation

Prostaglandins (PGE_1 > PGE_2)
Histamine
Bradykinin
Serotonin
Acetylcholine
Lactic acid
Hydrogen ions
Potassium ions

PGE_1, PGE_2, prostaglandins E_1 and E_2.

Table 40-3 Examples of Pain-Modulating Neurotransmitters
Excitatory
Glutamate
Aspartate
Vasoactive intestinal polypeptide
Cholecystokinin
Gastrin-releasing peptide
Angiotensin
Substance P
Inhibitory
Enkephalins
Endorphins
Somatostatin

Preemptive and Preventive Analgesia

The development of central or peripheral sensitization after traumatic injury or surgical incision can result in amplification of postoperative pain. Therefore, preventing the establishment of altered central processing by analgesic treatment may, in the short term, reduce postprocedural or traumatic pain and accelerate recovery. In the long term, the benefits may include a reduction in chronic pain and improvement in the patient's quality of recovery and life satisfaction. Although the concept of preemptive analgesia in decreasing postinjury pain is valid, the findings of clinical trials are mixed.[15-17]

The precise definition of preemptive analgesia is one of the major controversies in perioperative pain medicine, and contributes to the confusion regarding its clinical relevance. Preemptive analgesia can be defined as an analgesic intervention initiated before the noxious stimulus develops in order to block peripheral and central pain transmission. Preventive analgesia can be functionally defined as an attempt to block pain transmission prior to the injury (incision), during the noxious insult (surgery itself), *and* after the injury and throughout the recovery period. Unfortunately, the concept of preventive analgesia has not been completely examined in a rigorous fashion. Confining the definition of preemptive analgesia to only the immediate preoperative or early intraoperative (incisional) period may not be clinically relevant or appropriate because the inflammatory response may last well into the postoperative period and continue to maintain peripheral sensitization. However, preventive analgesia is a clinically relevant phenomenon. Katz and McCartney[5] described an analgesic benefit of preventive analgesia but no such benefit with the preemptive strategy. Maximal clinical benefit is observed when there is complete blockade of noxious stimuli, with extension of this blockade into the postoperative period. Central sensitization and persistent pain after surgical incision are predominantly maintained by the incoming barrage of sensitized peripheral pain fibers throughout the perioperative period,[18] which extend into the postsurgical recovery period. By preventing central sensitization and its prolongation by peripheral input, preventive analgesia along with intensive multimodal analgesic interventions could, theoretically, reduce acute postprocedure pain/hyperalgesia and chronic pain after surgery or trauma.[8]

Multimodal Approach to Perioperative Recovery

A multimodal approach to analgesia is a broad definition that may include a combination of interventional analgesic techniques (epidural catheter or peripheral nerve catheter analgesia) and a combination of systemic pharmacologic therapies (nonsteroidal anti-inflammatory agents [NSAIDs], α-adrenergic agonists, NMDA receptor antagonists, membrane stabilizers, and opioid administration) (also see Chapters 10 and 17). Postprocedural or posttraumatic pain is best managed through this multimodal approach.[19] For instance, basic perioperative therapy, such as including a single dose of the membrane stabilizer, gabapentin, can attenuate postoperative pain and decrease opioid dosage with minimal side effects in various types of surgeries.[20]

The principles of a multimodal strategy include a sufficient diminution of the patient's pain to instill a sense of control over their pain, enable early mobilization, allow early enteral nutrition, and attenuate the perioperative stress response. The secondary goal of this approach is to maximize the benefit (analgesia) while minimizing the risk (side effects of the medication being used). These goals are often achieved through regional anesthetic techniques (also see Chapters 17 and 18) and a combination of analgesic drugs (also see Chapter 10). The utilization of epidural anesthesia and analgesia is an integral part of the multimodal strategy because of the superior analgesia and physiologic benefits conferred by epidural analgesia.[21] A multimodal approach involving a combination of neuraxial analgesia and systemic analgesics during recovery from radical prostatectomy resulted in a reduction of opioid use, lower pain scores, and decreased length of stay.[22] Patients undergoing major abdominal or thoracic procedures and managed with a multimodal strategy have a reduction in hormonal and metabolic stress, preservation of total-body protein, shorter times to tracheal extubation, lower pain scores, earlier return of bowel function, and earlier achievement of criteria for discharge from the intensive care unit.[23,24] By integrating the most recent data and techniques for surgery, anesthesiology, and pain treatment, the multimodal approach is an extension of clinical pathways or fast track protocols by revamping traditional care programs into effective postoperative rehabilitation pathways.[23] This approach may potentially decrease perioperative morbidity, decrease the

V

length of hospital stay, and improve patient satisfaction without compromising safety. However, the widespread implementation of these programs requires multidisciplinary collaboration, changes in the traditional principles of postoperative care, additional resources, and expansion of the traditional acute pain service, all of which may be difficult in the current medical-economic climate.

ANALGESIC DELIVERY SYSTEMS

The traditional delivery systems for the management of perioperative pain have oral and parenteral on-demand administration of analgesics. More efficacious mechanisms, such as patient-controlled analgesia (PCA) are increasingly being used. A PCA mechanism can refer to oral, parenteral, neuraxial, or peripheral administration of an analgesic (Tables 40-4 to 40-6). This medication delivery technique is based on improved understanding of the neurophysiology of pain and the potential deleterious effects of postoperative pain. The formation of perioperative pain management services, directed by anesthesiologists with expertise in the pharmacology of analgesics

and regional analgesia, has facilitated the widespread application of these techniques and improved the care of the postoperative patient.

Patient-Controlled Analgesia

PCA can be delivered via oral, intravenous, subcutaneous, epidural, and intrathecal routes, as well as by peripheral nerve catheter. Upon activation of the delivery system, limits are placed on the number of doses per unit of time that will be administered to the patient. There is also a minimum time interval that must elapse between dose administrations (lockout interval). Also, a continuous background infusion superimposed on patient-controlled boluses can be implemented. Most patients determine a level of pain that is acceptable, and taper their dosage requirements as they recover. Patient acceptance of PCA is high because it restores the patient's feeling of having control of their therapy. When compared with traditional methods of intermittent intramuscular or intravenous injections of opioids to manage perioperative pain, PCA provides better analgesia with more safety, less total drug use, less sedation, fewer nocturnal sleep disturbances, and more rapid return to physical

Table 40-4 Oral and Parenteral Analgesics for Treatment of Perioperative Pain

Agent	Route of Administration	Dose (mg)	Half-Life (hr)	Onset	Analgesic Action (hr)	Peak Duration
Opioids and Opioid Derivatives						
Morphine	Intravenous	2.5-15	2-3.5	0.25	0.125	2-3
	Intramuscular	10-15	3	0.3	0.5-1.5	3-4
	Oral	30-60	3	0.5-1	1-2	4
Codeine	Oral	15-60	4	0.25-1	0.5-2	3-4
Hydromorphone	Intravenous	0.2-1.0	2-3	0.2-0.25	0.25	2-3
	Intramuscular	1-4	2-3	0.3-0.5	1	2-3
	Oral	1-4	2-3	0.5-1	1	3-4
Fentanyl	Intravenous	20-50 (μg)	0.5-1	5-10 min	5 min	1-1.5
	Transmucosal*	200-1600 (μg)	2-12	0.1-0.25	0.5-1	0.25-0.5
	Transdermal	12.5-100 (μg)	20-27	12-24	20-72	72
Oxymorphone	Oral	5-10	3.3-4.5	0.5	1	2-6
	Intravenous	0.5-1	3-5	0.15	0.25	3-6
	Subcutaneous	1-1.5	3-5	0.15	0.25	3-6
	Intramuscular	1-1.5	3-5	0.15	0.25	3-6
Hydrocodone	Oral	5-7.5	2-3	30	90	3-4
Oxycodone	Oral	5	3-5	0.5	1-2	4-6
Methadone	Oral	2.5-10	3-4	0.5-1	1.5-2	4-8
Propoxyphene	Oral	32-65	12-16	0.25-1	1-2	3-6
Other						
Tramadol†	Oral	50-100	5-6	0.5-1	1-2	4-6

*Transmucosal fentanyl is most appropriately reserved for breakthrough malignant (cancer) pain.
†Not classified by the U.S. Food and Drug Administration (FDA) as an opioid; however, tramadol possesses naloxone partial-reversal analgesia.

Table 40-5 Guidelines for Delivery Systems Used in Intravenous Patient-Controlled Analgesia

Drug Concentration	Size of Bolus*	Lockout Interval (min)	Continuous Infusion
Agonists			
Morphine (1 mg/mL)	0.5-2.5 mg	6-10	1-2 mg/hr
Fentanyl (0.01 mg/mL)	20-50 µg	5-10	10-100 µg/hr
Hydromorphone (0.2 mg/mL)	0.05-0.25 mg	10-20	0.2-0.4 mg/hr
Alfentanil (0.1 mg/mL)	0.1-0.2 mg	5-10	—
Methadone (1 mg/mL)	0.5-1.5 mg	10-30	—
Oxymorphone (0.25 mg/mL)	0.2-0.4 mg	8-10	—
Sufentanil (0.002 mg/mL)	2-5 µg	4-10	2-8 µg/hr
Agonist-Antagonists			
Buprenorphine (0.03 mg/mL)	0.03-0.1 mg	8-20	—
Nalbuphine (1 mg/mL)	1-5 mg	5-15	—
Pentazocine (10 mg/mL)	5-30 mg	5-15	—

*All doses are for a 70-kg adult patient. The anesthesiologist should proceed with titrated intravenous loading doses if necessary to establish initial analgesia. Individual patient's requirements vary widely, with smaller doses typically given for elderly or compromised patients. Continuous infusions are not recommended for opioid-naïve adult patients. Continuous opioid infusion doses often are considerably higher in the cancer pain population.

Table 40-6 Neuraxial Analgesics

Drug	Intrathecal Single Dose	Epidural Single Dose	Epidural Infusion
Opioid or Opioid Derivative*			
Fentanyl	5-25 µg	50-100 µg	25-100 µg/hr
Sufentanil	2-10 µg	10-50 µg	10-20 µg/hr
Alfentanil	—	0.5-1 mg	0.2 mg/hr
Morphine	0.1-0.3 mg	1-5 mg	0.1-1 mg/hr
Hydromorphone	—	0.5-1 mg	0.1-0.2 mg/hr
Meperidine	—	20-60 mg	10-60 mg/hr
Methadone	—	4-8 mg	0.3-0.5 mg/hr
ER morphine	—	5-15 mg	—
Local Anesthetics†			
Bupivacaine	5-15 mg	25-150 mg	1-25 mg/hr
Ropivacaine	—	25-200 mg	6-20 mg/hr
Adjuvant Drugs†			
Clonidine	—	100-900 µg	10-50 µg/hr

*Doses are based on use of a neuraxial opioid alone. No continuous intrathecal or subarachnoid infusions are provided. Smaller doses may be effective when administered to the elderly or when injected in the cervical or thoracic region. Units vary across drugs for single dose (mg versus µg) and continuous infusion (mg/hr versus µg/hr).
†Most commonly used in combination with an opioid, in which case the total dose of bupivacaine is reduced.
ER, extended release.

activity.[25] Some institutions employ pulse oximetry monitoring to assess the respiratory depression associated with opioid administration. Although better than having no specific monitor at all, pulse oximetry may not capture the relationship between respiratory depression and opioid administration.[26] Capnography and respiratory rate are more specific monitors of respiratory depression. However, capnography is not readily available in all institutions and is not needed universally for patients receiving opioid therapy. Capnography is best reserved for patients with substantial co-morbidities that increase the risks associated with opioid therapy.[26] Perhaps monitors that directly monitor respiratory rate will soon be available.

SYSTEMIC THERAPY

Oral Administration

Oral administration of analgesics is not optimal for the management of moderate to severe perioperative pain, primarily because of the NPO status of patients in the

V

immediate postoperative period. Traditionally, postoperative patients are switched to oral analgesics (aspirin, acetaminophen, COX-1/COX-2 inhibitors, weak opioids) when pain has diminished to the extent that the need for rapid adjustments of analgesia level is unlikely.

Perioperative administration of nonopioid analgesic medications is an integral component of multimodal analgesic treatment plans. The increased complexity of outpatient surgical procedures has introduced the need for perioperative analgesia plans that enable moderate to severe postoperative pain to be aborted or effectively treated in the outpatient setting. The use of NSAIDs and membrane stabilizers (gabapentin and pregabalin) in the preoperative setting decrease postoperative pain and opioid consumption.[20,27] However, preoperative clonidine or ketamine has no postoperative benefit.

Intramuscular Administration

Intramuscular (IM) administration of analgesics is the traditional method for treating moderate to severe postoperative pain because of a more rapid onset and time to peak effect than oral analgesics. Nevertheless, plasma concentrations of opioids achieved after IM administration may vary as much as three- to fivefold and, at a fixed time interval, can result in a cyclic period of sedation, analgesia, and, ultimately, in inadequate analgesia. The IM route of administering analgesics has been largely supplanted by the delivery of medications by intravenous or subcutaneous PCA.

Intravenous Administration

Intermittent intravenous (IV) administration of small doses of opioids (see Tables 40-4, 40-5) is commonly used to treat acute and severe pain in the postanesthesia or intensive care unit, where continuous nursing surveillance and monitoring are available. With a small IV dose of an opioid, the time delay for analgesia and the variability in plasma concentrations characteristic of IM injections are minimized. Rapid redistribution of the opioid produces a shorter duration of analgesia after a single IV administration than after an IM injection.

Ketamine is traditionally recognized as an intraoperative anesthetic; however, it is also effective in small doses for postoperative analgesia partly due to its NMDA antagonistic properties, which can attenuate central sensitization and opioid tolerance. Perioperative subanesthetic doses of ketamine reduced postoperative pain. In addition, intra- and postoperative ketamine decreases 24-hour PCA morphine consumption and postoperative nausea or vomiting, with minimal adverse effects.[28] Small-dose ketamine infusions do not cause hallucinations or cognitive impairment. The incidence of side effects, such as dizziness, itching, nausea, or vomiting, is comparable to that seen with opioids. The use of

ketamine in patients at high risk for the development of CPSP is warranted. Patients receiving large doses of opioids may experience hyperalgesia, resulting in increased excitatory amino acid release in the spinal cord. Ketamine directly inhibits the actions of the excitatory amino acids, and reverses opioid-induced hyperalgesia, leading to improved postoperative pain outcome.

Intraoperative administration of dexamethasone decreases postoperative pain scores and decreases opioid consumption. Intraoperative administration of clonidine decreases postoperative pain, but bradycardia and hypotension limit the benefits of its modest analgesic properties. Intraoperative magnesium, although it accentuates the blockade of the NMDA receptor, does not reduce postoperative pain or opioid requirements.

Subcutaneous Administration

Subcutanous (SC) administration of select medications (hydromorphone) is highly efficacious, and is a very practical approach for providing analgesia in patients without IV access or those in need of long-term, home-based analgesic care. The administration of hydromorphone exerts basically the same pharmacokinetics whether it is administered subcutaneously or intravenously. This modality is primarily utilized in oncology patients.

Transdermal/Iontophoretic Administration

The development of iontophoretic (ITD) fentanyl and the validation of its efficacy in postoperative patients may expand the possibilities of parenteral administration.[29] Traditional transdermal fentanyl is not ideal for acute pain because of its slow onset of analgesia. The full analgesic benefit of fentanyl can be 24 to 36 hours after application. Other important criterion for acute pain management includes reliability and predictability of analgesia. Unfortunately, there is wide intersubject and intrasubject variability in serum concentration and analgesic response after systemically administered opioids in the treatment of postoperative pain. The IM route of administration may result in wider variability than the IV or ITD routes, and therefore is a less ideal alternative. However, because the IM route possesses a rapid onset time, it may be the best alternative for patients who do not have the option of ITD or those without immediate IV access.

Transmucosal Administration

Transmucosal delivery of analgesics, such as fentanyl, may serve as an alternative to the oral administration of NSAIDs and opioids, especially when a rapid onset of drug effect is desirable. The primary candidates for this modality are opioid-tolerant, oncology adult patients with breakthrough pain, in whom the use of rescue medication can be significantly decreased.[30]

NEURAXIAL ANALGESIA (Also See Chapter 17)

A variety of neuraxial (intrathecal and epidural) and peripheral regional analgesic techniques are employed for postoperative pain. In general, when compared to systemic opioids, epidural and peripheral techniques can provide superior analgesia, especially when local anesthetics are applied;[31] furthermore, these techniques may decrease morbidity and mortality rates.[32] Clinical judgment is important with regard to the concerns regarding the use of these techniques in the presence of various anticoagulants (see later discussion).

Intrathecal Administration

Intrathecal administration of an opioid can provide short-term to intermediate length postoperative analgesia after a single injection. The intrathecal route offers the advantage of precise and reliable placement of low concentrations of the drug near its site of action. The onset of analgesic effects after intrathecal administration of an opioid is directly proportional to the lipid solubility of the drug. Duration of effect is longer with more hydrophilic compounds. Morphine produces peak analgesic effects in 20 to 60 minutes and postoperative analgesia for 12 to 36 hours. Adding a small dose of fentanyl to the morphine-containing opioid solution may speed the onset of analgesic effect. For lower abdominal procedures performed with spinal anesthesia (cesarean section, transurethral resection of the prostate), morphine may be added to the local anesthetic solution to increase the duration of analgesia.

The primary disadvantage of an intrathecal opioid injection is the lack of flexibility inherent to a single-shot modality. Clinicians must either repeat the injection or consider other options when the analgesic effect of the initial dose diminishes. The practical aspects of leaving a catheter in the intrathecal space for either continuous or repeated intermittent opioid injections is controversial, especially in view of reports of cauda equina syndrome after continuous spinal anesthesia with hyperbaric local anesthetic solutions injected through a small-diameter catheter.

Epidural Administration

Epidural administration of a local anesthetic as a continuous infusion through an epidural catheter is a common method of providing perioperative analgesia. Epidural infusions of local anesthetic alone may be used for postoperative analgesia, but in general, they are not as effective in controlling pain as local anesthetic-opioid epidural analgesic combinations.[21] This is due to the significant failure rate (from regression of sensory block and inadequate analgesia) and relatively frequent incidence of motor block and hypotension.[33]

The precise location of the action of local anesthetics in the epidural space has not been determined. Potential sites include the spinal nerve roots, dorsal root ganglion, or the spinal cord itself. Epidural infusions of local anesthetic alone may be warranted for postoperative analgesia, with the goal of avoiding opioid-related side effects.

The benefit of opioid monotherapy in epidural infusions is that they generally do not cause motor block or hypotension from sympathetic blockade. There are mechanistic differences between continuous epidural infusions of lipophilic (e.g., fentanyl, sufentanil) and hydrophilic (e.g., morphine, hydromorphone) opioids. The analgesic site of action (spinal versus systemic) for continuous epidural infusions of lipophilic opioids is not clear, although several randomized clinical trials suggest that it is systemic[34] because there were no differences in plasma concentrations, side effects, or pain scores between those who received intravenous or epidural infusions of fentanyl. A continuous infusion, rather than an intermittent bolus of epidural opioids, may provide superior analgesia with fewer side effects. Hydrophilic opioid epidural infusions have a spinal mechanism of action.[35] The impact of epidural analgesia is dependent upon the total dose administered rather than the volume or concentration.

Clinical efficacy of epidural analgesia (local anesthetic with and without opioids) for abdominal surgeries has demonstrated superior pain relief in the initial postoperative period, with fewer gastrointestinal-related side effects compared to systemic opioid therapy; however, there is an increased incidence of pruritus.[36] Epidural analgesia is beneficial for major joint surgery of the lower extremity, but has the associated disadvantages of neuraxial analgesia.[37] Thoracic epidural analgesia has been the mainstay of analgesia for thoracotomy, but paravertebral blockades may be just as effective with a more favorable side effect profile.[38] One of the primary benefits of epidural analgesia for traumatic rib fractures is the decreased required duration of mechanical ventilation when compared to using a local anesthetic alone.[39]

Side Effects of Neuraxial Analgesic Drugs

Many medication-related (opioid and local anesthetic) side effects can occur with postoperative epidural analgesia. When side effects are suspected, the patient's overall clinical status should be evaluated so that serious comorbidities are not inappropriately attributed to epidural analgesia. The differential diagnosis for a patient with neuraxial analgesia and hypotension should also include hypovolemia, bleeding, and a decreased cardiac output. Patients with respiratory depression should also be

V

evaluated for cerebrovascular accident, pulmonary edema, and evolving sepsis. Standing orders and nursing protocols for analgesic regimens, neurologic monitoring, treatment of side effects, and physician notification about critical variables should be standard for all patients receiving neuraxial and other types of postoperative analgesia.

MOST COMMON SIDE EFFECTS

The most frequent side effects of neuraxial analgesia include the following:

- *Hypotension* (0.3% to 7%)—Local anesthetics used in an epidural analgesic regimen may block sympathetic fibers and contribute to postoperative hypotension.
- *Motor block* (2% to 3%)—In most cases, motor block resolves within 2 hours after discontinuing the epidural infusion. Persistent or increasing motor block should be promptly evaluated, and spinal hematoma, spinal abscess, and intrathecal catheter migration should be considered as part of the differential diagnosis.
- *Nausea, vomiting, and pruritus* (15% to 18%)—Pruritus is one of the most common side effects of epidural or intrathecal administration of opioids, with an incidence of approximately 60% compared with about 15% to 18% for local epidural anesthetic administration or systemic opioids.
- *Respiratory depression* (0.1% to 0.9%)—Neuraxial opioids administered in appropriate doses are not associated with a more frequent incidence of respiratory depression than that seen with systemic administration of opioids. Risk factors for respiratory depression with neuraxial opioids include larger dose, geriatric age group, concomitant administration of systemic opioids or sedatives, the possibility of prolonged or extensive surgery, the presence of co-morbidities, and thoracic surgery.
- *Urinary retention* (10% to 30%)—Epidural administration of local anesthetics is also associated with urinary retention.

ANTICOAGULATION

The concurrent use of anticoagulants with neuraxial anesthesia and analgesia has always been a relatively controversial issue, but has been highlighted over the past decade with an increased incidence of spinal hematomas after the introduction of low-molecular-weight heparin in North America in 1993. Traditionally, the incidence of spinal hematoma is estimated at approximately 1 in 150,000 for epidural block, with a less frequent incidence of 1 in 220,000 for spinal blocks.[40] Before its introduction in North America, low-molecular-weight heparin was used in Europe without significant problems. However, the incidence of spinal hematoma increased to as frequent as 1 in 40,800 for spinal anesthetics and 1 in 6600 for epidural anesthetics (1 in 3100 for postoperative epidural analgesia) in the United States between 1993

and 1998.[41] The estimate of the more frequent incidence of spinal hematomas after epidural catheter removal is based in part on the Food and Drug Administration MedWatch data, which suggest that epidural catheter removal may be a traumatic event, although this is still a relatively controversial issue.

Different types and classes of anticoagulants vary in pharmacokinetic properties that affect the timing of neuraxial catheter or needle insertion and catheter removal. Despite a number of observational and retrospective studies investigating the incidence of spinal hematoma in the setting of various anticoagulants and neuraxial techniques, there is no definitive conclusion regarding the absolute safety of neuraxial anesthesia and anticoagulation. The American Society of Regional Anesthesia and Pain Medicine (ASRA) lists a series of consensus statements, based on the available literature, for the administration (insertion and removal) of neuraxial techniques in the presence of various anticoagulants, including oral anticoagulants (warfarin), antiplatelet agents, fibrinolytics-thrombolytics, standard unfractionated heparin, and low-molecular-weight heparin. The ASRA consensus statements include the concepts that (1) the timing of neuraxial needle or catheter insertion or removal should reflect the pharmacokinetic properties of the specific anticoagulant; (2) frequent neurologic monitoring is essential; (3) concurrent administration of multiple anticoagulants may increase the risk of bleeding; and (4) the analgesic regimen should be tailored to facilitate neurologic monitoring, which may be continued in some cases for 24 hours after epidural catheter removal. An updated version of the ASRA consensus statements on neuraxial anesthesia and anticoagulation[42] can be found on their web site (www.asra.com), with some of these statements addressing the newer anticoagulants.

INFECTION

Infection associated with postoperative epidural analgesia may result from exogenous or endogenous sources. Serious infections (e.g., meningitis, spinal abscess) associated with epidural analgesic are rare (<1 in 10,000), although some researchers report a more frequent incidence (approximately 1 in 1000 to 1 in 2000).[43] Closer examination of the studies that report a more frequent incidence of epidural abscesses reveal that the patients had a relatively longer duration of epidural analgesia, or the presence of coexisting immunocompromising or complicating diseases (e.g., malignancy, trauma). Use of epidural analgesia in the general surgical population, with a typical duration of postoperative catheterization of approximately 2 to 4 days, is generally not associated with epidural abscess formation. A trial of postoperative epidural analgesia (mean catheterization of 6.3 days) in more than 4000 surgical cancer patients did not reveal any abscesses.[44]

INTRA-ARTICULAR ADMINISTRATION

Intra-articular injection of opioids may provide analgesia for up to 24 hours postoperatively and prevent the development of chronic postsurgical pain. Opioid receptors are found in the peripheral terminals of primary afferent nerves, which may explain this improved analgesia, despite the lack of response with the addition of opioids to perineural anesthetic injections. The analgesic benefit of intra-articular opioids over systemic administration has not been demonstrated, and the systemic analgesic effect of these injections has not been excluded.[45] Glenohumeral intra-articular continuous catheters have been associated with chondrolysis when bupivacaine is used.[46]

INTRAPLEURAL REGIONAL ANALGESIA

Intrapleural regional analgesia is produced by the injection of a local anesthetic solution through a catheter inserted percutaneously into the intrapleural space. The local anesthetic diffuses across the parietal pleura to the intercostal neurovascular bundle and produces a unilateral intercostal nerve block at multiple levels. Effective postoperative pain relief requires intermittent intrapleural injections approximately every 6 hours of large volumes of local anesthetic (20 mL of 0.25% to 0.5% bupivacaine). This large bolus of local anesthetic into the intrapleural space produces significant side effects while providing minimal analgesia. Pleural drainage tubes placed after a thoracotomy will result in a large loss of the local anesthetic solution and, consequently, poor analgesia. This technique is recommended only if all other options have been exhausted.

PARAVERTEBRAL BLOCKS

The increased utilization of paravertebral blockade can be directly correlated with the beneficial effects for patients undergoing breast surgery. This block provides an effective mechanism for controlling acute pain associated with this procedure, but has also demonstrated benefit in decreasing the development of chronic postsurgical pain over other analgesic regimens.[47] This technique can be performed as a single-shot technique or as a continuous catheter infusion to provide ongoing perioperative analgesia.

PERIPHERAL NERVE BLOCK

Peripheral nerve blockade can provide analgesia as part of an autonomous or multimodal pain regimen. Single-shot injections can provide coverage for intraoperative pain control. However, many providers feel that the risk of the intervention warrants the prolonged benefit, which includes postoperative pain control, and have driven the need for flexible duration of action. Intermediate-term pain relief (<24 hours) can be achieved with a combination of a local anesthetic and adjuvant drugs in a single injection. Longer-acting pain control may be indicated by the surgical technique, rehabilitation needs, and patient comorbidities; and can be achieved by utilizing perineural catheters for continuous local anesthetic infusions.

Techniques

Nerve blocks can be inserted using anatomic landmarks, nerve stimulation, and ultrasound guidance. The efficacy between ultrasound-guided techniques and nerve stimulation vary, depending on the skill of the provider, primarily resulting in differences in comfort during placement and procedural time of the blockade. Nonetheless, these techniques provide a comparable quality of analgesia and similar complication profile.[48]

Adjuvant Drugs

Commonly used adjuvant drugs include epinephrine, clonidine, and opioids. Epinephrine for peripheral nerve blockade significantly increases the duration of the blockade, with minimal side effects. Epinephrine can also increase the sensitivity of intravascular injection; concentrations of 2.5 to 5 µg/mL are generally used. The mechanism of this effect is primarily through vasoconstriction. Opioids probably should not be added to a peripheral nerve blockade. Clonidine is beneficial in extending the duration of preoperative blockade, but has less utility with perineural catheters. The mechanism is most likely peripheral α_2-adrenergic receptor-mediated and dose-dependent. Clonidine is a better preemptive analgesic when added to a local anesthetic block than when used as a single drug. Side effects, including hypotension, bradycardia, and sedation, are less likely to occur in doses less than 1.5 µg/kg.[49] The use of clonidine increases the duration of analgesia and motor blockade by approximately 2 hours.[50]

REGIONAL ANALGESIA (Also See Chapter 18)

Efficacy and safety are primary limiting factors in the implementation of any therapeutic measure. Regional analgesia is becoming an increasingly popular technique for perioperative pain control, and has several specific advantages and disadvantages. The technical details of these blocks are covered in the regional anesthesia chapter; this section focuses on the utility and comparative efficacy of these blocks.

V

Catheter versus Single-Shot Techniques

UPPER EXTREMITY

Continuous interscalene blockade allows for longer duration of action compared with single-shot techniques. This technique has increased utility with the posterior interscalene approach for moderate to severely painful shoulder surgeries. The continuous administration allows for increased pain relief, with minimal opioid supplementation and increased patient satisfaction and sleep quality.[51]

LOWER EXTREMITY

Lower extremity orthopedic surgeries resulting in moderate to severe perioperative pain also benefit from long-acting regional techniques. Lower extremity perineural catheters are utilized for major joint surgery of the hip, knee, ankle, and foot. This type of catheter may decrease clinical signs of inflammation for some lower extremity procedures, although inflammation is not decreased at the cellular level.[52] Epidural catheters are utilized to provide good analgesia for major joint surgeries of the lower extremities, but expose patients to neuraxial analgesia risks, and generally have bilateral effects.[53] Lumbar plexus catheters have been utilized as part of a multimodal regimen, with better pain scores at rest and with physical therapy than multimodal regimens that include PCA with or without femoral catheters for unilateral hip repairs.[54] Patients undergoing major foot and ankle surgeries under continuous perineural blockade are not only potentially able to obtain pain relief comparable to single-shot and systemic analgesia, but also are discharged from postanesthetic care units in a shorter peroid of time.[55]

TRANSVERSUS ABDOMINIS PLANE BLOCK

Neuraxial analgesia techniques are starting to face competition from the transverse abdominis plane (TAP) block for many abdominal procedures. Theoretical advantages of this technique over other modalities include avoidance of both neuraxial involvement and lower extremity blockade, decreased urinary retention, and decreased systemic side effects. Compared with placebo blocks, TAP block provided increased analgesia and decreased systemic medication requirements as part of a multimodal analgesic regimen for total abdominal hysterectomy,[56] cesarean section,[57] and laparoscopic cholecystectomy.[58] Moreover, guidance by ultrasound has made this a more reliably efficacious treatment modality.[59]

QUESTIONS OF THE DAY

1. What is the difference between "preemptive analgesia" and "preventive analgesia"?
2. What are the principles of a multimodal approach to perioperative pain management?
3. What are the most common side effects of neuraxial analgesia? Which side effects can be life threatening?
4. What is the potential role of adjuvant drugs (e.g., epinephrine, opioids, clonidine) in peripheral nerve blockade?

ACKNOWLEDGMENT

The editors and publisher would like to thank Dr. Robert Stoelting for contributing a chapter on this topic to the prior edition of this work. It has served as the foundation for the current chapter.

REFERENCES

1. Ready LB: How many acute pain services are there in the United States, and who is managing patient-controlled analgesia? *Anesthesiology* 82:322, 1995.
2. Tuman KJ, McCarthy RJ, March RJ, et al: Effects of epidural anesthesia and analgesia on coagulation and outcome after major vascular surgery, *Anesth Analg* 73:696–704, 1991.
3. Rasmussen LS, Johnson T, Kuipers HM, et al: Does anaesthesia cause postoperative cognitive dysfunction? A randomised study of regional versus general anaesthesia in 438 elderly patients, *Acta Anaesthesiol Scand* 47:260–266, 2003.
4. Kiribayashi M, Inagaki Y, Nishimura Y, et al: Caudal blockade shortens the time to walking exercise in elderly patients following low back surgery, *J Anesth* 24:192–196, 2010.
5. Katz J, McCartney CJ: Current status of preemptive analgesia, *Curr Opin Anaesthesiol* 15:435–441, 2002.
6. Kehlet H, Jensen TS, Woolf CJ: Persistent postsurgical pain: Risk factors and prevention, *Lancet* 367:1618–1625, 2006.
7. Carr DB, Goudas LC: Acute pain, *Lancet* 353:2051–2058, 1999.
8. Perkins FM, Kehlet H: Chronic pain as an outcome of surgery. A review of predictive factors, *Anesthesiology* 93:1123–1133, 2000.
9. Merskey H: Pain and psychological medicine. In Wall PD, Melzack R, editors: *Textbook of Pain*, New York, 1994, Churchill Livingstone, pp 903–920.
10. Basbaum AI, Fields HL: Endogenous pain control systems: Brainstem spinal pathways and endorphin circuitry, *Annu Rev Neurosci* 7:309–338, 1984.
11. Julius D, Basbaum AI: Molecular mechanisms of nociception, *Nature* 413:203–210, 2001.
12. Basbaum AI: Spinal mechanisms of acute and persistent pain, *Reg Anesth Pain Med* 24:59–67, 1999.
13. Besson JM: The neurobiology of pain, *Lancet* 353:1610–1615, 1999.
14. Kissin I: Preemptive analgesia, *Anesthesiology* 93:1138–1143, 2000.
15. Moiniche S, Kehlet H, Dahl JB: A qualitative and quantitative systematic review of preemptive analgesia for postoperative pain relief: The role of timing of analgesia, *Anesthesiology* 96:725–741, 2002.

16. Dahl JB, Moiniche S: Pre-emptive analgesia, *Br Med Bull* 71:13–27, 2004.

17. Ong CK, Lirk P, Seymour RA, et al: The efficacy of preemptive analgesia for acute postoperative pain management: A meta-analysis, *Anesth Analg* 100:757–773, 2005.

18. Pogatzki-Zahn EM, Zahn PK: From preemptive to preventive analgesia, *Curr Opin Anaesthesiol* 19:551–555, 2006.

19. Kehlet H: Multimodal approach to control postoperative pathophysiology and rehabilitation, *Br J Anaesth* 78:606–617, 1997.

20. Hurley RW, Cohen SP, Williams KA, et al: The analgesic effects of perioperative gabapentin on postoperative pain: A meta-analysis, *Reg Anesth Pain Med* 31:237–247, 2006.

21. Block BM, Liu SS, Rowlingson AJ, et al: Efficacy of postoperative epidural analgesia: A meta-analysis, *JAMA* 290:2455–2463, 2003.

22. Ben-David B, Swanson J, Nelson JB, et al: Multimodal analgesia for radical prostatectomy provides better analgesia and shortens hospital stay, *J Clin Anesth* 19:264–268, 2007.

23. Kehlet H, Wilmore DW: Multimodal strategies to improve surgical outcome, *Am J Surg* 183:630–641, 2002.

24. Taqi A, Hong X, Mistraletti G, et al: Thoracic epidural analgesia facilitates the restoration of bowel function and dietary intake in patients undergoing laparoscopic colon resection using a traditional, nonaccelerated, perioperative care program, *Surg Endosc* 21:247–252, 2007.

25. Egbert AM, Parks LH, Short LM, et al: Randomized trial of postoperative patient-controlled analgesia vs. intramuscular narcotics in frail elderly men, *Arch Intern Med* 150:1897–1903, 1990.

26. Kopka A, Wallace E, Reilly G, et al: Observational study of perioperative PtcCO$_2$ and SpO$_2$ in non-ventilated patients receiving epidural infusion or patient-controlled analgesia using a single earlobe monitor (TOSCA), *Br J Anaesth* 99:567–571, 2007.

27. Elia N, Lysakowski C, Tramer MR: Does multimodal analgesia with acetaminophen, nonsteroidal antiinflammatory drugs, or selective cyclooxygenase-2 inhibitors and patient-controlled analgesia morphine offer advantages over morphine alone? Meta-analyses of randomized trials, *Anesthesiology* 103: 1296–1304, 2005.

28. Bell RF, Dahl JB, Moore RA, et al: Perioperative ketamine for acute postoperative pain, *Cochrane Database Syst Rev* CD004603, 2006 (online).

29. Viscusi ER, Reynolds L, Tait S, et al: An iontophoretic fentanyl patient-activated analgesic delivery system for postoperative pain: A double-blind, placebo-controlled trial, *Anesth Analg* 102:188–194, 2006.

30. Lennernas B, Lissbrant IF, Lennernas H, et al: Sublingual administration of fentanyl to cancer patients is an effective treatment for breakthrough pain: Results from a randomized phase II study, *Palliat Med* 24:286–293, 2010.

31. Dolin SJ, Cashman JN, Bland JM: Effectiveness of acute postoperative pain management: I. Evidence from published data, *Br J Anaesth* 89:409–423, 2002.

32. Wu CL, Fleisher LA: Outcomes research in regional anesthesia and analgesia, *Anesth Analg* 91:1232–1242, 2000.

33. Wheatley RG, Schug SA, Watson D: Safety and efficacy of postoperative epidural analgesia, *Br J Anaesth* 87:47–61, 2001.

34. Loper KA, Ready LB, Downey M, et al: Epidural and intravenous fentanyl infusions are clinically equivalent after knee surgery, *Anesth Analg* 70:72–75, 1990.

35. de Leon-Casasola OA, Lema MJ: Postoperative epidural opioid analgesia: What are the choices? *Anesth Analg* 83:867–875, 1996.

36. Werawatganon T, Charuluxanun S: Patient controlled intravenous opioid analgesia versus continuous epidural analgesia for pain after intra-abdominal surgery, *Cochrane Database Syst Rev* CD004088, 2005.

37. Choi PT, Bhandari M, Scott J, et al: Epidural analgesia for pain relief following hip or knee replacement, *Cochrane Database Syst Rev* CD003071, 2003.

38. Gulbahar G, Kocer B, Muratli SN, et al: A comparison of epidural and paravertebral catheterisation techniques in post-thoracotomy pain management, *Eur J Cardiothorac Surg* 37:467–472, 2010.

39. Carrier FM, Turgeon AF, Nicole PC, et al: Effect of epidural analgesia in patients with traumatic rib fractures: A systematic review and meta-analysis of randomized controlled trials, *Can J Anaesth* 56:230–242, 2009.

40. Tryba M: Epidural regional anesthesia and low molecular heparin: Pro, *Anasthesiol Intensivmed Notfallmed Schmerzther* 28:179–181, 1993.

41. Schroeder DR: Statistics: Detecting a rare adverse drug reaction using spontaneous reports, *Reg Anesth Pain Med* 23:183–189, 1998.

42. Horlocker TT, Wedel DJ, Rowlingson JC, et al: Regional anesthesia in the patient receiving antithrombotic or thrombolytic therapy: American Society of Regional Anesthesia and Pain Medicine Evidence-Based Guidelines, 3rd ed, *Reg Anesth Pain Med* 35:64–101, 2010.

43. Horlocker TT, Wedel DJ: Neurologic complications of spinal and epidural anesthesia, *Reg Anesth Pain Med* 25:83–98, 2000.

44. de Leon-Casasola OA, Parker BM, Lema MJ, et al: Epidural analgesia versus intravenous patient-controlled analgesia. Differences in the postoperative course of cancer patients, *Reg Anesth* 19:307–315, 1994.

45. Kalso E, Smith L, McQuay HJ, et al: No pain, no gain: Clinical excellence and scientific rigour—Lessons learned from IA morphine, *Pain* 98:269–275, 2002.

46. Busfield BT, Romero DM: Pain pump use after shoulder arthroscopy as a cause of glenohumeral chondrolysis, *Arthroscopy* 25:647–652, 2009.

47. Vila H Jr, Liu J, Kavasmaneck D: Paravertebral block: New benefits from an old procedure, *Curr Opin Anaesthesiol* 20:316–318, 2007.

48. Fredrickson MJ, Ball CM, Dalgleish AJ, et al: A prospective randomized comparison of ultrasound and neurostimulation as needle end points for interscalene catheter placement, *Anesth Analg* 108:1695–1700, 2009.

49. Neal JM, Gerancher JC, Hebl JR, et al: Upper extremity regional anesthesia: Essentials of our current understanding, 2008, *Reg Anesth Pain Med* 34:134–170, 2009.

50. Popping DM, Elia N, Marret E, et al: Clonidine as an adjuvant to local anesthetics for peripheral nerve and plexus blocks: A meta-analysis of randomized trials, *Anesthesiology* 111:406–415, 2009.

51. Mariano ER, Afra R, Loland VJ, et al: Continuous interscalene brachial plexus block via an ultrasound-guided posterior approach: A randomized, triple-masked, placebo-controlled study, *Anesth Analg* 108:1688–1694, 2009.

52. Martin F, Martinez V, Mazoit JX, et al: Antiinflammatory effect of peripheral nerve blocks after knee surgery: clinical and biologic evaluation, *Anesthesiology* 109:484–490, 2008.

53. Fowler SJ, Symons J, Sabato S, et al: Epidural analgesia compared with peripheral nerve blockade after major knee surgery: A systematic review and meta-analysis of randomized trials, *Br J Anaesth* 100:154–164, 2008.

54. Marino J, Russo J, Kenny M, et al: Continuous lumbar plexus block for postoperative pain control after total hip arthroplasty. A randomized controlled trial, *J Bone Joint Surg Am* 91:29–37, 2009.

V

661

55. Hunt KJ, Higgins TF, Carlston CV, et al: Continuous peripheral nerve blockade as postoperative analgesia for open treatment of calcaneal fractures, *J Orthop Trauma* 24:148–155, 2010.

56. Carney J, McDonnell JG, Ochana A, et al: The transversus abdominis plane block provides effective postoperative analgesia in patients undergoing total abdominal hysterectomy, *Anesth Analg* 107:2056–2060, 2008.

57. McDonnell JG, Curley G, Carney J, et al: The analgesic efficacy of transversus abdominis plane block after cesarean delivery: A randomized controlled trial, *Anesth Analg* 106:186–191, 2008.

58. Takahashi H, Suzuki T, Onda M: Postoperative analgesia for the laparoscopic cholecystectomy, *Masui* 58:1501–1505, 2009.

59. El-Dawlatly A, Turkistani A, Kettner C, et al: Ultrasound-guided transversus abdominis plane block: Description of a new technique and comparison with conventional systemic analgesia during laparoscopic cholecystectomy, *Br J Anaesth* 102:763–767, 2009.

Section VI

CONSULTANT ANESTHETIC PRACTICE

CRITICAL CARE MEDICINE

Lundy Campbell and Michael Gropper

C are of the critically ill patient is a core competency for anesthesiology. The practice of critical care medicine, which originated in the 1940s with anesthesiologists providing life support to patients with poliomyelitis, has undergone revolutionary change. The development of equipment, procedures, and medications has enabled intensivists to treat critically ill patients and support them through increasingly invasive procedures. In the past decade another revolution has taken place with the introduction of evidence-based medicine into the practice of critical care medicine (also see Chapter 2).

Ironically, anesthesiologists, who founded critical care medicine, represent a shrinking percentage of these specialists. Anesthesiologists are particularly well trained to manage critically ill patients in the intensive care unit (ICU) and do so on a regular basis in the operating room. Anesthesiologists may be required to care for patients in the operating room who either have been or will be admitted to the ICU, and familiarity with the unique challenges that these patients present may dramatically improve their care.

MECHANICAL VENTILATION

ICUs were developed to support patients in respiratory failure, and this function remains a major feature of modern critical care units. The availability of modern mechanical ventilators has made ventilatory support routine.

Indications

Mechanical ventilatory support is typically initiated for the treatment of respiratory failure (impaired oxygenation), ventilatory failure (impaired carbon dioxide excretion), and airway protection. Causes of respiratory failure include trauma, acute respiratory distress syndrome (ARDS), sepsis, pneumonia, and pulmonary edema (both cardiogenic and noncardiogenic). Ventilatory failure may be due to chronic obstructive pulmonary disease (COPD), asthma, and drug intoxication. Intubation plus mechanical ventilation for airway protection is usually limited to conditions such as acute airway edema, altered mental status, and significant neuromuscular disorders. Patients receive mechanical ventilatory support to (1) reduce the work of breathing, (2) reverse progressive respiratory acidosis or hypoxemia, (3) reduce the risk for aspiration of gastric contents, or (4) ensure a patent airway with severe neck and facial swelling or trauma.

Modes of Mechanical Ventilation

The goal of the several different modes of mechanical ventilation is to provide adequate oxygenation and removal of carbon dioxide. Yet, potentially lifesaving, mechanical ventilation may also propagate lung injury. Modern modes of mechanical ventilation have been developed with the goal of limiting the complication of ventilator-induced lung injury.

CONTINUOUS MANDATORY VENTILATION

Continuous mandatory ventilation (CMV) is present when the ventilator is programmed to deliver a set tidal volume at a set respiratory rate, thereby resulting in the delivery of a predictable minute ventilation. Regardless of patient effort, the ventilator will deliver its preset tidal volume at its preset time. If the patient makes additional efforts between delivered breaths, these breaths are unsupported. To regulate the amount of time that the ventilator spends cycling in inspiration and expiration, the inspiratory flow rate is set. By increasing inspiratory flow, the set tidal volume is delivered in a shorter time, which allows more time for exhalation.

A related mode of CMV is assist-control ventilation. Like intermittent mandatory ventilation (IMV), set tidal volume breaths are delivered at a set rate; however, additional breaths are detected by the ventilator and supported to full tidal volume. CMV is the most commonly used mode of mechanical ventilation in ICUs.

SYNCHRONIZED INTERMITTENT MANDATORY VENTILATION

In synchronized intermittent mandatory ventilation (SIMV), the tidal volume and respiratory rate are set as in IMV, but the ventilator attempts to synchronize the mandatory breaths that it delivers with the patient's own spontaneous breaths. If the patient does not initiate a breath within a set time, the ventilator delivers the set tidal volume machine breath as in the CMV mode. In this way, the ventilator ensures that the patient maintains the desired minimum ventilation. If a patient initiates additional breaths beyond those that are set in the SIMV mode to maintain the set minute ventilation, the ventilator can be programmed to deliver a pressure-supported breath. This combined mode of ventilation is known as SIMV with pressure support.

PRESSURE SUPPORT VENTILATION

In pressure support ventilation, the ventilator does not deliver a preset tidal volume but, instead, relies on the patient's intrinsic respiratory drive. When the machine senses the patient initiating a breath, the ventilator delivers a preset positive pressure to assist the patient in obtaining an adequate breath. Typically, the amount of pressure support is set between 5 and 20 cm H_2O to ensure adequate tidal volume and minute ventilation. In this mode, the ventilator stops its delivery of positive pressure when it senses that the patient's airflow has dropped below a preset level. Therefore, tidal volume will vary with patient effort. To use pressure support ventilation, the patient must possess an intact respiratory drive, and no residual neuromuscular blockade can be present (also see Chapter 12). However, as an added safety precaution, all modern ventilators with this mode also have a backup mode of emergency assist-control ventilation in the event that a patient's minute ventilation decreases to less than a set threshold.

POSITIVE END-EXPIRATORY PRESSURE

Positive end-expiratory pressure (PEEP) is constant positive airway pressure that is applied throughout the respiratory cycle. PEEP functions to increase mean airway pressure and thereby prevent atelectasis. It increases the functional residual capacity of the lungs and, in patients with lung injury, results in improved pulmonary compliance. The process of inflating collapsed alveoli is known as recruitment, and when properly applied, PEEP can improve oxygenation in a mechanically ventilated patient.

The typical PEEP range is between 5 and 20 cmH$_2$O. High levels of PEEP can overdistend and damage alveoli and may cause hemodynamic collapse by reducing preload to both the right and the left ventricles with a resultant fall in cardiac output. If sufficient time for exhalation of the delivered tidal breath is not allowed, a phenomenon known as intrinsic PEEP or auto-PEEP may occur. It results in a buildup of end-expiratory pressure, and when excessive, hemodynamic collapse may occur. Treatment of auto-PEEP entails disconnecting the patient from the ventilator to release the PEEP and increasing expiratory time to prevent recurrence.

Weaning from Mechanical Ventilation

To decrease the risks associated with continued mechanical ventilation, such as ventilator-associated pneumonia, patients are weaned from the ventilator as soon as possible. To be considered for weaning, a patient must have recovered from the process that originally required mechanical ventilatory support. In addition, the patient should be hemodynamically stable and receiving minimal vasopressor support because weaning may increase the work of breathing and thereby worsen cardiovascular strain.

Postsurgical as well as postpercutaneous coronary intervention (PCI) cardiac patients may be an exception to this rule. Although these patients still need to be hemodynamically stable to be considered for weaning, they may remain on relatively high-dose vasopressors during the weaning and tracheal extubation period. This select group is treated differently because patients who have undergone cardiopulmonary bypass often have myocardial dysfunction and peripheral vasodilatation that are not intrinsic to their disease state and will quickly resolve.

TRIAL OF WEANING

Generally, patients are not considered candidates for a trial of weaning and tracheal extubation until certain criteria are met. These criteria are discussed in the following paragraphs.

Inspired Oxygen Needed to Maintain Oxygenation

The patient's required inspired oxygen concentration to maintain adequate oxygenation saturation should be less than 40% to 50%. This amount of oxygen is chosen because this level can be reasonably and reliably delivered in the absence of a tracheal tube via face mask or nasal cannula. An oxygen requirement greater than this denotes that the patient still has a large shunt fraction through the lung and the underlying pulmonary process has not adequately resolved.

Tidal Volume

Patients must be strong enough to generate an adequate tidal volume. This can be ascertained by having the patient inhale as forcefully as possible. The negative inspiratory force of this breath (maximum negative inspiratory force) or the absolute size of the inhaled breath (vital capacity) can then be measured. For weaning, a negative inspiratory force of at least −20 cm H$_2$O pressure or a vial capacity of at least 10 mL/kg is required. In normal tidal breathing, a tidal volume of at least 5 mL/kg and a minute ventilation of no more than 10 L/min may also be used.

Protect the Airway against Aspiration of Gastric Contents

Patients must be able to protect their airway against aspiration of gastric contents and adequately clear their own pulmonary secretions. The ability to protect an airway usually requires an intact mental status and gag reflex. The ability to clear pulmonary secretions requires a strong cough. However, if a patient continues to have a large amount of pulmonary secretions, weaning from mechanical ventilation may be delayed despite the presence of an adequate cough because these patients may fatigue under the work of clearing copious thick secretions.

EVIDENCE-BASED WEANING STRATEGIES

A randomized controlled clinical trial comparing four modes of weaning (IMV, pressure support ventilation, intermittent trials of spontaneous breathing with continuous positive airway pressure [CPAP] or a T-piece, and once-daily trials of spontaneous breathing) found that patients were weaned successfully an average of 1 to 2 days sooner with spontaneous breathing trials versus IMV or pressure support weaning.[1] In addition, once-daily weaning trials are just as effective as intermittent (more than one trial per day) weaning trials.

In another trial, physician-directed weaning was compared with protocol-driven weaning managed by nurses and respiratory therapists.[2] When a patient met the criteria for tracheal extubation, a physician was notified and the trachea was subsequently extubated if the physician agreed. The patients in the protocol arm were weaned an average of 1.5 days sooner than the control

VI

(physician-directed) group did. From these trials, the most rapid and cost-effective weaning method is once-daily CPAP or T-piece weaning trials that are protocol driven by nurses and respiratory therapists.

NONINVASIVE POSITIVE-PRESSURE VENTILATION

Noninvasive positive-pressure ventilation (NIPPV) is frequently used in the ICU to provide support for both oxygenation and ventilatory failure. NIPPV is positive-pressure ventilation delivered without the use of an endotracheal tube. Positive airway pressure is delivered via a face mask that covers either the nose and mouth or the nose only or by "nasal pillows," which are similar to a large nasal cannula that fits into the nares. All NIPPV masks are held firmly in place by a tight-fitting strap.

Modes of Delivery

Noninvasive ventilation is typically administered as (1) CPAP or (2) bilevel positive airway pressure (BiPAP).

CONTINUOUS POSITIVE AIRWAY PRESSURE
CPAP is constant positive airway pressure that is applied throughout both the inspiratory and expiratory phases of ventilation. CPAP improves oxygenation and ventilation by recruitment of collapsed alveoli in acute lung injury, helps maintain a patent airway in the setting of airway obstruction such as sleep apnea, and increases mean airway pressure with respect to ambient atmospheric pressure in patients with COPD.

BILEVEL POSITIVE AIRWAY PRESSURE
BiPAP is similar to pressure support with PEEP ventilation because the ventilator cycles between two sets of positive-pressure settings. Positive pressure is delivered throughout the respiratory cycle, and higher positive pressure is applied during inspiration only. The ventilator is set by adjusting the level of both the inspiratory high pressure and the expiratory low pressure values.

Advantages

NIPPV has the advantage of being less invasive than traditional endotracheal intubation and ventilation, and reduces the risk of ventilator-associated pneumonia. Patients can be rapidly supported with NIPPV by simply fitting a proper face mask and can be removed from ventilatory support just as easily. NIPPV allows for ventilation during short periods only, such as while sleeping or immediately after discontinuation of traditional mechanical ventilation.

Indications

NIPPV is indicated in a patient who has a potentially rapidly reversible pulmonary process that requires ventilatory support. NIPPV reduces the morbidity associated with endotracheal intubation and allows the patient to remain awake and interactive during the period of ventilatory support.

In patients with acute exacerbations of COPD, NIPPV is an effective treatment that can reduce both the need for subsequent endotracheal intubation and the mortality rate for this group.[3] NIPPV can treat other forms of acute respiratory failure such as pneumonia, congestive heart failure, and postsurgical respiratory failure. NIPPV may be just as effective as conventional ventilation with respect to oxygenation and removal of carbon dioxide in these patients and is associated with fewer serious complications and shorter ICU stay.[4]

A multicenter study comparing the use of NIPPV with standard treatment (oxygen, bronchodilator therapy, tracheal reintubation when necessary) in postoperative patients who had undergone laparotomy, recently been tracheally extubated, and subsequently suffered postextubation respiratory failure concluded that both groups had the same reintubation rate but the NIPPV group had a significantly longer time to reintubation.[5] However, the NIPPV group also had a significantly higher mortality rate than did the standard medical treatment group (25% versus 14%). This study suggests that in those patients who fail extubation, the use of NIPPV as a means to improve ventilation or oxygenation and thereby hopefully avoid a reintubation, should be used with caution. A delay in reintubation is associated with an increase in mortality rate, and generally patients who fail extubation should be reintubated immediately.

Disadvantages

There are certain unique disadvantages to the use of NIPPV. The most frequently encountered problem is lack of patient compliance. Because NIPPV requires a tight-fitting mask for effective ventilation, many patients find it uncomfortable and it is poorly tolerated by those who are claustrophobic. Additionally, because NIPPV provides no airway protection, patients must be awake and able to follow commands and must possess an adequate cough and gag reflex such that it is certain that they will be able to protect their own airway against aspiration of gastric contents. Other problems associated with NIPPV include gastric distention from swallowing air when using high inspiratory pressure and difficulty delivering adequate enteral nutrition to patients while they are being ventilated. In patients who receive NIPPV for a prolonged period, an additional problem of pressure necrosis associated with a tight-fitting mask may be encountered. This usually occurs around the bridge of the patient's nose, and may be alleviated by discontinuing NIPPV, or by giving the patient periods of "rest" from NIPPV if he/she can tolerate it.

ACUTE RESPIRATORY DISTRESS SYNDROME

ARDS and acute lung injury (ALI) encompass a broad array of causes of respiratory failure and result in a similar clinical picture (Table 41-1).[6] ARDS may arise from an infectious insult such as pneumonia or sepsis, or it can develop from a noninfectious process such as trauma, pulmonary aspiration, burns, or transfusion-related acute lung injury (TRALI) (also see Chapter 24) (Table 41-2).[7] Typically, ARDS arising from causes such as trauma and TRALI has better outcomes and a less frequent mortality rate than does ARDS resulting from sepsis, pneumonia, and burns. Sepsis is associated with an unusually frequent occurrence of ALI or ARDS approximating 40%.[8]

Table 41-1 Acute Respiratory Distress Syndrome and Acute Lung Injury Definitions from the American-European Consensus Conference

Acute onset

Gas exchange
Acute lung injury: $Pao_2/Fio_2 \leq 300$ mm Hg
Acute respiratory distress syndrome: $Pao_2/Fio_2 \leq 200$ mm Hg

Bilateral infiltrates on the chest radiograph

Pulmonary artery occlusion pressure ≤ 18 mm Hg or clinical absence of left atrial hypertension

Data from Bernard GR, Artigas A, Brigham KL, et al. The American-European Consensus Conference on ARDS: Definitions, mechanisms, relevant outcomes, and clinical trial coordination. Am J Respir Crit Care Med 1994;149:818-824.

Table 41-2 Causes of Acute Respiratory Distress Syndrome

Causes of Direct Lung Injury	Causes of Indirect Lung Injury
Pneumonia	Sepsis
Aspiration of stomach contents	Severe trauma
Pulmonary contusion	Cardiopulmonary bypass
Reperfusion pulmonary edema	Drug overdose
Amniotic fluid embolus	Acute pancreatitis
Inhalational injury	Near-drowning Transfusion-related acute lung injury

Data from Ware LB, Matthay MA. The acute respiratory distress syndrome. N Engl J Med 2000;342:1334-1349.

Treatment

Treatment of ARDS remains supportive. There have been multiple clinical trials of pharmacotherapies targeting specific inflammatory mediators that are thought to be involved in the pathogenesis of ALI and ARDS, but thus far these treatments have generally been unsuccessful.

Ventilation Management

The ARDS Network (ARDSnet) trial of low-tidal volume ventilation in patients with ALI or ARDS showed decreased mortality rate in those receiving low tidal volumes (6 mL/kg) versus standard tidal volumes (12 mL/kg).[9] The hypothesis of the ARDSnet trial was that lower tidal volumes would "protect" the lung by preventing overdistention of normal regions of the lung. Consequently, the standard of care in critical care medicine is to ventilate all patients who have known or suspected lung injury with a low-tidal volume ventilation strategy.

When patients are ventilated with lower tidal volumes, they tend to have lower arterial oxygen tension and higher arterial carbon dioxide tension. This is termed permissive hypercapnia and hypoxemia, in recognition of the fact that to normalize arterial blood gas, significantly more harmful mechanical ventilation may be required. Although larger tidal volumes may improve oxygenation, they ultimately increase mortality rate. This is probably due to "volutrauma," in which excessive stretching of the lung releases injurious cytokines into the circulation.

SEDATION AND ANALGESIA IN THE INTENSIVE CARE UNIT

Sedation is used in the ICU to provide analgesia, anxiolysis, and amnesia and to protect the patient from dislodging or removing any indwelling lines, catheters, drains, or tubes. In certain instances, sedation is used to control or prevent seizures, reduce elevated intracranial pressure (ICP), and provide treatment for withdrawal from substances such as ethanol, benzodiazepines, and opioids. If patients are paralyzed with neuromuscular blocking drugs either as a result of a recent surgical procedure or for severe respiratory distress, effective and adequate sedation is essential.

Because of the risks associated with excessive sedation (prolonged mechanical ventilation, ventilator-associated pneumonia, pressure ulceration), sedation should be continuously evaluated with a sedation score and weaned as soon as possible (Table 41-3).[10] To achieve appropriate sedation, a variety of classes of sedative drugs (opioids, benzodiazepines, propofol, barbiturates, N-methyl-D-aspartate [NMDA] antagonists such as ketamine, and α_2-adrenergic receptor agonists) are used (Table 41-4).

VI

Table 41-3 The Ramsay Sedation Scoring System

Score	Response
1	Anxious and agitated or restless, or both
2	Cooperative, oriented, and tranquil
3	Responding to commands only
4	Brisk response to a light glabellar tap
5	Sluggish response to a light glabellar tap
6	No response to a light glabellar tap

Data from Ramsay MA, Savege TM, Simpson BR, et al. Controlled sedation with alphaxalone-alphadolone. BMJ 1974;2:656-659.

The choice of the specific drug used depends on the clinical situation and the drug effects that are desired. For example, an opioid is used to treat pain, whereas a benzodiazepine or propofol may be chosen to treat anxiety, withdrawal symptoms, seizures, or increased ICP.

Opioids (Also See Chapter 10)

Opioids (fentanyl, morphine, methadone, hydromorphone) are used primarily for analgesia and usually in combination with a sedative drug. As a class, opioids have very little effect on anxiolysis or amnesia unless the cause of anxiety is pain. Pain in the ICU may arise from many sources, including indwelling lines, catheters, and tubes; procedures performed in the ICU; recent surgeries; and simply lying in bed for an extended period. Fentanyl is most often used for its ease of administration, rapid pharmacokinetics, and lack of active or toxic metabolites. Opioids act via μ-receptors, and in patients receiving chronically large opioid doses, these receptors tend to become down-regulated and tolerance develops. As a result, progressively larger doses of opioids are required to achieve a desired effect. In this case, the addition of other non-narcotic pain medications may be helpful.

Methadone is a synthetic opioid that has some unique properties that make it especially useful in the ICU setting. Methadone has additional effects at the NMDA receptor, and because of this patients do not develop the same degree of tolerance to methadone as they do to other narcotics. Therefore, methadone is often used in patients with chronic pain who are already taking large doses of other narcotics and are quite tolerant to their effects. Methadone has a particularly long half-life, however, and care must be exercised when initiating this drug. Typically, the methadone dose is increased slowly to avoid oversedation.

Opioids are typically administered intravenously in the ICU, although certain drugs such as methadone have excellent bioavailability when given orally. When used intravenously, opioids may be administered by either repeated bolus injections or continuous infusion. Either method works satisfactorily to ensure adequate pain relief, provided that the bolus dosing interval is based on the drug's pharmacokinetics and pharmacodynamics and is titrated appropriately. If a continuous infusion is used, cumulation of the infused drug is a risk.

SIDE EFFECTS

The most dangerous side effects of opioids include respiratory and central nervous system (CNS) depression. Other side effects include constipation, urinary retention, and tolerance (manifested as increasing doses of drug to achieve the desired effect). It is important to note that a

Table 41-4 Commonly Used Sedatives and Analgesics

Drug	Elimination Half-Time	Peak Effect*	Suggested Dose
Morphine	2 to 4 hr	30 min	1- to 4-mg bolus 1 to 10 mg/hr
Fentanyl	2 to 5 hr	4 min	25- to 100-μg bolus 25 to 200 μg/hr
Hydromorphone	2 to 4 hr	20 min	0.2- to 1-mg bolus 0.2 to 5 mg/hr
Ketamine	2 to 3 hr	30 to 60 sec	1 to 20 mg/hr
Midazolam	3 to 5 hr	2 to 5 min	1- to 2-mg bolus 0.5 to 10 mg/hr
Lorazepam	10 to 20 hr	2 to 20 min	1- to 2-mg bolus 0.5 to 10 mg/hr
Propofol	20 to 30 hr	90 sec	25 to 100 μg/kg/min
Dexmedetomidine	2 hr	1 to 2 min	0.2 to 0.7 μg/kg/hr

*With intravenous administration.

patient never becomes tolerant to the constipating effects of opioids, and as the dose increases, this effect becomes even more pronounced. As a class, opioids are well tolerated with minimal effects on hemodynamics and organ perfusion and little impact on the metabolism of other drugs. However, when opioids are used in conjunction with other CNS depressants such as benzodiazepines or barbiturates, drug-induced CNS and respiratory depression may be amplified synergistically.

Benzodiazepines (Also See Chapter 9)

Benzodiazepines (midazolam, lorazepam) are administered to decrease anxiety and promote amnesia. In addition, they are often used to prevent or treat both seizures and alcohol withdrawal symptoms. Like opioids, benzodiazepines can be given either enterally or parenterally, but in the ICU they are most often given parenterally. Similar to opioids, a continuous infusion results in more stable and reliable plasma concentrations; however, the effects of the drug may accumulate. The effects become even more intensified when this class of drug is used in the elderly or patients with hepatic or renal failure. Weaning from mechanical ventilation after prolonged administration of these drugs must be done slowly because benzodiazepine withdrawal (as with ethanol withdrawal) can be life threatening.

Propofol (Also See Chapter 9)

Propofol is a hypnotic anesthetic with extremely rapid pharmacokinetics and pharmacodynamics, even when given by prolonged continuous infusion. It is this property that makes propofol so useful in the ICU. Propofol provides excellent amnesia and anxiolysis, but it has no significant analgesic effects. Therefore, an opioid is usually administered concomitantly with propofol. Propofol is especially useful in patients who require frequent neurologic examination. Because of its short elimination half-time and minimal accumulation, a patient can "wake up" a few minutes after discontinuation of a continuous propofol infusion and a reliable neurologic examination can be performed. It is also useful in preventing and treating seizures and in decreasing ICP.

SIDE EFFECTS

Hemodynamically, propofol has significant effects on decreasing myocardial contractility and reducing systemic vascular resistance. In hemodynamically unstable patients with low cardiac output or low afterload (or both), propofol must be used with caution. This property limits its usefulness in many unstable patients, such as postsurgical cardiac patients and those in profound shock.

Propofol is a profound respiratory depressant. Although most patients who receive propofol in the ICU are tracheally intubated and receiving mechanical ventilation, occasionally propofol may be used in patients whose tracheas are not intubated. An example is its use for procedural sedation (see Chapter 38). In this specific instance, extreme caution must be exercised to prevent severe respiratory depression with profound respiratory acidosis.

Propofol is formulated in a lecithin (egg white) solution, and as such, it is an excellent bacterial growth medium. Consequently, when a bottle is opened, it must be used relatively quickly to avoid contamination. Propofol also has a high fat content because of its lecithin base. Patients who are receiving long-term infusions of this drug must be periodically checked for hypertriglyceridemia. There have been many case reports of patients developing severe pancreatitis after prolonged propofol administration. Because of its high fat content, if a patient is receiving total parenteral nutrition (TPN) and then propofol is started, the Intralipid portion of the TPN needs to be reduced or eliminated altogether.

PROPOFOL INFUSION SYNDROME

This rare syndrome is associated with the prolonged use of propofol for sedation of a patient in the ICU setting. It is more common in children, and as a result, propofol is not approved for use in sedation of pediatric ICU patients,[11] although it continues to be widely and safely used in the operating room for pediatric sedation and anesthesia.

The definition of propofol infusion syndrome is controversial. In addition, this syndrome's rarity has contributed to difficulty in quantifying the actual risk of this syndrome in adult ICU patients. The occurrence of propofol infusion syndrome may be as frequent as 1% in the adult ICU population,[12] yet very few case reports have been published in adults. Generally, propofol infusion syndrome is defined as a relatively sudden onset of metabolic acidosis, with cardiac dysfunction, and at least one of the following findings: rhabdomyolysis, hypertriglyceridemia, and renal failure.[11] Hepatomegaly due to fatty liver infiltration and lipemia may be additional criteria.[13] The early cardiac findings include bradycardia and right bundle-branch block, both of which are relatively nonspecific findings. Of importance is that metabolic acidosis by itself is relatively common with prolonged high-dose (<5 mg/kg/day) propofol use, but it does not constitute propofol infusion syndrome. If propofol infusion syndrome is suspected, the propofol infusion should be discontinued immediately and another sedative drug should be chosen, as the mortality rate for this syndrome may be as high as 80%.[12]

Ketamine (Also See Chapter 9)

Ketamine is a dissociative anesthetic with profound analgesic effects even at low doses. Ketamine acts as an antagonist at NMDA receptors in the CNS. It produces potent psychomimetic effects with vivid hallucinations, similar to phencyclidine. As such, ketamine is usually

VI

prescribed along with a benzodiazepine or propofol, which will decrease its hallucinogenic effects. When given at small doses by continuous infusion (1 to 5 µg/kg/min), these adverse effects tend to be minimal, and ketamine may be given alone.

Ketamine is useful in the ICU because of its ability to produce profound analgesia without significant respiratory depression. This makes ketamine an excellent choice for patients with chronic pain who may require excessively large doses of opioids for pain relief, or in patients who are already on large doses of narcotics and in whom a further increase of narcotics will have minimal effects due to tolerance. Ketamine is also useful for patients who need to undergo brief, painful procedures (burn dressing changes) in the ICU.

Ketamine has intrinsic sympathomimetic properties that increase systemic blood pressure and heart rate during infusion. This may be useful when sedation and analgesia are required for a hemodynamically unstable patient. Ketamine is often combined with propofol in such patients to counteract the reduced blood pressure associated with propofol while providing adjuvant analgesia. However, ketamine is a direct myocardial depressant, and when given to a patient in shock, a decrease in arterial blood pressure should be anticipated. Ketamine increases ICP, increases the cerebral metabolic consumption of oxygen ($CMRO_2$), and decreases the seizure threshold. For these reasons, ketamine is infrequently used in neurosurgical patients or in any patients with an increased risk for seizures (also see Chapter 30).

Barbiturates

Barbiturates are used primarily to place patients in a "barbiturate coma" to suppress seizures in the setting of status epilepticus or to reduce ICP or $CMRO_2$ in the setting of brain injury. However, barbiturates also decrease arterial blood pressure and may therefore significantly decrease cerebral perfusion pressure. Because of its rapid metabolism, propofol has supplanted the use of barbiturates in the setting of pharmacologic neuroprotection. The frequency of inducing pharmacologic coma to reduce $CMRO_2$ may decrease because no significant benefit has been demonstrated.

α_2-Adrenergic Receptor Agonists

Examples of α_2-adrenergic receptor agonists are clonidine and dexmedetomidine. These drugs act by binding to α_2-receptors both centrally and peripherally. Central α_2-receptor binding at presynaptic neurons inhibits the release of norepinephrine. The central effects of these drugs produce analgesia, sedation, anxiolysis, and hypotension. With large doses, these drugs are anesthetics and induce a state that is very much like regular sleep. Patients will arouse when stimulated but rapidly fall back to sleep once the stimulation decreases. These properties make α_2-receptor agonists very effective drugs when patient cooperation is occasionally required, such as for frequent neurologic examinations.

At the level of the spinal cord, α_2-receptor activation is thought to modulate pain pathways, and this is the probable site of action for the analgesic effects of these drugs. These drugs also possess weak α_1-receptor affinity. With increasing doses, α_2-receptor agonists bind to peripheral α_1- and α_2-receptors, which induces vasoconstriction and hypertension with very large doses. Overall, in the recommended dosage range, their effect is to decrease systemic blood pressure by means of a decrease in both systemic vascular resistance and heart rate. Within the usual dose range, these drugs do not cause respiratory depression. However, because patients tend to fall asleep with larger dosages, these drugs can still cause upper airway obstruction and resultant hypoventilation. When comparing dexmedetomidine to midazolam for sedation of critically ill patients, dexmedetomidine is better because of reduced ventilator time, less delirium, and an improved quality of sedation.[14]

CLONIDINE

Clonidine can be administered by the oral, intravenous, intramuscular, transdermal, intrathecal, and epidural routes. It has a broad therapeutic index and as such is quite safe when given over a wide range of doses. Hypotension tends to be the limiting factor when administering this drug. At excessively large doses, essentially all α_2-receptors are saturated with agonist, and the less potent α_1-receptor effects tend to predominate.

DEXMEDETOMIDINE

Dexmedetomidine is an α_2-receptor agonist that is formulated for intravenous use only. It has a relatively short elimination half-time and is given by continuous infusion. Like clonidine, it has the same sedating and hemodynamic effects with smaller doses, with increasing systemic vascular resistance secondary to α_1 and α_2 effects at higher dosage ranges. However, dexmedetomidine has a much higher affinity for α_2-receptors than clonidine does, and as such it has an even broader therapeutic index. The usual dosage range for dexmedetomidine is 0.2 to 1.2 µg/kg/min. Bradycardia can be seen with larger doses or while rapidly escalating the dose of dexmedetomidine. This is due to a nodal blocking effect of α_2-receptor agonists along with decreased sympathetic tone and a corresponding increase in unopposed vagal tone.

Sedative Titration and Weaning from Mechanical Ventilation

As patients recover from their illness, they need to be weaned from mechanical ventilatory support and from sedation. Continuous sedative infusion is an independent risk factor for prolongation of mechanical ventilation. Patients who receive a continuous infusion have significantly longer periods of mechanical ventilation with correspondingly longer stays in both the ICU and hospital than do those who receive sedation by bolus administration or no sedation.[15] Nevertheless, continuous sedation is widely used because it is believed to provide improved patient comfort and hemodynamic control.

The preferred method for weaning from sedation is protocol driven.[16] Patients treated by daily interruption of their sedatives with retitration versus weaning only at the discretion of the ICU physician are successfully weaned from mechanical ventilation earlier and have shorter ICU lengths of stay. Rapid weaning of sedation does not increase complications such as inadvertent tracheal extubation. Protocol-driven weaning also decreases the length of ICU and hospital stay, which is not only cost effective but also likely to reduce time-dependent complications such as infection. Combining protocol-driven ventilator weaning with daily sedation interruption reduces both mortality rate and ICU length of stay, and should be developed as standing procedures in all ICUs.[17]

SHOCK

Shock is a common clinical condition in the ICU. Shock in any form results in inadequate tissue perfusion to end organs such as the brain, heart, liver, kidneys, and abdominal viscera. Shock represents an imbalance between oxygen demand and delivery. As such, when faced with inadequate oxygen delivery, organs begin to fail and multiorgan-system dysfunction and death result. Early in its course, shock may be reversible with proper diagnosis and effective treatment. However, if shock remains untreated, irreversible shock develops and death becomes inevitable.

Categories of Shock

The major categories of shock include hypovolemic, cardiogenic, septic, and other forms of vasodilatory shock (Table 41-5). Although all forms of shock are characterized by hypotension and inadequate tissue perfusion, the root cause of this hypotension is different in each case. In hypovolemic shock, hypotension is due to inadequate preload, whereas in cardiogenic shock, hypotension results from poor pump function and, in septic or vasodilatory shock, from low afterload.

HYPOVOLEMIC SHOCK
Hypovolemic shock is caused by decreased effective circulating blood volume and therefore inadequate ventricular preload. The most common cause of hypovolemic shock is major blood loss, such as occurs with trauma, surgery, or massive gastrointestinal hemorrhage.

Clinical Manifestations
With decreased preload, left ventricular end-diastolic volume and cardiac output decrease. In response to baroreceptor stimulation, the heart rate increases to maintain cardiac output. There is increased sympathetic nervous system outflow that constricts blood vessels, increases systemic vascular resistance, and diverts blood away from the skin and skeletal muscle beds to the brain and heart. As a result, the patient appears cool and clammy and has pale mucosa. Activation of the renin-angiotensin system ensues to increase sodium reabsorption and restore circulating blood volume. In addition, the release of catecholamines from the adrenal glands acts to inhibit insulin secretion and induce gluconeogenesis. The result is dramatically increased plasma glucose levels that help restore circulating blood volume by increasing the osmotic gradient for fluid reabsorption into the intravascular space.

Treatment
Treatment of hypovolemic shock involves restoration of circulating blood volume and treatment of the underlying cause of the hypovolemia. Treatment of the underlying cause of hypovolemic shock can be undertaken only when adequate intravenous access and aggressive fluid therapy are achieved. Vasopressor therapy may be used to increase systemic blood pressure, but it will probably be unsuccessful until intravascular volume is restored. Resuscitation can be guided with the use of data from central venous pressure or pulmonary artery catheters in concert with physical

VI

	Cardiac	Systemic Vascular	Central Venous	Pulmonary Capillary	Mixed Venous
Shock Type	**Output**	**Resistance**	**Pressure**	**Wedge Pressure***	**Oxygen Saturation**
Hypovolemic	↓	↑	↓	↓	↓
Cardiogenic	↓	↑	↑	↑*	↓
Vasodilatory	↑ or ↔	↓	↓	↓	↑ or ↔

Table 41-5 Characteristics of Various Shock States

*Pulmonary capillary wedge pressure is normal to low in right ventricular failure.

examination and measurement of metabolic variables. More recently, assessment of intravascular volume responsiveness using arterial blood pressure variation has attained widespread clinical usage as a more reliable assessment of circulating fluid volume.[18]

CARDIOGENIC SHOCK

Cardiogenic shock is characterized by failure of either or both ventricles. When the ventricle fails, preload increases and the ventricle cannot adequately eject the end-diastolic volume. This serves to further increase ventricular end-diastolic pressure, and eventually the ventricle becomes overdistended, which hastens the ventricular failure.

Clinical Manifestations

If the right ventricle is the initial site of failure, the increased right-sided preload will be noted as increased central venous pressure, detected clinically as distended neck veins, peripheral edema, or hepatic congestion. If the left ventricle fails, the increased preload can be detected as increased pulmonary capillary wedge pressure, which causes cardiogenic pulmonary edema and rales on physical examination. In this case, the right ventricle eventually fails under the increased pulmonary artery pressure afterload, and biventricular failure results.

In either scenario, cardiac output is low, and systemic blood pressure is therefore reduced. To counteract the hypotension, there is increased sympathetic outflow with resultant tachycardia and increased systemic vascular resistance. This compensatory mechanism initially works to increase blood flow to the brain and failing ventricle, but it simultaneously increases myocardial oxygen demand. Increased myocardial oxygen demand ultimately leads to worsening cardiac failure. On physical examination, a patient in cardiogenic shock appears cool and pale secondary to the high systemic vascular resistance and shunting of blood away from the skin and skeletal muscle beds.

Treatment

The goals in treatment of cardiogenic shock are to improve cardiac output and decrease afterload. These interventions allow the ventricle to eject more efficiently, decrease myocardial work, lower myocardial oxygen consumption, and reverse the dangerous spiral of cardiac failure. To oversee treatment, adequate monitoring is required, including the use of direct arterial and central venous pressure monitoring. In addition, echocardiographic and possibly pulmonary artery catheter measurements may be required to adequately treat these patients.

Depending on the type of cardiac failure and ventricular filling conditions, diuretics are generally indicated but must be used judiciously to avoid worsening the hypotension. Afterload and preload can be reduced with vasodilators and venodilators such as nicardipine, nitroglycerin, or nitroprusside. For inotropy, dobutamine is preferred because it improves cardiac output and reduces afterload with a minimal increase in myocardial oxygen demand. Additional interventions for left-sided cardiogenic shock include the use of intra-aortic balloon counterpulsation (IABP) and ventricular assist devices (VADs).

For right-sided failure, the goal of treatment is to reduce afterload with pulmonary vasodilators such as nitroglycerin, dobutamine, and even inhaled nitric oxide. An IABP may be placed for right-sided heart failure in order to improve coronary perfusion to the right side of the heart, despite the fact that no improvement of right-sided heart afterload will be gained with therapy. In extreme cases, a right-sided heart VAD may also be placed as a bridge to recovery or transplantation.

VASODILATORY SHOCK

Sepsis is the most common cause of vasodilatory shock, which is characterized by a low afterload state in which organ perfusion is impaired. Other major causes of this form of shock include anaphylaxis and neurologic dysfunction, such as stroke or spinal shock from a high spinal cord injury. Vasodilatory shock is often the final common pathway for the prolonged and severe hypotension resulting from late-stage shock of other causes, such as cardiogenic or hypovolemic shock. In all these conditions there is markedly reduced afterload with a redistribution of blood away from normally highly perfused organs (brain, heart, liver, and kidney) to large capacitance areas such as the skin and skeletal muscles.

Clinical Manifestations

Compensation for vasodilatory shock includes an increase in cardiac output mediated by increasing stroke volume and heart rate. Initially, increased cardiac output may provide adequate compensation. If left untreated, systemic vascular resistance continues to decrease with worsening metabolic acidosis. Myocardial perfusion becomes impaired, and the patient eventually progresses to cardiac failure as well. On physical examination, a patient in vasodilatory shock initially appears warm and vasodilated with increased peripheral blood flow secondary to vasodilatation in the skin and skeletal muscle beds. However, with progression to late, irreversible shock, the extremities become increasingly cold and poorly perfused.

Treatment

Treatment of vasodilatory shock involves initial intravenous fluid therapy until adequate preload is established, typically at a central venous pressure of approximately 8 to 12 cm H_2O. Vasopressors (phenylephrine, dopamine, epinephrine [especially for anaphylaxis], norepinephrine) are added if the patient remains hypotensive in an effort to increase systemic vascular resistance and cardiac output. The choice of drug depends on the specific clinical situation. As with all other forms of shock, the underlying cause of the disorder should be treated as soon as possible.

SEPSIS AND SEPTIC SHOCK

Septic shock is the final pathway of disseminated infection and, after respiratory failure, is the most common cause for admission to the ICU. The diagnosis of severe sepsis and septic shock is based on identifying the probable source of infection, the systemic inflammatory response to infection, and concomitant organ failure (Table 41-6).[19]

Patients with septic shock suffer an overwhelming systemic inflammatory response, with the final common pathway being multiple organ dysfunction and death. Essential for successful treatment of sepsis is early recognition, rapid resuscitation, early administration of broad-spectrum antibiotics, and identification of the source of infection, and prompt treatment of the infection.

Inotropic Drugs and Vasopressors

In the ICU patient population, shock is a common clinical disorder. As a result, inotropic drugs and vasopressors are often required to support cardiac output and systemic blood pressure. Many choices of vasopressors are available to the clinician, but there is little evidence regarding which vasopressor is preferred in a given clinical scenario.

DOPAMINE (Also See Chapter 7)

Dopamine has both direct and indirect agonist activity at the dopamine-1 (DA_1-), β_1-, and α_1-receptors. Its pharmacologic action varies with dose and within individuals as well. With small doses (0 to 5 µg/kg/min), dopamine has predominantly DA_1-receptor agonist activity, which causes dilatation of the renal arterioles and promotes diuresis. Small-dose dopamine may help convert oliguric renal failure to nonoliguric renal failure, which makes intravascular fluid management easier, but it does not protect the kidneys from ongoing failure.

At moderate doses (5 to 10 µg/kg/min), the β_1-adrenergic effects of dopamine begin to dominate. These β_1-adrenergic effects cause an increase in myocardial contractility, heart rate, and cardiac output. As a result, myocardial oxygen demand also increases. In fact, oxygen demand can increase more than myocardial oxygen delivery, with resultant myocardial ischemia.

At large doses (10 to 20 µg/kg/min), the α_1-agonist effects predominate and dopamine acts to increase vascular smooth muscle tone, which increases systemic vascular resistance. This causes a decrease in splanchnic and renal blood flow similar to the effects of large-dose phenylephrine. At all doses, dopamine mediates the indirect release of norepinephrine, which may be responsible for the tachycardia seen in some patients when dopamine is used at any dosage range.

Clinically, dopamine is regarded as a relatively weak vasopressor and is useful in mild hypotensive states. In patients who are in profound shock, dopamine is generally regarded as a second-line drug, and other more potent, direct-acting adrenergic agonists are preferred.

EPINEPHRINE (Also See Chapter 7)

Epinephrine causes direct stimulation of α_1-, β_1-, and β_2-receptors. At lower doses, epinephrine acts primarily as a β-receptor agonist, whereas at higher doses, it has increasing α_1-receptor effects. Increases in heart rate, myocardial activity, and cardiac output reflect β_1-receptor effects. The principal β_2-receptor effects are bronchial and vascular smooth muscle relaxation. With larger doses, the α_1-receptor effects of epinephrine act to increase systemic vascular resistance and reduce splanchnic and renal blood flow

Table 41-6 American College of Chest Physicians/Society of Critical Care Medicine (ACCP/SCCM) Consensus Conference Definitions for Sepsis

Definition	Criteria
Infection	Inflammatory response to microorganisms or invasion of normally sterile tissues SIRS (systemic inflammatory response syndrome) Clinical response to infection manifested by two of the following: Temperature >38° C or <36° C HR >90 beats/min Respirations >20 breaths/min or $Paco_2$ <32 mm Hg WBC count >12,000 cells/L or <4000 cells/L or 10% immature neutrophils
Sepsis	Confirmed or suspected infection plus two SIRS criteria
Severe sepsis	Sepsis and one organ dysfunction
Septic shock	Sepsis plus hypotension (<90 mm Hg) despite fluid resuscitation

HR, heart rate; WBC, white blood cell.
Data from Bone RC, Balk RA, Cerra FB, et al. Definitions for sepsis and organ failure and guidelines for the use of innovative therapies in sepsis: The ACCP/SCCM Consensus Conference Committee-American College of Chest Physicians/Society of Critical Care Medicine. Chest 1992; 101:1644-1655.

VI

while maintaining both cerebral and myocardial perfusion pressure.

Epinephrine also has anti-inflammatory effects by blocking the release of inflammatory mediators from mast cells and basophils. β-Activation in liver and skeletal muscle cells leads to increased gluconeogenesis via the adenylate cyclase signaling pathway. Both these actions function to increase blood glucose levels.

The main indications for epinephrine are in the management of cardiac arrest, severe cardiogenic shock, and anaphylactic and anaphylactoid reactions. When given as a continuous infusion, the usual range of epinephrine is between 1 and 20 μg/min. However, in patients with refractory, life-threatening shock, it may be necessary to administer epinephrine at even larger doses.

NOREPINEPHRINE (Also See Chapter 7)

Norepinephrine is a direct-acting adrenergic agonist with activity at both the α_1- and β_1-receptors. It is similar to epinephrine except that norepinephrine lacks the β_2-receptor effect of epinephrine and has much stronger α_1-receptor activity. As a result, norepinephrine increases arterial blood pressure through its α_1-effects on increasing systemic vascular resistance. The β_1-effects of norepinephrine also contribute to increased myocardial contractility and cardiac output.

Norepinephrine can be used for the treatment of septic shock. Its β_1-activity may help offset the myocardial dysfunction associated with severe sepsis and septic shock. Norepinephrine may even be the vasopressor of choice for patients in septic shock.

Norepinephrine must be given by continuous infusion, and the typical dose range is between 1 and 20 μg/min. At the lower end of this range there are more β_1-effects, whereas α_1-activity dominates with larger dosages.

PHENYLEPHRINE (Also See Chapter 7)

Phenylephrine is a direct-acting, highly selective α_1-receptor agonist which increases systemic vascular resistance and arterial blood pressure. Phenylephrine has no direct effect on myocardial function, but it can cause reflex bradycardia, which may decrease cardiac output. Phenylephrine is frequently used for the treatment of septic and other forms of vasodilatory shock to increase systemic blood pressure. However, it can also cause splanchnic ischemia, especially when used chronically with large doses.

Phenylephrine is often administered to brain-injured patients to improve cerebral perfusion pressure. Because it does not cross the blood-brain barrier, phenylephrine has no effect on the cerebral vasculature, but its ability to increase systemic blood pressure leads to increased cerebral blood flow. The typical dosage range for phenylephrine is up to 200 μg/min. Larger doses have little therapeutic effect, with only worsening of splanchnic ischemia.

DOBUTAMINE (Also See Chapter 7)

Dobutamine is a mixed β_1- and β_2-receptor agonist. As a result, the primary effect of dobutamine is to increase both heart rate and myocardial contractility. Dobutamine also relaxes vascular smooth muscle via binding at β_2-receptors. This combination acts to increase cardiac output by improving ventricular function (β_1-effect) and decreasing systemic vascular resistance (β_2-effect). Dobutamine is typically indicated for the treatment of patients in cardiogenic shock with high afterload and low cardiac output. It is one of the few drugs available to the clinician that will reduce pulmonary vascular resistance and possibly improve right-sided heart function.

Because of its β_2-effects, some patients may become hypotensive, particularly those with decreased intravascular volume. However, because dobutamine has a relatively short elimination half-time, its effects rapidly disappear once the infusion is discontinued. Dobutamine is given by continuous infusion only, and the usual dosage range is between 1 and 20 μg/kg/min.

VASOPRESSIN

Vasopressin is a potent vasoconstrictor that does not work via the adrenergic receptor system as do most other vasopressors. Rather, vasopressin binds to peripheral vasopressin receptors to induce potent vasoconstriction. Vasopressin provides a useful alternative to catecholamines, which do not function well in the setting of profound acidemia. Vasopressin remains efficacious as a vasoconstrictor even in the setting of severe acidosis.

Patients with severe sepsis and septic shock may have a relative deficiency of vasopressin. This group of patients is remarkably sensitive to the effects of vasopressin, and the usual dose ranges for vasopressin need to be reduced. For septic shock, the recommendation is to infuse vasopressin at 0.04 U/min. If the patient improves, the vasopressin infusion is discontinued, not weaned.

Vasopressin has been successfully used for cardiogenic shock. Patients who have recently been weaned from cardiopulmonary bypass may remain hypotensive secondary to a low afterload state. There is evidence that these patients also have a relative vasopressin deficiency, and vasopressin may be used to treat this form of vasodilatory shock. In these patients, the dose of vasopressin (0.1 U/min) is significantly larger than that used for septic shock.

ACUTE RENAL FAILURE

Acute renal failure (ARF) is a commonly encountered complication in the ICU. The consequences of ARF are devastating, possibly causing a higher mortality rate than does acute respiratory failure. The definition of ARF varies, but it is often described as an abrupt decrease in renal function, which is defined as urine output less than 0.5 mL/kg/hour or a 50% increase in serum creatinine over a 24-hour period.[20] Renal failure is normally categorized as prerenal (inadequate renal perfusion pressure), intrarenal (vascular, glomerular, or interstitial dysfunction), or postrenal (usually obstructive). In the management of ARF, prerenal failure must be recognized and treated by ensuring adequate intravascular fluid resuscitation and systemic arterial blood pressure Any postrenal obstruction can be detected by the use of ultrasound or other imaging techniques.

If the ARF is intrarenal, the cause is usually acute tubular necrosis. In addition to the history, which may include exposure to nephrotoxic drugs or prolonged hypotension, examination of urinary sediment may show renal tubular epithelial cells or granular casts. Management of ARF is supportive, with many patients ultimately requiring hemodialysis for the complications of ARF. Indications for acute hemodialysis include excessive intravascular volume, hyperkalemia, acidemia, uremia, toxins, or other electrolyte abnormalities. Hemodialysis may be intermittent or continuous (continuous renal replacement therapy, CRRT). Continuous hemodialysis has not been shown to be advantageous. Hypotensive patients often require continuous hemodialysis because of their inability to tolerate the intravascular volume shifts associated with intermittent hemodialysis, although the efficacy of intermittent hemodialysis is the same as that for CRRT.[21]

DELIRIUM

Delirium is a common and highly morbid condition in the adult ICU. Yet delirium is frequently not appropriately diagnosed or treated when it does arise.[22] Delirium is defined by the DSM-IV as a disturbance of consciousness with reduced ability to focus or sustain attention that is associated with a change in cognition or perceptual disturbances that are not accounted for by a preexisting dementia. These disturbances develop over a short period and tend to fluctuate throughout the course of the day.

Delirium can be divided into two different subtypes. Hyperactive delirium is the type with which most clinicians are familiar. It is characterized by periods of agitation, restlessness, and emotional lability, resulting in patients pulling out lines and catheters, or hitting and biting. Hypoactive delirium is the opposite form, and its hallmarks include a flat affect and apathy. Patients with this form may often seem calm and alert, although they suffer from the same cognitive changes as are in the hyperactive form. Both forms occur with equal frequency.

Delirium is widespread in the adult ICU population with estimated incidence between 48% and 87%.[23-25] Delirium is not a benign condition, or merely an inconvenience to patients and their care providers, as was once thought.

Delirium can be a cause of increased morbidity and mortality rates. Delirium is associated with an increased number of days a patient will spend mechanically ventilated, as well as increased days in the ICU and hospital.[23,24] In addition, delirium is associated with an increased risk of developing dementia in later life.[24] It is unclear whether delirium may actually cause dementia, or if patients who are at greatest risk of dementia or have an early subclinical form of dementia are more likely to have episodes of delirium in the ICU. Mortality rate among ICU patients is increased in those who develop delirium. These risks vary from a greater than threefold increase in 6-month mortality rate to a 10% increase in the risk of death for every day spent in a state of delirium in the ICU.[23]

The causes or conditions associated with delirium are numerous. Among these are preexisting cognitive impairment, advanced age, increasing severity of illness, multiorgan dysfunction, sepsis, immobilization, sleep deprivation, pain, mechanical ventilation, and the use of psychoactive drugs, especially benzodiazepines.[23-26] In order to actively prevent or treat delirium, it must be diagnosed first. The most widely used method of monitoring is the CAM-ICU assessment for delirium.[27] The CAM (confusion assessment method) should be used daily to assess for delirium in all ICU patients except those who are deeply sedated or comatose.

Once diagnosed, the treatment of delirium consists of several steps. First, prevention of the causes of delirium should be undertaken in all patients. Once delirium has occurred, active treatment to reduce the effects and duration of delirium must be accomplished as well. Prevention and treatment involve identification of possible causes and avoiding or reversing these causes as applicable. These actions may include improving pain control, preventing or reversing sleep deprivation, actively orienting a patient to the surroundings, avoiding the use of benzodiazepines, and minimizing the use of all sedatives if possible. Finally, if delirium still does occur, haloperidol may help improve orderly thought processes. Definitive data regarding the benefits of haloperidol do not exist.[28]

NUTRITIONAL SUPPORT

Critically ill patients require optimal nutrition for wound healing, maintenance of skeletal muscle mass, and prevention of infection. The nutritional status of most patients declines throughout the length of their ICU stay. Malnourished patients become increasingly catabolic and may have significant skeletal muscle wasting. Loss of skeletal muscle causes weakness, which may prolong ventilator weaning and decreases the ability to tolerate rehabilitation. Optimal nutrition may directly reduce infectious complications by maintaining immunocompetence, enhancing wound healing, and preventing bacterial translocation across gut mucosal cells.

VI

Enteral versus Parenteral Feeding

Patients may be fed either enterally (usually by a nasojejunal feeding tube) or parenterally (intravenously). It is always preferable to feed enterally. Advantages of enteral feeding include decreased cost, ease of administration, maintenance of normal gastrointestinal physiology, and less risk for infection. For example, parenteral nutrition formulas are easily infected, which greatly increases the risk for catheter-related blood stream infections. Additionally, without enteral feeding, the normal gastrointestinal tract begins to atrophy. Such atrophy causes loss of mucosal thickness, alteration of pH, and loss of gastrointestinal tract–associated lymphoid tissue. These changes can result in replacement of normal gastrointestinal tract flora with more pathologic organisms and increased translocation of these organisms across the increasingly atrophic gastrointestinal tissue.

Candidates for Enteral Feeding

Enteral feeding is often selected for patients with pancreatitis, enteric fistulas, inflammatory bowel disease, short-bowel syndrome, acute pancreatitis, hyperemesis gravidarum, and bone marrow transplants. Parenteral feeding is selected only for patients who cannot tolerate sufficient enteral feeding.

RAPID RESPONSE TEAMS

Patients who survive in-hospital cardiac arrest are typically admitted to the ICU. Because in-hospital cardiopulmonary arrests are relatively common, this patient group represents a significant percentage of all ICU admissions. Often, these patients have signs of physiologic instability long before the arrest event. Because of this, the Institute for Healthcare Improvement, as part of their 100,000 lives campaign, has recommended that hospitals utilize a system of rapid response teams to evaluate patients at risk of cardiopulmonary arrest prior to any significant clinical deterioration.[29]

Rapid response teams frequently utilize ICU professionals: physician intensivists, critical care nurse practitioners, ICU nurses, and respiratory therapists. These teams form a multidisciplinary group to evaluate and treat patients early in the course of a physiologic decline, and make interventions that will hopefully avert an impending cardiopulmonary arrest.

Despite the fact that the use of rapid response teams seems like it should improve patient care and outcome by making early interventions in unstable patients, and thereby reduce the number of in-hospital cardiac arrests, this has been difficult to demonstrate in clinical trials. Rapid response teams do function to decrease overall rates of cardiac arrests outside the ICU,[30,31] but based on numerous studies, the widespread use of rapid response teams does not reduce overall in-hospital cardiac arrests and overall in-hospital mortality rates.[31,32] Rapid response teams do find unstable patients earlier in the course of their decline, and these patients are then moved to the ICU earlier as well. However, these patients then seem to have their impending arrest in the ICU with no overall change in their mortality rates. The majority of published studies concerning the use of rapid response teams are single-center, unblinded, observational studies, and unless an actual treatment protocol is developed and implemented for these patients little actual results can be expected.

INTENSIVE INSULIN THERAPY

The optimal method of blood glucose control is not clear in critically ill patients. Initially, intensive insulin therapy to achieve a blood glucose level between 80 and 100 mg/dL was thought to be essential for improving survival in ICU patients.[33] However, intensive insulin therapy to keep very tight glucose control has recently been shown to not improve survival, but actually increases the risks of significant hypoglycemia.[34,35] Another recent multicenter study has shown that intensive insulin therapy actually increases mortality rate.[36] This is in part due to the increased episodes of hypoglycemia associated with strict control. Other factors such as increased insulin dosing to maintain tight glucose control may be important as well as insulin having pleiotropic effects. Currently, the best level at which blood glucose should be maintained in critically ill patients has not been precisely elucidated. Currently we suggest that a moderate range between 140 and 180 mg/dL should be maintained. This level minimizes the risks of severe hypoglycemia (less than 40 mg/dL) and hyperglycemia (more than 200 mg/dL).

END-OF-LIFE ISSUES

Despite delivering the best care possible, a large number of ICU patients will ultimately succumb to their illness. Approximately 1 in 5 Americans will die in the ICU.[37] Because of this fact, ICU physicians need to be as skilled in end-of-life care as they are in caring for critically ill patients. ICU physicians should regard death not as failure but as a normal part of life. Patients deserve the right to die with dignity and, if at all possible, in the manner that they see fit. Families deserve the right to assist in making decisions regarding their loved ones and to be treated with respect.

Occasionally, when a patient is suffering from a critical illness, the patient (or the family in accordance with the patient's wishes) may elect to stop treatment.

Sometimes only specific treatments are discontinued, and in other instances, all support (including mechanical ventilation, vasopressor support, and dialysis) is withdrawn. This is usually a difficult decision for patients and their families to make, and frequently the ICU physician is called on to help with this decision-making process.

In such patients, mechanical ventilatory support can be terminated and T-piece ventilation initiated with possible tracheal extubation, depending on family and physician preference. This can be accomplished in a peaceful and dignified manner. The patient is usually sedated during this process to relieve any discomfort that may be present. Patients should be given adequate sedation during the dying process, but the goal of sedation is always the relief of patient discomfort. Sedation is never given to hasten a patient's demise. Sedation that is given to relieve suffering may have the "double effect" of hastening death, but it is important that the intent of sedative or analgesic administration be the relief of discomfort. The ICU physician must convey to patients and their families that death is an inevitable part of life and can be approached with dignity.

QUESTIONS OF THE DAY

1. Which mechanical ventilation weaning strategies are most effective?
2. What are the diagnostic criteria for acute respiratory distress syndrome (ARDS)?
3. What are the manifestations of the propofol infusion syndrome?
4. What are the most important steps in the management of delirium in the ICU patient?
5. What is a rapid response team? What is the impact of rapid response teams on patient outcomes?
6. What is the optimal method of glucose control in the ICU patient?

ACKNOWLEDGMENTS

The editors and publisher would like to thank Drs. J.F. Tang and J.F. Pittet for contributing a chapter on this topic to the prior edition of this work. It has served as the foundation for the current chapter.

REFERENCES

1. Esteban A, Frutos F, Tobin MJ, et al: A comparison of four methods of weaning patients from mechanical ventilation, *N Engl J Med* 332:345–350, 1995.
2. Ely EW, Baker AM, Dunagan DP, et al: Effect on the duration of mechanical ventilation of identifying patients capable of breathing spontaneously, *N Engl J Med* 335:1864–1869, 1996.
3. Brochard L, Mancebo J, Wysocki M, et al: Noninvasive ventilation for acute exacerbations of chronic obstructive pulmonary disease, *N Engl J Med* 333:817–822, 1995.
4. Antonelli M, Conti G, Rocco M, et al: A comparison of noninvasive positive-pressure ventilation and conventional mechanical ventilation in patients with acute respiratory failure, *N Engl J Med* 339:429–435, 1998.
5. Esteban A, Frutos-Vivar F, Ferguson ND, et al: Noninvasive positive-pressure ventilation for respiratory failure after extubation, *N Engl J Med* 350:2452–2460, 2004.
6. Bernard GR, Artigas A, Brigham KL, et al: The American-European Consensus Conference on ARDS: Definitions, mechanisms, relevant outcomes, and clinical trial coordination, *Am J Respir Crit Care Med* 149:818–824, 1994.
7. Ware LB, et al: The acute respiratory distress syndrome, *N Engl J Med* 342:1334–1349, 2000.
8. Pepe PE, Potkin RT, Reus DH, et al: Clinical predictors of the adult respiratory distress syndrome, *Am J Surg* 144:124–130, 1982.
9. The Acute Respiratory Distress Syndrome Network: Ventilation with lower tidal volumes as compared with traditional tidal volumes for acute lung injury and the acute respiratory distress syndrome, *N Engl J Med* 342:1301–1308, 2000.
10. Ramsay MA, Savege TM, Simpson BR, et al: Controlled sedation with alphaxalone-alphadolone, *BMJ* 2:656–659, 1974.
11. Fudickar A, et al: Propofol infusion syndrome: Update of clinical manifestation and pathophysiology, *Minerva Anestesiol* 75:339–344, 2009.
12. Roberts RJ, Barletta JF, Fong JJ, et al: Incidence of propofol-related infusion syndrome in critically ill adults: A prospective, multicenter study, *Crit Care* 13:R169, 2009.
13. Kang TM: Propofol infusion syndrome in critically ill patients, *Ann Pharmacother* 36:1453–1456, 2002.
14. Riker RR, Shehabi Y, Bokesch PM, et al: Dexmedetomidine vs midazolam for sedation of critically ill patients: A randomized trial, *JAMA* 301(5):489–499, 2009.
15. Kollef MH, Levy NT, Ahrens TS, et al: The use of continuous IV sedation is associated with prolongation of mechanical ventilation, *Chest* 114:541–548, 1998.
16. Kress JP, Pohlman AS, O'Connor MF, et al: Daily interruption of sedative infusions in critically ill patients undergoing mechanical ventilation, *N Engl J Med* 342:1471–1477, 2000.
17. Girard TD, Kress JP, Fuchs BD, et al: Efficacy and safety of a paired sedation and ventilator weaning protocol for mechanically ventilated patients in intensive care (Awakening and Breathing Controlled Trial): A randomised controlled trial, *Lancet* 371(9607):126–134, 2008.
18. Marik PE, Cavallazzi R, Vasu T, et al: Dynamic changes in arterial waveform derived variables and fluid responsiveness in mechanically ventilated patients: A systematic review of the literature, *Crit Care Med* 37(9):2642–2647, 2009.
19. Bone RC, Balk RA, Cerra FB, et al: Definitions for sepsis and organ failure and guidelines for the use of innovative therapies in sepsis: The ACCP/SCCM Consensus Conference Committee-American College of Chest Physicians/Society of Critical Care Medicine, *Chest* 101:1644–1655, 1992.
20. Lameire N, et al: Acute renal failure, *Lancet* 365:417–430, 2005.
21. The RENAL Replacement Therapy Study Investigators: Intensity of renal-replacement therapy in critically ill

VI

patients, *N Engl J Med* 361:1627–1638, 2009.

22. Ely EW, Stephens RK, Jackson JC, et al: Current opinions regarding the importance, diagnosis, and management of delirium in the intensive care unit: A survey of 912 heath care professionals, *Crit Care Med* 32:106–112, 2004.

23. Thomason JW, Shintani A, Peterson JF, et al: Intensive care unit delirium is an independent predictor of longer hospital stay: A prospective analysis of 261 non-ventilated patients, *Crit Care* 9:R375–R381, 2005.

24. Ely EW, Shintani A, Truman B, et al: Delirium as a predictor of mortality in mechanically ventilated patients in the intensive care unit, *JAMA* 291:1753–1762, 2004.

25. Pisani MA, Murphy TE, Araujo KL, et al: Benzodiazepine use and the duration of ICU delirium in an older population, *Crit Care Med* 37(1):177–183, 2009.

26. Pandharipande P, Shintani A, Peterson J, et al: Lorazepam is an independent risk factor for transitioning to delirium in intensive care unit patients, *Anesthesiology* 104:21–26, 2006.

27. Ely EW, Inouye SK, Bernard GR, et al: Delirium in mechanically ventilated patients: validity and reliability of the Confusion Assessment Method of the Intensive Care Unit (CAM-ICU), *JAMA* 286:2703–2710, 2001.

28. Girard TD, et al: Delirium in the intensive care unit, *Crit Care* 12(Suppl 3):S3, 2008.

29. Berwick DM, Calkins DR, McCannon CJ, et al: The 100,000 lives campaign: Setting a goal and a deadline for improving health care quality, *JAMA* 295(3):324–327, 2006.

30. Offner PJ, et al: Implementation of a rapid response team decreases cardiac arrest outside of the intensive care unit, *J Trauma* 62:1223–1228, 2007.

31. Chan PS, Khalid A, Longmore LS, et al: Hospital-wide code rates and mortality before and after implementation of a rapid response team, *JAMA* 300(21):2506–2513, 2008.

32. Chan PS, Jain R, Nallmothu BK, et al: Rapid response teams, *Arch Intern Med* 170:18–26, 2010.

33. Van den Berghe G, Wouters P, Weekers F, et al: Intensive insulin therapy in critically ill patients, *N Engl J Med* 345:1359–1367, 2001.

34. The COIITSS Study Investigators: Corticosteroid treatment and intensive insulin therapy for septic shock in adults, *JAMA* 303(4):341–348, 2010.

35. Wiener RS, et al: Benefits and risks of tight glucose control in critically ill adults, *JAMA* 300(8):933–944, 2008.

36. The NICE-SUGAR Study Investigators: Intensive versus conventional glucose control in critically ill patients, *N Engl J Med* 360:1283–1297, 2009.

37. Angus DC, Barnato AE, Linde-Zwirble WT, et al: Robert Wood Johnson Foundation ICU End-of-Life Peer Group. Use of intensive care at the end of life in the United States: An epidemiologic study, *Crit Care Med* 32:638–643, 2004.

42 TRAUMA, BIOTERRORISM, AND NATURAL DISASTERS

Eric Y. Lin

Trauma remains one of the leading causes of morbidity and death in the world, with an estimated 5 million people dying each year from injuries. As the number one cause of death among those younger than 45 years old, trauma causes a disproportionate burden to society in terms of "quality-adjusted life years" lost and disability.[1] Over the last half-century, improved prehospital care and the establishment of specialized trauma centers have improved overall outcomes following trauma. The most specialized trauma centers (e.g., Level I hospitals) provide immediate coverage by providers from many disciplines, including anesthesia, critical care, emergency medicine, neurosurgery, orthopedic surgery, radiology, and trauma surgery. Resources such as emergency room space, operating rooms, radiology suites, intensive care unit (ICU) beds, and blood products are kept in a state of constant readiness at such Level 1 hospitals. Mass casualty events also occur frequently worldwide (e.g., Japan in 2011) and can produce large numbers of trauma patients that require substantial resources and preparedness. The anesthesia provider is a critical member of trauma and disaster response teams and must be immediately available to take care of severely injured patients from the moment they arrive.

BASIC PRINCIPLES OF TRAUMA CARE

Most trauma-related deaths occur within what has been termed "the golden hour" after injury, usually as a result of uncontrolled hemorrhage. Even beyond this first hour, delays in diagnosis or treatment lead to increased morbidity and mortality rates. The immediate goals in trauma care are therefore to (1) keep the patient alive; (2) identify life-threatening injuries; (3) stop any ongoing bleeding; and (4) complete definitive treatment as early as possible. Trauma response teams work to avoid all delays in the diagnosis and treatment of life-threatening injuries, even if the initial history and physical examination must be abbreviated to do so.

ACUTE MANAGEMENT OF TRAUMA PATIENTS

A standardized emergency trauma algorithm, such as that of the Advanced Trauma Life Support (ATLS) course,[2] is essential to providing timely and consistent care (Table 42-1). Acute management should proceed sequentially through the "ABCDEs" of trauma resuscitation: Airway, Breathing, Circulation, Disability, and Exposure/Environment. This initial assessment, termed the "Primary Survey," is performed rapidly to identify and treat any immediately life-threatening condition. Once these vital functions are intact, then a more detailed "Secondary Survey" should be performed that includes a complete physical examination and any necessary laboratory and diagnostic studies. If the patient becomes unstable at any point during management, providers should immediately return to the Primary Survey, again starting with the "Airway."

Airway and Breathing (Also See Chapter 16)

Evaluation always begins with an assessment of airway and breathing. If the trachea is already intubated, proper location of the endotracheal tube must be immediately confirmed. Upper airway obstruction can be relieved with simple jaw thrust or oral airway placement, but maneuvers such as head-tilt and mask ventilation should be avoided owing to cervical spine precautions and risk of aspiration. In most cases, physical examination and mechanism of injury are enough to initially determine the need for securing the airway.

Endotracheal intubation is indicated if a patient is not adequately oxygenating or ventilating, or if there is high risk of impending airway compromise (Table 42-2). Prior to endotracheal intubation, the patient should be breathing 100% oxygen, and a final check of resources should be performed (Table 42-3). Thoracostomy tube placement or pericardiocentesis should be considered prior to positive-pressure ventilation if pneumothorax or pericardial tamponade are suspected. All trauma patients require

Table 42-1 Algorithm for Initial Trauma Management

- Preparation—space, equipment, protection, personnel
- Assumption of care from prehospital providers—note mechanism of injury, interventions done
- Primary survey—ABCDEs, life support interventions
- Secondary survey*—detailed examination and history, laboratory and diagnostic studies
- Definitive care*

*Acute instability requires return to start of primary survey. ABCDEs, airway, breathing, circulation, disability, exposure/environment.

Table 42-2 Indications for Endotracheal Intubation in Trauma Patients

Inadequate airway protection
Loss of consciousness
High spinal cord injury
Aspiration
Impending loss of airway
Severe maxillofacial fractures
Neck hematoma
Inhalational (burn) injury
Laryngeal or tracheal injury
Stridor
Inadequate ventilation
Severe closed head injury (Glasgow Coma Scale score ≤8)
Poor respiratory efforts
Inadequate oxygenation

Table 42-3 Preparations for Endotracheal Intubation

- **S**uction (functioning and turned on)
- **O**xygen (breathing circuit and ventilator connected to oxygen sources)
- **A**irway equipment (face mask, oropharyngeal airways, laryngoscopes, endotracheal tubes, laryngeal mask airways, video laryngoscope, circothyrotomy kit, fiberoptic scopes)
- **P**harmaceuticals (hypnotics, neuromuscular blocking drugs, vasopressors)
- **I**ntravenous access
- **M**onitors (blood pressure, pulse oximeter, electrocardiogram, capnography devices)
- **S**pecial equipment
- Personal protection (eye protection, masks, gloves, gown)
- Assistants to help with cervical spine and aspiration precautions
- Tension pneumothorax supplies (angiocatheters, thoracostomy tube trays)
- Tracheotomy tray

full stomach precautions (i.e., evacuation and alkali), with a rapid sequence induction of anesthesia and application of cricoid pressure to prevent aspiration of gastric contents (see Chapter 14). Etomidate (0.1 to 0.3 mg/kg IV) or ketamine (1.0 to 3.0 mg/kg IV) are often used for induction of anesthesia because these drugs have few cardiovascular effects. Opiates and benzodiazepines are also frequently used (see Chapter 25). Doses of anesthetics should be reduced in most trauma patients, as blunting of

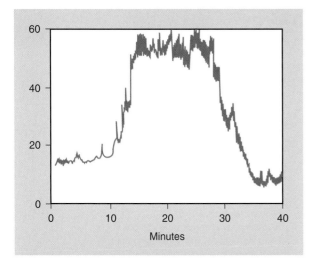

Figure 42-1 Diagram of a plateau wave causing severe intracranial hypertension. A plateau wave is an abrupt and sustained (10 to 20 minutes) increase in intracranial pressure followed by a rapid decrease, often to a level lower than the previous baseline.

compensatory sympathetic tone can lead to cardiovascular collapse in severely hypovolemic patients. Succinylcholine (1.5 mg/kg IV) is most commonly used for neuromuscular blockade and can be used safely in the first 24 hours following trauma or burn if no other contraindications exist. In most cases, large-dose rocuronium (1.2 mg/kg IV) is a suitable alternative (also see Chapter 12). If patients have suspected intracranial hypertension, lidocaine or fentanyl can be given to blunt the risk of plateau waves with stimulation (Fig. 42-1). The cervical spine should be stabilized for most trauma patients with altered mental status or distracting injury to avoid neck extension during direct laryngoscopy.[3] Despite increased use of video laryngoscopy for endotracheal intubation, no clear benefit over direct laryngoscopy has been demonstrated. Therefore, it should not be routinely used as the initial technique.[4] Alternative emergency supplies for tracheal intubation must always be available, including cricothyrotomy and tracheotomy kits. For patients who are likely to be difficult to tracheally intubate or unable to tolerate positive-pressure ventilation, securing the airway may be most safely done in the operating room, possibly via awake fiberoptic bronchoscopy. Vital signs should be continually monitored throughout airway management, with aggressive intravascular fluid and vasopressor therapy if needed.

Circulation and Shock

Once airway and breathing are stable, circulation is evaluated next. Adequate circulation is confirmed quickly by checking for mentation and a palpable pulse. Cardiac arrest requires immediate intervention as per ACLS algorithms (see Chapter 44) and will usually be due to uncontrolled hemorrhage. Pericardial tamponade, tension pneumothorax, and myocardial contusion should also be considered, particularly in patients with chest injuries. Emergent bedside thoracotomy is indicated for pulseless electrical activity following penetrating chest trauma. Hypotension with bradycardia can be a sign of neurogenic shock in patients with brain or spinal cord injuries.

Shock is defined as inadequate perfusion to vital organs. Tachycardia and hypotension, changes in mental status, and cool skin are traditional markers of shock and must be noted. However, these signs may be absent in patients with early or compensated shock. Increased base deficit or lactate levels are more sensitive and specific markers of shock after trauma, and one or both should be checked at the time of admission in all patients with severe injuries.[5]

Trauma patients with identified shock should be suspected of having ongoing bleeding until proven otherwise. The mechanism and location of injury are important clues in identifying sources of bleeding. Massive hemorrhage can occur into the thoracic, abdominal, or pelvic cavities. In patients with suspected hemothorax, a thoracostomy tube should be placed and can help diagnose active intrathoracic bleeding. Chest tube output of more than 1500 mL immediately or 200 mL/hour warrants emergent surgical exploration. Abdominal trauma often results in splenic rupture or liver laceration, both of which can result in profound hemorrhage. Early Focused Assessment with Sonography in Trauma (FAST) examination is increasingly being used in all trauma patients to detect free intra-abdominal fluid or pericardial effusion. Continued hematuria after placement of a bladder catheter indicates a possible bladder injury and the need for a cystogram or intravenous pyelogram. Pelvic instability indicates pelvic ring disruption; a pelvic binder or similar device should immediately be applied. Long bone fractures should similarly be placed on traction and splinted. Computed tomography (CT) is often the diagnostic test of choice to better evaluate injuries and hemorrhage within the head, thorax, abdomen, and pelvis. CT angiography can be used to identify vascular injuries. Only hemodynamically stable patients should be transported to CT, however; unstable patients require immediate definitive intervention.

Intravenous fluid resuscitation is the initial therapy for shock following injury. Even in critically ill trauma patients without ongoing hemorrhage, early and aggressive fluid replacement is associated with improved outcomes[6] (also see Chapter 23). ATLS-based guidelines dictate 2 L of warmed isotonic crystalloid on arrival for all trauma patients. Among the different crystalloid solutions available, lactated Ringer's is generally preferred over normal saline to avoid causing a hyperchloremic metabolic acidosis. Resuscitation with colloid fluids, such as albumin, is not commonly used. Persistent or worsening shock despite crystalloid therapy should prompt resuscitation with

VI

primarily blood products, starting with emergency type O packed red blood cells (PRBCs) until typed and crossmatched products are ready for the patient (also see Chapter 24). If available, whole blood with a short storage duration is effective. Arterial and central venous catheters should be inserted early in unstable patients, and the use of pressurized infusion devices may be helpful. Overzealous resuscitation, however, can increase blood loss, cause hemodilution, and disrupt early hemostatic clots. Hypotensive fluid resuscitation to a target systolic blood pressure of 80 to 100 mm Hg has become the widely accepted goal until hemorrhage control is achieved, particularly for penetrating trauma victims.[5,6] Higher arterial blood pressure may be targeted, using intravenous vasopressors or fluids, in patients with head or spinal cord injury if necessary to maintain adequate perfusion pressure.

In patients requiring massive transfusion (>10 units in 24 hours), the risk of death from uncontrolled hemorrhage remains high. This fact, coupled with recent recognition that 25% to 30% of major trauma patients have coagulopathy at the time of admission, early and empiric administration of either fresh whole blood or a "balanced resuscitation" fluid of PRBCs, fresh frozen plasma (FFP), platelets, and cryoprecipitate is becoming the standard practice for massive transfusion[5] (also see Chapter 24). Many trauma centers now target an FFP-to-PRBC unit ratio of 1:1 to 1:3 with minimal crystalloid administration and early use of platelets and cryoprecipitate. Because the benefit of "balanced resuscitation" in massive transfusion is largely undefined, however, blood product transfusion after hemorrhage control should be based on evidence of coagulopathic bleeding and abnormal laboratory values to avoid complications such as transfusion-related acute lung injury and abdominal compartment syndrome.[7]

Disability (Neurologic Injury)

The "D" in the "ABCDEs" of trauma resuscitation stands for disability, or neurologic injury (in contrast to the acronym used in ACLS). The basic level of consciousness is rapidly noted in the primary survey, while a more complete neurologic examination is performed as part of the secondary survey to assess the presence of traumatic brain, spine, or spinal cord injuries. A critical part of this evaluation is calculation of a patient's Glasgow Coma Score (GCS) (Table 42-4), as a GCS of 8 or less suggests severe traumatic brain injury (TBI) and a higher risk of death. Loss of consciousness, history of severe blow to the head, pupillary dilatation, and altered mental status may also indicate TBI. Early CT of the head should be performed to assess for intracranial hypertension or hemorrhage and the need for emergent intervention.

Hypotension, hyperthermia, hypoxia, and increased intracranial pressure predict worse outcome in patients with TBI (also see Chapter 30). Arterial blood pressure should be maintained to support a cerebral perfusion

Table 42-4 Glasgow Coma Scale	
Eye opening (E4)	
Spontaneous	4
To speech	3
To painful stimulation	2
No response	1
Verbal response (V5)	
Oriented to person, place, and date	5
Converses but is disoriented	4
Says inappropriate words	3
Says incomprehensible sounds	2
No response	1
Motor response (M6)	
Follows commands	6
Makes localizing movements to pain	5
Makes withdrawal movements to pain	4
Flexor (decorticate) posturing to pain	3
Extensor (decerebrate) posturing to pain	2
No response	1

pressure greater than 60 mm Hg. Mild hypothermia is permitted, but induced hypothermia does not benefit in TBI. One hundred percent oxygen is initially administered at high levels, and early endotracheal intubation is associated with improved outcomes in severe TBI. If increased intracranial pressure (ICP) is suspected, methods to decrease ICP should be employed (see Chapter 30). These methods include optimal position (see Chapter 19), hyperosmolar therapy with mannitol (0.25 to 1.4 g/kg IV over a period of 15 to 30 minutes) or hypertonic saline (2 mg/kg of 7.5% or 30 mL of 23%), intravascular fluid restriction and diuretic administration, drainage of cerebrospinal fluid, and drug therapy to decrease both cerebral blood flow and metabolic requirements.[8,9] Glucose-containing solutions should not be administered because of the potential for hyperglycemia and hypotonicity. Steroids have no benefit in TBI.[10] Hyperventilation should be performed only in cases of impending herniation, prior to decompressive craniectomy. Although decreases in $Paco_2$ can decrease ICP through cerebral vasoconstriction and reduced cerebral blood flow, this also increases the likelihood of ischemia and prolonged hyperventilation leads to worse neurologic outcomes. If emergent hyperventilation is needed, $Paco_2$ should not be decreased to below 30 mm Hg.[8,9]

Spinal fractures and spinal cord injuries are assessed through neurologic examination and palpation of the spine. Trauma patients with unclear history or loss of consciousness must be treated with cervical spine precautions until clinically cleared. CT has replaced plain films as the best way to diagnose cervical spine fractures. This can frequently be done in conjunction with torso scanning to save time and also assess the thoracic and lumbar spine. The cervical spine collar should not be removed until the patient can reliably deny pain with neck motion, as ligamentous injury is still possible despite normal CT results. If there is evidence of unstable fracture or cord compression, providers should immediately consult neurosurgery, maintain adequate perfusion pressures, and consider steroid therapy.

Exposure/Environment

The last of the "ABCDEs" refers to exposure and environment. Exposure of the patient is necessary in order to perform a complete examination. All clothing and prehospital dressings are removed to avoid missing any injuries. This also separates the patient from potentially contaminated material. Examination of the back and neck, often hidden by the hard backboard and cervical spine collar, must also not be forgotten.

Environment refers to both the current hospital environment and any environmental agents that contributed to injury. Hypothermia can cause coagulopathy and cardiac dysfunction and is associated with increased mortality rate following trauma. The room temperature should always be kept warm, the patient should be re-covered with warm blankets or external warming devices, and all administered fluids should be warmed.

Environmental agents that cause injury include thermal, chemical, radiation, and biologic agents. In cases of known radiation or chemical injury, removal of clothing should be followed by warm irrigation of the skin and open wounds. Because detection of certain agents may be difficult on initial survey, a high index of suspicion must be maintained. Early isolation of select patients and the use of specialized protective clothing and respirators by health care providers can be critical to minimizing casualties. The management of mass casualty situations and specific agents is described later in this chapter. Regardless of the specific agent involved, providers should always adhere to basic principles of trauma care and treat associated life-threatening injuries as early as possible.

Thermal Injuries (Burns)

Special considerations for burn patients should be taken into account on arrival. Initial prognostic factors in burn patients include extremes of age, larger total body surface area (BSA) burns, and coexisting inhalational injury. Presence of all three factors predicts a mortality rate approaching 90%.[11] Patients burned in a closed space are at higher risk for both carbon monoxide poisoning and inhalational injury, and 100% oxygen should be initially administered while determining carboxyhemoglobin levels and need for intubation. Inhalational injury should also be suspected if patients have facial burns, singed nasal hair, voice changes, or carbonaceous sputum. Mild edema can progress rapidly to complete airway obstruction and require an emergent surgical airway. Patient stridor, supraglottic swelling, or fiberoptic visualization of soot or inflammation

in the trachea all dictate immediate endotracheal intubation.[12] Soon after arrival, the patient's percentage of BSA with second- and third-degree burns is estimated using the rule of nines: 9% for each upper extremity and the head and neck region, 18% for each lower extremity and each side (anterior and posterior) of the trunk, and 1% for the perineal area. Special burn charts are used to estimate pediatric burns. The initial rate of fluid administration is then calculated by the Parkland formula (recently renamed the Consensus formula): 4 mL/kg body weight per percent of BSA burned equals the volume of lactated Ringer's solution to be given in the first 24 hours, half of which should be given within the first 8 hours since time of injury (not arrival) and the other half over the next 16 hours. More important, this calculated fluid rate should be continuously adjusted (e.g., to target a urine output of 0.5 mL/kg/hour) because complications occur from both under-resuscitation and over-resuscitation. Colloids have no advantage over lactated Ringer's solution and may worsen outcomes.[13] Intravenous or intraosseous access should be established early and ideally away from burned skin, but can be done through third-degree burns if necessary. Emergent escharotomies may be necessary in cases of compartment syndrome or decreased thoracic compliance, and burn wounds are later managed with excision and skin grafting. Early transfer to a burn center improves outcomes for patients with significant burn injury.[13]

EMERGENCY SURGERY FOR TRAUMA

Through initial assessment and management, patients with ongoing hemorrhage or neurologic emergencies are identified and transported directly to the operating room or angiography suite for definitive treatment. Surgical treatment of life-threatening injuries should precede any treatment of associated burn, chemical, or radiation injuries. Delays in transfer to the operating room and hemorrhage control are considered major and preventable causes of intraoperative death, and anesthesia providers play a major role in the early achievement of definitive care for these patients.

Preoperative Preparation

A "trauma operating room" should always be available and appropriately equipped (Table 42-5). There is no ideal anesthetic plan for a trauma patient, but general anesthesia is almost always necessary for those requiring emergency surgical intervention. In addition to standard ASA monitoring, patients should have an intra-arterial catheter for continuous blood pressure and serial blood gas monitoring. Two large-bore peripheral intravenous catheters and a central venous catheter, all ideally above the diaphragm, are used for monitoring and administration of fluids and drugs. Transesophageal echocardiography

VI

Table 42-5 Devices and Equipment Needed in a Trauma Operating Room

Well-equipped anesthesia machine and carts
Pressure transducer lines setup and zeroed
Ventilator able to deliver volume-control and pressure-control modes
Rapid fluid infusion and warming devices
Cell saver machine
Forced air warmer and warm ambient environment
Eye protection, masks, gloves, gowns
Anesthesia records, laboratory slips
Difficult airway cart with bronchoscopes
Echocardiography machine and probes
Ultrasound machine for vascular access
Direct telephone lines to the clinical laboratory/blood bank
Emergency resuscitation cart with defibrillator, pacer
Arterial blood gas machine, hemoglobin machine, glucometer
Crystalloid and colloid solutions
Emergency type O-negative blood (preferred)

should be available and can be used to diagnose injury and guide fluid therapy. Blood products should be available prior to incision if possible, with activation of the massive transfusion protocol if necessary. All fluids should be run through fluid warmers or rapid infusion devices. Cell saver technology may also be helpful.

Management of Anesthesia

If the trachea was not already intubated prior to surgery, the airway should be secured with rapid sequence induction of anesthesia and appropriate precautions as described earlier. Maintenance of anesthesia is typically accomplished with small doses of inhaled anesthetic or benzodiazepines, depending on hemodynamic stability. The level of anesthesia tolerated by the patient is often too small to prevent movement, necessitating maintenance of neuromuscular blockade throughout surgery. Intravenous antibiotics should be administered prior to incision and redosed at regular intervals or with excessive blood loss. Because of coexisting lung injury and potential for long-term critical care needs, patients should be ventilated with a low tidal volume lung protective strategy.

Intraoperative fluid management follows the same principles as discussed earlier for circulation management, maintaining adequate blood volume while optimizing

conditions for hemorrhage control. Acidosis and hypothermia can contribute to coagulopathy, and therefore, respiratory compensation and active warming is routine practice. In cases of more severe acidosis, trishydroxymethyl amino methane (THAM) is increasingly being used in massive transfusion cases. Drugs such as recombinant factor VIIa and antifibrinolytics may be considered early in profound coagulopathic bleeding but have not demonstrated benefit in clinical trials, should not be used routinely, and are unlikely to help as last-line approaches. Arterial blood gases, hematocrit and platelet count, coagulation factors, and electrolytes should be measured at frequent intervals to assess the progress of resuscitation and surgery. Restoration of base deficit to normal predicts better outcome, but persistence or worsening of base deficit suggests under-resuscitation and increased blood loss. As a general rule, opening of an enclosed space (pleural, peritoneal, retroperitoneal, or dural) with recent hemorrhage can precipitate cardiovascular collapse as the decrease in extravascular pressure can trigger uncontrolled hemorrhage. Good communication between the anesthesia and surgical teams is therefore essential. Temporizing measures such as packing, aortic cross-clamping, and the use of agents such as vasopressin may be needed periodically to restore perfusion pressure and circulating volume. Once hemorrhage control is achieved, hemodynamic values typically improve and greater levels of anesthesia and analgesia can be tolerated. Control of hemorrhage should also signal a transition to more long-term critical care management of the patient, including more restrictive strategies of blood transfusion. This should also be the management for stable trauma patients undergoing urgent but not life-saving procedures.

SPECIAL CONSIDERATIONS
Abdominal Injuries

High-energy penetrating injuries to the abdomen such as gunshot wounds require surgical exploration. Low-energy injuries such as stab wounds can be managed medically if local exploration reveals no violation of the peritoneum. Blunt trauma is generally caused by collisions or falls and the need for emergent surgery is determined by the severity of injury. Blunt splenic and liver injuries are increasingly managed with a nonoperative approach of ICU monitoring and sequential hematocrit measurements if there are no signs of ongoing bleeding. Patients with active hemorrhage are now increasingly managed through "damage control" surgery, whereby the initial operation is shortened and focused primarily on rapid hemorrhage control, with delay of definitive repair until the patient is fully resuscitated and stabilized in the ICU. For patients with intra-abdominal bleeding, the technique of abbreviated laparotomy with therapeutic packing has gained worldwide adoption over the last 20 years with reported improvement in survival.[14]

Pelvic Fractures

Pelvic fractures are most commonly seen following motor vehicle accidents and are found in as much as 25% of victims with multiple injuries. The overall mortality rate from pelvic fractures is between 15% and 50%, depending on the extent of the injuries. The initial treatment of unstable pelvic fractures is closure of the ring with a pelvic binder. The pelvic ring can also be closed with a bed sheet or pelvic C-clamp. Unlike other sources of bleeding that are treated emergently in the operating room, patients with ongoing pelvic bleeding are taken emergently for angiogram and possible embolization, as extraperitoneal packing has traditionally worse outcomes but can be performed if angioembolization is not available or possible.[15] Following embolization, patients often undergo external fixation of the fractures. The optimal algorithm for a multitrauma patient requiring both pelvic angioembolization and operating room intervention is unclear and largely dependent on the patient's injuries and institutional bias.

Postoperative Care (Also See Chapters 39 and 41)

Severely injured patients usually require continued postoperative support and monitoring in an ICU environment. Patients with hemodynamic instability or resuscitation with large volumes of fluid typically have their endotracheal intubation, sedation, and paralysis sustained during transport to the ICU. Appropriate and necessary drugs and equipment should accompany the patient to the ICU. A transport ventilator is preferred if oxygenation or ventilation (or both) needs to be continuously supported. Drain and chest tube output should be closely monitored for evidence of recurrent hemorrhage and need for return to the operating room. All patients with abdominal injury should be monitored for abdominal compartment syndrome (intra-abdominal pressure greater than 20 mm Hg associated with new organ dysfunction) because of the large fluid shifts and increased vascular permeability.

MASS CASUALTY DISASTERS

Large numbers of patients can suddenly require critical care at any time due to natural, unintentional, and intentional disasters (Table 42-6). In recent years, events such as the World Trade Center attacks of September 11, 2001, Hurricane Katrina in 2005, the H1N1 influenza pandemic of 2009-2010 and the earthquake and tsunami in Japan in early 2011 have served as vivid reminders of the constant and real threat of catastrophic incidents. These types of disasters require substantial resources, preparedness, and organization at many different levels to minimize morbidity and mortality rates. Governments, communities, and individual providers, particularly

Table 42-6	Disasters That Result in Mass Casualties
Natural	
Hurricanes	
Tornados	
Floods	
Earthquakes	
Fires	
Unintentional	
Public transportation accident	
Boat accident	
Nuclear accident	
Industrial accident	
Building collapse/sports stadium disaster	
Intentional	
Bombing	
Nuclear attack	
Biologic attack	
Chemical attack	

Adapted from Murray MJ. Disaster preparedness and weapons of mass destruction. In Barash PG, Cullen BF, Stoelting RK (eds). Clinical Anesthesia, 5th ed. Philadelphia, Lippincott Williams & Wilkins, 2006, pp 1521-1537.

anesthesia providers,[16,17] must be well prepared and well informed in order to protect their own welfare and save the lives of others.

Role of Government

If an incident has widespread effects or requires more than local agencies can manage, state or federal emergency management systems are activated. In the United States, state governors can activate disaster plans utilizing national resources, and nearly all federal agencies have predefined responsibilities in the event of national disasters (Table 42-7). Many governments maintain a national pharmaceutical stockpile program with resources ready for prompt deployment to disaster sites if needed. The U.S. Centers for Disease Control and Prevention, for example, continuously monitor domestic and international threats to public health and have the capability of delivering medications, equipment, and personnel at any time via aircraft within 2 to 6 hours of notification. Military services may also be needed to contain exposures, ensure public safety, or establish field hospitals if local hospitals are compromised.

Community Preparedness

The initial response to any mass casualty incident will start at the local level. Community preparedness for disasters is critical because additional resources are unlikely to arrive within the first 24 to 72 hours. Communities must assess and maintain a "surge capacity" on a daily basis in order

VI

Table 42-7 Key United States Government Agencies and Responsibilities in Mass Casualty Disasters

Agency	Responsibility
Federal Bureau of Investigation	Domestic terrorism and crisis management
Federal Emergency Management Agency (FEMA), now part of the Department of Homeland Security	Coordinates national emergency response. Provides assistance to local and state governments, emergency relief to affected persons and businesses, and support for public safety.
Department of Health and Human Services	Provides health-related and medical services.
Department of Defense	Assists with biologic or chemical terrorism, bomb disposal, and decontamination.
Centers for Disease Control and Prevention	Coordinates response to public health threats and provides resources to local and state organizations.

Table 42-8 Emergency Management Standards for Hospitals*

Develop a management plan that addresses emergency management:
- Mitigation
- Preparedness
- Response
- Recovery

Perform a hazard vulnerability analysis:
- Establish emergency procedures in response to a hazard vulnerability analysis.
- Define the organization's role with that of other community agencies.
- Notify external authorities of emergencies.
- Notify hospital personnel when emergency procedures are initiated.
- Assign available personnel to cover necessary positions.
- Manage the following activities:
  - Patient/resident activities
  - Staff activities
  - Staff/family support
  - Logistics of critical supplies
  - Security
  - Evacuation of the facility if necessary
- Establish internal/external communication systems.
- Establish an orientation/education program.
- Monitor ongoing drills and real emergencies.
- Determine how an annual evaluation will occur.
- Provide alternative means of meeting essential building and utility needs.
- Identify radioactive and biologic isolation and decontamination sites.
- Clarify alternative responsibility of personnel.

Involve the community in the response.

Reestablish and continue operations after a disaster.

*Requirements for hospital accreditation by The Joint Commission (www.jcrinc.com/).
Adapted from Murray MJ. Disaster preparedness and weapons of mass destruction. In Barash PG, Cullen BF, Stoelting RK (eds). Clinical Anesthesia, 5th ed. Philadelphia, Lippincott Williams & Wilkins, 2006, pp 1521-1537.

to handle the potentially thousands of patients produced by disasters. Recent experience with terrorist attacks and natural disasters, especially the 2011 earthquake in Japan, has also shown that better communication is needed to improve outcomes in future disasters. Law enforcement agencies, fire and rescue services, and health care organizations must have a coordinated emergency response plan in place and familiarity with the command and control structure. This plan should include protection of personnel, continual assessment of resources, and means for expanding surge capacity. All hospitals are expected to meet published standards of emergency management (Table 42-8) and create or participate in such community preparedness plans.[18]

Role of the Anesthesia Provider

Anesthesia providers must be familiar with their hospital's disaster plan in anticipation of what their roles may be should a disaster occur. Like all physicians, they need to recognize and maintain the clinical competencies needed for emergency preparedness in the event of a large disaster (Table 42-9). It is difficult to predict all possible roles that anesthesia providers may be required to fulfill in managing victims of terrorist attacks or natural disasters. Although they will be needed in the operating room, their knowledge of physiology and pharmacology, combined with expertise in airway management and acute resuscitation, will likely be important in the triage area, emergency department, and intensive care unit as well (Table 42-10).[16,17] Because anesthesia providers are at increased risk for inhaled exposure, direct contact with pathogens, and spread of blood-borne infection, familiarity with basic isolation and decontamination techniques is essential to prevent secondary exposures.

Triage of Victims

Triage of mass casualty victims must be done early and rapidly, ideally at the scene, in order to maximize resources and patient survival. Because patients may outnumber the available resources, triage in mass casualty events is designed to classify individuals not only on severity of

Table 42-9 Clinical Competencies for Clinicians and Emergency Preparedness

Clinicians should be able to:

- Describe their role in the emergency response
- Respond to an emergency event within the emergency management system
- Recognize an illness or injury as potentially resulting from exposure to weapons of mass destruction
- Report identified cases or events through the public health care system
- Recognize that their institution may be a target
- Be prepared to diagnose and treat victims of bioterrorism
- Be familiar with the characteristics of (investigational) vaccines (efficacy, side effects/benefits) offered to potential first responders
- Identify and manage expected stress and anxiety
- Participate in postevent feedback (after-action report)

Table 42-10 Role of the Anesthesia Provider in Mass Casualty Disasters

- Decontamination
- Triage
  - Immediate—life-saving care needed acutely
  - Delayed—hospitalization, but survival expected even if treatment is delayed
  - Minimal—minor injuries, no hospitalization
  - Expectant—not expected to survive or already dead
- Operating room—intervention
- Intensive care unit—burns, flail chest, traumatic amputations

Adapted from Murray MJ. Disaster preparedness and weapons of mass destruction. In Barash PG, Cullen BF, Stoelting RK (eds). Clinical Anesthesia, 5th ed. Philadelphia, Lippincott Williams & Wilkins, 2006, pp 1521-1537.

illness but also on the likelihood of benefit from emergency intervention and surgery. A number of mass casualty triage systems exist (e.g., SALT, START, SAVE, MASS) and providers should be aware of the structure used in their particular health care system.[19,20] All triage systems seek to accomplish the same goals: prioritize injuries and apply limited resources to achieve the greatest benefit from surgical or medical intervention. Critically injured patients who are expected to die of their injuries (classified as "expectant") should be separated from the main patient flow and kept in a quiet, reassuring environment with attention to providing analgesia and comfort. The remaining victims are classified based on whether they require immediate, urgent, or delayed treatment.

Prehospital Care

Prior to hospital admission, patients are stabilized per usual trauma principles but with greater consideration given to resource limitations, crush or blast injuries, and possible exposures to chemical, biologic, or radioactive agents. All providers must wear full protective gear. Contaminated clothing is removed and the victim's skin decontaminated at the scene before transportation. Soap and water are effective decontaminants, and if available, a dilute solution (0.5% to 2%) of hypochlorite (household bleach) can be used to decontaminate the skin.[21] Patients may require on-scene establishment of intravenous access for fluid resuscitation and appropriate antidotes.

Tracheal intubation at the injury scene may be necessary in some cases, particularly with chemical agent exposure. The conditions themselves may make intubation even more difficult, and the technique to facilitate the process is based on the expertise of the health care provider and the availability of drugs.[22] An awake, blind nasal intubation may be the preferred technique for securing the airway, as these patients may be difficult to position and have a high risk of aspiration. Ketamine is often used, with or without benzodiazepines, for procedures such as limb amputation that may be required to facilitate extraction of trapped victims. If intubation attempts are unsuccessful, supraglottic devices such as a laryngeal mask airway or an esophageal-tracheal combitube have good success as rescue devices.

Hospital Care

Though prehospital decontamination is ideal, hospitals should still have decontamination facilities as part of their disaster preparedness plan. When possible, patients should be met on arrival and taken to a well-demarcated decontamination-treatment area that is isolated from the main hospital. Due to limitations in resources, surgeries are typically limited to life-saving or limb salvage procedures. Frequently, there is no time for preoperative evaluation, and resuscitation strategies may need to be altered because of scarce supplies.[23]

ANESTHETIC TECHNIQUES

Like the prehospital setting, an awake intubation may still be the preferred method for securing the airway in the hospital. Induction agents are not needed and spontaneous ventilation is preserved, which is significantly beneficial if there will be more intubated patients than available ventilators. Airway nerve blocks are helpful in facilitating intubation while the patient is awake. Induction of anesthesia is often accomplished with ketamine or etomidate, with or without a benzodiazepine. The choice of agent for maintenance of anesthesia depends largely on the condition of the patient and hospital resources. Regional anesthesia with a peripheral nerve

VI

block may be appropriate for select surgeries, but a central neuraxial block is usually avoided because of hypovolemia and the risk of severe hypotension.

POSTOPERATIVE CARE

As with the management of any trauma victim, these patients may require continued intravascular fluid volume resuscitation, mechanical ventilation, and frequent assessment. Invasive monitoring is continued, and provision of additional sedation and analgesia may be required. The postoperative period may also be the first time available to document the patient's name and injuries and complete the anesthetic record.

NUCLEAR EXPOSURE

Exposure of large populations to ionizing radiation is most likely to result from (1) nuclear power plant or reactor accidents, (2) terrorist actions, or (3) detonation of nuclear bombs. This chapter is being edited soon after the huge 2011 Japan earthquake and tsunami, which clearly indicates the potential dangers for the future. There is no doubt that much will be learned from the experience in Japan. Radiation exposure may result from external sources (beta particles, gamma rays), contaminated debris, or inhaled gases. Predictable injuries from nuclear accidents include radiation burns, bone marrow suppression, destruction of the gastrointestinal tract mucosa and bleeding with translocation of bacteria, and septic shock.[24] Although the effects of a blast, crush, or thermal injury are readily apparent, the effects of ionizing radiation are not usually evident.

Like other disaster victims, patients exposed to radiation are stabilized and decontaminated, preferably at the site of exposure if possible to avoid bringing radioactive material into the hospital. External decontamination is done by removing all clothing and rinsing the skin with warm soapy water. The skin is impermeable to most radionuclides, but open wounds should also be decontaminated with copious irrigation. Internal decontamination may be equally important to remove and isolate all biologic materials contaminated with radioisotopes. This is accomplished with methods such as gastric lavage, emetics, laxatives, and diuretics. Because radiologic contamination poses little risk to health care providers, standard trauma protocols are followed and interventions for life-threatening injuries must precede any treatment of associated radiation injury.[24]

Once stabilized, radiation-exposed victims should be admitted to the ICU and monitored for signs of acute radiation syndrome (thrombocytopenia, granulocytopenia, nausea, vomiting, diarrhea). Potassium iodide (Lugol's solution) can prevent radiation-induced thyroid effects (e.g., cancer), but it must be given within 24 hours to be effective.[25] Granulocyte colony-stimulating factor may be helpful for the management of postirradiation sepsis.[24] Ammonium chloride, calcium gluconate, and diuretics may be administered to facilitate renal excretion. Chelation therapy may include calcium and zinc diethylenetriamine penta-acetic acid.[26] All body orifices (nostrils, ears, mouth, rectum) should be swabbed and a 24-hour stool and urine collection performed if internal contamination is considered. The white blood cell counts should be serially checked, with neutropenic precautions taken when appropriate.

CHEMICAL AND BIOLOGIC TERRORISM

Chemical-biologic terror attacks, more so than other mass disasters, place the medical responders at significant risk of secondary exposure. Specific chemical or biologic weapons are selected in large part on their ability to rapidly and widely cause morbidity, death, and panic (Table 42-11).[27,28] Such agents include viruses, bacteria, toxins, neuropeptides, nerve agents, vesicants (e.g., mustard gas), cyanogens, and lung-damaging agents (e.g., phosgene). A cluster of casualties with similar exposure and symptoms is the first clue to detection, and may include emergency medical personnel who were exposed when participating in rescue attempts. Once a chemical or biologic exposure is suspected, it is critical to (1) clearly demarcate the contaminated zone, (2) establish entry and exit points, and (3) institute existing procedures to provide self-protection and decontaminate victims.[21] Antidotes to specific chemicals do exist, although treatment of nerve agent and cyanide toxicity would require the administration of antidote within minutes to be effective. Proper

Table 42-11 Characteristics of Effective Biologic Weapons
Easy to produce in large quantities
Inexpensive
Readily transported and disseminated (inhalational more effective than oral forms)
Odorless and tasteless
Survives drying and aerosolization
Highly infectious and contagious
Results in widespread morbidity and mortality
Lacks natural immunity
Places significant demands on public health and governmental resources
Results in panic and social disruption

Adapted from Coursin DB, Ketzler JT, Kumar A, et al. Bioterrorism may overwhelm medical resources. Anesth Patient Safety Found Newsletter Spring 2002, pp 4-8; available at http://www.apsf.org.

protection must be worn at all times and measures must be taken to limit the toxicity and latency of the exposure agent.[16] Even after on-scene decontamination, providers should wear protective suits to prevent cutaneous absorption. A pressure demand, self-contained breathing apparatus should also be used if pulmonary chemical agents (e.g., phosgene or chlorine gas) are involved or if the agent is unknown.[29]

The most common chemical and biologic agents are discussed here. Because of the rapidly changing nature of chemical and biologic terrorism, updated detection and treatment information about these and other agents should be reviewed regularly. Such information can be accessed from the web sites of agencies such as the Centers for Disease Control and Prevention, public health organizations, and the Department of Defense.

BIOTERRORISM AGENTS

Biologic weapons are divided into three categories, A through C, based on their potential to cause widespread harm (Table 42-12).[17] The Category A agents, which pose the greatest threat to public health, will be discussed in greater detail in this section. Health care providers must remain alert to illness patterns and diagnostic clues that might signal a bioterrorist attack (Tables 42-13 and 42-14).[27]

Anthrax

Anthrax is a gram-positive, spore-forming bacillus that is transmitted to humans from contaminated animals or their by-products (Table 42-15).[30] The three primary types of anthrax are cutaneous, inhalational, and gastrointestinal. Weaponized anthrax is intended to infect by

Table 42-13 Epidemiologic Features Suggesting Exposure or Infection with Biologic Weapons
Unusually high incidence or mortality rate from a disease cluster
Single case of an unusual pathogen (inhaled anthrax, smallpox)
Cluster of patients with a suspicious clinical illness Flulike illness leading to acute respiratory distress syndrome, shock, meningitis (anthrax) Acute febrile illness with pustular lesions (smallpox)
Occurrence of a disease outside its natural geographic boundaries (hemorrhagic fever, tularemia, plague)
Cluster of patients with acute flaccid paralysis (botulism)
Clustering of diseases that affect animals as well as humans

Adapted from Coursin DB, Ketzler JT, Kumar A, et al. Bioterrorism may overwhelm medical resources. Anesth Patient Safety Found Newsletter Spring 2002, pp 4-8, available at http://www.apsf.org.

inhalation. Inhalational anthrax initially presents with typical influenza-like symptoms followed by seeming recovery. Unlike typical viral illnesses, however, patients then develop profound respiratory failure and chest pain (Table 42-16).[30] The most notable radiographic finding is a widened mediastinum due to central lymphadenopathy (Fig. 42-2).[30] Usually, when profound dyspnea develops, death ensues within 1 to 2 days. Weaponized anthrax has been engineered to be resistant to penicillin G. Ciprofloxacin or doxycycline is an effective treatment of anthrax.

Table 42-12 Bioterrorism Agents and Diseases		
Category A	**Category B**	**Category C**
(Highest priority; easily disseminated or transmitted, high mortality rate, public panic)	(Second-highest priority; moderate dissemination and morbidity rates, low mortality rate)	(Third-highest priority; emerging pathogens, not yet mass-engineered)
Bacillus anthracis (anthrax)	*Coxiella burnetii* (Q fever)	Various equine encephalitic viruses
Variola major (smallpox)	*Brucella* species (brucellosis)	
Yersinia pestis (plague)	*Burkholderia mallei* (glanders)	
Clostridium botulinum (botulism)	Enteric pathogens (*Escherichia coli, Salmonella, Shigella*)	
Francisella tularensis (tularemia)	Pathogens associated with water safety threats (*Vibrio cholerae, Cryptosporidium*)	
Hemorrhagic fever viruses (e.g., Ebola, Lassa, Marburg)	Various encephalitic viruses Various biologic toxins (e.g., ricin)	

Categories defined by the United States Centers for Disease Control and Prevention. Available at bt.cdc.gov/bioterrorism/.

VI

Table 42-14 Initial Management of Suspected Victims of Bioterrorism

- High index of suspicion based on clustering of unusual illnesses
- Protection of health care workers—gowns, gloves, masks
- Notification of hospital, public health, and governmental officials
- Decontamination of sick and exposed persons
- Triage (some patients will require isolation):
  - Designate a hospital ward and selected health care workers to care for patients with suspected infectious diseases.
  - Stable and noninfectious patients should be discharged to reduce the risk of exposure to contagious diseases.
- Labeling of all materials from affected patients with bioterrorist/biohazard tags
- Supportive therapy—fluids, ventilation, circulatory support
- Antimicrobial agents (if indicated)

Adapted from Coursin DB, Ketzler JT, Kumar A, et al. Bioterrorism may overwhelm medical resources. Anesth Patient Safety Foundat Newsletter Spring 2002, pp 4-8, available at http://www.apsf.org.

Smallpox

Routine vaccination for smallpox was discontinued in 1972 in the United States, and in 1980 the World Health Organization announced that the world was free of the variola virus.[31] Smallpox is highly infective, with only 10 to 100 organisms required to infect an individual. The clinical manifestations of smallpox in an unvaccinated individual include a prodrome of malaise, headache, and fever as high as 40° C (Table 42-17).[27,31] The fever decreases over the next 72 to 96 hours, at which time the rash appears. This pattern contrasts with chickenpox, in which the rash and fever develop simultaneously. All cutaneous lesions of smallpox are at the same stage, whereas chickenpox lesions are at multiple stages (papules, vesicles, pustules, scabs). Most cases of smallpox are transmitted through aerosolized droplets that are inhaled, but clothes and blankets that have come in contact with pustules are infectious. Strict isolation of patients with smallpox is critically important. Vaccination of contacts is effective in the first 3 to 7 days after exposure.

Plague

Rodents and fleas are the natural hosts for the gram-positive bacillus that causes plague (Table 42-18).[27] Humans are accidental hosts and most commonly acquire the disease from a flea bite. As an aerosolized weapon the bacillus is viable for approximately 60 minutes. The two types of plague are bubonic and pneumonic. With bubonic plague, there is a 2- to 6-day incubation period

Table 42-15 Pathophysiology of Anthrax (*Pasturella anthracis* Infection)

Infectivity	High if weaponized airborne type
Incubation period	1-7 days
Clinical features	Inhalational: flu-like illness followed by respiratory distress, shock, meningitis Gastrointestinal: abdominal pain, peritonitis, shock Cutaneous: painless ulcers progressing to a black eschar
Mortality rate	Inhalational or gastrointestinal: 80%-95% Cutaneous: 25%
Chance of secondary infection or spread	Little or none from a victim with an established infection
Diagnosis	Gram-positive bacilli on Gram stain and blood culture Widened mediastinum on chest radiograph or computed tomography scan
Precautions	Avoid contact Bleach environmental surfaces Wash contaminated clothes and individuals
Treatment	Ciprofloxacin Doxycycline Penicillin (likely ineffective against weaponized form)
Prophylaxis for exposed patients	Antibiotics alone: Ciprofloxacin, doxycycline, or levofloxacin for 60 days Combined: Vaccine plus 30-day anitibiotic course

Adapted from Coursin DB, Ketzler JT, Kumar A, et al. Bioterrorism may overwhelm medical resources. Anesth Patient Safety Found Newsletter Spring 2002, pp 4-8, available at http://www.apsf.org.

after exposure, followed by a sudden onset of fever, chills, weakness, and headache. Intense painful swelling occurs in the lymph nodes, and this swelling ("buboes") is typically oval (1 to 10 cm in diameter) and extremely tender. Without treatment, patients develop septic shock with cyanosis and gangrene in peripheral tissues ("black death"). Pneumonic plague presents as a rapidly developing pneumonia, is highly contagious, and must be treated early to prevent death. The diagnosis is made by Gram stain or culture of organisms from blood, sputum, or buboes. Streptomycin, gentamicin, tetracycline, and chloramphenicol are all effective therapies and can also be used as prophylaxis in those directly exposed.

Table 42-16 Differentiation of Viral Flu-like Illness from Inhalational Anthrax

Clinical Manifestation	Viral Flu	Inhalational Anthrax
Fever, chills, myalgia	Yes	Yes
Nasal coryza	Yes	No
Pharyngitis	Common	Occasional
Cough	Yes	Yes
Substernal chest pain	Rare	Common
Dyspnea	Rare	Common
Abdominal pain	Rare	Common
Leukocytosis	No	Yes
Arterial hypoxemia	Rare	Common
Sepsis syndrome	Rare	Common
Mediastinal adenopathy on chest radiograph	No	Yes

Adapted from Coursin DB, Ketzler JT, Kumar A, et al. Bioterrorism may overwhelm medical resources. Anesth Patient Safety Found Newsletter Spring 2002, pp 4-8, available at http://www.apsf.org.

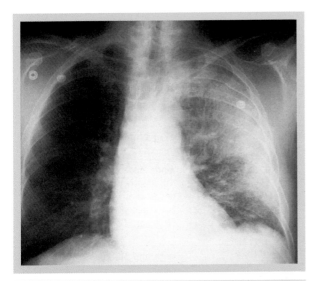

Figure 42-2 Chest radiograph showing a widened mediastinum in a patient with inhalational anthrax. (From Coursin DB, Ketzler JT, Kumar A, et al. Bioterrorism may overwhelm medical resources: New and different patient safety challenges must be anticipated. Anesth Patient Safety Found Newsletter, Spring 2002, pp 4-8; available at http://www.apsf.org, used with permission.)

Tularemia

Tularemia as a result of bioterrorism is caused by aerosolization of the gram-negative coccobacillus *Francisella tularensis*, and causes acute respiratory symptoms 3 to

Table 42-17 Pathophysiology of Smallpox (*Variola Major*)

Infectivity	High
Incubation period	7-14 days
Clinical features	Fever Headache Cough Centripetal pustules, all at the same stage of development, involving the palms and soles
Mortality rate	Overall: 35% No previous vaccination: >50% Vaccination >20 years before exposure: 11.1% Vaccination within 10 years of exposure: 1.4%
Chance of secondary infection or spread	Very high
Diagnosis	Electron microscopic evaluation of pustular material Culture
Precautions	Strict isolation (negative-pressure room)
Treatment	Supportive Cidofovir or ribavirin (?) Antibiotics for secondary bacterial infections
Prophylaxis for exposed patients and health care workers	Vaccination within 4 days of exposure (may prevent or significantly ameliorate infection)

Adapted from Coursin DB, Ketzler JT, Kumar A, et al. Bioterrorism may overwhelm medical resources. Anesth Patient Safety Found Newsletter Spring 2002, pp 4-8, available at http://www.apsf.org.

5 days after exposure, often accompanied by pleuritic pain and hilar lymphadenopathy (Table 42-19).[27,32] Transmission of tularemia from person to person has not been documented, so isolation of tularemia patients is not recommended. Streptomycin is the treatment of choice for isolated cases, but oral doxycycline or ciprofloxacin is the recommended treatment in mass casualty situations.[32]

Botulism

Botulism is a neuroparalytic disease caused by *Clostridium botulinum* toxin, the most potent known poison. Unlike other bioterrorism agents, botulism is caused by the toxin and not by the live organism; it is therefore

VI

Table 42-18 Pathophysiology of Plague (*Yersinia pestis* Infection)

Infectivity	Moderate to high for the pneumonic form
Incubation period	2-8 days
Clinical features	Pneumonic form: Fever Mucopurulent sputum Chest pain Hemoptysis Bronchopneumonia on chest radiograph Severe toxicity (shock common)
Mortality rate	Nonpneumonic form: 50% Pneumonic form: 100% if treatment is delayed
Chance of secondary infection or spread	High with the pneumonic form
Diagnosis	Sputum Blood culture
Precautions	Respiratory and contact isolation for 48 hours after initiation of antibiotics or negative sputum culture
Treatment	Streptomycin Gentamicin Tetracycline Chloramphenicol
Prophylaxis for exposed patients and health care workers	Postexposure prophylaxis for 7 days with tetracycline, doxycycline, sulfonamides, or chloramphenicol

Adapted from Coursin DB, Ketzler JT, Kumar A, et al. Bioterrorism may overwhelm medical resources. Anesth Patient Safety Found Newsletter Spring 2002, pp 4-8, available at http://www.apsf.org.

Table 42-19 Pathophysiology of Tularemia (*Francisella tularensis* Infection)

Infectivity	High
Incubation period	3-5 days
Clinical features	Acute onset of nonspecific febrile illness—dry cough, pleuritic chest pain Atypical pneumonia on chest radiograph
Mortality rate	Undiagnosed: 30%
Chance of secondary infection or spread	None
Diagnosis	High index of suspicion Blood and sputum cultures Serology
Precautions	No isolation required
Treatment	Streptomycin
Prophylaxis for exposed victims	Streptomycin

Adapted from Coursin DB, Ketzler JT, Kumar A, et al. Bioterrorism may overwhelm medical resources. Anesth Patient Safety Found Newsletter Spring 2002, pp 4-8, available at http://www.apsf.org.

Table 42-20 Pathophysiology of Botulism (*Clostridium botulinum* Infection)

Infectivity	Moderate to high with intentional inhalational or gastrointestinal exposure
Incubation period	12-36 hours after inhalation or ingestion
Clinical features	Acute onset of bilateral neuropathy with symmetric descending weakness No sensory deficit No fever No hemodynamic instability
Mortality rate	With appropriate supportive care: <5%
Chance of secondary infection or spread	None
Diagnosis	Toxin detection in blood or stool
Precautions	Toxin is not contagious
Treatment	Trivalent equine antitoxin
Prophylaxis for exposed victims	Trivalent equine antitoxin if signs or symptoms are present

Adapted from Coursin DB, Ketzler JT, Kumar A, et al. Bioterrorism may overwhelm medical resources. Anesth Patient Safety Found Newsletter Spring 2002, pp 4-8, available at http://www.apsf.org.

not contagious (Table 42-20).[27,33] Ingestion or inhalation of *C. botulinum* is followed by distribution of the toxin to cholinergic receptors, where it blocks the release of acetylcholine by inhibiting the intracellular fusion of acetylcholine vesicles to the membranes for release. Skeletal muscle weakness (diplopia, dysphagia, dyspnea, paralysis) occurs between 12 and 36 hours after ingestion or inhalation of the toxin.[34] There is decreased salivation, ileus, and urinary retention. The toxin can be removed by gastric lavage and the use of cathartics. Tracheal intubation and mechanical ventilation of the patient's lungs may be required. Administration of trivalent antitoxin is indicated.

Viral Hemorrhagic Fever Syndrome

Viral hemorrhagic fever syndrome describes a viral process that is spread in nature by arthropod vectors but becomes highly infectious when weaponized as an aerosol (Table 42-21).[21] There is an abrupt onset of a febrile illness that may later evolve to shock and generalized mucous membrane hemorrhage. A high index of suspicion and early isolation is required to prevent rapid spread of the disease. Strict precautions must be taken by providers, and suspected or confirmed cases must be reported early to hospital and public health officials. Initial treatment involves supportive care and administration of ribavirin while awaiting diagnostic confirmation.

CHEMICAL TERRORISM AGENTS

The use of chemical agents in warfare was introduced during World War I and has recurred during isolated conflicts since that time. Chemical weapons are inexpensive in comparison to conventional and nuclear weapons and, when used against populations, create fear and panic combined with overwhelming demands on the health care system.[21,35] Most chemical agents are liquid at room temperature and heavier than air when vaporized (hydrogen cyanide is an exception). If exposed, one should ascend to higher levels, and even standing up provides some protection. Onset latency is longest with phosgene and chlorine, while nerve and blood agents have short latency times (seconds to minutes).

Nerve Agents

Nerve agents are military-grade chemicals similar to organophosphate pesticides. They act by inhibiting acetylcholinesterase (AChE), resulting in an accumulation of acetylcholine at nerve terminals. They were originally developed as pesticides but their toxicity made them unsafe for public use. Clinical manifestations include skeletal muscle fasciculations, weakness, and hyperthermia (nicotinic effects), as well as vomiting and diarrhea, bronchoconstriction, urinary and fecal incontinence, bronchorrhea, lacrimation, and salivation (muscarinic effects). The effect on heart rate is unpredictable, as it may be slow due to muscarinic effects, increased from nicotinic stimulation, or normal. Nerve agents are lipophilic, clear liquids that vaporize at room temperature and are absorbed through skin, mucous membranes, lungs, or gastrointestinal tract. Most nerve agents can be referred to by either a common name (e.g., Sarin) or its two-letter military designation (e.g., GB) (Table 42-22).[21] VX is the most potent known nerve agent; contact with as little as one drop can be fatal.

Table 42-21 Pathophysiology of Viral Hemorrhagic Fevers (Ebola, Marburg, Lassa Viruses)

Infectivity	Modest (inhalational)
Incubation period	5-10 days
Clinical features	Typical—acute onset of fever, myalgia, and headache Common—chest pain, cough, pharyngitis, nausea, vomiting, diarrhea Maculopapular rash on trunk after ~5 days of illness Hemorrhagic complications—petechiae, ecchymoses
Mortality rate	25% to 90%
Chance of secondary infection or spread	Modest
Diagnosis	High index of suspicion Enzyme-linked immunosorbent assay
Precautions	Respiratory and contact isolation
Treatment	Ribavirin Immune serum
Prophylaxis for exposed victims or health care workers	Ribavirin Immune serum

Adapted from Coursin DB, Ketzler JT, Kumar A, et al. Bioterrorism may overwhelm medical resources. Anesth Patient Safety Found Newsletter Spring 2002, pp 4-8, available at http://www.apsf.org.

Table 42-22 Examples of Chemical Weapons

Common Name	U.S. Military Code
Nerve Agents	
Tabun	GA
Sarin	GB
Soman	GD
Cyclosarin	GF
VX	VX
Pulmonary Agents	
Chlorine	CL
Phosgene	CG
Skin Agents (Vesicants)	
Sulfur mustard	HD
Nitrogen mustard	HN$_1$
Lewisite	L
Phosgene oxime	CX
Blood Agents	
Hydrogen cyanide	AC
Cyanogen chloride	CK
Arsine	SA

Adapted from Murray MJ. Chemical weapons compromise provider safety. Anesth Patient Safety Found Newsletter Spring 2002, pp 12-14, available at http://www.apsf.org.

VI

Nerve agent exposure is treated with atropine (2 to 6 mg IV or IM) and pralidoxime (600 to 1800 mg IM). Atropine is administered every 5 to 10 minutes (in extreme cases, doses of atropine may exceed 100 mg) until secretions begin to decrease and ventilation is improved. Pralidoxime is a longer-acting anticholinergic drug that unbinds the nerve agents from AChE and reactivates the enzyme. Automatic injectors are available and allow self-administration of 2 mg of atropine and 600 mg of pralidoxime IM. Pyridostigmine, which reversibly binds to AChE, can provide protection from nerve agents if administered 30 minutes before exposure.

Pulmonary Agents

Phosgene is a colorless gas with an odor of recently cut hay and is the most deadly of the pulmonary agents. Because of a vapor density of 3.4, it stays in the air for prolonged periods and accumulates in low-lying areas. It is highly soluble in lipids and can easily penetrate pulmonary epithelium and cells lining the alveoli. Phosgene reacts with water to form hydrochloric acid and carbon dioxide. Hydrochloric acid is irritating to tissues and causes capillary leak and the development of acute lung injury. Coughing, nausea, vomiting, choking, and chest tightness occur. After initial exposure there may be a brief symptom-free period (1 to 24 hours), but lung injury is occurring and pulmonary edema follows. Gas masks provide the best protection against the effects of phosgene and other pulmonary agents such as chlorine gases. When sufficient quantities of phosgene are inhaled to cause acute lung injury, management is similar to that for patients with noncardiogenic pulmonary edema (acute respiratory distress syndrome). The patient's airway, oxygenation, and ventilation must be supported, and hemodynamics monitored closely.

Blood Agents

Blood agents used in chemical terrorism are typically cyanogens. When inhaled, these agents release hydrogen cyanide that impairs cytochrome oxidase and aerobic metabolism at the level of the mitochondria. The resulting metabolic acidosis and the sequelae of cellular hypoxemia are lethal. Symptoms depend on the exposure dose and range from dyspnea and restlessness to convulsions, coma, and cardiac arrest. Hydrogen cyanide itself is a colorless liquid that can be absorbed through the skin, but its high volatility makes it difficult to use as a biologic weapon. Treatment is with thiosulfate, similar to the treatment of nitroprusside toxicity. Administration of thiosulfate provides the necessary sulfur substrate for the enzyme rhodanese to convert cyanide to thiocyanate. Supportive care is necessary, often requiring tracheal intubation, supplemental oxygen, and support of hemodynamics with vasopressors and inotropes.

Vesicants

Sulfur mustard, nitrogen mustard, lewisite, and phosgene oxime are the most notable vesicants. These compounds, also known as "blister agents," produce burns and blisters on contact with the skin and eyes. When inhaled, they cause damage to the lungs and multiple organ dysfunction syndrome. Symptoms are immediate with lewisite and phosgene oxime, whereas mustard exposure may not produce symptoms for 2 to 24 hours. Mild poisoning (tearing, erythema, cough, hoarseness) does not require treatment other than supportive care. More severe poisoning may result in blindness, nausea, vomiting, diarrhea, leukopenia, severe respiratory difficulty, or central nervous system effects. A protective suit and gas mask provide the best protection against vesicants. Exposed individuals should be decontaminated as though they were exposed to a nerve agent (remove clothing and wash with warm soapy water with or without 0.5% to 2% hypochlorite). Tracheal intubation and mechanical ventilation of the patient's lungs may be required. There are no specific antidotes for sulfur mustard. Dimercaprol is a specific antidote for lewisite.[21]

INFECTIOUS DISEASE DISASTERS

In addition to biologic and chemical terrorism, anesthesia providers need to be familiar with contagious diseases (influenza, severe acute respiratory syndrome, West Nile virus). Influenza has killed more people in the twentieth century than any other infectious disease. Only subtypes of influenza A virus normally infect people. Typically, birds do not get sick when they are infected, but avian viruses can transform and infect humans, with subsequent human-to-human transmission and a resulting pandemic. The airway and ventilator management skills possessed by anesthesia providers may become essential for the care of these patients. The risk for exposure is high and providers must always maintain a high level of suspicion and wear the appropriate protective gear when managing these patients. Public health authorities should always be notified to assist with confirmation and containment of such cases.

QUESTIONS OF THE DAY

1. What are the "ABCDEs" of trauma resuscitation?
2. What is the Consensus formula for the initial fluid management of a patient with significant burn injury?
3. What is "damage control" surgery in a patient who has sustained abdominal trauma?

4. What is the potential role of the anesthesia provider in a mass casualty disaster?

5. What are the clinical manifestations of exposure to nerve agents such as Sarin? What is the appropriate initial management?

ACKNOWLEDGMENT

The editors and publisher would like to thank Drs. J. F. Tang, J. F. Pittet, Robert K. Stoelting, and Ronald D. Miller for contributing a chapter on this topic to the prior edition of this work. It has served as the foundation for the current chapter.

REFERENCES

1. Krug EG, et al: The global burden of injuries, *Am J Public Health* 90: 523–526, 2000.

2. Kortbeek JB, Al Turki SA, Ali J, et al: Advanced trauma life support, 8th ed: The evidence for change, *J Trauma* 64:1638–1650, 2008.

3. Crosby ET: Airway management in adults after cervical spine trauma, *Anesthesiology* 104:1293–1318, 2006.

4. Robitaille A, Williams SR, Tremblay MH, et al: Cervical spine motion during tracheal intubation with manual in-line stabilization: Direct laryngoscopy versus GlideScope videolaryngoscopy, *Anesth Analg* 106:935–941, 2008.

5. Spahn DR, Cerny V, Coats TJ, et al: Management of bleeding following major trauma: A European guideline, *Crit Care* 11:R17, 2007.

6. Moore FA, McKinley BA, Moore EE, et al: Inflammation and the host response to injury, a large-scale collaborative project: Patient-oriented research core—standard operating procedures for clinical care. III. Guidelines for shock resuscitation, *J Trauma* 61:82–89, 2006.

7. Snyder CW, Weinberg JA, McGwin G Jr, et al: The relationship of blood product ratio to mortality: Survival benefit or survival bias? *J Trauma* 66:358–362, 2009; discussion 62–64.

8. Vincent JL, et al: Primer on medical management of severe brain injury, *Crit Care Med* 33:1392–1399, 2005.

9. Bratton SL, Chestnut RM, Ghajar J, et al: Guidelines for the management of severe traumatic brain injury, *J Neurotrauma* 24:S7–S95, 2007.

10. Alderson P, et al: Corticosteroids for acute traumatic brain injury, *Cochrane Database Syst Rev* Jan 25:CD000196, 2005.

11. Ryan CM, Schoenfeld DA, Thorpe WP, et al: Objective estimates of the probability of death from burn injuries, *N Engl J Med* 338:362–366, 1998.

12. Mlcak RP, et al: Respiratory management of inhalation injury, *Burns* 33:2–13, 2007.

13. Latenser BA: Critical care of the burn patient: the first 48 hours, *Crit Care Med* 37:2819–2826, 2009.

14. Shapiro MB, Jenkins DH, Schwab CW, et al: Damage control: Collective review, *J Trauma* 49:969–978, 2000.

15. Hak DJ: The role of pelvic angiography in evaluation and management of pelvic trauma, *Orthop Clin North Am* 35:445–449, 2004.

16. Baker DJ: Chemical and biologic warfare agents: The role of anesthesiologists. In Miller RD, editor: *Anesthesia*, ed 6, Philadelphia, 2005, Churchill Livingstone, pp 2497–2526.

17. Murray MJ, et al: Anesthesiologists must now prepare for biologic, nuclear, or chemical terrorism, *Anesth Patient Safety Found Newsletter* Spring:1–3, 2002. Available at http://www.apsf.org.

18. Joint Commission on Accreditation of Healthcare Organizations: *Healthcare at the Crossroads: Strategies for Creating and Sustaining Community Wide Emergency Preparedness Systems.* Available at http://www.jcaho.org.

19. Lerner EB, Schwartz RB, Coule PL, et al: Mass casualty triage: An evaluation of the data and development of a proposed national guideline, *Disaster Med Public Health Prep* 2:S25–S34, 2008.

20. SALT mass casualty triage: Concept endorsed by the American College of Emergency Physicians, American College of Surgeons Committee on Trauma, American Trauma Society, National Association of EMS Physicians, National Disaster Life Support Education Consortium, and State and Territorial Injury Prevention Directors, *Disaster Med Public Health Prep* 2:245–246, 2008.

21. Murray MJ: Chemical weapons compromise provider safety, *Anesth Patient Safety Found Newsletter* Spring:12–14, 2002. Available at http://www.apsf.org.

22. Lockey D, et al: Survival of trauma patients who have prehospital tracheal intubation without anaesthesia or muscle relaxants: Observational study, *BMJ* 323:141–146, 2001.

23. Dutton RP, et al: Anesthesia for trauma. In Miller RD, editor: *Miller's Anesthesia*, ed 6, Philadelphia, 2005, Churchill Livingstone, pp 2451–2496.

24. Mongan PD, et al: Threat of radiologic terrorism increases, *Anesth Patient Safety Found Newsletter* Spring:9–11, 2002. Available at http://www.apsf.org.

25. American Academy of Pediatrics Committee on Environmental Health: Radiation disasters and children, *Pediatrics* 111:1455–1461, 2003.

26. Reeves GI: Radiation injuries, *Crit Care Clin* 15:457–462, 1999.

27. Coursin DB, Ketzler JT, Kumar A, et al: Bioterrorism may overwhelm medical resources: New and different patient safety challenges must be anticipated, *Anesth Patient Safety Found Newsletter* Spring:4–8, 2002. Available at http://www.apsf.org.

28. Lane HC, Fauci AS: Bioterrorism on the home front: A new challenge for American medicine, *JAMA* 286: 2595–2597, 2001.

29. *Managing Hazardous Material Incidents. Volume III. Agency for Toxic Substances and Disease Registry (ATSDR)*, Atlanta, GA, 2001, U.S. Department of Health and Human Services. Public Health Service.

30. Swartz MN: Recognition and management of anthrax—An update, *N Engl J Med* 345:1621–1626, 2001.

31. Breman JG, et al: Diagnosis and management of smallpox, *N Engl J Med* 346:1300–1306, 2002.

32. Dennis DT, Inglesby TV, Henderson DA, et al: Tularemia as a biological weapon: Medical and public health management, *JAMA* 285:2763–2773, 2001.

33. Arnon SS, Schechter R, Inglesby TV, et al: Botulinum toxin as a biological weapon: Medical and public health management, *JAMA* 285:1059–1070, 2001.

34. Bhalla KD, et al: Biological agents with potential for misuse: A historical perspective and defensive measures, *Toxicol Appl Pharmacol* 199:71–77, 2004.

35. Evison D, et al: Chemical weapons, *BMJ* 324:332–337, 2002.

VI

43 CHRONIC PAIN MANAGEMENT

Pankaj Mehta and James P. Rathmell

Anesthesiologists first ventured into the treatment of patients with chronic pain as an extension of regional anesthesia in the operating room. Pain medicine is now a well-established subspecialty of anesthesiology, with many practitioners dedicating their entire clinical practice to caring for patients with chronic pain and employing a wide range of diagnostic and therapeutic modalities that now extend far beyond the scope of regional anesthesia. The International Association for the Study of Pain (IASP) defines pain as "an unpleasant sensory and emotional experience associated with actual or potential tissue damage, or described in terms of such damage" and chronic pain as "pain without apparent biological value that has persisted beyond the normal tissue healing time usually taken to be 3 months."[1] Chronic pain leads to enormous personal and societal costs in lost productivity and prolonged and all too often seemingly futile medical treatment.

CLASSIFICATION OF CHRONIC PAIN

Chronic pain is often classified as cancer-related pain or noncancer pain, to distinguish the former, which is often associated with the issues that arise near the end of life. However, as more effective treatments for many cancers have emerged, many more patients are surviving for prolonged periods of time on treatment or emerging as long-term survivors, and some of these patients suffer from persistent pain. Chronic pain is often divided into *nociceptive pain* in which activity in peripheral pain neurons due to ongoing tissue injury is present, such as the pain of osteoarthritis, and *neuropathic pain* in which abnormal function of the nervous system causes ongoing pain, such as the pain associated with postherpetic neuralgia or painful diabetic peripheral neuropathy. Neuropathic pain is often associated with signs and symptoms of abnormal nerve function. The abnormal sensations associated with neuropathic pain include shooting or burning pain often accompanied with *hyperalgesia* (severe pain to a normally minimally painful stimulus, e.g., pinprick causes severe pain) and *allodynia* (pain to a normally nonpainful stimulus, e.g., light touch causes pain).

MULTIDISCIPLINARY PAIN MANAGEMENT

Chronic pain is a complex disorder and patients suffering with chronic pain often have biologic disease that is inextricably intertwined with cognitive, affective, behavioral, and social factors. Thus, managing patients with chronic pain necessitates employing the expertise of practitioners from a range of medical disciplines to address the physical and psychological aspects of their illness to allow them to regain control over their lives and optimize their overall level of function. Such a multidisciplinary team approach is the most efficacious and cost-effective means for the treatment of chronic pain.[2] The core of the multidisciplinary pain team consists of a physician, a psychologist, and a physical therapist often working in conjunction with an occupational therapist and nurse specialists. The physician coordinates diagnosis and medical treatment, including drug therapy and appropriate pain-relieving interventions; the psychologist typically incorporates patient education, cognitive-behavioral therapy, and relaxation training; and the physical therapist plans various exercise regimens, including muscle conditioning and aerobics, aimed at optimizing the patient's overall function.

COMMON PAIN SYNDROMES

Low Back Pain

DEFINITIONS

Low back pain, a nonspecific term, refers to pain centered over the lumbosacral junction. The diagnosis and treatment must be as precise as possible. Pain can be differentiated primarily over the axis of the spinal column from that which refers primarily to the leg (Fig. 43-1).[1] *Lumbar spinal pain* is pain inferior to the tip of the twelfth thoracic spinous process and superior to the tip of the first sacral spinous process. *Sacral spinal* pain is inferior to the first sacral spinous process and superior to the sacrococcygeal joint. *Lumbosacral spinal pain* is pain in either or both regions and constitutes "low back pain." Other patients present with "sciatica," or pain predominantly localized in the leg. The proper term is *radicular pain* because stimulation of the nerve roots or the dorsal root ganglion of a spinal nerve evokes the pain.

Pain is a normal physiologic process and serves as a signal of actual or impending tissue injury. Pain from tissue injury is usually well localized and associated with sensitivity in the region. Pain signals are carried toward

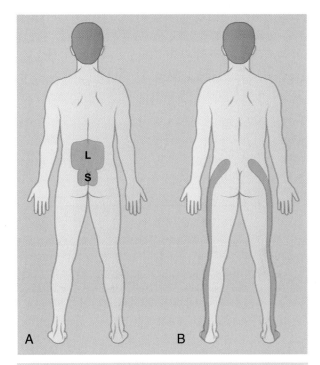

Figure 43-1 The definition of low back pain. **A,** "Low back pain" is more precisely termed lumbosacral spinal pain, which encompasses both lumbar spinal pain (L) and sacral spinal pain (S). **B,** Radicular pain describes pain that is referred to the lower extremity and is caused by stimulation of a spinal nerve.

the central nervous system (CNS) via the peripheral sensory nerves. This type of pain is termed *nociceptive pain*, or *physiologic pain*. In contrast, persistent pain following injury to the nervous system is termed *neuropathic pain*.

EPIDEMIOLOGY

Low back pain is among the most common problems leading patients to seek medical attention. The majority of episodes of acute low back pain, with or without radicular pain, resolve without treatment. Overall, 60% to 70% of those affected recover by 6 weeks, and 80% to 90% recover by 12 weeks (Fig. 43-2).[3] However, recovery after 12 weeks is slow and uncertain. Fewer than half of patients disabled for longer than 6 months will return to work. The return-to-work rate for those absent for 2 years is near zero. Low back pain is frequently recurrent; the vast majority of patients with a single episode experience another episode at some later time. Risk factors for developing chronic low back pain include age, gender, socioeconomic status, education level, body mass index, tobacco use, perceived general health status, physical activity (e.g., bending, lifting, twisting), repetitive tasks, job dissatisfaction, depression, spinal anatomic variations, and imaging abnormalities.[4]

VI

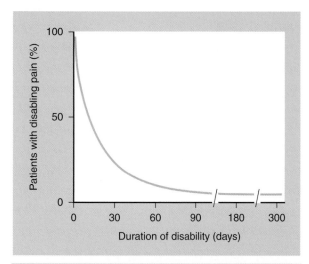

Figure 43-2 The time course of acute low back pain. (Redrawn with permission from Andersson GB. Epidemiological features of chronic low-back pain. Lancet 1999;354(9178):581-585.)

PATHOPHYSIOLOGY

The basic functional unit of the spine is the *functional spinal unit* and comprises two adjacent vertebral bodies with two posterior facet joints, an intervertebral disk, and the surrounding ligamentous structures. The intervertebral disk absorbs energy and distributes weight evenly from one spinal segment to the next while allowing movement of the protective bony elements. Lifting, bending, twisting, or whole body vibration can damage elements of the spine. With injury and aging, progressive degenerative changes appear in each element of the functional spinal unit, along with the onset of characteristic symptoms (Fig. 43-3). The earliest change in the lumbar facet joints is synovitis, which progresses to degradation of the articular surfaces, capsular laxity and subluxation, and finally enlargement of the articular processes (facet hypertrophy). Progressive degeneration also occurs within the intervertebral disks, starting with loss of hydration of the nucleus pulposus followed by the appearance of circumferential or radial tears within the annulus fibrosis (internal disk disruption).

Lumbosacral pain can arise from the facet joints or the annulus fibrosis.[5] With internal disruption of the annulus, some of the gelatinous central nucleus pulposus can extend beyond the disk margin, as a disk herniation (herniated nucleus pulposus, or HNP). When HNP extends to the region adjacent to the spinal nerve, it incites an intense inflammatory reaction. Patients with HNP typically present with acute radicular pain. Hypertrophy of the facet joints and calcification of the ligamentous structures can reduce the size of the intervertebral foramina and central spinal canal (spinal stenosis), with onset of radicular pain and neurogenic claudication.

Patients with prior lumbar surgery and either recurrent or persistent low back pain, often termed *failed back surgery syndrome*, often require a more complex evaluation. Knowing the type of surgery performed, the indications for and results of the surgery, and the time course and characteristics of any changes in the pattern and severity of postoperative pain, is essential. Recurrent pain or progressive symptoms signal the need for further diagnostic evaluation.

INITIAL EVALUATION AND TREATMENT

In first evaluating a patient with low back pain, several features in the history ("red flag" conditions) require prompt investigation, including new onset or worsening back pain after trauma, infection, or previous cancer. Patients with progressive neurologic deficits (typically worsening numbness or weakness) or bowel or bladder dysfunction, also warrant immediate radiologic imaging to rule out a compressive lesion.[6]

Diagnosis and treatment usually rely on location and duration of symptoms, and determining if the pain is acute or chronic and primarily radicular or lumbosacral in nature. *Acute* low back pain is pain that is present for less than 3 months, and *chronic* low back pain is defined as being present for a longer period of time.

ACUTE RADICULAR PAIN

HNP typically causes acute radicular pain, with or without radiculopathy (signs of dysfunction including numbness, weakness, or loss of deep tendon reflexes referable to a specific spinal nerve). In elderly patients and those with extensive lumbar spondylosis, acute radicular symptoms caused by narrowing of one or more intervertebral foramina can occur. Initial treatment is symptomatic, and following HNP, symptoms resolve without specific treatment in about 90% of patients.[7] For those with persistent pain after HNP, lumbar diskectomy may be indicated. A controlled trial of surgical versus nonoperative treatment showed significant improvement in both groups over 2 years, but remained inconclusive about the superiority of either approach.[8]

CHRONIC RADICULAR PAIN

Persistent leg pain in the distribution of a spinal nerve may occur in patients with a disk herniation with or without subsequent surgery. In those with persistent pain, a search for a reversible cause of nerve root compression is warranted. In many individuals, scarring around the nerve root at the operative site show on magnetic resonance imaging and electrodiagnostic studies as a pattern suggesting chronic radiculopathy. This patient group has characteristics similar to those suffering from other nerve injuries, and initial management should consist of pharmacologic treatment for neuropathic pain.[9]

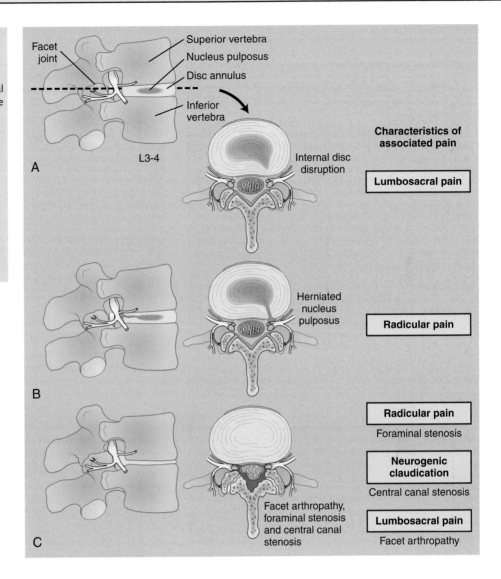

Figure 43-3 The functional spinal unit and the degenerative changes that lead to lumbosacral and radicular pain. **A,** The normal functional spinal unit. **B,** The degenerative changes leading to lumbosacral (disk disruption, facet joint arthropathy) pain and radicular pain (herniated nucleus pulposus). **C,** The degenerative changes of lumbar spondylosis leading to lumbosacral (facet joint) pain, radicular (foraminal stenosis) pain, and neurogenic claudication (central canal stenosis).

ACUTE LUMBOSACRAL PAIN

Most patients presenting with acute onset of lumbosacral pain without radicular symptoms have no obvious abnormal physical findings,[10] and radiologic imaging is unlikely to be helpful.[11] Traumatic sprain of the muscles and ligaments of the lumbar spine or the zygapophyseal joints, and early internal disk disruption, are significant causes of acute lumbosacral pain. As with patients with acute radicular pain, this group is best managed symptomatically.

CHRONIC LUMBOSACRAL PAIN

There are many causes of chronic lumbosacral pain, and identification of the anatomic cause cannot be done with certainty in up to 90% of cases.[6] The structures most commonly implicated include the sacroiliac joint, lumbar facets, and lumbar intervertebral disks.[12] In chronic low back pain, the incidence of internal disk disruption has been estimated to be 39% (range 29% to 49%), facet joint pain 15% (10% to 20%), and sacroiliac joint pain 15% (7% to 23%). The gold standard for diagnosing sacroiliac and facet joint pain is injection of local anesthetic at the site. However, the use of uncontrolled local anesthetic blocks for diagnostic purposes is plagued by placebo response. For patients achieving significant short-term pain relief with diagnostic blocks, radiofrequency treatment offers a simple, minimally invasive intervention that can provide pain reduction for 3 to 6 months in those with facet-related pain. Pain from degenerating intervertebral disks is also a source of chronic axial back pain. Diagnostic provocative diskography may identify symptomatic disks prior to management with therapies such as intradiscal electrothermal therapy (IDET) or surgical fusion.

VI

Neuropathic Pain

Persistent pain following injury to the nervous system is termed *neuropathic pain* and has unique characteristics:

- Spontaneous pain–pain that occurs with no stimulus (e.g., sudden lancinating pain described with postherpetic neuralgia)
- Hyperalgesia–an exaggerated painful response to a normally mildly noxious stimulus (e.g., light pinprick leading to extreme, prolonged pain)
- Allodynia–a painful response to a normally nonnoxious stimulus (e.g., light touch causing pain)

Neuropathic pain is believed to arise when the normal protective physiologic systems of the nervous system that produce sensitization of the peripheral and central nervous systems (sensitization that affords protection during the healing process) persist after the injured tissue has healed. Three of the most common forms of neuropathic pain include postherpetic neuralgia, painful diabetic neuropathy, and complex regional pain syndrome.

POSTHERPETIC NEURALGIA

The varicella-zoster virus produces a highly contagious primary viral infection called chickenpox that is common in childhood, characterized by the appearance of a diffuse vesicular rash that typically heals without scarring.[13] The varicella-zoster virus lies dormant in the dorsal root ganglia following resolution of the primary infection. In individuals with immunosuppression or with aging of the immune system, the virus can produce a secondary infection called shingles in which the virus replicates and travels from the ganglia along one or more spinal nerves erupting in an acute vesicular rash that is typically limited to one or two dermatomes on one side of the body. This secondary infection leads to damage to small unmyelinated nerve fibers and can lead to severe and persistent pain, termed postherpetic neuralgia (PHN). PHN is characterized by episodic lancinating pain and severe allodynia in the affected dermatome. The incidence of PHN has been reduced in recent years with the emergence of an effective vaccine. Antiviral therapy with acyclovir, famcyclovir, or valacyclovir started within the first few days after eruption of vesicles also appears to reduce the incidence of PHN. The incidence rate of herpes zoster ranges from 1.2 to 3.4 per 1000 person-years among healthy individuals, increasing to 3.9 to 11.8 per 1000 person-years among those older than 65 years. Sympathetic blockade during acute herpes zoster can produce excellent analgesia, but is ineffective in treating established PHN.[14] Treatment of established PHN is difficult. Topical lidocaine can reduce pain in those with marked allodynia. Tricyclic antidepressants and anticonvulsants remain the primary treatment for PHN.

PAINFUL DIABETIC PERIPHERAL NEUROPATHY

Diabetes mellitus is the most common cause of neuropathic pain and is caused by damage to small unmyelinated nerve fibers.[15] Diabetic peripheral neuropathy (DPN) can result in painless sensory loss or painful neuropathy. DPN typically begins with symmetrical numbness in the toes associated with paresthesias, dysesthesias, and pain. The pain is often described as burning but equally common is a simple deep aching pain in the area affected. The neuropathy progresses slowly over many years. As the sensory changes reach the proximal portion of the feet, the same symptoms often appear in the hands. The incidence of painful DPN is directly related to glycemic control, with marked reduction in the incidence, severity, and rate of progression of the neuropathy in those with the tightest control of blood glucose levels. Similar to other forms of neuropathic pain, patients with DPN report modest improvements in pain with tricyclic antidepressants and anticonvulsants.

COMPLEX REGIONAL PAIN SYNDROME

Complex regional pain syndrome (CRPS) refers to a constellation of signs and symptoms that emerge in a subset of patients with injury to peripheral nerves (Table 43-1).[16] CRPS typically begins with a traumatic event, most often involving an extremity. As the traumatized area heals, patients who develop CRPS are left with persistent pain that has the characteristics of neuropathic pain associated with signs and symptoms of dysfunction of the sympathetic nervous system (swelling, edema, erythema or bluish discoloration, temperature asymmetry when compared with the contralateral limb). CRPS is divided into two subgroups: CRPS type 1 (formerly called reflex sympathetic dystrophy) is present when persistent pain accompanied by sympathetic dysfunction occurs without an identifiable nerve injury, such as following a severe ankle sprain; CRPS type 2 (formerly called causalgia) is present when the same signs

---

Table 43-1 International Association for the Study of Pain (IASP) Diagnostic Criteria for Complex Regional Pain Syndrome (CRPS)*

1. The presence of an initiating noxious event, or a cause of immobilization
2. Continuing pain, allodynia, or hyperalgesia in which the pain is disproportionate to any known inciting event
3. Evidence at some time of edema, changes in skin blood flow, or abnormal sudomotor activity (sweating, piloerection) in the region of pain (can be sign or symptom)
4. Diagnosis of CRPS excluded by existence of other conditions that would otherwise account for the degree of pain

*CRPS type 1: no identifiable nerve lesion; CRPS type 2: identifiable nerve lesion.

and symptoms occur following an identifiable nerve injury such as a gunshot wound to the brachial plexus.

CRPS can lead to long-term, severe, persistent pain and loss of function related to loss of use of the painful extremity. Successful management requires a multimodal approach. The central tenant of managing patients with CRPS is to focus on maintenance and restoration of function through aggressive physical therapy. Pain reduction can facilitate functional restoration. By extension from their use in treating other forms of neuropathic pain, tricyclic antidepressants and anticonvulsants are often the first-line analgesics used to treat CRPS. Sympathetic nerve blocks have been used for many years in managing patients with CRPS; they can produce dramatic pain reduction that facilitates physical therapy, but they are rarely useful in the long-term management of these patients.[16] Spinal cord stimulation has emerged in recent years as a more effective long-term means to produce pain reduction and facilitate functional restoration in patients with CRPS.[16] Multidisciplinary treatment teams that include a provider that oversees medical management working in close coordination with a physical therapist and a psychologist appear to be the most effective means to help this group of patients.

Cancer-Related Pain

Pain related to cancer and its treatment is common; indeed, pain is the most common presenting symptom of undiagnosed malignancy. The pain may be due to direct invasion of the malignancy or result from cancer treatment; chronic pain of various types often coexists with cancer-related pain. The primary focus of pain reduction in those with cancer is direct treatment of the malignancy; indeed, successful treatment often leads to complete pain resolution. Nonetheless, ongoing pain during the course of treatment or as the disease progresses is all too common. More than three decades ago, the World Health Organization (WHO) revolutionized the treatment of cancer pain by introducing a simple, three-step analgesic ladder (Table 43-2). This approach has been adopted worldwide, and promotes the aggressive treatment of cancer-related pain by tailoring the analgesic used to the severity of the pain, starting with nonopioids and moving toward more potent opioid analgesics as necessary to control pain.[17]

Anesthesiologists are often called upon to apply their knowledge of regional anesthesia and neuraxial drug delivery in caring for a small group of patients whose pain cannot be controlled with the more conservative approaches laid out in the WHO approach. One of the more common nerve blocks that has been used to successfully treat patients with pain associated with abdominal malignancy is the neurolytic celiac plexus block (described later). With the advent of implantable intrathecal drug delivery systems, long-term treatment of patients with

Table 43-2 World Health Organization (WHO) Analgesic Ladder for the Treatment of Cancer Pain

Step 1: Mild Pain
Nonopioid analgesics (acetaminophen, NSAIDs)
± adjuvant analgesics (TCAs, anticonvulsants) for neuropathic pain

Step 2: Moderate Pain
Use of short-acting opioids (e.g., hydrocodone, oxycodone) in starting doses
± nonopioid analgesics (acetaminophen, NSAIDs)
± adjuvant analgesics (TCAs, anticonvulsants) for neuropathic pain

Step 3: Severe Pain
Use of potent opioids (e.g., morphine, hydromorphone) in higher doses
± nonopioid analgesics (acetaminophen, NSAIDs)
± adjuvant analgesics (TCAs, anticonvulsants) for neuropathic pain

NSAIDs, nonsteroidal anti-inflammatory drugs; TCAs, tricyclic antidepressants.

intractable cancer-related pain using intrathecal opioids and other drugs (local anesthetics, clonidine, ziconotide) has become routine.

PHARMACOLOGIC MANAGEMENT OF CHRONIC PAIN

Acetaminophen and Nonsteroidal Anti-inflammatory Drugs

Acetaminophen and the nonsteroidal anti-inflammatory drugs (NSAIDs) are among the most common agents used to treat mild to moderate pain, ranging from headache to acute muscle sprain and strain. The NSAIDs have also proved useful in the long-term reduction of pain and stiffness associated with osteoarthritis. Acetaminophen is a novel nonopioid analgesic with a poorly understood mechanism of action; the aspirin and the NSAIDs produce potent inhibition of the enzyme cyclooxygenase, resulting in decreased levels of prostaglandins. The long-term use of NSAIDs in other chronic painful conditions such as low back pain is common but poorly supported by scientific evidence, which shows little utility in use of these agents.[18] These two groups of analgesics also represent the first step in the WHO analgesic ladder and are recommended as the initial drugs to treat mild to moderate cancer-related pain. During the last decade, the COX-2-selective analgesics have emerged; celecoxib is currently the only drug that remains available in the United States. Celecoxib has a lesser risk of gastrointestinal complications (gastric and duodenal ulcers, including perforated ulcers) than do the nonselective NSAIDs, but the analgesia from nonselective NSAIDs and the COX-2-selective analgesics is similar. Many of the COX-2-selective agents (valdecoxib, rofecoxib) have been removed from the market due to a slight increase in thromboembolic (stroke and myocardial infarction) events in patients on long-term therapy.[19]

Antidepressants

Tricyclic antidepressants (TCAs, such as nortriptyline, desipramine) and newer selective norepinephrine reuptake inhibitors (SNRIs, such as venlafaxine, duloxetine) are effective in the treatment of neuropathic pain, including PHN and painful DPN.[20] Secondary amine tricyclic antidepressants (TCAs) nortriptyline and desipramine are preferred because they are better tolerated than tertiary amine TCAs (amitriptyline and imipramine). Common side effects of the TCAs include dry mouth and urinary retention; TCAs can also worsen preexisting heart block. The SNRIs have a more favorable side effect profile and similar efficacy when compared with the TCAs.

Anticonvulsants

Antiepileptic drugs (e.g., gabapentin, pregabalin) also are effective for the treatment of neuropathic pain.[20] These drugs are generally well tolerated; the most common side effects are dizziness, somnolence, and peripheral edema.

Decisions regarding pharmacologic treatment of neuropathic pain (Table 43-3) may be based on an analysis of the number needed to treat (NNT); the NNT (with 95% confidence interval [CI]) are TCA 3.1 (2.7 to 3.7); SNRI 6.8 (3.4 to 4.41); and gabapentin/pregabalin 4.7 (4.0 to 5.6).[20]

Chronic Opioid Therapy

Chronic opioid therapy in the long-term management of noncancer-related pain remains controversial.[21] Advocates point to long-term efficacy and improvement in function in patients with chronic painful conditions, including low back pain. Opponents cite difficulties in prescribing these drugs over the long term. Although aberrant drug-related behavior (e.g., losing prescriptions, escalating drug use) is relatively common in patients receiving the opioids for chronic pain, overt addiction is unusual. However, treating acute pain in the opioid-tolerant patient is difficult, and it is becoming evident that chronic opioid use can worsen pain by inducing hyperalgesia. There remain few high-quality RCTs (randomized controlled trials) to guide the use of opioids in treating chronic low back pain. A Cochrane Review identified only three trials deemed methodologically sufficient; all compared tramadol with placebo.[21] Pooled results showed that tramadol was more effective than placebo for pain relief, with a standardized mean difference (SMD) of 0.71

Table 43-3	Stepwise Pharmacologic Management of Neuropathic Pain

Step 1: Assessment and diagnosis of the neuropathic pain syndrome followed by detailed explanation of the pain management plan setting realistic goals.

Step 2: Initial pharmacologic therapy including one of the following agents:
First-Line Medications
TCAs (nortriptyline, desipramine) or SNRIs (duloxetine, venlafaxine)
Anticonvulsants, either gabapentin or pregabalin
Topical lidocaine
Second-Line Medications
Opioid analgesics and tramadol, which can be used alone or in combination for acute exacerbations, neuropathic cancer pain or when prompt relief is required

Step 3: If follow-up evaluation demonstrates substantial pain relief with tolerable side effects (pain <3/10), treatment is continued. If the relief is partial after an adequate trial (pain >4/10), another first-line drug is added. If pain relief is inadequate at the target dosage (<30% reduction), an alternative first-line medication is started.

Step 4: If the initial trial fails, a second-line or third-line medication is considered.
Third-Line Medications
Certain other antiepileptic agents (carbamazepine, oxcarbazepine) and antidepressants (citalopram, paroxetine), NMDA receptor antagonists, topical capsaicin

NMDA, *N*-methyl-D-aspartic acid; SNRIs, serotonin-norepinephrine reuptake inhibitors; TCAs, tricyclic antidepressants.
Adapted with permission from Dworkin RH, O'Connor AB, Backonja M, et al. Pharmacologic management of neuropathic pain: Evidence-based recommendations. Pain 2007;32:237-251.

(95% CI, 0.39 to 1.02), and for improving function, SMD 0.17 (95% CI 0.04 to 0.30).

When treating a patient with long-term opioids, many drugs are available. The traditional paradigm for opioid treatment is based on cancer pain management. In this approach, patients with significant chronic pain are given a long-acting opioid for continuous analgesia; short-acting opioids may cause fluctuations in pain control. A small dose of a short-acting drug is also available for intermittent pain that occurs with activity and "breaks through" the control provided by the long-acting drug alone.

Nearly every available opioid has been used successfully in treating chronic low back pain, including short-acting agents (e.g., hydrocodone, oxycodone) alone or in combination with ibuprofen or acetaminophen, and long-acting agents (e.g., methadone, controlled-release morphine, transdermal fentanyl, controlled-release oxycodone). A new type of "ultrafast onset" opioid (e.g., oral transmucosal fentanyl citrate, fentanyl buccal tablet) has emerged for the rapid treatment of breakthrough pain. As with the patient selection process, choosing the opioid drug and the appropriate dose remains empiric. The decision to use short- or long-acting drugs alone or in combination should be tailored to the individual patient's pattern of pain.

INTERVENTIONAL PAIN THERAPIES

Interventional pain therapy refers to a group of targeted treatments used for specific spine disorders, ranging from epidural injection of steroids to percutaneous intradiscal

techniques. Some have been rigorously tested in RCTs, and others are in widespread use without critical evaluation. When these treatment techniques are used for the disorders they are most likely to benefit (Table 43-4), they can be highly effective; however, when used haphazardly, they are unlikely to be helpful and may cause harm.

Epidural Injection of Steroids

Numerous RCTs have examined the efficacy of epidural corticosteroid injection for acute radicular pain.[22] Such injections into the epidural space are thought to combat the inflammatory response that is associated with acute

---

Table 43-4   Application of Medical Therapies in Treating Low Back Pain

Level of evidence is based on the Oxford Evidence-Based Medicine Levels for Treatment: Level I, high-quality RCTs or systematic reviews of RCTs; Level II, low-quality RCTs, cohort studies, or systematic reviews of cohort studies; Level III, case-control studies or systematic reviews of case-control studies; Level IV, case-series; Level V, expert opinion.

Acute radicular pain	**Initial therapy:** • A 7- to 10-day course of an oral analgesic (NSAID or acetaminophen, ± opioid analgesic) with a relaxant drug, for those with superimposed muscle spasm. (Level I)	**Persistent acute radicular pain:** • Between 2 and 6 weeks after onset of acute radicular pain, consider lumbar epidural steroid injection to has attenuation of radicular symptoms. (Level II)
Chronic radicular pain	**Initial therapy:** • Initial treatment of chronic radicular pain is similar to treatment of other types of neuropathic pain and should begin with a trial of a tricyclic antidepressant, SNRI, or anticonvulsant. (Level 1) • Chronic radicular pain may respond to treatment with chronic opioids, but neuropathic pain is less responsive to opioids than nociceptive pain. (Level II)	**Persistent chronic radicular pain:** • Consider evaluation for a trial of spinal cord stimulation. (Level II)
Acute lumbosacral pain	**Initial therapy:** • A 7- to 10-day course of an oral analgesic (NSAID or acetaminophen, ± opioid analgesic) with a relaxant drug, for those with superimposed muscle spasm. (Level I)	**Persistent acute lumbosacral pain:** • Between 2 and 6 weeks after onset of chronic radicular pain, consider referral for physical therapy for stretching, strengthening, and aerobic exercise in conjunction with patient education. (Level I)
Chronic lumbosacral pain	**Initial therapy:** • Diagnostic medial branch blocks of the nerves to the facet joints. If >50% pain relief is obtained with the diagnostic blocks, radiofrequency treatment may be effective. (Level II)	**Persistent chronic lumbosacral pain:** • Consider enrollment in a formal pain program that incorporates medical management, behavioral therapy, and physical therapy. (Level I) • Consider cognitive-behavioral therapy. (Level I) • If no response is obtained with diagnostic facet blocks and MRI shows evidence of early degenerative disk disease affecting fewer than two intervertebral disks, consider diagnostic provocative diskography. (Level III) If diskography is concordant (pain is reproduced at anatomically abnormal level[s] and no pain is present at an adjacent anatomically normal level), consider treatment with intradiscal electrothermal therapy (IDET) at the symptomatic level(s). (Level II)

MRI, magnetic resonance imaging; RCTs, randomized controlled trials.
Adapted with permission from Rathmell, JP. A 50-year-old man with chronic low back pain. JAMA 2008;299:2066-2077.

VI

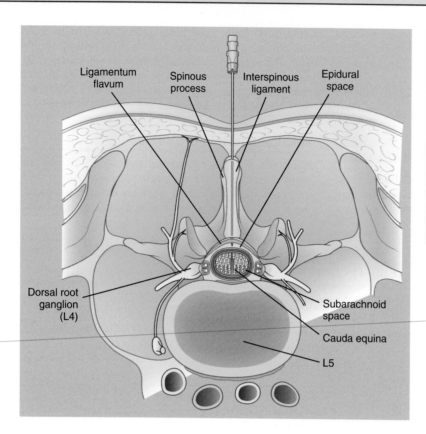

Figure 43-4 Axial diagram of interlaminar lumbar epidural injection. The epidural needle is advanced in the midline between adjacent spinous processes to traverse the ligamentum flavum and enter the dorsal epidural space in the midline. The normal epidural space is approximately 4 to 6 mm wide (from the ligamentum flavum to the dura mater in the axial plane). Note the proximity of the underlying cauda equina during lumbar epidural injection. (Redrawn with permission from Rathmell JP. Atlas of image-guided intervention in regional anesthesia and pain medicine. Lippincott Williams & Wilkins, Philadelphia, 2006, p 47.)

disk herniation. In acute radicular pain with HNP, epidural steroids reduce the severity and duration of leg pain if given between 3 and 6 weeks after onset. Adverse effects, such as injection site pain and transient worsening of radicular pain, occur in less than 1% of treated subjects. Beyond 3 months from treatment, there are no long-term reductions in pain or improvements in function. This therapy has never proved helpful for lumbosacral pain without radicular symptoms. Epidural injection of steroids can be accomplished by the interlaminar route (Fig. 43-4) or the transforaminal route (Fig. 43-5). The rationale for use of the transforaminal route is to place the steroid in high concentration directly adjacent to the spinal nerve close to the site of inflammation. The transforaminal approach may be more effective than the interlaminar approach, but additional studies are needed.

Facet Blocks and Radiofrequency Treatment

Pain from the lumbar facet joints affects up to 15% of chronic low back pain patients.[12] Patients are identified based on typical patterns of referred pain, with maximal pain located directly over the facet joints and patient report of pain on palpation over the facets; radiographic findings are variable, but some degree of facet arthropathy is typically present. The intra-articular injection of anesthetics and corticosteroids may lead to intermediate-term (1 to 3 months) pain relief in patients with an active inflammatory process. Radiofrequency denervation delivers energy through an insulated, small-diameter needle positioned adjacent to the sensory nerve to the facet joint (Fig. 43-6), creating a small area of tissue coagulation that denervates the facet joint. Radiofrequency denervation probably provides better pain relief than sham intervention for facet-related pain.[23] Approximately 50% of patients treated report at least 50% pain reduction. Pain typically returns 6 to 12 months after treatment, and denervation can be repeated without lessening of efficacy. Adverse events are uncommon; in 1% of treated patients, pain at the treatment site lasted 2 weeks or less.

Lumbar Diskography and Intradiscal Treatments

The intervertebral disk is probably involved in 29% and 49% of patients with chronic low back pain.[12] Provocative diskography is a controversial diagnostic test that employs a series of needles placed in the central portion of the intervertebral disks; a small volume of saline or radiographic contrast material is then introduced to try to reproduce the patient's typical pain to determine the offending disk.[24] This test has been used to select patients for surgical fusion,

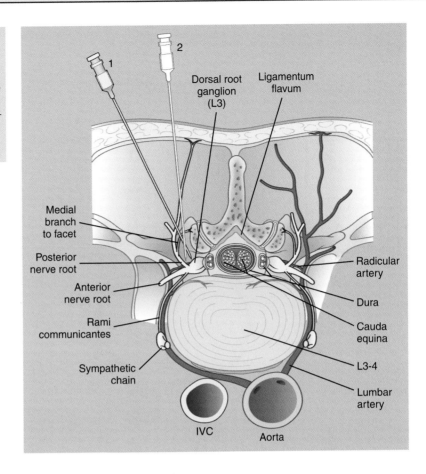

Figure 43-5 Axial view of lumbar transforaminal and selective nerve root injection. The anatomy and proper needle position (axial view) for right (1) L3-L4 transforaminal injection and (2) L3 selective nerve root injection. (Redrawn with permission from Rathmell JP. Atlas of image-guided intervention in regional anesthesia and pain medicine. Lippincott Williams & Wilkins, Philadelphia, 2006, p 58.)

Dorsal root ganglion (L3)

Ligamentum flavum

Medial branch to facet

Posterior nerve root

Anterior nerve root

Rami communicantes

Sympathetic chain

Radicular artery

Dura

Cauda equina

L3-4

Lumbar artery

IVC

Aorta

but its ability to predict outcome is questionable. Diskography has also been used to select patients for a procedure called Intradiscal Electrothermal Therapy (IDET), which is used to treat discogenic chronic lumbosacral pain. IDET employs a steerable thermal resistance wire placed along the posterior annulus fibrosus. Thermal energy is applied to destroy penetrating nociceptive fibers and to change the cross-linking of glycosaminoglycans, thereby stiffening the intervertebral disk. Clinical study results are mixed. Probably, a 50% reduction in pain may occur, as is improvement in sitting and standing tolerance in 45% to 50% of patients receiving IDET at a single level with concordant diskography and well-preserved disk height.[25] Percutaneous plasma disk decompression is a minimally invasive means designed to remove a portion of the central nucleus pulposus to treat persistent radicular pain associated with focal disk bulges. This technique reduces pain and increases the long-term functional status for patients with small (<3 mm) disk bulges.[26] Unfortunately, most patients with disabling radicular pain have large disk herniations that are not amenable to this approach. Minimally invasive techniques for treating both lumbosacral and radicular forms of low back pain are emerging rapidly, but most remain of unproven efficacy.

Sympathetic Blocks

Blockade of sympathetic nerve fibers can produce pain relief in specific pain syndromes, including complex regional pain syndrome (CRPS) and ischemic pain produced by microvascular insufficiency. These chronic pain states are often referred to as *sympathetically maintained pain* because they share the characteristic of pain relief following blockade of the regional sympathetic ganglia.[27] There is little scientific evidence to support long-term reductions in pain or improvements in physical function associated with the use of sympathetic blocks; nonetheless, they are still widely used to produce short-term pain reduction in order to facilitate active involvement in physical therapy.[16] One exception to this rule is the use of neurolytic celiac plexus block for the treatment of pain associated with abdominal malignancies, where significant pain reduction can extend over weeks to months after treatment.[28]

STELLATE GANGLION BLOCK
Stellate ganglion block is an established method for the diagnosis and treatment of sympathetically maintained pain of the head, neck, and upper extremity. Sympathetic

VI

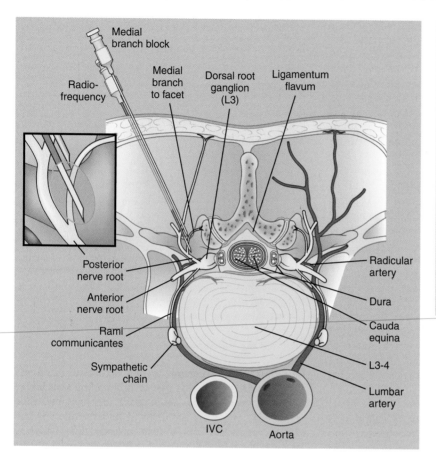

Medial branch block

Radio-frequency

Medial branch to facet

Dorsal root ganglion (L3)

Ligamentum flavum

Posterior nerve root

Anterior nerve root

Rami communicantes

Sympathetic chain

IVC

Aorta

Radicular artery

Dura

Cauda equina

L3-4

Lumbar artery

Figure 43-6 Axial diagram of lumbar medial branch nerve blocks and radiofrequency treatment. A 22-gauge, 3½-inch spinal needle (or 22-gauge, 10-cm radiofrequency cannula with a 5-mm active tip) is advanced toward the base of the transverse process, where it joins with the superior articular process. Cannula placement for conventional radiofrequency treatment should be carried out with 25 to 30 degrees of caudal angulation of the C-arm to bring the axis of the active tip parallel to the course of the medial branch nerve in the groove between the transverse process and the superior articular process. (Redrawn with permission from Rathmell JP. Atlas of image-guided intervention in regional anesthesia and pain medicine. Lippincott Williams & Wilkins, Philadelphia, 2006, p 89.)

fibers to and from the head, neck, and upper extremities pass through the stellate ganglion. In most individuals, the stellate ganglion is formed by fusion of the inferior cervical and first thoracic sympathetic ganglia. The ganglion is commonly found just lateral to the lateral border of the longus colli muscle, anterior to the neck of the first rib and the transverse process of the seventh cervical vertebra (Fig. 43-7). In this position, the ganglion lies posterior to the superior border of the first part of the subclavian artery and the origin of the vertebral artery posterior to the dome of the lung. Although several approaches to stellate ganglion block have been described, the most common is the anterior paratracheal approach at C6 using surface landmarks. Performing the block at C6 reduces the likelihood of pneumothorax, which is more likely when the block is carried out close to the dome of the lung at C7. The anterior tubercle of the transverse process of C6 (Chassaignac's tubercle) is readily palpable in most individuals. To perform the block without radiographic guidance, the operator palpates the cricoid cartilage, and then slides a finger laterally into the groove between the trachea and the sternocleidomastoid muscle, retracting the muscle and adjacent carotid and jugular vessels laterally.

Chassaignac's tubercle is typically palpable in this groove at the C6 level. Once the tubercle has been identified, a needle is advanced through the skin and seated on the tubercle, where local anesthetic is injected. The local anesthetic spreads along the prevertebral fascia in a caudal direction to anesthetize the stellate ganglion, which lies just inferior to the point of injection in the same plane. In practice, there is marked variation in the size and shape of Chassaignac's tubercle that reduces the rate of successful block. Signs of successful stellate ganglion block include the appearance of Horner's syndrome (miosis [pupillary constriction]); ptosis (drooping of the upper eyelid); and enophthalmos (recession of the globe within the orbit). Other signs of successful block include anhidrosis (lack of sweating), nasal congestion, venodilation in the hand and forearm, and increase in temperature of the blocked limb by at least 1 degree Celsius degree. The adjacent vertebral artery and C6 nerve root must be avoided to safely conduct this block. A simple modification of technique in which the needle is directed medially toward the base of the transverse process using radiographic guidance is a safe and simple means of improving the reliability of stellate ganglion block (see Fig. 43-7).

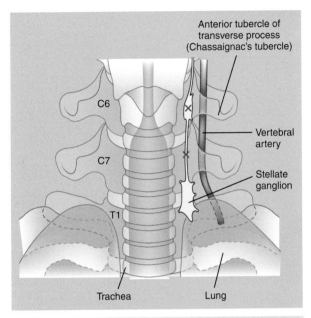

Anterior tubercle of
transverse process
(Chassaignac's tubercle)

C6

C7

T1

Vertebral
artery

Stellate
ganglion

Trachea

Lung

Figure 43-7 Anatomy of the stellate ganglion. The stellate ganglion conveys sympathetic fibers to and from the upper extremities and the head and neck. The ganglion comprises the fused superior thoracic ganglion and the inferior cervical ganglion and is named for its fusiform shape (in many individuals, the two ganglia remain separate). The stellate ganglia lies over the head of the first rib at the junction of the transverse process and uncinate process of T1. The ganglion is just posteromedial to the cupola of the lung and medial to the vertebral artery. Stellate ganglion block is typically carried out at the C6 or C7 level to avoid pneumothorax, and a volume of solution that will spread along the prevertebral fascia inferiorly to the stellate ganglion is employed (usually 10 mL). When radiographic guidance is not used, the operator palpates the anterior tubercle of the transverse process of C6 (Chassaignac's tubercle), and a needle is seated in the location. With radiographic guidance it is simpler and safer to place a needle over the vertebral body just inferior the uncinate process of C6 or C7. Particular care should be taken when performing the block at the C7 level to assure that the needle does not stray lateral to the uncinate process, as the vertebral artery courses anterior to transverse process at this level and is often not protected within a bony foramen transversarium. (Redrawn with permission from Rathmell JP. Atlas of image-guided intervention in regional anesthesia and pain medicine. Lippincott Williams & Wilkins, Philadelphia, 2006, p 116.)

Stellate ganglion block has long been the standard approach to diagnosis and treatment of sympathetically maintained pain syndromes involving the upper extremity, such as CRPS. Other neuropathic pain syndromes, including ischemic neuropathies, herpes zoster (shingles), early postherpetic neuralgia, and postradiation neuritis may also respond to stellate ganglion block. Blockade of the stellate ganglion has also proved successful in reducing pain and improving blood flow in vascular insufficiency conditions

such as intractable angina pectoris, Raynaud's disease, frostbite, vasospasm, and occlusive and embolic vascular disease. Finally, the sympathetic fibers control sweating; thus, stellate ganglion block can be quite effective in controlling hyperhidrosis (recurrent and uncontrollable sweating of the hands).

There are many structures within the immediate vicinity of the needle's tip once it is properly positioned for stellate ganglion block (see Fig. 43-7). Diffusion of local anesthetic can block the adjacent recurrent laryngeal nerve. This often leads to hoarseness, a feeling of having a lump in the throat, and a subjective feeling of shortness of breath and difficulty swallowing. Bilateral stellate ganglion block should not be performed because bilateral recurrent laryngeal nerve blocks may well lead to loss of laryngeal reflexes and respiratory compromise. The phrenic nerve is also commonly blocked by direct spread of local anesthetic and will lead to unilateral diaphragmatic paresis. Diffusion of local anesthetic as well as direct placement of local anesthetic adjacent to the posterior tubercle will result in somatic block of the upper extremity. This may take the form of a small area of sensory loss due to diffusion of local anesthetic or a complete brachial plexus block when the local anesthetic is placed within the nerve sheath. Patients with significant somatic block to the upper extremity should be sent home with a sling in place and counseled to guard their limb, just as one would instruct a patient who had received a brachial plexus block.

Major complications associated with stellate ganglion block include neuraxial block (spinal or epidural) and seizures. Extreme medial angulation of the needle from a relatively lateral skin entry point may lead to needle placement into the spinal canal through the anterolaterally oriented intervertebral foramen. In this manner, local anesthetic can be deposited in the epidural space, or if the needle is advanced far enough, it may penetrate the dural cuff surrounding the exiting nerve root and lie within the intrathecal space. More likely is placement of the needle tip on the posterior tubercle and spread of local anesthetic proximally along the nerve root to enter the epidural space. In this case, partial or profound neuraxial block, including high spinal or epidural block with loss of consciousness and apnea, may ensue. Airway protection, ventilation, and intravenous sedation should be promptly administered and continued until the patient regains airway reflexes and consciousness. Because the maximal effects of epidural local anesthetic may require 15 to 20 minutes to develop when using longer acting local anesthetics, it is imperative that patients are monitored for at least 30 minutes after stellate ganglion block.

Intravascular injection during stellate ganglion block will likely result in immediate onset of generalized seizures. The carotid artery lies just anteromedial to Chassaignac's tubercle, and the vertebral artery lies within the bony transverse foramen just posteromedial to the tubercle.

VI

If injection occurs into either structure, the local anesthetic injected enters the arterial supply traveling directly to the brain, and generalized seizures typically begin rapidly and after only small amounts of local anesthetic (as little as 0.2 mL of 0.25% bupivacaine have led to seizure). However, because the local anesthetic rapidly redistributes, the seizures are typically brief and do not require treatment. In the event of seizure, halt the injection, remove the needle, and begin supportive care.

CELIAC PLEXUS BLOCK

Neurolytic celiac plexus block (NCPB) is among the most widely applicable of all neurolytic blocks. NCPB has a long-lasting benefit for 70% to 90% of patients with pancreatic and other intra-abdominal malignancies.[29] Several techniques have been described for localizing the celiac plexus. The classic technique employs a percutaneous posterior approach using surface and bony landmarks to position needles in the vicinity of the plexus. Numerous reports have described new approaches for celiac plexus block using guidance from plain radiographs, fluoroscopy, computed tomography (CT), or ultrasound (an endoscopic transgastric technique). No single methodology has proved clearly superior in either its safety or success rate. In recent years, general agreement has arisen that radiographic guidance is necessary to perform celiac plexus block. Some practitioners have turned to routine use of CT, taking advantage of the ability to visualize adjacent structures when performing this technique.

The celiac plexus comprises a diffuse network of nerve fibers and individual ganglia that lie over the anterolateral surface of the aorta at the T12-L1 vertebral level. Sympathetic innervation to the abdominal viscera arises from the anterolateral horn of the spinal cord between the T5 and T12 levels. Nociceptive information from the abdominal viscera is carried by afferents that accompany the sympathetic nerves. Presynaptic sympathetic fibers travel from the thoracic sympathetic chain toward the ganglion, traversing over the anterolateral aspect of the inferior thoracic vertebrae as the greater (T5 to T9), lesser (T10 to T11), and least (T12) splanchnic nerves (see Fig. 43-1). Presynaptic fibers traveling via the splanchnic nerves synapse within the celiac ganglia, over the anterolateral surface of the aorta surrounding the origin of the celiac and superior mesenteric arteries at approximately the L1 vertebral level. Postsynaptic fibers from the celiac ganglia innervate all of the abdominal viscera with the exception of the descending colon, sigmoid colon, rectum, and pelvic viscera.

Celiac plexus block using a transcrural approach places the local anesthetic or neurolytic solution directly on the celiac ganglion anterolateral to the aorta (Fig. 43-8). The needles pass directly through the crura of the diaphragm en route to the celiac plexus. Spread of the solution toward the posterior surface of the aorta may thus be

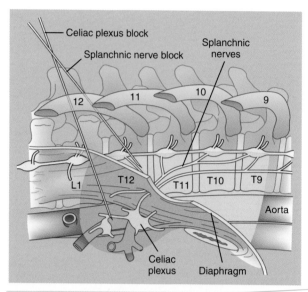

Figure 43-8 Anatomy of the celiac plexus and splanchnic nerves. The celiac plexus comprises a diffuse network of nerve fibers and individual ganglia that lie over the anterolateral surface of the aorta at the T12-L1 vertebral level. Presynaptic sympathetic fibers travel from the thoracic sympathetic chain toward the ganglion, traversing over the anterolateral aspect of the inferior thoracic vertebrae as the greater (T5-T9), lesser (T10-T11), and least (T12) splanchnic nerves. Celiac plexus block using a transcrural approach places the local anesthetic or neurolytic solution directly on the celiac ganglion anterolateral to the aorta. The needles pass directly through the crura of the diaphragm to the celiac plexus. In contrast, for splanchnic nerve block the needles remain posterior to the diaphragmatic crura in close apposition to the T12 vertebral body. Shading indicates the pattern of solution spread for each technique. (Redrawn with permission from Rathmell JP. Atlas of image-guided intervention in regional anesthesia and pain medicine. Lippincott Williams & Wilkins, Philadelphia, 2006, p 124.)

limited, perhaps reducing the chance of nerve root or spinal segmental artery involvement. In contrast, splanchnic nerve block (see Fig. 43-8) avoids the risk of penetrating the aorta, uses smaller volumes of solution, and the success is unlikely to be affected by anatomic distortion caused by extensive tumor or adenopathy within the pancreas. Because the needles remain posterior to the diaphragmatic crura in close apposition to the T12 vertebral body, this has been termed the retrocrural technique. Splanchnic nerve block is a minor modification of the classic retrocrural celiac plexus block, the only difference being that for splanchnic block, the needles are placed over the midportion of the T12 vertebral body rather than the cephalad portion of L1. Retrocrural celiac plexus block at the superior aspect of the L1 vertebral body and splanchnic nerve block at the mid T12 vertebral body have both been described, and they are essentially the same technique relying on cephalad spread of solution to block the splanchnic nerves in a retrocrural location. In most cases, celiac plexus (transcrural or retrocrural) and splanchnic nerve block can be used interchangeably to effect the same results. Even though there are those who strongly advocate one approach or the other, there is no evidence that either approach results in superior clinical outcomes.

Celiac plexus and splachnic nerve block are used to control pain arising from intra-abdominal structures. These structures include the pancreas, liver, gallbladder, omentum, mesentery, and alimentary tract from the stomach to the transverse colon. The most common application of neurolytic celiac plexus block is to treat pain associated with intra-abdominal malignancy, particularly pain associated with pancreatic cancer. Neurolysis of the splanchnic nerves or celiac plexus can produce dramatic pain relief, reduce or eliminate the need for supplemental analgesics, and improve quality of life in patients with pancreatic cancer and other intra-abdominal malignancies. The long-term benefit of neurolytic celiac plexus block in those with chronic nonmalignant pain, particularly those with chronic pancreatitis, is debatable. Many patients with pancreatic cancer have a short life span left. Analgesia sometimes lasts the rest of their lives.

Several physiologic side effects are expected following celiac plexus block and include diarrhea and orthostatic hypotension. Blockade of the sympathetic innervation to the abdominal viscera results in unopposed parasympathetic innervation of the alimentary tract and may produce abdominal cramping and sudden diarrhea. Likewise, the vasodilation that ensues often results in orthostatic hypotension. These effects are invariably transient, but may persist for several days after neurolytic block. The hypotension seldom requires treatment other than intravenous hydration.

Complications of celiac plexus and splanchnic nerve block include hematuria, intravascular injection, and pneumothorax. The kidneys extend from between T12 and L3 with the left kidney slightly more cephalad than the right. The aorta lies over the left anterolateral border of the vertebral column. The celiac arterial trunk arises from the anterior surface of the aorta at the T12 level and divides into the hepatic, left gastric, and splenic arteries. Using the transaortic technique, caution must be used to avoid needle placement directly through the axis of the celiac trunk as it exits anteriorly. The inferior vena cava lies just to the right of the aorta over the anterolateral surface of the vertebral column. The medial pleural reflection extends inferomedially as low as the T12-L1 level.

Neurolytic celiac plexus block carries small but significant additional risk. Intravascular injection of 30 mL of 100% ethanol will result in a blood ethanol level well above the legal limit for intoxication, but below danger of severe alcohol toxicity. Intravascular injection of phenol is associated with clinical manifestations similar to

that of local anesthetic toxicity: CNS excitation, followed by seizures, and in extreme toxicity, cardiovascular collapse. The most devastating complication associated with neurolytic celiac plexus block using either alcohol or phenol is paraplegia. The theoretical mechanism is spread of the neurolytic solution toward the posterior surface of the aorta to surround the spinal segmental arteries. At the level of T12 or L1, it is common to have a single, dominant spinal segmental artery, the artery of Adamkiewicz. In some individuals, this artery is the dominant arterial supply to the anterior two thirds of the spinal cord in the low thoracic region. Neurolytic solution may cause spasm or even necrosis and occlusion of the artery of Adamkiewicz leading to paralysis. The actual incidence of this complication is unknown, but appears to be less than 1:1000.

LUMBAR SYMPATHETIC BLOCK

The sympathetic nervous system is involved in the pathophysiology that leads to a number of different chronic pain conditions, including CRPS and ischemic pain.

The lumbar sympathetic chain consists of four to five paired ganglia that lie over the anterolateral surface of the L2 through L4 vertebrae (Fig. 43-9). The cell bodies that travel to the lumbar sympathetic ganglia lie in

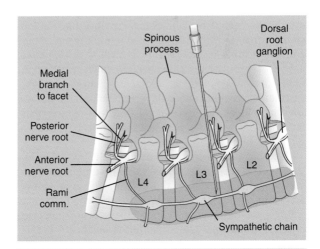

Figure 43-9 Anatomy of the lumbar sympathetic chain. The lumbar sympathetic ganglia are variable in number and location from one individual to another. Most commonly, the ganglia lie over the anteromedial surface of the vertebral bodies between L2 and L4. Temporary lumbar sympathetic block using local anesthetic is best performed by advancing a single needle cephalad to the transverse process of L3 in order to avoid the exiting nerve root. The needle tip is placed adjacent to the superior portion of the anteromedial surface of the L3 vertebral body. Use of 15 to 20 mL of local anesthetic solution will spread to cover multiple vertebral levels (*shaded region*). (Redrawn with permission from Rathmell JP. Atlas of image-guided intervention in regional anesthesia and pain medicine. Lippincott Williams & Wilkins, Philadelphia, 2006, p 136.)

VI

the anterolateral region of the spinal cord from T11 to L2, with variable contributions from T10 and L3. The preganglionic fibers leave the spinal canal with the corresponding spinal nerve root, join the sympathetic chain as white communicating rami, and then synapse within the appropriate ganglion. Postganglionic fibers exit the chain to join either the diffuse perivascular plexus around the iliac and femoral arteries or via the gray communicating rami to join the nerve roots that form the lumbar and lumbosacral plexuses. Sympathetic fibers accompany all of the major nerves to the lower extremities. The majority of the sympathetic innervation to the lower extremities passes through the L2 and L3 lumbar sympathetic ganglia, and blockade of these ganglia results in near complete sympathetic denervation of the lower extremities.

Lumbar sympathetic blockade has been used extensively in the treatment of sympathetically maintained pain syndromes involving the lower extremities. The most common of these are the CRPS type 1 (reflex sympathetic dystrophy) and type 2 (causalgia). The local anesthetic block can produce marked pain relief of long duration, and this block is used as part of a comprehensive treatment plan to provide analgesia and facilitate functional restoration.

Patients with peripheral vascular insufficiency due to small vessel occlusion may also be treated effectively with lumbar sympathetic blockade. Proximal fixed lesions are best treated with surgical intervention using bypass grafting or intra-arterial stent placement to restore blood flow. In those patients with diffuse, small vessel occlusion, lumbar sympathetic block can improve microvascular circulation and reduce ischemic pain. If local anesthetic block improves blood flow and reduces pain, these patients will often benefit from surgical or chemical sympathectomy.

Other patients with neuropathic pain involving the lower extremities have shown variable response to lumbar sympathetic block. In those with acute herpes zoster and early postherpetic neuralgia, sympathetic block may reduce pain. However, once postherpetic neuralgia is well established (beyond 3 to 6 months from onset), sympathetic blockade is rarely helpful. Likewise, deafferentation syndromes such as phantom limb pain and neuropathic lower extremity pain following spinal cord injury have shown variable and largely disappointing responses to sympathetic blockade.

Significant and potentially toxic levels of local anesthetic can result from direct needle placement into a blood vessel and intravascular injection during lumbar sympathetic block. Hematuria can follow direct needle placement through the kidney, and is usually self-limited. Nerve root, epidural, or intrathecal injection can arise when the needle is advanced through the intervertebral foramen and is usually avoided entirely with proper use of radiographic guidance. Following neurolytic lumbar sympathetic block, significant postsympathectomy pain arises in the L1 and L2 nerve root distribution over the anterior thigh in as many as 10% of treated patients. This observation stems from the results following open surgical sympathectomy, but such postsympathectomy neuralgia has also been reported after both chemical and radiofrequency sympathectomy. Postsympathectomy neuralgic pain in the anterior thigh has been postulated to result from partial neurolysis of adjacent sensory fibers, most often the genitofemoral nerve.

Spinal Cord Stimulation

Based on the theory that non-noxious sensory input interferes with the perception of pain, direct activation of the ascending fibers within the dorsal columns of the spinal cord that transmit nonpainful stimuli is used to treat chronic back pain. Modern systems make use of pacemaker-like, implanted pulse generators connected to a small electrode array positioned within the dorsal epidural space of the spinal column. These systems are implanted in a simple, brief surgical procedure. There is evidence from systematic review of observational trials that spinal cord stimulation (SCS) is effective, particularly in patients with chronic lumbosacral or radicular pain following lumbar surgery.[29] The quality of the available trials is generally low, but suggests that more than half of patients report at least 50% pain relief 5 years after device implantation. Use of SCS for chronic lumbosacral pain has been less satisfactory, but results have improved with new dual-lead systems and electrode arrays providing a broad area of stimulation. Spinal cord stimulation is less expensive and more effective than reoperation in the management of persistent postoperative radicular pain. Adverse effects are declining with the advent of newer devices and improved surgical techniques; in the most recent RCT, one or more complications occur in 32% of patients, with lead displacement requiring reoperation in 10% and infection or wound breakdown in 8%. Based on more than a decade of observational studies and two recent, high-quality RCTs, SCS has the most favorable outcomes in unilateral radicular pain; significant reduction in long-term pain occurs in patients with CRPS treated with spinal cord stimulation.

Intrathecal Drug Delivery

Evidence that direct application of morphine to the spinal cord produces spinally mediated analgesia first appeared in the mid-1970s. Intrathecal opioids, the most common being morphine, are now widely used in treating acute and chronic pain. Some nonopioid drugs with spinal selectivity also show promise, including ziconotide, a selective N-type calcium channel blocker. The advent of small, programmable pumps that can be implanted in the abdominal wall and deliver precise, continuous drug infusions has allowed application of this technology to patients with chronic noncancer-related pain.[30] Intrathecal drug delivery is usually reserved for patients with severe pain that does not respond to conservative management. A comparison of maximal medical therapy (oral or parenteral opioids) with intrathecal drug delivery for cancer-related pain showed similar improvement in analgesia and reduction in opioid-related side effects (less somnolence and fatigue) in those who received intrathecal therapy, and intrathecal drug delivery is now commonly used to treat severe cancer-related pain that is unresponsive to more conservative treatments.[29] Morphine is currently the only opioid that is approved for intrathecal use by the Food and Drug Administration, but other drugs singly and in combination are also used. Ziconotide delivered intrathecally demonstrated significant analgesia in patients with severe chronic pain, but side effects were common, the most common being CNS side effects. Intrathecal drug delivery in non-cancer-related pain has not been subject to controlled trials and remains controversial, but numerous observational studies suggest it provides significant pain reduction in some patients whose chronic low back pain fails to respond to more conservative management.

SUMMARY

A brief overview of the most common chronic pain problems and treatments used in the modern practice of the anesthesiology subspecialty of pain medicine is presented. Our understanding of chronic pain as a discrete disease of the nervous system continues to evolve, as does our understanding of the link between acute and chronic pain. Indeed, the anesthesiologist is well poised

in the perioperative arena to help with gaining a better understanding of how new approaches to the treatment of acute pain following surgery can be used to effectively reduce the incidence and severity of chronic pain and to provide precise delivery of new therapeutics to the neuraxis.

QUESTIONS OF THE DAY

1. How do the signs and symptoms of neuropathic pain differ from those of nociceptive pain?
2. A patient presents for evaluation of back pain. What features on the history and physical examination would warrant urgent radiologic evaluation?
3. What are the diagnostic criteria for complex regional pain syndrome (CRPS)?
4. What is the role of epidural steroid injection in a patient with lumbosacral pain?
5. What are the expected physiologic effects after celiac plexus blockade? What are the potential complications of celiac plexus blockade, including neurolytic celiac plexus blockade?
6. What is the rationale for spinal cord stimulation in patients with chronic back pain? What patient population is most likely to benefit?

ACKNOWLEDGMENT

The editors and publisher would like to thank Dr. David J. Lee for contributing a chapter on this topic to the prior edition of this work. It has served as the foundation for the current chapter.

REFERENCES

1. International Association for the Study of Pain Task Force on Taxonomy: In Merskey NB, editor: *Classification of Chronic Pain*, ed 2, Seattle, 1994, IASP Press, pp 209–214.
2. Gatchel RJ, Okifuji A: Evidence-based scientific data documenting the treatment and cost-effectiveness of comprehensive pain programs for chronic nonmalignant pain, *J Pain* 7:779–793, 2006.
3. Andersson GB: Epidemiological features of chronic low-back pain, *Lancet* 354:581–585, 1999.
4. Rubin DI: Epidemiology and risk factors for spine pain, *Neurol Clin* 25:353–371, 2007.
5. Schwarzer AC, Aprill CN, Derby R, et al: The prevalence and clinical features of internal disc disruption in patients with chronic low back pain,

Spine (Phila Pa 1976) 20:1878–1883, 1995.
6. Koes BW, van Tulder MW, Thomas S: Diagnosis and treatment of low back pain, *BMJ* 332:1430–1434, 2006.
7. Saal JA, Saal JS: Nonoperative treatment of herniated lumbar intervertebral disc with radiculopathy, *Spine (Phila Pa 1976)* 14:431–437, 1989.
8. Weinstein JN, Lurie JD, Tosteson TD, et al: Surgical vs. nonoperative treatment for lumbar disk herniation: the Spine Patient Outcomes Research Trial (SPORT) observational cohort, *JAMA* 296:2451–2459, 2006.
9. Chen H, Lamer TJ, Rho RH, et al: Contemporary management of neuropathic pain for the primary care physician, *Mayo Clin Proc* 79:1533–1545, 2004.

10. Deyo RA, Weinstein JN: Low back pain, *N Engl J Med* 344:363–370, 2001.
11. Jarvik JG, Deyo RA: Diagnostic evaluation of low back pain with emphasis on imaging, *Ann Intern Med* 137:586–597, 2002.
12. Bogduk N, McGuirk B: Causes and sources of chronic low back pain. In Bogduk N, McGuirk B, editors: *Medical Management of Acute and Chronic Low Back Pain. An Evidence-Based Approach: Pain Research and Clinical Management*, Amsterdam, 2002, Elsevier Science BV, pp 115–126.
13. Sampathkumar P, Drage LA, Martin DP: Herpes zoster (shingles) and postherpetic neuralgia, *Mayo Clin Proc* 84:274–280, 2009.
14. Benzon HT, Chekka K, Darnule A, et al: Evidence-based case report: The prevention and management of postherpetic neuralgia with emphasis

VI

on interventional procedures, *Reg Anesth Pain Med* 34:514–521, 2009.

15. Guastella V, Mick G: Strategies for the diagnosis and treatment of neuropathic pain secondary to diabetic peripheral sensory polyneuropathy, *Diabetes Metab* 35:12–19, 2009.

16. Tran de QH, Duong S, Bertini P, et al: Treatment of complex regional pain syndrome: A review of the evidence, *Can J Anaesth* 57:149–166, 2010.

17. Christo PJ, Mazloomdoost D: Cancer pain and analgesia, *Ann N Y Acad Sci* 1138:278–298, 2008.

18. Machado LA, Kamper SJ, Herbert RD, et al: Analgesic effects of treatments for non-specific low back pain: A meta-analysis of placebo-controlled randomized trials, *Rheumatology (Oxford)* 48:520–527, 2009.

19. Farkouh ME, Greenberg BP: An evidence-based review of the cardiovascular risks of nonsteroidal anti-inflammatory drugs, *Am J Cardiol* 103:1227–1237, 2009.

20. Dworkin RH, O'Connor AB, Audette J, et al: Recommendations for the pharmacological management of neuropathic pain: An overview and literature update, *Mayo Clin Proc* 85(Suppl 3):S3–S14, 2010.

21. Noble M, Treadwell JR, Tregear SJ, et al: Long-term opioid management for chronic noncancer pain, *Cochrane Database Syst Rev* (1): CD006605, 2010.

22. Sethee J, Rathmell JP: Epidural steroid injections are useful for the treatment of low back pain and radicular symptoms: Pro, *Curr Pain Headache Rep* 13:31–34, 2009.

23. Bogduk N, Dreyfuss P, Govind J: A narrative review of lumbar medial branch neurotomy for the treatment of back pain, *Pain Med* 10:1035–1045, 2009.

24. Cohen SP, Hurley RW: The ability of diagnostic spinal injections to predict surgical outcomes, *Anesth Analg* 105:1756–1775, 2007.

25. Appleby D, Andersson G, Totta M: Meta-analysis of the efficacy and safety of intradiscal electrothermal therapy (IDET), *Pain Med* 37:308–316, 2006.

26. Gerszten PC, Smuck M, Rathmell JP, et al: Plasma disc decompression compared with fluoroscopy-guided transforaminal epidural steroid injections for symptomatic contained lumbar disc herniation: A prospective, randomized, controlled trial, *J Neurosurg Spine* 12:357–371, 2010.

27. Gibbs GF, Drummond PD, Finch PM, et al: Unravelling the pathophysiology of complex regional pain syndrome: Focus on sympathetically maintained pain, *Clin Exp Pharmacol Physiol* 35:717–724, 2008.

28. Christo PJ, Mazloomdoost D: Interventional pain treatments for cancer pain, *Ann N Y Acad Sci* 1138:299–328, 2008.

29. Turner JA, Loeser JD, Deyo RA, et al: Spinal cord stimulation for patients with failed back surgery syndrome or complex regional pain syndrome: A systematic review of effectiveness and complications, *Pain* 108:137–147, 2004.

30. Prager JP: Neuraxial medication delivery: The development and maturity of a concept for treating chronic pain of spinal origin, *Spine (Phila Pa 1976)* 27:2593–2605, 2001.

44 CARDIOPULMONARY RESUSCITATION

David Shimabukuro and Linda L. Liu

Cardiopulmonary resuscitation (CPR) is a term that was first used in the early 1960s by Safar and Kouwenhoven to describe a combined technique of mouth-to-mouth ventilation and closed cardiac chest compressions in a pulseless patient. Over the past 40 years, significant advances in CPR and cardiovascular life support have been made, especially in its application in the out-of-hospital setting. Today, the early descriptions of CPR would be considered basic life support (BLS), whereas adult advanced cardiovascular life support (ACLS) and pediatric advanced cardiovascular life support (PALS) include the more sophisticated use of pharmacotherapy and other definitive techniques. Out-of-hospital resuscitation has been well described in the literature. Yet, in-hospital life support including resuscitation has only occasionally been described.

In 1986 the American Heart Association published the first ACLS algorithms. In 2000, the International Liaison Committee on Resuscitation assembled the first international conference to produce worldwide guidelines for emergency cardiovascular care and CPR. These expert panels meet every few years so that the guidelines and algorithms for CPR and ACLS can be revised and updated based on newly published studies. The most recent guidelines were released in October 2010 and will be covered in this chapter.[1,2]

BASIC LIFE SUPPORT

For any patient having cardiac arrest, the most important steps are (1) immediate recognition of unresponsiveness, (2) checking for lack of breathing or lack of normal breathing (3) activating an emergency response system and retrieving an automated external defibrillator (AED), (4) checking for a pulse (no more than 10 seconds), and (5) starting cycles of 30 chest compressions followed by 2 breaths (Fig. 44-1).

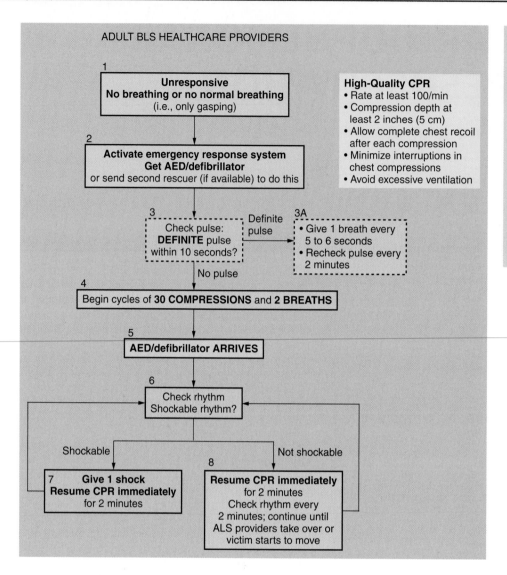

ADULT BLS HEALTHCARE PROVIDERS

1
Unresponsive
No breathing or no normal breathing
(i.e., only gasping)

2
Activate emergency response system
Get AED/defibrillator
or send second rescuer (if available) to do this

High-Quality CPR
• Rate at least 100/min
• Compression depth at least 2 inches (5 cm)
• Allow complete chest recoil after each compression
• Minimize interruptions in chest compressions
• Avoid excessive ventilation

3
Check pulse:
DEFINITE pulse within 10 seconds?

Definite pulse →

3A
• Give 1 breath every 5 to 6 seconds
• Recheck pulse every 2 minutes

No pulse

4
Begin cycles of **30 COMPRESSIONS** and **2 BREATHS**

5
AED/defibrillator ARRIVES

6
Check rhythm
Shockable rhythm?

Shockable

Not shockable

7   Give 1 shock
Resume CPR immediately
for 2 minutes

8
Resume CPR immediately
for 2 minutes
Check rhythm every 2 minutes; continue until ALS providers take over or victim starts to move

Figure 44-1
Resuscitation algorithm for basic life support (BLS). AED, automated external defibrillator; ALS, advanced life support; cm, centimeter; min, minute. (From Berg RA, Hemphill R, Abella BS, et al. Part 5: Adult Basic Life Support: 2010 American Heart Association Guidelines and Cardiopulmonary Resuscitation and Emergency Cardiovascular Care, *Circulation* 122:S689 2010.)

Responsiveness

Prior to approaching a victim, the rescuer should make sure that the scene is safe; then the victim is assessed for responsiveness by tapping or questioning ("Are you OK?"). A quick check for presence of breathing or lack of normal breathing should occur simultaneously. If distress is present, then the emergency response system should be activated, and an AED should be quickly retrieved.

Circulation

Because a pulse can be very difficult to assess, other clues should be used, such as whether the patient is breathing spontaneously or moving. The health care provider should take no more than 10 seconds to check for a definitive pulse either at the carotid or femoral artery. If

the patient has no pulse, no signs of life, or the rescuer is unsure, chest compressions should be started immediately. The heel of the hand should be placed longitudinally on the lower half of the sternum, between the nipples (Fig. 44-2). The sternum should be depressed at least 5 cm (2 inches) at a rate of at least 100 compressions per minute. Complete chest recoil is necessary to allow for venous return and is important for effective CPR. The pattern should be 30 compressions to 2 breaths (30:2 equals 1 cycle of CPR), regardless of whether one or two rescuers are present.

Airway

With the new 2010 BLS guidelines, the importance of definitive airway management has taken a secondary role. The old mnemonic ABCD (airway, breathing,

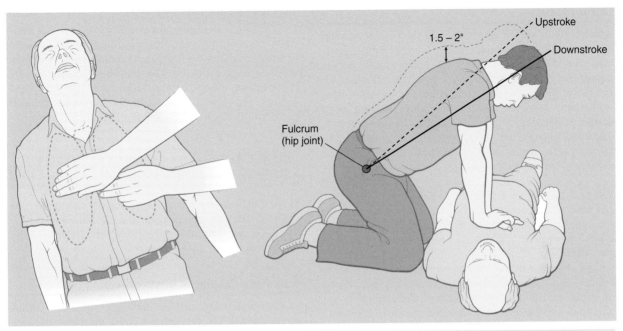

Figure 44-2 Proper hand and body position for performance of closed-chest (external) cardiac compressions in an adult. (From Guidelines for cardiopulmonary resuscitation and emergency cardiac care. JAMA 1999;268:2171-2295, used with permission.)

circulation, and defibrillation) with "look, listen, and feel" has been changed to CAB (compression, airway, breathing). This change is due to evidence proving the importance of chest compressions and the need to quickly restore blood flow to improve the likelihood of a return of spontaneous circulation (ROSC). Airway maneuvers should still be attempted, but they should occur quickly, efficiently, and minimize interruptions in chest compressions. Opening of the airway can be achieved by a simple head tilt–chin lift technique (Fig. 44-3). A jaw thrust maneuver can be used in patients with suspected cervical spine injury. Simple airway devices, such as nasal or oral airways, can be inserted to displace the tongue from the posterior oropharynx.

Breathing

Although several large out-of-hospital studies have demonstrated that chest compression-alone CPR is not inferior to traditional compression-ventilation CPR, health care providers are still expected to provide assisted ventilation.[3] A lone rescuer, if not an expert in airway management, should not use a bag-mask for ventilation, but should use mouth-to-mouth or mouth-to-mask. Care should be taken to avoid rapid or forceful breaths. Delivered tidal volumes are given over 1 second and should produce visible chest rise. A lower than normal minute ventilation (cardiac output is much less than normal) should be the goal because hyperventilation has been proved to be detrimental for neurologic recovery.

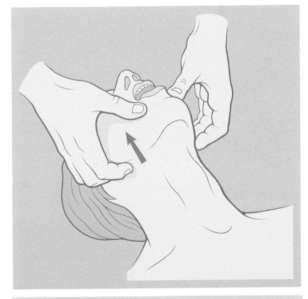

Figure 44-3 The head tilt–jaw thrust maneuver provides a patent upper airway by tensing the muscles attached to the tongue, thus pulling the tongue away from the posterior pharynx. Forward displacement of the mandible is accomplished by grasping the angles of the mandible and lifting with both hands, which serves to displace the mandible forward while tilting the head backward.

VI

Defibrillation

A defibrillator should be attached to the patient as soon as possible. Proper electrode pad placement on the chest wall should be to the right of the upper sternal border below the clavicle and to the left of the nipple with the center in the midaxillary line (Fig. 44-4). Most electrode pads now come with diagrams showing their correct positioning. Alternative locations include anterior-posterior, anterior-left infrascapular, and anterior-right infrascapular. Right anterior axillary to left anterior axillary is not recommended.

ENERGY USED FOR DEFIBRILLATION

The amount of energy (joules) delivered is dependent on the type of defibrillator used. Two major defibrillator types (monophasic and biphasic) are available. Monophasic waveform defibrillators deliver a unidirectional energy charge, whereas biphasic waveform defibrillators deliver an in-series bidirectional energy charge. Based on evidence from implantable defibrillators, bidirectional energy delivery is probably more successful in terminating ventricular tachycardia (VT) and ventricular fibrillation (VF). In addition, biphasic waveform shocks require less energy than traditional monophasic waveform shocks (120 to 200 J versus 360 J, respectively) and may therefore cause less myocardial damage.

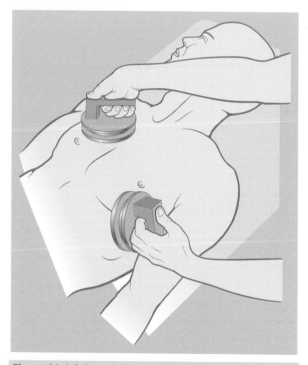

Figure 44-4 Schematic depiction of the proper placement of paddle electrodes in an adult.

TIME TO DEFIBRILLATION

The time until defibrillation is critical to survival, especially because the most frequent initial cardiac rhythm in adult patients is VT/VF. Survival rates after VF cardiac arrest decrease by 7% to 10% with every passing minute. If adequate chest compressions are provided, this decrease in survival rate improves to 3% to 4% with every minute of delay until defibrillation.[4]

ADULT ADVANCED CARDIOVASCULAR LIFE SUPPORT: ALGORITHMS

Three ACLS algorithms relevant to the anesthesia provider in the operating room are (1) pulseless cardiac arrest, (2) symptomatic bradycardia, and (3) symptomatic tachycardia (Figs. 44-5 to 44-7).[2]

Pulseless Cardiac Arrest

Cardiac dysrhythmias that produce pulseless cardiac arrest are (1) VF, (2) rapid VT, (3) pulseless electrical activity (PEA), and (4) asystole (see Fig. 44-5). During pulseless cardiac arrest, the primary goals are to provide effective chest compressions and early defibrillation if the rhythm is VF or VT. Drug administration is of secondary importance because the efficacy of pharmacologic interventions has been difficult to measure or prove. After initiating CPR and defibrillation, rescuers can then establish intravenous access, obtain a more definitive airway, and consider drug therapy, all while providing continued chest compressions and ventilation.

AIRWAY MANAGEMENT

Bag-mask ventilation and ventilation through an advanced airway (endotracheal tube, supraglottic airway) are acceptable methods of ventilation during CPR. Because chest compressions are not performed during tracheal intubation, the rescuer has to weigh the need for compressions against the need for definitive airway management. Perhaps insertion of an advanced airway should be deferred until after the patient fails to respond to several cycles of CPR and defibrillation. However, this decision is not always absolutely correct. For example, a patient in severe pulmonary edema may benefit from endotracheal intubation sooner rather than later.

With the presence of a more definitive airway, the adequacy of ventilation should be evaluated again. The chest should rise bilaterally and breath sounds should be auscultated. In addition, proper positioning of the endotracheal tube should be confirmed with a second test to decrease false positive and false negative findings. Capnography to measure end-tidal carbon dioxide (P_{ETCO_2}) is the most ideal test and is highly recommended. Alternative tests include pH paper (color change) and an

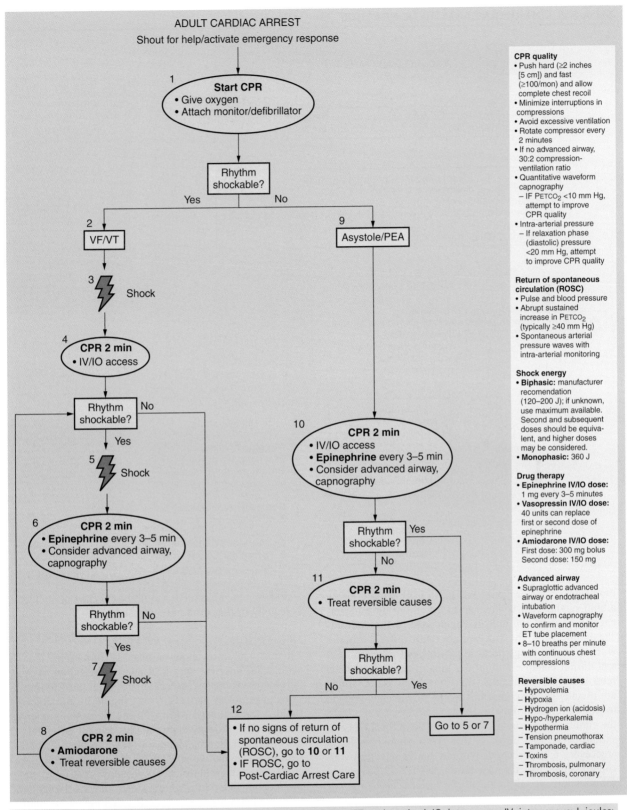

Figure 44-5 Resuscitation algorithm for pulseless arrest. cm, centimeter; ET, endotracheal; IO, intraosseus; IV, intravenous; J, joules; mg, milligram; min, minute; mm Hg, milliliters of mercury; PEA, pulseless electrical activity; PETCO$_2$, partial pressure of end-tidal carbon dioxide; VF, ventricular fibrillation; VT, ventricular tachycardia. (From Neumar RW, Otto CW, Link MS, et al. Part 8: Adult Advanced Cardiovascular Life Support: 2010 American Heart Association Guidelines and Cardiopulmonary Resuscitation and Emergency Cardiovascular Care, *Circulation* 122:S736, 2010.)

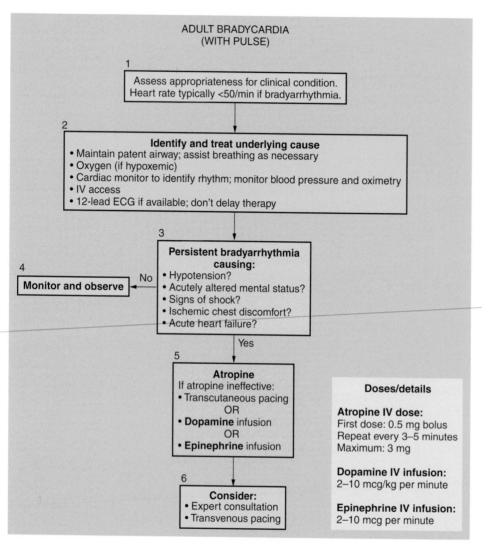

**ADULT BRADYCARDIA
(WITH PULSE)**

1
Assess appropriateness for clinical condition.
Heart rate typically <50/min if bradyarrhythmia.

2
Identify and treat underlying cause
• Maintain patent airway; assist breathing as necessary
• Oxygen (if hypoxemic)
• Cardiac monitor to identify rhythm; monitor blood pressure and oximetry
• IV access
• 12-lead ECG if available; don't delay therapy

3
**Persistent bradyarrhythmia
causing:**
• Hypotension?
• Acutely altered mental status?
• Signs of shock?
• Ischemic chest discomfort?
• Acute heart failure?

4
Monitor and observe ← No

Yes

5
Atropine
If atropine ineffective:
• Transcutaneous pacing
OR
• **Dopamine** infusion
OR
• **Epinephrine** infusion

6
Consider:
• Expert consultation
• Transvenous pacing

Doses/details

Atropine IV dose:
First dose: 0.5 mg bolus
Repeat every 3–5 minutes
Maximum: 3 mg

Dopamine IV infusion:
2–10 mcg/kg per minute

Epinephrine IV infusion:
2–10 mcg per minute

Figure 44-6 Resuscitation algorithm for bradycardia with a pulse. ECG, electrocardiogram; IV, intravenous; kg, kilogram; mcg, microgram; mg, milligram; min, minute. (From Neumar RW, Otto CW, Link MS, et al. Part 8: Adult Advanced Cardiovascular Life Support; 2010 American Heart Association Guidelines and Cardiopulmonary Resuscitation and Emergency Cardiovascular Care, *Circulation* 122:S749, 2010.)

esophageal detector device (EDD). An EDD involves using a bulb suction that is attached to the end of the endotracheal tube once the bulb is compressed. If the endotracheal tube is in the trachea, the bulb quickly inflates with air in the lungs because the tracheal rings are stiff and do not collapse around the tube. If the endotracheal tube is in the esophagus, the esophageal walls, which are pliable, collapse around the end of the endotracheal tube, and the bulb remains in the compressed state. Once the endotracheal tube is confirmed to be in the trachea, it should be secured in place. One breath should be delivered every 6 to 8 seconds without synchronization with compressions. Failed resuscitation may reflect poor chest compressions or migration of the endotracheal tube out of the trachea. Continuous monitoring of P$_{ETCO_2}$ can be extremely beneficial during the resuscitation. Although values have not been correlated with ROSC, it does guide the rescuers in adequacy of pulmonary blood flow. If continuous end-tidal carbon dioxide monitoring is not available, tube placement should be checked periodically, especially during prolonged resuscitation.

MEDICATIONS

Establishing intravenous access is important, but it should not interfere with CPR and defibrillation. A large peripheral venous catheter is sufficient in most resuscitations of pulseless patients. Drugs should be administered rapidly and followed with a 20-mL fluid bolus if given peripherally. If intravenous access cannot be obtained or is lost, certain drugs (epinephrine, lidocaine, vasopressin, atropine, naloxone) can be given via the endotracheal tube. The endotracheal tube dose is 2 to 10 times the recommended intravenous dose, and the drug should be diluted in 5 to 10 mL of sterile water before instillation down the endotracheal tube. A preferable alternative to the intravenous route is the intraosseus route. Kits are now commercially available to rapidly place these lines. No dose changes are required from the IV route.

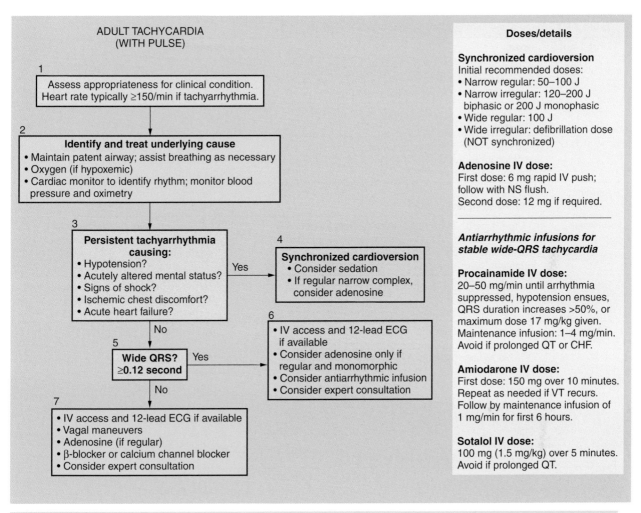

ADULT TACHYCARDIA
(WITH PULSE)

1
Assess appropriateness for clinical condition.
Heart rate typically ≥150/min if tachyarrhythmia.

2
Identify and treat underlying cause
• Maintain patent airway; assist breathing as necessary
• Oxygen (if hypoxemic)
• Cardiac monitor to identify rhythm; monitor blood pressure and oximetry

3
Persistent tachyarrhythmia causing:
• Hypotension?
• Acutely altered mental status?
• Signs of shock?
• Ischemic chest discomfort?
• Acute heart failure?

Yes →

4
Synchronized cardioversion
• Consider sedation
• If regular narrow complex, consider adenosine

No

5
Wide QRS?
≥0.12 second

Yes →

6
• IV access and 12-lead ECG if available
• Consider adenosine only if regular and monomorphic
• Consider antiarrhythmic infusion
• Consider expert consultation

No

7
• IV access and 12-lead ECG if available
• Vagal maneuvers
• Adenosine (if regular)
• β-blocker or calcium channel blocker
• Consider expert consultation

Doses/details

Synchronized cardioversion
Initial recommended doses:
• Narrow regular: 50–100 J
• Narrow irregular: 120–200 J biphasic or 200 J monophasic
• Wide regular: 100 J
• Wide irregular: defibrillation dose (NOT synchronized)

Adenosine IV dose:
First dose: 6 mg rapid IV push; follow with NS flush.
Second dose: 12 mg if required.

Antiarrhythmic infusions for stable wide-QRS tachycardia

Procainamide IV dose:
20–50 mg/min until arrhythmia suppressed, hypotension ensues, QRS duration increases >50%, or maximum dose 17 mg/kg given. Maintenance infusion: 1–4 mg/min. Avoid if prolonged QT or CHF.

Amiodarone IV dose:
First dose: 150 mg over 10 minutes. Repeat as needed if VT recurs. Follow by maintenance infusion of 1 mg/min for first 6 hours.

Sotalol IV dose:
100 mg (1.5 mg/kg) over 5 minutes. Avoid if prolonged QT.

Figure 44-7 Resuscitation algorithm for tachycardia with a pulse. CHF, congestive heart failure; ECG, electrocardiogram; IV, intravenous; J, joules; kg, kilogram; min, minute; mg, milligram; NS, normal saline; VT, ventricular tachycardia. (From Neumar RW, Otto CW, Link MS, et al. Part 8: Adult Advanced Cardiovascular Life Support: 2010 American Heart Association Guidelines and Cardiopulmonary Resuscitation and Emergency Cardiovascular Care, *Circulation* 122:S751, 2010.)

VENTRICULAR FIBRILLATION/VENTRICULAR TACHYCARDIA

If the cardiac arrest was witnessed, the health care provider should immediately place the defibrillator pads on the patient's chest, determine the rhythm, and deliver a shock if VF or VT is present (see Fig. 44-5). In unwitnessed arrests, rescuers may give five cycles of CPR before checking the rhythm and attempting defibrillation. CPR should be resumed immediately after delivery of the shock and continued for five cycles or about 2 minutes, followed by reevaluation of the cardiac rhythm. If the patient remains in VF/VT, the defibrillator should be charged to the appropriate energy level (360 J for monophasic or 120 to 200 J for biphasic) while CPR is still being performed.

If VF or VT persists after one to two sets of CPR-defibrillation cycles, a vasopressor should be given (Table 44-1). Epinephrine, 1 mg IV, may be administered every 3 to 5 minutes. One dose of vasopressin, 40 units IV, may replace either the first or second dose of epinephrine. Drug administration should be timed to minimize interruptions in chest compressions. If VF/VT persists after another set of CPR-defibrillation and vasopressor administration, an antiarrhythmic medication, amiodarone, is recommended for VF/VT. Lidocaine can be considered if amiodarone is not available, but a survival benefit for lidocaine over amiodarone is not clear. Magnesium sulfate can be considered if torsades de pointes is suspected.

ASYSTOLE AND PULSELESS ELECTRICAL ACTIVITY

Asystole is usually an agonal rhythm, whereas PEA is often caused by a reversible condition and can be treated if the inciting cause is identified (Table 44-2). These two

VI

Table 44-1 Drugs Used During Adult Cardiopulmonary Resuscitation

Drug Name	Dose	Indication
Adenosine	6 mg IV May repeat 12 mg IV (cut dose in half if using central line)	For stable narrow QRS tachycardia or monomorphic VT (contraindicated with preexcitation syndrome)
Amiodarone	300 mg IV May repeat 150 mg IV	For pulseless VT/VF
	150 mg IV over a 10-minute period Maintenance infusion of 1 mg/min for 6 hours, then 0.5 mg/min Maximum total dose of 2.2 g/24 hr	For stable VT or uncertain wide QRS tachycardia and narrow QRS tachycardias
Atropine*	0.5 mg IV May repeat to total dose of 3 mg	For bradycardia
Diltiazem	15 to 20 mg (0.25 mg/kg) IV over a 2-minute period May repeat 20 to 25 mg (0.35 mg/kg) in 15 minutes Maintenance infusion of 5- to 15- mg/hr, titrated to heart rate	For stable narrow QRS tachycardia (contraindicated with preexcitation syndrome)
Dopamine	2 to 10 µg/kg/min by infusion	For bradycardia instead of a pacer, while awaiting a pacer, or if a pacer is ineffective or not tolerated
Epinephrine*	1 mg IV Repeat every 3 to 5 minutes 2 to 10 µg/min by infusion	For pulseless cardiac arrest For bradycardia instead of a pacer, while awaiting a pacer, or if a pacer is ineffective or not tolerated
Esmolol	0.5 mg/kg IV load, followed by an infusion at 0.05 mg/kg/min May repeat the 0.5-mg/kg bolus and increase the infusion to 0.1 mg/kg/min Maximum infusion of 0.3 mg/kg/min	For stable narrow QRS tachycardias (contraindicated with preexcitation syndrome)
Lidocaine*	1 to 1.5 mg/kg IV May repeat 0.5 to 0.75 mg/kg IV Maximum total of 3 doses or 3 mg/kg	For pulseless VT/VF when amiodarone is NOT available
Magnesium	1 to 2 g IV	For torsades de pointes
Metoprolol	5 mg IV May repeat every 5 minutes Maximum total dose of 15 mg	For stable narrow QRS tachycardias (contraindicated with preexcitation syndrome)
Procainamide	20 to 50 mg/min IV (max 17 mg/kg) until arrhythmia suppressed Maintenance infusion of 1 to 4 mg/min	For stable wide QRS tachycardia
Sotalol	100 mg (1.5 mg/kg) IV over 5 minutes	For stable wide QRS tachycardia
Vasopressin*	40 U IV	For pulseless cardiac arrest to replace the first or second dose of epinephrine
Verapamil	2.5 to 5 mg IV over a 2-minute period May repeat 5 to 10 mg over a 15- to 30-minute period Maximum total dose of 20 mg	For stable narrow QRS tachycardia (contraindicated with preexcitation syndrome)

*Also effectively delivered by tracheal mucosal absorption when administered through an endotracheal tube.
g, gram; hr, hour; IV, intravenous; kg, kilogram; mcg, microgram; mg, milligram; min, minute; U, unit; VF, ventricular fibrillation; VT, ventricular tachycardia.

cardiac rhythms have been combined as the second part of the pulseless arrest algorithm because of similarities in their management (see Fig. 44-5). Neither will benefit from defibrillation, so the focus should be on performing effective CPR with minimal interruptions, identifying reversible causes, and establishing an advanced airway. A vasopressor may be administered after initiation of CPR. Epinephrine, 1 mg IV, may be given every 3 to 5 minutes. Alternatively, a single dose of vasopressin, 40 units IV, may replace either the first or second dose of

Table 44-2 Major Causes of Cardiovascular Collapse in the Perioperative Period

8 Hs	8 Ts
Hypovolemia	**T**oxins (anaphylaxis/anesthesia)
Hypoxia	**T**amponade
Hydrogen ion (acidosis)	**T**ension pneumothorax
Hyperkalemia/hypokalemia	**T**hrombosis in coronary artery
Hypoglycemia	**T**hrombus in pulmonary artery
Hypothermia	**T**rauma
Malignant **h**yperthermia	Q**T** interval prolongation
Hypervagal response	Pulmonary hyper**t**ension

Adapted from the 5 Hs and 5 Ts proposed by the American Heart Association (AHA).

epinephrine. Atropine has been removed from the algorithm because studies show that routine use of atropine is unlikely to provide any benefit. Cardiac rhythm checks should be performed after every five cycles or 2 minutes of CPR. If an organized cardiac rhythm is present, the rescuer should check for a pulse. If there is no pulse, CPR should be continued. If a pulse is present, the rescuer should identify the rhythm and treat accordingly. Given the poor survival and neurologic recovery rates of patients in asystole, the length and effort of resuscitation should be carefully considered.

Bradycardia

Bradycardia is defined as a heart rate slower than 60 beats/min (see Fig. 44-6). Some patients, especially young athletes, may have a resting heart rate slower than 60 beats/min yet continue to exhibit signs of adequate perfusion. Asymptomatic patients do not require treatment. Intervention by pharmacologic treatment or electrical pacing should be based on signs and symptoms of inadequate perfusion. Symptoms cannot be obtained under anesthesia, so the anesthesia provider should use discretion in determining whether end-organ perfusion is compromised by the slow heart rate. Initial treatment of symptomatic bradycardia should focus on support of airway, breathing, and circulation. Supplemental oxygen should be delivered, and continuous cardiac rhythm, systemic blood pressure, and pulse oximetry should be monitored. Further therapies include atropine (0.5 mg IV every 3 to 5 minutes; no more than 3 mg), an infusion of β-adrenergic agonists (dopamine, epinephrine), or transcutaneous pacing.

Tachycardia

Regardless of the underlying origin of the tachycardia, unstable or symptomatic patients should be immediately shocked via synchronized cardioversion (see Fig. 44-7).

A trial of adenosine before cardioversion can be considered in select cases of unstable regular narrow-complex tachycardia. In stable patients with fast ventricular rates, determining whether the underlying rhythm has a narrow or wide QRS complex (>0.12 second) on the electrocardiogram is important. Patients with asymptomatic tachycardias, especially those with wide-complex tachycardias, should be evaluated by a consultant to help determine whether the rhythm is ventricular or atrial in origin. Treatment should be guided by the consultant's opinion, which often can include the use of antidysrhythmic medication or atrioventricular (AV) nodal blocking drugs. If the rhythm is an irregular narrow-complex tachycardia, the underlying rhythm is probably atrial fibrillation, and heart rate control should be attempted with AV nodal blocking drugs. If the rhythm is a regular narrow-complex tachycardia, conversion back to sinus rhythm should be attempted by vagal maneuvers or the administration of adenosine, or both. Cardiac rhythm conversion signifies probable reentry supraventricular tachycardia, and recurrence can be treated with adenosine or longer-acting AV nodal blocking drugs. If cardiac rhythm conversion does not occur, the underlying rhythm is possibly atrial flutter or junctional tachycardia. In this case, effort should be made to achieve rate control with the use of AV nodal blocking drugs.

ADULT ADVANCED CARDIOVASCULAR LIFE SUPPORT: DRUG THERAPY (Also See Chapter 7)

Epinephrine, vasopressin, and amiodarone are among the most commonly used drugs in the ACLS algorithms (see Table 44-1) and deserve special attention.

Epinephrine

Epinephrine is a combined direct α- and β-adrenergic receptor agonist. It increases myocardial oxygen consumption by increasing heart rate and afterload. In multiple animal studies, epinephrine has shown to be of benefit in establishing return of spontaneous circulation. Epinephrine can increase diastolic pressure and thereby restore coronary perfusion pressure and blood flow back to the myocardium.

Vasopressin

Vasopressin is a naturally occurring antidiuretic hormone with a half-life of 10 to 20 minutes. It is a nonadrenergic peripheral vasoconstrictor that acts by direct stimulation of smooth muscle vasopressin-1 receptors and leads to intense vasoconstriction of the vasculature in the skin, skeletal muscles, intestine, and fat. Vasopressin has also been found in animals to selectively vasodilate the cerebral, coronary, and pulmonary vascular beds. Like epinephrine, vasopressin is believed to increase diastolic

VI

pressure and therefore increase coronary perfusion pressure with restoration of blood flow to the myocardium. Given its relatively long half-life, it is recommended that vasopressin be given only once during the resuscitation of a pulseless patient.

There are no significant differences in rates of hospital admission or survival between patients with out-of-hospital arrest who receive vasopressin or epinephrine. When compared with epinephrine in patients with asystole, vasopressin is associated with more frequent hospital admission and hospital discharge rates, but not neurologically intact survival.[5] A recent study has shown no improvement in hospital admissions with the addition of vasopressin to epinephrine during asystole.[6] Because the effects of vasopressin and epinephrine in patients with cardiac arrest are not significantly different, one dose of vasopressin may substitute for either the first or second dose of epinephrine in the treatment of pulseless cardiac arrest.

Amiodarone

Amiodarone was initially developed as an antianginal drug in the 1950s but was abandoned because of its side effects. Because it has effects on cardiac sodium and potassium channels, as well as α- and β-receptors, amiodarone has been reinvestigated for its antiarrhythmic effects. In this regard, amiodarone prolongs repolarization and refractoriness in the sinoatrial node, the atrial and ventricular myocardium, the AV node, and the His-Purkinje cardiac conduction system. Amiodarone can exacerbate or induce arrhythmias, especially torsades de pointes. This drug may interact with volatile anesthetics to produce heart block, profound vasodilation, myocardial depression, and severe hypotension. It has many drug interactions, and can prolong the effects of oral anticoagulants, phenytoin, digoxin, and diltiazem. Despite its multiple disadvantages, amiodarone has been shown in adults with out-of-hospital VF/VT arrest to improve survival to hospital admission when compared with placebo and lidocaine.[7,8] The recommended dose of amiodarone for VF/VT is 300 mg IV. An additional dose of 150 mg IV may be given for persistent VF/VT.

PEDIATRIC ADVANCED LIFE SUPPORT (Also See Chapter 34)

Resuscitation of infants and children follows the same basic principles as those for adults. It is important to remember that most pediatric cardiac events are a result of arterial hypoxemia and respiratory compromise, and thus, airway management and breathing are critical to successful pediatric resuscitation. In contrast, adults tend to experience cardiac arrest as a result of VT or VF secondary to myocardial ischemia. Defibrillation is the more important early intervention in these cases. Regardless, pediatric BLS follows the same algorithm as for adults: C-A-B. Naturally, there are several specific differences between adult and pediatric patients because children are much smaller. For the health care provider, infants are considered to be younger than 1 year, whereas children are considered to be between 1 year old and adolescence. Adult BLS resuscitation guidelines can be used for adolescent children (Table 44-3).

Airway

The airway of pediatric patients is slightly different from that of an adult, but head tilt–chin lift is still the technique of choice to open the airway. Children tend to have a larger tongue and epiglottis in relation to the mouth and larynx. In addition, they have a larger head in relation to the body. Over extension or excessive flexion of the head can lead to difficulty visualizing the glottic opening during direct laryngoscopy. Straight laryngoscope blades may be preferred over curved blades to lift the epiglottis anteriorly and away from the glottic opening in young children.

Circulation

Pulse checks and closed chest compressions are performed slightly differently, depending on whether the patient is a child or an infant. In children, the pulse is palpated at the carotid or femoral artery, similar to adults. In infants, the pulse is checked at the brachial or femoral artery.

External Compressions

In a child, the heel of one or both hands should be placed on the lower half of the sternum, between the nipples, while keeping the fingers off the rib cage and staying above the xiphoid process. In an infant, chest compressions are delivered via the two-finger technique. Two fingers of one hand are placed over the lower half of the sternum approximately one fingerwidth below the intermammary line while keeping above the xiphoid process. For both infants and children, the sternum should be depressed at least one third to one half the anterior-posterior diameter of the chest at a rate of at least 100 compressions per minute. The pattern should be 30 compressions to 2 breaths (30:2) if there is a single rescuer and 15 compressions to 2 breaths (15:2) if there are two rescuers.

Defibrillation

In children, defibrillation should be performed when a pulseless rhythm (VT, VF) is present. An initial energy of 2 to 4 J/kg should be attempted, regardless of the waveform type. Subsequent defibrillations should be at least 4 J/kg, but should not exceed 10 J/kg. Biphasic automated external defibrillators can be used in children older than 1 year outside the hospital setting. American Heart Association guidelines recommend the use of a

Table 44-3 Comparative Resuscitation Techniques between Adults, Children, and Infants (Summary of Key BLS Components for Adults, Children, and Infants*)

Component	Recommendations		
	Adults	*Children*	*Infants*
Recognition	Unresponsive (for all ages)		
	No breathing or no normal breathing (i.e., only gasping)	No breathing or only gasping	
	No pulse palpated within 10 seconds for all ages (HCP only)		
CPR sequence	C-A-B		
Compression rate	At least 100/min		
Compression depth	At least 2 inches (5 cm)	At least ⅓ AP diameter About 2 inches (5 cm)	At least ⅓ AP diameter About 1½ inches (4 cm)
Chest wall recoil	Allow complete recoil between compressions HCPs rotate compressors every 2 minutes		
Compression interruptions	Minimize interruptions in chest compressions Attempt to limit interruptions to <10 seconds		
Airway	Head tilt – chin lift (HCP suspected trauma: jaw thrust)		
Compression-to-ventilation ratio (until advanced airway placed)	30:2 (1 or 2 rescuers)	30:2 (Single rescuer) 15:2 (2 HCP rescuers)	
Ventilations: when rescuer untrained or trained and not proficient	Compressions only		
Ventilations with advanced airway (HCP)	1 breath every 6-8 seconds (8-10 breaths/min) Asynchronous with chest compressions About 1 second per breath Visible chest rise		
Defibrillation	Attach and use AED as soon as available. Minimize interruptions in chest compressions before and after shock; resume CPR beginning with compressions immediately after each shock.		

AED, automated external defibrillator; AP, anterior-posterior; CPR, cardiopulmonary resuscitation; HCP, healthcare provider.
*Excluding the newly born, in whom the etiology of an arrest is nearly always asphyxial.
(From Hazinski MR, ed. Highlights of the 2010 American Heart Association Guidelines for CPR and ECC, 2010, p 8)

pediatric dose attenuator system that will decrease the amount of delivered energy. If one is not available, a standard external defibrillator can be substituted.

Drugs

Most drug dosages are calculated by using current known weight or ideal body weight based on height. Most pediatric units have resuscitation carts divided by weight to facilitate drug administration in an emergency so that calculations do not need to be performed and valuable time is not wasted.

POSTRESUSCITATION CARE

After successful resuscitation with return of spontaneous circulation, patients should be admitted to the intensive care unit (if not already there) for further definitive and supportive treatment (Fig. 44-8).[9] Postcardiac arrest care should be focused to optimize cardiopulmonary function to ensure organ perfusion is adequate. It should be consistent, integrated, and multidisciplinary. When possible, therapies are administered concurrently. Specifically, percutaneous coronary interventions (PCI) should not be delayed to institute hypothermia, and the institution of hypothermia should not delay PCI. Often, vasopressors and inotropes need to be administered during the immediate postresuscitation period because of the presence of myocardial stunning and hemodynamic instability. Central venous access for drug administration may be necessary, along with an intra-arterial catheter to facilitate hemodynamic monitoring.

In addition to cardiac recovery, neurologic recovery is of vital importance. This is especially true during the immediate postresuscitation phase. Hypothermia protocols should be established to facilitate institution. Consequently, due to the widespread use of mild hypothermia, traditional

VI

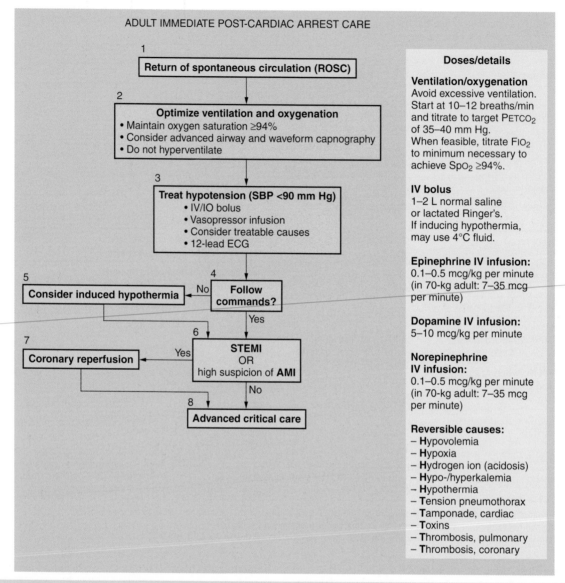

ADULT IMMEDIATE POST-CARDIAC ARREST CARE

1 Return of spontaneous circulation (ROSC)

2 Optimize ventilation and oxygenation
- Maintain oxygen saturation ≥94%
- Consider advanced airway and waveform capnography
- Do not hyperventilate

3 Treat hypotension (SBP <90 mm Hg)
- IV/IO bolus
- Vasopressor infusion
- Consider treatable causes
- 12-lead ECG

4 Follow commands?

5 Consider induced hypothermia ← No

Yes

6 STEMI OR high suspicion of AMI

7 Coronary reperfusion ← Yes

No

8 Advanced critical care

Doses/details

Ventilation/oxygenation
Avoid excessive ventilation. Start at 10–12 breaths/min and titrate to target P_{ETCO_2} of 35–40 mm Hg. When feasible, titrate F_{IO_2} to minimum necessary to achieve SpO_2 ≥94%.

IV bolus
1–2 L normal saline or lactated Ringer's. If inducing hypothermia, may use 4°C fluid.

Epinephrine IV infusion:
0.1–0.5 mcg/kg per minute (in 70-kg adult: 7–35 mcg per minute)

Dopamine IV infusion:
5–10 mcg/kg per minute

Norepinephrine IV infusion:
0.1–0.5 mcg/kg per minute (in 70-kg adult: 7–35 mcg per minute)

Reversible causes:
– Hypovolemia
– Hypoxia
– Hydrogen ion (acidosis)
– Hypo-/hyperkalemia
– Hypothermia
– Tension pneumothorax
– Tamponade, cardiac
– Toxins
– Thrombosis, pulmonary
– Thrombosis, coronary

Figure 44-8 Algorithm for postcardiac arrest care. AMI, acute myocardial infarction; C, centigrade; ECG, electrocardiogram; FIO_2, fraction of inspired oxygen; IO, intraosseous; IV, intravenous; kg, kilogram; L, liters; mcg, microgram; min, minute; mm Hg, millimeters of mercury; $PETCO_2$, partial pressure of end-tidal carbon dioxide; SBP, systolic blood pressure; SpO_2, pulse oximeter oxygen saturation; STEMI, ST-elevation myocardial infarction. (From Peberdy M, Callaway CW, Neumar RW, et al. Part 9: Post Cardiac Arrest Care: 2010 American Heart Association Guidelines and Cardiopulmonary Resuscitation and Emergency Cardiovascular Care, *Circulation* 122:S769, 2010.)

means to determine neurologic prognosis in patients who have been cooled have not been validated and should be interpreted accordingly.

Mild Hypothermia

Temperature should be monitored closely, and hyperthermia should be avoided at all times. Mild hypothermia for the first 24 to 48 hours may be beneficial to the neurologic recovery of patients after out-of-hospital VF/VT arrest.[10,11] Recommendations are to cool comatose (defined as inability to follow verbal commands) patients who are successfully resuscitated from out-of-hospital VF/VT arrest to 32° C to 34° C for the first 12 to 24 hours. Hypothermia has not been well studied in patients with an initial rhythm of asystole or PEA. However, given recent technologic advances in cooling patients quickly and easily, mild hypothermia has been expanded to all comatose patients following return of spontaneous circulation regardless of the initial pulseless rhythm and whether it occurred out of hospital or in hospital.[12] Warming is allowed to occur passively unless it is beyond the 48-hour window.

Glucose Levels

Increased blood glucose concentrations after resuscitation from cardiac arrest are associated with poor neurologic outcome. However, studies have not shown that tight control of serum glucose improves neurologic outcome. Regardless, glucose levels after resuscitation should be monitored closely to avoid hypoglycemia and hyperglycemia.

Normocapnia

Hyperventilation does not protect the brain or other vital organs after resuscitation from cardiac arrest. In fact, iatrogenic hyperventilation can lead to increased airway pressure, intrinsic positive end-expiratory pressure ("auto-PEEP"), increased intrathoracic pressure, and increased intracranial pressure. In patients with brain injury, hyperventilation may worsen the neurologic outcome. There are no data to support targeting a specific partial pressure of arterial carbon dioxide $PaCO_2$ after resuscitation, so ventilation to normocapnic levels is recommended.

SPECIAL PERIOPERATIVE CONSIDERATIONS

Anesthesia providers sometimes encounter unique situations and experiences that are rarely seen by other medical practitioners. Cardiac arrest during anesthesia is distinct from cardiac arrest in other settings in that our patients have a different pathophysiology. Cardiac arrests under anesthesia are usually witnessed, and frequently anticipated. The traditional guidelines don't often translate well into the perioperative setting. Because of that, the American Society of Anesthesiologists (ASA) Committee on Critical Care Medicine published a monograph specific to advanced life support for anesthesia. They expanded the traditional 5 Hs and 5 Ts as established by the American Heart Association (AHA) to the 8 Hs and 8 Ts. Included in the list is hypoglycemia, malignant hyperthermia, hypervagal response, trauma, QT interval prolongation, and pulmonary hypertension (see Table 44-2). Four unique circumstances to the general anesthesia providers are detailed in the next paragraphs.[13]

Anaphylaxis

Minor drug reactions such as a rash are not an uncommon occurrence in the operating room. Major reactions, like anaphylactic shock, occur much less often, but will happen at least once to every anesthesiologist. Common agents associated with anaphylaxis are latex, beta-lactam antibiotics, succinylcholine, nondepolarizing muscle relaxants (i.e., rocuronium; also see Chapter 12), and intravenous contrast material. The treatment of anaphylaxis involves giving epinephrine to interrupt the cascade

Table 44-4   Treatment of Anaphylaxis
Stop or remove inciting agent or drug
Oxygen at FIO_2 1.0
Intravenous fluids
CPR/ACLS if pulseless

Epinephrine, intravenous
  ■ *Bolus*: 10 to 100 µg—if not pulseless
  ■ *Bolus*: 1-3 mg—if pulseless
  ■ *Infusion*: 4-10 µg/min

Vasopressin, intravenous
  ■ *Bolus*: 0.5 to 2 units—if not pulseless
  ■ *Bolus*: 40 units—if pulseless

H_1 blocker, intravenous: diphenhydramine 50 mg
H_2 blocker, intravenous: famotidine 20 mg
Steroid, intravenous: hydrocortisone 50 to 150 mg

ACLS, adult advanced cardiovascular life support; CPR, cardiopulmonary resuscitation; H_1, H_2, histamine receptor types.

of profound vasodilation and significant vascular leak. If possible, the offending drug should be removed or stopped. Epinephrine and vasopressin can be used to support blood pressure, while steroids and antihistamines are administered to further attenuate the response. Intravenous fluid administration is essential secondary to the vascular leak. CPR and ACLS should be immediately instituted if there is no pulse. In the event of complete cardiovascular collapse, much larger doses of epinephrine may be required (Table 44-4).

Gas Embolism (Also See Chapter 30)

Although a very rare event, the incidence of gas embolism has the potential to increase in parallel with the worldwide increase in laparoscopic surgical procedures, posterior spine surgery, and endobronchial laser procedures. The initial management should be to stop the cause (i.e., halt insufflation), occlude open veins, and flood the surgical field with saline. Patients should be placed in Trendelenburg position with left side down to keep the gas in the apex of the ventricle and allow for filling. Complete circulatory collapse should be treated with CPR and ACLS.

Local Anesthetic Toxicity (Also See Chapter 11)

Local anesthetics affect sodium channels throughout the body, including the brain and the heart. In general, toxicity occurs in a dose-dependent fashion with cardiovascular collapse occurring at the end of the spectrum. In nonanesthetized patients, central nervous system symptoms are vital to recognize as they tend to precede cardiac manifestations. Cardiac rhythms can range from premature

VI

Table 44-5 Treatment of Local Anesthetic Toxicity

Stop local anesthetic
CPR/ACLS if pulseless
20% Intralipid IV: ■ *Load*: 1.5 mL/kg ■ *Infusion*: 0.25 mL/kg/hr
Sodium bicarbonate to maintain pH >7.25 in a prolonged resuscitation
Consider transcutaneous or transvenous pacing for bradycardic rhythms
Continue CPR for at least 60 min

ACLS, adult advanced cardiovascular life support; CPR, cardiopulmonary resuscitation.

ventricular contractions to asystole. If possible, the administration of the local anesthetic should be stopped. Intralipid should be given for cardiovascular toxicity.[14] There have been reports of good neurologic recovery in these patients despite the prolonged resuscitation (Table 44-5).

Neuraxial Anesthesia (Also See Chapter 17)

Cardiovascular collapse from neuraxial anesthesia has been described, but is a poorly understood.[15] It seems to occur in younger, otherwise healthy patients undergoing routine surgical procedures with neuraxial anesthesia. Proposed mechanisms causing the arrest include a shift in autonomic balance toward the parasympathetic system, a decrease in venous return from pooling in the splanchnic circulation, and activation of baroreceptors that stimulate a paradoxical Bezold-Jarisch response. A high spinal anesthesia seems to be the biggest culprit. Regardless, treatment follows standard CPR and ACLS recommendations.

QUESTIONS OF THE DAY

1. What is the impact of time to defibrillation on the survival from ventricular fibrillation?
2. What ACLS medications can be administered by endotracheal tube? How should they be prepared and delivered?
3. What is the proper hand placement for external cardiac compression in children and infants? What is the proper depth and frequency of compression?
4. Which postcardiac arrest patients with neurologic injury are most likely to benefit from therapeutic hypothermia?

REFERENCES

1. Berg RA, Hemphill R, Abella BS, et al: Part 5: Adult Basic Life Support: 2010 American Heart Association Guidelines for Cardiopulmonary Resuscitation and Emergency Cardiovascular Care, *Circulation* 122: S685–S705, 2010.
2. Neumar RW, Otto CW, Link MS, et al: Part 8: Adult Advanced Cardiovascular Life Support: 2010 American Heart Association Guidelines for Cardiopulmonary Resuscitation and Emergency Cardiovascular Care, *Circulation* 122:S729–S767, 2010.
3. SOS-KANTO Study Group: Cardiopulmonary resuscitation by bystanders with chest compression only (SOS-KANTO): An observational study, *Lancet* 369:920–926, 2007.
4. Valenzuela TD, Roe DJ, Cretin S, et al: Estimating effectiveness of cardiac arrest interventions: A logistic regression survival model, *Circulation* 96:3308–3313, 1997.
5. Wenzel V, Krismer AC, Arntz HR, et al: A comparison of vasopressin and epinephrine for out-of-hospital cardiopulmonary resuscitation, *N Engl J Med* 350:105–113, 2004.
6. Gueugniaud PY, David JS, Chanzy E, et al: Vasopressin and epinephrine vs. Epinephrine alone in cardiopulmonary resuscitation, *N Engl J Med* 359:21–30, 2008.
7. Kudenchuk PJ, Cobb LA, Copass MK, et al: Amiodarone for resuscitation after out-of-hospital cardiac arrest due to ventricular fibrillation, *N Engl J Med* 341:871–878, 1999.
8. Dorian P, Cass D, Schwartz B, et al: Amiodarone as compared with lidocaine for shock-resistant ventricular fibrillation, *N Engl J Med* 346:884–890, 2002.
9. Peberdy M, Callaway CW, Neumar RW, et al: Part 9: Post Cardiac Arrest Care: 2010 American Heart Association Guidelines for Cardiopulmonary Resuscitation and Emergency Cardiovascular Care, *Circulation* 122: S768–S786, 2010.
10. Hypothermia after Cardiac Arrest Study Group: Mild therapeutic hypothermia to improve the neurologic outcome after cardiac arrest, *N Engl J Med* 346:549–556, 2002.
11. Bernard SA, Gray TW, Buist MD, et al: Treatment of comatose survivors of out-of-hospital cardiac arrest with induced hypothermia, *N Engl J Med* 346:557–563, 2002.
12. Bernard S: Hypothermia after cardiac arrest: Expanding the therapeutic scope, *Crit Care Med* 37:S227–S233, 2009.
13. Gabrielli A, O'Connor M, Maccioli G: *Anesthesiology/Perioperative ACLS by the American Society of Critical Care Anesthesiologists and the American Society of Anesthesiologists, Committee on Critical Care Medicine. Anesthesia advanced circulatory life support (monograph)*, Feb. 2008. Available at http://www.asahq.org/clinical/Anesthesiology-CentricACLS.pdf.
14. Rosenblatt MA, Abel M, Fischer GW, et al: Successful use of a 20% lipid emulsion to resuscitate a patient after a presumed bupivacaine-related cardiac arrest, *Anesthesiology* 105:217–218, 2006.
15. Kopp SL, Horlocker TT, Warner ME, et al: Cardiac arrest during neuraxial anesthesia: Frequency and predisposing factors associated with survival, *Anesth Analg* 100:855–865, 2005.

45 OPERATING ROOM MANAGEMENT

Amr E. Abouleish

"Healing is an Art, Medicine is a Science, and Healthcare is a Business"

Author unknown

Anesthesiologists are in a unique position among physicians. Anesthesiologists bridge medical and surgical specialties. In providing care, we must work directly with many specialties, including surgeons, obstetricians and gynecologists, emergency physicians, and other proceduralists including, but not limited to, interventional radiology, gastrointestinal specialists, cardiologists, and hematologists-oncologists. Further, in evaluating patients, anesthesiologists work with primary care physicians and medical specialists to understand underlying co-morbidities and how to optimize care for these conditions. Because of these many varied relationships with other physicians, anesthesiologists are often identified to help with administrative tasks within a hospital or medical school. Although these positions can be at all levels of administration, the most common administrative role for an anesthesiologist is that of medical director of the operating room (OR), which can include the postanesthesia care unit (PACU) (also see Chapter 39) and day surgery unit (also see Chapter 37). Traditionally, this role has not included administrative roles over OR purchasing and materials management or nursing staff. On the other hand, the role involves day-to-day case flow management as well as overall governance of block scheduling and staffing. The role also overlaps with anesthesiology group management with decisions of the OR management impacting staffing, billing, income, and ultimately, the success of the anesthesiology group. The goal of this chapter is to provide a basic discussion of OR management issues that impact the anesthesiology group and that an OR medical director faces daily: (1) staffing, (2) efficiency and utilization, and (3) turnover and OR throughput. At the end of this chapter, additional resources and references are supplied that allow for more in-depth exploration of these issues and other topics.

ANESTHESIOLOGY STAFFING

In today's economic situation, the cost of anesthesia staffing an OR often exceeds the revenue generated from anesthesia care, creating the need for medical facilities to provide funds for staffing.[1,2] This situation requires an examination of staffing needs and how such needs are determined. The medical center facility, which may be paying for part of the anesthesia staffing, wants to minimize the number of staff members needed, and the anesthesiology group that provides the services wants to ensure that the staff numbers are adequate. This variance leads to a desire from both sides to have an objective manner to determine the actual staff needs.

The most logical process is to determine the workload and the average workload per full-time equivalent (FTE). Then simple division will lead to the number of FTEs needed on any given day. (See later discussion about converting FTEs to actual number of providers.)

This logic is often applied to anesthesia-provider staffing. The workload is often used to determine the staffing needs. The problem with this approach becomes evident when simply answering the following question: "For your OR tomorrow, how many people do you need to provide anesthesia at the start of the day?"[3] Unfortunately, the answer rarely includes the number of cases to be done. Instead, the primary determinants of staffing needs are the number of clinical sites to be staffed and the staffing ratio (i.e., concurrency). Other determinants include whether or not a second shift is needed in the evening and the number of staff members who are on-call or post-call. In other words, if an anesthesiology group needs to provide care for 20 operating rooms at 7:30 AM, the number of anesthesia providers required is no different if all the ORs finish at noon or 3 PM! Therefore, instead of determining staffing needs, workload should be used to determine the appropriate number of ORs needed—assuming this decision is based solely on workload.

A staffing grid, utilizing a spreadsheet, is used to determine the staffing needs.[3] (An online example spreadsheet can be downloaded from reference 3.) The spreadsheet has in the first column the types of clinical sites/duties, and in the second column the number of anesthesiologists; for care-team model groups, the third and fourth columns are used for the number of anesthesia providers (resident, certified registered nurse anesthetist [CRNA], anesthesia assistant [AA]) that are supervised or medically directed by the anesthesiologists (Table 45-1). Several factors will impact the staffing ratio. First, for residents, the accrediting rules limit staffing ratio to a maximum of two; that is, one anesthesiologist can cover only two rooms. For Medicare billing of medical direction, the limit is four rooms. Second, the type of surgery may determine the safety of staffing a second room. For example, a neonatal surgery case may not allow the anesthesiologist to cover another room. Third,

location of clinical site may not allow for a second room to be covered. Finally, other duties must be considered; for example, the schedule runner (anesthesiologist in charge of the schedule) may be able to cover only one room. All these factors on staffing ratio will need to be examined before a final number is determined. For instance, the anesthesiology group might argue that the schedule runner, the anesthesiologist covering radiology, and two other anesthesiologists must be planned for covering only one room with a resident or CRNA, resulting in four clinical sites covered one-on-one. The hospital might argue that only the schedule runner and the radiology anesthesiologist need one-on-one coverage.

The next part of the grid includes the non-OR locations, such as labor and delivery, pain management clinic and procedures, preoperative clinic and consults, and intensive care unit, and for academic departments, resident away rotations. In addition, the number of call providers coming in later in the day and the number who are not available because of post-call status are also listed. The final numbers need to be agreed upon by the anesthesiology group and the hospital.

The staffing grid determines the number of FTEs needed each day. But this number of FTEs cannot be simply converted to determine the number of staff required. For example, 1 FTE anesthesiologist does not work 52 weeks of the year or even all 50 weeks of weekdays remaining after the typical 10 weekday holidays or 2 weeks vacation during a year. Therefore, if 1 FTE is needed, then more than one anesthesiologist will be needed on staff. An estimate can be made by determining the number of weeks a full-time anesthesia provider works in the year, or in other words, determining how many weeks off the typical anesthesiologist has in that group. To illustrate with a hypothetical example, suppose each anesthesiologist takes off 2 weeks for hospital holidays, 4 weeks for vacation, 1 week for CME (continuing medical education) activity, and 1 week for sick leave, for a total of 8 weeks. Therefore, the typical anesthesia provider in this group works 44 of 52 weeks (or 86%). One way to look at this number is to say that each anesthesiologist represents 0.86 FTE. So if 6 FTEs are needed, then seven anesthesiologists will be needed. In addition, for academic departments, the issue of nonclinical rotations also needs to be factored into the calculations. (In Table 45-1, these calculations are at the end of the staffing grid. For more details, see reference 3 and the downloadable Excel workbook with instructions.)

The preceding processes describe only the first steps in determining staffing needs. With daily hour limits, types of shifts people work, the usual inability to hire a fraction of an FTE, and special considerations of the facility, the staffing grid can become complex. But the final message is the same as the initial point: staffing needs are determined by the clinical sites to be covered, not by the workload!

Table 45-1 Example Staffing Grid for An Academic Anesthesiology Department Covering 22 ORs Model: Single Day Shift with Single In-house Call Shift

	ORs Covered	Faculty	Resident	CRNA/AA
Clinical FTEs needed				
Medical direction main OR (includes Remotes)	18.0	9.0	13.0	5.0
One-on-one rooms	1.0	1.0	1.0	
Faculty rooms in main OR	2.0	2.0		
Schedule runner main OR	1.0	1.0		1.0
Total OR sites covered	**22.0**			
Preoperative clinic		1.0	1.0	
Labor and delivery		1.0	3.0	
Pain management clinic and consults		1.0	2.0	
Critical care services		1.0	3.0	
Post call		2.0	6.0	
Daily Clinical FTEs needed		**19.0**	**29.0**	**6.0**
Nonclinical FTEs				
Average Clinical FTE % of FTE		0.75	0.89	0.80
Number of providers that are non-clinical		**6.50**	**4.00**	**1.50**
Away FTEs				
Meeting		1.15	0.21	0.19
Vacation		2.31	1.38	0.77
Sick		1.00	1.00	0.50
Total Away FTEs		**4.46**	**2.59**	**1.46**
Total FTEs needed in dept.		29.96	35.59	8.96
Total on Staff				
Current		30	36	10
Departures		5	12	1
Hires		6	12	0
Total Available FTEs		**31**	**36**	**9**
Excess (or deficit) expected		**1.04**	**0.41**	**0.04**

See text for details of the department. Results based on calculations found in the Excel workbook that can be downloaded from the ASA Web site. Initial estimates utilized no faculty rooms, but results showed a deficit in residents and nurse anesthetists/AAs. Final estimates include two faculty rooms. OR = operating room, FTE = full-time equivalent, AA=anesthesiologists assistant.

OPERATING ROOM EFFICIENCY

Because the staffing needs and costs are determined by number of sites to be covered and not by the actual work being done in those sites, then a goal of any OR management is to use the staff efficiently. In other words, if one is going to pay for a person to be there, then the goal is to have that person working rather than just simply being available. This is true for the anesthesiology group as well as for the hospital staff (OR nurses and surgical technicians).

This idea that one wants the staff working every minute of their shift can actually lead to unintended consequences. The concept of underutilized and overutilized hours is important to understand. An underutilized hour occurs when the staff (and the OR) is not working during the scheduled shift. That is, if the staff is supposed to work until 5 PM, but finishes the last case at 4 PM, then there is 1 underutilized hour. On the other hand, if the last case finishes at 6 PM, there is 1 overutilized hour. In this latter case, one may at first think this is good because the staff worked all of the shift and then some! Unfortunately, that overutilized hour can be costly. For scientific studies a factor of 1.75 to 2.0 is used to multiply the cost of a regular shift to determine the cost of the overutilized hour. This increased cost may be in direct costs (in compensation) or in indirect costs (for recruitment of new staff to replace former staff members who left because of having to stay late frequently). Therefore, 1 underutilized hour costs less than 1 overutilized hour. A measurement of efficiency would be the sum of underutilized hours and overutilized hours (multiplying by the factor). An efficient OR would be one in which this sum is minimized.[4] Consequently, one of the goals of an efficient staffing system is to match staffing shifts to the actual demand. The work shifts should be aligned among anesthesiologists, the OR staff,

VI

and the schedule. For example, if the OR allows for surgeons to schedule cases to finish at 5 PM, then inefficient staffing practice would be to staff the OR until 3 PM and then make staff stay late. On the other hand, an efficient staffing approach would be to increase staffing by either increasing individual shift hours or plan for a second shift to start later in the day.

Alternatively, efficiency of an OR can be evaluated by how well the OR is running. Macario recommended seven performance measurements in scoring OR efficiencies (Table 45-2).[5] In addition to staffing costs, the measurements also include OR function costs and scheduling costs. Factors such as first-start tardiness, prolonged turnover times, delays, and PACU holds all contribute to an inefficient OR. An infrequent case cancellation and a good prediction of case length are signs of an efficient OR. Finally, measurement of contribution margin (revenue minus costs, including staffing costs) is the best measurement of efficiency for the hospital.

Operating Room Utilization

Unlike efficiency, utilization is easier to measure and better reported and followed. The simplest definition of utilization is the percentage of time the OR is used for patient care by dividing the time the patient is in the OR by the time that is available for patient care. A more accurate numerator would include setup and cleanup as well as the time the patient is in room time. In addition, determining the denominator correctly—the available time for patient care—is very important. Unfortunately, this definition is not always the same among the OR nursing staff, the hospital administration, the anesthesiology group, and surgeons. From an operational perspective, the utilization of regularly scheduled time is the important number. So inclusion of after-hour shifts can confuse the final calculations. The exercise of determining what the regularly scheduled hours are may in fact point out that staffing shifts do not match the available hours of patient care. For example, surgeons may feel that every OR is staffed and available for surgery till 5 PM each weekday. But in reality, nursing staffs only 40% of the ORs after 3 PM. That is, nursing does not plan or have staff for 60% of ORs from 3 PM to 5 PM. Further, the anesthesia staff may turn over cases to the call team at 4:30 PM with the plan of only staffing a few rooms after this time. Without a consensus of the hours of operation, confusion, dissatisfaction, and frustration will occur. Coming to an agreement of the definition is essential to any OR management team.

But what is a good utilization percentage? Again, this depends on who is answering the question. For example, hospital administrators may feel that 100% utilization should be the goal, while nursing and the anesthesiology group would like 75%. Also, the surgeons can benefit from a low utilization. (Remember that when a surgeon has an add-on case, the surgeon would like to do it when he/she wants, in the OR he/she wants, and with the staff he/she wants; therefore, a low utilization means the OR is more likely to be open for add-ons). As discussed

Table 45-2 A Scoring System for Operating Room (OR) Efficiency*

Metric	Points Scored		
	0	1	2
Excess staffing costs	>10 %	5-10%	<5%
Start-time tardiness—mean tardiness of start times for elective cases per OR per day	>60 min	45-60 min	<45 min
Cancellation rate	>10%	5-10%	<5%
PACU admission delays—% of workdays with at least one delay in PACU admission	>20 %	10-20%	<10%
Contribution margin (mean) per OR per hour	<$1000/hr	$1000-$2000/hr	>$2000/hr
Turnover times—mean setup and cleanup turnover time for all cases	>40 min	25-40 min	<25 min
Prediction bias—bias in case duration estimates per 8 hours of OR time	>15 min	5-15 min	<5 min
Prolonged turnovers—% of turnovers that take longer than 60 minutes	>25 %	10-25%	<10%

*Efficiency scoring system for an OR that takes into account staffing costs, scheduling costs, and functioning costs. For full details of how to use this system, see cited source.
PACU, postanesthesia care unit.
From Macario A. Are your hospital operating rooms "efficient"? A scoring system with eight performance indicators. Anesthesiology 2006;105:237-240.

previously, 100% of regular hours means that no under-utilized time exists, but because not all the rooms will finish at the end of regular hours, overutilized hours must exist. This will lead to costly direct staff compensation or indirect costs of having to recruit new staff to replace those that leave in frustration of always working over-time. On the other hand, a utilization of 70% to 80% reflects some underutilized hours that actually might mean a better managed OR. Also, it allows for some lee-way for emergency cases.

The most common method of analyzing utilization is by determining block time; that is, the amount of time a surgeon has to schedule cases. Unfortunately, simply relying on utilization for determination of block time can result in poor OR management decisions. For exam-ple, if Surgeon A has utilization of 120% and Surgeon B has utilization of 75%, then the OR management deci-sion based on utilization alone is to give more time to Surgeon A and take time away from Surgeon B. But what if Surgeon A and B are doing the same exact surgical procedures and the same number of patients each day? Surgeon B obviously has shorter surgical durations. If one assumes both surgeons have the same payer mix, then revenue is the same for each, but the costs of Sur-geon A would be higher due to more OR time and over-time of OR staff. So the contribution margin (i.e., net profit = revenue minus costs) is better for Surgeon B. An additional benefit of Surgeon B is that there is regular time available for an add-on case. (Complete discussion for determining proper block scheduling is beyond the scope of this chapter. See reference 6 for more details.)

Another use of utilization is to determine if hospital funding is needed to cover costs of anesthesia staffing. This is often seen in negotiated agreements between hospital and an anesthesiology group when expanding into new clinical sites. The average revenue per hour of care (average revenue per unit and ASA units billed per hour care) can be used to estimate the number of hours of patient care that is needed to cover the staffing costs for one OR. By dividing the number of hours needed by the agreed-upon scheduled staffing hours, a break-even utilization can be estimated. The hospital agreement can state that if utilization is less than this point, the facility will need to help fund the staff-ing costs. On the other hand, if utilization is above the break-even mark, no facility funding will be necessary.

Operating Room Throughput and Turnover Time

Once the hospital or facility and the anesthesiology group have agreed to staff a clinical site or an OR, then the goal is to maximize the output for that OR (efficiency) without increasing costs further (e.g., with overtime). Therefore, a common focus of OR management is how to perform more cases per OR, or in other words, how to maximize OR throughput.

A complete examination of OR throughput starts at the beginning of the process, which begins at the time of referral to the surgeon's office. Then, scheduling (including block scheduling), properly predicting surgical duration, and preoperative evaluation and testing (the preoperative clinic) all occur prior to the day of surgery. On the day of surgery, the day surgery unit must prepare the patient and have the patient transported to the OR in a timely fashion. The surgery is completed and then the patient is admitted to the PACU and then either dis-charged from day surgery or admitted to the hospital. The whole process ends back in the surgeon's office dur-ing the postoperative outpatient visit. As one can see, the OR throughput process involves many other departments and personnel than simply the OR staff and anesthesia providers on the day of surgery.[6]

Prolonged turnover times is often stated as the reason more cases cannot be performed. As the previous descrip-tion of OR throughput demonstrates, this criticism about turnover time is an oversimplification. But why is this criticism so prevalent? The answer is that turnover time is easy to measure and understand. Many of the other parts of OR throughput are complex or involve many dif-ferent parties, but turnover time is focused on one OR and those small number of staff, including the anesthesia provider in that one OR. Therefore, OR managers must understand the issues of turnover time, especially as it relates to OR throughput.

TURNOVER TIME

A commonly stated theme is, "if turnover time were shorter, we could do more cases." Intuitively, it is clear that this is usually not true, and research has established the fact that further reducing reasonable turnover times usually does not increase the number of cases that can be done in a workday.[7,8] The exception would be if the anesthesia providers and/or surgeons are unavailable for some reasons. In these instances an excessively long turnaround could result. For example, if the surgical and/or anesthesia personnel are different than in the first case, they may not be readily available. Turnover time is defined as the time beginning when the preceding patient leaves the OR and the next one enters the OR. For instance, for an OR in a nonambulatory surgical center hospital, a reasonable maximum turnover time between procedures might be 35 minutes. Reducing this number by 20% would only result in a 7-minute time saving between cases. If three cases were done per OR per day, this would mean a 14-minute time saving per day, which is only a fraction of the duration of one case. Therefore, even a good effort of reducing turnover time by 20% will not allow for one more surgical case to be done. Obvi-ously, in an OR where more cases are being performed in a day (e.g., 7 to 10 cataract or pediatric otolaryngology surgeries), reducing turnover time by 7 minutes per case may be significant. But in these specific ORs, the turnover

VI

time is already much shorter than in the rest of the ORs (e.g., 15 minutes) and further reduction may not be possible.

Despite the foregoing discussion, evaluation of turnover times has merit. Instead of working on all turnovers, which will result in few benefits, emphasis should be on reducing delays. A delay is a prolonged turnover time that is longer than the reasonable maximum turnover time. Focusing on delays and not all turnovers allows for more potential improvement in the process. For instance, suppose it is decided that the maximum allowed turnover is 35 minutes. Then when a turnover is longer than 35 minutes (a delay), the reasons for the delay must be reported. Avoidable delays are analyzed and often identify system issues that occur not just in this one case, but multiple times during the week and even each day. Examples of system issues include (but are not limited to) the preoperative preparation process (anesthesia evaluation), proper surgical paperwork (history and physical examination, informed consent) not completed or available, delayed process of preparing the patient on the day of surgery (from arrival to the hospital to being ready for transport to the holding room), transportation issues, equipment issues (including proper procedure posting), and processes in the OR. By focusing on the delays, more than a handful of minutes per case can be saved that add up over a multitude of cases, in contrast to when all turnovers are examined.

THROUGHPUT ON THE DAY OF SURGERY
Traditional Approach

Traditionally, OR throughput initiatives have focused on how to improve the work processes of the current staff.[9,10] Successful initiatives have involved an interdisciplinary team that includes all personnel involved from physicians (surgeons and anesthesia providers) and nursing staff to transportation staff and environmental service personnel. Surgeons who are technically efficient intraoperatively facilitate throughput of surgical cases. The improvement process looks at work flow assessment and redesign of work. This process works, at least over the short run. Unfortunately, to maintain any gains, the improvement process must include continuous and repeated educational efforts and monitoring. Further, potential gains are limited by the existing staffing levels.

Parallel Processing

Additional approaches can improve OR throughput even more, but additional staff and a paradigm shift in the work flow will be needed. Most OR work flow is performed in series. Specifically, one task is completed before the next task is started. For instance, setup for the next case is not performed until the preceding patient is in the PACU and the OR is cleaned. Further, induction

of anesthesia in the next patient cannot be performed before the OR surgical equipment is completely set up. In parallel processing, tasks done during the nonoperative time are not done faster or reduced, but are done at the same time. By doing them at the same time, the total nonoperative time is reduced (see Fig. 45-1). Parallel processing can be successful in allowing an additional case to be performed.[11-16] In practice, all parallel process solutions will require additional staffing, with the type of staffing dependent on the solution. Parallel processing is used on an increasing frequency in busy tertiary care hospitals.

One example of parallel processing is the practice of providing a surgeon with two ORs. In these situations, the surgeon's operative time should be the same or less than the nonoperative time (emergence, clean up/setup, and induction) and the surgeon's case load is sufficient to justify two ORs. In other words, while the surgeon is working in OR A on patient 1, the next patient (patient 2) is induced in OR B. While patient 1 is emerging in OR A and then OR A is cleaned and set up and patient 3 is induced in OR A, the surgeon is completing the procedure on patient 2 in OR B. The surgeon then moves to OR A and begins surgery on patient 3 while patient 2 is emerging in OR B.

Another example of parallel processing is the use of a regional block room. In this situation, the surgeon is working in the OR, but the induction of anesthesia with regional blocks is done in the block room. While the surgeon is finishing the surgery in the preceding patient, regional anesthesia is performed on the next patient. When the OR is cleaned and ready, then the next patient is taken in the OR and the prep begins immediately. Further, the emergence time period is minimal and time is saved there as well.

Another example is to utilize not another OR but an alternative space to complete tasks. This space may allow for induction of general anesthesia and invasive monitoring to be placed. Alternatively (or in addition), a sterile space is provided to allow for the surgical equipment to be set up on a movable table. Both of these solutions will allow for tasks to be performed while the preceding patient is still in the OR or while the OR is being cleaned.

Several limitations to parallel processing exist. First, all the solutions require additional resources—sometimes physical space, but always additional staff. Economically, these solutions may make sense if the additional revenue is larger than the incremental staffing costs. On the other hand, if overutilized time exists, staffing cost savings may occur even if additional staff are hired. For instance, hiring an assistant to help the surgical technician set up the surgical equipment may be less costly than having the whole OR staff (including a registered nurse) work overtime. The second limitation is that to do an additional case, the surgical duration

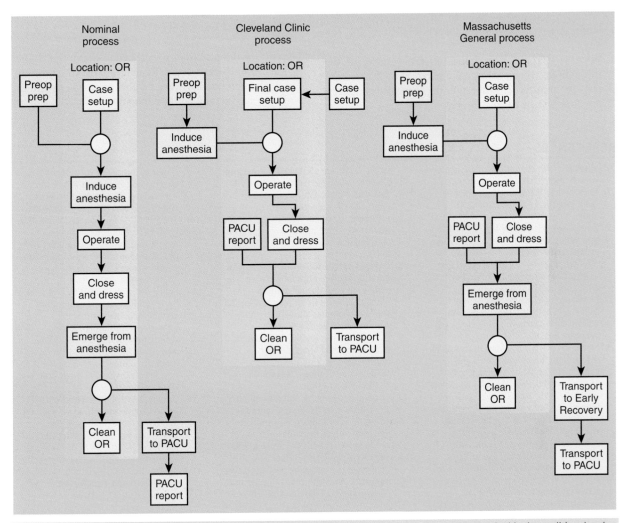

Figure 45-1 Flow diagrams of parallel processing for OR throughput. Three processes are illustrated. Nominal is the traditional series process in which all activity is done sequentially. The Cleveland Clinic Process (see reference 14) and the Massachusetts General Process (see reference 11) are examples of parallel processes. In both of these processes, nonoperative tasks are not done in series, but can be done at the same time (i.e., in parallel) but may require additional staff and space. (Redrawn from Sandberg WS. Engineering parallel processing perioperative systems for improved throughput. Am Soc Anesthesiol Newsletter 2010;74(1):26-27, 30-31. Available at www.asahq.org/For-Members/Publications-and-Research/Periodicals/ASA-Newsletter-Landing.aspx; last accessed Feb. 22, 2010.)

must not be long. For example, it makes no sense to implement parallel processing for surgical duration cases of 12 hours, but it may make sense in cases of less than 1 hour. In addition, the surgeon should have the additional patients to fill freed-up OR time. For example, a surgeon may request two rooms. The operative time needs to be short. Providing a second room seems reasonable. But if the patient volume is too small, then the surgeon will go from one OR with a full schedule to two ORs with a partial schedule in each OR. Finally, the last limitation may occur if the "time-out briefing" is changed. Currently, the process is done immediately before incision. But if the process requires the surgeon to be present prior to induction of anesthesia or

regional block, then some of the solutions noted here may not be possible. The technical and clinical skills of all providers, including surgeons, anesthesia providers, nurses and other operating room personnel, are essential components of efficiently managed operating rooms.

QUESTIONS OF THE DAY

1. What information is needed to determine the number of anesthesia providers required for 10 full-time equivalent (FTE) positions?

VI

2. What is the impact of reduced turnover time on number of cases completed in an operating room (OR) per day?

3. What is "parallel processing" in the context of OR throughput? Under what circumstances will throughput be improved? What are the limitations to the effectiveness of parallel processing?

ACKNOWLEDGMENT

The editors and publisher would like to thank Drs. Jeffrey A. Katz, Eric Huczko and J. Renee Navarro for contributing a chapter on this topic to the prior edition of this work. It has served as the foundation for the current chapter.

REFERENCES

1. Sandberg WS: Barbarians at the gate, *Anesth Analg* 109:695–699, 2009.
2. Kheterpal S, Tremper KK, Shanks A, et al: *Anesth Analg* 109:263–272, 2009.
3. Abouleish AE, Zornow MH: Estimating how many anesthesia providers do our group needs? *Am Soc Anesthesiologists Newsletter* 65:14–16, 2001. Available at http://www.asahq.org/home/For%20Healthcare%20Professionals/Publications%20and%20Research/Other%20Publications/Estimating%20Staffing%20Requirements.aspx; last accessed Feb. 22, 2010.
4. Strum DP, Vargas LG, May JH: Surgical subspecialty block utilization and capacity planning. A minimal cost analysis model, *Anesthesiology* 90:1176–1185, 1999.
5. Macario A: Are your hospital operating rooms "efficient"? A scoring system with eight performance indicators, *Anesthesiology* 105:237–240, 2006.
6. McIntosh C, Dexter F, Epstein RH: Impact of service-specific staffing, case scheduling, turnovers, and first-case starts on anesthesia group and operating room productivity: A tutorial using data from an Australian hospital, *Anesth Analg* 103:1499–1516, 2006.
7. Dexter F, Abouleish AE, Epstein RH, et al: Use of operating room information system data to predict the impact of reducing turnover times on staffing, *Anesth Analg* 97:1119–1126, 2003.
8. Dexter F, Macario A: Decrease in case duration required to complete an additional case during regularly scheduled hours in an operating room suite: A computer simulation study, *Anesth Analg* 88:72–76, 1999.
9. Overdyk FJ, Harvey SC, Fishman RL, et al: Successful strategies for improving operating room efficiency at academic institutions, *Anesth Analg* 86:896–906, 1998.
10. Cendan JC, Good M: Interdisciplinary work flow assessment and redesign decreases operating room turnover time and allows for additional caseload, *Arch Surg* 141:65–69, 2006.
11. Sandberg WS, Daily B, Egan M, et al: Deliberate perioperative systems design improves operating room throughput, *Anesthesiology* 103:406–418, 2005.
12. Hanss R, Buttgereit B, Tonner PH, et al: Overlapping induction of anesthesia: An analysis of costs and benefits, *Anesthesiology* 103:391–400, 2003.
13. Torkki PM, Marjamaa RA, Torkki MI, et al: Use of anesthesia induction rooms can increase the number of urgent orthopedic cases completed within 7 hours, *Anesthesiology* 103:401–405, 2005.
14. Smith MP, Sandberg WS, Foss J, et al: High-throughput operating room system for joint arthroplasties durably outperform routine processes, *Anesthesiology* 109:25–35, 2008.
15. Abouleish AE: Increasing operating room throughput: Just buzzwords for this decade? *Anesthesiology* 109:3–4, 2008.
16. Sandberg WS: Engineering parallel processing perioperative systems for improved throughput, *Am Soc Anesthesiologists Newsletter* 74(1):26–27, 30–31, 2010. Available at http://www.asahq.org/For-Members/Publications-and-Research/Periodicals/ASA-Newsletter-Landing.aspx; last accessed Feb. 22, 2010.

Additional Resources

Sperry RJ: Principles of economic analysis. Basic economic principles written with an anesthesiologist's perspective, *Anesthesiology* 86:1197–1205, 1997.

A bibliography of OR management articles can be found at http://www.franklindexter.net/bibliography_TOC.htm; last accessed Feb. 22, 2010.

Resident Practice Management Education Web page with podcasts, lectures, and a primer on practice management. Available at: www.asahq.org: sign-in in the members-only section, choose "Resident PM" page; last accessed Feb. 22, 2010.

46 AWARENESS UNDER ANESTHESIA

Karen B. Domino and Daniel J. Cole

During interventional/therapeutic procedures, patients may receive drugs that affect the central nervous system (CNS) along a continuum from the awake state to general anesthesia. Dependent upon the nature of the procedure and patient wishes, anesthetic drugs may be given with the intent to produce different levels of sedation or general anesthesia. Patients consenting to receive drugs with the intent to produce only sedation should do so with the understanding that they may have recall of intraoperative events. Conversely, a fundamental component of general anesthesia is unconsciousness and subsequent amnesia, and patients consenting for general anesthesia do so with the expectation that they will not see, hear, feel or remember intraoperative events.

Although amnesia has been a fundamental tenet of training and continuing medical education in anesthesia, recently there has been increased public concern regarding intraoperative awareness. A large percentage of patients who undergo general anesthesia report preoperative fears of intraoperative awareness,[1] and awareness is the most important cause of patient dissatisfaction with anesthesia.[2]

INCIDENCE

Memory consists of explicit, or conscious, memory and implicit, or unconscious, memory. Explicit memory refers to the conscious recollection of previous experiences and is equivalent to remembering. Awareness during anesthesia describes conscious recall (explicit memory) of intraoperative events. However, many more anesthetized patients may respond to commands, yet lack conscious recall of intraoperative events (implicit memory). The anesthetic depth required to block implicit memory is probably more frequent than that required to block explicit memory (intraoperative recall).

The incidence of intraoperative awareness is more common than most practitioners believe.[3] The incidence of intraoperative awareness is probably best estimated by formally interviewing patients postoperatively, well after discharge from the postanesthesia recovery room. Moreover, memory formation for intraoperative awareness may be delayed beyond the immediate recovery period. Sandin and associates[3] reported that only one third of cases of awareness were identified before the patient left the postanesthesia care unit. Often, patients will not voluntarily report awareness if they were not disturbed by it, or if embarrassed to do so. Therefore, a structured interview is recommended to evaluate the incidence of awareness:[4]

1. What was the last thing you remember before you went to sleep?
2. What is the first thing you remember after your operation?
3. Can you remember anything in between?
4. Can you remember if you had any dreams during your procedure?
5. What was the worst thing about your procedure?

The methodologies used to assess the incidence of intraoperative awareness are inconsistent, and the results have predictable variation (Table 46-1).[2–3,5–11] However, in prospective studies when a structured interview was used, intraoperative awareness occur red with surprising frequency. A prospective evaluation of awareness in nearly 12,000 patients undergoing general anesthesia conducted in Sweden revealed an incidence of awareness of 0.18% in cases in which neuromuscular blocking drugs were used and 0.10% in the absence of such drugs, for an overall incidence of 0.13% (see Table 46-1).[3] A similar incidence (1 per 1000 patients) has been observed in the United States in tertiary care centers. Patients with coexisting morbidities tend to have a more frequent incidence of awareness.[8] The risk for intraoperative awareness and subsequent recall is more frequent with a light level of anesthesia, such as occurs during obstetric and cardiac anesthesia.[12] The incidence of awareness is underestimated when assessed retrospectively using quality improvement and patient self-reporting (see Table 46-1).[2,9–11]

ETIOLOGY AND RISK FACTORS FOR INTRAOPERATIVE AWARENESS

The three major causes of intraoperative awareness of anesthesia are light anesthesia, increased patient anesthetic requirements, and anesthetic delivery problems.[12,13] Light anesthesia due to reduced anesthetic doses generally occurs because of hemodynamic intolerance of anesthetic drugs or during procedures in which the anesthetic dose is kept deliberately low, such as in cesarean delivery or open heart surgery. Reduced anesthetic doses may be necessary for optimal physiology and safety in hypovolemic patients or those with limited cardiac reserve. Patients with American Society of Anesthesiologists (ASA) physical status 3 to 5 undergoing major surgery are at increased risk for intraoperative awareness and indeed have a more frequent incidence of awareness.[8] Patients who have experienced intraoperative awareness are more likely to have impaired cardiovascular status, undergo emergency surgery, receive smaller doses of volatile anesthetics, and have experienced an anesthetic with technical difficulties.[14] Anesthetic technique is important in the pathogenesis of awareness during anesthesia. Intraoperative awareness is more likely to occur during anesthetics based on nitrous oxide and intravenously administered anesthetics, and is less likely to occur when volatile anesthetics are used.[15] Use of volatile anesthetics in concentrations at or above 0.7 MAC (minimum alveolar concentration) prevent conscious recall in anesthetized patients similar to that achieved by a brain function monitor of anesthetic depth.[16] Neuromuscular blockade prevents an early sign of light anesthesia, namely patient movement. Lower anesthetic concentrations are needed to prevent awareness than to render immobility; therefore, an inadequately anesthetized, nonparalyzed patient usually moves first.[17]

Some patients, such as those using alcohol, opioids, amphetamines, and cocaine may require an increase in anesthetic dose.[12] Moreover, although incompletely defined, genetic factors may influence anesthetic requirements.[18] Finally, equipment problems with the vaporizer or intravenous infusion devices may lead to awareness, although these are less common causes of awareness, especially with use of end-tidal anesthetic gas analysis.[14]

Table 46-1 Reported Incidence of Intraoperative Awareness

Incidence	N*	Prospective Design	Reference
0.0065%	384,786	No	11
0.007%	211,842	No	10
0.1%	10,811	No	2
0.13%	19,575	Yes	8
0.15%	11,785	Yes	3
0.2%	1000	Yes	7
0.23%	44,006	No	9
0.41%	11,101	Yes	6
0.6%	4001	Yes	5

*Number of patients in reported series.

PSYCHOLOGICAL SEQUELAE

Awareness under general anesthesia can be a traumatic experience, with approximately one third of patients experiencing late psychological sequelae.[19] Some of the most common recalled awareness experiences include auditory sounds, feelings of paralysis, seeing lights, and feelings of helplessness, fear, or anxiety. Pain is less common, although it does occur in some patients, particularly those with complete neuromuscular blockade and who are unable to move. Psychological sequelae of recalled memories may include flashbacks, anxiety/nervousness, loneliness, nightmares, and fear/panic attacks that vary from bothersome to distressing.[19] Some patients develop severe, persistent symptoms (posttraumatic stress disorder) that profoundly interfere with interpersonal relationships and daily activities.[20] Many patients also complain of psychological sequelae after awareness during regional anesthesia or monitored anesthesia care.[9,19]

The risk factors for developing severe psychological consequences after awareness during general anesthesia are not completely known. An acute emotional reaction to the experience significantly predicted the development of late psychological sequelae,[19] whereas pain during surgery does not.[21] The role of premorbid depression and other psychological conditions is also unclear.[22] Recurrence of trauma can trigger previous psychological symptoms.

Early psychotherapeutic intervention may reduce the likelihood of acute and long-term psychological sequelae. An explanation or validation of the awareness incident may affect the presence and duration of the psychological consequences.[23] However, if patients do not inform their anesthesia provider of their recall from general anesthesia, they are less likely to know that they should seek psychological therapy. More reporting from patients also increases the understanding of the experiences. The American Society of Anesthesiologists (ASA) established a registry where patients can report their experiences (www.awaredb.org) and others can learn more about patients' experiences of awareness during general anesthesia and psychological sequelae.

PREVENTION OF AWARENESS

Conventional monitoring of anesthetic depth has included rudimentary signs such as patient movement, autonomic changes, tearing, perspiration, and subjective clinical instinct. Autonomic changes, such as an increase in arterial blood pressure and heart rate, do not reliably predict intraoperative awareness.[24,25] Indeed, intraoperative awareness can occur in the absence of tachycardia or hypertension.[26] With the advent of anesthetic gas analyzers, anesthetic depth has also been assessed by surrogate data such as determining the dose of volatile anesthetic administered to the patient.[16] In addition, considerable effort has been devoted to establishing a monitor that will reliably determine a patient's depth of anesthesia and hence the risk for intraoperative awareness. Several different devices are commercially available, yet none are 100% effective. These monitors typically collect spontaneous or evoked brain electrical activity, and then process the raw data by a proprietary algorithm and display data to the clinician as a quantitative data point (e.g., number from 0 to 100).

At present there are at least three inherent obstacles to the development of a "foolproof" monitor of anesthetic depth, which is based on electrical activity of the brain and its ability to detect intraoperative awareness. First, at present we have not comprehensively validated a unitary mechanism of general anesthesia, and thus various anesthetics are likely to produce unique electrical activity at a given anesthetic depth.[27] Consequently, a unique algorithm to each specific anesthetic regimen would likely be required for optimal correlation between electrical signals in the brain and anesthetic depth. Second, general anesthesia occurs on a continuum without a quantitative dimension, and there is considerable interpatient pharmacodynamic variability to a specific anesthetic. Attempting to translate a conscious or unconscious state into a quantitative number can at best be limited to the art of probability with an expectation of false positive and false negative data (Fig. 46-1).[28] Finally, there is the likelihood of cortical electric activity having sensitivity and

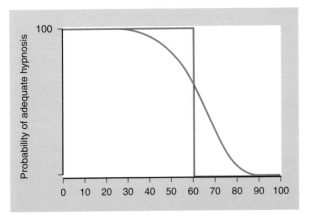

Figure 46-1 Probability of adequate hypnosis based upon brain function monitoring index. The straight line is the ideal probability curve with 100% sensitivity and specificity. The curved line is a more realistic expectation of monitoring in which a progressive decrease of the monitored index value correlates with increased probability of adequate hypnosis. (From Cole DJ, Domino KB. Depth of anesthesia: Clinical applications, intraoperative awareness and beyond. In Schwartz AJ (ed). ASA Refresher Courses in Anesthesiology. Philadelphia, Lippincott, Williams & Wilkins, 2007.)

VI

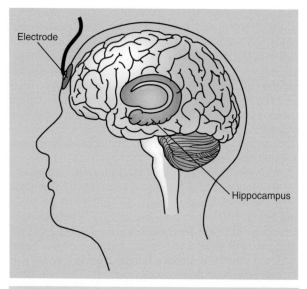

Figure 46-2 A brain function monitor typically records cortical electrical activity from a sensor placed on the forehead. Memory is a biochemical function that occurs in the hippocampus, which is some distance from the recording of brain electrical activity.

specificity to a biochemical event which occurs at a distant subcortical structure (hippocampus) which forms memory (Fig. 46-2).

Published suggestions for the prevention of awareness include premedication with an amnesic drug such as a benzodiazepine, giving adequate doses of drugs to induce anesthesia, avoiding muscle paralysis unless necessary, and administering a volatile anesthetic at a dose of 0.7 MAC or more with monitoring of end-tidal levels to ensure delivery of adequate levels of volatile anesthetics.[16,29]

In 2004, the Joint Commission issued a *Sentinel Alert* that contains suggestions for preventing and managing intraoperative awareness.[30] Their recommendations included the development and implementation of an anesthesia awareness policy, including staff education, informed consent for high-risk patients, and timely maintenance of anesthesia equipment. Also advised were postoperative follow-up of all patients who have undergone general anesthesia, and postoperative counseling for patients with awareness.

Brain Function Monitoring

In general, devices that monitor brain electrical activity for the purpose of assessing depth of anesthesia record electroencephalographic (EEG) activity. Some devices process spontaneous EEG and electromyographic activity and others measure evoked responses to auditory stimuli. Most of the research concerning depth of anesthesia has

been performed on the bispectral index (BIS, Aspect Medical Systems) monitor.

The bispectral index uses a proprietary algorithm to convert a single channel of frontal EEG into an index of hypnotic level, ranging from 100 (awake) to 0 (isoelectric EEG). Specific ranges of 40 to 60 are recommended to reduce the risk of consciousness during general anesthesia. Although many investigators have assessed the effect of brain function monitors on intraoperative awareness, the best evidence in support of a reduction in awareness during general anesthesia with BIS monitoring is derived from four sources: a randomized controlled trial in high-risk patients,[31] a nonrandomized cohort comparison with historical control subjects,[32] a prospective nonrandomized study,[8] and a randomized trial that compared BIS to end-tidal gas monitoring.[16]

Myles and coworkers[31] reported on a randomized controlled trial of BIS monitoring in 2500 patients at high risk for intraoperative awareness (e.g., high-risk cardiac surgery, impaired cardiovascular status, trauma surgery, cesarean section, and patients with chronic benzodiazepine or opioid use, heavy alcohol intake, or prior history of awareness). Intraoperative awareness occurred in two patients (0.17%) when BIS monitors were used to guide anesthesia and in 11 patients (0.91%) managed by routine clinical practice ($p < 0.02$).[31] It is important to realize that if only one extra patient had reported awareness in the BIS group, the difference would have no longer been statistically significant. This is particularly relevant as the end point "awareness" has no "gold standard," unlike death, myocardial infarction, or stroke. Other limitations of the study included unresolved issues such as difficulties in determining "possible" compared to "definite" awareness and the optimal time to interview a patient for the presence or absence of awareness.

Ekman and associates[32] determined the incidence of awareness in a prospective cohort of 5057 patients and compared these data to the incidence in a historical control group of 7826 patients.[3] In this study, BIS was used to guide anesthetic administration. Explicit recall occurred in 0.04% of the BIS patients versus 0.18% in the historical control group ($p < 0.038$). Once again, if just one extra patient were classified with awareness in the BIS-monitored cohort and one less in the historical cohort, the difference would not have been statistically significant. In addition, anesthetic practice may have been changed unrelated to BIS monitoring and affected by the "Hawthorne effect" (the effect of performing a study leads to better performance). Another prospective nonrandomized cohort study ($n = 19{,}575$) was reported by Sebel and associates.[8] In this study, the intent was to determine the incidence of intraoperative awareness, but the authors reported that BIS was monitored in 38% of the patients. The authors found no difference in the incidence of awareness in the BIS-monitored patients as compared to those who were not monitored with a BIS device, although this study did not use BIS values to alter anesthetic concentrations.

Finally, in 2008 Avidan and coworkers[16] reported the effect of BIS and end-tidal anesthetic gas monitoring on the incidence of intraoperative awareness. Patients were randomly assigned to either BIS-guided therapy ($n = 967$) where the intent was to maintain the BIS level between 40 to 60, or end-tidal anesthetic gas therapy ($n = 974$) where the intent was to maintain the end-tidal anesthetic gas concentration between 0.7 and 1.3 MAC. There was no difference in the incidence of definite awareness between the two groups (two for each group).

The predictive positive and negative values of brain monitors for awareness are low due to the infrequent occurrence of intraoperative awareness. Accordingly, the cost of monitoring low-risk patients undergoing general anesthesia is high.[33]

THE ASA'S PRACTICE ADVISORY ON INTRAOPERATIVE AWARENESS AND BRAIN FUNCTION MONITORS

The ASA approved a practice advisory on "Intraoperative Awareness and Brain Function Monitoring" in 2005 which was subsequently published in 2006.[29] A practice advisory is a systematically developed report that is intended to assist clinical decision making in areas in which scientific evidence is insufficient to compel a specific decision matrix. Advisories are approved only after a synthesis and analysis of expert opinion, clinical feasibility data are obtained, open-forum commentary is provided, and consensus surveys are acquired. Advisories are not intended as standards or guidelines. Each practitioner should read and be familiar with the entire document,[29] and apply the information as he/she deems in the best interests of the patient. The authors of this chapter and the Editor-in-Chief of this text had significant input into this practice advisory. This was a very intense and complete analysis. The four areas of advice pertain to preoperative evaluation, preinduction phase of anesthesia, intraoperative monitoring, and intraoperative and postoperative management as summarized in Table 46-2.[29]

The preoperative evaluation should involve review of past medical records for potential risk factors for intraoperative awareness. In addition, the patient interview should assess the presence of other potential anesthetic and surgical risk factors. Finally, the advisory recommends that an informed consent discussion include the potential for intraoperative awareness in high-risk patients.[29]

The routine for the preinduction phase of anesthesia should include a checklist protocol for anesthesia machine and equipment and verification of the proper functioning of intravenous access and infusion equipment, including the presence of appropriate backflow

Table 46-2 ASA Practice Advisory Summary[29]

Preoperative Evaluation
- Identify potential risk factors for awareness.
- Interview patient.
- Obtain informed consent for patients at increased risk for awareness.

Preinduction Phase of Anesthesia
- Use checklist for machine/equipment check.
- Verify function of intravenous access and infusion equipment.
- Consider preoperative benzodiazepine.

Intraoperative Monitoring
- Use multiple modalities to monitor depth of anesthesia.
  - Clinical (e.g., purposeful or reflex movement)
  - Conventional monitors (e.g., end-tidal anesthetic analyzer, HR, BP)
  - Brain function monitoring on a case-by-case basis

Intraoperative and Postoperative Management
- Consider benzodiazepine if patient unexpectedly becomes conscious.
- Speak with patient postoperatively.
- Consider structured interview or Brice questionnaire to determine patient's experience.
- Report occurrence for continuous quality improvement.
- Offer patient psychological counseling.

ASA, American Society of Anesthesiologists; BP, blood pressure; HR, heart rate.
Adapted from the Practice advisory for intraoperative awareness and brain function monitoring: A report by the American Society of Anesthesiologists Task Force on Intraoperative Awareness. Anesthesiology 2006;104:847-864.

check valves. Finally, the anesthesia provider should consider administration of a benzodiazepine on a case-by-case basis for selected patients, especially in patients at increased risk for intraoperative awareness. This recommendation was made even though the data supporting the ability of preoperative benzodiazepines to reduce the incidence of intraoperative awareness are not evident, and preoperative benzodiazepines may convey some risk of postoperative delirium in geriatric patients.

The advisory recommended that multiple modalities should be used to monitor depth of anesthesia. These modalities include clinical techniques such as checking for purposeful or reflex movement, conventional monitoring systems (e.g., ECG, blood pressure monitoring, heart rate), and finally, analysis of the dose of volatile anesthetic delivered to the patient by an end-tidal anesthetic analyzer.[29] The advisory did not recommend routine brain function monitoring for the purpose of preventing awareness.[29] The advisory recommended use of a brain function monitor on a case-by-case basis determined by the individual practitioner for selected patients.[29]

VI

Regarding the intraoperative and postoperative management, the decision to administer a benzodiazepine intraoperatively after a patient unexpectedly becomes conscious should be made on a case-by-case basis.[29] Although a benzodiazepine may be given after such an event, little scientific evidence exists that supports such treatment. The anesthesia provider should speak with patients who report intraoperative awareness to obtain details of the event and to discuss possible reasons for its occurrence. A questionnaire or structured interview may be used to obtain a detailed account of the patient's experience. Once an episode of intraoperative awareness has been reported, an occurrence report concerning the event should be completed for the purpose of continuous quality improvement. And finally, the anesthesia provider should offer counseling or psychological support to those patients who report an episode of intraoperative awareness.

MEDICOLEGAL SEQUELAE OF AWARENESS

As with most complications of anesthesia, the occurrence of an episode of intraoperative awareness does not necessarily mean that a malpractice claim will follow. Only 1 out of 25 patient injuries from negligent care results in a malpractice claim, with even fewer claims arising from injuries due to standard care.[34-36] For intraoperative awareness, there is an enormous disparity between the number of patients who might suffer awareness (based upon incidence statistics), and the few awareness claims (approximately 10 per year) that enter the ASA Closed Claims database. This database captures claims from liability insurers, which insure approximately one third of anesthesiologists in the United States.[26]

This large disparity between the incidence of awareness and malpractice claims is likely due to both the nature and severity of the injuries associated with awareness, as well as the medicolegal and injury compensation systems. Episodes of awareness that do not result in severe short-term or significant long-term sequelae will not enter the malpractice system. Empathetic explanation of the cause of an awareness episode or an apology may not only be therapeutic, but also helpful in preventing escalation of problems to the point of initiation of a malpractice claim.[37,38] In addition, malpractice claims are biased by the large prevalence of negligent or substandard care, an essential component of the tort system.

Factors influencing a patient's decision to initiate a claim are poor communication, unmet expectations, and financial pressures on the patient.[39] A study by Huycke and Huycke surveying individuals who had contacted law firms regarding the initiation of malpractice claims found that 50% of these potential plaintiffs felt they had a poor relationship with their physician.[39] Anesthesia providers have a very brief window of opportunity for establishing a good relationship with a patient preoperatively. Compounding the problem of brief preoperative contact are descriptions from closed claims of patient complaints of not having had an opportunity to discuss their intraoperative awareness with their anesthesiologist postoperatively. In addition, their concern regarding awareness may have been dismissed by health care providers. An insensitive reception to a patient's report of awareness by anesthesiologists and other health care providers may exacerbate injury and contribute to a patient's initiation of a malpractice claim.[38,40,41]

Patients with awareness may avoid situations that trigger painful memories, which the litigation process will certainly bring out.[15,21] In addition, most plaintiffs' lawyers work on a contingency-fee basis, taking a percentage of the award as a fee and earning nothing if the plaintiff loses the case.[42] In a system in which plaintiffs' lawyers must bear the initial costs of the litigation, they will weigh the merits of any potential case. It would be poor business practice to take cases with either a low probability of success or with historically limited financial compensation. In a U.S. survey, attorneys are reluctant to take on cases in which expected financial compensation was less than $61,700 (adjusted to 2007 dollars)[39] and a Canadian study indicated a threshold of $107,000 U.S. (adjusted to 2007 dollars).[43] This threshold would decrease the total number of awareness claims, as the median payments for awareness damages have historically been lower than this threshold. Therefore, lawyers are the de facto gatekeepers to the legal system.

Data from the ASA Closed Claims Project

The Closed Claims Project is an ongoing structured evaluation of adverse anesthetic outcomes obtained from the files of 37 participating liability insurance companies in the United States. The project was established in 1985 and now contains almost 9000 medical malpractice claims.

Recent claims ($n = 71$) for awareness during general anesthesia in the Closed Claims database were compared to those previously published by Domino and associates[26] in 1999 ($n = 80$).[44] Claims for both "awake paralysis" and "recall during general anesthesia" were included as awareness claims. Awake paralysis claims are medication errors, such as syringe swaps, mislabeled medications, errors with succinylcholine infusions, and other out-of-sequence neuromuscular blockade administration resulting in a paralyzed but awake patient. Recall during general anesthesia claims represented awareness in the absence of a classic medication error.[26]

Claims for awareness represent 2% of all claims in the Closed Claims database in both time periods. In both time periods, the majority of patients were female, ASA 1-2, less than 60 years old, and underwent elective surgery. Half of the patients were described as obese.[44] The association with female gender may reflect a greater tendency among females to file malpractice claims for emotional injuries. However, females also have increased requirements for opioids and hypnotics and their anesthetic requirement may have been underestimated.[45,46]

The surgical procedures were different in the two time periods. In the newer claims, the proportion of patients undergoing cardiac surgery increased 21% versus 5%.[44] Although anesthetics for patients undergoing cardiac procedures have long been recognized as among the highest risk for the occurrence of awareness,[47] they have not been previously associated with awareness malpractice claims. This occurrence may signal a change in patient expectations regarding outcomes of cardiac surgery. Interestingly, although trauma surgery also has a high risk for awareness, there were no malpractice claims for awareness in these procedures in the Closed Claims database.

Liability characteristics of awareness claims differed in the two time periods in that the distribution of payment (adjusted for inflation to 2007 dollars) was increased in the recent claims (Table 46-3).[44] The median payment in recent claims was $71,500, with a range of $924 to $1,050,000. Why payment amounts for awareness were increased in recent times is unclear, particularly because these trends have not been observed for other anesthesia complications. However, increased publicity concerning awareness and the possibility of a preventive monitor may increase awards. Higher payments are associated with the existence of a monitor that might prevent the complication in other anesthetic malpractice claims.

The two main causes of awareness in the closed claims were light anesthesia and anesthetic delivery problems (Fig. 46-3).[48] Specific causes of light anesthesia included low dose of induction or maintenance drug (17%) and hemodynamic instability limiting volatile anesthetics (8%). Causes of anesthetic delivery problems included ventilator- and vaporizer-related problems (17%) and medication errors (8.5%). Anesthetic delivery problems were more prevalent among malpractice claims owing to the importance of negligence in liability. No single cause of awareness could be found in 35% of claims, either due to insufficient information or the multiplicity of factors included in the description of the claim.[44] Examination of records generated by an automated anesthesia information management system (AIMS) has revealed that some occurrences of awareness are associated with low doses of volatile anesthetics as captured by the AIMS, but not recognized or reported by the anesthesiologist.[49]

Future Medicolegal Trends for Awareness

It is likely that payments for awareness claims will continue to increase in the future. Changes in public perception of a medicolegal problem can increase the liability burden.[25] The wave of media publicity focusing on awareness in recent years is likely related to the development of brain function monitors. The public in their role as jury members and the court may choose to ignore the uncertainty among anesthesiologists regarding the role of brain function monitors, and consider their use to be part of the standard of care. Once a monitor that may prevent a condition becomes available, the payments for damages are larger when the monitor is not used. These factors might contribute to an increase in what has been a low burden of liability with regard to awareness in the United States for the last three decades.

SUMMARY

Amnesia is a fundamental component of general anesthesia. Accordingly, monitoring for depth of anesthesia is an important factor in the anesthetic management of patients. The issue of intraoperative awareness continues to generate opinions. The most recent editorial was by Nickalls and Mahajan[50] in which they emphasized the importance of anesthetic dose. When considering depth of anesthesia as it relates to the risk of intraoperative awareness, the following points are key:

- The incidence as defined by prospective trials is generally accepted to be 1 to 2 per 1000 patients.
- There is the potential for serious psychological and medicolegal sequelae when a patient suffers an episode of awareness under general anesthesia.
- An equipment check is paramount to the prevention of intraoperative awareness.

Table 46-3 Liability Characteristics of Awareness[44]

Characteristic	Reported Findings	
	Claims from Domino et al., 1999[26] (N = 80)	Newer Claims (N = 71)
Substandard care	44 cases (67%)	32 cases (54%)
Payment made	45 cases (62%)	39 cases (59%)
Median payment*	$26,065[†]	$71,500[†]
Range of payments	$1,520-$1,050,000	$924-$1,050,000

*Payments adjusted to 2007 dollars using consumer price index.
[†]The distribution of payments differed between published claims[26] and newer claims based on Kolmogorov-Smirnov test (p = 0.007). Adapted from original published in Kent CD, Domino KB. Medicolegal consequences of intraoperative awareness. In Mashour GA (ed). Consciousness, Awareness, and Anesthesia. New York, Cambridge University Press, 2010.

VI

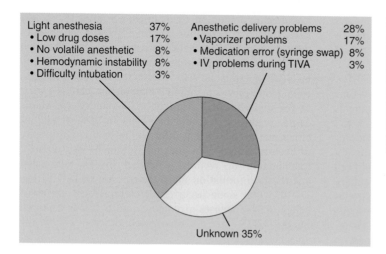

Light anesthesia	37%	Anesthetic delivery problems	28%
• Low drug doses	17%	• Vaporizer problems	17%
• No volatile anesthetic	8%	• Medication error (syringe swap)	8%
• Hemodynamic instability	8%	• IV problems during TIVA	3%
• Difficulty intubation	3%		

Unknown 35%

Figure 46-3 Causes of awareness during anesthesia in recent closed malpractice claims ($n = 71$). (Excerpted from Kent CD. Awareness during general anesthesia: ASA Closed Claims Database and Anesthesia Awareness Registry. (Reprinted with permission from the American Society of Anesthesiologists Newsletter 2010;74:14-16. A copy of the full text can be obtained from ASA, 520 N. Northwest Highway, Park Ridge, IL 60068-2573.)

■ Amnestic drugs might be considered for both preventive treatment of intraoperative awareness and as a treatment for patients who have had an episode of inadequate anesthesia (although it should be noted that data supporting such treatment are not available).

■ It is advisable to re-dose hypnotics in clinical situations that carry a risk for intraoperative awareness (e.g., difficult airway).

■ Hemodynamics are unreliable as a predictor of inadequate anesthesia.

■ There is no proven awareness monitor that has 100% sensitivity and specificity. Multimodality monitoring is recommended. This should include clinical signs, end-tidal volatile anesthetic gas monitor, and the consideration of a brain function monitor.

■ Consider at least a 0.7 MAC level of a volatile anesthetic.

■ Neuromuscular blockers will mask an important indicator of inadequate anesthesia.

QUESTIONS OF THE DAY

1. What are the risk factors for intraoperative awareness after general anesthesia?

2. What are the inherent limitations to the use of brain electrical monitoring for assessment of anesthetic depth?

3. According to an American Society of Anesthesiologists (ASA) practice advisory, how should depth of anesthesia be monitored during surgery?

4. What are the main causes of awareness reported in the ASA Closed Claims database?

REFERENCES

1. McCleane GJ, Cooper R: The nature of pre-operative anxiety, *Anaesthesia* 45:153–155, 1990.

2. Myles PS, Williams DL, Hendrata M, et al: Patient satisfaction after anaesthesia and surgery: Results of a prospective survey of 10,811 patients, *Br J Anaesth* 84:6–10, 2000.

3. Sandin RH, Enlund G, Samuelsson P, et al: Awareness during anaesthesia: A prospective case study, *Lancet* 355:707–711, 2000.

4. Brice DD, Hetherington RR, Utting JE: A simple study of awareness and dreaming during anaesthesia, *Br J Anaesth* 42:535–542, 1970.

5. Errando CL, Sigl JC, Robles M, et al: Awareness with recall during general anaesthesia: A prospective observation evaluation of 4001 patients, *Br J Anaesth* 101:178–185, 2008.

6. Xu L, Wu AS, Yue Y: The incidence of intra-operative awareness during general anaesthesia in China: A multicenter observational study, *Acta Anaesthesiol Scand* 53:873–882, 2009.

7. Nordstrom O, Engstrom AM, Persson S, et al: Incidence of awareness in total i.v. anaesthesia based on propofol, alfentanil and neuromuscular blockade, *Acta Anaesthesiol Scand* 41:978–984, 1997.

8. Sebel PS, Bowdle TA, Ghoneim MM, et al: The incidence of awareness during anesthesia: A multicenter United States study, *Anesth Analg* 99:833–839, 2004.

9. Mashour GA, Wang LY, Turner CR, et al: A retrospective study of intraoperative awareness with methodological implications, *Anesth Analg* 108:521–526, 2009.

10. Pollard RJ, Coyle JP, Gilbert RL, et al: Intraoperative awareness in a regional medical system: A review of 3 years' data, *Anesthesiology* 106:269–274, 2007.

11. Ross KG, Hilmi I: The incidence of intraoperative awareness during a nine-year period at a tertiary medical center, *ASA Annual Meeting* A621, 2009.

12. Ghoneim MM, Block RI, Haffarnan M, et al: Awareness during anesthesia: Risk factors, causes and sequelae: A review of reported cases in the literature, *Anesth Analg* 108:527–535, 2009.

13. Orser BA, Mazer CD, Baker AJ: Awareness during anesthesia, *Can Med Assoc J* 178:185–188, 2008.

14. Myles PS: Prevention of awareness during anaesthesia, *Best Pract Res Clin Anaesthesiol* 21:345–355, 2007.

15. Moerman N, Bonke B, Oosting J: Awareness and recall during general anesthesia. Facts and feelings, *Anesthesiology* 79:454–464, 1993.

16. Avidan MS, Zhang L, Burnside BA, et al: Anesthesia awareness and the bispectral index, *N Engl J Med* 358:1097–1108, 2008.

17. Ghoneim MM: Drugs and human memory (Part 2). Clinical, theoretical, and methodologic issues, *Anesthesiology* 100:1277–1297, 2004.

18. Weber B, Schaper C, Bushey D, et al: Increased volatile anesthetic requirement in short-sleeping *Drosophila* mutants, *Anesthesiology* 110:313–316, 2009.

19. Samuelsson P, Brudin L, Sandin RH: Late psychological symptoms after awareness among consecutively included surgical patients, *Anesthesiology* 106:26–32, 2007.

20. Leslie K, Chan MT, Forbes A, et al: Posttraumatic stress disorder in aware patients from the B-Aware Trial, *Anesth Analg* 110:823–828, 2010.

21. Lennmarken C, Bildfors K, Enlund G, et al: Victims of awareness, *Acta Anaesthesiol Scand* 46:229–231, 2002.

22. Ranta SO, Laurila R, Saario J, et al: Awareness with recall during general anesthesia: Incidence and risk factors, *Anesth Analg* 86:1084–1089, 1998.

23. Mashour GA, Wang LY, Esaki RK, et al: Operating room desensitization as a novel treatment for post-traumatic stress disorder after intraoperative awareness, *Anesthesiology* 109:927–929, 2008.

24. Ghoneim MM: Awareness during anesthesia, *Anesthesiology* 92:597–602, 2000.

25. Domino KB, Aitkenhead AR: Medicolegal consequences of awareness during anesthesia. In Ghoneim MM, editor: *Awareness during Anesthesia*, Woburn, MA, 2001, Butterworth Heinemann, pp 155–172.

26. Domino KB, Posner KL, Caplan RA, et al: Awareness during anesthesia: A closed claims analysis, *Anesthesiology* 90:1053–1061, 1999.

27. Akrawi WP, Drummond JC, Kalkman CJ, et al: A comparison of the electrophysiologic characteristics of EEG burst-suppression as produced by isoflurane, thiopental, etomidate, and propofol, *J Neurosurg Anesthesiol* 8:40–46, 1996.

28. Cole DJ, Domino KB: Depth of anesthesia: Clinical applications, intraoperative awareness and beyond. In Schwartz AJ, editor: *ASA Refresher Courses in Anesthesiology*, vol 35, Philadelphia, 2007, Lippincott, Williams & Wilkins, pp 51–52.

29. Practice advisory for intraoperative awareness and brain function monitoring: A report by the American Society of Anesthesiologists Task Force on Intraoperative Awareness, *Anesthesiology* 104:847–864, 2006.

30. The Joint Commission: Preventing, and managing the impact of, anesthesia awareness, *Sentinel Event Alert* 1–3, 2004. Oct. 6. Available at http://www. jointcommission.org/SentinelEvents/ SentinelEventAlert/sea_32.htm; accessed Feb. 4, 2010.

31. Myles PS, Leslie K, McNeil J, et al: Bispectral index monitoring to prevent awareness during anaesthesia: The B-Aware randomised controlled trial, *Lancet* 363:1757–1763, 2004.

32. Ekman A, Lindholm ML, Lennmarken C, et al: Reduction in the incidence of awareness using BIS monitoring, *Acta Anaesthesiol Scand* 48:20–26, 2004.

33. O'Connor MF, Daves SM, Tung A, et al: BIS monitoring to prevent awareness during general anesthesia, *Anesthesiology* 94:520–522, 2001.

34. Studdert DM, Mello MM, Gawande AA, et al: Claims, errors, and compensation payments in medical malpractice litigation, *N Engl J Med* 354:2024–2033, 2006.

35. Studdert DM, Thomas EJ, Burstin HR, et al: Negligent care and malpractice claiming behavior in Utah and Colorado, *Med Care* 38:250–260, 2000.

36. Localio AR, Lawthers AG, Brennan TA, et al: Relation between malpractice claims and adverse events due to negligence. Results of the Harvard Medical Practice Study III, *N Engl J Med* 325:245–251, 1991.

37. Blacher RS: On awakening paralyzed during surgery. A syndrome of traumatic neurosis, *JAMA* 234:67–68, 1975.

38. Payne JP: Awareness and its medicolegal implications, *Br J Anaesth* 73:38–45, 1994.

39. Huycke LI, Huycke MM: Characteristics of potential plaintiffs in malpractice litigation, *Ann Intern Med* 120:792–798, 1994.

40. Cass NM: Medicolegal claims against anaesthetists: A 20 year study, *Anaesth Intensive Care* 32:47–58, 2004.

41. Cobcroft MD, Forsdick C: Awareness under anaesthesia: The patients' point of view, *Anaesth Intensive Care* 21:837–843, 1993.

42. Studdert DM, Mello MM, Brennan TA: Medical malpractice, *N Engl J Med* 350:283–292, 2004.

43. Robertson GB: The efficacy of the medical malpractice system: A Canadian perspective, *Ann Health Law* 3:167–178, 1994.

44. Kent CD, Domino KB: Medicolegal consequences of intraoperative awareness. In Mashour GA, editor: *Consciousness, Awareness, and Anesthesia*, New York, 2010, Cambridge University Press, pp 204–220.

45. Gan TJ, Glass PS, Sigl J, et al: Women emerge from general anesthesia with propofol/alfentanil/nitrous oxide faster than men, *Anesthesiology* 90:1283–1287, 1999.

46. Drover DR, Lemmens HJ: Population pharmacodynamics and pharmacokinetics of remifentanil as a supplement to nitrous oxide anesthesia for elective abdominal surgery, *Anesthesiology* 89:869–877, 1998.

47. Phillips AA, McLean RF, Devitt JH, et al: Recall of intraoperative events after general anesthesia and cardiopulmonary bypass, *Can J Anaesth* 40:922–926, 1993.

48. Kent CD: Awareness during general anesthesia: ASA Closed Claims Database and Anesthesia Awareness Registry, *ASA Newsl* 74:14–16, 2010.

49. Driscoll WD, Columbia MA, Peterfreund RA: Awareness during general anesthesia: Analysis of contributing causes aided by automatic data capture, *J Neurosurg Anesthesiol* 19:268–272, 2007.

50. Nickalls RW, Mahajan RP: Awareness and anaesthesia: Think dose, think data, *Br J Anaesth* 104:1–2, 2010.

VI

47 QUALITY OF CARE AND PATIENT SAFETY

Vinod Malhotra and Patricia Fogarty Mack

Safety is not just a priority but should be of paramount significance in the daily care of patients in the perioperative arena. Preventing mishaps such as patient falls, positioning injuries, wrong-site (person, site, or side) surgery, medication errors, and surgical fires that should never occur (never events) must be our goal. This approach gets to the basic tenet of medical care, which is "first, do no harm."

In 2009, HealthGrades reviewed 41 million CMS (Center for Medicare and Medicaid Services) hospitalizations over the years 2004 to 2006 and determined that over 150,000 lives may have been saved over this period because of processes and systems initiated to improve patient safety and outcomes. Based on these and similar findings from the Institute of Medicine (IOM) and various other organizations, The Joint Commission introduces National Patient Safety Goals (NPSG) every year (Table 47-1).

Further, surgical outcomes can be improved by appropriate interventions that are evidence based. These have been introduced via the Surgical Care Improvement Project (SCIP) and are tracked by CMS as core measures (Table 47-2). The performance of hospitals in compliance with these core measures is reported on the government website www.hospitalcompare.hhs.gov.

Patient satisfaction is another measure of quality of care and should be a goal for any facility that provides surgical care. Patient safety, improved outcomes, and improved patient satisfaction in health care constitutes the triad of excellence in clinical care. Many agencies such as the CMS and Press Ganey National Surveys report on patient satisfaction with perioperative care, which are frequently the basis upon which Medical Centers are judged (Fig. 47-1).

Quality of care includes not only the clinical care indicators, but also the measures of efficiency such as timely starts, short turnaround times between cases, appropriate access for emergencies, and effective utilization of the operating rooms, equipment, and staff. Operational

Table 47-1 The Joint Commission National Patient Safety Goals: 2010

- Improve the accuracy of patient identification
- Improve the effectiveness of communication among caregivers
- Improve the safety of using medications
- Reduce the risk of health care–associated infections
- Accurately and completely reconcile medications across the continuum of care
- Reduce the risk of patient harm resulting from falls
- Reduce the risk of influenza and pneumococcal disease in older adults
- Reduce the risk of surgical fires
- Encourage patients' active involvement in their own care as a safety strategy
- Prevent health care–associated pressure ulcers
- Identify safety risks inherent in the organization's patient population
- Improve recognition and response in a patient's condition
- *Universal protocol*: Prevent wrong person–wrong site–wrong procedure surgery

Table 47-2 SCIP Core Measures: 2010

SCIP-Inf-1: Prophylactic antibiotic received within 1 hour before surgical incision
SCIP-Inf-2: Prophylactic antibiotic selection for surgical patients
SCIP-Inf-3: Prophylactic antibiotic discontinued 24 hours after surgery end time (48 hours for cardiac surgery)
SCIP-Inf-4: Cardiac surgery with controlled 6 AM postoperative serum glucose
SCIP-Inf-6: Surgery patients with appropriate hair removal
SCIP-Inf-9: Urinary catheter removed on postoperative day 1 or 2, with day of surgery being day 0
SCIP-Inf-10: Surgery patients with perioperative temperature management
SCIP-Card-2: Surgery patients on β-blocker before admission received β-blockers during perioperative period
SCIP-VTE-1: Surgery patients with recommended VTE prophylaxis ordered
SCIP-VTE-2: Surgery patients who received appropriate VTE prophylaxis within 24 hours before and after surgery

Inf, infection; Card, cardiac; SCIP, Surgical Care Improvement Project; VTE, venous thromboembolism.

benchmark data are recorded and reported by several outfits. Some are private such as Benchmark International, and others are professional organizations.

The American Association of Clinical Directors (AACD) has developed a Procedural Times Glossary to measure

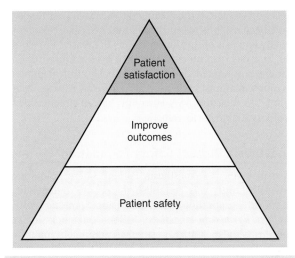

Figure 47-1 The triad of quality of care.

and compare operating room (OR) efficiency benchmarks.[1] The American Society of Anesthesiologists (ASA) has embraced this terminology through the Standard Nomenclature in Medicine (SNOMED). The ASA also created the Anesthesia Quality Institute (AQI) in 2009 to establish standardized quality measures, promote research, and obtain useful data to improve quality of patient care.

ANESTHESIOLOGY AND PATIENT SAFETY

Anesthesiology has often been cited as an example of how a medical specialty has systematically improved patient safety. In 1954, Beecher and Todd's review of mortality rate during anesthesia, finding a frequency of 1 death in every 1561 operations, was one of the first to scientifically identify and quantify risks associated with anesthesia.[2] At first, patient safety efforts focused on the anesthesia delivery systems utilized in patient care. For example, many of the features of the anesthesia machine, such as Pin Index Safety Systems, oxygen fail-safe controls, and the elimination of hanging bellows, were all developed to enhance patient safety by avoiding critical technical failures.

ASA Closed Claims Database

In 1985 American Society of Anesthesiologists (ASA), with the cooperation of several law firms, established the ASA Closed Claims Database. Through review of closed malpractice claims, sources of technical failure and human error that may lead to patient injury could be identified and shared with the anesthesia community. Most claims initially reviewed were due to unrecognized esophageal intubation or other reasons for inadequate oxygenation.[3,4] These findings accelerated the requirement for pulse oximetry and capnography as standard monitors for patients undergoing general anesthesia. Several additional ASA

VI

Task Forces such as the Postoperative Visual Loss Registry have been established to further address concerns identified by analysis of the Closed Claims Database.[5] For example, analysis of problems identified by the Closed Claims Database prompted the ASA to publish clinical practice recommendations such as ASA Difficult Airway Algorithm.[6] In fact, the ASA currently has 23 practice advisories available on its website.

Anesthesia Patient Safety Foundation

Also in 1985, the Anesthesia Patient Safety Foundation (www.apsf.org) was established as an independent, nonprofit corporation with the vision "*that no patient shall be harmed by anesthesia*." Board members include anesthesiologists, nurse anesthetists, equipment manufacturers, lawyers, and engineers. Its current mission statement identifies safety research and education, patient safety programs and campaigns, and the national and international exchange of information and ideas as its continuing goals. In fact, its quarterly newsletter is the most widely circulated anesthesia publication in the world, providing a forum to publicize not only advances in technology, but also concerns regarding medications, patient factors, and common anesthesiology practices.

Advances in equipment technology over the past 30 years have made the provision of anesthesia care safer and facilitated providing anesthesia and surgical care to patients who years ago would have been deemed too sick to undergo major surgery. Through the implementation of technical advances and practitioner education, mortality rate from anesthesia has improved to 1:250,000.[7] However, as the population has aged and patients with more severe medical problems are undergoing surgery, mortality rate for the very ill may be as frequent as 1:10,000 to 1:1500.[8]

PATIENT SAFETY, MEDICAL ERROR, ADVERSE AND SENTINEL EVENTS

Patterned after the APSF, the National Patient Safety Foundation (NPSF) was established in the late 1990s. The NPSF has defined patient safety and health care error as the following:

Patient Safety

Patient safety is defined as the prevention of health care errors, and the elimination or mitigation of patient injury caused by health care errors.

Health Care or Medical Error

A health care or medical error is defined as an unintended health care outcome caused by a defect in the delivery of care to a patient. Health care errors may be errors of *commission* (doing the wrong thing), *omission* (not doing the right thing), or *execution* (doing the right thing incorrectly). Errors may be made by any member of the health care team in any health care setting (www.npsf.org).

Other important definitions key to understanding various patient safety initiatives are as defined by the Association for Healthcare Research and Quality (www.ahrq.org):

Adverse Event

An adverse event is any injury caused by medical care. The label of an "adverse event" does not imply "error," "negligence," or poor quality care. An adverse event simply indicates that an undesirable clinical outcome resulted from some aspect of diagnosis or therapy, not an underlying disease process.

Sentinel Event

A sentinel event is an unexpected occurrence involving death or serious physical or psychological injury, or the risk thereof. Serious injury specifically includes loss of limb or function. The phrase "or the risk thereof" includes any process variation for which a recurrence would carry a significant chance of a serious adverse outcome.

- Such events are called "sentinel" because they signal the need for immediate investigation and response.
- The terms "sentinel event" and "medical error" are not synonymous; not all sentinel events occur because of an error and not all errors result in sentinel events.

Since January 1995, The Joint Commission has reviewed 6600 sentinel events through December 31, 2009. Sixty-eight percent of these patients died. Among the 10 most frequently reported sentinel events were wrong-site surgery, operative/postoperative complications, medication errors, and unintended retention of a foreign body (data available at www.jointcommission.org/sentinel/events/statistics/).

Root Cause Analysis

Root cause analysis (RCA) is a structured process for identifying the causal or contributing factors underlying adverse events or critical incidents.[9] The release of the Institute of Medicine's reports "To Err is Human: Building a Safer Health System" (Nov. 1, 1999)[10] and "Crossing the Quality Chasm: A New Health System for the 21st Century" (March 1, 2001)[11] indicated that 98,000 patients in the United Stated die annually as a result of medical errors. Contained in these reports were also recommendations regarding many nationally based patient safety initiatives with the goal of reducing the number of errors by 50% within 5 years. The development of many patient safety initiatives by both governmental and private non-profit organizations has been sanctioned by the government and compliance with some of these initiatives is required for Medicare and Medicaid reimbursement.

In addition to the IOM-based initiatives regarding specific errors that need to be prevented, there are many opportunities for improving the delivery of medical care at a systems level rather than at an individual level.[12] This is supported by the work of the National Surgical Quality Improvement Program (NSQIP), which began at the Veterans Administration hospitals and has expanded through the American College of Surgeons to many private institutions throughout the nation. The NSQIP initiative is credited with improving postoperative surgical mortality rate by 31% and the morbidity rate by 45%.[13] NSQIP has demonstrated that while obvious errors can be detected on the local (hospital) level, subtle systems errors or deficiencies cannot be appreciated without comparison to data from peer institutions.[13] NSQIP has identified three important patient safety observations:

1. Safety is indistinguishable from overall quality of (surgical) care and should not be addressed independent of (surgical) quality.
2. During an episode of (surgical) care, adverse outcomes, and hence patient safety, are primarily determined by quality of systems of care.
3. Reliable comparative outcome data are imperative for the identification of system problems and the assurance of patient safety from adverse outcomes.

Anesthesiology has also been at the forefront of patient safety in the intensive care unit (ICU). Peter Pronovost, MD, PhD, at Johns Hopkins developed a simple checklist that practitioners should perform while placing central venous catheters in patients.[14] Although seemingly simple, institution of this practice without exception in ICUs in Michigan led to a sustained 68% reduction in infection rate. During an 18-month study period, 1500 lives and $100 million were probably saved.

The checklist requires that practitioners should:

1. Wash their hands with soap.
2. Clean the patient's skin with chlorhexidine antiseptic.
3. Put sterile drapes over the entire patient.
4. Wear a sterile mask, hat, gown, and gloves.
5. Put a sterile dressing over the catheter site.

THE JOINT COMMISSION NATIONAL PATIENT SAFETY INITIATIVE

The Joint Commission is an independent, not-for-profit organization that accredits and certifies more than 17,000 health care organizations and programs in the United States. According to their web site, The Joint Commission accreditation and certification are recognized nationwide as a symbol of quality that reflects an organization's commitment to meeting certain performance standards. The web site www.jointcommission.org states the organization's mission statement as, "To continuously improve health care for the public, in collaboration with other stakeholders, by evaluating health care organizations and inspiring them to excel in providing safe and effective care of the highest quality and value." Over the past two decades the federal government (Department of Health and Human Services and Center for Medicare and Medicaid Services) has recognized The Joint Commission's accreditation as deeming hospitals, laboratories, and other medical care providers able to participate in Medicare and Medicaid programs.

The Joint Commission conducts unannounced surveys of hospitals on a regular basis with the goal of assessing structural attributes, policies, and staff to ensure patient safety and quality of care. In addition, The Joint Commission develops annual National Patient Safety Goals (NPSGs), which form the focus for its reviews of hospitals and other institutions (see Table 47-1).

Preventing Wrong-Site Surgery

By definition, wrong-site surgery involves all surgical procedures performed on the wrong patient, wrong body part, wrong side of the body, or the wrong level of a correctly identified anatomic site. From 1995 through December 31, 2009, wrong-site surgery was the most frequently reported sentinel event (13.5%) to The Joint Commission.

According to The Joint Commission, the reports of wrong-site surgery or procedures is steadily increasing, although the Pennsylvania State Patient Safety Reporting System (PSPSRS) has observed a modest decline. However, the PSPSRS reports that 50% (7 of 14) of the wrong-site incidents in the last quarter of 2009 were wrong-site anesthesia blocks. (www.patientsafetyauthority.org/ADVISORIES/AdvisoryLibrary/2010/Mar7%281%29/Pages/26.aspx—accessed April 14, 2010). The actual incidence of wrong-site surgery is unknown but has been estimated to be 1:15,000 to 1:112,000.[15]

To prevent this "never event," The Joint Commission has issued a universal protocol that requires three steps: (1) preoperative verification of the patient, which uses two patient identifiers, the procedure, and the site/side or vertebral level and involves at least two health care providers (one of whom is the surgeon); (2) site marking of the operative site by the surgeon using his/her initials or "yes" with patient involvement; and (3) "time-out" right before starting the procedure.

The "checklist" theory has been applied to facilitate the process of "time-out" or universal protocol, when all the services involved in caring for the patient

VI

Table 47-3 Universal Protocol: Time-Out—10 Elements

1. Identification of the patient using two identifiers
2. Correct side/site
3. Correct procedure
4. Correct position
5. Verification that implants, devices, and special equipment are available
6. Relevant images are properly labeled and displayed
7. Allergies
8. Antibiotics administered
9. Safety precautions based on fire, hazards, patient history, or medication use
10. Verbal agreement that all time-out criteria have been met

(surgery, anesthesiology and nursing) pause before beginning a procedure or surgery to ensure that the correct patient is undergoing the correct procedure on the correct location of the body and that all the necessary imaging studies and equipment necessary to safely complete the procedure are available. The essential elements for a preprocedural "time-out" are listed in Table 47-3. The World Health Organization has taken this concern of patient safety during the perioperative period to a global level by introducing an implementation manual and a "WHO Surgical Safety Checklist." Verification of elements is done (a) before induction of anesthesia, (b) before the beginning of surgery, and (c) before the patient leaves the room (available at www.who.int/patientsafety/safesurgery/tools_resources/SSSL_Checklist_finalJun08.pdf).

Improving Patient Identification

In addition to preventing wrong-site or wrong-side surgery, another NPSG has focused on improving patient identification by checking two independent identifiers such as name and date of birth or name and medical record number. These patient identifiers must be checked every time a patient is to undergo a diagnostic test or procedure or is to receive medication.

Improving Communication

Improving communication between caregivers is also a National Patient Safety Goal.[16] When a patient is transferred from the care of one practitioner to another, whether it be from floor nurse to anesthesiologist in the operating room, anesthesia provider to postanesthesia care unit nurse or within services from daytime team to on-call team, structured systems to facilitate the transfer of vital patient information are essential to avoid errors. The Joint Commission has termed these transfers of patient care as "handoffs."

Among the several structured communication tools available, one that is becoming widely accepted is the SBAR communication tool. Originally developed for U.S. Navy communications, it has been adapted by many health care organizations and is internationally accepted as an effective communication regarding a change in a patient's condition either from nurse to physician or among physicians.

The elements of SBAR communication are as follows:

Situation: The notifying health care practitioner identifies the patient and the problem or the change in the patient's condition.
Background: Relevant background information specific to the situation is presented by the practitioner. For example, this information could include the patient's diagnosis, mental status, current vital signs, complaints, pain level, and physical assessment findings.
Assessment: This step of the communication provides the practitioner with the opportunity to offer an analysis of the problem or to convey more extensive data about the patient, such as changes from prior assessments.
Recommendation: This step covers what the practitioner believes would help resolve the situation or what is the desired response.

More information regarding SBAR may be found on the Institute for Healthcare Improvement website (www.ihi.org/ihi).

Improving Medication Safety

Medication safety is a critical aspect of the NPSGs. Anesthesia providers are instrumental in assuring the safe delivery of medication in the perioperative arena. A critical step in patient transfer of care is "medication reconciliation," which refers to the process by which the medications the patient is on preoperatively are reviewed for any possible adverse reactions with any medications the patient might receive intra- and postoperatively. Medication reconciliation occurs whenever the patient is admitted, transferred to another unit or service, or discharged home.

LABELING SYRINGES

Proper medication labeling is extremely important in the operating room and procedure suites. Medications should not be drawn into syringes until immediately prior to patient use, and the syringes must be labeled with the drug name, drug concentration, and the time medication is drawn up. Anesthesia providers have long adopted the use of color-coded labels to distinguish among different classes of medications in an effort to avoid medication administration errors. The Joint Commission recommends against the labeling of empty syringes in anticipation of future medication preparation because this practice does not obviate drawing the incorrect medication into a differently labeled syringe.

AVOIDING ABBREVIATIONS AND DECIMAL POINTS

Additional requirements in assuring medication safety are avoiding the use of abbreviations both with regard to drug name and unit of dose. $MgSO_4$ (magnesium sulfate) and MSO_4 (morphine sulfate) might be confused for each other, as might the handwritten abbreviations for microgram and milligram (μg and mg). The use of decimal points followed by a trailing zero is also to be avoided. For example, if an order is written "morphine sulfate 1.0 mg" and the decimal point is missed, the patient might be given 10 mg in error. The order should be written "morphine sulfate 1 mg." Similarly, a zero must be placed in front of a decimal point to avoid dosing errors. For example hydromorphone 0.2 mg/mL is the appropriate concentration for patient-controlled analgesia infusion. An order entry of .2 mg might be mistaken for 2 mg, resulting in a tenfold overdose.

THE DO NOT USE LIST

The official Do Not Use List also prohibits the use of "U" for units, "IU" for international units and Q.D. or Q.O.D. for daily or every other day dosing. Also endorsed by The Joint Commission for annual review and possible future inclusion are the following abbreviations and symbols:

The symbols > and <
All abbreviations for drug names
Apothecary units
The symbol @
The abbreviation cc
The abbreviation μg
Look-alike and sound-alike drugs

Finally, a list of look-alike and sound-alike drugs is available from several sources. Care must be taken to avoid using vials of drugs from manufacturers that look alike (for example, 1-mL pop-top vials with blue lids—atropine and ondansetron—should not be placed near one another in any pharmacy drawer). In addition, tall-man lettering may be utilized on preprinted labels, and thus, EPInephrine may be distinguished from EPHedrine.

Improving Fire Safety

Another source of patient injury is the occurrence of a surgical fire. In order for a fire to start, each element of the fire triangle—heat, fuel, and oxygen—must be present. Heat is the by-product of electrocautery units, lasers, and endoscopes. Paper drapes and fabric towels and gauze sponges provide ample fuel. Oxygen is often present at high concentrations in localized areas such as during facial plastic surgery or tracheotomy. The newer, more effective skin preparation solutions often contain alcohol, which is highly flammable and must be allowed to dry completely prior to placement of surgical drapes. There probably are 100 surgical fires each year, resulting in 20 serious injuries and two patient deaths.[17] Effective communication between all perioperative team members is essential in combating this devastating threat. Prep solutions must be completely dried prior to surgical draping, and lasers and endoscopes should be turned off or to standby when not in use. When there is a possibility that oxygen may come into direct contact with electrocautery, as in airway surgery or when oxygen is administered in a nonclosed circuit and may build up under surgical drapes, oxygen should be utilized at the lowest possible concentrations necessary for the patient to maintain oxygenation.

Reducing Hospital-Acquired Infection

Because perioperative care is a part of the continuum of hospital care meticulous attention to sterility and cleanliness is essential to prevention of hospital-acquired infections. This goal requires strict adherence to hand hygiene protocols, prevention of central line infections, preventing surgical site infections, and preventing the spread of multidrug-resistant organisms.

In addition to The Joint Commission's National Patient Safety Goals, guidance for health care practitioners is provided by numerous other national governmental and private organizations.

SURGICAL CARE IMPROVEMENT PROJECT

Of specific relevance to anesthesiology is the formation of the Surgical Care Improvement Project (SCIP), a national quality partnership of organizations interested in improving surgical care by significantly reducing surgical complications. In 2003 an article was published in the Journal of the American Medical Association (JAMA) that determined that postoperative complications, including infections, cardiac events, thromboembolism, and respiratory complications, accounted for 22% of preventable deaths.[18]

SCIP was initiated that year with the goal of reducing surgical complications by 25% by 2010. The Steering Committee is composed of 10 national organizations that have pledged their commitment and full support for SCIP:

- Agency for Healthcare Research and Quality
- American College of Surgeons
- American Hospital Association
- American Society of Anesthesiologists
- Association of Perioperative Registered Nurses
- Centers for Disease Control and Prevention
- Centers for Medicare & Medicaid Services
- Institute for Healthcare Improvement
- The Joint Commission
- Veterans Health Administration

VI

SCIP Core Measures

The SCIP has focused on improving and standardizing perioperative practices based on evidence from scientific studies. Current SCIP quality measures are listed in Table 47-2 and include the following evidence-based outcome improvement interventions:

Measures to reduce surgical site infection:

- Prophylactic antibiotics: The appropriate antibiotic is to be selected based upon evidence from scientific studies as to what is effective antibiotic prophylaxis for specific procedures in specific body areas. Antibiotics are to be administered within 1 hour of skin incision, with the exception of vancomycin and fluoroquinolones, which may be administered within 2 hours of skin incision. Finally, prophylactic antibiotics should be discontinued within 24 hours of surgery (48 hours for cardiac surgery patients). The benefit of this protocol is not only to reduce infection but also to reduce the development of antibiotic-resistant strains of microorganisms.
- Appropriate hair removal preoperatively: Depilatory cream or hair clippers should be used rather than razors to remove hair at the surgical site.
- Glycemic control in cardiac surgery patients: Patients should have a serum glucose value of less than 200 mg/dL at 6 AM the morning after surgery.
- Removal of urinary catheter: Catheter is removed on day 1 or 2 postoperatively, with daily reassessment of necessity. Placement of a urinary catheter is not necessary in most surgical cases, and the indications for urinary catheters should be carefully scrutinized.
- Maintenance of perioperative normothermia: Patients should have a core temperature of 36.0° C upon arrival to the postanesthesia care unit. Unplanned perioperative hypothermia is associated with impaired wound healing, adverse cardiac events, altered drug metabolism, coagulopathy, increased likelihood of blood transfusion, prolonged hospitalization, and increased health care expenditures. Therefore, the requirement is that in all patients, regardless of age, undergoing surgical procedures under general or neuraxial anesthesia of longer than 60 minutes' duration, there must be documentation of either active warming to maintain normothermia or a body temperature of 36.0° C or warmer recorded within 30 minutes immediately prior to or 15 minutes immediately after anesthesia end time.

Venous thromboembolism (VTE) prophylaxis:

- VTE prophylaxis will be administered to appropriate patients within 24 hours before and continuing 24 hours after surgery.

Measures to reduce perioperative myocardial infarction:

- Appropriate β adrenergic-blocker therapy is continued perioperatively in patients already receiving β-blocker therapy.

NEVER EVENTS

The National Quality Forum (NQF) has defined 28 *never events*; these are events that should at no time occur. CMS has a list of never events (Table 47-4), some of which correspond to the NQF list. If these events occur, CMS will not pay the hospital for the added cost of the extra care incurred as a result.

In order to successfully implement the many initiatives aimed at improving patient safety, a culture change in the "hierarchy" of medicine has been developing. After the worst commercial aviation accident occurred in Tenerife, Canary Islands in 1977, the postaccident review concluded that the junior officer in one of the planes did not speak up to object to an improper decision made by the pilot. This led to a change in culture in commercial aviation so that any member of the flight crew is empowered to speak up if they sense something is amiss. This culture of safety is present in many high-reliability organizations. These are critical concepts to the improvement of patient safety.

Culture of Safety

A culture of safety requires a commitment at all levels of a health care institution characterized by the following:

- A blame-free environment in which individuals are able to report errors or close calls without fear of reprimand or punishment.

Table 47-4 Never Events of Significance in Perioperative Period
Foreign object left in patient after surgery
Surgery on wrong patient
Surgery on wrong body part
Wrong surgery on a patient
Death/disability associated with intravascular air embolism
Death/disability associated with incompatible blood
Death/disability associated with hypoglycemia
Death/disability associated with a fall within facility
Death/disability associated with electric shock
Death/disability associated with a burn incurred within facility

- An expectation of collaboration across ranks to seek solutions to vulnerabilities.
- A willingness on the part of the organization to direct resources for addressing safety concerns.[19]

High-Reliability Organizations

High-reliability organizations refer to organizations or systems that operate in hazardous conditions but have nearly failure-free performance records, not simply better than average. Commonly discussed examples include air traffic control systems, nuclear power plants, and naval aircraft carriers.[20]

Compliance with patient safety initiatives involves either voluntary or mandatory reporting of adverse events. Reporting requirements are different in each state and for federal government programs as well. In 2002, Pennsylvania became the first state to establish a mandatory reporting system for not only serious adverse events but "incidents" (near-misses) as well. The Patient Safety Authority analyzes and evaluates those reports so it can learn from the data reported in order to advise facilities and make recommendations for changes in health care practices and procedures that may be instituted to reduce the number and severity of serious events and incidents.

OPERATING ROOM EFFICIENCY (Also See Chapter 45)

Beyond the markers of excellence in clinical care are the measures of operating room efficiency that further determine the quality of care in high-quality organizations. Anesthesiologists can be leaders in facilitating punctuality, on-time starts, keeping turnaround times between cases to a minimum, and promoting expeditious surgery to improve the utilization of resources in the operating rooms. The operating rooms are the most expensive units to run in a hospital and, if run inefficiently, can become a major cost drain. Yet, they are also the best source of revenue for most hospitals.

A systems approach and standardization of equipment and processes will not only streamline operations and improve efficiency but also improve patient safety, staff satisfaction, and patient satisfaction.

PATIENT AND STAFF SATISFACTION

According to the National Surveys (Press Ganey) about one third of patients surveyed would not recommend the facility where they received care to friends or family. Also, about one third of health care employees at the hospitals surveyed were dissatisfied with their jobs. These surveys have tracked a close link between staff satisfaction and patient satisfaction at health care facilities. Consequently, a goal for every facility should be to promote staff satisfaction and be intolerant of disruptive behavior so that the safest and best of care is rendered to all patients. Clearly, assessing and achieving safety and quality are of prime importance in all aspects of patient care.

QUESTIONS OF THE DAY

1. What is the difference between an adverse event and a sentinel event?
2. What is the SBAR communication tool?
3. What are the quality measures addressed in the Surgical Care Improvement Project (SCIP)?
4. What is a "never event" as defined by the National Quality Forum? List examples of never events in the perioperative period.

REFERENCES

1. Donham RT, Mazzei WJ, Jones RL: Association of Anesthesia Clinical Director's Procedural Times Glossary, *Am J Anesthesiol* 23(5S):1–12, 1996. (updated 2007 at www.aacdhq.org).
2. Beecher HK, Todd DP: A study of the deaths associated with anesthesia and surgery: Based on a study of 599,548 anesthesias in ten institutions 1948-1952, inclusive, *Ann Surg* 140:2–35, 1954.
3. Cheney FW, Posner KL, Lee LA, et al: Trends in anesthesia-related death and brain damage: A closed claims analysis, *Anesthesiology* 105:1081–1086, 2006.
4. Cheney FW: The American Society of Anesthesiologists Closed Claims Project: What have we learned, how has it affected practice, and how will it affect practice in the future? *Anesthesiology* 91:552–556, 1999.
5. Lee LA, Roth S, Posner KL, et al: The American Society of Anesthesiologists Postoperative Visual Loss Registry: Analysis of 93 spine surgery cases with postoperative visual loss, *Anesthesiology* 105:652–659, 2006.
6. ASA Task Force on Management of the Difficult Airway: Practice guidelines for management of the difficult airway, an updated report, *Anesthesiology* 98:1269–1277, 2003.
7. Lienhart A, Auroy Y, Pequignot F, et al: Survey of anesthesia-related mortality in France, *Anesthesiology* 105:1087–1097, 2006.
8. Lagasse RS: Anesthesia safety: Model or myth? A review of the published literature and analysis of current original data, *Anesthesiology* 97:1609–1617, 2002.
9. Wald H, Shojania KG: Root cause analysis. In Shojania KG, Duncan BW, McDonald KM, et al, editors: *Making Health Care Safer: A Critical Analysis of Patient Safety Practices*, Evidence Report/Technology Assessment No. 43 from the Agency for Healthcare Research and Quality, AHRQ Publication No. 01-E058, 2001; available at http://www.ahrq.gov/clinic/ptsafety/chap5.htm.
10. Kohn LT, Corrigan JM, Donaldson MS, editors: *To Err Is Human: Building a Safer Health System. Institute of*

VI

Medicine, Board on Health Care Services, Washington, DC, 1999, National Academy Press.

11. Committee on Quality of Health Care in America, Institute of Medicine: *Crossing the Quality Chasm: A New Health System for the 21st Century*, Washington, DC, 2001, National Academy Press.

12. Stoelting RK, Khuri SF: Past accomplishments and future directions: Risk prevention in anesthesia and surgery, *Anesthesiol Clin North Am* 24:235–253, 2006.

13. Neumayer L, Mastin M, Vanderhoof L, et al: Using the Veterans Administration National Surgical Quality Improvement Program to improve patient outcomes, *J Surg Res* 88:58–61, 2000.

14. Pronovost P, Needham D, Berenholtz S, et al: An intervention to decrease catheter-related bloodstream infections in the ICU, *N Engl J Med* 355:2725–2732, 2006.

15. Patient Safety Advisory: *Pennsylvania Patient Safety Reporting System*, vol 4, No. 2, June 2007, pp 29–45.

16. Patterson ES, Wears RL: *Continuity of Care. Patient Handoffs: Standardized and Reliable Measurement Tools Remain Elusive*, vol 36, Feb. 2010, Joint Commission on Accreditation of Healthcare Organizations, pp 52–61.

17. ECRI: A clinician's guide to surgical fires: How they occur, how to prevent them, how to put them out [guidance article]. *Health Devices*, 2003; 32:5–24.

18. Zhan C, Miller MR: Excess length of stay, charges, and mortality attributable to medical injuries during hospitalization, *JAMA* 290:1868–1874, 2003.

19. Pizzi L, Goldfarb N, Nash D: Promoting a culture of safety. In Shojania KG, Duncan BW, McDonald KM, et al, editors: *Making Health Care Safer: A Critical Analysis of Patient Safety Practices*, Evidence Report/Technology Assessment No. 43 from the Agency for Healthcare Research and Quality, AHRQ Pub. No. 01-E058, 2001; available at:http://www.ncbi.nlm.nih.gov/books/bv.fcgi?rid=hstat1.section.61719.

20. Bierly III PE, Gallagher S, Spender JC: Innovation and Learning in High-Reliability Organizations: A case study of United States and Russian Nuclear Attack Submarines, 1970–2000; IEEE, TEM August 2008;393–408.

INDEX

Note: Page numbers followed by *f* indicate figures and *t* indicate tables.